Davidson's Principles and Practice of Medicine

The Editors

JOHN MACLEOD

Formerly: Consultant Physician, Western General Hospital, Royal Edinburgh Hospital, and Clinic for Rheumatic Diseases, Royal Infirmary, Edinburgh

CHRISTOPHER EDWARDS

Professor of Clinical Medicine and Chairman, University Department of Medicine, Western General Hospital, Edinburgh, and Honorary Consultant Physician, Western General Hospital, Edinburgh

IAN BOUCHIER

Professor of Medicine, University of Edinburgh, and Honorary Consultant Physician, Royal Infirmary, Edinburgh

Davidson's Principles and Practice of Medicine

A TEXTBOOK FOR STUDENTS AND DOCTORS

EDITED BY

John Macleod

Christopher Edwards

Ian Bouchier

FIFTEENTH EDITION

CHURCHILL LIVINGSTONE
EDINBURGH LONDON MELBOURNE AND NEW YORK 1987

CHURCHILL LIVINGSTONE
Medical Division of Longman Group UK Limited

Distributed in the United States of America by Churchill
Livingstone Inc., 1560 Broadway, New York, N.Y. 10036,
and by associated companies, branches and representatives
throughout the world.

First Edition 1952
Second Edition 1954
Third Edition 1956
Fourth Edition 1958
Fifth Edition 1960
Sixth Edition 1962
Seventh Edition 1964
Eighth Edition 1966
Ninth Edition 1968
Tenth Edition 1971
Eleventh Edition 1974
Twelfth Edition 1977
Thirteenth Edition 1981
Fourteenth Edition 1984
Fifteenth Edition 1987

ISBN 0 443 03824 4 (paper)
ISBN 0 443 03823 6 (cased)

British Library Cataloguing in Publication Data
Davidson, *Sir* Stanley
  Davidson's principles and practice of medicine: a textbook
  for students and doctors.—15th ed.
  1. Pathology   2. Medicine
  I. Title   II. MacLeod, John. *1915-*
  III. Edwards, Christopher R.W.
  IV. Bouchier, Ian A.D.
  616   RB111

Library of Congress Cataloging in Publication Data
Davidson, Leybourne Stanley Patrick (Sir), 1894-
  Davidson's principles and practice of medicine.
  Includes bibliographies and index.
  1. Internal medicine.   I. MacLeod, John.
  II. Edwards C. R. W. (Christopher Richard Watkin)
  III. Bouchier, Ian A. D. (Ian Arthur Dennis)
  IV. Title.   V. Title: Principles and practice of medicine.
  [DNLM: 1. Medicine. WB 100 D252p]
  RC46.D24   1987   616   87-8044

Produced by Longman Group (FE) Ltd
Printed in Hong Kong

Preface to the Fifteenth Edition

With this new production, *Davidson's Principles and Practice of Medicine* will have appeared in 15 editions since it was first published 35 years ago. The book has established an international reputation; it is used extensively throughout the English speaking world and has also been translated into Spanish, Portuguese, Italian, Greek, Malay and Serbo-Croat. Since 1965 it has been published in Africa and Asia in a paperback edition under the auspices of the English Language Book Society. This continuing success is a remarkable tribute to the genius and vision of the late Sir Stanley Davidson and the progressive editorial policy he instituted, but we are acutely aware that, if the book is to retain its unique place in the field of medical education it must be kept completely up to date in relation to the evolution of medical science and technology.

In pursuit of this aim, the regular recruitment of younger authors in place of those who have retired from clinical practice has always been a main feature of editorial policy. On this occasion there are three new contributors, namely Professor I.A.D. Bouchier and Drs R.E. Cull and A.M. Davison.

There are more changes in this than in any previous edition. Prominent among them is extensive rewriting of the chapters dealing with immunology, nutrition and diseases of the kidney, and a very thorough revision of water and electrolytes, respiratory, pancreatic, liver and biliary diseases and of disorders of the pituitary gland, blood and nervous system. All other chapters have been amended with particular reference to updating. New figures and tables have been introduced. Nevertheless the size of the book has been contained, mainly by discarding material that has been superseded.

The opening chapters provide an overall view of fundamental general factors such as genetics, immunology, infection, nutrition, electrolyte balance and oncology. This is followed by accounts of diseases of the various systems and by outlines of psychiatry and acute poisoning. Emphasis has been placed on the more important (i.e. commoner) conditions and on those of educational value. A chapter on tropical disease and climatic disorders is included so that Western readers will have at least some knowledge of medical problems and human needs in countries other than their own and will be alerted to the dangers of imported disease. Next there is a major chapter on diseases due to infection with particular reference to those encountered in the tropics. A final short chapter deals on a global basis with the promotion of health and prevention of disease, re-emphasising the prominence given to prophylaxis throughout the book. In recognition of the fact that education must be a continuing process, many of the chapters conclude with brief comments on problems and prospects for the immediate future. Guidance is given about further reading, most of the references being briefly annotated to encourage students to use medical libraries and to consult more comprehensive books such as the *Oxford Textbook of Medicine* or *Cecil's* or *Harrison's Textbook of Medicine*. A close interrelationship has been maintained with the 7th edition of *Clinical Examination*.

A major change in this edition has been the introduction of two additional editors, Professor Christopher Edwards and Professor Ian Bouchier.

This is the last occasion in which I shall participate. Having been associated with his book from the outset, I am sure that Sir Stanley Davidson would have approved of it continuing to be sponsored by the Departments of Medicine from which it originated.

Our primary objective, as in previous editions, has been to ensure that the book provides a rational and easily comprehensible basis for the practice of medicine. We hope that 'Davidson' will continue to make as substantial a contribution to the education of medical students, both undergraduate and postgraduate, in the future as it has done in the past.

Edinburgh, 1987   John Macleod

Acknowledgements

We have had generous help from many colleagues, and students and doctors from all over the world have provided the challenge of constructive criticism. We are particularly indebted to Professor Ivan Roitt, Drs Jonathan Brostoff and David Male, and Gower Medical Publishing for giving us permission to use illustrations from their textbook *Immunology*. Other acknowledgements are made in the text.

List of Contributors

N.C. Allan MB ChB FRCP(Edin) FRCPath
Senior Lecturer, University Department of Medicine, Western General Hospital, Edinburgh; formerly Senior Lecturer, University of Ibadan, Nigeria; Consultant Haematologist, Western General Hospital, Edinburgh
Diseases of the blood

Joyce D. Baird MA MB ChB FRCP(Edin)
Senior Lecturer, University Department of Medicine, Western General Hospital, Edinburgh; Honorary Consultant Physician, Western General Hospital, Edinburgh
Diabetes mellitus and other metabolic disorders
Obesity

I.A.D. Bouchier MD FRCP(Edin) FRCP(Lond)
Professor of Medicine, University of Edinburgh; Honorary Consultant Physician, Royal Infirmary, Edinburgh
Diseases of the biliary system
Promotion of health and prevention of disease

A.D.M. Bryceson MD FRCP(Edin) DTM & H
Senior Lecturer, London School of Hygiene and Tropical Medicine; Consultant Physician, Hospital for Tropical Diseases, London; Consultant in Tropical Dermatology, St John's Hospital for Diseases of the Skin, London
Tropical diseases and climatic disorders
Diseases due to infection

G.P. Crean PhD FRCP(Edin) FRCP(Glasg)
Honorary Lecturer in Medicine, University of Glasgow (Western Infirmary); Consultant Physician,. Southern General Hospital, Glasgow; Physician-in-charge, Gastrointestinal Centre, Southern General Hospital, Glasgow
Diseases of the alimentary tract and pancreas

G.K. Crompton MB ChB FRCP(Edin)
Senior Lecturer, University Department of Medicine, Western General Hospital, Edinburgh; Senior Lecturer, University Department of Respiratory Medicine, City Hospital, Edinburgh; Consultant Physician, Respiratory Unit, Northern General Hospital, Edinburgh
Diseases of the respiratory system

R.E. Cull BSc PhD MB ChB FRCP(Edin)
Consultant Neurologist, Royal Infirmary, Edinburgh; Senior Lecturer in Neurology, University of Edinburgh
Diseases of the nervous system

A.M. Davison BSc MD FRCP(Edin) FRCP(Lond)
Consultant Renal Physician, St James's University Hospital, Leeds
Diseases of the kidney and genito-urinary system

D.P. de Bono MD(Cantab) FRCP(Edin)
Consultant Physician, Department of Cardiology, The Royal Infirmary, Edinburgh
Diseases of the cardiovascular system

C.R.W. Edwards MA MD(Cantab) FRCP(Edin) FRCP(Lond)
Professor of Clinical Medicine and Chairman, University Department of Medicine, Western General Hospital, Edinburgh; Honorary Consultant Physician, Western General Hospital, Edinburgh
Diseases of the hypothalamus, pituitary and parathyroid glands and sexual disorders
The promotion of health and prevention of disease

A.E.H. Emery MD PhD(Johns Hopkins) DSc FRCP(Edin) MFCM FLS FRSE
Professor Emeritus (Human Genetics), University of Edinburgh
Genetic factors in disease

N.D.C. Finlayson PhD MB ChB FRCP(Edin) MRCP(Lond)
Physician, Gastrointestinal and Liver Service, The Royal Infirmary, Edinburgh
Diseases of the liver and biliary system

A.M. Geddes MB ChB FRCP(Edin) FRCP(Lond)
Honorary Professor of Infectious Diseases, University of Birmingham; Consultant Physician, Department of Communicable and Tropical Diseases, East Birmingham Hospital
Infection and disease
Diseases due to infection

W.J. Irvine DSc MB ChB FRCP(Edin) FRCPath FRSE
Reader, Department of Medicine, University of Edinburgh; Consultant Physician, Royal Infirmary, Edinburgh
Immunological factors in disease
Disease of the thyroid and adrenal glands

D.G. Julian MA MD FRCP(Edin) FRCP(Lond) FRACP
Consultant Medical Director, British Heart Foundation; Professor Emeritus of Cardiology, University of Newcastle upon Tyne; Visiting Professor, Royal Postgraduate Medical School, London
Diseases of the cardiovascular system

Anne T. Lambie MB ChB FRCP(Edin) FRCP(Lond)
Senior Lecturer in Medicine and Consultant Physician, Royal
Infirmary, Edinburgh
*Disturbances in water and electrolyte balance and in hydrogen
ion concentration*
Diseases of the kidney and genito-urinary system

A.A.H. Lawson MD FRCP(Edin)
Honorary Senior Lecturer in Medicine, University of Edinburgh; Consultant Physician, Milesmark Hospital, Dunferm-
line, and to associated hospitals in West Fife District, Fife
Acute poisoning

G.J.R. McHardy MA BSc BM FRCP(Edin) FRCP(Lond)
Senior Lecturer, Department of Respiratory Medicine, Univ-
ersity of Edinburgh; Consultant Physician, Chest Unit, City
Hospital, Edinburgh; Consultant Clinical Respiratory Physiol-
ogist, City Hospital and Western General Hospital, Edinburgh
Diseases of the respiratorty system

George Nuki MB BS FRCP(Edin) FRCP(Lond)
Professor of Rheumatology, University of Edinburgh; Honor-
ary Consultant Physician, Northern General Hospital and
Royal Infirmary, Edinburgh
Diseases of connective tissues, joints and bones

John Richmond MD FRCP(Edin) FRCP(Lond)
Professor of Medicine, University of Sheffield; Honorary
Consultant Physician, Sheffield Area Health Authority
(Teaching)
Diseases of the liver

D.J.C. Shearman PhD MB ChB FRCP(Edin) FRACP
Mortlock Professor of Medicine, University of Adelaide; Head
of the Professorial Medical Unit, Royal Adelaide Hospital,
Australia
Diseases of the alimentary tract and pancreas

J.A. Simpson MD(Glasg) FRCP(Edin) FRCP(Glasg)
FRCP(Lond) FRSE
Professor of Neurology, University of Glasgow; Senior Neur-
ologist, Institute of Neurological Sciences, Southern General
Hospital; Consultant Neurologist, Western Infirmary, Glas-
gow
Diseases of the nervous system

J.F. Smyth MA MD(Cantab) MSc(Lond) FRCP(Edin)
FRCP(Lond)
Imperial Cancer Research Fund Professor of Medical
Oncology, University of Edinburgh; Honorary Consultant
Physician, Western General Hospital and Royal Infirmary,
Edinburgh
Introduction to oncology

R.N. Thin MD FRCP(Edin)
Consultant Physician, Department of Genito-urinary Medi-
cine, St Thomas' Hospital, London
Sexually transmitted diseases

A.S. Truswell MD FRCP(Lond) FFCM
Boden Professor of Human Nutrition, Sydney University;
Head of Nutrition Section, School of Public Health and
Tropical Medicine, Sydney; Honorary Consultant in
Nutrition, Royal Prince Alfred Hospital, Sydney, Australia
Nutritional factors in disease

Henry Walton PhD MD MD(Hon) (Uppsala) FRCP(Edin)
DPM
President, World Federation for Medical Education; Professor
Emeritus (Psychiatry), University of Edinburgh
Psychiatry

Contents

Note to readers. The policy regarding administration of
drugs and advice about their dosage is given on page 820.

1

Genetic factors in disease

Nowadays there is an increasing awareness of the importance of genetic factors in the aetiology and pathogenesis of many disorders affecting man. Perhaps of more importance is that this knowledge has also led to possible means of prevention of such disorders through genetic counselling and antenatal diagnosis.

At the turn of the century morbidity and mortality in infancy and childhood could largely be attributed to environmental factors such as infections and nutritional deficiencies. With advances in medicine these problems are decreasing, at least in the developed countries, while others, in which genetic factors are largely or even entirely responsible, are becoming more obvious. In a survey carried out in Newcastle a few years ago, no less than 42% of childhood deaths could be attributed to diseases which are genetic in causation. The contribution of genetic factors to mortality and morbidity in adults is more difficult to assess but is also increasing.

It is useful to consider human disease as forming a spectrum at one end of which we have those diseases which are entirely genetic in origin and in which environmental factors play little if any part. This group of disorders includes *chromosomal abnormalities* and so-called *unifactorial disorders*. The latter are due to single gene defects (Mendelian factors); though individually rare there are over 3 thousand of them. They are usually serious disorders; they often present at birth or in childhood, though notable exceptions are Huntington's chorea, myotonic dystrophy and polyposis coli. The mode of inheritance is straightforward and

follows Mendelian principles, and the risks of occurrence in relatives are high. For the vast majority of these unifactorial disorders there is as yet no effective treatment and prevention is the main approach to the problem.

At the other end of the spectrum are those diseases such as infections and nutritional deficiencies which are entirely environmental in aetiology. In the middle of the spectrum are many common conditions which are partly genetic and partly environmental in causation, so-called *multifactorial disorders*. These include many congenital malformations (such as congenital dislocation of the hip, club foot, congenital pyloric stenosis, congenital heart disease, anencephaly and spina bifida), 'diseases of modern society' (diabetes mellitus, essential hypertension, coronary artery disease) and possibly certain psychiatric disorders (such as schizophrenia and manic-depressive psychosis). In multifactorial disorders the genetic component is complex, probably involving in each case many genes. The risks to relatives are usually low.

In this chapter, after a review of the chemical basis of inheritance, an outline is given of chromosomal abnormalities, unifactorial and multifactorial disorders and the prevention of genetic disease.

CHEMICAL BASIS OF INHERITANCE

In the nucleus of every cell are the chromosomes containing the genes composed of segments of deoxyribonucleic acid (DNA) within which genetic information is stored.

DNA is made up of two polynucleotide chains, twisted together to form a double helix (Fig.1.1). Each nucleotide is composed of a nitrogenous base, a sugar molecule (deoxyribose) and a phosphate molecule. The nitrogenous bases in DNA are adenine and guanine (purines) and cytosine and thymine (pyrimidines). A purine in one chain always pairs with a pyrimidine on the other chain. There is also specific base pairing: guanine in one chain always pairs with cytosine in the other chain and adenine always pairs with thymine. At nuclear division the two strands of the DNA molecule separate and as a result of specific base pairing each chain then builds its complement. In this way, when a cell divides, genetic information is conserved and transmitted to each daughter cell.

The primary action of the gene is to synthesise protein by various combinations of 20 different amino acids. Genetic information is stored within the DNA molecule in the form of a triplet code such that a sequence of three bases specifies the structure of one amino acid.

Whereas DNA is found mainly in the chromosomes, ribonucleic acid (RNA) is found mainly in the nucleolus and the cytoplasm. RNA has a structure similar to DNA (Fig.1.1): both nucleic acids contain adenine, guanine and cytosine but thymine is replaced by uracil in RNA and the latter contains the sugar ribose.

The information stored in the DNA code of the gene is transmitted from one strand to a particular type of RNA, so-called messenger-RNA (m-RNA). Each m-RNA is formed by a particular gene, such that every base in the m-RNA molecule is complementary to a corresponding base in the DNA of the gene: cytosine with guanine, thymine with adenine but adenine with uracil since the latter replaces thymine in RNA. The m-RNA then migrates into the cytoplasm where it becomes associated with the ribosomes which are the site of protein synthesis. In the ribosomes the m-RNA forms the template for arranging particular amino acids in sequence.

In the cytoplasm there is yet another form of RNA referred to as transfer-RNA (t-RNA). Each amino acid in the cytoplasm becomes attached to a particular t-RNA. The other end of the t-RNA molecule consists of three bases which combine with complementary bases on the m-RNA. Thus a particular triplet in the m-RNA is related through t-RNA to a specific amino acid. The ribosome moves along the m-RNA in a zipper-like fashion, the assembled amino acids linking up to form a polypeptide chain.

A change (mutation) of a base pair of the DNA molecule may result in any one of a number of possible effects. If the altered triplet codes for the same amino acid then of course the change will go undetected. Possibly 20 to 25% of all possible single base changes are of this type. Alternatively a single base mutation may result in a triplet which codes for a different amino acid resulting in an altered protein. The latter may retain its biological activity (e.g. enzyme activity) but have altered physico-chemical properties such as electrophoretic mobility or stability so that it is more rapidly broken down. This is the case in many of the abnormal haemoglobinopathies in which the aberrant haemoglobin may be detected by its altered electrophoretic mobility. However the substitution of a different amino acid may result in reduced or even absent biological activity. In inborn errors of metabolism therefore the level of a particular enzyme may be reduced because it is not synthesised, or it is synthesised but has reduced activity or because of its instability it is more rapidly broken down.

CHROMOSOMES AND CHROMOSOMAL DISORDERS

Chromosome structure and number. Among higher animals each species bears within the nucleus of its cells a set of chromosomes which is characteristic both in number and in morphology for that species. Each nucleus in the somatic cells of man contains a set of 46 chromosomes. Two of these chromosomes determine the sex of the individual and are therefore known as *sex chromosomes*; the remaining 44 chromosomes are known as *autosomes*.

The DNA of higher organisms is coated with histone and non-histone proteins. This produces a deoxyribonucleoprotein fibre (chromatin) which forms the basic unit of chromosome structure. Chromosomes are in a suitable state for detailed study only during specific intervals within the

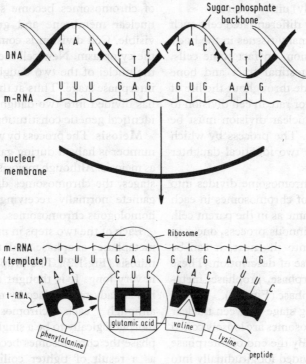

Fig.1.1 Protein synthesis. Sequences of bases in nuclear DNA (genes) send instructions via messenger RNA (m-RNA), to transfer RNA (t-RNA) on ribosomes in the cytoplasm, whereby amino acids are linked to form polypeptides. In these processes guanine (G) pairs with cytosine (C) and adenine (A) with thymine (T) or uracil (U).

period of cell division, for it is during these periods that the chromosomes become contracted, thicker and more readily stained. Chromosomes in the resting nucleus do not take up most stains in a satisfactory way.

Each chromosome has a point along its length, a constriction, known as the *centromere* which divides the chromosomes into two arms which are usually unequal in length. The chromosomes also differ in their overall length. Further, by using certain stains each chromosome can be shown to have a specific banding pattern. By these criteria it is now possible to identify individual chromosomes.

The chromosomal complement of any nucleus is composed of two sets of chromosomes which are arranged in pairs. Because the two members of any given pair (with the exception of the sex chromosomes) resemble one another they are said to be *homologous*. One homologue of any pair is derived from one parent and its partner from the other parent. Thus man has 22 pairs of homologous chromosomes (autosomes) and one pair of sex chromosomes.

During gametogenesis the number of chromosomes is halved in order that the number of chromosomes remains constant and is not doubled at each conception. Thus somatic cell nuclei contain twice as many chromosomes as gametes and with respect to their chromosome complement are said to be *diploid*, whereas gametes are said to be *haploid*.

The two sex chromosomes of the female are identical and are referred to as *X chromosomes*. The sex chromosomes of the male, however, are not identical. One of the pair resembles the X chromosomes seen in females while the other is much smaller, differs considerably in morphology and is referred to as a *Y chromosome*. Thus the sex chromosome constitution is XX in a female and XY in a male. In the female each ovum bears one or other of the X chromosomes, whereas in the male the sperms bear either an X or a Y chromosome. At fertilisation an ovum therefore has an equal chance of being fertilised by either an X or a Y bearing sperm. It is for this reason that the sex ratio is approximately (not exactly) unity at birth.

Mitosis. Unlike highly differentiated cells such as neurones, the cells of many tissues in the body repeatedly undergo division. In fact some cells, such as those of the intestinal tract and bone marrow, continue to divide throughout the life of an individual. For the error rate in cell division to remain as low as it is, nuclear division must be extremely well regulated. The process by which nuclei divide to produce two identical daughter nuclei is known as mitosis.

During mitosis each chromosome divides into two so that the number of chromosomes in each daughter nucleus is the same as in the parent cell. Though mitosis is a continuous process, one step merging imperceptibly into the next, it can be divided into stages for ease of description. These stages are known as interphase, prophase, metaphase, anaphase and telophase (Fig.1.2).

Interphase is the resting stage between nuclear divisions when the chromosomes are loosely coiled and difficult to visualise. By the end of interphase each chromosome has divided longitudinally into two daughter chromosomes, or *chromatids*, which remain attached to each other at the centromere.

During *prophase*, the chromosomes take up stains more readily and therefore become easier to visualise. By the end of prophase the nucleoli are no longer visible and each chromatid is a tightly coiled structure which is closely aligned to its partner.

Metaphase begins with the disappearance of the nuclear membrane and the formation of the spindle apparatus, which consists of a number of minute 'threads' which run from one pole (centriole) of the spindle to the other. The chromosomes become orientated around the centre of the cell in the equatorial plane. Each chromosome is attached to the spindle by means of its centromere. The spindle is responsible for the movement of the chromosomes during mitosis.

During *anaphase* the centromere of each chromosome divides into two, each half 'repels' the other and the chromatids move apart towards opposite poles of the spindle. When the chromatids reach the poles they form two separate but identical groups.

Telophase begins as the daughter chromosomes arrive at the poles of the spindle. The two groups of chromosomes become surrounded by a new nuclear membrane and gradually become less visible. Cell division is completed by cleavage of the cytoplasm. New cell membranes develop and the nuclei of the two daughter cells re-enter the interphase stage. Thus at the end of mitosis a cell has divided into two daughter cells each with an identical genetic constitution.

Meiosis. The process by which the chromosome number is halved during gametogenesis is known as meiosis. Although meiosis involves two division stages, the chromosomes divide only once, each gamete normally receiving either of a pair of homologous chromosomes.

Each of the two steps in meiosis has a prophase, metaphase, anaphase and telophase stage as in mitosis (Fig.1.2). The prophase of the first stage is very long. It is thought that DNA replication has already taken place by the onset of this stage, although each chromosome still appears morphologically to be a single thread. During prophase the chromosomes become more contracted, as a result of tighter coiling, and homologous chromosomes come together and pair along their length. Then a process known as *crossing-over* may occur in which there is an exchange of genetic material between chromatids of homologous chromosomes.

Following prophase the sequence of events is essentially similar to that occurring in mitosis, except that during this first meiotic division the centromere does not divide. Instead the members of each pair of homologous chromosomes migrate to opposite poles of the nucleus so that each daughter nucleus receives only one member of each pair and therefore bears a haploid chromosome complement.

In the second stage of meiosis the centromere divides and the chromatids of each chromosome separate and migrate into different nuclei. Thus each daughter cell from the first meiotic division has in turn divided to form two identical cells. Meiosis therefore results in each gamete having a haploid number of chromosomes and receiving one or the other member of each homologous pair of chromosomes and the genes it bears. This forms the cytological basis for Mendelian inheritance.

Methods of studying chromosomes. There are a variety of ways in which the study of

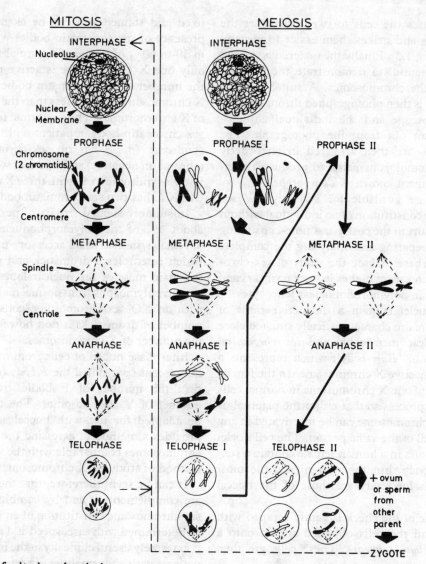

Fig.1.2 Stages of mitosis and meiosis.

chromosomes can be approached. Broadly these fall into two categories: those techniques which are used to study the complete chromosome complement of an individual, or those which enable information to be gained about the sex chromosome constitution of a person without having to do a complete chromosome analysis.

Since it is only during critical stages of the mitotic or meiotic cycle that the chromosomes are in a suitable state to study, chromosome analysis requires the provision of a large number of cells which are actively dividing. Meiotic studies can of course be done only on specimens of tissue

obtained from the gonads. Mitotic studies, on the other hand, can be made on a variety of different and more easily available tissues, e.g. directly from cells which are rapidly dividing in vivo, as in bone marrow. More commonly, however, specimens are obtained from tissues which are not rapidly dividing in vivo but are much more accessible to study, such as skin and blood leucocytes, and the cells are stimulated to divide in vitro by the addition of phytohaemagglutinin. The addition of colchicine arrests cell division at the metaphase stage when the chromosomes are most suitable for study. The use of hypotonic solutions causes the cells to swell, disperses the chromosomes and makes them easier to identify and count (Fig.1.3). Finally the material is stained (e.g. with Giemsa) to demonstrate the banding patterns of the chromosomes. A suitable metaphase spread is then photographed through a high power microscope and the individual chromosomes are cut out from the photograph. The chromosomes are then arranged in an orderly fashion, in homologous pairs, to produce a standard arrangement known as a *karyotype*.

Methods are available for studying the sex chromosome constitution of an individual without having to resort to the costly and time-consuming process of preparing and analysing the complete karyotype. These include the study of sex-chromatin and fluorescent bodies in buccal smears and 'drumsticks' in polymorphonuclear leucocytes.

Female nuclei contain a distinctive mass of nuclear chromatin characteristically situated close to the nuclear membrane, the *sex chromatin*, *X-chromatin* or '*Barr-body*', which represents a genetically inactive X chromosome. In the female inactivation of one X chromosome in normal cells is a random process so that either the paternal or maternal X chromosome can be inactivated in any particular cell of the same person. The cell nuclei of all the tissues in a human female contain a sexchromatin body, but for convenience the most suitable cells for study are those of the buccal mucosa.

The inside of the cheek is gently scraped with a spatula and the cells obtained spread onto a glass slide (*buccal smear*). These cells are then fixed and stained and can be examined for the presence of sex-chromatin bodies which are seen in 30 to 60% of nuclei of a normal female. Since only one X chromosome is active per cell, then the number of sex-chromatin bodies (inactivated X chromosomes) is one less than the total number of X chromosomes. Thus a normal female has one sex chromatin body, a patient with XO Turner's syndrome (p. 9) has no sex-chromatin bodies (chromatin negative) and a patient who has Klinefelter's syndrome (p. 9) with three X chromosomes (XXXY) has two sex chromatin bodies.

In suitably stained smears of peripheral blood about 3% of the polymorphonuclear leucocytes of females show a small accessory nuclear lobule, which resembles a drumstick and projects from the main mass of the nuclear lobes. This is not seen in polymorphs from normal males, or females with an XO sex-chromosome constitution. The number of drumsticks is not, however, related to the number of X chromosomes.

Interphase nuclei of cells from males exhibit a fluorescent spot called the *F body* (or Y chromatin); the number of F bodies represents the number of Y chromosomes. The technique can be adapted for use with buccal smears and so provides a method of assessing the number of Y chromosomes comparable with the sex-chromatin method of studying X chromosomes.

It can be seen, therefore, that these techniques are complementary and by combining them the sex chromosome constitution of an individual can be determined with ease, speed and accuracy. This is extremely useful clinically in the investigation of patients with abnormalities of sexual development or infertility, or for use in large-scale population surveys.

Chromosome nomenclature. A shorthand notation is used to describe a karyotype in the simplest way. This consists first of the total number of chromosomes (in numerals), followed by the sex chromosome constitution, and finally by any abnormalities that are present. Thus a normal male is 46, XY; a normal female is 46, XX. A girl with Turner's syndrome may be 45, XO and a boy with Klinefelter's syndrome, 47, XXY. The short and long arms of any chromosome are designated 'p' and 'q' respectively. A (+) or (−) sign is placed before an appropriate

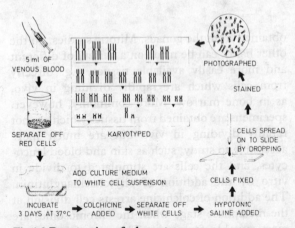

Fig.1.3 Preparation of a karyotype.

symbol where it means an additional or missing whole chromosome, but after a symbol when it refers only to part of a chromosome. Thus a boy with Down's syndrome is 47,XY,+21 and a boy with part of the short arm of chromosome 5 missing is 46,XY,5p−.

Chromosomal disorders

Specific chromosomal abnormalities are associated with recognised diseases or clinical syndromes in man. These include Down's syndrome (mongolism), abnormalities of sexual development (Turner's and Klinefelter's syndromes), syndromes of multiple congenital malformations (13- and 18-trisomies), spontaneous abortions, personality disorders (XYY and XXX etc.), chronic myeloid leukaemia and ataxia telangiectasia.

It has been found that 1 in every 200 live-born babies has a gross abnormality of chromosome number or structure. High as this figure is, it does not indicate fully the frequency with which chromosomal anomalies occur at fertilisation, for in a study of early spontaneous abortions chromosomal aberrations occurred in over 50%. Many of these chromosomal anomalies are rarely found in live-born babies and are therefore presumably lethal and the cause of a significant number of early abortions.

Chromosomal abnormalities can be divided into those which involve the autosomes and those which involve the sex chromosomes. These can be further divided into abnormalities of number and of structure. Numerical abnormalities arise when one or more chromosomes are either lost or gained, a phenomenon referred to as *aneuploidy*. When a whole set of chromosomes is gained the phenomenon is known as *polyploidy* and is not compatible with survival in man. The loss of a whole autosome, *monosomy*, also appears to be lethal in man. The addition of an extra chromosome, so resulting in three chromosomes instead of two (*trisomy*), seems, however, to result in less severe effects.

Autosomal abnormalities. Trisomy of a number of different autosomes have now been reported in man; the most common is trisomy-21 which results in Down's syndrome. The two other well-recognised syndromes (trisomy-13 and trisomy-18) occur far less frequently than Down's syndrome. They are both more severe in effect and usually result in death within the infant period.

DOWN'S SYNDROME occurs in about 1 in 700 live-births and is characterised by a flat face with widely spaced and upward slanting eyes, epicanthic folds, brachycephaly, malformed ears, broad and/or short neck, and a single, transverse palmar crease. Patients with Down's syndrome are invariably mentally retarded, but have a pleasant, quiet personality and show a great fondness for music. The condition is also associated with an increased frequency of both congenital visceral anomalies, particularly congenital heart disease, and acute leukaemia. Although the mortality rate of these patients is high within the first year of life, many now survive into adulthood and there are several reports of women with Down's syndrome having children; on average half their offspring are normal and half have Down's syndrome.

About 95% of cases of Down's syndrome are due to regular trisomy-21 which arises as a result of non-disjunction during meiosis. Normally during meiosis the two homologous chromosomes of any pair separate and pass into different gametes. Occasionally an accident occurs and the chromosomes fail to separate, both members of the pair passing into the same gamete. If such a gamete is then fertilised by a normal gamete the resulting zygote will possess an additional chromosome.

All the trisomy syndromes are found to have a significant relationship to maternal age, the frequency of trisomic births increasing with increasing maternal age. It is thought that perhaps some effect of ageing in the ova of older mothers makes them more prone to non-disjunction. There have been reports, however, of trisomy-21 recurring in some families, which suggests that the phenomenon of non-disjunction may be under genetic control at least in these rare families.

About 1% of cases of Down's syndrome are *mosaics*, that is, they possess two different cell lines, one of which has a normal chromosome constitution, the other an extra chromosome 21. This arises as a result of non-disjunction occurring at or after the first zygotic division and is very rarely inherited. The clinical picture may often be considerably modified in some of these cases.

About 4% of cases of Down's syndrome result from a phenomenon known as *translocation*, in which there is an exchange of segments between different chromosomes. The mechanism is thought to be that two chromosomes lying close to one another suffer simultaneous breaks followed by an exchange of chromosomal material. For example, in Down's syndrome a large part of chromosome 21 may be united with part of chromosome 15. A carrier of such a translocation (who has only 45 chromosomes) produces four types of gametes. A gamete may contain a normal chromosome 15 and a normal chromosome 21, in which case the resulting offspring will be normal. Or a gamete may contain a translocation (15/21), in which case the resulting offspring will have only 45 chromosomes and will be a carrier like the parent. Or a gamete may contain the translocation and a normal chromosome 21, in which case the offspring will have 46 chromosomes but in effect will be trisomic for chromosome 21 and will therefore have Down's syndrome. Finally a gamete may contain a chromosome 15 but no chromosome 21; this would produce a zygote monosomic for chromosome 21 which is lethal and would presumably result in an abortion. Theoretically, therefore, a carrier of such a translocation has a 1 in 3 chance of having a child with Down's syndrome, but for reasons which are not clear, the actual risk is much less. In Down's syndrome the translocation usually involves an exchange of material between chromosomes 13, 14 or 15 and chromosome 21. Rarely there may be an exchange between chromosomes 21 and 22 or even between two 21s. In the case of a parent who carries a translocation involving two 21s, all the offspring will have Down's syndrome.

OTHER AUTOSOMAL ABNORMALITIES. *Deletions* arise when a segment of a chromosome has been lost. New techniques have led to the demonstration of deletions involving a number of autosomes and an increasing number of these are being associated with clinically recognisable syndromes, examples of which are given in Table 1.1. Other rarer forms of chromosomal abnormalities are *ring chromosomes* and *isochromosomes*. Ring chromosomes involving both autosomes and sex

Table 1.1 Examples of autosomal abnormalities associated with recognised clinical syndromes.

Chromosome abnormality	Syndrome	Clinical features
Trisomy-21 Translocation 13-15/21 Translocation 22/21 Translocation 21/21	Down's	Characteristic facies Mental retardation Hypotonia Congenital heart disease Simian palmar crease
Trisomy-13	Patau's	Motor and mental retardation Microcephaly Microphthalmia Cleft palate/hare lip Polydactyly Congenital heart disease
Trisomy-18	Edwards'	Motor and mental retardation Flexion deformities of fingers Micrognathia 'Rocker-bottom' feet Congenital heart disease
4p-	Wolf's	Mental retardation Abnormal facies Cleft palate Coloboma Epilepsy Hypospadias Scalp defects
5p-	Cri du chat	Mental retardation Microcephaly Hypertelorism Characteristic cry

chromosomes have been described; they are thought to be formed when two ends of a chromosome have been deleted and the broken (more 'sticky') ends fuse to form a ring. In effect ring chromosomes are manifest as deletions and in shorthand they are represented as an 'r'. An isochromosome is formed when the centromere divides horizontally instead of longitudinally resulting in a chromosome consisting of either two long arms or of two short arms.

The *Philadelphia chromosome* (Ph') is an *acquired* chromosomal abnormality associated with chronic myeloid leukaemia. It is a deleted chromosome 22, the long arm being translocated to another autosome, usually chromosome 9.

Sex chromosome abnormalities. Numerical abnormalities of the sex chromosomes are more common than with the autosomes, and in general they produce less severe effects. They are brought about by the same phenomenon of non-disjunction. As with the autosomes, abnormalities of structure also occur although they are far less common than the numerical anomalies.

KLINEFELTER'S SYNDROME was the first sex chromosome aneuploidy to be demonstrated in man. Affected males have an extra X chromosome resulting in an XXY sex chromosome constitution or as many as four X chromosomes may be present; an extra Y chromosome may also be present on occasions resulting in an XXYY sex chromosome constitution. The main clinical features are eunuchoid body proportions, sterility (due to azoospermia), hypogonadism, gynaecomastia and often mental retardation.

There appears to be a relationship between mental retardation and the number of X chromosomes in both males and females. In Klinefelter's syndrome all individuals with an XXXY sex chromosome constitution are mentally retarded, whereas this is so in only about one-quarter of those with XXY sex chromosome constitution. Like the autosomal trisomies, Klinefelter's syndrome is found to occur more frequently in the sons of older mothers.

THE XYY CONSTITUTION is another sex chromosome aneuploidy in the male. Such men are reported to occur with increased frequency amongst inmates of institutions for the mentally retarded with criminal tendencies. It has been shown by various surveys that between 2 and 5% of such populations may be XYY. However, the exact relationship of this chromosomal anomaly with either mental retardation or criminal tendencies is uncertain especially as XYY individuals have been found amongst the normal general population.

TURNER'S SYNDROME was the first aneuploidy to be described in females. An XO sex chromosome constitution is the commonest abnormality, but clinical features of Turner's syndrome may also result from iso-chromosomes, deletions, and rings involving the X chromosome. This abnormality also arises by non-disjunction, but unlike Klinefelter's syndrome, Turner's syndrome does not show a relationship with maternal age.

The main clinical features are shortness of stature, primary amenorrhoea, lack of secondary sex characteristics and a variety of congenital abnormalities such as webbing of the neck, increased carrying-angle of the forearm (cubitus valgus) and coarctation of the aorta. Although, overall, patients with Turner's syndrome have a significantly lower I.Q. than normal, marked retardation is uncommon and the discrepancy is mainly in the performance aspect of their I.Q.

Females have also been described with three or even four X-chromosomes (XXX, XXXX); they may occasionally be mentally subnormal or have psychiatric disorders, but in all other respects appear to be healthy. Usually children born to XXX females are normal.

UNIFACTORIAL INHERITANCE

These disorders are due to defects of a single gene, i.e. to a primary error in the DNA code. They are inherited in a simple fashion, following Mendelian laws. The risk of their recurring in a family may therefore be accurately predicted on theoretical grounds making genetic counselling more straightforward.

These disorders may be subdivided according to the chromosome on which the abnormal (or mutant) gene is situated and also by the nature of the trait itself. Thus a trait which is determined by a gene situated on an autosome is said to be inherited as an *autosomal* trait, and this may be either *dominant* or *recessive*. A trait determined by a gene situated on one of the sex chromosomes is said to be *sex-linked* and may also be either dominant or recessive.

Autosomal dominant inheritance. A dominant trait is one which is manifested in the *heterozygote*. In other words a person exhibiting an autosomal dominant trait possesses both the mutant gene and the normal gene, the presence of only one mutant gene being necessary for the trait to be manifested in the carrier. If the disorder is common, then some affected individuals could be *homozygotes* (i.e. have a 'double dose' of the mutant gene), but if the disorder is rare (as is usually the case), then affected individuals are almost always heterozygotes. It should be noted that the normal and abnormal genes are known as *alleles*, i.e. they are alternative forms of the same gene.

Usually persons affected with an autosomal dominant trait are found to have an affected parent, the trait being transmitted from one generation to the next in a family, as illustrated in Figure 1.4.

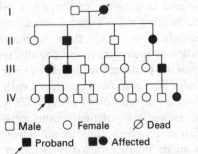

☐ Male   ○ Female   ⊘ Dead
■ Proband   ■● Affected

Fig.1.4 Characteristic pedigree: autosomal dominant trait.

This is not always the case, however; sometimes the disorder may appear suddenly in a family when no members of previous generations have been affected. This may be due to illegitimacy, to one parent being minimally affected and the disorder not recognised, or more commonly to the occurrence of a new mutation. This may complicate genetic counselling and is a problem which arises particularly in conditions inherited in a dominant fashion.

In diseases which are severe, affected individuals seldom have children because they are either infertile or do not survive to reach reproductive age. In such conditions the disease will eventually become extinct in affected families and is maintained in the population only by fresh mutations. Achondroplasia is one of the forms of short-limbed dwarfism and is inherited as an autosomal dominant trait. In one large study it was shown that affected individuals exhibited a marked reduction in reproductive fitness. It is not surprising, therefore, that a high proportion of cases are the result of new mutations.

In conditions which do not have much effect on survival it is often possible to trace the conditions through many generations of a family. Such a condition is the adult form of polycystic disease of the kidneys. Although affected individuals may eventually die from chronic renal failure, they often show no symptoms or signs of the disease until early middle life when they have already had their family and run the risk of transmitting the trait to their children.

In autosomal dominant conditions, if an affected individual marries a normal person, then on aver-age half their children will be similarly affected. This arises because the affected individual produces gametes, half of which contain the normal gene and the other half contain the mutant gene. The normal partner produces gametes all of which contain the normal gene. Thus at fertilisation the normal partner's gametes have an equal chance of uniting with a gamete carrying either a normal or an abnormal gene with the result that at conception there is a 1 in 2 chance of producing an affected individual. Because of the smaller size of modern families, by chance all the children of an affected individual may be normal, or similarly by chance again all his children may be affected. It is on average that half the offspring of an affected individual will be affected.

Some autosomal dominant traits are extremely variable in severity, this variability in clinical manifestation being referred to as *expressivity*. Osteogenesis imperfecta, for example, is an auto-somal dominant condition in which affected individuals may have only blue sclerae, whereas others may exhibit the full syndrome of blue sclerae, deafness and multiple fractures.

Occasionally an individual may carry a mutant gene and yet not exhibit any of its effects; the gene is then said to be non-penetrant, *penetrance* being the probability that an individual with the genetic predisposition will express clinical disease. This phenomenon explains situations where dominant mutant traits appear to have 'skipped' generations in certain families. This variation in expression of a mutant gene results both from the modifying influence of other genes and from environmental factors. The degree of penetrance of a gene is that proportion of heterozygotes who express the gene in any degree, however mild. For a gene to be *fully penetrant* its effects must be manifest to some degree in all individuals who carry the gene.

The phenomenon of varying penetrance can give rise to problems when estimating recurrence risks in order to give genetic advice. For example, tuberous sclerosis (epiloia) is inherited as a dominant trait but is not always penetrant. This condition is characterised by adenoma sebaceum (small papules over the cheeks and nose), epilepsy and mental retardation of varying severity. Some individuals carrying the gene may be so mildly affected as to pass as normal and so produce an apparently 'skipped' generation. However, it is unusual to find a proven carrier (e.g. with an affected child and an affected parent) who does not show at least some evidence of the disease, such as a few typical papules on the face.

Autosomal recessive inheritance. Autosomal recessive traits also affect both males and females. Unlike dominant traits, recessive traits are manifest only in the homozygous state, that is, in those individuals who possess a double dose of the mutant gene. Heterozygotes who possess only one mutant gene are usually perfectly healthy. Similarly the offspring of an affected person are usually normal, because most recessive conditions are so rare that it would be most unlikely that an affected person would marry a person heterozygous for the same mutant gene. In the even more unlikely event of two persons homozygous for the same recessive trait marrying, all their children would be affected. In general, however, both parents and offspring of a person homozygous for a rare recessive gene will be healthy. Characteristically in recessive traits, affected individuals cannot be traced from one generation to the next and if more than one member of a family is affected they are usually sibs, i.e. brothers and sisters. The pedigree of an autosomal recessive trait (Fig.1.5), therefore, differs from that of a dominant trait.

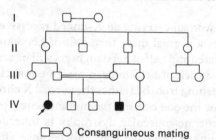

☐—○ Consanguineous mating

Fig.1.5 Characteristic pedigree: autosomal recessive trait.

At conception there is a 1 in 4 chance that any child of two heterozygous parents will be affected. Each parent produces gametes of two types, one bearing the normal gene and the other bearing the mutant gene. At conception, therefore, one-quarter of the offspring will be normal, one-half will be healthy heterozygotes and one-quarter will be affected. These are average figures; by chance all the offspring of such a couple might be affected, or similarly all their offspring might be normal. It

has been calculated theoretically that in marriages between two heterozygotes, in 75% of families with only one child that child will be unaffected, in 56% of families with two children both children will be unaffected, but in only 32% of families with four children will all four children be unaffected.

When dealing with rare recessive diseases the parents of affected individuals are often found to be related, because such individuals are more likely to have inherited the same mutant gene from an ancestor they have in common. The chance that first cousins will carry the same recessive gene is 1 in 8, but the chance that two unrelated individuals will carry the same recessive gene is very much lower and depends on the frequency of the particular gene in the population. In general the rarer the gene the greater the frequency of consanguinity amongst the parents of affected individuals.

At present roughly 1 in 200 marriages in Britain is between first cousins, so that giving advice on the genetic consequences of cousin marriages is a problem with which geneticists are frequently faced. Several extensive studies have shown that among the offspring of consanguineous matings there is an increased perinatal mortality rate together with an increased frequency of both congenital abnormalities and mental retardation, but the actual risks are small and in fact only slightly greater than in the general population. The situation is quite different, however, if there is a family history of a recessive disorder, when the risks will be greatly increased.

Many conditions show an autosomal recessive mode of inheritance and include, for example, many inborn errors of metabolism, some types of deaf-mutism and some types of congenital blindness. The commonest autosomal recessive trait known in Western Europe is cystic fibrosis which affects one in every 2000 births.

Sex-linked inheritance. Conditions determined by genes situated on either of the sex chromosomes are said to be inherited as sex-linked traits. Genes carried on the X chromosome are said to be X-linked, those on the Y chromosomes being Y-linked. Y-linkage of a gene implies that only males would be affected and that all the sons of an affected male would inherit the gene. There are no proven examples of Y-linked single gene disorders in man. Thus all known sex-linked conditions are due to genes on the X chromosome. As with autosomal traits these conditions may be either dominant or recessive.

X-linked dominant conditions are manifest both in females who are heterozygous for the mutant gene and in males who carry the mutant gene on their single X chromosome. The pedigree of an X-linked dominant trait (Fig.1.6) can superficially resemble that of an autosomal dominant trait, but there is a fundamental difference. Although an affected female will transmit the trait to half her offspring of either sex, an affected male will transmit the trait to all of his daughters but to none of his sons. There will therefore be an excess of affected females in families exhibiting such conditions. There are few X-linked dominant disorders but a notable example is one form of vitamin D resistant rickets.

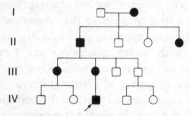

Fig.1.6 Characteristic pedigree: X-linked dominant trait.

An *X-linked recessive condition* is caused by a gene carried on the X chromosome and is manifest in females only when the gene is in the homozygous state. In males, a mutant gene present on the single X chromosome is always manifest because it is unopposed by the modifying effect of a normal gene on the second X chromosome, as happens in females. As with autosomal recessive conditions, the heterozygous carrier is usually healthy. Conditions inherited in this way therefore predominantly affect males and are transmitted by healthy female carriers (Fig.1.7). In those conditions where affected males may survive to have children, the condition will also be transmitted by affected males (Fig.1.8).

Haemophilia is the best known example of an X-linked recessive trait. Whereas in the past most boys with this disease died at an early age, with improvements in treatment most now survive. If an affected man marries a normal woman, then all his daughters will be carriers but none of his

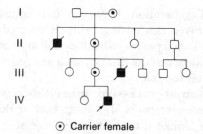

⊙ Carrier female

Fig.1.7 Characteristic pedigree: X-linked recessive trait—when affected males do not reproduce (e.g. Duchenne muscular dystrophy).

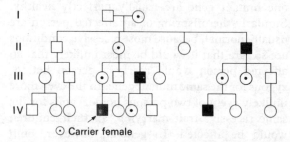

⊙ Carrier female

Fig.1.8 Characteristic pedigree: X-linkled recessive trait—when affected males do reproduce (e.g. haemophilia).

sons will be affected. An X-linked trait is never transmitted from father to son. This is because a man transmits his only X chromosome (which if he is affected bears the mutant gene) to each of his daughters but his Y chromosome to each of his sons.

If a woman carrying an X-linked recessive trait marries a normal man, then half of her sons will be affected and half of her daughters will be carriers because each of her children has an equal chance of inheriting from her either the normal X chromosome or the one bearing the mutant gene.

Duchenne muscular dystrophy is inherited as an X-linked recessive trait and because affected boys die young, it is transmitted solely by healthy female carriers.

Very rarely a female may exhibit an X-linked recessive trait. This situation may arise in several different ways. Firstly, she may have an abnormal chromosomal constitution resulting in her having only one X chromosome, such as in Turner's syndrome (XO). Secondly, she may be homozygous for the mutant gene, but this is very unlikely with rare recessive disorders because she would have to have inherited the disorder from both her parents. The third possibility is that she may be a 'manifesting heterozygote'. If, by chance, in the majority of her cells it is the normal X chromosome which is inactivated, then a female heterozygote may exhibit the trait. Careful examination of carriers of Duchenne muscular dystrophy sometimes reveals varying degrees of weakness in the same group of muscles that are weak in affected boys.

The modes of inheritance for some unifactorial disorders are given in Table 1.2.

MULTIFACTORIAL INHERITANCE

Many human characteristics can be measured and if the values are plotted against the number of individuals in the population with each particular value then a bell-shaped or normal frequency distribution curve is found (Fig.1.9). This applies to such characteristics as intelligence, stature, weight, skin colour and blood pressure. Some of these traits may be largely environmentally determined, such as weight, whereas others are largely genetically determined, such as stature and intelligence. In each case many genes are probably involved. Characteristics which are due to many genes plus the effects of environment are said to be inherited on a multifactorial basis.

It is now believed that many common disorders

are inherited in this way. In such conditions it is assumed that there is some underlying graded attribute which is related to causation. This is referred to as the individuals' *liability*, which includes not only their genetic predisposition but also the environmental factors which render them more or less likely to develop the disease. It is assumed that the curve of liability has a normal distribution in the general population.

In one simple model (Fig.1.9), it is believed that there is a *threshold* value such that all affected individuals have a liability above this value and all unaffected individuals have a liability below this value. Relatives of affected individuals have a higher average liability than the population average so the curve of liability for relatives is shifted to the right. In the general population the proportion above the threshold is the population incidence and among relatives the proportion above the threshold is the familial incidence. Such a model can be used to explain the familial incidence of such disorders as essential hypertension, coronary artery disease, peptic ulceration and many of the commoner congenital malformations.

There are several consequences of such a model. Familial incidence will be greater among the relatives of more severely affected individuals because presumably they are more extreme devi-

Table 1.2 Mode of inheritance of some unifactorial disorders.

Autosomal dominant	Autosomal recessive	X-linked recessive
Achondroplasia	Albinism	Christmas disease
Facioscapulohumeral	Ataxia telangiectasia	Duchenne muscular dystrophy
muscular dystrophy	Congenital adrenal	Glucose-6-phosphate
Gilbert's syndrome	hyperplasia	dehydrogenase deficiency
Hereditary spherocytosis	Congenital goitrous	Haemophilia
Huntington's chorea	cretinism	Hunter's syndrome
Hyperlipoproteinaemia	Crigler-Najjar syndrome	Lesch-Nyhan syndrome
Type II	Cystic fibrosis	Nephrogenic diabetes
Marfan's syndrome	Dubin-Johnson syndrome	insipidus
Myotonia congenita	Fanconi's syndrome	
Myotonic dystrophy	Friedrich's ataxia	
Neurofibromatosis	Galactosaemia	
Osteogenesis imperfecta	Gaucher's disease	
Polycystic disease	Glycogen storage diseases	
of kidneys (adult	Hurler's syndrome	
form)	Limb girdle muscular	
Polyposis of colon	dystrophy (Erb)	
Porphyria, acute	Niemann-Pick disease	
intermittent	Phenylketonuria	
Tuberous sclerosis	Pendred's syndrome	
von Willebrand's disease	Tay-Sachs disease	
	Wilson's disease	

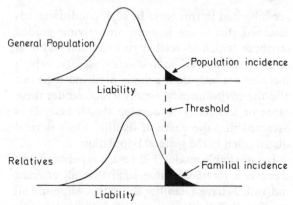

Fig.1.9 Liability. Hypothetical curve of liability in the general population and in relatives for a hereditary disorder in which the genetic predisposition is multifactorial.

ants along the curve of liability and the number of abnormal genes segregating in such families is greater than in families in which individuals are less severely affected. Thus in hare lip with or without cleft palate the proportion of affected sibs and children is roughly 6% when the index patient has double hare lip and cleft palate, but only 2.5% if the index patient has a single hare lip. By similar reasoning it would be expected that the incidence among sibs born subsequent to the index patient would be greater the more affected relatives there were in the family. In spina bifida, for example, the incidence of this condition, or the related disorder anencephaly, in sibs born after one affected child is roughly 5%, but the incidence rises to 10% after the birth of two affected children. This is quite different from the situation in unifactorial disorders where the risk to subsequent sibs remains constant irrespective of the number of affected individuals in the family (e.g. 1 in 4 for an autosomal recessive trait). Finally as a consequence of this model it might be expected that when there is a sex difference in the population incidence, the relatives of the less frequently affected sex would be more often affected. The reason for this is that in the less frequently affected sex, when individuals are affected they are presumably more extreme deviants along the curve of liability and possess more abnormal genes. Thus in congenital pyloric stenosis, which is 5 times commoner in boys than girls, the proportions of affected relatives of male index patients are roughly 5.5% for sons and 2.4% for daughters, but 19.4%

for sons and 7.3% for daughters when the index patient is a female.

Though it is not possible to measure liability to a particular disease it is possible to estimate how much of the aetiology can be ascribed to genetic factors as opposed to environmental factors. This is referred to as the *heritability* which is calculated from the known incidences of the disorder in the general population and in relatives. Some estimates of heritability are given in Table 1.3. The values, though approximate, do indicate that genetic factors are of more importance in aetiology in asthma and schizophrenia than in, for example, peptic ulcer.

Table 1.3 Estimates for heritability for various multi-factorial disorders.

Disorder	Incidence (%)	Heritability (%)
Schizophrenia	1	85
Asthma	4	80
Cleft lip ± cleft palate	0.1	76
Pyloric stenosis (congenital)	0.3	75
Ankylosing spondylitis	0.2	70
Club foot (congenital)	0.1	68
Coronary artery disease	3	65
Hypertension (essential)	5	62
Dislocation of hip (congenital)	0.1	60
Anencephaly and spina bifida	0.5	60
Peptic ulcer	4	37
Congenital heart disease (all types)	0.5	35

PREVENTION OF GENETIC DISEASE

Since there is at present no effective treatment for most genetic disorders the role of the medical practitioner lies mainly in the prevention of such conditions through genetic counselling. This involves providing advice on the chances of recurrence of a genetic disorder in the children of either healthy parents who already have an affected child, or when one of the parents or a near relative is affected with a disease which is known to be inherited.

In chromosomal disorders if the parents have normal karyotypes, i.e. do not carry a translocation which in the unbalanced state would cause abnormality, then the chances of recurrence are usually low. The most important chromosomal disorder from this point of view is Down's syndrome. The risk of having a child with Down's syndrome is about 1 in 100 in women who have previously had an affected child, and at least 1 in 50 in women over the age of 40. However, the risks are higher if one of the parents carries a chromosome translocation (Table 1.4).

Table 1.4 Recurrence risks of Down's syndrome (C = Carrier, N = Normal).

Patient	Father	Mother	Recurrence risk (%)
Translocation			
21/13-15	N	C	10-15
	C	N	5
21/22	N	C	10-15
	C	N	5
21/21	N	C	100
	C	N	100
Trisomy 21	N	N	1
Translocation or mosaic	N	N	1

In unifactorial disorders the chances of recurrence are based on Mendelian principles. As we have seen, for example, for a fully penetrant autosomal dominant disorder there is a 1 in 2 chance of recurrence in any child of an affected parent. However, if both parents are healthy an affected child is most likely to be the result of a new mutation and the chances of recurrence in subsequent children are negligible. If parents have had a child with an autosomal recessive disorder the chance of recurrence in subsequent children is 1 in 4. Should such a child survive there is very little chance of its having affected children. Finally, with X-linked recessive disorders there is a 1 in 2 chance that any son of a known carrier will be affected and a 1 in 2 chance that any daughter will be a carrier. All the daughters of an affected male will be carriers. A major advance in the prevention of X-linked disorders has been the development of tests for detecting healthy female carriers of such disorders as Duchenne muscular dystrophy and haemophilia. An important problem is the need for reliable methods of detecting symptomless, preclinical cases of autosomal dominant disorders such as Huntington's chorea, polyposis coli, polycystic kidney disease and myotonic dystrophy in which symptoms often do not develop until the third or fourth decade of life. Such tests would make it possible to identify individuals who carry

the mutant gene and are therefore likely to transmit the disease to their children. Developments in recombinant DNA may soon make possible preclinical detection of many of these disorders (p. 17).

In multifactorial disorders risk of recurrence cannot be predicted from Mendelian principles but have to be determined by studying the frequency of the condition among the relatives of affected individuals. Examples of risk figures, derived in this way (*empiric risks*), are given in Table 1.5.

Genetic advice

The procedure for giving genetic advice is first to establish a precise diagnosis, second to be certain that the disorder in question is genetic and third to verify the presence or absence of the disease in relatives. Without a precise diagnosis it is not possible to give reliable genetic counselling since certain disorders though superficially similar may be inherited differently. For example Hunter's syndrome and Hurler's syndrome both present similar clinical features of 'gargoylism' but whereas clouding of the cornea does not occur in the former condition it is present in the latter. Further, Hunter's syndrome is an X-linked recessive trait and therefore the unaffected sister of an affected boy may be at risk of having affected children. Hurler's syndrome on the other hand is an autosomal recessive disorder and only affects sibs. In this latter condition there is therefore no chance of an unaffected sister having affected children, provided she does not marry a near relative who might also carry the mutant gene.

It is always advisable to check that the disease in question is in fact genetic and not due to some environmental factor (i.e. a *phenocopy*). For example congenital deafness is often due to a rare recessive gene but it may also result from intrauterine infection with rubella during the first three months of pregnancy which may also cause abnormalities in the fetus such as congenital heart disease and eye defects. If it can be shown in a particular case that congenital deafness was due to maternal rubella then there would be no chance of recurrence in subsequent children. It is therefore important before giving genetic advice to ask about the possibility of maternal exposure to radiation,

Table 1.5 Examples of empiric risks (in percent).

Disorder	Incidence	Sex ratio M:F	Normal parent having a second affected child	Affected parent having an affected child	Affected parent having a second affected child
Asthma	3–4	1:1	10	26	—
Congenital heart disease (all types)	0.50	1:1	1–4	1–4	10
Diabetes mellitus (juvenile, insulin-dependent)	0.20	1:1	6	1–2	—
Epilepsy ('idiopathic')	0.50	1:1	5	5	10
Manic-depressive psychosis	0.40	2:3	10–15	10–15	—
Mental retardation ('idiopathic')	0.30–0.50	1:1	3–5	10	20
Schizophrenia	1–2	1:1	10	16	—
Tracheo-oesophageal fistula	0.03	1:1	1	1	—

drugs or infections during pregnancy and details of any birth trauma which might possibly account for the disorder in question.

Factors which influence the parents' decision whether or not they will accept a risk of having an affected child include the severity of the abnormality, whether or not there is an effective treatment, the actual risk, their religious attitude and possibly their socioeconomic status. In general, however, parents usually accept the risk of having an affected child if this is less than 1 in 20 but do not accept a risk of greater than 1 in 10 if the disease is serious.

Antenatal diagnosis. Family limitation is not the only course of action open to parents who are found to be at high risk of having a child with a serious genetic disorder. Other possibilities include (1) artificial insemination by donor (if the father is affected with a dominant disorder or carries a chromosome translocation or if both parents are heterozygous for a rare recessive gene) and (2) antenatal diagnosis with selective abortion of affected fetuses. The second procedure is possible by studying cells present in amniotic fluid or the amniotic fluid itself. About 5 to 10 ml of fluid is removed by transabdominal amniocentesis around the 16th week of gestation. The specimen is centrifuged and the cells removed and cultured for cytogenic or biochemical studies.

Fetal sexing is valuable in X-linked disorders which cannot yet be diagnosed *in utero*. In this way a known carrier mother can be guaranteed a daughter who will not be affected (though she might be a carrier), for if the fetus is a male the parents may decide on termination since there is a one in two chance the fetus could be affected. It is possible not only to sex the fetus but also to diagnose cytogenetic abnormalities and certain inborn errors of metabolism in the fetus. At present the main application of such studies is in the antenatal diagnosis of Down's syndrome and many centres now offer amniocentesis to all pregnant women over the age of 40 because of their increased risk of having a child with this disorder. Anencephaly and open spina bifida are associated with raised levels of alpha-fetoprotein in amniotic fluid and these disorders may therefore also be diagnosed in utero. More recently the technique of chorionic biopsy has been introduced and from the study of chorionic tissue various cytogenetic and biochemical disorders can now be diagnosed as early as 8 to 10 weeks' gestation.

Conclusion. The main contribution which genetics can make to medicine is in understanding more about the aetiology of certain disorders and in preventing such disorders through genetic counselling. But it is not sufficient merely to quote risk figures. As far as possible the nature and cause of the disease should be explained to parents and any feelings of guilt should be removed. Since genetic counselling may have profound long-term effects on a family such advice must never be given without careful appraisal of all the factors involved if the needs of the individual are to be met. Genetic counselling, like many other aspects of medicine, is as much an art as a science.

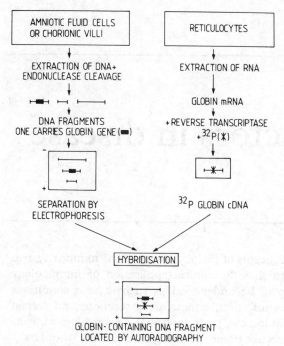

Fig.1.10 Technique used in the antenatal diagnosis of haemoglobinopathies. The probe used here is a complementary DNA copy (cDNA) produced from mRNA using RNA-dependent DNA polymerase (reverse transcriptase) and labelled with ^{32}P ($\star$).

RECOMBINANT DNA TECHNOLOGY

A major advance in the last few years has been the introduction of genetic engineering, or more precisely recombinant DNA technology which consists essentially of generating fragments of DNA containing specific genes of interest. This is done by using enzymes called restriction endonucleases which cleave DNA at sequence-specific sites. These fragments are incorporated into the DNA of a vector such as a plasmid which is a small circle of DNA. This is the recombinant part of the process. The vector is then introduced into a microbial host, usually *Escherichia coli*, which is grown in culture to produce clones with multiple copies of the incorporated gene. The cloned gene may be labelled with ^{32}P and used as a probe to detect homologous DNA sequences in various tissues. This is done by hybridisation (fusion of 2 different single strands of DNA by

complementary base pairing) and autoradiography on electrophoresis gels, a method known as the Southern blot.

These techniques have wide applications in medicine, the most important being the synthesis of biologically important molecules (such as human insulin, growth hormones and interferon), carrier detection, preclinical diagnosis and the antenatal diagnosis of certain genetic diseases. In the case of several disorders, including the haemoglobinopathies, antenatal diagnosis is possible because it has been found that the normal and abnormal genes are carried on DNA fragments of unequal size which can be recognised by their different mobilities on an electrophoresis gel (Fig.1.10).

PROSPECTS IN GENETICS

There is little doubt that recombinant DNA technology will have considerable impact on the clinical applications of genetics over the next few years. It will help us to understand more about the molecular basis of disease and its prevention through antenatal diagnosis. Furthermore the treatment of certain genetic diseases by the direct replacement of defective genes (gene therapy) may soon become a reality. There is also the possibility of developing presymptomatic treatments for those who are healthy but would otherwise develop a genetic disorder and perhaps one day even to treat the affected fetus before birth.

A.E.H. EMERY

FURTHER READING:
Emery A E H 1983 Elements of medical genetics, 6th edn. Churchill Livingstone, Edinburgh. An introductory text-book
Emery A E H, Rimoin D 1983 Principles and practice of medical genetics. Churchill Livingstone, Edinburgh. A more detailed textbook
Emery A E H 1986 Methodology in medical genetics, 2nd edn. Churchill Livingstone, Edinburgh. A textbook concerned with the more statistical aspects of medical genetics
Emery A E H 1984 An introduction to recombinant DNA. Wiley, Chichester

2

Immunological factors in disease

The science of immunology arose from the study of man's resistance to infection. The most striking feature of this resistance is the specific nature of its enhancement in individuals following infection. Thus, antigenic stimulation and antibody production began to be elucidated in the context of infectious disease and immunity to it. Terms such as 'immunology', 'immunisation' and 'immune response' are derived from these origins.

It soon appeared that such specific 'immune' responses might also confer unpleasant and sometimes dangerous hypersensitivity to subsequent exposure to the provoking antigen. Resistance to infection is not an essential feature of the immune response; for example, bacteria may induce antibodies which have no obvious protective value and immune responses are evoked by injection of intrinsically harmless non-living organic substances, such as serum protein from another individual or species. After exposure to antigen the individual develops a changed reactivity or *allergy*, a term which originally included immunity and hypersensitivity but which is now restricted to the latter.

The ability to develop specific immunity to infection is only one consequence of a wider capacity in the individual to recognise and to respond specifically to the foreignness of an extensive range of biological substances that are not normally present. Immunology is the study of what this 'changed reactivity' is in terms of molecular biology and cellular biochemistry, how it is brought about, and how it is regulated.

In this chapter an account is given of current concepts of the physiology of the immune system so that the clinical application of immunology may be understood in such diverse conditions as infection, asthma, drug reactions and certain endocrine, gastrointestinal, haematological, connective tissue, neurological and other disorders.

THE IMMUNE SYSTEM

The immune system is divided into two functional components, namely the innate and the adaptive immune systems. Innate immunity acts as a first line of defence against infectious agents and most pathogens are checked before they establish an overt infection. If these first defences are breached the adaptive immune system is called upon. This system produces a specific reaction to each infectious agent which normally eradicates that agent. Furthermore, the adaptive immune system remembers that particular infectious agent and can prevent it causing disease later. The innate and adaptive immune systems consist of a variety of molecules and cells distributed throughout the body (Table 2.1). The most important cells are leucocytes, which fall into two broad categories: (1) phagocytes, which form part of the innate immune system, and include neutrophil polymorphs, monocytes and macrophages; and (2) lymphocytes, which mediate adaptive immunity.

INNATE IMMUNE SYSTEM

Phagocytes. If an organism penetrates the exterior defences of an epithelial surface it encounters neutrophil polymorphs and monocytes whose

Table 2.1 Main features of the innate and adaptive immune systems. There is considerable overlap between the two. (Based on Roitt, Brostoff and Male.)

Immune system	Innate	Adaptive
Humeral immunity	Lysozyme Acute phase protein Interferon	Antibody
Complement pathway	Alternative	Classical
Cellular immunity	Phagocytes NK cells	T and B lymphocytes K cells
Repeated infection	Efficacy not improved	Efficacy improved

function is to engulf particles, including infectious agents, and destroy them. These phagocytes migrate out of the blood vessels into the tissues in response to a suitable chemotactic stimulus. They differ in that the polymorph is a short-lived cell while the monocyte develops into a tissue macrophage. The central role of macrophages and their products in the induction phase of inflammation, tissue damage and repair and the killing of bacteria and tumour cells is illustrated in Figure 2.1 and discussed on page 24.

Natural killer cells and soluble factors. When a cell becomes infected by a virus, or transforms into a cancerous cell its surface molecules are altered. These alterations can sometimes be recognised by natural killer (NK) cells which engage the cell and kill it. Virally infected cells produce *interferons* which can signal to neighbouring tissue cells and put them into a state capable of resisting viral replication, so preventing spread of the virus. Interferons can activate NK cells and amplify their cytotoxic action. Interferons, which can also be released by T lymphocytes as a lymphokine (p. 24), are produced very early in infection and are a first line of defence against many viruses.

Acute phase proteins. The serum concentration of a number of proteins increases rapidly during infection. These acute phase proteins include C-reactive protein, so-called because of its ability to bind the C protein of pneumococci. C-reactive protein then promotes the binding of complement. This process enhances phagocytosis

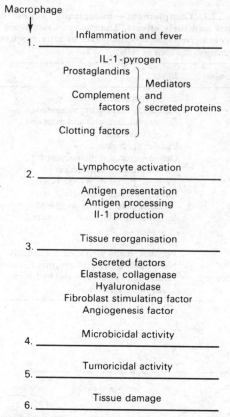

Fig. 2.1 Role of macrophages and their products in the induction of inflammation, lymphocyte activation and tissue reorganisation and repair. Their microbicidal and tumoricidal functions may also cause tissue damage as in delayed hypersensitivity reactions. (Adapted from Roitt, Brostoff and Male).

and is known as opsonisation.

Complement is a group of about 20 proteins in the blood which interact with each other and with other components in the innate and adaptive immune systems. The complement system is spontaneously activated by the surface of a number of micro-organisms via the alternative complement pathway (Fig. 2.3). Various complement components have important roles in chemotaxis, opsonisation and lysis (Table 2.2). The complement system is further described on page 22.

ADAPTIVE IMMUNE SYSTEM

Problems arise when the phagocytes are unable to recognise the infectious agent either because they lack a suitable receptor for it or because the

Table 2.2 Complement—biologically active components and their effects. The main end results are activation of macrophages, opsonisation of bacteria, mediation of inflammation and lysis of cells.

Component	Effect
C3a	Smooth muscle contraction
	Vascular permeability increased
	Eosinophil, basophil and mast cell degranulation
	Platelet aggregation
C3b	Opsonisation and phagocytosis
C4a	Smooth muscle contraction
	Vascular permeability increased
C5a	Smooth muscle contraction
	Vascular permeability increased
	Eosinophil, basophil and mast cell degranulation
	Platelet aggregation
	Polymorph and monocyte chemotaxis
	Neutrophil hydrolytid enzymes released
C5a-des-arg	Neutrophil chemotaxis and hydrolytic enzymes released

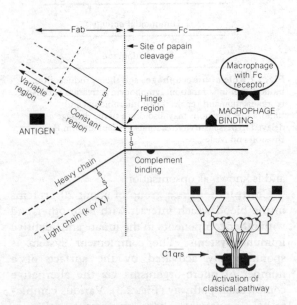

Fig. 2.2 The central role of antibody — a flexible link between specific antigen and complement. The structure of IgG is shown. Disulphide bond cleavage produces two light chains and two heavy chains. Papain cleavage produces two Fab fractions and one Fc fragment. The amino acids that vary in sequence for different antibodies are shown as interrupted ends of the light and heavy chains representing the antigen binding sites. The binding of antigen to antibody activates the Fc segment of the antibody with subsequent binding and activation of the first components of complement.

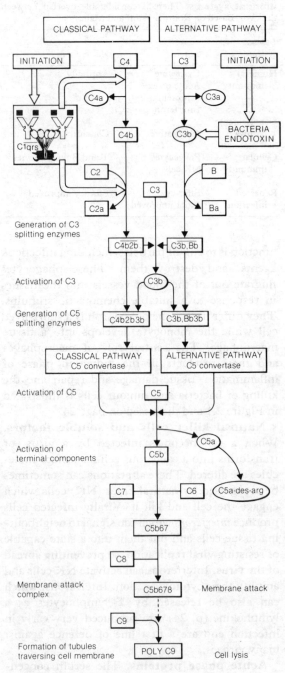

Fig. 2.3 Role of complement and its classical and alternative pathways. The main biologically active products are encircled. Their actions are given in Table 2.2. A horizontal bar above indicates an activated state. Both pathways generate a C3 convertase—C4b2b (classical pathway) and C3b,Bb (alternative pathway. (Adapted from Roitt, Brostoff and Male).

micro-organism does not activate complement and so cannot become attached to the phagocyte via the C3b receptor. What is needed is a flexible adaptor that can attach at one end to the micro-organism and at the other to the phagocyte. Antibody, as part of the adaptive immune system, fulfils this function (Fig. 2.2).

Immunoglobulin

Antibodies are immunoglobulins and are secreted by plasma cells, characterised by their rich endo-plasmic reticulum and derived through activation, proliferation and transformation of B lymphocytes (p. 23), which in turn are derived from the bone marrow. It is believed that the population of antibody-producing cells arises by random mutation and that a single cell will then react to produce a family of cells (clone) with a specific function. Essential to this concept is that random mutation of lymphocytes allows the genesis of cells that are capable of responding to all antigens, although a single cell can react to only one antigen. Antibody production is a special example of pro-tein synthesis, i.e. the putting together of amino acids to form protein molecules, in this instance, immunoglobulins, and the replication of this pro-cess according to a pattern. It can be varied on demand to produce different antibodies capable of reacting to any of the many different antigenic determinants. The immunological classes (IgG, IgM, IgA, IgD and IgE) and subclasses (IgG 1, 2, 3 and 4) differ in their biological properties.

Structure. Immunoglobulins are made up of distinct sub-units held together in the whole molecule by disulphide (S-S) bonds (Fig. 2.2). The bonds can be broken by reducing agents, so that the molecule falls apart into pairs of polypeptide chains called light and heavy chains as determined by their molecular weights. Two types of light chain exist, kappa and lambda, of which individual immunoglobulins have only one type.

The enzyme papain splits the immunoglobulin molecule into two antigen binding (Fab) fractions (Fig. 2.2) and one Fc fragment which fixes and activates the first component of complement (C1q). The Fc component also binds macrophages and is responsible for the antigenic differences between the classes of immunoglobulin which enables their ready quantitation by antisera.

Within the variable (V) regions of the Fab components are many hypervariable areas, each of approximately 5 amino acids, where the major differences between V regions are localised. The unique antigenic structures within the variable region are called idiotypes. An individual can develop anti-idiotype responses and these deter-mine, at least in part, the magnitude and duration of antibody production to a given antigen.

Classification and functions. IgG. In healthy adults, the total IgG accounts for 73% of the immunoglobulins in normal serum and is distri-buted equally between the blood and interstitial fluids, about a quarter passing across the capillary walls each day and the same amount returning via the thoracic duct. In man, IgG is the only immunoglobulin that is transported across the placenta (IgG2) to reach the fetal circulation and provide the baby with passive immunisation during its early life. IgG is particularly suited to neutralising soluble toxin such as that of Clostri-dium diphtheriae. IgG also has an opsonic effect on bacteria, coating them so that their ingestion by phagocytes is facilitated.

IgM. The macro-molecular IgM is predomin-antly intravascular. It constitutes only 7% of the serum immunoglobulins and is made up of five immunoglobulin units linked with disulphide bonds to provide ten identical combining-sites instead of the two of IgG. IgM is especially effective in activating complement to produce immune lysis of foreign cells by creating tubules penetrating the cell membranes at the sites where antibody has reacted. IgM antibodies are much more efficient than IgG antibodies in linking particulate antigens together for agglutination and phagocytosis and would seem to be specially adapted for dealing with cell debris or bacteria in the bloodstream.

IgA accounts for 19% of the total serum im-munoglobulins and is preferentially secreted into colostrum, saliva, intestinal juice and respiratory secretions. The major sites of IgA synthesis are the laminae propriae underlying the mucous mem-branes throughout the respiratory tract and the gut. The monomer produced locally by plasma cells is taken up as a dimer by the epithelial cells of the gut, and a secretory piece is added which protects the immunoglobulin from digestive enzymes. Secretory IgA is available right though to the colon and these antibodies are vital in the defence of the gut against enteroviruses, e.g. poliomyelitis. In general, IgA plays a major role as part of an antiseptic secretion over the mucous surfaces of the body.

IgD has some of the properties of IgG. It is almost exclusively found on the surface of B lymphocytes and may be involved in their regulation.

IgE has a very low serum level, a distinctive affinity for cell surfaces and constitutes an integral part of immediate hypersensitivity reactions such as occur in hay fever. The physiological function of IgE antibodies is obscure but they may possibly have a role in the defence against helminths.

Complement system

The principle activities of the complement system are directed at protection against infection. Complement belongs to the group of plasma systems termed 'triggered enzyme cascades', which also include the coagulation and fibrinolytic systems. They are all effector mechanisms which can produce a rapid and amplified response to a specific stimulus.

Two pathways, the classical and the alternative (Fig. 2.3), lead to the formation of enzymes (convertases) splitting C3 and C5. Thereafter there is a single pathway leading to the production of the membrane attack complex. This leads to the polymerisation of C9 (polyC9) to form tubules traversing the cell membrane, with resultant free exchange of solutes across the membrane and cell lysis.

The activation of C3 brought about by the C3 convertases is the central event of the complement sequence. The two routes leading to the cleavage of C3 are interrelated enzyme cascades that amplify the effect of the initial triggering reaction. Most complement components of the classical pathway are β globulins and consist mainly of one peptide chain or two peptide chains joined by disulphide bonds. The main exception is C1q which is a collagen-like protein with a unique structure resembling a bunch of six tulips when seen under the electron microscope (Figs. 2.2 and 2.3). The classical pathway is triggered by immune complexes combining with C1q.

The alternative pathway generates a C3 convertase without the need for antibody, C1, C2 or C4. Instead, the most important activators are bacterial cell walls and endotoxin. The alternative pathway may therefore be particularly relevant before a primary immune response has been mounted. The initial cleavage of C3 in the alternative pathway happens continuously and independently, generating a low level of C3b. This is an unstable substance and if a suitable acceptor surface is not available, the attachment site in Cb decays. If an acceptor surface is nearby, the C3b molecules can bind and remain active. They are able to use factor B of the alternative pathway to produce the active enzyme C3bBb. This can break down more C3, providing still more C3b, or become stabilised in the presence of properdin to form the C5 convertase of the alternative pathway.

The biologically active complement activation products are shown in Figure 2.3 and their effects in Table 2.2. The generation of a C3b macromolecular coating on target particles is the major biological function of complement. C3b receptors are present on neutrophils, eosinophils, monocytes and macrophages and on B lymphocytes, where they also act as receptors for the EB virus.

Control and deficiency. The complement pathway is controlled by two mechanisms. A number of the activated components are inherently unstable; if the next protein in the cascade is not immediately available, the active substance decays. There are also a number of specific inhibitors, e.g. C1 inhibitor and factor H (a competitor for factor B). The interaction between the complement system and the clotting, fibrinolytic and kinin pathways is illustrated in the condition of angio-oedema resulting from a deficiency of C1 inhibitor. Nephritic factor is an unusual IgG3 subclass autoantibody against the alternative pathway C3 convertase. The clinical consequence is marked C3 hypocomplementaemia as found in Type 2 mesangiocapillary glomerulonephritis (p. 387).

In the inherited complement deficiencies there is usually a total absence of the complement protein implying the lack of a functional gene.

The association of C1, 4 and 2 deficiencies with immune complex-like or lupus-like disorders is probably due to the failure to eliminate immune complexes. The importance of C3 and subsequently C5–8 in dealing with infection is emphasised.

Cellular components of adaptive immunity

Lymphoid cells. Stem cells originating in the bone marrow differentiate to form two main lymphocyte populations (T and B) and a third group of large granular lymphocytes, which does not consistently carry markers of either T or B cells, sometimes referred to as 'null cells' (Table 2.3).

Table 2.3 Lymphocytes: functional classification.

T cells
　Helper (T_H)
　Suppressor (T_S)
　Cytotoxic (T_C)
　Mediators of delayed hypersensitivity T_D)
　Memory

B cells
　Secretory (plasma cells)
　Memory

Large granular lymphocytes ('null cells')
　Natural killer (NK) cells
　Killer (K) cells

T lymphocytes are dependent on a hormone or factor produced by the epithelial cells of the thymus for becoming immunologically competent from non-competent precursors originating in the bone marrow. Given appropriate stimulation they proliferate and differentiate into a range of subsets with differing functions—helper (T_H), suppressor (T_S), cytotoxic (T_C) and T cells that mediate delayed hypersensitivity reactions (T_D).

B lymphocytes are independent of the thymus but are dependent on the bursa of Fabricius in birds; its equivalents in man are probably the tonsils and the lymphoid tissue of the gut, or simply the bone marrow itself. B lymphocytes undergo proliferation during stimulation to form plasma cells, responsible for the synthesis of antibodies.

Cell markers. Although both T and B cells are small lymphocytes of similar appearance, they can be distinguished by the different proteins on the cell membrane which act as 'markers'. The development of monoclonal antibodies has greatly facilitated this task, but so far there is no antibody that can distinguish between T_C and T_S surface antigens, and these cells have to be identified by their functional characteristics. Other monoclonal antibodies can be used to identify T and B cells in different stages of differentiation in the diagnosis of lymphoid malignancies.

Killer cells. The mechanisms of action of the effector cells leading to the death of the respective target cells are illustrated in Figure 2.4. Killer (K) cells along with the natural killer (NK) cells are considered to be part of the third population of lymphoid cells that have the morphological appearance of large granular lymphocytes (LGL). The cytotoxic action of K cells is initiated through contact of the K cell with the Fc portion of the antibody-antigen complex on the surface of the target cell. It is possible that K cells may also be 'armed' through the Fc receptor with antigen-antibody complex which, when present in antibody excess, will be cytotoxic to target cells coated with that specific antigen. Should immune complexes be produced in the presence of excess antigen, there would be no free combining sites left on the antibody moiety to react with antigen on the target surfaces so that this type of K cell would be ineffective (blocked).

MHC restriction. The description of how T_C cells attack their targets introduces the concept of major histocompatibility (MHC) restriction. The MHC (HLA) antigens are grouped in three classes (p. 29). T_C cells recognise antigen in association with MHC class 1 antigens (Fig. 2.4) while T_H cells use class 2 MHC antigens. The fact that antigen requires to be presented to T_H cells along with MHC class 2 antigen on the surface of the antigen presenting cell means that the T_H cells ignore antigens in the free state, and recognise them only after processing by the specialised antigen presenting cells (APC). In this way the lymphocytes could be forced to take note of the message left on these APC by other lymphocytes. It also appears that APC in different sites have different properties, so that the Langerhans cells of the skin seem particularly adapted towards mediation of delayed hypersensitivity, while the

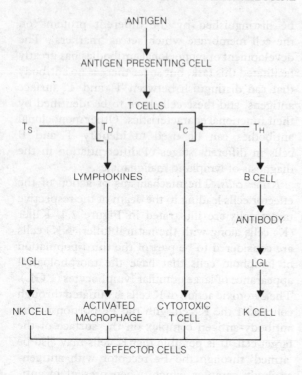

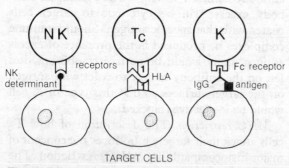

Fig. 2.4 Effector cells of the immune response and their mode of action on target cells. The role of the macrophage is shown in Figure 2.1. LGL = large granular lymphocytes.

dendritic cells of lymphoid follicles probably mediate priming of B cells for antibody production.

Regulation. Among other factors, the immune system is regulated by the balance between T_H and T_S cells. T_S cells have been found to release specific factors in vitro. The failure to find these factors in serum suggests that they normally act over a very short range. It may be that T_H and T_S cells migrating through lymphoid tissue leave their messages behind as factors adhering to APC where they can serve to activate or suppress the next lymphocytes of appropriate specificity which

come along. The balance of helper and suppressor factors on any particular APC may then determine whether it does or does not activate other lymphocytes.

Lymphokines. The T_D cells mediating delayed hypersensitivity reactions are activated by antigen presenting cells. The T_D cell releases a variety of lymphokines which activate macrophages and attract them to the site of antigen challenge and amplify the local response (Fig. 2.4). The effects of some lymphokines are shown in Table 2.4. Activated macrophages are primarily involved in the intracellular killing of organisms.

Table 2.4 Examples of lymphokines and their effects.

Lymphokine	Effect
Migration inhibition factor	
Chemotactic factor for macrophages	Macrophage localisation
Macrophage activating factor	Macrophage activation
Interleukin-2	T cell clone proliferation
Interferons	Antiviral. Immunoregulation
Transfer factor	Antifungal
Lymphotoxin	? Tumour inhibition

Myeloid cells. The role of *macrophages* and their derivation from monocytes has been described. Although *neutrophils* do not show any specificity for antigens they play an important part in acute inflammation and, together with antibodies and complement, in protection against micro-organisms. The predominant role of neutrophils is emphasised by the great increase in susceptibility to infections found in individuals with neutropenia.

Mast cells. These 'tissue basophils' are of central importance in immediate hypersensitivity reactions in which IgE bound to receptors on mast cells are cross-linked by appropriate antigens (Fig. 2.5). This triggers degranulation, releasing preformed mediators such as histamine. Other mediators are also synthesized. Mast cells can be activated also by complement components C3a and C5a and by certain drugs, e.g. morphine. Different newly formed mediators arise from different populations of mast cells, so that the clinical effects of mast cell activation vary according to the population of mast cells in the organ concerned. *Basophils,* which are found in very small numbers in the circulation, have properties similar to mast cells.

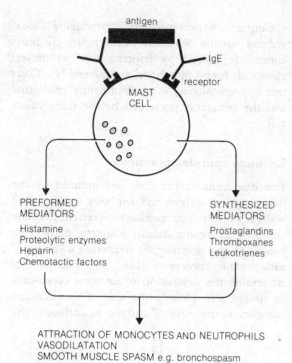

PREFORMED
MEDIATORS

Histamine
Proteolytic enzymes
Heparin
Chemotactic factors

SYNTHESIZED
MEDIATORS

Prostaglandins
Thromboxanes
Leukotrienes

ATTRACTION OF MONOCYTES AND NEUTROPHILS
VASODILATATION
SMOOTH MUSCLE SPASM e.g. bronchospasm

**Fig. 2.5 Role of mast cell in immediate
hypersensitivity.**

Eosinophils are attracted by products released
from T cells, mast cells and basophils and, in
the same way as mast cells and basophils, are
degranulated by appropriate stimuli, releasing
histaminase and other substances which inactivate
mast cell products. The effect is to suppress the
inflammatory response. Eosinophils are thought
to play a specialised role in helminthic infections
especially during the invasive phase. Thus they
bind schistosomulae (p. 783) coated with IgG
antibody, degranulate and release a toxic protein.
Common causes of eosinophilia include drug
allergies and a range of allergic diseases such as
hay fever, asthma, angio-oedema, serum sickness,
vasculitis, eczema and pemphigus. Other
examples are bronchopulmonary and tropical pulmonary eosinophilia (p. 241).

IMMUNE MECHANISMS IN DISEASE

1. IN RESPONSE TO FOREIGN ANTIGENS

Immediate (anaphylactic) hypersensitivity

Previously the term anaphylaxis emphasised the
clinically severe form, anaphylactic shock, but
current usage refers to the underlying mechanism
and not to clinical severity. Anaphylactic reactions
depend on whether the portal of entry of the
antigen is local, systemic or via the intestine.
Relatively mild symptoms occur when antigen-
antibody reactions take place on an exposed mucosal surface. These reactions occur most commonly
to pollens or animal dander and the symptoms
may be limited to rhinorrhoea and conjunctivitis.
However, intense bronchospasm may be produced
as a result of inhalation of the antigen. Patients
with asthma induced by contact with antigens in
this manner have levels of IgE that may be much
higher than those found in patients with asthma
that is not induced in this way.

Systemic anaphylaxis consists of a group of
much more severe reactions which may occur
rapidly if the antigen is injected, as in the case of
a drug such as penicillin, foreign sera, or the sting
of an insect. The features are bronchospasm,
laryngeal oedema resulting in extreme dyspnoea
and cyanosis and a marked fall in blood pressure
(anaphylactic shock). There may also be nausea,
vomiting and diarrhoea. Systemic anaphylaxis is
a potentially fatal condition if not treated promptly
with adrenaline (500–1000 μg i.m.) and an antihistamine (e.g. chlorpheniramine 10–20 mg slowly
i.v.) followed, in severely ill patients, by intravenous corticosteroids.

Urticaria, the formation of weal and flare lesions
in the skin, is an anaphylactic phenomenon which
can develop as a result of absorption of antigen
through the intestinal tract. Common allergens are
present in strawberries, nuts, eggs and shellfish.
Urticaria often occurs alone, but may be associated
with other signs of anaphylaxis. Not all urticaria
is caused by an immune reaction; the pharmacological agents which cause urticaria can be released
by other means, especially physical agents such
as trauma or cold.

Delayed hypersensitivity

In the classification of hypersensitivity suggested
by Gell and Coombs in 1963 delayed hypersensitivity (cell-mediated or type IV) was used as a
general category to describe all those hypersensitivity reactions that took more than 12 hours to
develop. It is now evident that several different
types of reaction can produce delayed hypersensi-

tivity, and that although T_D cells are implicated they can act by recruiting other cell types to the site of the reaction, e.g. macrophages.

Reactions effected by T_D lymphocytes are characteristically induced by infectious agents which are predominantly intracellular in the infected host, e.g. many viral infections and some bacterial infections such as tuberculosis and syphilis. The classical example of this reaction is the tuberculin test (p. 227).

Granulomatous hypersensitivity is clinically the most important form of delayed hypersensitivity, causing many of the pathological effects in diseases which involve T cell mediated immunity. It results from the presence of a persistent antigen within macrophages which the cell is unable to destroy. A dramatic example of delayed hypersensitivity occurs in the borderline leprosy reaction (p. 757).

Contact hypersensitivity, producing local eczema usually maximal at 48 hours, is most commonly caused by haptens such as nickel, chemicals found in rubber, and poison ivy. Contact hypersensitivity is predominantly epidermal and the antigen is presented by the Langerhans cell.

Immune complex reactions

Immune complex reactions are induced by the deposition of antigen and antibody in the vessel walls as a result of interaction between the immune complex and complement, platelets, mast cells, basophils and polymorphs triggering a variety of inflammatory processes (Fig. 2.6). Factors that determine the deposition of immune complexes in tissues also include the size of the immune complexes, the ratio of antigen to antibody, the

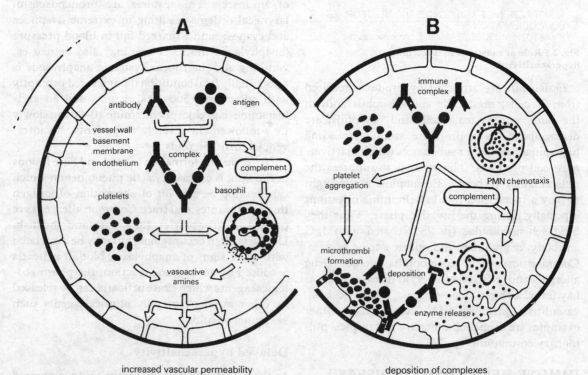

Fig. 2.6 Deposition of immune complexes in blood vessel walls. A. Antibody and antigen combine to form immune complexes which act on complement (to release C3a and C5a) which in turn acts on basophils to release vaso-active amines. The complexes also act directly on basophils and platelets to release amines including histamine and 5-hydroxytryptamine which cause endothelial cell retraction and permeability. B. With increased vascular permeability, complexes become deposited in the vessel wall. The complexes induce platelet aggregation and complement activation. The platelets form microthrombi on the exposed collagen of the basement membrane of the endothelium. Polymorphonuclear leucocytes (PMN) attracted to the site by chemotactic peptides, cannot phagocytose the complexes and so release their lysosomal enzymes causing damage to the vessel wall. (From Roitt, Brostoff and Male).

nature of the antigen, and local haemodynamics.

Diseases resulting from immune complex formation can be placed broadly into the following five groups:

1. Persistent infection (e.g. infective endocarditis, malaria or viral hepatitis) together with a weak antibody response leads to the chronic formation of immune complexes and their deposition in the tissues.

2. Immune complexes may be formed at body surfaces, for example in the lungs, following repeated inhalation of antigenic materials from moulds, plants or animals. In farmer's lung and pigeon fancier's lung (which are examples of extrinsic allergic alveolitis) there are circulating IgG antibodies to fungi following repeated exposure to mouldy hay or to pigeon antigens. When antigen enters the body again by inhalation, local immune complexes are formed in the alveoli leading to inflammation.

3. An Arthus reaction may occur when an antigen is injected into the skin of a subject who has previously been sensitised to that antigen. The reaction of preformed antibody with this antigen results in a high concentration of local immune complexes. The reaction develops in some 6–24 hours with oedema, haemorrhage and necrosis at the injection site.

4. In serum sickness IgG antibody produced in response to the injection of foreign antigen in large quantity, e.g. for immunisation, reacts with remaining antigen to form circulating, soluble immune complexes. Local swelling at the injection site, urticaria, fever, enlargement of the lymph nodes, arthralgia and sometimes glomerulonephritis occur about 10 days after the initial exposure to the antigen. As the immune complexes are formed, the antigen concentration is rapidly lowered. Since the process continues only as long as the antigen persists, the condition is usually self-limiting.

5. In autoimmunity immune complexes are frequently deposited in the kidneys, joints, arteries and skin.

2. IMMUNE MECHANISMS IN RESPONSE TO AUTOANTIGENS

Normally a person or animal does not mount a significant immune response against its own body constituents because intricate controlling and suppressor mechanisms exist to prevent this happening. A defect in immunological tolerance may either occur spontaneously or be induced by some exogenous factor. The concept that autoantibodies arise through spontaneous mutation is no longer tenable as they are so seldom monoclonal. In general autoantibodies occur in related groups reflecting the spectrum of autoimmune disease, ranging from the organ specific to the non-organ specific (Table 2.5). Thus there are a number of autoantibodies formed to different thyroid antigens in autoimmune thyroid disease, and patients with one of the diseases in the organ-specific group tend to have an increased prevalence of autoantibodies to the target organs of other diseases in the group.

Table 2.5 Spectrum of autoimmune diseases. (From Roitt, Brostoff and Male.)

Organ specific

- Hashimoto's thyroiditis
- Primary myxoedema
- Thyrotoxicosis
- Pernicious anaemia
- Autoimmune atrophic gastritis
- Autoimmune Addison's disease
- Premature menopause (few cases)
- Type I diabetes mellitus
- Goodpasture's syndrome
- Myasthenia gravis
- Male infertility (few cases)
- Pemphigus vulgaris
- Pemphigoid
- Sympathetic ophthalmia
- Phacogenic uveitis
- Multiple sclerosis (?)
- Autoimmune haemolytic anaemia
- Idiopathic thrombocytopenic purpura
- Idiopathic leucopenia
- Primary biliary cirrhosis
- Active chronic hepatitis negative for HB_s antigen
- Cryptogenic cirrhosis (some cases)
- Ulcerative colitis
- Sjögren's syndrome
- Rheumatoid arthritis
- Dermatomyositis
- Systemic sclerosis
- Discoid LE
- Systemic lupus erythematosus (SLE)

Non-organ specific

Aetiology. *Loss of* T_S *control.* There is some evidence to suggest that in the autoimmune diseases there is a loss of suppressor T cell control of the T helper cells. The observation that T_S cell function diminishes with age provides an attractive explanation for the rising incidence of subclinical and clinical organ-specific auto-immune disease with advancing years.

Sequestrated antigen. There are some antigens that do not normally come into contact with the immunological system so that there has been no opportunity for immunological tolerance of self-recognition to develop. For example, sperm, if extravasated following unilateral blockage of the vas deferens, may induce antibody formation and contribute to sterility. Sperm antibodies may also be produced following vasectomy in normal men.

Infection. In the hypersensitive host, invading micro-organisms may share antigen with certain of the host's tissues and induce the formation of antibodies which cross-react with these tissues. Thus the sharing of antigen between some Group A haemolytic streptococci and the heart may be relevant to rheumatic carditis. Likewise, the sharing of antigen between *Esch. coli* 014 and colonic epithelium may be relevant to the patho-genesis of ulcerative colitis.

Drugs such as methyldopa seem to alter the immunological system so that antibodies develop that are reactive with red cells occasionally pro-ducing haemolytic anaemia which is reversible on withdrawal of the drug. Other drugs are associated with the development of antinuclear antibodies (p.575).

Genetic factors are important in autoimmune disease as can be seen from experimental animal models, from family (including twin) studies and from the association of many autoimmune diseases with the MHC system (p. 29). As described on page 23, MHC class 2 antigens are involved in the presentation of antigen on the surface of the antigen-presenting cells and are of central importance in the regulation of the immune response. In certain autoimmune diseases (such as thyroiditis and type 1 diabetes) the thyroid cells and the islet cells express MHC class 2 antigens on their surfaces. This abnormal present-ation of such MHC antigens may facilitate sen-sitisation and activation of the T_H cells with the augmentation of an autoimmune response of the normal control mechanism. It may be that viruses are implicated in the expression of MHC antigens on the surface of tissue cells.

Immunological mechanisms. Some examples of different immunological mechanisms producing autoimmune diseases are shown in Table 2.6.

Antibodies in the serum as predictive markers. While particular antibodies may play a crucial role in the pathogenesis of disease, others seem to have little pathological function but may be useful markers indicating some degree of auto-immunity in the corresponding organ. Many auto-immune diseases can be compared to icebergs, with clinical manifest disease showing above the waterline, and characteristically a large amount of subclinical disease below it. The rate of pro-gression of autoimmune disease may be highly variable in different subjects. In the organ-specific group of disorders, antibody in the serum may act as a marker or indicator that immunological damage of some degree may be occurring in the corresponding tissue even although there is at that time no clinical evidence. Most tissues have a

Table 2.6 Immunological mechanisms in autoimmune disease.

Mechanism	Effect	Examples of disease
Antibody reactive with cell bound antigen	Complement activation	Autoimmune haemolytic anaemias Myasthenia gravis Idiopathic thrombocytopenia
	Cell stimulation Blocking antibody	Graves' disease (Type I thyrotoxicosis) Pernicious anaemia Infertility (some cases)
Deposition of immune complexes in tissues	Complement activation in tissues	SLE
Mixture of cytotoxic antibody, immune complex deposition and various cell-mediated mechanisms (T_C, T_D, and K)	Lymphocyte infiltration Atrophy	Thyroiditis Autoimmune Addison's disease

substantial reserve of function that must be eroded before clinical disease is manifest. The antibody that is most readily detectable and useful as a marker in the serum may or may not be implicated as a damaging agent. The rate of progression of that disease process may be over many years or more rapid, and it has as yet not been possible to determine what factors in an individual patient determine that rate of progression. Such markers, however, have great potential usefulness in that they indicate subjects at risk for the development of serious disease for which current modes of therapy are not optimal (such as type 1 diabetes). For immunologically-mediated diseases this offers the opportunity of intervening with immuno-suppressive methods that may prevent the progression of the disorder to its irrevocable end-stage, provided a form of immunosuppression can be found that is sufficiently specific so as not to compromise the normal immune resources of the body.

The major histocompatibility complex

The antigens causing the immune response that results in the rejection of a tissue allograft are known as major histocompatibility antigens. In man the major histocompatibility complex (MHC) is the HLA gene cluster on chromosome 6 (Table 2.7). As MHC antigens were originally described on human leucocytes, they are still referred to as human leucocyte antigens (HLA). Although the MHC was identified by its role in transplantation rejection, it is now recognised that proteins encoded in this region are involved in many aspects of immunological recognition, including interaction between different lymphoid cells, as well as between lymphocytes and antigen-presenting cells.

The HLA antigens are cell surface glycoproteins of three classes (Table 2.7). They are remarkable for the extensive degree of genetic polymorphism; i.e. the variability between individuals is very great and most unrelated persons possess different HLA antigens. HLA class 1 antigens come in three series, A, B and C and like class 2 are defined by appropriate antisera. Rapid progress is now being made into the better definition of class 2 antigens using monoclonal anti-

sera, e.g. DP, DQ and DR. The HLA specificities currently detected at each of these subregions are shown in Table 2.8. Class 1 antigens are distributed on all nucleated cells and platelets while class 2 antigens are restricted to B lymphocytes, macrophages, monocytes, epithelial cells, melanoma cells and activated T cells. Class 3 consists of complement proteins.

Table 2.7 Major histocompatibility complex (MHC)— short arm of chromosome 6.

Genes	HLA - DR - DQ - DP - C2 - C4 - FB - B - C - A		
Antigens	Class 2	Class 3	Class 1
Result	Regulation via T_H	Activation of C3	Cytotoxicity via T_C

Table 2.8 HLA specificities currently detected at each subregion. Those not unequivocally established are designated 'w' (workshop). Examples of recognised associated diseases are given in the text.

DR	DQ	DP	B	C	A
DR1	Dw1	DQw1 DPw1	Bw4	Bw47	Cw1 A1
DR2	Dw2	DQw2 DPw2	B5	Bw48	Cw2 A2
DR3	Dw3	DQw3 DPw3	Bw6	B49	Cw3 A3
DR4	Dw4	DPw4	B7	Bw50	Cw4 A9
DR5		DPw5	B8	B51	Cw5 A10
DRw6		DPw6	B12	Bw52	Cw6 A11
DR7	Dw7		B13	Bw53	Cw7 Aw19
DRw8	Dw8		B14	Bw54	Cw8 A23
DRw9			B15	Bw55	A24
DRw10			B16	Bw56	A25
DRw11	Dw5		B17	Bw57	A26
DRw12			B18	Bw58	A28
DRw13	Dw6		B21	Bw59	A29
DRw14	Dw9		Bw22	Bw60	A30
DRw52			B27	Bw61	A31
DRw53			B35	Bw62	A32
			B37	Bw63	Aw33
			B38	Bw64	Aw34
			B39	Bw65	Aw36
			B40	Bw67	Aw43
			Bw41	Bw70	Aw66
			Bw42	Bw71	Aw68
			B44	Bw72	Aw69
			B45	Bw73	
			Bw46		

Skin grafts between HLA identical siblings show a marked prolongation of survival, while renal allographs between HLA identical siblings have very few rejection episodes and a 95% survival at 3 years. However, in unrelated cadaver renal transplantation, true HLA identity is rare and a partial matching for HLA can offer only a modest improvement in survival figures.

HLA and disease. Some strong associations between HLA and susceptibility to certain diseases have been described, especially to the autoimmune diseases and to certain other conditions with a probably allergic basis. Examples are ankylosing spondylitis (B27), rheumatoid arthritis (DR4), autoimmune Addison's disease (B8, DR3), insulin-dependent diabetes (B8, DR3, DR4), Type 1 thyrotoxicosis (B8, Dw3) and myasthenia gravis (B8). Other HLA disease associations are not related to autoimmunity, e.g. haemochromatosis (A3) and the strongest of all, narcolepsy (DR2).

Certain HLA antigens occur together more commonly than would be expected by chance (alleleic association or linkage disequilibrium). In some instances the presence of an HLA antigen, or group of antigens in linkage disequilibrium, is protective as in insulin-dependent diabetes (p. 462).

SUPPRESSION OF IMMUNE REACTIONS OR OF THEIR EFFECTS

Antihistamines. When anaphylaxis presents as an acute clinical problem the immediate aim is to give drugs which antagonise the effects of the mediators. These antagonists are the antihistamines and various drugs which have opposite actions to the mediators.

The antihistamines occupy the same tissue receptors as histamine without providing any stimulus to the effector cells. The intravenous injection of an antihistamine quickly produces adequate tissue concentrations. The weal, the erythema and the itch of acute urticaria are reduced but there is no consistent improvement in lung function in acute bronchial asthma.

The failure of the antihistamines to relieve airway obstruction caused by an anaphylactic reaction has been attributed to high concentrations of histamine close to the smooth muscle cells. It may also be due to the presence of other mediators of the anaphylactic response. Bradykinin is rapidly inactivated in plasma by a kininase but its effects are not inhibited by antihistamines.

Sodium cromoglycate is believed to inhibit the release of the mediators from mast cells following the interaction of antigens with IgE antibodies (Fig. 2.5). It is partially effective in preventing the induction of asthma by specific antigens. If inhaled by an asthmatic subject before exposure to the antigen, protection may last for several hours, but if given after exposure to the antigen it has little effect.

Adrenaline and related drugs act by producing effects which oppose the mediators and are more effective in emergencies than the antihistamines. Adrenaline, isoprenaline and aminophylline are efficient bronchodilators in bronchial asthma. Urticaria is relieved and where oedema threatens the airway, the risk of asphyxia is lessened.

Despite their effectiveness these non-specific antagonists have serious disadvantages. They act on receptors which differ from those occupied by the mediators, and their effects never precisely counteract those of the mediators. The dose of a sympathomimetic amine which relieves airflow obstruction may produce tachycardia and palpitations even when the amine is administered as an aerosol. Salbutamol does not have these disadvantages as it is more specific in its actions on β-adrenergic receptors in the bronchi.

Corticosteroids such as prednisolone interfere at many points in the immune response, affecting lymphocyte recirculation and cytotoxic effector cells. The anti-inflammatory effect of steroids is due to their inhibition of neutrophil adherence to vascular endothelium in an inflammatory area and suppression of monocyte/macrophage functions such as microbicidal activity and response to lymphokines.

Hyposensitisation. Anaphylactic individuals can be made less sensitive by multiple subcutaneous injections of antigen in gradually increasing dosage. Pollen antigens can be used to prevent the development of hay fever and asthma in some patients. The patient develops IgG antibodies against the antigen; these antibodies have a higher avidity for the antigen than do IgE antibodies and are able to compete successfully for the antigen sites on the pollen, or whatever has induced the anaphylactic response. The amount of IgG antibodies produced is not sufficient to cause an immune complex reaction. In this context the IgG antibodies are referred to as blocking antibodies.

Immunosuppressive drugs. The production of immunoglobulins and the cellular immune response are dependent upon the division of lymphoid cells. Drugs which interfere with dividing cells are therefore all potentially immunosuppressive and were originally developed as anti-tumour agents. Of these azathioprine, cyclophosphamide and methotrexate have been used for immunosuppression. Such drugs may have serious adverse effects, including bone marrow suppression and the promotion of tuberculous, viral or fungal infection. A further possible hazard is an increased incidence of malignant tumours, such as lymphomas, possibly on account of the suppression of immunological surveillance of the body tissues in relation to infection with oncogenic viruses (below).

Cyclosporin is a naturally occurring fungal metabolite. It suppresses both humoral and cell mediated immunity, and has been shown to have a direct suppressive (but non-cytotoxic) effect on B cells and T helper cells. Resting cells which carry the vital memory of immunity to microbial infections are spared and there is little toxicity for dividing cells in the gut and bone marrow. Cyclosporin must be used at doses below those causing nephrotoxicity so that blood levels have to be monitored regularly by radioimmunoassay. Cyclosporin-treated patients may also be susceptible to EB viral induced lymphomas. However, the latest results suggest that the incidence of lymphoma is relatively low in patients treated with cyclosporin compared with that reported for allografted patients treated with drugs such as azathioprine or cyclophosphamide.

Anti-D immunoglobulin. The clearest example of interference with a specific immune response is the use of human anti-D immunoglobulin to prevent haemolytic disease of the newborn (p. 518).

Plasmapheresis. Apheresis is the generic term for removal of a component from the blood; a prefix indicates whether this is plasma, leucocytes etc. Plasmapheresis (plasma exchange) has been used beneficially in myasthenia gravis and Goodpasture's syndrome, removing acetylcholine-receptor and glomerular basement membrane antibodies respectively. It is used in conjunction with cytotoxic drugs and corticosteroids in order to check the rate of resynthesis of antibody.

Thymectomy as a treatment for autoimmune diseases other than myasthenia gravis may be effective only in childhood when the influence of the thymus on the immunological system is particularly important. It is seldom advocated.

Cancer immunology. Cancer cells lose some of the normal tissue-specific antigens and appear to gain some tumour-associated antigens which were not previously present in the cells from which they were derived. It used to be thought that the process of immunological surveillance destroys many early cancers by virtue of the recognition by the normal immune system of the 'foreignness' of tumour-associated antigens. However, immunodeficiency, either primary or induced by immunosuppressive drugs is mainly associated with lymphomas and not with cancer generally. It is more likely that the immune system is important in relation to the control of oncogenic viruses, rather than immune surveillance *per se*.

IMMUNODEFICIENCY DISORDERS

So important are the immunological mechanisms for survival that it is not surprising that patients are rarely seen suffering from major defects. Deficiencies of the humoral and cellular components of the immunological system may occur separately or together. Figure 2.7 shows the probable sites of the primary defects in the immune system for a number of clinical patterns that have been recognised. The more precise analysis of immunodeficiencies is being greatly aided by the monoclonal antibody markers for the different T cell subsets, for the different stages of maturity of B cells, and for monocytes.

Combined deficiency states

A block in the development of the stem-cell leads to deficiency in both the T and B lymphocyte systems and therefore to impairment of cell-mediated hypersensitivity and of synthesis of humoral antibody (Fig. 2.7, lesion 1). A failure of stem-cell development at an even earlier stage leads to the additional feature of agranulocytosis although the red cells and platelets are normal. About half the infants with the autosomal recessive

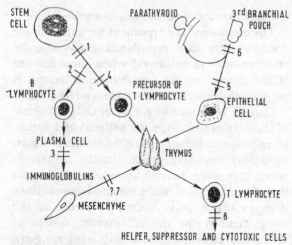

Fig. 2.7 Immunodeficiency syndromes. Sites of some of the developmental and other defects.

Site of Defect	Clinical Syndrome
1	*Severe combined immunodeficiency*: thymic hypoplasia, lymphopenia and agammaglobulinaemia. Autosomal recessive or X-linked inheritance. Do not survive infancy, but variable therapeutic success has been achieved with fetal liver cell or fetal thymus transplants.
2	*X-linked recessive agammaglobulinaemia*: normal thymus, no lymphopenia and normal cell-mediated hypersensitivity. Recurrent infection with extracellular pyogenic pathogens. Treated effectively with gammaglobulin.
3	*Defective synthesis of immunoglobulins.*
4 & 5 & 6	*Thymic hypoplasia and lymphopenia*: normal immunoglobulins. Frequently fungal or viral infections. Usually die in infancy. In 5, Di George syndrome, absence of parathyroids presenting as tetany in the newborn can be dramatically reversed by transplants of fetal thymic tissue.
7	*Thymic hypoplasia-ataxia telangiectasia.*May be part of a more widespread mesenchyme deficiency. Thymus fails to develop. Autosomal recessive inheritance. Difficult to classify.
8	*Various defects of helper, suppressor and cytotoxic cells.* These include impaired suppressor T cells in autoimmunity and excessive suppressor T cell activity resulting in hypogammaglobulinaemia.

form of severe combined immunodeficiency have a concomitant deficiency of adenosine deaminase which has enabled prenatal diagnosis by finding the enzyme deficiency in cultured amnion cells. Infants with either the autosomal or the X-linked type are incapable of limiting the most benign viral infections. Death has resulted from generalised chickenpox, or measles or from cytomegalic or other viral infections. Vaccination results in pro-gressive, ultimately fatal vaccinia infection. Following successful bone marrow transplantation, 10 year survivals with maintenance of normal T and B cell function have been recorded.

Deficiency of immunoglobulins

Primary immunoglobulin deficiency. Selective deficiency of the B lymphocyte system occurs in X-linked recessive hypo- or agamma-globulinaemia (Fig. 2.7, lesion 2). The lack of immunoglobulins is not absolute but the patient fails to respond to antigenic stimuli. However, cell mediated hypersensitivity is normal. This disorder is not incompatible with survival for many years, though the patient is very susceptible to bacterial infections.

Most patients with immunoglobulin deficiency have 'acquired' or 'late onset' agammaglobulin-aemia known as '*common, variable, unclassifiable immunodeficiency*'. B lymphocytes are usually, but not always present in contrast to their absence in the X-linked form of agammaglobulinaemia. Deterioration of T cell function may also be observed. Primary acquired agammaglobulin-aemia is associated with an unusually high incidence of autoimmune disease, such as pernicious anaemia or haemolytic anaemia. A prominent and frequent complication is a sprue-like syndrome and *Giardia intestinalis* infection (p. 776) is common. Another distinguishing feature of the acquired form is the frequent occurrence of non-caseating granulomas, e.g. in lungs, liver, and skin.

As the different immunoglobulins have different functions, deficiencies might be expected to produce clinical pictures. Thus IgM deficiency is possibly associated with meningococcal meningitis and lack of IgA with gastrointestinal or respiratory tract infections. The absence of IgA permits invasion of the normally sterile upper gut by bacteria, some of which could produce decomposition of bile salts and thus affect the absorption of fat.

Immunoglobulin injections consisting mainly of IgG can provide effective protection against severe, recurrent pyogenic infections in patients with various types of hypo- or agammaglobulin-aemia. Since the half-life of the gamma globulin injected is 30 days or more, these patients must receive at least a monthly injection of 100 mg per kg.

Secondary immunoglobulin deficiency. Maternal IgG2 is transferred across the placenta by active secretion to the fetus during the third trimester of pregnancy. Premature babies may thus have some degree of hypogammaglobulin-aemia and prophylactic IgG treatment may reduce the incidence of infections. The production of immunoglobulins in the early years of life is well below that of adults and this may well explain the greatly increased susceptibility of the young to infection, particularly gastrointestinal and respiratory tract infection because of IgA deficiency. IgA is present in colostrum and there is evidence that breast feeding provides the infant with intestinal immunity.

Immunoglobulin deficiency may arise also in adults as a result of abnormal metabolism of serum proteins as occurs in uraemic patients in whom susceptibility to infection is increased. Drugs may also depress the immune system; for example phenytoin or penicillamine may induce IgA deficiency.

Deficiency of cellular immunity

Primary cellular deficiency. This condition is a selective primary deficiency of T lymphocytes (Fig. 2.7, lesions 4, 5 and 6). There is severe lymphocytopenia and a predominance of reticulum cells in the lymphoid tissue. The patient's lymphocytes are unable to respond by transformation into lymphoblasts following stimulation with antigens. On account of the deficiency in cell-mediated hypersensitivity, affected children do not respond in the normal way to antigens such as monilia. Infants with thymic aplasia in whom the cell-mediated aspect is completely lacking are highly susceptible to viral infections, which usually prove fatal.

The fact that there are deficient humoral antibody responses to some antigens in conditions associated with lesions at sites 4, 5 and 6 of Figure 2.7 exemplifies the existence of co-operation between T and B lymphocytes in relation to certain antigens.

The transplantation of fragments of human fetal thymus has been effective in replacing the cellular immune deficiency in congenital thymic aplasia. Tissue matched bone marrow transplantation or transfer factor (p. 24) has been used in the Wiskott-Aldrich syndrome; this is a hereditary cellular immunodeficiency disorder, characterised by thrombocytopenia, but difficult to classify.

Secondary cellular deficiency. Secondary T cell defects may occur in Hodgkin's disease or sarcoidosis, following infections such as leprosy, miliary tuberculosis or measles, or may be induced by cytotoxic drugs. The *acquired immunodeficiency syndrome* (AIDS) is described on page 726.

PROSPECTS IN IMMUNOLOGY

Exciting developments can be anticipated in terms of the better understanding of the physiology of the immune system and how it may be modified in disease and in the treatment of such diseases. Thus the use of monoclonal antibody technology should further define and quantify the different lymphocyte subclasses and the involvement of the MHC system in the initiation of the immune response both in health and disease. Better understanding of the amplification mechanisms (e.g. lymphokines such as interleukin 2 and interferon) should lead to improved ways of reducing or increasing the immune response. The threat of an epidemic of AIDS has provided a strong stimulus to the study of immunodeficiency and this may well yield useful new information about the involvement of the immune system in disease in general.

The improvements in immunological knowledge that have occurred since the last edition of this book have taken us appreciably closer to the goal of antigen-specific suppression of the immune response. The further study of anti-idiotype antibodies are likely to lead to advances in this direction. With improved genetic and immunological markers for disease susceptibility, it should be possible within the not too distant future to initiate effective immunosuppressive therapy at an earlier stage in a range of disabling immunological disorders.

W. J. IRVINE

FURTHER READING:

Roitt I M 1987 Essential immunology, 6th edn. Blackwell Scientific Publications, Oxford

Weir D M 1988 Immunology. An outline for students of medicine and biology, 6th edn. Churchill Livingstone, Edinburgh

More detailed texts

Roitt I M, Brostoff J, Male D 1985 Immunology. Churchill Livingstone, Edinburgh. A profusely illustrated book with a concise text dealing with clinical immunology in depth

Stites D P, Stobo J D, Fudenberg H H, Wells J C (eds) 1984 Basic and clinical immunology, 5th edn. Lange, Los Altos

3

Infection and disease

General aspects of infection

Infection can involve any organ or system of the body and thus embraces all medical disciplines. It will therefore be referred to in each chapter. In this introductory chapter an account is given of general aspects, spread, diagnosis, prevention and treatment of infection. The term infectious disease is commonly used to denote infections that are contagious or communicable, i.e. transmissible from man to man. However, there has been a trend, especially in North America, to refer to all diseases caused by micro-organisms as infectious diseases.

Infection differs from other diseases in a number of aspects; the most important is that it is caused by a living micro-organism, which can frequently be identified, thus establishing the aetiology of the disease early in the illness. Many of these organisms, including all bacteria, are sensitive to antibiotics and most infections are therefore curable, unlike many non-infective diseases such as those of the cardiovascular or nervous systems which frequently become chronic and are not amenable to specific therapy. The communicability of infections is another factor which differentiates them from non-infective diseases; this leads to the transmission of pathogenic organisms to other people and if large numbers are involved an epidemic may result. Finally, many infections are preventable by hygienic measures or by vaccines. In certain circumstances, infection may be prevented by the judicious use of antibiotics (chemoprophylaxis).

During the past 50 years there has been a dramatic fall in the incidence of communicable diseases in developed countries. This is due to several factors such as immunisation, anti-microbial chemotherapy, improved nutrition, and better sanitation and housing. Infections which have decreased, and in some instances almost disappeared in these countries include diphtheria, poliomyelitis, tuberculosis, brucellosis and bacillary dysentery. In less advanced countries, however, especially in the tropics, infection continues to be one of the commonest causes of death, particularly in children; measles, for example, has a high mortality in malnourished infants in many African countries.

Even in developed countries certain infections continue to pose problems and some are even increasing in incidence. Sexually transmitted diseases have become common as a result of sexual 'liberation' and promiscuity both heterosexual and homosexual. Food poisoning caused by Salmonellae and Campylobacter species has increased due commonly to the modern practice of battery-rearing and deep-freezing of poultry. Patients in hospitals have always been at risk of acquiring infection as Lord Lister and Florence Nightingale recognised over a hundred years ago. In spite of the availability of antiseptics and antibiotics, however, hospital-acquired (nosocomial) infection remains a major problem which has increased in recent years in parallel with the introduction of new techniques of patient care, the grouping together of susceptible patients in specialized units, and the number of patients with decreased resistance to infection (compromised hosts).

A patient's resistance to infection may be reduced as a result of extremes of age, disease, medical or surgical therapeutic regimes, or a combination of several of these factors. A person whose resistance to infection is decreased as a result of abnormality in the immune response is referred to as an immunocompromised host.

Examples of immunocompromised patients are provided by a recipient of a renal transplant or a patient suffering from leukaemia. Both have serious diseases and are usually being treated with immunosuppressive and corticosteroid drugs and are thus very susceptible to infection which is not infrequently fatal. Infections in immunocompromised patients are caused by a wide variety of micro-organisms including those which are common human pathogens such as *Staphylococcus aureus* and the varicella/zoster virus. However, these patients are also very susceptible to organisms which rarely cause serious infections in healthy people, for example *Staphylococcus epidermidis* and *Pseudomonas aeruginosa* and fungi such as *Candida albicans* (opportunist organisms).

By the end of the present decade, approaching one thousand million passengers will travel by air each year, and it is now possible to circumnavigate the world in less than 48 hours. As a result there has been an increase in the number of imported infections in developed countries. These commonly originate in areas of the world with tropical or sub-tropical climates. Returning travellers may suffer from a wide variety of infections, the commonest being diarrhoeal diseases and malaria.

Within the past 10 years a number of 'new' infections have been recognised, principally as a result of new laboratory diagnostic techniques, but also due to improved epidemiological methods including the establishment of national centres for the surveillance of communicable disease. These centres monitor incidents and outbreaks of infection and exchange information with similar oganizations in other countries. The main 'recently recognized' infections are: *Campylobacter enteritis* (p. 752), *rotavirus enteritis* (p. 321), *non-A, non-B and delta viral hepatitis* (p. 346), *legionnaires' disease* (p. 219), *viral haemorrhagic*

fevers (p. 733), *Chlamydia urethritis* (p. 418), *antibiotic-associated colitis* (p. 44), *group B streptococcal neonatal infections* (p. 741), *toxic shock syndrome* (p. 743), *Lyme disease* (p. 572), and the *acquired immune deficiency syndrome* (AIDS, p. 726).

Source and spread of infection

Infection may originate from the patient (autogenous) usually from the skin, nasopharynx or colon, or from outside sources (exogenous), commonly from another person who may either be suffering from an infection or carrying a pathogenic micro-organism. Carriers are usually healthy and may harbour the organism in the throat (diphtheria) or stool (salmonella).

Micro-organisms may be transmitted by several routes. Autogenous infection may develop as a result of local spread, e.g. from bowel to peritoneum, or by the blood-stream. An example of the latter is infective endocarditis caused by *Streptococcus sanguis* originating in the patient's mouth and entering the blood during meals or dental procedures. Exogenous infection may be acquired directly or indirectly by one of the following routes.

1. *Direct contact*. Venereal and skin infections are transmitted by contact between body surfaces.
2. *Airborne transmission*. This includes transmission by droplets and dust particles. Infected droplets originate in the nasopharynx and mouth and are expelled during talking, breathing and sneezing, carrying micro-organisms with them. Respiratory tract infections and many of the common infectious diseases of childhood such as measles are airborne-spread.
3. *Faecal–oral spread*. Infections transmitted by this route are usually acquired by the ingestion of food and drink contaminated by human faeces. This often occurs during preparation of meals as a result of a low standard of personal hygiene in kitchen workers. Large outbreaks of hepatitis or cholera may follow pollution of domestic water supplies. Other diseases spread by the faecal–oral route include dysentery and enteroviral infections such as poliomyelitis.
4. *Mammal, bird or insect borne*. Certain infections (zoonoses) may be contracted directly or

indirectly from animals. Examples include rabies (dog bite), leptospirosis (rat's urine), brucellosis (goat's milk) and salmonellosis (poultry meat). Blood sucking insects are vectors in the transmission of many important infections such as malaria, yellow fever, plague and rickettsial diseases.

5. *Transmission by medical and nursing procedures.* Infection may be transmitted by inadequately sterilized instruments, faulty nursing techniques or contamination of transfused blood or other liquid.

Incubation period is the period of time which elapses between the invasion of the tissues by pathogens and the appearance of clinical symptoms and signs of infection.

Diagnosis of infectious disease

A knowledge of infections prevailing in the locality may be a valuable guide to diagnosis. It is wise to enquire about contacts among the family, friends and workmates. Persons following certain occupations may be exposed to infection, e.g. leptospirosis occurs in abbatoir and farm workers (p. 761) and anthrax in handlers of hides and bone meal (p. 745).

A recent history of laparotomy or of obscure abdominal pain should suggest subphrenic or intrahepatic abscess as a cause of unexplained fever.

Residence or travel abroad raises the possibility of malaria, amoebic abscess of the liver or other exotic disease.

In many infections a diagnosis beyond all reasonable doubt may be made on clinical grounds, e.g. measles or chickenpox. In others a diagnosis may require confirmation by bacteriological, immunological or haematological examination, radiography or scanning.

Occasionally the cause of a febrile illness remains uncertain in spite of investigation and such a case is categorised PUO (pyrexia of unknown origin). In order to establish the diagnosis the following measures should be undertaken.

1. Retake the history; a symptom may have been overlooked or misinterpreted; enquire again whether the patient has lived or travelled overseas.
2. Repeat the examination of the patient; new signs may have appeared while others could have been missed or their significance not appreciated.
3. Examine the urine repeatedly for protein, white and red blood cells and micro-organisms.
4. Review the results of laboratory investigations, thoroughly rescrutinise any radiographs and repeat such examinations as may seem necessary.

If the diagnosis is still uncertain further tests will be required. These will be indicated by any new information obtained as a result of the clinical reassessment. It should be borne in mind that most causes of PUO are due to a common disorder with an unusual presentation. In Britain the most frequent causes of PUO are tumours (especially lymphomas), infections (among which tuberculosis is important), connective tissue disorders and drug hypersensitivity. In the tropics and elsewhere a wide variety of infections must be considered, as a glance at the map on page 717 will demonstrate.

Mysterious fevers, particularly in patients who have some knowledge of medicine or nursing, may be due to deceit (factitious fever). Doubts should be raised if the skin of a supposedly febrile patient does not feel hot or if the general health does not deteriorate in spite of persistent fever. The occurrence of some bizarre symptom or sign may arouse suspicion that the temperature is being falsified. There are both subtle and simple techniques for doing this. The latter include holding the thermometer close to a hot water bottle or other source of heat, dipping it into a hot drink, applying friction to the bulb, or shaking it in a retrograde manner.

If the diagnosis remains obscure another opinion should be obtained, as reconsideration of the evidence by an unbiased observer may throw new light on the problem.

When a diagnosis still cannot be established and the patient's condition is deteriorating, various remedies, e.g. antibiotics, may be tried empirically in the hope of influencing the course of the disease. A therapeutic trial should not be regarded as a satisfactory diagnostic test and it can further obscure the diagnosis by suppressing but not curing the infection. It is most useful in suspected tuberculosis.

The prevention of infection

The prevention of infection depends on three concepts which may be interrelated:

1. *Elimination of the source*. Successful examples of this include the eradication of tuberculosis and brucellosis from cattle in many countries and the world-wide elimination of smallpox. The laboratory screening of donated blood for syphilis and hepatitis B virus has virtually eliminated these sources of infection.
2. *Prevention of transmission of infection*. This may be accomplished by the isolation of infected patients (source isolation) and of those such as the immunosuppressed who are particularly susceptible to infection (protective isolation). Strict antisepsis in operating theatres and good nursing practices in wards are essential if transmission of infection is to be prevented. Hand-washing is of paramount importance.

Insect control, by the elimination of breeding grounds and the use of insecticides, is a major factor in malaria prevention programmes. Individuals who have been in close contact with serious infectious diseases such as diphtheria or Lassa fever are placed in quarantine — a term derived from the period of 40 days of compulsory isolation of ships after leaving a port where life-threatening infections such as plague were rife. The duration of quarantine depends on the incubation period of the disease.

3. *Protection of susceptible persons*. This involves the judicious use of prophylactic antibiotics (p. 47) and of active or passive immunisation.

Active immunisation. In Britain parents should be advised to have their children immunised against whooping-cough, diphtheria, tetanus, measles and poliomyelitis (Table 3.1). Because of the risk of damage to the developing embryo or fetus if rubella should occur during pregnancy, it is recommended that rubella vaccine be given to all girls between 11 and 14 years and to non-pregnant women of child-bearing age who are found to be serologically negative for this antigen.

The indications for immunisation against influenza, hepatitis B, enteric fevers, cholera, plague, typhus, yellow fever and rabies depend upon the likelihood of exposure or international health regulations (p. 802). Acute demyelinating encephalomyelitis (p. 648) and polyneuropathy are rare complications of immunisation.

Passive immunisation. An injection of immunoglobulin will provide temporary protection against certain infectious diseases. Human normal immunoglobulin (pooled) is indicated for prevention of measles (p. 728) and virus A hepatitis (p. 344), and human specific immunoglobulin for chickenpox (p. 731), virus B hepatitis (p. 346), tetanus (p. 745) and rabies (p. 732).

Diseases due to infection

Diseases due to infection are the commonest cause of ill health throughout the world. The organisms involved are viruses, chlamydia, rickettsia, bac-

Table 3.1. Immunisation schedule recommended in Britain.

Age	Visits	Vaccine	Intervals
3–12 months	3	Three administrations of DTP + OPV	6–8 weeks and 4–6 months
12–24 months	1	Measles vaccination	
First year at school	1	Booster DT + OPV	
10–13 years	1	BCG for the tuberculin negative	
Girls: 11–13 years	1	Rubella vaccination	
15–19 years or on leaving school	1	TT + OPV	

DTP = Diphtheria, tetanus, pertussis ('triple') vaccine.
OPV = Oral poliomyelitis vaccine.
DT = Diphtheria, tetanus vaccine.
TT = Tetanus toxoid.

teria, spirochaetes, fungi, protozoa and helminths. The term infestation is limited to ectoparasites, usually arthropods such as lice and fleas, which remain on the surface of the body but which may transmit a systemic infection.

As yet few specific therapeutic measures are available for viral diseases, among which are the exanthemata — chickenpox, measles and rubella; mumps and infectious mononucleosis; respiratory illnesses such as the common cold and influenza; viral hepatitis and diseases of the nervous system such as rabies, poliomyelitis and meningitis. The number of viral infections for which prophylaxis, using vaccines, is available in increasing parallel with modern advances in virology and now there is preventative treatment for rabies, hepatitis B, yellow fever, poliomyelitis, measles, mumps and rubella. Several viral infections may be prevented temporarily by passive immunisation with human immunoglobulin.

Organisms smaller than true bacteria, the rickettsiae which cause typhus fevers, and the chlamydia of psittacosis, lymphogranuloma, urethritis and trachoma are widespread and susceptible to antimicrobial therapy.

The range of diseases caused by bacteria is large; streptococci and staphylococci are widespread and produce similar diseases throughout the world. Other such as the cholera vibrio and plague bacillus are locally endemic but may produce epidemics from time to time. Some bacterial infections may be acute such as meningitis and tetanus, others chronic such as tuberculosis, syphilis and leprosy.

Fungi causing ringworm and thrush occur all over the world but systemic infections with other fungi, such as coccidioidomycosis, histoplasmosis and the blastomycoses, are rare except in certain geographic locations (p. 44–45).

Protozoal infections such as malaria, amoebic dysentery, sleeping sickness and leishmaniasis and helminthiasis (worms) are of great importance in the tropics and are discussed in Chapters 18 and 19.

Most bacterial, fungal and protozoal infections can be successfully treated with antimicrobial agents provided that the appropriate drug is prescribed early in the disease. This emphasises the need for rapid and accurate diagnosis supplemented where necessary by specific tests to indicate the most effective therapeutic agent.

Diseases due to infection which involve one system predominantly are described in the appropriate chapters of this book, e.g. infective endocarditis (p. 160), respiratory infections (p. 214), viral hepatitis (p. 342), sexually transmitted disease (p. 415), infectious mononucleosis (p. 522), and meningitis (p. 638). Other infectious diseases are described in Chapter 19.

Students should familiarise themselves first with infections which are common in their own countries. In Britain these include streptococcal and staphylococcal infections (p. 741), the childhood infectious diseases such as measles (p. 728), whooping cough (p. 747), and chickenpox (p. 750), food poisoning (p. 751) and the serious imported infections, e.g. typhoid fever (p. 750) and malaria (p. 770).

ANTIMICROBIAL THERAPY

The ability of one micro-organism to interfere with the growth of another is called antibiosis and is due to specific diffusible metabolic products termed *antibiotics*. Since the introduction of penicillin in 1940, research has produced a wide range of antibiotics. A variety of chemotherapeutic agents such as metronidazole, trimethoprim, dapsone and isoniazid has also followed the demonstration of the therapeutic effect of sulphanilamide in 1935. A general term for all of these substances is *antimicrobial agent*.

Effective therapy is now available against all known bacteria, rickettsiae, mycoplasmas and chlamydia. Specific antiprotozoal compounds are used in the treatment of diseases such as sleeping sickness, kala azar, malaria and amoebic dysentery. Topical antifungal agents are widely prescribed, but fully effective, non-toxic, anti-fungal drugs have not yet been found for use in systemic infection. Antimicrobial agents active against viruses have also been discovered but few have been successful therapeutically.

THE BETA-LACTAM ANTIBIOTICS

These are the *penicillins* and *cephalosporins* and are so called because of the 4 membered beta-lactam ring which forms part of their basic structure. Resistance is commonly due to bacterial enzymes called beta-lactamases (pencillinases and cephalosporinases) which can inactivate the antibiotics by opening the beta-lactam ring. The plasmids (p. 17) which code for these enzymes are transmissible between bacteria.

The penicillins

All penicillins are bactericidal and the range of activity of the group is wide as both Gram-positive and certain Gram-negative organisms are sensitive to individual penicillins. The outstanding adverse effect is the risk of inducing a hypersensitivity reaction. Even so the penicillins are the most useful antibiotics at present available. The principal penicillins are:

1. *Benzylpenicillin,* which is the original and most active penicillin; it must be given by injection. Its action can be prolonged by combining it with procaine — *procaine penicillin.* An even longer-acting form is *benzathine penicillin.*
2. *Phenoxymethylpenicillin* is absorbed when administered by mouth.
3. *Cloxacillin* and *flucloxacillin* are not inactivated by staphylococcal penicillinase and are used for the treatment of staphylococcal infections resistant to benzylpenicillin.
4. *Ampicillin,* its esters and its analogue *amoxycillin* are effective against Gram-negative bacilli, in contrast to most other penicillins whose activity is largely limited to Gram-positive organisms and Gram-negative cocci.
5. The *acylureidopenicillins,* mezlocillin, azlocillin and piperacillin are ampicillin derivatives which have a broader spectrum than ampicillin but, like ampicillin, are susceptible to beta-lactamases.
6. *Ticarcillin* and *azlocillin* are used in pseudomonas infections.

Benzylpenicillin is rapidly absorbed following intramuscular injection and is excreted by the kidneys within a few hours. A dose of 300 mg (half a million units) 6- or 8-hourly will suffice for most infections due to sensitive organisms. Large intramuscular or intravenous doses (up to 12 million units daily) may be required to achieve therapeutic concentrations within deep-seated or walled-off foci of infection, as occurs in infective endocarditis or lung abscess. The intramuscular injection of large doses is painful. Probenecid, 2 g daily by mouth, will raise the blood level of penicillin by delaying its excretion by the kidney and allow smaller doses to be used.

Benzylpenicillin remains the antibiotic of choice for the treatment of pneumococcal, meningococcal and streptococcal infections, gonorrhoea and syphilis, yaws, diphtheria, tetanus, gas gangrene, anthrax and actinomycosis. It is also indicated for infections caused by penicillin-sensitive strains of *Staph. aureus.*

Penicillin is also used prophylactically. Benzylpenicillin is given to patients with valvular heart disease before a dental extraction to reduce the risk of infective endocarditis (p. 160). It is also given to prevent gas gangrene and tetanus after high amputations of ischaemic legs and for wounds containing dirt and devitalised tissue.

Procaine penicillin and benzathine penicillin. These are long-acting penicillins given by injection and used in the treatment of gonorrhoea and the treponemal diseases, syphilis and yaws. *Procaine penicillin* in aqueous suspension, in a dose of 300 mg once a day intra-muscularly, will maintain an adequate blood level for 24 hours.

Benzathine penicillin has a duration of action of 3 to 4 weeks. It can be used for the prophylaxis of rheumatic fever in patients who cannot be relied upon to take oral penicillin. The dose varies from 229–916 mg once a week. For rheumatic fever prophylaxis the dose is 916 mg every 3 weeks.

Phenoxymethylpenicillin is incompletely absorbed from the stomach and frequent oral administration will produce reasonable blood levels. The usual dose is 500 mg every 4 to 6 hours, taken half an hour before meals to ensure maximum absorption.

Phenoxymethylpenicillin is indicated for minor streptococcal infections and for pneumococcal pneumonia after initial therapy with benzylpenicillin. It is used prophylactically on a long-term basis following an attack of rheumatic fever to prevent recurrences.

Cloxacillin and flucloxacillin. These semi-synthetic penicillins are stable to staphylococcal beta-lactamases. The only indications for their use are infections caused by penicillin-resistant *Staph. aureus* and *Staph. epidermidis* (p. 742). For oral therapy flucloxacillin is superior to cloxacillin as it is almost twice as well absorbed from the gut. The dose is 500 mg 6-hourly but this can be increased to 1 g every 4 hours for seriously ill patients.

Ampicillin. This is a semisynthetic penicillin which is effective by mouth and which has a bactericidal action against Gram-positive organisms and also a variety of Gram-negative organisms, including salmonellae, shigellae, *Haemophilus influenzae* and certain strains of *Esch. coli* and *Proteus*. It is inactivated by staphylococcal penicillinase. Ampicillin is of value in urinary tract infections due to *Esch. coli* and *Proteus* and in exacerbations of chronic bronchitis.

The dose is 250 mg to 1 g, 4- to 8-hourly by mouth. Preparations for injection are also available. Maculopapular rashes occur in approximately 5% of all patients given ampicillin and in over 90% of patients with infectious mononucleosis; this antibiotic should not therefore be prescribed for sore throats which may be due to infectious mononucleosis.

There are a number of ampicillin esters including talampicillin, bacampicillin and pivampicillin. These improve the absorption of ampicillin thus producing higher blood levels of the antibiotic.

Amoxycillin is an analogue of ampicillin which has a similar antibacterial range but is better absorbed from the gastrointestinal tract. It is effective in typhoid fever.

Clavulanic acid is a new beta-lactam agent with only weak antibacterial activity. It is, however, a potent inhibitor of many beta-lactamases and can protect beta-lactamase-susceptible antibiotics, such as amoxycillin, from inactivation by these enzymes. A combination of amoxycillin plus sodium clavulanate is available. (Augmentin)

Ticarcillin. Carbenicillin was initially the only penicillin with activity against *Ps. aeruginosa*. This organism, however, is only moderately sensitive to carbenicillin which has been replaced by its more active analogue ticarcillin.

Mezlocillin, azlocillin and piperacillin. These acylureidopenicillins have a wider range of activity than ampicillin and are also more effective against many Gram-negative bacilli. They are used in combination with other antibiotics for the treatment of undiagnosed infections in immunocompromised patients.

Azlocillin is more active than ticarcillin against *Ps. aeruginosa*, an organism which is usually of relatively low virulence but is an important cause of disease in patients with impaired defence mechanisms. Treatment is with either ticarcillin or azlocillin but in pseudomonas septicaemia an aminoglycoside is also required; tobramycin plus azlocillin is probably the best choice.

Adverse effects of the penicillins. An increasing number of patients have acquired hypersensitivity to the systemic administration of the penicillins. This takes the form of urticaria and pyrexia or of an acute anaphylactic reaction which has occasionally proved fatal. Ampicillin commonly produces a maculopapular rash which differs from penicillin-induced urticaria and is specific for ampicillin. It is almost certainly unrelated to true penicillin allergy and is not a contraindication to future treatment with other penicillins. The patient should always be asked about previous allergy to any form of penicillin before treatment is commenced as a severe reaction may be provoked by the administration of only a few milligrams. Patients who suffer from bronchial asthma or are hypersensitive to other drugs are particularly liable to become allergic to penicillin.

Skin sensitisation may result from topical applications of any antibiotic, but is so frequent with penicillin that it should never be applied locally.

Although penicillin is otherwise a safe antibiotic, its accumulation in patients with renal failure may lead to encephalopathy, so that dosage in these circumstances must be modified and guided by the blood levels. The injectable preparations of all penicillins are formulated as sodium or potassium salts and hypernatraemia or hyperkalaemia can also result if large doses are given to patients with renal failure. Penicillin should never be given intrathecally.

It is important to avoid accidental intravenous administration when injecting procaine penicillin intramuscularly as this may result in a sensation of impending death, paraesthesiae and confusion lasting up to an hour The reaction may be fatal.

The cephalosporins

The cephalosporins have a wide range of activity against many, but not all, important Gram-positive and Gram-negative bacteria and are therefore of value for the initial 'blind' therapy of undiagnosed infections. *Cephalexin, cefaclor* and *cephradine* are all absorbed from the gut but the other available cephalosporins such as *cefuroxime, cephamandole* and *cephazolin* must be given by injection. *Cefoxitin*, a cephamycin antibiotic, has the additional advantage of activity against *Bacteroides fragilis*, an anaerobic bacillus which is a common cause of intra-abdominal sepsis (p. 321). Cefuroxime and cefoxitin are very resistant to degradation by many beta-lactamases.

Cefotaxime, latamoxef, ceftizoxime and *ceftazidime* are expensive cephalosporins which are especially stable in the presence of beta-lactamases and have greater intrinsic activity against many Gram-negative bacilli than the earlier cephalosporins. They also have varying degrees of activity against *Ps. aeruginosa* and *B. fragilis* but are less active than cefuroxime or cephamandole against Gram-positive organisms, especially *Staph. aureus. Cefsulodin* is a cephalosporin with only one indication, i.e. infection caused by *Ps. aeruginosa*.

The dose of the cephalosporins ranges from 250–1000 mg 6-hourly depending on the size of the patient, renal function, and severity of infection. For abdominal sepsis the dose of cefoxitin is 2 g. Cefuroxime is probably the best cephalosporin for general use and ceftazidime is the most active against Gram-negative bacilli.

Adverse reactions are similar to those of the penicillins. A small number of penicillin-sensitive patients may also be allergic to the cephalosporins which should be avoided if there is a history of significant hypersensitivity to the penicillins. Latamoxef can cause bleeding. Nephrotoxicity is discussed on page 412.

Other beta-lactam agents

Aztreonam is a new monocyclic beta-lactam antibiotic the efficacy of which is limited to Gram-negative aerobic bacteria including *Ps. aeruginosa, N. gonorrhoea* and *H. influenzae*. Side-effects are similar to those of other beta-lactam antibiotics.

THE TETRACYCLINES

Tetracycline, oxytetracycline and chlortetracycline are very closely related bacteriostatic agents which for practical purposes have an identical range of activity. The adult dose is 250–500 mg 6-hourly before meals because the absorption of most tetracyclines is reduced by chelation with calcium (e.g. in milk). *Doxycycline* is an exception and also has the advantage that it is given only once daily, 200–300 mg on the first day and 100–200 mg thereafter.

The tetracyclines inhibit the growth of a wide range of Gram-positive and Gram-negative bacteria and are particularly useful in the treatment of exacerbations of chronic bronchitis, but their value is limited by an increase in tetracycline-resistant pneumococci and *H. influenzae*. The tetracyclines are also active against rickettsiae (typhus fevers), *Coxiella burneti* (Q-fever), *Mycoplasma pneumoniae* and chlamydia (lymphogranuloma venereum, psittacosis and non-gonococcal urethritis) and are effective in brucellosis.

The tetracyclines are employed systemically in acne vulgaris and rosacea where their beneficial effect is almost certainly not due solely to their antibacterial action. Chlortetracycline is used for the local treatment of skin infections as it does not cause cutaneous sensitisation.

Adverse effects. The tetracyclines are safe with few side-effects. The commonest is diarrhoea which usually stops when the antibiotic is discontinued. Tetracyclines chelate with calcium and are deposited in developing bone and teeth causing a brown discoloration. They should not therefore be given to children or pregnant women. With the exception of doxycycline, the tetracyclines can exacerbate renal failure and should not be given to patients with kidney disease.

THE AMINOGLYCOSIDE ANTIBIOTICS

Streptomycin, kanamycin, gentamicin, tobramycin, netilmicin, amikacin and neomycin have similar chemical structures, pharmacological actions and adverse effects. They are not absorbed and for systemic treatment must be given by injection. The outstanding property of *streptomycin* is its bactericidal effect on the tubercle bacillus. It is given with two other antituberculous drugs and this triple therapy prevents the emergence of resistant strains (p. 230). For long-term therapy the daily dose of streptomycin should not exceed 1 g.

Kanamycin is active against many Gram-negative bacilli but has been mainly replaced by gentamicin for infections caused by Gram-negative bacilli.

Gentamicin has a range of activity similar to kanamycin but has the very important additional advantage of being effective against *Ps. aeruginosa*. It is also active against penicillin-resistant staphylococci but inactive against anaerobes and streptococci with the exception of *Strep. faecalis*; in serious infections caused by this organism gentamicin is combined with ampicillin. The dose of gentamicin depends on renal function and the age and weight of the patient. Up to 7.5 mg per kilogram body weight per 24 hours in divided doses is required for serious infections but 2 mg per kg is sufficient for uncomplicated urinary tract infections. Therapeutic blood concentrations of gentamicin are given on page 818.

Tobramycin is more active than gentamicin against *Ps. aeruginosa* but has no other advantage.

Netilmicin, a gentamicin derivative, is stable to three of nine aminoglycoside-inactivating enzymes, and like amikacin, should be reserved for infection caused by gentamicin-resistant organisms. Netilmicin is slightly less nephrotoxic than gentamicin to which it is preferred in the elderly and if renal function is impaired.

Amikacin, a derivative of kanamycin, has less intrinsic antibacterial activity than gentamicin, but has the advantage of being stable to eight of nine aminoglycoside-inactivating enzymes, in contrast to gentamicin which is susceptible to six of the nine. For this reason amikacin is active against many gentamicin-resistant Gram-negative bacilli and should be reserved for the treatment of infections caused by these organisms. The dose is 500 mg 12-hourly — this may have to be increased for serious infections.

Neomycin is too toxic to be given parenterally but local applications containing neomycin are used in infections of the skin and eye. Neomycin is used in hepatic encephalopathy to reduce the numbers of colonic bacteria.

Adverse effects. The aminoglycosides are all nephrotoxic (p. 412) and ototoxic. The commonest adverse effect of the aminoglycosides is on the eighth cranial nerve. With streptomycin and gentamicin the vestibular division is initially affected with resultant vertigo and incoordination. Later, deafness may also occur. Kanamycin tends to cause deafness first. Aminoglycosides, especially gentamicin, should not be administered together with the diuretic frusemide, as both can cause eighth nerve damage and additive ototoxicity may result from the combination.

The ototoxicity of the aminoglycosides is related to the age of the patient, the serum level of the antibiotic and the duration of administration. The aminoglycosides are principally excreted from the body by the kidneys and the risk of toxicity is increased when there is impairment of renal function. In such cases serum levels of the antibiotic must be monitored and the frequency of dosage adjusted accordingly. Serum concentrations of the antibiotic must be measured in all seriously ill patients to prevent toxicity and also to ensure therapeutic blood levels.

OTHER ANTIBIOTICS AND CHEMOTHERAPEUTIC AGENTS

Chloramphenicol

Chloramphenicol has a range of activity similar to that of the tetracyclines with the important difference that it is effective in enteric fever. It is more active than the tetracyclines against *H. influenzae* and is the antibiotic of choice in meningitis due to this organism. The daily dose for an adult is 1–3 g. Preparations for parenteral administration are also available. Chloramphenicol eye drops and ointment are indicated for purulent conjunctivitis.

Adverse effects. Chloramphenicol has in its chemical structure a benzene ring of the type known to cause bone marrow aplasia. Although pancytopenia due to chloramphenicol is very uncommon, it is almost invariably fatal; this antibiotic should be used systemically only for the treatment of typhoid fever and *H. influenzae* infections and in other conditions if there is no alternative therapy.

Chloramphenicol should never be given to premature infants and very rarely to the newborn because of the risk of the development of the frequently fatal *'grey baby syndrome'*. This is a state of acute circulatory failure caused by the very high blood levels of chloramphenicol due to its inadequate conjugation in the liver at this age.

Clindamycin

Clindamycin (7-chlorolincomycin) has a similar antibacterial spectrum to penicillin against most Gram-positive organisms including penicillin-resistant staphylococci. It penetrates well into bone and is therefore useful for osteomyelitis caused by *Staph. aureus*. The other principal indication is for the treatment of infections caused by *B. fragilis* (p. 321). The dose is 300 mg 6-hourly, orally or by injection.

Clindamycin is the commonest cause of *antibiotic-associated colitis*. This adverse reaction, which can also complicate treatment with other antibiotics, especially ampicillin, is due to selective overgrowth of *Clostridium difficile* which produces a toxin detectable in the faeces and is the direct cause of the disease. Treatment is with vancomycin or metronidazole, the latter being less costly.

Erythromycin

Erythromycin has a similar although not identical antibacterial spectrum to penicillin and is commonly used to treat infections caused by Gram-positive organisms in penicillin-allergic patients. It is also effective in whooping cough, Campylobacter enteritis and Legionnaires' disease provided it is given early enough in the course of these illnesses. It is a safe and effective antibiotic for the treatment of respiratory infections in children in domiciliary practice. Erythromycin is prescribed in a dosage of 250–500 mg by mouth every 6 hours. There is a preparation for intravenous injection. Diarrhoea is the principal side effect although cholestatic jaundice may rarely develop if the course of treatment exceeds 10 days.

Sodium fusidate

This sodium salt of fusidic acid is highly bactericidal against *Staph. aureas* and is useful in infections caused by penicillin-resistant staphylococci. Like clindamycin it is well concentrated in bone. Sodium fusidate is given orally in doses of 250–500 mg thrice daily, is rapidly absorbed, attains high tissue levels and is reasonably well tolerated, although nausea and vomiting are not uncommon during therapy. An intravenous preparation is available. Jaundice has occasionally been associated with its use. This antibiotic is expensive and is indicated for serious infections due to staphylococci, especially osteomyelitis and endocarditis.

Spectinomycin

Spectinomycin is an aminocyclitol compound with certain structural similarity to streptomycin although it is not an aminoglycoside. Its only clinical use is for the treatment of gonorrhoea if penicillin is contraindicated because of allergy or bacterial resistance.

Vancomycin

Vancomycin is a bactericidal antibiotic with a limited but important antibacterial spectrum. It is particularly active against: (1) staphylococci and streptococci and is an alternative to the penicillins for the treatment of serious infections such as endocarditis caused by these organisms in penicillin-allergic patients; (2) highly resistant staphylococci such as the multiply-resistant organisms (p. 743) which are serious causes of hospital infection; (3) *Clostridium difficile* which causes antibiotic-associated colitis.

Parenteral administration is by slow intravenous infusion over 60 minutes. Side-effects include fever, rash and, rarely, nephrotoxicity and ototoxicity. The daily dose for injection is 1-2 g which must be reduced in renal failure when serum levels should be monitored. 125 mg 6-hourly is given by mouth for antibiotic-associated colitis.

The sulphonamides and trimethoprim

Although the sulphonamides have been superseded in many countries by antibiotics, their usefulness has been extended by the introduction of co-trimoxazole, a combination of sulphonamide and trimethoprim. The sulphonamides most suitable for clinical use are the short-acting preparations, e.g. sulphadimidine, which is rapidly absorbed and quickly excreted in the urine in a soluble form.

The most common indication for the use of sulphonamides is cystitis. A dose of 1 g, 8 hourly by mouth is adequate. Sulphonamides have long been used in the treatment of meningococcal infection, particularly meningitis but the incidence of resistant strains is increasing and therefore penicillin is now used in treating this condition.

Adverse effects. Sulphonamides have a wide range of potential hazards including rashes, fever and agranulocytosis. Serious but rare complications are haemolytic anaemia, purpura, pancytopenia and renal lesions (p. 412). Glucose-6-phosphate dehydrogenase deficiency (p. 512) is a contraindication to the use of sulphonamides, as haemolysis may be induced. The Stevens-Johnson syndrome (erythema multiforme and ulceration of mucous membranes) may be induced by sulphonamide and can be fatal. When any of the above complications develop the drug must be stopped immediately.

Sulphonamides can detach protein-bound drugs such as warfarin and sulphonylurea antidiabetic agents and thereby cause overdosage.

Sulphonamide preparations applied to the skin are liable to cause light sensitivity; they should not be used topically.

Co-trimoxazole. The two components of this compound, trimethoprim and sulphamethoxazole, act by inhibiting enzymes at two successive stages in the synthesis of para-aminobenzoic acid to folic acid and DNA. Co-trimoxazole is particularly useful in exacerbations of chronic bronchitis and infections of the urinary tract. It is also effective in the treatment of invasive salmonella infections and typhoid carriers. The adult dose is 2 tablets twice daily and there is a preparation for injection. High-dose co-trimoxazole is used to treat pneumonia caused by *Pneumocystis carinii* (p. 220).

The adverse effects are those of the sulphonamides but the clinician must also be on the alert for possible haematological reactions to trimethoprim including thrombocytopenia and megaloblastic anaemia due to folate deficiency (p. 000). Side-effects due to co-trimoxazole are commonest in the elderly.

Trimethoprim. This is now available alone for the treatment of urinary tract infection for which it is given in a dose of 200 mg twice a day, or 100 mg each evening for long-term chemoprophylaxis. It is also used for the treatment of respiratory tract infections. Side-effects are less than with co-trimoxazole especially in the elderly.

Metronidazole

This imidazole compound has high activity against anaerobic bacteria and protozoa but none against aerobic organisms. It is the drug of choice for infections due to *Trichomonas vaginalis, Giardia lamblia* and *Entamoeba histolytica* (p. 774) and is widely used for the treatment and prophylaxis of infections caused by anaerobic bacteria, notably *B. fragilis* (p. 321). It is active against *Clostridium tetani* and *Cl. difficile*.

Metronidazole is a non-toxic drug but should not be given to women during the first trimester of pregnancy as fetal abnormalities have been reported in animals given high doses for prolonged periods. Alcohol should be avoided during therapy with metronidazole which has a similar action to disulfiram (p. 696). The oral dose varies from 200–400 mg given 3 or 4 times a day. Up to 800 mg 3 times a day is required for amoebic infections. There is a preparation for intravenous infusion.

Tinidazole is similar to metronidazole but has a longer serum half-life (12 hours as compared with 7 hours) allowing less frequent administration.

Antituberculous drugs

These are discussed on page 230.

Antifungal drugs

For therapeutic purposes, fungal infections are classified as superficial (skin or mucous membranes) and systemic. The former are commonly caused by *Candida albicans* and usually respond readily to topical applications of any anti-fungal agent. Systemic fungal infections often occur in a compromised host and can be extremely difficult to cure.

Nystatin is the most commonly prescribed agent for the treatment of Candida infections of skin and mucous membranes (thrush). It is not absorbed when given by mouth and cannot be administered parenterally because of its low solubility and toxicity. A suspension, tablets and pessaries are available for the treatment of oral, intestinal and vaginal thrush.

Imidazole antifungal agents. These include *clotrimazole, econazole, miconazole* and *ketoconazole.* They are effective against a wide range of fungi. The first two agents are used for the topical therapy of superficial fungal infections. Miconazole and ketoconazole are absorbed from the gut and have been successfully used for the treatment of systemic fungal infections as well as for superficial mycoses. There is also an intravenous formulation of miconazole. Hepatotoxicity has been reported during ketoconazole therapy. Liver function tests should, therefore, be carried out during long-term therapy.

Amphotericin remains the most important antibiotic for the treatment of systemic fungal infections. It is a moderately toxic drug and side-effects are relatively common. These include fever, vomiting, thrombophlebitis and nephrotoxicity (p. 412). The antibiotic is given by intravenous infusion in increasing daily doses usually commencing with 1 mg.

Flucytosine is well absorbed from the gut and side-effects are relatively uncommon although bone-marrow depression can occur. It is active only against yeasts and has been used for the treatment of systemic candidosis, sometimes in combination with amphotericin. *C. albicans* can develop resistance to flucytosine.

Griseofulvin is selectively concentrated in keratin and is the drug of choice for widespread or chronic dermatophyte infections such as ringworm. It is well absorbed from the gut and is given in a daily dose of 250 mg (child) and 500 mg (adult). Skin lesions respond quickly but infection of the nails requires several months of therapy. Localised and minor ringworm lesions usually respond to topical application of Whitfield's ointment or miconazole.

Antiviral drugs

The main problem with antiviral chemotherapy is to find an agent which will arrest the replication of the virus without interfering with the metabolism of the host cell. Another difficulty is that by the time a viral infection has been diagnosed much of the damage has already been done to the host tissues. The following is an outline of the present position.

Idoxuridine is effective in herpes zoster (shingles) and *H. simplex* keratitis if applied early; it is too toxic for parenteral administration.

Acyclovir is an antiviral agent which is highly active against herpes simplex viruses types I and II (p. 729) and varicella-zoster virus (p. 645). It is indicated for the treatment of *H. simplex* infections and has been used successfully for life-threatening chickenpox and shingles in immuno-compromised patients. There is a preparation for intravenous injection and eye drops for ophthalmic herpes infections. Oral and topical formulations are also available for the treatment of *H. simplex* infections of the skin and mucous membranes including genital herpes. Side-effects are uncommon, the only notable adverse reaction being a rise in serum urea if the intravenous injection is given too quickly.

Interferon (p. 19). Possible uses include the treatment of hepatitis and influenza. It also has anti-tumour activity.

Ribavirin is a 'broad spectrum' antiviral agent, being active *in vitro* against DNA and RNA viruses. It can be effective in Lassa fever (p. 732).

Zidovudine (Retrovir – formerly known as azidothymidine or AZT) is used in the treatment of AIDS (p. 726).

Antiprotozoal drugs and anthelmintics

These are discussed in Chapter 19.

SELECTION OF ANTIMICROBIAL AGENT

In addition to knowledge about the properties of the available antimicrobial agents, important considerations in the choice of effective chemo-therapy are the nature and site of the infection, adverse effects and cost.

The nature and site of the infection. In instances where the nature of the infection can usually be predicted from the clinical features of the illness, treatment can proceed without isola-tion of the causative organism as in acute follicular tonsillitis and lobar pneumonia. In exacerbations of chronic bronchitis the causative organisms are almost always pneumococci and *H. influenzae* and the use of ampicillin or co-trimoxazole is indicated without specific laboratory diagnosis.

If the patient is seriously ill, antibiotic therapy must be started on a 'best guess' (empirical) basis. The presentation of the illness may assist in the selection of the most appropriate agent. If there are no clues as to the nature of the infection, treatment should be started with a combination of antibiotics such as gentamicin plus a penicillin, or with a cephalosporin such as cefuroxime.

Where there is uncertainty about the nature of the infection a bacteriological diagnosis should be made, if possible, so that the appropriate antibiotic can be given. If the organism is one such as *Streptococcus pyogenes*, which has a predictable susceptibility to the generally used antimicrobial agents, no further laboratory sensitivity tests are necessary.

Sensitivity tests will be required for bacteria known to vary in their susceptibility to anti-microbial agents. The acquisition of resistance occurs particularly with staphylococci, Gram-negative bacilli and tubercle bacilli. Once the sensitivity of the organism has been determined, it is relatively rare for this to change in the course of treatment.

When sensitivity tests indicate that several anti-microbial agents are effective it is advisable in the first instance to select one that is bactericidal in order that the organisms are killed rapidly; bacteriostatic drugs suppress the growth of the organism while the natural defence mechanisms of the body dispose of it. The choice is probably of no great significance in the majority of infec-tions but may be important in the treatment of bacteraemia and in patients with deficient defence mechanisms.

Antibiotics with a relatively limited range of activity such as benzylpenicillin are usually prefer-able to broad-spectrum compounds like one of the new cephalosporins, so as to reduce the danger of superinfection.

The use of two or more antibacterial drugs is only occasionally of proven value in other than the seriously ill. Thus in tuberculosis three agents are prescribed, at least initially, so as to reduce the emergence of resistant strains. Drugs with differing ranges of activity may also be used when it has been shown that the effect of the combination is more potent than an equivalent amount of any one of the compounds acting alone. Co-trimoxazole is an example of such synergy.

The selection of an antimicrobial agent is also determined by the site of the infection. This is discussed with the treatment of individual diseases and in the management of bacteraemia (p. 48).

Selection of antimicrobial agents in relation to adverse effects. Before prescribing an antimicrobial agent enquiry should be made about any previous allergic reactions. Pregnant women and children should not be given tetra-cyclines. Co-trimoxazole is also best avoided in pregnancy and this compound, together with other sulphonamides, must not be given to patients with glucose-6-phosphate dehydrogenase deficiency as haemolysis may be precipitated (p. 512). Chloramphenicol should be prescribed only in the circumstances described on page 42 and is contraindicated in the neonate. Ampicillin must not be given to patients suffering from infectious mononucleosis and the aminoglycoside antibiotics should be used with caution in patients with renal disease and in the elderly. Clindamycin should not be used for trivial infection because of the risk of colitis.

Prophylactic use of antibiotics. The indi-cations for this are limited. They include the prevention of tuberculosis (p. 233), meningococcal infections (p. 747) and diphtheria (p. 744) in susceptible contacts. Chemoprophylaxis is also indicated in patients with heart valve lesions undergoing dental or urological procedures (p. 162), for the prevention of tetanus (p. 745) and gas gangrene, and to prevent infective complications following gastrointestinal and gynaecological surgery.

Cost. The chemotherapy of infections can be very expensive, especially when newly introduced preparations are used. Unusual antibiotics should not be prescribed without good reason as the difference in cost can be over a hundred-fold.

Bacteraemia, septicaemia and bacteraemic (septic) shock

Spread of infection to the blood-stream is known as *bacteraemia* and, if the organisms multiply there, as *septicaemia*. Further dissemination may result in 'metastatic' foci of infection especially in bone, liver, brain or heart valves. The site of the primary infection varies but can be in diverticular disease, the gall bladder or the urinary tract, especially in the compromised host.

Bacteraemic shock occurs in up to one third of episodes of Gram-negative septicaemia: it is due to potent bacterial endotoxins which affect cell walls, promote the release of vasoactive substances such as histamine and bradykinin and cause endothelial damage.

Initially there is a hyperdynamic reaction with high cardiac output, vasodilatation and low peripheral resistance followed by fluid loss from the vascular compartment as a result of extensive capillary leakage; this leads to hypovolaemia, peripheral vasoconstriction and acute circulatory failure (p. 143). The endotoxin may initiate disseminated intravascular coagulation (DIC, p. 551) by endothelial injury activating the clotting mechanisms and leading to tissue damage and organ failure.

Clinical features. The pyrexia of the infection may be overtaken by the hypothermia of acute circulatory failure. Leucopenia, thrombocytopenia and a prolonged bleeding time point to DIC. Progressive impairment of blood flow may

then lead to organ failure, particularly of the brain, kidneys, liver and lungs. Mortality can be over 60% in Gram-negative sepsis causing severe hypotension and a low cardiac output.

Treatment. Antimicrobial therapy must be commenced immediately with a combination such as gentamicin and an agent active against Gram-positive cocci (e.g. penicillin or flucloxacillin) plus possibly a third against anaerobes (e.g. metronidazole). This is adjusted when the nature of the infection has been determined.

When Gram-positive cocci are the cause of the infection, benzylpenicillin should be given if the organism is known to be sensitive to penicillin. Flucloxacillin is indicated if penicillinase-producing staphylococci are responsible for the infection. If the patient is allergic to penicillin or the organism is resistant to cloxacillin, the next choice is clindamycin. Metronidazole is indicated for anaerobic infections. Gentamicin alone will suffice for other Gram-negative infections but not for pseudomonas (p. 41). Amikacin is reserved for gentamicin-resistant organisms.

Two doses of corticosteroid (e.g. dexamethasone 1.5 mg/kg) given early may be beneficial by suppressing the damage caused by the exaggerated inflammatory response. They inhibit prostaglandin production and possibly act as endotoxin mediators. Acute circulatory failure (p. 143) and DIC (p. 551) must also be treated.

A.M. GEDDES

FURTHER READING:
British National Formulary 1987 An invaluable source of reference regarding the prescription of all drugs including antimicrobial agents.
Christie A B 1980 Infectious diseases : epidemiology and clinical practice, 3rd edn. Churchill Livingstone, Edinburgh.
Garrod L P, O'Grady F, Lambert H P 1981 Antibiotic and chemotherapy, 5th edn. Churchill Livingstone, Edinburgh.
Shanson D C 1982 Microbiology in clinical practice. Wright, Bristol.

4

Nutritional factors in disease

No medical history is complete without enquiring about the patient's food and drink intake. What people eat is one of the major environmental influences that can sooner or later contribute to disease. Lack of food or of essential nutrients in food also leads to disease. The word nutrition comes from the Latin *'nutrire'* which means to breast feed or nurse and from the time of Hippocrates diet has been a primary part of the management of sick people. Modern physicians can in addition use purified nutrients and parenteral formulas and they advise healthy people about prudent eating to suit the individual.

Study and clinical applications of nutrition

Origins of scientific knowledge about nutrition. For at least 99% of the time *homo sapiens* has been evolving from his primate precursors he has been a hunter-gatherer (Table 4.1). Agriculture started only 10 000 years ago, so that our bodies have presumably evolved well adapted for eating hunter-gatherers' food. We have information from archaeological records and from studies of the few fast-disappearing groups of contemporary hunter-gatherers. From peoples who eat different foods from us, under stable conditions or during a disaster, we can form hypotheses about the physiological effects of different food patterns. For example we have learnt about the role of very long chain polyunsaturated fatty acids from the Eskimos and about deficiency diseases from nutritional observations by medical prisoners of war.

Knowledge has also been derived from food analysis, studies in humans and experiments in animals.

Food analysis. Food constituents are the independent variables in nutritional epidemiology and in the dietetic treatment of disease. Food analysis is work that is never finished; foods keep changing and demand develops for constituents not measured before such as certain fatty acids, trace elements or natural toxicants.

Human experiments and trials last from hours to years; many different variables can be measured. Examples include: (1) absorption and uptake studies, e.g. glycaemic index (blood glucose over 3 hours) after different foods containing carbohydrates; (2) metabolic balance studies, e.g. nitrogen or sterol balances on different diets; (3) experiments measuring energy expenditure; (4) experimental depletion of a single nutrient in volunteers; (5) intervention trial of low saturated fat diet against control affluent diet in middle-aged men for prevention of coronary heart disease; (6) long-term testing of the value and safety of novel protein foods; (7) pharmacokinetic studies of the metabolism of food additives; and (8) trials of vitamin C against placebo for preventing colds during winter.

Clinical records have been informative about the role of diet in disease, including some of the inborn errors of metabolism. Information about requirements for trace elements has come recently from experiences with total parenteral nutrition.

Epidemiological studies. These range in the power of their design. Associations and corre-

Table 4.1 Nutrition at 5 stages of technical development.

Stage	People and their food	Characteristic nutritional disorders
Hunter-gatherers	Our ancestors till 10 000 years ago or less. Few contemporary HGs left, e.g. !Kung Bushmen. Collect wide range of veg foods; also eat meat (lean if terrestrial) and fish. No salt, alcohol, milk (other than mother's), little cereal or sugar (wild honey)	Lean (no obesity) Malnutrition unlikely No coronary disease, hypertension, no dental caries or alcoholism
Pastoralists	Follow their grazing animals where adequate pasture, e.g. Lapps, Tibetans, Mongols, Tuareg, Fulani, Masai. Diet high in animal foods and milk	Least studied of all groups Some groups are tall Persistence of adult lactase
Peasant agriculturalists	Nearly all rural people in Third World and in industrial countries till this century. Tend to rely on one crop which yields best. Vulnerable to crop disease, crop toxin and to drought. Seasonal shortages. Milling and refining cereals increases risk of malnutrition.	Famine in areas with unreliable rainfall Malnutrition from lack of some nutrient(s) in staple food, e.g. kwashiorkor, pellagra, beri beri Mycotoxins. Hypertension but no coronary disease
Urban slum and periurban shanty	The poor masses in and round the rapidly growing cities of today's Third World. Similar situation in London, New York, etc. in 19th century. Loss of food traditions, no home gardens, mothers often have to work, poor food hygiene, food expensive	Children most vulnerable; not breast fed, gastroenteritis and marasmus Rickets in high latitudes Alcoholism. Adults may be obese. Hypertension but no coronary disease
Affluent societies	Favourite food year round. High fat diet. Processed, convenience and take-away food. Tower of Babel of nutritional breakthroughs, scares and advice. Alternative and unorthodox advice. 'Health foods.' Many take vitamin tablets	Malnutrition confined to hospital patients and the elderly disabled Coronary heart disease common 'Nutritional hypochondriasis' Hypersensitivity to foods apparently common Obesity unfashionable but difficult to avoid Anorexia nervosa

lations of disease characteristics and dietary variables do not prove cause and effect, but prospective (cohort) studies, especially if repeated in different groups, give valuable information on the relation between usual diets and chronic diseases, e.g. dietary fat and coronary heart disease.

Animal experiments were the principal technique for working out the vitamins. The right animal model has to be used, for example the guinea pig in the study of vitamin C (p. 68).

Nutrition and disease. Like immune reactions and infections, nutrition can affect any organ of the body or several at once. Different parts of the whole field of human nutrition are used regularly by different specialists. Cardiologists are interested in dietary fats and plasma cholesterol, nephrologists in protein deficiency and in potassium excess and gastroenterologists in multiple deficiencies from malabsorption, in dietary fibre and in hypersensitivity to wheat and milk; neurol-

ogists are interested in alcohol excess and thiamin deficiency, haematologists in deficiencies of iron, folate and vitamin B_{12}, psychiatrists in anorexia nervosa, geriatricians in the effects of drugs on nutritional status and general practitioners in dietary advice for pregnancy and middle age and in infant feeding. Consequently some nutritional disorders are dealt with in this chapter; others have their main description elsewhere in the book.

There are differences also between Third World and industrial countries in the nutritional knowledge used in everyday practice. Which nutritional disorders are common depends where and with whom one is working (Table 4.1), but the study of human nutrition has grown because some workers have taken a global view. Our understanding of protein deficiency and of dietary fibre originated in Africa; human zinc deficiency was first described in the Middle East and selenium deficiency in China. On the other hand some

'Western diseases' like diabetes mellitus are now increasingly occurring in tropical countries.

Uses of nutritional knowledge in clinical medicine.

1. Some diseases result primarily from disturbed nutrition — the major deficiency diseases and obesity. These are described in this chapter.

Deficiency diseases seldom present in pure form. More often than not they are secondary to some other illness. Even where food is short all the members of a community are not equally affected. Individuals with some physical or mental abnormality usually show clinical manifestations first.

When malnutrition occurs it is unlikely to involve only one nutrient. Even if the clinical features suggest a single deficiency, biochemical tests usually reveal depletion of other nutrients. Treatment should therefore never be confined to large intakes of the nutrient whose deficiency is indicated by the clinical signs. Furthermore, malnourished patients are liable to complications, especially certain infections which may be the presenting illness or may occur in modified form because malnutrition has suppressed some of their characteristic signs. Thus complications of malnutrition must be looked for and treated. Much of the skill in diagnosing patients with malnutrition is being aware of and disentangling predisposing illnesses, other associated malnutrition and complicating diseases.

2. In developed countries, patients in hospital for long periods with a serious illness are very likely to develop some degree of nutritional depletion such as protein-calorie malnutrition and/or other deficiencies, e.g. of folate, potassium or iron. It is important to monitor patients' nutrition and provide appropriate support because nutritionally-depleted patients are weaker and have impaired wound healing and reduced resistance to infection. The principles of nutritional diagnosis and management for hospital patients are summarised in this chapter.

3. Modification of the diet in coeliac disease, hepatic encephalopathy and phenylketonuria is the principal treatment and may be life saving. In other conditions, e.g. diabetes mellitus and mild hypertension, the appropriate diet is useful treatment, alternative or complementary to drugs. In other chapters therapeutic diets are outlined under the diseases concerned. Examples of diet sheets for obesity, diabetes and hypercholesterolaemia appear in the Appendix. Space does not allow inclusion of others; the reader is referred to a textbook of nutrition and dietetics (p. 83).

4. Evidence is accumulating that the habitual diet is one of the multiple causative factors in many chronic degenerative diseases (e.g. coronary heart disease, hypertension, diabetes mellitus, dental caries and diverticular disease) and even in some carcinomas (e.g. stomach, liver and large bowel). These diseases take a long time to develop; exactly which dietary components are involved, and how closely, needs discussion and is often controversial. Details are not appropriate to a clinical primer. Elsewhere in this book the role of diet is mentioned briefly in the paragraphs on aetiology of the different diseases, and the final chapter on health promotion contains a number of measures related to food and nutrition.

Classification of nutritional disorders

1. **Undernutrition** is not enough food energy (calories or joules). Severe forms are *starvation* in adults or *marasmus* in children. Undernutrition secondary to disease may be called cachexia (wasting). Epidemic undernutrition is famine.

2. **Malnutrition** is a deficiency of protein or of one or more of over 30 other essential nutrients (Table 4.2). Most individual foods lack several of these nutrients; the full number is normally provided by a variety of different foods. Deficiency diseases like kwashiorkor and rickets are examples of malnutrition. It can also be subclinical.

3. **Obesity.** Excess of body fat results from a prolonged positive energy balance, an energy (calorie or joule) intake greater than energy expenditure.

4. **Nutrient excess** is due to too much of one nutrient. For many nutrients a very high intake in the short term or a chronic high intake can be harmful. The nutrient may be an essential one, e.g. hypervitaminosis D or siderosis (iron overload) or non-essential, e.g. alcohol or saturated fat.

5. **Effects of toxicants.** Foods, unless very refined, contain hundreds of substances other than nutrients, most in tiny amounts (Table 4.3). Some can cause illness if people rely too heavily on a

Table 4.2 Size of adult requirements for different nutrients.

Adult daily requirement in foods	Essential nutrients for man
2–10 μg	Vit B_{12}, vit D, vit K, Cr
c.100 μg	Biotin, I, Se
200 μg	Folate, Mo
1–2 mg	Vit A, thiamin, riboflavin, vit B_6, F, Cu
5–10 mg	Pantothenate, Mn
c.15 mg	Niacin, vit E, Fe, Zn
c.50 mg	Vit C
300 mg	Mg
c.1 g	Ca, P
1–5 g	Na, Cl, K, essential fatty acids
c.50 g	Protein (8–10 essential amino acids)
50–100 g	Available carbohydrate
1 kg (l)	Water

Figures are approximate, in places rounded to fit with others on a line. The range of requirements for different nutrients is about 10^9. In addition sulphur is required in the form of the amino acids, methionine and cysteine. Cobalt is required in the form of vitamin B_{12}.

single foodstuff, e.g. tropical spinal ataxia (p. 657). Other substances affect only a few hypersensitive individuals, e.g. coeliac disease (p. 304), favism (p. 512), urticaria (p. 25) and migraine (p. 627).

Nutrients can be subdivided into four groups:
1. Energy-yielding nutrients (carbohydrates, fats, proteins and alcohol)
2. Water, electrolytes and other essential (inorganic) elements
3. Vitamins
4. Fibre.

In this chapter the related disorders will be described under these headings and thereafter obesity will be considered.

ENERGY-YIELDING NUTRIENTS

Carbohydrates (4 kcal/g) usually provide the greater part of the energy in a normal diet. No individual carbohydrate is an essential nutrient in the sense that the body needs it but cannot make it for itself from other nutrients. If the carbohydrate intake is less than 100 g per day ketosis is likely to occur.

The major carbohydrates in food are:

1. Available sugars

a. Monosaccharides — ribose, glucose and fructose

b. Disaccharides — sucrose, lactose and maltose

2. Available polysaccharides — starch, glycogen and synthetic glucose polymers.

3. Unavailable polysaccharides — most forms of dietary fibre (p. 75).

Fats. With their high calorie value (9 kcal/g) fats are useful to people with a large energy expenditure. On the other hand they are an insidious cause of obesity for sedentary people. Saturated fats, especially those containing palmitic (16:0) and myristic (14:0) acids increase plasma low-density lipoproteins and total cholesterol. Polyunsaturated fats are in two main groups, depending on the distance of their first double bond, counting from the methyl (ω) end of the molecule. The principal fatty acid in plant seed oils is linoleic acid (18:2 ω6). This and its elongated ω6 derivatives linolenic acid (18:3 ω6) and arachidonic acid (20:4 ω6) are the essential fatty acids (EFAs), precursors of the prostaglandins and part of the structure of lipid membranes in all cells.

Essential fatty acid deficiency is rare in man but it has been reported in patients fed solely by vein for long periods without fat emulsions. If sufficient glucose and amino acids are given they inhibit free fatty acid mobilisation from adipose tissue (where there is usually a moderate store of linoleic acid) and tissues in the rest of the body become depleted. There is a scaly dermatitis and the diagnosis can be confirmed biochemically by an increased ratio of eicosatrienoic acid (20:3 ω9) to arachidonic in plasma lipids.

The ω3 series of polyunsaturated fatty acids, e.g. eicosapentaenoic (20:5 ω3) and docosahexaenoic (22:6 ω3) occur in fish oils. Though not essential they are inhibitors of thrombosis and appear to act by competitively antagonising thromboxane A2 formation (p. 550).

Proteins provide some 20 amino acids, of which eight are essential for normal protein synthesis and for maintaining nitrogen balance in adults. These *essential amino acids* are methionine, lysine, tryptophan, phenylalanine, leucine, isoleucine, threonine, and valine. Histidine and per-

Table 4.3 Potentially toxic substances in foods.

Natural

Inherent, naturally occurring	Usually present in the food and affects everyone if they eat enough, e.g. solanine in potatoes (green sprouts); tropical spinal ataxia from cassava
Toxin resulting from abnormal conditions of animal or plant used for food	e.g. Neurotoxic mussel poisoning; ergotism
Consumer abnormally sensitive	e.g. Coeliac disease from wheat gluten; allergy to particular food; or drug-induced, e.g. cheese reaction
Contamination by pathogenic bacteria	Acute illness, usually gastro-intestinal, e.g. toxins produced by *Staphylococcus aureus* or *Clostridium botulinum*
Mycotoxins	Food mouldy or spoiled, e.g. aflatoxin B_1 from *Aspergillus flavus* is a liver carcinogen

Man made

Unintentional additives — man-made chemical used in agriculture and animal husbandry	e.g. Fungicides on grain, insecticides on fruit, antibiotics or hormones given to animals
Environmental pollution	e.g. Organic mercury, cadmium, lead, PCB and radioactive fall-out can affect any stage of food chain
Intentional food additives— preservatives, emulsifiers, flavours, colours, etc.	The most thoroughly tested and monitored of all chemicals in foods. Occasional individuals hypersensitive, e.g. to some azo colours

haps arginine are also needed for growth in infants.

The 'biological value' of different proteins depends on the relative proportions of essential amino acids they contain. Proteins of animal origin, particularly from eggs, milk and meat, are generally of higher biological value than the proteins of vegetable origin which are deficient in one or more of the essential amino acids. However it is possible to have a diet of mixed vegetable proteins with high biological value if the principle of *complementation* is used. For example cereals, e.g. wheat, contain about 10% protein and are relatively deficient in lysine. Legumes contain around 20% of protein which is relatively deficient in methionine. If two parts of wheat are mixed (or eaten) with one part of legume, a food results which contains 13% protein of high biological value. This happens because cereals contain enough methionine and legumes enough lysine to supplement the other component of the mixture.

The usual recommended allowance for an adequate protein intake is 10% of the total calories, i.e. about 65 g per day for the average adult. The minimum requirement is around 40 g of protein

of good biological value.

Energy requirements. The largest component of energy expenditure is the basal metabolic rate (BMR). This increases with lean body mass (which is related to weight and height); it declines with age and is less in women than men. Extra energy is required for growth, pregnancy and lactation, for muscular activity and for pyrexia. There is also considerable variation between individuals of the same size, age, sex and activity. Adaptation occurs to an inadequate energy intake and to a lesser degree to superfluous energy intake.

Apyrexial male patients in bed in industrial countries need about 2000 kcal per day. Male office workers in affluent countries need around 2700 kcal and subsistence farmers in a Third World country (who have a smaller body size) require around 2800 kcal; about 3500 kcal are needed for men doing heavy work. Female patients in bed require about 1600 kcal if apyrexial. A healthy housewife in Britain requires around 2000 kcal and a rural woman in a developing country about 2250 kcal per day.

Individuals in Britain, including children, probably need somewhere around 2500 kcal per day. The food moving into consumption has to provide more to allow for wastage, pets, tourists, etc. This gross value, around 3000 kcal, is easier to estimate. It is this higher figure that is discussed in the press and parliament and often confused with average physiological requirements.

There are two units in use for energy: kilocalories and kilo-joules (1 kcal = 4.184 kJ). Though both are metric, joules are SI units and are gradually replacing calories in scientific usage.

Starvation

Starvation is severe undernutrition from a prolonged negative energy balance. What follows here describes the features seen in adults and older children. In infants and pre-school children a similar process (marasmus) is described on page 55.

Aetiology. The main causes of undernutrition and starvation are: (1) not enough food, as in famine; (2) persistent vomiting or oesophageal or pyloric obstruction; (3) anorexia, which is a major factor in many patients with wasting secondary to another disease; (4) malabsorption from disease of the small intestine; (5) increased BMR, e.g. in thyrotoxicosis, prolonged infections; (6) loss of calories in urine, as glucose, in diabetes mellitus; and (7) cachexia in malignant disease. There appears to be a circulating antimetabolite in some cases.

Clinical features. Children stop growing and adults lose weight. The symptoms include craving for food, thirst, weakness, feeling cold, nocturia, amenorrhoea and impotence.

The face at first looks younger but later becomes old, withered and expressionless. The skin is lax, pale and dry and may show pigmented patches. Hair becomes thinned or lost except in adolescents. The extremities are cold and cyanosed and there may be pressure sores. Subcutaneous fat disappears, skin turgor is lost, and muscles waste. The arm circumference is subnormal. Oedema may be present in famine victims without hypoalbuminaemia ('famine oedema'). Body temperature is subnormal. The pulse is slow, blood pressure low and the heart small. The abdomen is distended and diarrhoea is common. Tendon jerks are diminished. Psychologically, starving people lose initiative; they are apathetic, depressed and introverted but become aggressive if food is nearby.

Under-nourished individuals are susceptible to infections. With respiratory muscles weakened by wasting, bronchopneumonia carries an increased mortality. Starving groups in famines have often had high mortalities from epidemics, e.g. typhus or cholera. The usual signs of infection may not appear. In advanced starvation patients become completely inactive and may assume a flexed, fetal position. Death comes quietly and often quite suddenly in the last stage of starvation. The very old are most vulnerable. All the organs are atrophied at necropsy except the brain which tends to maintain its weight.

Investigation. Plasma free fatty acids are increased; there is ketosis and may be a mild metabolic acidosis. Plasma glucose is low but albumin concentration is often normal. Insulin secretion is diminished, glucagon and cortisol concentrations tend to increase, reverse T_3 replaces normal triiodothyronine. The resting metabolic rate goes down considerably. The urine has a fixed specific gravity and creatinine excretion becomes low. There may be mild anaemia, leucopenia and thrombocytopenia. The ESR is normal unless there is infection. Tests of delayed skin sensitivity, e.g. to tuberculin, are falsely negative. The ECG shows sinus bradycardia and low voltages.

Treatment. Whether in a famine or dealing with wasting secondary to disease, people or patients need to be graded:

1. Mild starvation = weight for height 90–81% of standard, or body mass index (BMI, p. 813) = 20–18
2. Moderate starvation = weight for height 80–71% of standard (BMI = 18–16)
3. Severe starvation = weight for height ⩽ 70% of standard (BMI < 16).

People with mild starvation are in no danger; those with moderate starvation need extra feeding. People who are severely underweight need hospital type care. 1500 to 2000 kcal/day will prevent the downward progress of undernutrition.

In severe starvation there is atrophy of the

intestinal epithelium and of the exocrine pancreas and bile is dilute. When food becomes available the extra should be given in small amounts at first. Food should be bland and preferably similar to the usual staple meal, for example a cereal with some sugar, milk powder and oil. Salt should be restricted and a multivitamin preparation is desirable. A refeeding schedule of 1 month to replace every 5% loss of weight is a good guide.

Circumstances and resources are different in every famine. The problems are mainly non-medical, e.g. organising transport and repair of trucks and shelters, co-ordinating relief from different organisations, reconciling international workers with local politicians and administrators, arranging security of food stores, ensuring that food is distributed on the basis of need and trying to procure the right food and appropriate medical supplies. Civil disturbances do not occur during severe famine. They may happen at an early stage (food riots) or afterwards (revolution). Lastly, plans must be made for the future; for example, agricultural workers will be needed with enough strength to plough and plant the next crop when the rains return.

PROTEIN-ENERGY MALNUTRITION (IN YOUNG CHILDREN)

Aetiology and classification. Protein-energy malnutrition (PEM) in early childhood is a spectrum of disease. At one end there is *kwashiorkor* in which the essential feature is deficiency of protein with relatively adequate energy intake. At the other end is *nutritional marasmus* which is total inanition of the infant, usually under 1 year of age, and which is due to a severe and prolonged restriction of all food, i.e. energy sources and other nutrients in addition to protein. In the middle of the spectrum is *marasmic kwashiorkor* in which there are clinical features of both disorders.

Some children adapt to prolonged energy and/or protein shortage by *nutritional dwarfism.* The most prevalent of all the varieties is *mild to moderate PEM* or the underweight child (Table 4.4). Children with one form of PEM often shift to another form. Thus a child with mild to moderate PEM may develop kwashiorkor after an infection. Such a child, when treated, loses oedema and may look marasmic. In marasmus there is a major loss of muscle, the body's main mass of protein; in kwashiorkor anorexia is characteristic and leads to inadequate secondary energy intake. For reasons like these, marasmus, kwashiorkor and milder forms are grouped together as protein-energy malnutrition.

The incidence of PEM in its various forms is high in India and S.E. Asia, in most parts of Africa and the Middle East, in the Caribbean islands and in South and Central America. PEM is the most important dietary deficiency disease in the world. Severe forms affect around 2% and mild to moderate PEM affects around 20% of young children in the Third World.

Nutritional marasmus

Aetiology. This is the commoner form of severe protein-energy malnutrition. It is the childhood version of starvation. It usually occurs in the second 6 months of life. The cause is a diet very low in both calories and protein. Typically the child was weaned early and fed with dilute cows' milk formulae. This is a disease of infants of poor women in the cities of developing countries. The mother may have to go out to work and

Table 4.4 Classification of PEM in young children.

	Body weight as percentage of international standard	Oedema	Deficit in weight for height
Kwashiorkor	80–60	+	+
Marasmic kwashiorkor	<60	+	+ +
Marasmus	<60	0	+ +
Nutritional dwarfing	<60	0	minimal
Underweight child	80–60	0	+

leave her baby with its grandmother, older sister or a neighbour. She has difficulty paying for the feeds and has neither the kitchen equipment nor the knowledge to prepare them without bacterial contamination. Poor hygiene leads to gastroenteritis and a vicious cycle starts. Diarrhoea leads to poor appetite and the decision to give more dilute feeds. In turn further depletion leads to intestinal atrophy and more susceptibility to diarrhoea.

Clinical features. The child is very thin with no subcutaneous fat, and looks wizened and shrunken; its muscles are severely wasted. The head is large for the body, the ribs stand out, the abdomen may be distended (with gas), the limbs look like sticks and the buttocks are baggy. Diarrhoea is usual. In contrast to kwashiorkor, there is no oedema and skin and hair changes are mild or absent. The child is not usually anorexic but the weight is reduced below 60% of standard. Although the child has not been growing, weight is reduced more than length.

A search must be made for chronic infection like tuberculosis or other major disease (cardiac, renal, intestinal) that could produce secondary marasmus. Dehydration frequently occurs as a result of diarrhoea or vomiting. There may be associated deficiencies of vitamins, such as vitamin A causing keratomalacia and of inorganic nutrients such as potassium and magnesium.

Patients with PEM (marasmus and kwashiorkor) have increased susceptibility to many infections, e.g. (1) gastroenteritis and Gram-negative bacteraemia, (2) respiratory infections, (3) certain viral diseases, especially measles and herpes simplex, (4) tuberculosis, (5) streptococcal and staphylococcal skin infections and (6) helminthic infections.

Treatment of marasmus is substantially the same as for kwashiorkor (p. 57).

Kwashiorkor

Aetiology. The name comes from Ghana where the condition was first described by Cicely Williams in 1933. This form of malnutrition occurs most often in the second year of life when the child is weaned from the breast on to a diet low in protein such as cassava, plantain or yam or to a cereal that has been refined and diluted. There is little milk and custom, sometimes reinforced by taboos, determines that the limited foods of animal origin are given to the men of the family, or the small amount of protein-rich food is in a sauce made with hot peppers or spices and unsuitable for young children. If the customary diet of a population is limited in protein and in calories to around the levels of minimum requirements, a child may be in moderate health until the protein requirements are increased by an infection. Gastroenteritis, measles and malaria are all notorious precipitants of kwashiorkor.

Pathogenesis. There is oedema with a fatty liver and characteristic changes in skin, hair and mucosa. The pathogenesis appears to be that very low dietary protein with more adequate carbohydrate maintains insulin secretion (unlike marasmus). Insulin spares muscle protein but at the expense of liver protein. With loss of all liver proteins, plasma albumin concentration falls and hence there is oedema. Low density lipoprotein synthesis is also impaired so that free fatty acids coming to the liver from adipose tissue accumulate as triglycerides and produce a fatty liver. Some of the features of kwashiorkor may be due to zinc deficiency.

Clinical features. The child is not very thin. There is oedema which tends to be generalised. The child is miserable and apathetic and has a characteristic cry. The skin shows symmetrical changes, maximally in the napkin (diaper) area. At first it is pigmented and thickened as if varnished, then it cracks and leads to denuded areas of shallow ulceration. In moderate cases the areas of dermatosis resemble crazy paving; when severe the desquamated area can look as if the child has been burnt. The hair alters in colour from black to blond, reddish or grey; it becomes thin and sparse. Mucosal changes, such as angular stomatitis, may be seen. Anorexia is present and diarrhoea is common. The liver may be palpable. The characteristic laboratory finding is a very low plasma albumin concentration.

Treatment of severe PEM whether kwashiorkor or marasmus, is in three phases.

1. *Resuscitation* consists of correction of dehydration, electrolyte disturbances, acidosis, hypoglycaemia and hypothermia and also treatment of infections (p. 56).

2. *Start of cure* consists of refeeding, gradually working up the calories to 150 kcal/kg with protein about 1.5 g/kg. The major units with research experience of PEM have each evolved somewhat different dietary formulas, depending on local availability and preferences for weaning foods. They are usually based on dried skimmed milk mixed with some flour or sugar and some oil and given 5 to 6 times a day. Because of anorexia, children often have to be hand fed, preferably in the lap of their mother or a nurse they know. Potassium, magnesium and a multi-vitamin mixture are also needed.

3. *Nutritional rehabilitation.* After about 3 weeks the child should be obviously better. If there was oedema this will have cleared, any skin lesions are healing and diarrhoea has ceased. The child is stronger, mentally bright and has a good appetite but is still underweight for his or her age. During this stage of rehabilitation and catch-up growth, the child should be looked after in a convalescent home or by the mother who should have been educated about nutrition and helped to obtain extra food. The diet should be based on nutritious combinations of local, familiar foods.

Prognosis. Severe PEM has a mortality around 20% even in well equipped hospitals. Most deaths occur in the first 10 days. Follow-up studies have shown that the fatty liver of acute kwashiorkor resolves quickly and does not go on to cirrhosis. Physical growth of the brain is retarded in children who suffer severe PEM in the first two years of life (usually marasmus). There is circumstantial evidence that intelligence may be impaired, particularly if the child goes home to a poor environment.

Mild to moderate PEM (the underweight child)

For every florid case of kwashiorkor or marasmus there are likely to be 7 or 10 in the community with mild to moderate PEM. The situation is like an iceberg; there is more malnutrition below the surface than is recognisable on clinical inspection. Even the mothers themselves do not notice most of these cases because their children are similar in size and vitality to many others of the same age. Most children with subclinical PEM can,

however, be detected by their weight for age, which is less than 80% of the international standard (Table 21.1, p. 812). In parts of many developing countries surveys may show that up to 50% of children under 5 are underweight. Because scales are difficult to carry, a convenient screening test for mild to moderate malnutrition is to measure the mid-upper arm circumference with a simple piece of tape. From 12 to 60 months of age over 13.5 cm is a normal circumference (coloured green on the tape), 12.5 to 13.5 cm suggests mild malnutrition (coloured amber) and under 12.5 indicates probable malnutrition (red part of the tape). The normal arm circumference stays the same for those 4 years.

In areas where kwashiorkor is the predominant florid form of PEM, subclinical cases have reduced plasma albumin and sometimes other biochemical signs of protein deficiency ('prekwashiorkor'). Sometimes a child is seen who has adapted to chronic inadequate feeding by reduced linear growth but who looks like a normal child a year or two younger. This is known as *nutritional dwarfism*.

The great importance of mild to moderate PEM is that these children are growing up smaller than their potential and they are very susceptible to gastroenteritis and respiratory infections, which in turn can precipitate frank malnutrition. Mild to moderate PEM is probably the major underlying reason why the 1 to 4 year mortality in a developing country can be 30 to 40 times higher than in Europe or North America. Official statistics record most of these deaths as due simply to infections.

Prevention. The principle of prevention of kwashiorkor is by education of mothers, by advice to farmers and by provision of supplements in clinics to increase the protein intake of young children in those areas where kwashiorkor is common. Animal foods, milk powder or eggs are good if available but not essential. Locally produced high protein plant foods, especially legumes, nuts and seeds may well be more reliable and economical. Cameron and Hofvander (p. 83) recommend nutritious weaning mixtures suitable for the conditions of various developing countries.

Prevention of marasmus is more complex. It is a product of poverty and overcrowding in Third World cities. Family planning, immunisation, encouragement of breast feeding and a campaign for adequate maternity leave can all help to reduce the problem. A network of maternity and child health clinics, run mostly by an experienced nurse with a periodic medical visit is much better value for the restricted health budget in a poor developing country than a prestigious teaching hospital in the capital.

UNICEF has drawn world-wide attention to four relatively simple and inexpensive methods, abbreviated as 'GOBI', which they believe could halve the present death rate of children in developing countries:

G for growth monitoring. The mother keeps the simple growth chart — the Road to Health card — in a cellophane envelope and brings the child to a clinic regularly for weighing and advice.

O for oral rehydration. The UNICEF formula (NaCl 3.5 g, NaH CO₃ 2.5 g, KCl 1.5 g, glucose 20 g or sucrose 40 g and clean water to 1 litre) is saving many lives from gastroenteritis.

B for breast feeding. This is a matter of life and death in a poor community with no facilities for hygiene. Additional food prepared from locally available products is not usually needed until 6 months of age.

I for immunisation. For $5 a child can be protected against measles, diphtheria, pertussis, tetanus, tuberculosis and poliomyelitis. In a rational world the money for this could be taken from a small part of the $800 billion spent on armaments each year.

WATER, ELECTROLYTES AND MINERALS

The normal distribution of water and electrolytes in the body and the disturbances which result when their intake or output is diminished or increased are discussed in detail on pages 84 to 95.

Twelve or more elements are essential for man, as they are for other animals; deficiency disease is known for each due to inadequate diet or from excessive losses. The elements are sodium (p. 85), potassium (p. 87), magnesium (p. 91), calcium, phosphorus, iron, sulphur, iodine, zinc, copper, chromium, selenium, manganese and molybdenum. Fluoride appears to be essential for rats

and optimal intakes reduce dental caries in man. Cobalt is physiologically active only in the form of vitamin B_{12}.

In addition tin, vanadium, nickel and silicon have been shown, by artificial isolator systems, to be essential for animals. Human deficiency disease is not known for any of these minor trace elements.

Elements of importance in human nutrition

Calcium. The body of an adult normally contains about 1200 g of calcium. At least 99% of this is present in the skeleton, where calcium salts (chiefly hydroxyapatite), held in a cellular matrix, provide the hard structure of the bones and teeth.

Obviously all of this calcium comes from the diet. Among common foods, the calcium-containing protein of milk (caseinogen) is much the richest source, which is one reason why milk and cheese are especially valuable for growing children. Half a litre of cow's milk contains about 0.6 g of calcium. Most other foods contribute much smaller amounts. However, peas, beans, other vegetables and particularly cereal grains are frequently the chief contributors because of the large amounts eaten.

Drinking water can provide significant amounts of calcium ranging from none in water from peaty, acidic hill lochs in Scotland to 200 mg or even more in water obtained from wells sunk in chalk or limestone.

Absorption. 70 to 80% of the calcium in the food is normally excreted in the faeces. Calcium absorption may be impaired either by lack of vitamin D, by any condition causing small intestinal hurry, by the combination of calcium with excess fatty acids to form insoluble soaps in steatorrhoea, or by certain substances in the diet which can form insoluble salts with calcium. These include foods rich in oxalic acid (e.g. spinach) and phytic acid which is present in the outer layers of cereal grains. Hence 'wholemeal' bread contains more phytic acid than white.

Recommended intakes of calcium. The amount of calcium which has to be added to the bones to produce the final adult amount averages 180 mg/day from 0 to 18 years but reaches 400 mg/day at the peak of adolescent growth. Since calcium absorption is inefficient the recommended intake in Britain is 600 mg for children and 700 mg in adolescents. Expert opinion is divided on the safe minimum intake in adults. WHO recommended 500 mg/day because in many parts of Africa and Asia children develop and adults maintain healthy bones on this intake or lower. The USA recommends 800 mg for adults and 1000 mg have been advised for post-menopausal women. These figures are based on calcium balances. It appears that calcium is handled less economically in developed countries. Possible explanations include less skin synthesis of vitamin D from sunshine and increased obligatory urinary calcium because of high animal protein and sodium intakes. In pregnancy and lactation extra calcium is needed — 1200 mg per day.

Calcium is the most obvious and persistent of the micro-nutrients, the fifth most abundant element, and the most abundant cation, in the body, yet it is more difficult to measure adequacy of intake for calcium than for other nutrients. Any reduction of absorbed calcium does not show in the plasma concentration, which is immediately reset by increased parathyroid secretion and formation of 1,25 dihydroxy-vitamin D, probably because any change of ionised plasma concentration would disturb neuromuscular irritability and blood coagulation. Likewise intracellular plasma concentration, which affects activities of many enzymes, is also tightly controlled. If calcium intake is inadequate, therefore a little less will go into the bones in children or a little will be removed from the bones in adults. Small changes in total bone calcium can be measured only as research procedures at present.

The two major questions about calcium nutrition are (1) Will a high intake during the growing phase of life contribute to taller adult height or heavier bones. If so, how much is optimal? (2) Will a high intake from about 45 years onwards delay the onset of osteoporosis (p. 67)?

Phosphorus. This is of course used by the body in the form of phosphate which is present in all cells and so in all unrefined plant and animal foods and in milk. Dietary deficiency is rare. Usual dietary intakes are rather higher than for calcium, about 1.5 g/day. Total body phosphorus

is about 700 g, most being in the bones.

Phosphate deficiency occurs in premature infants fed on human milk, in patients with Fanconi's syndrome and other forms of renal tubular phosphate loss, from prolonged high dosage of aluminium hydroxide antacids, sometimes when alcoholics are re-fed with high carbohydrate foods and in patients on total parenteral nutrition if not enough phosphate is provided. The features of deficiency are hypophosphataemia (subnormal plasma inorganic phosphorus) and muscle weakness.

Iron. A good mixed diet with average amounts of meat and vegetable contains about 12–15 mg of iron. Cheap, monotonous high carbohydrate diets based on refined wheat flour contain much less. Foods rich in iron are meat, liver, wholemeal cereals, oatmeal, peas, beans and lentils. Iron absorption from food is inefficient, averaging 10% from a mixed diet but much less from many plant foods and from eggs. Absorption of haem iron (e.g. meat) is better than that of non-haem iron. The latter is enhanced by vitamin C eaten at the same time and reduced by the binding of iron to substances such as tannins (e.g. in tea) and phytates. There is no physiological mechanism for secretion of iron so maintenance of its homeostasis depends on iron absorption. Normally body iron loss from desquamated surface cells adds up to about 1 mg daily. Assuming 10% absorption, about 10 mg are therefore required in the diet daily in men, but if there is any bleeding this brings with it much more loss of iron. Blood is the tissue richest in iron; 1 ml contains 0.5 mg of iron so that a regular blood loss of only 2 ml/day doubles the iron requirement. At menstruation 30 mg of iron can be lost and considerably more in a few women.

An account of iron metabolism and of the measures for the prevention and treatment of iron deficiency anaemia is given on page 500. This is one of the most important nutritional causes of ill-health in Britain and other prosperous countries.

Siderosis. Dietary iron overload is seen in South African black men who cook and brew beer in iron pots. They may ingest as much as 100 mg of iron per day. Iron accumulates in the liver and when severe can lead to cirrhosis. A similar condition has been described in other countries following excessive indulgence in cheap wines which can contain 30 mg of iron per litre.

Iodine has the heaviest atomic weight of the essential elements. It is present in the sea, in seafoods and in trace amounts in soil and water over most of the land and in foods grown there. Iodine is lacking in the major mountainous areas of the world, e.g. the Alps, Himalayas, Rockies, Andes and the mountains of central America and Papua New Guinea. About 400 000 000 people living in these areas are estimated to have an inadequate iodine intake and they show endemic goitre and other iodine deficiency disorders.

The great majority of endemic goitres are only a cosmetic nuisance but when just visible goitres are found in 5% or more of adolescents this indicates that the whole community is deficient in iodine and other iodine deficiency disorders can be expected, of which the most serious is cretinism (p. 442). Where most women have endemic goitre, 1% or more of the babies are born with cretinism and the other 'normal' people in the community show a higher prevalence than usual of deafness, slowed reflexes and poor learning.

Endemic goitre has now almost disappeared from most of the low iodine regions of Europe and North America due to the use of iodised salt and inter-regional trade of foods. In remote mountainous parts of the Third World without roads, shops and a cash economy, iodised salt will not reach enough people and the best way of preventing cretinism is by injecting all women of child-bearing age with 1 to 2 ml of iodised poppyseed oil every 5 years.

Fluoride. The regular presence of fluoride in minute amounts in human bones and teeth and its influence on the prevention of dental caries justifies its inclusion as an element of importance in human nutrition.

Sources. Most adults ingest between 1 and 3 mg of fluoride daily. The chief source is usually drinking water, which, if it contains 1 part per million (p.p.m.) of fluoride, will supply 1–2 mg/day. Soft waters usually contain no fluoride, whilst very hard waters may contain over 10 p.p.m.

Compared with that in water, the fluoride in foodstuffs is of little importance. Very few contain more than 1 p.p.m.; the exceptions are sea-fish which may contain 5–10 p.p.m. and tea. In Britain, Australia and China, where people drink tea frequently, the adult intake from this source may be as much as 3 mg daily.

Use of fluoride in the prevention of dental caries. Epidemiological studies in many parts of the world have established that where the natural water supply contains fluoride in amounts of 1 p.p.m. or more, the incidence of dental caries is lower than in comparable areas where the water contains only traces of the element.

Fluoride becomes deposited in the enamel surface of the developing teeth of children. Such teeth are unusually resistant to caries. Fluoride is not deposited in fully developed adult teeth, so that less benefit to adults can be expected when they begin for the first time to drink water containing traces of fluoride.

The deliberate addition of traces of fluoride (at 1 p.p.m.) to those public water supplies which are deficient is now a widespread practice throughout North America where about 100 million people are now drinking fluoridated water. In at least 30 other countries similar projects have been started. In Britain regrettably some local authorities are not yet adding fluoride to their water supplies in those areas in which the element is lacking.

Fluorosis. In parts of the world where the water fluoride is high (over 3 to 5 p.p.m.) mottling of the teeth is common. The enamel loses its lustre and becomes rough, pigmented and pitted. The effect is purely cosmetic; fluorotic teeth are resistant to caries and not usually associated with any evidence of skeletal fluorosis, or impairment of health.

Chronic fluoride poisoning occurs in several localities in India, China, Argentina, East and South Africa, where the water supply contains over 10 p.p.m. fluoride. Fluorine poisoning has also occurred as an industrial hazard among workers handling fluorine-containing minerals such as cryolite, used in smelting aluminium. The main clinical features are in the skeleton which shows sclerosis of bone, especially of the spine, pelvis and limbs, and calcification of ligaments and tendinous insertions of muscles.

Zinc. Although human deficiency was not clearly established before 1972, zinc is emerging as a nutrient of clinical importance. In PEM, associated zinc deficiency causes thymic atrophy and zinc supplements may accelerate the healing of skin lesions.

In adults a negative zinc balance and low plasma zinc can occur in intestinal disease, chronic alcoholism, anorexia nervosa, diabetes mellitus, nephrotic syndrome, burns, haemodialysis and chronic febrile illness. In some cases poor wound healing has responded to treatment with zinc.

Acute zinc deficiency has been reported in patients receiving prolonged intravenous alimentation without added zinc. Diarrhoea, mental apathy, a moist eczematoid dermatitis especially round the mouth and loss of hair were accompanied by a very low plasma zinc concentration.

Chronic deficiency has been described in association with dwarfism and hypogonadism.

The recommended intake in adults is 15 mg/day. The best dietary sources are meats, whole grain cereals and legumes. Oysters are outstandingly rich in zinc, while white bread, fats and sugar contain negligible amounts.

Selenium content of soil varies. In some areas farm animals develop disease from too much selenium, in others they will thrive only when given a selenium supplement. In Keshan in N.E. China a cardiomyopathy was described in children in 1979. Soil and blood seleniums are very low and Keshan disease can be prevented by giving small selenium supplements. A little selenium must be included in the fluid for total parenteral nutrition; myopathy has occurred when it was not. Selenium is part of the enzyme glutathione peroxidase which helps prevent hydroperoxides accumulate in lipids of cell membranes. Some of the functions of selenium and vitamin E overlap.

Other minerals. *Sulphur* is mainly supplied by the S-containing amino acids in the diet — methionine and cysteine; effects of its deficiency are therefore inseparable from those of protein. *Copper* metabolism is abnormal in Wilson's disease (p. 359). Deficiency occasionally occurs in young children, the main features are anaemia, retarded growth and skeletal rarefaction. *Chromium* facilitates the action of insulin. Deficiency has been reported in some children with PEM and as a rare complication of prolonged parenteral nutrition, presenting as hyperglycaemia.

The roles of *sodium, potassium* and *magnesium* are discussed in the next chapter.

THE VITAMINS

Deficiencies of vitamins still occur in affluent countries, e.g. of folate, thiamin and vitamins D and C. Some of these are induced by diseases or drugs. In the Third World deficiency diseases are more prevalent, e.g. vitamin A deficiency (xerophthalmia) is a major cause of blindness.

Some vitamins have pharmacological actions above the intake that prevents classic deficiency disease, e.g. vitamins A, C and B_6; nicotinic acid is a standard treatment for some types of hyperlipidaemia.

Taking vitamin tablets is fashionable in affluent countries and a few unorthodox practitioners recommend 'megavitamin therapy'. Doctors therefore need to know the features of both deficiency and of overdosage of the major vitamins.

Vitamins are organic substances in food which are required in small amounts but which cannot be synthesised in adequate quantities. 12 vitamins have, so far, been demonstrated to have clinical effects in man. These are:

Fat-soluble	Water-soluble
Vitamin A	Vitamin C—Ascorbic acid

Fat-soluble		Water-soluble
Vitamin D		Thiamin (B_1)
Vitamin E		Riboflavin
Vitamin K		Niacin
	Vitamin B complex	Pyridoxine (B_6)
		Biotin
		Folate
		Cobalamins (B_{12})

Pantothenic acid, a major component of coenzyme A, also appears to be essential, but human deficiency disease has not been reported, perhaps because the vitamin is widely distributed in foods, as its name implies.

Factors influencing the utilisation of vitamins

Availability. Fat-soluble vitamins may be deficient if dietary fat is not eaten or absorbed.

Not all of a vitamin may be in absorbable form; for instance niacin in maize is bound in such a way that it is not absorbed from the gut unless the food is specially treated.

Antivitamins are known to be present in some natural foods, e.g. thiaminase in raw fish. Some synthetic antagonists of the vitamins are used as drugs in the therapy of neoplasms (e.g. methotrexate, p. 109) or of infections (e.g. pyrimethamine, p. 773). Neoplastic cells and micro-organisms are much more sensitive than normal cells but with high doses of the antivitamin a secondary vitamin deficiency can occur in the host.

Provitamins. Substances occur in foods which are not themselves vitamins but are capable of conversion into vitamins in the course of digestion or metabolism. Thus some of the carotenes are provitamins of vitamin A and the amino acid tryptophan can be converted to niacin.

Bacteria in the gut. The normal bacterial flora of the gut is capable of synthesising significant amounts of vitamin K. Bacteria are also capable of extracting vitamins from the ingested food and retaining them until excreted in the faeces. Except for vitamin K and probably biotin, for both of which the requirements are very small (about 0.1 mg per day) bacteria are more likely to reduce than to increase the amounts of vitamins available for absorption, as is demonstrated in bacterial colonisation of the small intestine (p. 305).

Biosynthesis in the skin. Vitamin D need not be provided in the diet if the skin is regularly exposed to adequate sunlight (p. 64).

Interactions of nutrients. If the diet is rich in carbohydrates or alcohol more thiamin is needed for their metabolism. The requirement for vitamin E is increased when the intake of polyunsaturated fats is high.

These considerations indicate how difficult it may be in practice to define the nutritive value of a diet simply from the chemical analysis of its vitamin content.

VITAMIN A (RETINOL)

Retinol has a place in the function of the retina and of epithelial and probably other cells. It may be a protective factor against cancer of the lung and possibly other epithelial sites. On the world scale vitamin A deficiency is one of the seven most common causes of blindness (the others being trachoma, onchocerciases, gonococcal ophthalmia, accidents, cataract and glaucoma). WHO estimates that 250 thousand children become blind every year from keratomalacia.

Dietary sources. Retinol is found only in foods of animal origin. Herbivores obtain the vitamin from its precursors or provitamins — some of the carotenoid pigments in plants. The conversion of even the best of these, β carotene, into retinol in the human small intestinal wall is only 30% efficient. The absorption of both retinol and carotene is facilitated by fats and bile salts.

Retinol is chiefly found in milk, butter, cheese, egg yolk, liver and some of the fatty fish. The liver oils of fish are the richest natural sources but these are used as nutritional supplements rather than foods. Carotene is found chiefly in dark green leafy vegetables. Other useful sources are some of the yellow and red fruits and red palm oil. In Britain and some other countries retinol is added artificially to margarine to provide the same concentration as in good quality summer butter. Healthy adults in Britain have large stores of retinol in their livers (pp. 326 and 330).

Recommended daily intakes of retinol are 300 μg for infants and young children, 750 μg for adolescents and adults, and 1200 μg for lactating women (1 μg retinol = 3 of the old i.u.). In many parts of the world most or all of the requirements are obtained from carotenoids in vegetable foods. Because only approximately $\frac{1}{3}$ of β carotene is absorbed into the intestinal wall and then only $\frac{1}{2}$ of this is converted into retinol, 1 μg retinol equivalent (= 1 μg retinol) is now taken as = 6 μg β carotene.

Night blindness

Retinol is an essential component of the pigment rhodopsin (visual purple) on which rod vision in dim light depends. Hence lack of retinol may result in impairment of dark adaptation. Night blindness is common, as also is vitamin A deficiency, in poor people living in underdeveloped countries; it can occur in the malabsorption syndrome in affluent countries. The diagnosis of vitamin A deficiency is supported by low plasma vitamin A concentration and is confirmed by marked improvement in dark adaptation following therapeutic doses of retinol.

Xerophthalmia

The earliest sign is xerosis conjunctivae — a dry, thickened and pigmented bulbar conjunctiva with a peculiar smoky appearance. Bitôt's spots are glistening white plaques of desquamated thickened conjunctival epithelium, usually triangular in shape and firmly adherent to the underlying conjunctiva. Xerosis conjunctivae and Bitôt's spots are certainly common in children whose diet is deficient in vitamin A but they can also occur in children whose intake of the vitamin is satisfactory. When dryness spreads to the cornea it takes on a dull, hazy, lacklustre appearance due to keratinisation, and xerophthalmia is said to be present.

In young children, xerophthalmia is almost always attributed to recent vitamin A deficiency and is usually associated with PEM. In older children and in adults its interpretation is less simple. Exposure to dust and glare may produce similar changes. They should, however, always call attention to the diet. Recognition of xerophthalmia is very important in young children because once the cornea is involved the process can rapidly progress to keratomalacia.

Keratomalacia

This disease causes blindness among Indians, Indonesians and other rice-eating people of Asia; it also occurs in parts of Africa, the Middle East and Latin America. In Europe and North America it is very rare. Children between the ages of 1 and 5 years are most commonly affected. It occurs only in persons who have been living for a long period on diets almost entirely devoid of vitamin A. The disease is frequently associated with PEM.

The earliest manifestations are night blindness and xerophthalmia. Later the cornea undergoes necrosis and ulceration. Unless early and adequate treatment is given, there is a grave risk of blindness or death from associated diseases.

Treatment. Immediately on diagnosis 60 mg retinol as palmitate or acetate (200 000 i.u.) should be given orally, or, if there is vomiting or severe diarrhoea 55 mg retinol palmitate by intramuscular injection. The oral dose should be repeated the next day and again prior to discharge or at a follow-up visit.

Underlying conditions such as PEM and other nutritional disorders, diarrhoea, dehydration and electrolyte imbalance and infections must be treated appropriately.

For the secondary bacterial infection, antibiotics are of value. Local treatment of the eye will be required only if disorganisation is already present, in which case the services of an ophthalmic surgeon should be obtained.

Prevention. Doctors and nurses working in the tropics, who may have been trained in Europe or North America, should make sure they are familiar with the appearances of xerophthalmia. If in doubt it is better to give a short course of vitamin A treatment.

Pregnant women should be advised to eat dark green leafy vegetables. This helps to build up stores of retinol in the fetal liver. They should also be taught to give such vegetables or locally available carotene-rich fruits to their babies. In some countries where keratomalacia is a major cause of blindness, e.g. in India, single prophylactic oral doses of 60 mg retinol (200 000 i.u.) are being tried in young children.

VITAMIN D

The material originally described as *vitamin D₁* was subsequently found to be an impure mixture of sterols. *Vitamin D₂ (ergocalciferol)* is manufactured by the action of ultraviolet light on ergosterol, a sterol found in fungi and yeasts. Although used in therapeutics, it occurs very rarely in nature. *Vitamin D₃ (cholecalciferol)* is the natural form of the vitamin which occurs in man and other animals. It is formed in the skin by the action of ultraviolet light on 7-dehydrocholesterol.

Cholecalciferol is not the active form of the vitamin. It is converted in the liver to 25-hydroxycholecalciferol (25-OH-D_3) which is further hydroxylated in the kidney, mainly to 1,25 dihydroxycholecalciferol (1,25 $(OH)_2D_3$). Most of the hydroxylated forms of vitamin D in human plasma are based on vitamin D_3 (cholecalciferol) derived from synthesis in the skin or from fish liver oils. A smaller proportion is based on vitamin D_2 (ergocalciferol) from calciferol tablets or fortified milk (e.g. in USA). Though plasma 25-OH-D_3 and 25-OH-D_2 can be distinguished by immunoassay, they and their corresponding derivatives appear to have identical activities.

1,25$(OH)_2D_3$ is many times more potent than cholecalciferol and can be regarded as a hormone. It is transported in the blood to target organs, notably gut and bone and is regulated by a complex feedback system. The main function of 1,25$(OH)_2D_3$ is, by inducing a specific transport protein in the enterocyte, to increase calcium absorption to meet the demands of growth, pregnancy and lactation. An adequate concentration of calcium is thus ensured for the formation of calcium phosphate in bone where calcium comes in contact with inorganic phosphates, liberated from organic phosphates under the influence of phosphatase produced by osteoblasts.

Alfacalcidol, 1α hydroxycholecalciferol (1α OH-D_3), is a synthetic analogue which is converted into 1,25 $(OH)_2D_3$ in the liver without the need for hydroxylation in the kidney. It is used in treating hypocalcaemia and osteomalacia due to renal disease.

The main reasons for impaired production of 1,25 $(OH)_2D_3$ are: (1) deficiency of 25-OH-D_3 due to lack of sunlight, an inadequate diet or malabsorption; (2) disturbed metabolism in liver or renal disease, notably chronic renal failure and (3) depression of the feedback system as in hypoparathyroidism.

Dietary sources. The richest sources are fatty fish and their liver oils, some of which contain thousands of micrograms of vitamin D per 100 g. Vitamin D is also present in much smaller quantities in dairy products such as butter and eggs. In Britain vitaminised margarine is the most reliable food source of the vitamin for adults: 28 g (1 oz) contains nearly the daily requirement. Milk has a very small content of vitamin D; meat and white fish have insignificant amounts and cereals, vegetables and fruit have none. Unlike vitamin A, stores of vitamin D in the body are not large; only a little is stored in the liver and moderate amounts in adipose tissue.

People who regularly have adequate exposure of their skin to sunlight do not normally need vitamin D in their diet. Otherwise the recommended daily intake (WHO) for infants and children up to 5 years of age and for pregnant or lactating women is 10 μg. For older children and adults about 2.5 μg is adequate (1 μg = 40 i.u.).

Rickets

Rickets is the characteristic result of deficiency of vitamin D in children. When the epiphyses have fused the corresponding deficiency disease is oestomalacia. Both mainly affect the bones but they differ in details.

Infants in their first year are susceptible to rickets because of the low content of vitamin D in both human and animal milk and if they are not given a supplement of vitamin D and if, for various social and cultural reasons, their mothers wrap them up in clothes which prevents their exposure to sunlight. By the second year the infant is able to crawl about in the sunshine and spontaneous healing usually occurs.

The disease is now uncommon in countries where vitamin D is freely available. In Britain clinical rickets occurs in Asian immigrant children, often of schoolgoing age, from a combination of little exposure of the skin to sunlight and very low dietary intakes of vitamin D. High phytate intake in chapatti flour may contribute by inhibiting calcium absorption. The disease is also liable to occur in premature babies.

Clinical features. The infant with rickets has often received sufficient calories and may appear well nourished, but is restless, fretful and pale, with flabby muscles and is prone to respiratory and gastrointestinal infections. Development is delayed; the teeth often erupt late and there is failure to sit, stand, crawl and walk at the normal ages.

The bony changes are the most characteristic signs of rickets. The earliest lesion is often craniotabes — small round unossified areas in the membranous bones of the skull, yielding to the pressure of the finger, with a crackling feeling. This sign is of particular value in the diagnosis of rickets in developing countries where the disease is common in infants under 1 year of age. It usually disappears within 12 months of birth.

Two other early signs are enlargement of the epiphyses at the lower end of the radius and swelling of the costochondral junctions of the ribs ('rickety rosary'). Later there may be 'bossing' of the frontal and parietal bones and delayed closure of the anterior fontanelle. Later still, there may be deformities of the chest such as pigeon chest and Harrison's sulcus.

If rickets continues into the second or third year of life, deformities such as kyphosis develop as a result of the new gravitational and muscular strains caused by sitting up and crawling. At the same time there may be enlargement of the epiphyses at the lower ends of the femur, tibia and fibula. When the rachitic child begins to walk, deformities of the shafts of the leg bones develop, so that 'knock knees' or 'bow legs' are seen. Pelvic deformities may follow and lead later to serious difficulties at childbirth.

When there is a reduction in ionised plasma calcium, infantile tetany may result, with spasm of the hands and feet and of the vocal cords. The latter causes a high-pitched distressing cry and difficulty in breathing. Epileptic fits may also occur.

Investigation. *Radiological examination* of the wrist will show characteristic changes in the epiphyses at the lower ends of the radius. The zones of epiphyseal cartilages are thickened and the distal ends of the shafts are widened. When fully developed this shows as a typical 'saucer' deformity.

Chemical pathology. Plasma calcium tends to fall from its normal level (p. 814). More commonly the serum phosphate falls due to the parathyroid glands responding to a slight reduction in calcium by increasing the excretion of phosphate in the urine.

Clinical rickets may occur when the levels of calcium and phosphorus in the plasma are still within normal limits but an increase in alkaline phosphatase is of diagnostic value. This enzyme is formed by the osteoblasts which, unable to make bone without a sufficient supply of calcium, liberate into the circulation the excess of this enzyme which they cannot use. Plasma 25-hydroxycholecalciferol, the main circulating form of vitamin D, is absent or very low.

Treatment. The two essentials of treatment are the provision of a supplement of vitamin D and an ample intake of calcium, the best source of which is milk.

A therapeutic dose of vitamin D varies from 25 to 125 μg (1000–5000 i.u.) daily, depending on the severity of the disease and age of the child. In contrast, the prophylactic dose is 10 μg (400 i.u.) or less daily depending on the sunlight. The daily administration of small doses is the method recommended for normal practice, because of the danger of overdosage (p. 66).

In times of social upheaval, such as may be occasioned by war or disasters, when a young child may be seen once by an emergency medical service and perhaps not again for months, a single massive dose of vitamin D, e.g. 3 mg, can be given by mouth with reasonable safety and curative effects.

Treatment of tetany is described on page 448.

PROGRESS. The earliest evidence of healing in rickets is provided by radiological examination of the growing ends of the bones. Serum calcium and phosphorus provide an unreliable guide. The raised serum alkaline phosphatase does not usually fall for several weeks after treatment is initiated. The therapeutic dose of vitamin D should be continued so long as the alkaline phosphatase remains elevated; thereafter it can be reduced to the prophylactic dose of 10 μg daily.

Rickets is not a fatal disease *per se,* but the untreated rachitic child is always at risk of infections, notably bronchopneumonia. The skeletal changes, if mild in degree, usually tend to heal spontaneously as the child gets older, but in severe cases pigeon chest, spinal curvature, knock knees, bow legs or contracted pelvis persist.

SECONDARY AND RESISTANT RICKETS. In malabsorption, e.g. in coeliac disease, rickets is common. Children on long-term anti-epileptic drugs are liable to develop rickets; these drugs induce changes in liver microsomal enzymes which convert vitamin D to inactive metabolites.

Occasional cases of rickets are encountered which are resistant to ordinary therapeutic doses of vitamin D. The commonest type of vitamin D resistant rickets is familial hypophosphataemic rickets, an X-linked dominant condition in which there is renal tubular loss of phosphate. There are also two types of 'vitamin D dependent rickets', in one of which 1α hydroxylation of 25 OH vitamin D is impaired; in the other form there appears to be end-organ resistance to the active metabolite. Alfacalcidol is useful in these conditions.

HYPERVITAMINOSIS D. In the case of vitamin D it is possible to have too much of a good thing. Large doses are toxic and cause hypercalcaemia. The symptoms include nausea, vomiting, constipation, drowsiness and signs of renal failure; metastatic calcification in the arteries, kidneys and other tissues may occur.

Since renal damage may occur before clinical signs of toxicity appear, all patients on large doses of vitamin D should have their serum calcium level checked regularly at 3 monthly intervals and if this is found to be above 2.6 mmol/l (10.5 mg/100 ml) it is an early indication of overdosage.

Prevention. The provision of adequate milk for children, the clearing of slums, the building of new housing estates and smoke abatement schemes are basic prophylactic measures in high latitude countries. In addition mothers must be educated in the need to keep their infants and children in the sunshine as much as possible.

None of the common foods in a child's diet is a good source of vitamin D and children may benefit from a daily supplement of about 10 μg from cod-liver oil, continued at least in the winter for the first 5 years of life or more. Not only is there no advantage in giving children more than 10 μg of vitamin D daily for prophylactic purposes, but higher doses over a long period could predispose to infantile hypercalcaemia, a form of hypervitaminosis D.

OSTEOMALACIA AND OSTEOPOROSIS

Osteomalacia, which means softening of bone, is primarily due to a deficiency of vitamin D. This results in a failure to replace the turnover of calcium and phosphorus in the organic matrix of bone. Hence the bone content is demineralised and bony substance becomes replaced by soft osteoid tissue.

Osteoporosis, which is atrophy of bone, is believed to be due to predominance of resorption over formation of the cellular matrix of bone which leads to a reduction in the total mass of bone. In other words osteoporosis is too little

bone of normal mineral content. In contrast to osteomalacia the ratio of calcium phosphate to matrix is normal.

Osteomalacia

Aetiology. Osteomalacia is the adult counterpart of rickets. It was formerly common in women in purdah in oriental countries, living on poor cereal diets devoid of milk, kept indoors and seldom seeing the sun. Symptoms occurred with pregnancy.

In Scotland and in other countries where osteomalacia is a relatively common disease in old people, especially women, the disease may be due to malabsorption from any cause, including operations like partial gastrectomy, or to direct dietary deficiency of vitamin D. Chronic renal disorders are a less important cause. Adults who have to take antiepileptic drugs for years are likely to develop osteomalacia (p. 65).

Clinical features. Skeletal discomfort is usually present and persistent and ranges from backache to severe pain. Bone tenderness on pressure is common. Muscular weakness is often present and the patient may find difficulty in climbing stairs or getting out of a chair. A waddling gait is not unusual. Tetany may be manifested by carpopedal spasm and facial twitching. Spontaneous fractures may occur, independent of the pseudo-fractures described below. The biochemical changes in the blood are the same as in rickets.

Radiological examination shows rarefaction of bone and commonly translucent bands (pseudo-fractures or Looser's zones), often symmetrical, at points submitted to stress. Common sites are the ribs, the axillary border of the scapula, the pubic rami and the medial cortex of the upper femur. Pseudo-fractures are pathognomonic when well developed.

Histological examination of stained undecalcified sections of bone obtained by biopsy shows the presence of excess osteoid tissue.

Treatment. When osteomalacia is primarily due to defective intake, treatment is essentially the same as for rickets, namely 25 to 125 μg vitamin D daily. The response is usually dramatic. If there is evidence of malabsorption the dose should be increased or given intramuscularly at weekly intervals. If the disease is secondary to renal disorders alfacalcidol (p. 64) should be used.

Maintenance treatment with vitamin D will be required for all cases of osteomalacia in which the cause cannot be removed. In addition a good diet should be given which includes milk.

Prevention. Free access to sunshine and an adequate intake of dairy produce, supplemented when necessary with prophylactic vitamin D (10 μg/day), will prevent nutritional osteomalacia. Particular attention to these prophylactic measures should be given to inmates of geriatric and mental hospitals and to old people living alone whose exposure to sunshine is limited and also to those who have had gastric surgery. Patients on long-term antiepileptic therapy should be given prophylactic doses of vitamin D.

Osteoporosis

Osteoporosis is the commonest metabolic disease of bone and is found most frequently in elderly women when it is known as postmenopausal osteoporosis. It may occur in elderly men (senile osteoporosis) and rarely in younger people (idiopathic osteoporosis). There is a wide variation in the geographical and racial incidence of generalised osteoporosis. For example, in the United States it is more prevalent in Caucasians than in Negroes.

Aetiology. Bone mass reaches a peak early in adult life and thereafter declines. Weight of bone at maturity is lower in women than men and the rate of decline tends to be faster. When bone mass is sufficiently reduced the clinical features of osteoporosis are to be expected. This may result from either lighter bones at maturity or from an accelerated rate of bone loss with ageing or both. In post-menopausal women the loss of calcium in the urine is increased. It is not yet established whether this is primary and depletes bones of calcium or secondary to bone resorption. High sodium and animal protein intakes increase urinary calcium loss and hence the calcium requirement. There is considerable support for the calcium hypothesis that either (1) a low intake of calcium (for an individual's requirements) early and/or later in life leads to osteoporosis or (2) that a generous intake of calcium can delay its

appearance. But it is still puzzling why osteoporosis has a higher prevalence in Britain and North America than it does in Africa and Asia where there is little or no milk and calcium intakes are lower.

Inadequate physical activity promotes generalised osteoporosis and may, in part at least, account for the high incidence of this condition in affluent societies. Immobilisation by splinting, inflammation or pain is the main cause of local osteoporosis.

Generalised osteoporosis may be secondary to prolonged treatment with adrenal corticosteroids; it occurs in various endocrine disorders, notably Cushing's syndrome and hypogonadism, and also in severe malnutrition and chronic renal disease. Osteoporosis, like anaemia, may therefore be the end result of a number of diverse processes.

Clinical features. The patient is usually an elderly woman who is otherwise healthy. There may be no disability despite obvious radiological abnormality. In others there are episodes of severe pain usually due to fractures of the brittle bones often occurring after minimal trauma. The lumbar and thoracic vertebrae, the neck of the femur, the upper end of the humerus and the lower end of the radius are the commonest sites of fracture. Healing is not impaired and as it occurs pain usually subsides. More persistent backache is a later feature of osteoporosis due to progressive compression or collapse of several vertebrae. This may result in loss of stature and in kyphosis. Persistent pain elsewhere is not a feature of osteoporosis but is more characteristic of osteomalacia, Paget's disease or skeletal metastases. In contrast to these conditions there is also a tendency for spontaneous improvement to occur in osteoporosis. Idiopathic osteoporosis is occasionally found in younger persons in whom it also tends to be self-limiting.

The radiological changes are more marked in the bones of the axial skeleton than in the limbs; they consist of loss of bone density, reduction in the number and size of trabeculae and thinning of the cortex. The upper and lower surfaces of the lumbar and thoracic vertebral bodies become biconcave, and later compression or collapse causes anterior wedging.

The calcium, phosphorus and alkaline phosphatase levels in the blood are normal in contrast to osteomalacia.

Treatment. Any primary factor such as excessive corticosteroid therapy or endocrine disease should be corrected if possible. The physiological decline in skeletal mass, the obscure aetiology of idiopathic osteoporosis and its tendency to remission, together with the need for long-term assessment, make therapeutic measures very difficult to evaluate.

The patient should know that the natural history of the disease is characterised by spontaneous improvement and that suitable regular exercise is beneficial. The patient should remain ambulant if symptoms permit. The use of spinal supports is undesirable. Immobilisation following a fracture should be limited to the part involved and accompanied by graduated remedial exercises. It should be borne in mind that osteomalacia can coexist with osteoporosis especially in patients with a fracture of the neck of the femur. Obesity must be avoided and, if present, corrected.

Cyclical oestrogen therapy may be prescribed for otherwise healthy post-menopausal women. At least an adequate intake of vitamin D and calcium should be ensured. Cows' milk is the best source of the latter, half a litre providing about 600 mg of calcium. There is evidence that calcium supplements may be beneficial. The use of sodium fluoride to stimulate osteogenesis and also 1α OH-D are under investigation.

VITAMIN E

Alpha-tocopherol is the most potent of eight related substances with vitamin E activity. Good sources include vegetable oils, wholegrain cereals and nuts.

Vitamin E prevents oxidation of polyunsaturated fatty acids in cell membranes. The first feature of human deficiency is a mild haemolytic anaemia which has been described only in premature infants and in a few cases of malabsorption. In chronic deficiency, e.g. in cystic fibrosis, ataxia and visual scotomas occur which respond to vitamin E. Early oral administration reduces the severity of retrolental fibroplasia in premature infants given oxygen.

There is no scientific justification for self-medication with vitamin E in the belief that this will increase energy or virility. Pharmacological doses of vitamin E have produced surprisingly few side effects but they do appear to interfere with thyroid function and potentiate the action of coumarin anticoagulants.

VITAMIN K

Vitamin K is required for the formation in the liver of factors necessary for the normal clotting of blood (p. 549). It exists in nature in two forms, vitamin K_1 and vitamin K_2. Vitamin K_1 (phytomenadione) is found in leafy vegetables. Adequate amounts are normally supplied in the average diet and absorbed with other lipids. Bacterial synthesis of vitamin K_2 occurs within the colon.

Primary vitamin K deficiency is not uncommon in the newborn when there is no formation of vitamin K in the gut and hypoprothrombinaemia occurs. 1 mg vitamin K_1 at birth is a safe prophylactic measure against the development of haemorrhagic disease of the newborn.

Secondary vitamin K deficiency and its clinical features and treatment are discussed on page 549.

VITAMIN C (ASCORBIC ACID)

Ascorbic acid is a simple sugar. It is the most active reducing agent found in the aqueous phase of living tissues and is easily and reversibly oxidised to dehydro-ascorbic acid. Its highest concentrations are in the adrenal cortex and in the eye. Stress and corticotrophin secretion lead to a loss of ascorbic acid from the adrenal cortex. The presumption, therefore, is that ascorbic acid is somehow concerned in bodily reactions to stress.

Dietary sources. Blackcurrants, guavas, citrus fruits, berries and green vegetables are the richest sources. Foods of animal origin contain very little except for liver and glandular tissue. Dried cereals and pulses contain no ascorbic acid.

Ascorbic acid is very easily destroyed by heat, alkalies such as sodium bicarbonate, traces of copper or by an oxidase liberated by damage to plant tissues. Ascorbic acid is very soluble in water. For these reasons many traditional methods of cooking reduce or eliminate it from the diet.

The recommended intake is 30–60 mg in different countries. Body stores last for about $2\frac{1}{2}$ to 3 months on a deficient diet.

Scurvy

Aetiology. In 1497 when Vasco de Gama sailed round the Cape of Good Hope 100 out of his 160 men died of scurvy. For the next 300 years scurvy was a major factor determining the success or failure of all sea ventures even after it was recognised by Lind (1753) and by Cook (1755) that it results from the prolonged consumption of a diet devoid of fresh fruit and vegetables. Final proof and isolation of vitamin C were not possible until the guinea pig was found (1907) to provide a suitable animal model because, like man and unlike most animals, it cannot synthesise ascorbic acid from glucose.

Sporadic cases of scurvy continue to arise in infants as a result of ignorance, poverty and maternal neglect and also amongst old people, especially men living alone who are not feeding themselves properly. Scurvy appears to be rare in most tropical countries but is more likely to occur in arid regions in times of drought.

Pathology. Ascorbic acid deficiency results in defective formation of collagen in connective tissue because of failure of hydroxylation of proline to hydroxyproline, the characteristic amino acid of collagen. There is in consequence delayed healing of wounds. There are also capillary haemorrhages and subnormal platelet stickiness.

Clinical features. ADULT SCURVY. The pathognomic sign is the swollen and spongy gums particularly of the papillae between the teeth, sometimes producing the appearance of 'scurvy buds'. These bleed easily. The teeth may become loose and even fall out in severe cases. There is always some infection; indeed this seems necessary for the production of the scorbutic gingival appearances since volunteers suffering from experimental deficiency did not develop it if their gums were previously healthy. In patients without teeth the gums appear normal.

The first sign of cutaneous bleeding is often found on the lower thighs. These are perifollicular haemorrhages — tiny points of bleeding around the orifice of a hair follicle. There is a heaping-up of keratin-like material on the surface around the mouth of the follicle, through which a deformed 'corkscrew' hair characteristically projects. Perifollicular haemorrhages are often followed by petechial haemorrhages, developing independently of the hair follicles, which are usually first seen on the feet and ankles. Thereafter large spontaneous bruises (ecchymoses) may arise almost anywhere in the body, but usually first in the lower extremities, producing the characteristic 'woody leg'. Haemorrhage may occur into joints, into a nerve sheath, under the nails or conjunctiva or into the gastrointestinal tract; there may be epistaxis. Scurvy can present with any of these features. By the time the disease is fully developed the patient is usually anaemic.

Before the changes in the gums and skin appear, the patient has usually felt feeble and listless for some weeks. Another characteristic of scurvy is that fresh wounds fail to heal — a possibility that the surgeon has to bear in mind. A patient with scurvy may die suddenly without warning, apparently from cardiac failure.

The dietary and social history is helpful in doubtful cases. Old, solitary people may insist that they fend very well for themselves, but careful questioning will reveal that they do not buy fresh fruit or vegetables. In other instances the proper foods may be purchased but they are so badly cooked that the diet loses all its vitamin C.

Plasma ascorbate is very low (p. 814); a fresh sample of plasma is needed because the vitamin can decompose in a few hours at warm room temperatures. Probably a better index of tissue reserves of the vitamin is its concentration in the buffy layer or in the platelets.

INFANTILE SCURVY. The main clinical features are lassitude, anaemia, painful limbs and enlargement of the costochondral junctions. Until the teeth have erupted, scorbutic infants do not develop gingivitis. The first sign of bleeding is usually a large subperiosteal haemorrhage in one of the long bones. This gives rise to intense pain, especially on movement.

Treatment. The normal body contains about 1.5 g of the vitamin, so that a dose of 250 mg by mouth four times daily should saturate the tissues quickly. Attention should be paid to correcting the general deficiencies of the patient's former diet. A liberal mixed diet should be given. If the patient is anaemic iron and sometimes folic acid are indicated. With adequate treatment no patient dies of scurvy and recovery is usually rapid and complete.

Prevention. In breast milk the vitamin C content responds to maternal intake. Fruit juice should be given to bottle-fed infants.

No simple administrative means has been found of preventing scurvy among the old and solitary. Should the physician be unable to persuade such a person to eat fruit or vegetables, 50 mg synthetic ascorbic acid should be taken daily.

Trauma, surgery and burns, infections, smoking and certain drugs — adrenocortical steroids, aspirin, indomethacin and tetracycline — all increase the requirement for vitamin C. Consequently such persons require considerably more than the recommended allowance of 30–60 mg/d.

ASCORBIC ACID AND THE COMMON COLD. It has been claimed that ascorbic acid in doses of 1–2 g daily, or even more, will prevent the common cold. If it does, this is a pharmacological and not a vitamin effect as coryza is not a manifestation of scurvy. In the largest controlled trial, in Toronto, two placebo groups were included. One of these had fewer colds than those taking 0.25, 1 or 2 g vitamin C per day prophylactically. It is inadvisable for people to dose themselves with large quantities of ascorbic acid as this favours the formation of oxalate stones in the urinary tract.

THIAMIN (VITAMIN B₁)

Thiamin pyrophosphate (TPP) is an essential coenzyme for the decarboxylation of pyruvate to acetyl coenzyme A. This is the bridge between anaerobic glycolysis and the tricarboxylic acid (Krebs) cycle. TPP is also the coenzyme for transketolase in the hexose monophosphate shunt pathway and for decarboxylation of α-ketoglutarate to succinate in the Krebs cycle. Consequently when thiamin is deficient (1) the cells cannot utilise glucose aerobically; this is likely to affect the nervous system first, since it depends entirely on glucose for its energy requirements; (2) there is accumulation of pyruvic acid and of lactic acid derived from it, which produce vasodilatation and increase cardiac output. Thiamin deficiency can produce high output cardiac failure and/or peripheral neuropathy and/or encephalopathy. These occur in various combinations in wet and dry beriberi, infantile beriberi and Wernicke's encephalopathy.

High carbohydrate diets, heavy alcohol intake or intravenous glucose infusions predispose to and aggravate thiamin deficiency. The body contains only 30 mg of thiamin — 30 times the adult daily requirement — and deficiency starts after about a month on a thiamin-free diet, sooner than for any other vitamin.

Dietary sources. Legumes, pork, liver, nuts, the germ of cereals and yeast, are the only good sources. Green vegetables, roots, fruits, fresh foods and dairy produce (except butter) contain small amounts of the vitamin. It is not found in fats or oils. In sugar and many cereal products (wheat, rice) nearly all the naturally occurring vitamin may be removed; there is little or none in most alcoholic drinks. Thiamin is more sensitive to heat than other B vitamins, especially at alkaline pH, i.e. if baking soda is used. The loss of thiamin is usually around 25% in cooking an ordinary mixed diet.

Beriberi

Beriberi is a nutritional disorder formerly widespread in South and East Asia. The word comes from the Singhalese language and means 'I cannot' (said twice), signifying that the patient is too ill to do anything. Beriberi has almost disappeared from prosperous Asian countries such as Japan, Taiwan and Malaysia and from big cities such as Hong Kong, Manila and Singapore.

Oriental beriberi is usually caused by eating diets in which most of the calories are derived from polished, i.e. highly milled, rice. The disorder is often precipitated by infections, hard physical labour or pregnancy and lactation. In Britain and North America occasional cases of beriberi heart disease are seen, usually in alcoholics who have been consuming little but alcohol for some weeks.

Owing to a lack of thiamin, glucose is incompletely metabolised and pyruvic and lactic acids accumulate in the tissues and body fluids. These metabolites cause dilatation of peripheral blood vessels, as in normal exercise. In beriberi this vasodilatation may be extreme, so that fluid leaks out through the capillaries, producing oedema. At the same time the blood flows rapidly through the dilated peripheral circulation. There is a high cardiac output and as the disease progresses the heart dilates because the myocardium is both overworked and unable to use glucose efficiently as an energy substrate. Cardiac failure accentuates the oedema. Sudden death may result. Microscopic examination usually shows loss of striation of myocardial fibres, which are also finely vacuolated and often fragmented and separated by oedema.

Clinical features. WET BERIBERI. Oedema is the most notable feature and may develop rapidly to involve not only the legs but also the face, trunk and serous cavities. Palpitations are marked and there may be pain in the legs after walking, probably due to the accumulation of lactic acid. There is usually tachycardia and an increase in pulse pressure. The heart is enlarged and the jugular venous pressure rises.

While the circulation is well maintained, the skin is typically warm owing to the vasodilatation; as heart failure advances, the skin of the extremities can become cold and cyanotic. The mind is usually clear. Electrocardiograms often show no changes except sinus tachycardia but in some cases there are inverted T waves or conduction defects.

DRY BERIBERI is characterised by a polyneuropathy resulting in severe wasting of muscles. In long-standing cases there is degeneration and demyelination of both sensory and motor nerves. The vagus and other autonomic nerves may also be affected. In dry beriberi the level of blood pyruvate is usually within normal limits.

The disease is essentially a chronic one, which may be arrested at any stage by improving the diet. Bedridden patients and those with severe cachexia are very susceptible to infections. Patients with dry beriberi are always liable to a sudden onset of oedema which may be due to a variety of dietary causes, e.g. lack of thiamin or protein, or to starvation.

INFANTILE BERIBERI. This was formerly the chief cause of death between 2 to 6 months of age in rice-eating rural areas in S.E. Asia. It appears to be uncommon now but it may still occur in isolated areas. It is found in breast-fed infants, usually between the second and fifth months. Although the mothers of such infants have been eating a diet and secreting milk with a low thiamin content, classical signs of beriberi are stated to be absent in 50% of them.

The illness usually starts acutely and is rapidly fatal, it not promptly treated. The mother may have noticed that the infant is restless, often cries, is passing less urine than normal and shows signs of puffiness. The infant then may suddenly become cyanosed with dyspnoea and the physical signs of acute cardiac failure and die within 24 to 48 hours. Other serious signs are convulsions and coma. In severe cases partial to complete aphonia is characteristic and is usually preceded by the infant's cry becoming thin with a plaintive whine.

WERNICKE'S ENCEPHALOPATHY AND KORSAKOFF'S PSYCHOSIS. This cerebral form of thiamin deficiency occurs in Europe and North America. It often presents acutely, usually in an alcoholic but it is sometimes seen in people with malnutrition, e.g. persistent vomiting; it occurred in prisoners of war on small rations of polished rice.

In *Wernicke's encephalopathy* there are foci of congestion and petechial haemorrhage in the upper part of the mid-brain, the hypothalamus, and the walls of the third ventricle. Involvement of the mamillary bodies is a pathognomonic finding at post-mortem. The patient is quietly confused and the most valuable clinical sign is some form of bilateral, symmetrical ophthalmoplegia. This may be in one or more than one direction and accompanied by abnormal pupillary reflexes and/or nystagmus. Ataxia is also present. The confusion is liable soon to progress to stupor or death if treatment is delayed.

Korsakoff's psychosis. In some cases the predominant change in mental function is a memory defect, the characteristic bedside feature of which is confabulation. Psychological tests show a severe defect in storing new information.

Wernicke's encephalopathy and Korsakoff's psychosis are often associated with polyneuropathy and/or with superior midline cerebellar degeneration (p. 657) but it is surprising how uncommon these cerebral forms are in S.E. Asia and that beriberi cardiomyopathy is seldom seen with Wernicke/Korsakoff disease.

Investigation. Plasma pyruvic or lactic acids are not elevated in the more chronic forms of beriberi and if they are increased are not specific. The best laboratory test is measurement of trans-ketolase activity in red cells with and without added thiamin pyrophosphate (TPP) in vitro. The test requires fresh heparinised whole blood and this must be taken before thiamin treatment is started. A TPP effect above 30% is to be expected in beriberi or Wernicke's encephalopathy.

Treatment. *Wet beriberi.* Treatment must be started as soon as the diagnosis is made, because fatal heart failure may occur suddenly. Complete rest is essential and 50 mg thiamin should be given intramuscularly for 3 days. Thereafter 10 mg 3 times a day should be continued by mouth until convalescence is established.

The response of a patient with beriberi to thiamin is one of the most dramatic therapeutic events. Within a few hours the breathing is easier, the pulse rate slower, the extremities cooler and a rapid diuresis begins to dispose of the oedema. In a few days the size of the heart is restored to normal. Muscular pain and tenderness are also dramatically improved.

Dry beriberi. The treatment is that of a nutritional polyneuropathy as described on page 664.

Wernicke's encephalopathy should be treated without delay with 50 mg thiamin hydrochloride by slow intravenous injection followed by 50 mg intramuscularly daily for a week. Confusion, disorientation and ophthalmoplegia should respond within 2 to 3 days. Indeed this response to thiamin helps to confirm the diagnosis. The memory disorder takes longer to improve; it may become more obvious as confusion clears and the patient's general condition improves. Some degree of memory impairment may persist.

Prevention. In Western countries the prevention of beriberi and Wernicke's encephalopathy is related to the control of alcoholism. In a chronic alcoholic vitamin B complex tablets can at least prevent the complications of thiamin deficiency. Beriberi is much less common in Asia than it used to be.

NIACIN *(nicotinic acid and nicotinamide)*

Nicotinamide is an essential part of the two important pyridine nucleotides, NAD and NADP which are hydrogen-accepting coenzymes for dehydrogenases at many steps in the pathways of glucose oxidation. NAD is also the coenzyme for alcohol dehydrogenase. Nicotinic acid is readily converted in the body into the amide. For nutritional purposes the two have equal biological activity and are considered together in foods under the generic term 'niacin'. Both are water-soluble and resistant to heat.

Dietary sources. Niacin is widely distributed in plant and animal foods, but only in relatively small amounts, except in meat (especially the organs), fish, wholemeal cereals and pulses. Removal of the bran in milling cereals reduces their niacin to low levels. A cup of good coffee provides about 1 mg of niacin. In a normal Western European diet about half the nicotinic acid content is provided by meat and fish.

A special feature of this vitamin is that it is normally synthesised in the body in limited amounts from the amino acid tryptophan; 60 mg of tryptophan yields 1 mg of nicotinamide. For this reason niacin equivalents in a diet are calculated by adding together the niacin plus 1/60 of the tryptophan intake (in mg). As a rule of thumb it can be assumed that tryptophan is about 1/100th of the protein intake. Therefore a protein intake of 60 g provides 10 mg ($60 \times 1/100 \times 1/60$ g) of the adult daily requirement of 18 mg niacin equivalents (pre-formed niacin + that from tryptophan).

Pellagra

Pellagra is a nutritional disease formerly endemic among poor peasants who subsisted chiefly on maize (American corn). The greater part of the niacin in maize is in a bound form, niacytin, which is unavailable to the consumer. In areas where pellagra remains, e.g. in parts of Africa, the incidence is much less than formerly. It is occasionally seen in alcoholics and in the malabsorption syndrome. In the rare inborn error of metabolism, *Hartnup disease,* tryptophan absorption is impaired and there is a pellagrous dermatitis with neurological abnormalities which respond to nicotinamide.

Clinical features. Pellagra can develop in only 6 to 8 weeks on diets very deficient in niacin and tryptophan. It has been called the disease of the three Ds: dermatitis, diarrhoea and dementia.

Skin. The diagnosis is usually first suggested by the appearance of the skin. Characteristically, there is an erythema resembling severe sunburn, appearing symmetrically over the parts of the body exposed to sunlight and especially on the neck. Local trauma or irritation of the skin may also determine the site of the lesion. The affected areas are well demarcated from normal skin. In acute cases the skin lesions may progress to vesiculation, cracking, exudation and crusting with ulceration and sometimes secondary infection. In chronic cases the dermatitis occurs as a roughening and thickening of the skin with a brown pigmentation. Dermatitis of the vulva, perineum and perianal area is usually present.

Alimentary tract. There may be anorexia, nausea and dysphagia. Glossitis is an early symptom and may precede the skin lesions. The mouth is sore and often shows angular stomatitis and cheilosis (p. 74). It is probable that a non-infective inflammation extends throughout the gastrointestinal tract and accounts for the diarrhoea which is usually present.

Nervous system. In severe cases delirium is the most common mental disturbance in the acute form of the disease and dementia in the chronic form. Because of these changes, chronic pellagrins have in the past been admitted to mental hospitals.

Treatment. Nicotinamide is given in a dose of 100 mg every 6 hours by mouth, although a smaller dose is likely to be effective. The vitamin is well absorbed but can be given parenterally. The response is usually rapid; within 24 hours the erythema of the skin diminishes and the diarrhoea ceases. Often there is also striking improvement in the patient's behaviour and mental attitude.

Nicotinamide alone is usually insufficient to restore health. There are likely to be associated nutritional deficiencies. A relatively low intake of protein including tryptophan is an essential condition for development of the disease, and hypoalbuminaemia is common. Deficiencies of other B complex vitamins are to be expected. Nicotinamide treatment should therefore be supplemented with a nutritious diet, high in protein. Vitamin B complex tablets should be given and

iron, folic acid and vitamin B_{12} may be necessary in addition for some cases. Alcohol should be forbidden.

Prevention. The disappearance from the southern states of America of pellagra which before the Second World War afflicted tens of thousands of poor country folk, demonstrates that the disease is preventable. Fortification of bread and maize meal with nicotinic acid, is only one of several factors which have produced this satisfactory result. General improvement in the economic state, education and nutrition of the population appears to have had more effect.

In Central America the peasants eat a staple diet of maize but pellagra is unusual. This appears to be because the traditional method of boiling the maize in lime water (dilute calcium hydroxide) before they make tortillas hydrolyses the indigestible niacytin to free niacin.

RIBOFLAVIN

Riboflavin is a constituent of the flavoproteins which are concerned with tissue oxidation. It is a yellow-green fluorescent compound soluble in water. Though stable to boiling in acid solution, in alkaline solution it is decomposed by heat. It is also destroyed by exposure to light.

Dietary sources. The best sources of riboflavin are liver, kidney, milk, meat, cheese and eggs. Green vegetables contain moderate amounts. It differs from other components of the vitamin B complex in that it occurs in good amounts in dairy produce, but is relatively lacking in cereal grains, especially when highly milled. Ordinary methods of cooking do not destroy the vitamin. If foods, especially milk, are left exposed to sunshine, large losses may occur.

Disorders due to riboflavin deficiency

When human volunteers have been given diets very low in riboflavin, the most consistent clinical manifestations were angular stomatitis, cheilosis and nasolabial seborrhoea; these responded to the addition of pure riboflavin in the deficient diet.

Angular stomatitis is not specific for lack of riboflavin. Deficiencies of niacin, pyridoxine and iron can all produce it. It can follow herpes febrilis at the angle of the mouth. A common cause is ill-fitting dentures, associated with candidosis.

Cheilosis is a zone of red, denuded epithelium at the line of closure of the lips. It has occurred in experimental pure niacin deficiency. It is often associated with angular stomatitis and frequently seen in pellegra.

Nasalabial seborrhoea consists of enlarged follicles around the sides of the nose which are plugged with dry sebaceous material. This occurs in primates on a diet deficient only in riboflavin. It is seen in some patients with pellagra.

Other abnormalities. Vascularisation of the cornea, scrotal dermatitis, a magenta-coloured tongue and anaemia have been attributed to riboflavin deficiency but they may have alternative explanations.

Riboflavin clearly plays a vital role in cellular oxidation and there are communities and individuals who have both low dietary intakes and very low concentrations in urine or blood. Yet it is surprising that the clinical effects of riboflavin deficiency are trivial and mainly non-specific. Features of riboflavin deficiency are most likely to be found in pellagrins and in malnourished rice-eaters in S.E. Asia. In the first situation they are overshadowed by niacin deficiency and in the second by thiamin or protein deficiency.

Treatment. The therapeutic dose of riboflavin is 5 mg 3 times a day by mouth. It gives the patient's urine a green fluorescence. As discussed above, other B complex vitamins should also be given.

PYRIDOXINE (VITAMIN B₆)

Pyridoxine, pyridoxal and pyridoxamine are three closely related compounds with similar physiological actions. The active form of the vitamin in man is pyridoxal phosphate, the coenzyme for a large number of different enzyme systems involved in the metabolism of the amino acids including aminotransferases. Vitamin B_6 is widely distributed in plants and animal tissues. Liver, whole grain cereals, peanuts and bananas are good sources. The normal adult requirement is 2 mg per day.

Disorders due to vitamin B₆ deficiency

Although a series of pathological changes in the skin, liver, blood vessels, nervous tissue and bone marrow have been produced experimentally in various animals, disorders due to deficiency of vitamin B_6 rarely occur in man, and then very seldom as a result of dietary deficiency.

A minor epidemic of convulsions in infants in the USA in the 1950s was traced to a milk formula which provided little vitamin B_6 because of a manufacturing error. In adults dermatitis, cheilosis, glossitis and angular stomatitis have been produced by means of the pyridoxine inhibitor, 4-desoxy-pyridoxine. The peripheral neuropathy associated with isoniazid therapy is due to a secondary vitamin B_6 deficiency. Certain drugs such as isoniazid and penicillamine, act as chemical antagonists to pyridoxine. Some cases of sideroblastic anaemia respond to treatment with pyridoxine (p. 503).

Biochemical features suggesting vitamin B_6 deficiency can occur in women taking oral contraceptives, and the mild depression which affects a small proportion of such women may be relieved by pyridoxine.

Megavitamin doses of vitamin B_6 (200 mg/day) have been reported to cause a sensory polyneuropathy.

BIOTIN

Biotin functions as coenzyme for several carboxylases. It is present in a number of different foods; the requirement is small (about 100 μg/day) and it can be synthesised by intestinal bacteria. Human deficiency is rare; it has occurred in adults who have taken for long periods large amounts of raw egg-white which contain the antagonist avidin, and an otherwise poor diet. The clinical features include dermatitis and hypercholesterolaemia. A form of seborrhoeic dermatitis of infants responds to biotin.

VITAMIN B₁₂ AND FOLATE

These vitamins and disorders due to their deficiency are discussed on page 504 and page 507.

DIETARY FIBRE

This is the natural packing of plant foods. It can be defined as those parts of foods which are not digested by human enzymes. The principal classes of dietary fibre are cellulose, hemicelluloses, lignins, pectins and gums. These are all polysaccharides (i.e. carbohydrates) except lignin, which occurs with cellulose in the structure of plants. Pectins and gums are viscous, not fibrous.

Some types of dietary fibre, notably the hemicellulose of wheat, increase the water-holding capacity of colonic contents and the bulk of the faeces. They relieve simple constipation, appear to prevent diverticulosis and may reduce the risk of cancer of the colon. Other, viscous indigestible polysaccharides like pectin and guar gum have more effect in the upper gastrointestinal tract. They tend to slow gastric emptying, contribute to satiety, may flatten the glucose tolerance curve and reduce plasma cholesterol concentration.

Dietary fibre is in fact partly digested in the large intestine, by resident bacterial flora, not endogenous enzymes, with flatus formation, and a small quantity of volatile fatty acids is absorbed through the colonic mucosa. There are as yet no official recommended intakes because analyses for the different types of dietary fibre in foods are not complete, but the present average intakes of about 15 to 20 g/day in affluent countries are thought to be too low.

NUTRITION OF PATIENTS IN HOSPITAL

Malnutrition does not occur only in poor children in developing countries. It affects a substantial proportion of seriously ill people in the hospitals of affluent countries. This was fully recognised only after the deficiency diseases in the Third World had been well delineated and approaches established to their management. During the 1970s it was realised that: (1) some degree of malnutrition affects an important minority of patients in hospital; it may be obscured by the primary illness; (2) malnourished patients have a worse prognosis; and (3) with modern technology something can be done to maintain or improve patients' nutrition even when the gastrointestinal tract is not functioning.

Disease leads to nutritional depletion. A few patients are admitted to hospital in a malnourished state but more become nutritionally depleted in hospital. Serious illness, major operations and long stay are all associated with a greater chance of depletion partly because patients may be unable to ingest, digest or absorb their food but also because nutritional requirements and/or losses are increased in a number of diseases.

Factors leading to nutritional depletion include anorexia, unfamiliar food, 'nil per mouth' (because of tests), failure to feed (because of neurological or psychological disease), vomiting, gastrointestinal diseases (e.g. malabsorption), increased protein catabolism (due to trauma, infections or other stress), increased metabolic rate (because of fever), antagonism of certain nutrients by particular drugs and, lastly, losses (from burns, bleeding, discharges, diarrhoea or in urine).

Functional consequences of nutritional depletion. These depend on the degree and type of depletion, but sooner or later malnutrition will have some or even all the following effects: (1) reduced cellular or humoral responses to infections, (2) weakness, reduced ability to cough and susceptibility to bronchopneumonia, (3) impaired healing of wounds (whether traumatic or surgical), (4) surface epithelium atrophic with reduced protective secretions is more easily penetrated by bacteria, (5) bedsores and ulcers, (6) reduced haemopoiesis, (7) reduced ability to metabolise drugs, (8) mental impairment, (9) dehydration and its consequences, (10) specific types of malnutrition, e.g. Wernicke's encephalopathy.

Controlled prospective studies show that patients with features of malnutrition have more postoperative complications, more infections, longer stay in hospital and a higher mortality. In some diseases nutritional support has been demonstrated in controlled trials to improve the outcome significantly, e.g. in inflammatory bowel disease, in burns and in patients with enterocutaneous fistulae. In other conditions clinical trials are insufficient to allow generalisations and it is sensible to assess each patient's status and if this is subnormal, to consider the indications for the different types of nutritional support.

Patients at increased nutritional risk. Before using technical methods to work out a detailed nutritional profile, the first step is to recognise the high-risk patient. A patient in any of the categories below is at increased risk of malnutrition though it may not yet have developed:

1. Severely underweight, weight (for height) below 80% of standard
2. Recent weight loss of 10% or more of usual body weight
3. Alcoholism
4. Malabsorption syndromes
5. Increased metabolic needs: burns, severe infection or trauma or prolonged fever
6. Increased losses, e.g. fistulae, draining wounds, renal dialysis
7. No food by mouth for over a week while receiving simple intravenous infusions
8. Antinutrient or catabolic drugs, e.g. immunosuppressants, adrenocortical steroids, cancer chemotherapy.

Systematic nutritional assessment consists of four components :

1. THE HISTORY. In medical use this is usually qualitative; has the patient been eating too little food, or omitted any major foods? Is an unusual diet being taken? Quantitative nutrient intake first elicits estimates of weights of all foods eaten by one of four methods — dietary history, 24 hour recall, food diary or food frequency. By using food tables (p. 00), usually in computer form, the daily intake of the major nutrients is obtained. These can then be compared against the recommended dietary allowance (RDA), a more detailed version of Table 4.2. An intake just below the RDA shows there is a risk of malnutrition but does not establish it because (1) the days on which food intake was estimated may have been unrepresentative, (2) the physiological requirements between individuals for different nutrients range by a factor of about 2 and the RDAs are set to cover the requirements of nearly all healthy people and (3) for some nutrients, e.g. vitamins A and B_{12}, there are considerable reserves in the body.

2. CLINICAL EXAMINATION. Thinness, oedema, pallor, weakness and other signs described in this chapter may be found, but one should not wait for the classic clinical features of deficiency disease before intervening with nutritional support in a seriously ill patient in hospital. The primary illness may obscure or confuse signs of malnutrition.

3. ANTHROPOMETRY. Changes of body weight reflect the water and/or energy (calorie) balance. If there is no unusual loss of water, each kilogram lost corresponds to 6000 to 7000 kcal of energy (i.e. mostly adipose tissue), unless there is increased protein catabolism when the energy values of weight lost is less. Regular weighing of patients in hospital is valuable in management but it is difficult in paralysed, deformed, and very sick patients, those nursed at strict bed rest, or with splints, fluid lines, catheters and drains. Weighing beds are scarce in most hospitals. The patient should in addition be watched for wasting of both subcutaneous fat and of muscles. If weighing is impractical these observations are more critical. Clinical estimation can be made more objective by measuring mid-arm circumference with a tape. The relative contributions of fat and muscle can be calculated (mid-arm muscle circumference = arm circumference $-\pi \times$ triceps skinfold), but accurate measurement of skinfold thickness requires special calipers.

4. LABORATORY INVESTIGATIONS consist of (1) those that indicate the protein status and (2) biochemical tests for micronutrient deficiencies. Plasma albumin concentration provides the most reliable assessment of protein depletion. Urinary nitrogen (or urea nitrogen) shows the degree of protein catabolism. Reduced total lymphocyte count indicates the possibility of impaired cell-mediated immunity of which protein depletion is one cause. Biochemical tests for vitamins are listed in Table 4.5. As with other tests in chemical pathology there can be both false positives and negatives. Each result needs to be evaluated with critical understanding; for example serum vitamin B_{12} is increased in acute hepatitis and alkaline phosphatase may not be elevated if rickets is accompanied by PEM.

In general when the dietary intake of a nutrient is inadequate (less than obligatory losses) the individual goes through three stages. The first stage is that of adaptation to the low intake. For example, urine excretion falls but there is no

Table 4.5 Biochemical methods for diagnosing vitamin deficiencies.

Nutrient	Principal methods		Supplementary methods
	Indicating reduced intake	Indicating impaired function or cell depletion	
Vitamin A	Plasma carotene		
Thiamin	Urinary thiamin	RBC transketolase and TTP effect	
Riboflavin	Urinary riboflavin	RBC glutathione reductase and FAD effect	RBC riboflavin
Niacin	Urine N'methyl nicotinamide		Fasting plasma tryptophan
Vitamin B$_6$	Urinary 4-pyridoxic acid and/or plasma pyridoxal phosphate	RBC glutamic oxal-acetic transaminase and PP effect	Urinary xanthurenic acid after tryptophan load
Folate	Plasma folate	Red cell folate	Urinary FIGLU after histidine load
Vitamin B$_{12}$	Plasma vitamin B$_{12}$	Reduced vitamin B$_{12}$ or transcobalamin	Schilling test
Vitamin C	Plasma ascorbate	Leucocyte ascorbate	Urinary ascorbate
Vitamin D	Plasma 25-hydroxy-cholecalciferol	Plasma alkaline phosphatase	Plasma 1,25 di OH vitamin D
Vitamin E	Plasma tocopherol	RBC haemolysis with H$_2$O$_2$ in vitro	
Vitamin K	PIVKA II	Plasma prothrombin	

evidence of abnormal function or of depletion of the cells. In the second stage there are in addition biochemical changes indicating either impaired function, e.g. reduced red cell transketolase activity in thiamin deficiency, or cellular depletion, e.g. reduced white cell ascorbic acid. But clinical manifestations of deficiency are absent or non-specific. The third stage is that of clinical deficiency disease.

Most clinical biochemistry laboratories provide only some of the methods as a routine but others could be set up in special circumstances or, alternatively, a laboratory specialising in nutrition research could be asked to help.

Types of nutritional depletion in hospital patients. *Protein-energy malnutrition* is the most important but is not always obvious and tends to be overshadowed by the primary disease. These nutrients cannot be given as capsules or an injection and providing sufficient energy and protein parenterally is expensive.

As in poorly fed children, there are varying degrees of PEM in hospital patients. At one end of the range is *semi-starvation* seen, for example, in anorexia nervosa or obstruction of the oesophagus. There is neither increased catabolism nor increased losses of body protein. There is loss of weight, decrease of arm circumference and skinfolds and normal plasma albumin.

At the other end of the range is *hypoalbuminaemic malnutrition,* which is sometimes called adult kwashiorkor. This form is to be expected in a patient with increased protein catabolism, e.g. after burns or severe trauma, who has been receiving only intravenous glucose and water. This stimulates insulin which causes disproportional loss of visceral protein. Plasma albumin is low, there can be oedema and cell-mediated immunity is impaired so resistance to infection is reduced.

Types of *micronutrient deficiency* in hospitals include:

Folate. Reserves small; proliferative disorders increase requirements.

Vitamin K from biliary obstruction or intestinal antibiotics.

Iron from bleeding.

Vitamin C losses increased by stress; requirements increased for wound healing.

Zinc as for vitamin C.

Vitamin B$_{12}$ destroyed by prolonged nitrous oxide anaesthesia.

Potassium and sodium – see Chapter 5.

Nutritional support. Intake of vitamins and other micronutrients can be boosted by giving these in one or other pharmaceutical preparation, by mouth or by injection. When a multivitamin preparation is given it is important to check that it contains all the major vitamins (e.g. some omit folic acid).

As micronutrients can be provided fairly easily in hospital the main purpose of nutritional support is to get water, calories and protein into the patient. There are four principal routes and more than one can be used together:

1. *Oral feeding.* The ordinary diet can be reinforced with calorie-dense or protein-rich supplements.

2. *Tube (enteral) feeding* is usually given by fine bore plastic nasogastric tubes but sometimes a gastrostomy or jejunostomy is used. Feeding can be continuous or intermittent and there is a wide range of enteral preparations. The 'polymeric' ones are mixtures, for example, of casein, maltodextrin, oils and micronutrients. Chemically-defined, 'monomeric' or 'elemental' preparations (amino acids, glucose, oil and micronutrients) are intended for patients who cannot take whole foods, e.g. for those with inflammatory bowel disease.

3. *Parenteral feeding* by a peripheral vein is easily established and is used for supplementary calorie and/or fluid support. Glucose infusions must be at not more than 10% concentration. Full energy requirements cannot be achieved unless intravenous lipid emulsion is given daily.

4. *Parenteral feeding by central venous alimentation* allows more concentrated glucose infusions (25–35%). Although it is possible to provide all a patient's calorie needs in this way, there are disadvantages to such a high carbohydrate intake such as high insulin levels and essential fatty acid deficiency. It is probably best to give about 30% of energy as intravenous fat emulsion, along with glucose, amino acids and micronutrients. The day's prescription can be made up sterile in the pharmacy in a 3 l bag container.

INDICATIONS. Total enteral nutrition is indicated in patients who cannot eat or drink because of unconsciousness, dysphagia, oesophageal obstruction, head and neck surgery and general weakness. Total parenteral nutrition is life-saving in patients with major disease of the small intestine.

A.S. TRUSWELL

OBESITY

Obesity is the most common nutritional disorder in affluent societies. Its significance requires constant emphasis because it is associated with increased mortality, predisposes to the development of important diseases and diminishes the efficiency and happiness of those affected.

Obesity may be defined as a condition in which there is an excessive amount of body fat. This simple definition gives rise to two questions: how can body fat be measured, and what is 'excessive'?

All methods of measuring the fat content in the living subject are, to a greater or lesser degree, indirect. The simplest, but also the least direct, is the measurement of body weight and this is the method almost exclusively used in clinical practice. In the clinical context the 'desirable' or 'ideal' weight for height (p. 813) is that associated with the lowest mortality in actuarial terms and excessive weight that associated with increased mortality.

Aetiology. Excess fat accumulates because there is imbalance between energy intake and expenditure. This can arise in different ways and obesity is a clinical sign with several possible causes. There is no satisfactory aetiological classification of obesity, but a number of factors are known to be associated with its development.

Age. Obesity is most prevalent in middle-age, but can occur at any stage of life. Obesity in childhood and adolescence is likely to be followed by obesity in adult life.

Socio-economic. In affluent countries obesity is more common in the lower socio-economic groups. In developing countries it can occur only in the prosperous elite. Some occupations predispose to obesity, e.g. cooks and barmen, whilst jockeys, fashion models and airline pilots have to keep themselves slim. In some societies fat men are respected and fat women considered beautiful; in others they are not.

Heredity. A familial tendency exists in many cases, but it is difficult to disentangle environmental and genetic components. Patterns of eating and activity are influenced by social, cultural and economic factors which may be handed on from one generation to another. However, studies involving twins and adopted children indicate the importance of genetic factors in influencing both total body fat and its distribution. There is no evidence in man of obesity produced by a single gene, as in the genetically obese strains of rodents.

Endocrine factors. An endocrine influence on body fat is seen both in normal physiological situations and in pathological states. The normal fat content of young adult women is about twice that of young men and pregnancy is characterised by an increase in body fat. Obesity in women commonly begins at puberty, during pregnancy or at the menopause. Obesity frequently, but not invariably, accompanies hypothyroidism, hypogonadism, hypopituitarism and Cushing's syndrome. However, the overwhelming majority of obese patients show no clinical evidence of an endocrine disorder. The plasma concentration of insulin and cortisol is commonly raised and that of growth hormone reduced in obese subjects, but these changes probably result from, rather than cause the obesity, since they disappear when weight is lost.

Energy balance. A very small excess of calories, if habitual, can lead eventually to a large accumulation of fat. If a person eats a slice (20 g) of bread that is not needed each day or goes by car instead of walking for 20 minutes, the daily extra 48 kcal (200 kJ) will build up over 10 years to 20 kg of fat deposited.

Social factors, such as advertising and business lunches, may contribute to overeating and some people overeat because they are unhappy. There is some evidence that in obese people eating is determined less by 'internal cues', i.e. hunger and satiety, than by external influences like the availability, appearance and taste of food or the environment in which the food is served.

Physical inactivity has an important role in the development of obesity. Affluence is commonly associated with reduced energy expenditure. It is well recognised that physical activity is less in the obese than in the lean, but this may result from, rather than cause, the obesity. Moreover, the amount of energy expended by an obese person on most tasks is likely to be more because of the extra weight to be moved.

Many obese people believe that they do not eat more than their lean counterparts and frequently report an inability to lose weight on a low energy diet. These claims together with the failure of most dietary surveys to demonstrate a significant difference in the daily energy intake of obese and non-obese subjects have led to the hypothesis that in many instances the development of obesity is due to a metabolic defect causing reduced energy expenditure. The recent development of a new non-invasive technique (the doubly labelled water method) in conjunction with whole body calorimetry to measure total energy expenditure has made it possible to study, for the first time, unrestricted living subjects over an extended period. Such studies have shown that not only the basal metabolic rate but also the thermic response to food and the energy cost of activity are identical in lean and obese subjects when corrected for differences in fat-free mass and total body mass. Moreover while self-recorded monitoring of energy intake was accurate for lean subjects, those who were obese consistently under-reported their actual consumption of food. Thus it is clear that relatively mild but significant overeating may remain undetected in surveys employing standard techniques and is probably sufficient to account for the development of obesity without the need to invoke energy sparing mechanisms.

Drugs. The use of steroids, oral contraceptives, phenothiazines and insulin is commonly followed by obesity, mainly because appetite is stimulated.

Clinical features. In most cases the diagnosis will be apparent from the patient's appearance but the degree of obesity should also be assessed, usually by measurement of height and weight and reference to a table such as that on page 813. In addition, the skinfold thickness over the triceps muscle can be measured using special spring-loaded calipers. Obesity is indicated by a reading above 20 mm in a man, and above 28 mm in a woman.

This very common disorder is frequently overlooked because the doctor is preoccupied by one of its many complications or ignores it because it is so familiar.

Obesity must be distinguished from a gain in weight due to fluid retention associated with cardiac, renal or hepatic disease, bearing in mind the fact that oedema does not become manifest clinically until the extracellular fluid has increased by about 15%.

Complications. *Psychological.* Obese patients often have psychological problems, but it is difficult to distinguish between cause and effect. Depressed or anxious patients or the emotionally deprived may seek solace in food. Many obese people, especially younger adult females, are ashamed of their unattractive appearance and develop psychosocial and sexual problems.

Mechanical disabilities. Flat feet and osteo-arthrosis of the knees, hips and lumbar spine are more common in obese people. The abdominal muscles supporting the viscera and the leg muscles, whose contractions promote venous return, are less efficient, predisposing to the development of abdominal and diaphragmatic hernias and varicose veins. Adipose tissue around the trunk interferes with the mechanics of respiration resulting in exertional dyspnoea and increased susceptibility to respiratory infection. Fat people are more likely to suffer from accidents.

Metabolic disorders. Non-insulin dependent diabetes mellitus, hyperlipidaemia (elevation of cholesterol and triglyceride), gallstones, hyperuric-aemia and gout are all more common among the obese than in the general population.

Cardiovascular disorders. Obesity increases the work done by the heart, which enlarges with rising body weight. Cardiac output, stroke volume, and blood volume all increase. Hypertension is common but, in the obese, blood pressure recorded with a standard sphygmomanometer cuff may be higher than direct intra-arterial measurements. The major source of error is failure of the cuff completely to encircle the arm.

The contribution which obesity alone makes to the aetiology of ischaemic heart disease is controversial. There is little doubt that obesity is associated with this disease, but it is difficult to separate the contribution of obesity from that of other risk factors which may be causally associated, such as diabetes, hypertension and hyperlipidaemia, or from that of independent risk factors, such as smoking. Special mention should also be made of physical inactivity, which may be both a cause and an effect of obesity and also plays an important role in the genesis of ischaemic heart disease.

Life expectancy. With all these possible complications it is not surprising that overweight is associated with an increased rate of mortality at all ages. The level of excess mortality varies more or less in proportion to the degree of obesity. Thus subjects 30% overweight incur a 50% increase in mortality.

There is also evidence that a substantial reduction of the body weight of obese people is alone sufficient to diminish the greater death rate. In the Society of Actuaries Build and Blood Pressure Study of 1979, the mortality was reduced to near normal in those who successfully lost and maintained weight within the desirable range. Thus the diagnosis and effective treatment of obesity is literally of vital importance, and recording the patient's weight and height must be just as much a routine part of clinical examination as taking the blood pressure or testing the urine.

Treatment. Whatever the ultimate cause of obesity in the individual case the immediate cause is energy imbalance, and weight reduction can be achieved only by reducing energy intake or by increasing output, or by a combination of the two. This involves change in the individual's way of life. Thus treatment is difficult and the patient needs motivation. Rewards must be seen ahead and psychological understanding and behavioural advice are essential weapons. It is most important for success that patients should be educated and informed about their disorder and misconceptions corrected. There are no 'slimming foods' or 'slimming tablets', which do not depend on a reduced energy intake.

Long-term results are best where patients are well motivated and educated, follow structured diets designed to provide 800 to 1600 kcal daily (p. 809) and are being seen and weighed regularly, every 1 to 2 weeks initially, by the same person. The number of patients requiring supervision is so great, the need for support is so prolonged and the success of some lay organisations such as 'Weight Watchers' compares so favourably with conventional medical methods, that it is justifiable to take advantage of the facilities provided by these groups. Most refer members to their own doctors at the first suggestion of any untoward developments.

However supervision is arranged, it is most important for success that obese patients should be given precise instructions as to how they should reorganise their dietary and other habits, a target weight to aim for and an indication of the rate of weight loss expected.

Among the important lessons to be learned by obese people is the need to manage the disorder themselves. Unlike many conditions for which patients seek help, success does not depend upon operations, drugs, injections or other manipulations undertaken by the therapist but rather on the ability of the patient to accept advice, to act upon it, and to persist indefinitely with some restriction on dietary freedom.

The physician's role is to provide advice and continuing support. Many doctors find obese people unattractive, have difficulty in sympathising with their problems and fail to establish satisfactory rapport with them. Such attitudes contribute to the frequent lack of success in treatment.

THE CONSTRUCTION OF A WEIGHT REDUCING DIET. A weekly weight loss of 0.5 to 1 kg should be the general aim. An obese middle-aged housewife will usually lose weight satisfactorily on a diet providing 800 to 1000 kcal per day, such as the example on page 809. An obese man engaged in active physical work will not tolerate a diet as low as 1000 kcal per day but a satisfactory weight loss can be expected from a diet containing about 1500 kcal per day.

Protein. Dietary protein of 50 g/day is sufficient to maintain nitrogen balance. High protein diets may satisfy appetite more effectively than high carbohydrate diets, but they are expensive, may not be particularly palatable after a time, or may have a high incidental content of fat, and are therefore seldom practicable.

Carbohydrate. Obese people seldom develop more than a trace of ketosis and never sufficient to cause symptoms as long as they consume small amounts of carbohydrate. In a diet of 1000 kcal/day, 100 g of carbohydrate is a suitable allowance and this should be taken as foods providing complex carbohydrates and dietary fibre (such as fruits and vegetables and whole grain cereals) rather than as foods containing glucose and sucrose.

Fat. A 1000 kcal diet containing 100 g of carbohydrate and 50 g of protein, cannot include more than 40–45 g of fat. This allowance of fat, though small, is sufficient to make the diet palatable.

Vitamins. The diet should contain plenty of green vegetables and fruits, since they contain few calories, while their bulk helps to fill the stomach and relieve hunger; they also help to minimise the constipation common with a low food intake. Their vitamin A activity and vitamin C content will be sufficient to meet the body's needs. With meat, fish and eggs and fruit and vegetables in the diet there should be enough of the other vitamins.

Minerals. The only minerals that need serious consideration are calcium and iron. Provided the diet includes 300 ml of skimmed milk, there is little likelihood of a negative calcium balance developing in an adult. The supply of iron is less sure and may call for the prescription of iron supplements.

Fluids and salt. Sweetened 'soft drinks' must be avoided, except those sold for diabetic patients or weight reduction, which have a low caloric content.

The obese are susceptible to water and salt retention but diuretics must be used with care because potassium depletion is particularly liable to occur while patients are on a reducing regimen. Salt restriction alone may be sufficient to alleviate oedema, but if diuretics are considered essential, potassium supplements should be given.

Alcoholic drinks are also a source of calories and hence are best avoided, but if taken, a corresponding reduction in the diet is necessary. A 100 ml glass of dry wine or 30 ml whisky and water provide 70 kcal and half a pint of lager 80 kcal.

General. This diet is suitable for treatment of obese persons in Britain but it may be unsuitable in other circumstances and in other climates. Dietitians with knowledge of local eating customs can devise diets which are socially acceptable and which provide about 1000 kcal made up from about 100 g carbohydrate, 50–60 g protein and 40–45 g fat.

In the absence of oedema or any endocrine disorder, failure to respond to such a diet nearly always indicates non-compliance, despite protestations to the contrary! In such cases, treatment in hospital under strict supervision for 1 to 2 weeks may be beneficial to demonstrate that the prescribed regimen is effective if carefully followed and to allow a period of intensive education.

THERAPEUTIC STARVATION. A period of several weeks of starvation in hospital with only water, non-caloric drinks with vitamin and mineral supplements being allowed, has been recommended for very obese patients who have failed to respond to orthodox treatment.

Although the initial loss of weight may be marked, the long-term results are no more satisfactory than with other systems since many patients regain most of the weight lost when strict measures are discontinued. Such a regimen is contraindicated for older patients, especially if they have cardiovascular complications, since deaths have occasionally occurred. Ketosis may be troublesome in the early stages and hyperuricaemia, sometimes accompanied by gout, can develop.

EXERCISE. Most obese people lead sedentary lives and benefit from physical activity such as walking, swimming and gardening, provided it does not exceed their cardiovascular capacity. Regular daily exercise is much more valuable than episodic activity.

An hour's walk at 3 miles per hour will expend about 240 kcal above basal (or more for a heavy person). This may seem a small amount, equivalent to about 30 g of fat, but if the daily walk becomes a habit it will add up, other things being equal, to a weight loss of 10 kg in a year. Doctors should suggest, discuss and work out with each patient an increasing programme of exercise which is within the physical capacity and which will add to the quality of life of the individual.

DRUG THERAPY. This is no substitute for a dietary regimen but has a limited use as an adjunct in carefully selected patients with refractory obesity. Some of the more effective drugs used in the past, notably amphetamine, are addictive and have been so widely abused that they should not be prescribed for the treatment of obesity.

Amphetamine-like drugs with similar anorectic properties but causing less central nervous stimulation include diethylpropion (75 mg in a single dose daily) and phentermine (15–30 mg before breakfast). They may be given intermittently for periods of about a month to help attain a short-term goal. They should not be used in patients with hypertension or coronary heart disease.

Fenfluramine, which increases release of serotonin in the brain, probably acts by stimulating satiety rather than inducing anorexia. It may cause nausea, diarrhoea, lethargy, breathlessness due to pulmonary hypertension, excessive dreaming and, particularly if withdrawn, depression. It must be given only under careful medical supervision in a dose of 20 mg b.d., gradually increased to a maximum of 120 mg daily, unless adverse effects intervene. Treatment can be continued as long as weight is being lost.

These drugs must not be given to a patient with a history of psychiatric illness.

The administration of thyroxine to euthyroid patients is not only useless but is potentially dangerous, especially if heart disease is present. It should be prescribed only if hypothyroidism coexists with obesity.

FIBRE-RICH PRODUCTS. There is evidence that some foods rich in fibre have an effect on satiety. Methylcellulose is an indigestible substance which adds bulk to the diet. It distends the stomach and so may help to allay hunger. In clinical trials it has been shown to have little if any effect in promoting weight loss.

SURGICAL TREATMENT. Wiring the jaws together to prevent eating has been used to treat those who have found it impossible to adhere to a low-energy diet. Although this usually results in marked loss of weight, many patients regain weight when the procedure is reversed. An alternative and fairly safe operation (though a major one) is to reduce the size of the stomach, for example by stapling, which can be undone. Small intestine bypass, aimed at inducing malabsorption, has been undertaken in some centres for the treatment of severe 'morbid' obesity but complications can be severe and sometimes fatal. It should be emphasised that surgery should be considered only for those with gross intractable obesity.

Prognosis. It is easy for an obese person to lose up to 5 kg in weight. This accounts for the temporary successes of numerous popular 'slimming cures'. How difficult it is to achieve further losses is not generally realised. The published records of seven obesity clinics in the USA showed that satisfactory results ranged only from 12 to 28% if the index of success was the loss of 12 kg or more.

Experience in many clinics has also shown that it is difficult for patients to maintain their reduced weight since this requires some restriction of energy intake on a long-term basis.

Prevention. This must depend in part on the doctor who discerns when patients, be they infants, children or adults, are gaining too much weight. For this purpose alone, among the most useful information that a doctor can keep about patients is a record of body weight, measured at regular intervals. The doctor's responsibility with an overweight patient, at any time, is advisory and educational; the attention of patients must be drawn to the dangers of obesity and to the appropriate methods of correcting it.

All the health agencies available should be mustered to support a steady campaign of education and persuasion of patients and potential patients on the need to avoid obesity. The antenatal services, infant welfare clinics, school health authorities, health visitors and many others to whom the public look for advice should contribute to this educational programme. The media also play an increasingly important role.

JOYCE D. BAIRD
A.S. TRUSWELL

FURTHER READING:

General nutrition
Truswell A S 1986 ABC of nutrition. British Medical Journal. A series of 20 articles that appeared in the BMJ in the second half of 1985.
Passmore R, Eastwood M A 1986 Davidson's Human nutrition and dietetics, 8th edn. Churchill Livingstone, Edinburgh. A well established standard textbook.
Olson R E et al (eds) 1984 Nutrition reviews' present knowledge in nutrition, 5th edn. The Nutrition Foundation, Washington DC. 900 pages of authoritative reviews on each of the nutrients, concentrating on biochemical aspects.
Paul A A, Southgate D A T 1978 McCance & Widdowson's The composition of foods, 4th edn. HMSO, London. British food tables but used in other countries because there is so much data in a single volume.
Silk D B A 1983 Nutritional support in hospital practice. Blackwell Scientific Publications, Oxford.
Cameron M, Hofvander Y 1983 Manual on feeding infants and young children (for application in the developing areas of the world with special reference to home-made weaning foods), 3rd edn. Oxford University Press, Delhi.

Obesity
Garrow J S 1981 Treat obesity seriously. A clinical manual. Churchill Livingstone, Edinburgh. The author has translated his research and clinical practice on obesity into a book with emphasis on management.
Royal College of Physicians 1983 Obesity. Royal College of Physicians, London. A comprehensive report.
Burton B T, Foster W R 1985 Health implications of obesity: an NIH consensus development conference. Journal of the American Dietetics Association 85: 1117–1120.

5

Disturbances in water and electrolyte balance and in hydrogen ion concentration

The chemical events collectively called metabolism require the concentration of hydrogen ions and electrolytes to remain within narrow limits in the tissue cells and in the fluid which bathes them. Derangement of water and electrolyte balance and disturbances in hydrogen ion concentration, $[H^+]$, occur in a wide variety of clinical conditions which are separately described in the appropriate chapters of this book. It is convenient, however, to summarise here the relevant physiological facts and to describe briefly the more common abnormalities.

The kidney plays an important part in maintaining water, electrolyte and acid base balance; the details of the movements of ions that occur in the nephron are given on pages 370 and 371.

NORMAL DISTRIBUTION OF WATER AND ELECTROLYTES

Water. The body of a normal man of 65 kg contains approximately 40 litres of water. About 28 litres of this is intracellular, and 12 litres extracellular. The latter is composed of 9–10 litres of interstitial fluid and 2–3 litres of plasma. Water passes freely through almost all cell membranes and thus moves readily from one body compartment to another, its final distribution being determined by osmotic and hydrostatic forces. Under normal conditions total body water remains remarkably constant despite wide variations of the intake of solute and water.

Electrolytes. The inorganic ions dissolved in the body water include sodium, potassium, calcium, magnesium, chloride, phosphate, bicarbonate and sulphate. These are not dispersed in the same concentrations throughout the various body fluid compartments.

Sodium and chloride are confined mainly to the extracellular fluids where they are present in average concentrations of 142 mmol/l and 100 mmol/l respectively. These ions contribute the major part of the osmotic activity of plasma and extracellular fluids.

Potassium, magnesium, phosphate and sulphate which are present in highest concentration in cells maintain intracellular osmotic activity in a manner analogous to sodium and chloride in the extracellular fluids. In extracellular fluid potassium is present in a mean concentration of only 4.5 mmol/l and magnesium in a concentration of about 1 mmol/l.

Bicarbonate is found in the extracellular fluid and in the tissue cells in concentrations of 25 mmol/l and 10 mmol/l respectively.

Hydrogen ions are present in the extracellular fluids in a concentration of only 40 nmol/l. They are present within cells at a higher concentration. The differences in ionic composition between the cells and the fluid that bathes them are essential to life and are maintained by the activity of ionic pumps within the cell membrane. Despite these differences in ionic pattern, the osmotic activity in health is believed to be identical in intracellular and extracellular fluids.

Because of the permeability of the capillaries, the concentration of electrolytes in the plasma and in the extracellular fluids in the tissue spaces is very similar. Interchange between these extracellular compartments is limited, however, in respect of protein molecules, the concentration of which is many times greater in the plasma than in the interstitial fluid. The volume of the plasma is largely determined by the balance between capillary hydrostatic pressure which tends to force water and electrolytes outwards, and the colloid osmotic pressure of the plasma proteins which draws the water and salts back into the vascular bed.

DISTURBANCES IN WATER AND ELECTROLYTE BALANCE

Changes in the volume and composition of body fluids occur both as a result of disease and as a consequence of treatment. Such disturbances not only contribute to the clinical picture of many diseases, but can themselves hinder recovery or even endanger life. For this reason it is important to maintain the volume and the chemical composition of the body fluids and if necessary to correct any derangements that may arise. Specific disturbances should be recognised and appropriately treated; the non-specific labelling of abnormalities of water and electrolyte balance as 'dehydration' and their indiscriminate treatment with isotonic NaCl solution, i.e. 'normal' saline, is to be deprecated. The more important disturbances of water and electrolyte balance are described below. It is convenient to discuss the disorders separately but in practice two or more often coexist.

Sodium depletion

Normal sodium balance depends upon equality between the amounts of sodium excreted and ingested. In health in temperate climates negligible amounts of sodium are lost in the stools and from the skin. Provided the kidneys are healthy, and the amount of solute excreted in the urine is not very large, renal conservation of sodium is extremely efficient and normal sodium balance can be maintained with a very small daily intake.

Sodium depletion therefore occurs because of excessive loss of salt from the body rather than because of inadequate intake.

Because of the intimate relation of sodium balance to water balance, loss of sodium is usually accompanied by a reduction in the water content of the body. *Pure sodium depletion* unattended by significant water deficit is uncommon and occurs only when there has been abnormal loss of salt and water and fluid loss has been replenished by salt-free liquids. In these circumstances the change in total body water may be negligible in spite of a considerable deficit of body salt. More commonly, however, conditions giving rise to sodium depletion are attended by some degree of water loss and a *mixed depletion* exists, though the sodium loss may predominate.

Causes of sodium depletion. In temperate regions sodium depletion usually arises as a result of excessive loss of sodium in the urine or because of increased loss of sodium-containing fluids from the gastrointestinal tract.

Failure of the kidney to conserve sodium may develop because of intrinsic renal disease or inadequate hormonal control. Examples are found in some patients with chronic pyelonephritis (i.e. 'salt-losing nephritis'), or cystic disease of the kidney, in the diuretic phase of acute renal failure, and sometimes immediately after the relief of obstruction of the urinary tract. It also occurs in Addison's disease. Excessive loss of sodium and water in the urine occurs in the osmotic diuresis of chronic uraemia and uncontrolled diabetes mellitus. If diabetic ketoacidosis develops, urinary sodium loss is further increased because sodium is excreted along with the anions of the ketoacids until the production of renal ammonia increases (p. 372). Sodium depletion may also result from the excessive or prolonged use of diuretics.

Gastrointestinal causes of sodium and water depletion include all conditions involving external loss of sodium-containing fluids, i.e. acute or chronic diarrhoea, intestinal fistulae, aspiration of gastrointestinal contents and vomiting. Considerable losses of sodium and water also occur if gastrointestinal secretions are sequestered in dilated loops of intestine as in ileus or in the peritoneal cavity in ascites or peritonitis.

Sweating is a well-known cause of sodium

depletion in tropical countries and often aggravates the degree of sodium depletion caused by disease (p. 723). Loss of sodium and water from the skin also occurs in extensive burns, severe generalised dermatitis and cystic fibrosis.

Consequences of sodium depletion. As sodium is mainly extracellular, depletion reduces the volume of the extracellular fluids. When proportionately more sodium than water is lost, the extracellular fluids become hypotonic and the plasma sodium concentration falls. This trend is mitigated by two events, (1) initially secretion of antidiuretic hormone (ADH) is inhibited and the proportion of water relative to solute excreted in the urine is increased, and (2) some extracellular water migrates into the cells. As a result there is a further diminution in the volume of extracellular fluid, including plasma, while the water content of the cells may increase.

The fact that sodium depletion chiefly affects the volume of the extracellular fluid is responsible for many of the clinical features such as loss of elasticity of the skin, diminution of intra-ocular pressure and dryness of the tongue. Thirst is not a prominent complaint, and its absence may be due to the hypotonicity of the body fluids. With progressive reduction of blood volume there is a reduction in cardiac output and a fall in blood pressure. The pulse rate rises. Glomerular filtration falls and oliguria occurs; the capacity to excrete urea diminishes and uraemia develops. Selective vasoconstriction diminishes the circulation through the skin so that the extremities become pale and cold. Although the plasma sodium concentration may be within normal limits, it may be reduced to 120 mmol/l or less in severe cases or in those in whom the deficit of water has been partly made good; in such patients muscle cramps are common.

Treatment. Administration of water or of glucose in water in conditions associated with sodium depletion is dangerous because the hypotonicity may be further aggravated. Moreover, much of the administered water passes into cells and initially the kidneys respond by excreting dilute urine in an attempt to restore extracellular tonicity; thus the extracellular fluid volume remains low. The ill-effects of such treatment are all too easily obscured by the conventional fluid balance chart which records only fluid intake and urine output, without reference to sodium balance.

Adequate treatment consists of giving salt and water by mouth or an isotonic NaCl solution intravenously. The latter is required in all but mild cases with normal recumbent blood pressure. In adults with moderately severe depletion 2–4 litres of isotonic NaCl solution intravenously in 6–12 hours represents the usual requirements.

In severe cases with marked circulatory impairment, deficits equivalent to 4–8 litres of isotonic NaCl solution occur. Such deficits should be corrected largely by isotonic sodium chloride solution but when acidosis is present some of the sodium may be given as isotonic $NaHCO_3$ (p. 97). The first 2–3 litres should be given rapidly within the first 2–3 hours and the remainder within 24–48 hours.

The best guides to the amount required are the disappearance of the signs of extracellular fluid depletion and the restoration of normal blood pressure and pulse rate. Plasma sodium determinations are useful in controlling the treatment of severe cases, especially when the causative disease is likely to lead to a continued salt loss, (e.g. severe and persisting diarrhoea), and in regulating the relative amounts of sodium and water to be given. Excessive administration of sodium salts is to be avoided; the bases of the lungs should be frequently examined for crepitations, and the jugular venous pressure assessed. In severe cases it is often helpful to monitor the right atrial (central venous) pressure or the pulmonary capillary (wedge) pressure.

Severe sodium and water depletion is commonly associated with disturbances in acid-base balance. Frequently potassium balance, and occasionally magnesium metabolism, are also disturbed. In these circumstances appropriate amounts of other electrolytes need to be added to the intravenous fluid once the circulation has been restored (p. 145).

Primary water depletion

Pure or predominant water depletion is one of the simplest of chemical disorders. The water content of the body is reduced both absolutely and relative to the sodium content, and the osmolal concentration of the extracellular fluids rises.

In a temperate climate an adult loses between 0.5–1 litre of water daily in the expired air and by evaporation from the skin. This loss continues irrespective of the water intake. The urine is the other main channel of excretion of water but the volume of urine can be reduced if water is in short supply by increasing its concentration up to a limit determined by renal concentrating ability and the amount of solute to be excreted.

Causes of water depletion. Primary water depletion occurs less commonly in clinical practice than sodium depletion and usually arises because water intake is reduced below an amount necessary to maintain balance.

Water deficiency is liable to occur in patients who suffer from dysphagia or have obstructive lesions of the oesophagus or in those who are comatose, depressed or apathetic, as is common for example in the aged. It then occurs because the intake falls below the amount being lost from the lungs, skin and urine. This obligatory daily loss of water from the lungs and skin is increased by hyperpnoea, hyperthyroidism and in fever.

Excessive loss of water in the urine is a less common cause of water depletion but occurs in patients in whom the renal power of concentration is markedly restricted, as for example in diabetes insipidus, hyperparathyroidism or certain uncommon renal tubular lesions.

Water deficiency may be induced by giving patients liquid feeds containing large amounts of protein or salt mixed with insufficient water. Newborn infants are especially susceptible to this danger as their power to concentrate the urine is not fully developed.

Consequences of water depletion. As water is lost from the body the extracellular fluid becomes hypertonic and the concentration of plasma sodium rises. Water then migrates from the cells until osmotic equilibrium is re-established and intracellular dehydration occurs. The overall body water loss is thus shared by the extracellular and intracellular fluids. For this reason the circulatory signs of dehydration are not so obvious as those of salt depletion.

Thirst is usual unless the patient is senile or confused. The migration of water from the cells to the extracellular fluids mitigates the reduction of the volume of the extracellular fluid so that the blood pressure, haemoglobin, and plasma electrolyte concentrations change little until considerable depletion has occurred. The patient, however, may exhibit mental confusion or complain of vertigo and have difficulty in swallowing. In severe cases the skin and tissues acquire a curious 'doughy' consistency and there is marked muscle weakness possibly due to loss of potassium from dehydrated cells. When the kidneys are healthy a small amount of highly concentrated urine is passed. Ultimately renal blood flow is reduced and the blood urea concentration rises. By this stage the plasma sodium concentration and the haemoglobin concentration are elevated.

Treatment. Water depletion can often be prevented if the need to maintain an adequate intake is recognised in patients who are unable to swallow or who do not drink enough of their own accord.

Established depletion should be treated by giving salt-free fluids. The use of isotonic NaCl solution is contraindicated. If the patient is conscious and is not vomiting, water should be given by mouth until thirst is quenched and thereafter amounts of between 1.2 to 2.5 litres per day are usually sufficient. If the patient is unable to swallow fluids in sufficient amounts, 5% glucose in water should be given by intravenous infusion.

The amount required varies with the degree of depletion. In moderately severe cases 2–4 litres of 5% glucose in the course of 24 hours is usually sufficient. In severe water depletion 5–10 litres may be needed and such a deficit should be replaced over 2–3 days to avoid sudden shift of water into cells which can cause severe disturbances of cerebral function. The best guides to the amount of fluid required are the clinical improvement of the patient and the increase in the volume of urine, which should rise to at least 1.5 litres per 24 hours.

When water depletion coexists with sodium loss, isotonic NaCl solution and water are both required and should both be given in amounts determined by clinical assessment of the relative degrees of the two deficiencies.

Potassium depletion

Maintenance of potassium balance depends largely on the regulation of urinary excretion of this ion, since in health over 85% of the daily potassium intake is excreted in the urine and the remainder in the stools. The extracellular fluid contains less than 2% of body potassium at a concentration of 3.5–5 mmol/l. Most of the remainder is in cells where a concentration of between 140 and 150 mmol/l is maintained by the operation of active transport mechanisms including the sodium/potassium pump. The large concentration gradient across the cell membrane is the primary determinant of the resting membrane potential and small changes in the ratio result in severe disturbances of neuromuscular function. Cellular uptake of potassium is enhanced by insulin, adrenaline and aldosterone and influenced by the blood $[H^+]$ and plasma tonicity. In health both total body potassium and the distribution of the ion between cells and extracellular fluid are closely regulated.

Causes of potassium depletion. Potassium depletion usually occurs as a result of excessive loss of potassium from the gastrointestinal tract or in the urine. Alimentary losses occur as a result of severe acute or chronic diarrhoea, vomiting, fistulous drainage or gastric aspiration. The habitual use of laxatives which is sometimes a factor is easily missed and a potassium secreting villous adenoma of the large bowel is an important but uncommon cause. In the malabsorption syndrome excessive potassium loss can occur even when the stools are well formed.

Renal wastage of potassium is more complex. Since most filtered potassium is reabsorbed in the upper nephron, urinary potassium is largely determined by the rate at which the ion enters the tubular fluid in the distal nephron into which it diffuses passively down a luminal negative, transepithelial, electrochemical gradient. The magnitude of this gradient increases (1) when the intracellular concentration of potassium rises, (2) when the rate of flow through the distal nephron increases, (3) when the rate of reabsorption of sodium in the distal tubule increases and (4) when poorly reabsorbed anions are present in excess in the distal tubules. In most cases in which renal wastage of potassium occurs, one or more of these factors augment diffusion of potassium into the urine. The clinical conditions in which these factors operate are considered in two categories,

extrarenal and renal.

1. Disorders in which extrarenal factors increase the rate of potassium excretion. In primary aldosteronism, Cushing's syndrome and in patients receiving corticosteroids the uptake of potassium into distal tubular cells, the intracellular potassium concentration and the permeability of the luminal membrane to this ion are increased; this encourages the diffusion of potassium into the tubular lumen. A similar mechanism probably operates in secondary aldosteronism occurring in the course of heart failure, liver disease, the nephrotic syndrome or renovascular hypertension.

In metabolic or respiratory alkalosis (p. 98) loss of potassium in the urine is due mainly to its increased concentration in the tubular cells. This loss is further augmented by the presence of poorly reabsorbed, negatively charged bicarbonate ions in distal tubular fluid. Cell potassium is reduced in acidosis but paradoxically in long-standing metabolic acidosis, urinary potassium is often increased because of an accompanying increase in the delivery of sodium and water to the distal nephron. Diuretics and osmotically active substances such as mannitol and glucose, which increase delivery of sodium and water to the distal nephron, also facilitate potassium loss by this means.

In diabetic ketoacidosis the delivery of both poorly reabsorbable anions of ketoacids and increased amounts of sodium and water to the distal tubule result in loss of potassium in the urine.

2. Renal diseases in which the rate of potassium excretion is increased. Occasionally potassium is lost in the urine as a result of a primary renal disease. Thus, renal potassium wastage occurs in renal tubular acidosis, probably because of a change in the potassium permeability of the luminal membrane of the distal tubular cells and because of the alkaline urine. Loss of potassium also occurs in the recovery phase of acute tubular necrosis and after relief of severe urinary tract obstruction.

Circumstances which encourage transfer of potassium from the cells to the extracellular fluid lead to increased urinary loss and ultimately to potassium depletion. These include lack of insulin, severe water depletion, shock, hypoxia and metabolic or respiratory acidosis in which buffering of H^+ in cells leads to loss of potassium ions from them.

Many elderly people who take a diet inadequate in potassium become mildly potassium-depleted. The precise mechanism is unknown but it is most likely due to inappropriate urinary loss.

Consequences and clinical features of potassium depletion. In the presence of severe extracellular fluid depletion or of any factor which reduces cell uptake of potassium, clinically significant potassium depletion occurs without a change in the plasma concentration of this ion. This is often seen in patients with untreated diabetic ketoacidosis. Conversely administration of insulin or beta-adrenergic agonists which stimulate uptake of potassium by cells may cause hypokalaemia despite a normal total body potassium. The plasma potassium often falls following the start of treatment of patients with severe megaloblastic anaemia due to vitamin B_{12} deficiency as potassium is taken up by newly-formed red cells. Mild metabolic alkalosis may accompany potassium depletion (p. 98).

The most important features of potassium depletion are due to changes in electrical potential difference across cell membranes. Deficits of less than 300 mmol potassium give rise to few, if any, clinical features. Larger deficits are associated with progressive development of generalised weakness of skeletal muscle, depression of tendon reflexes and paresis or flaccid paralysis. Reduction of intestinal motility results in constipation, abdominal distension and eventual ileus. The ECG commonly shows a small T wave and ST depression. Potassium depletion may induce cardiac arrhythmias such as atrial tachycardia; it also increases susceptibility to intoxication with digitalis. Severe potassium depletion lowers the cardiac output. Paraesthesiae are frequently present and there is often apathy and loss of memory which may progress to disorientation and confusion. Severe chronic potassium deficiency is associated with polyuria and thirst due to inability of the kidney to concentrate urine. Death may occur from respiratory paralysis or cardiac arrest if potassium depletion is unrelieved or treatment is inadequate.

Treatment. Potassium depletion should be treated by giving a potassium salt orally or intravenously. The former route is more commonly used and carries less risk of inducing hyperkalaemia than parenteral administration. The normal daily intake of potassium is about 2–3 g (50–80 mmol).

1. Established deficiencies of moderate severity (about 400 mmol) can be remedied by giving 10–15 g/day (134–201 mmol) of potassium chloride, in divided doses, for some days and a diet rich in potassium, i.e. containing fruit juices, coffee, milk based food and meat.

Potassium chloride tablets sometimes cause gastrointestinal ulceration especially if there is delay in intestinal transit. 'Slow release' tablets of potassium chloride are less troublesome in this respect; each tablet contains 600 mg (8 mmol) of KCl. Some patients tolerate effervescent potassium tablets more readily as these appear to be less nauseating. Each tablet contains 250 mg (6.4 mmol) of potassium and some also contain chloride. The latter is useful in correcting the metabolic alkalosis which is associated with potassium depletion and which is frequently due to concurrent chloride depletion (p. 98).

2. Intravenous infusions of potassium chloride are needed for patients who are unable to take potassium by mouth, but should be given only when hypokalaemia is established by chemical analysis. Such infusions should rarely be used in the presence of significant sodium depletion, anuria or oliguria and only when facilities for repeated chemical analysis are available. Associated water and salt depletion should be treated first.

For intravenous administration, potassium chloride (1.5 g in sterile ampoules) can be conveniently added to 500 ml of isotonic NaCl or 5% glucose solution. The solution then contains 40 mmol/l and should be given slowly over 2 to 3 hours. Repeated measurements of the plasma potassium are necessary to determine whether further infusions are required.

Administration of potassium by mouth should be started as soon as possible, as most of the deficit is best corrected by this means. When the depletion of potassium has arisen because of persistent vomiting and is associated with alkalosis due to loss of gastric hydrochloric acid, potassium is sometimes given with sodium and ammonium chloride as described on page 99.

Prophylactic administration of potassium chloride (3–4 g daily) or effervescent potassium tablets should be given to patients who are being treated by drugs known to increase urinary loss of potassium. These include corticosteroids and many diuretics.

Potassium excess

Causes. When the ability to excrete potassium in the urine is impaired, hyperkalaemia may develop, particularly if large amounts of potassium are released from cells or if the intake of the ion is unrestricted. It is therefore common in severe circulatory failure and in established acute renal failure. The plasma potassium is often high in severe untreated diabetic ketoacidosis despite an overall deficit of the ion. Lack of insulin, metabolic acidosis and increased extracellular fluid tonicity all reduce cellular uptake of potassium and contraction of the volume of the extracellular fluid exacerbates matters. Some patients with severe chronic renal failure develop hyperkalaemia especially if potassium supplements, spironolactone or potassium-conserving diuretics are given. Since aldosterone stimulates distal tubular secretion of potassium, any interference with the function of the renin-angiotensin-aldosterone axis can cause hyperkalaemia—a fact which has been recognised for many years in patients with adrenal insufficiency. Drugs, such as captopril, the prostaglandin inhibitors and beta-blockers, which interfere with normal operation of the renin-aldosterone axis can cause hyperkalaemia in patients with reduced renal function. Release of renin is impaired in some chronic renal diseases, notably interstitial nephritis and diabetic glomerulosclerosis, and patients with these disorders may have hyperkalaemia at a time when their overall renal function is still moderately good.

Consequences of potassium excess. Patients with hyperkalaemia develop muscular weakness which may progress to flaccid paralysis with loss of tendon reflexes. Abdominal distension due to ileus also occurs. In addition tingling of the face, hands and feet is common. These features are indistinguishable from those of severe hypokalaemia.

Cardiac disturbances are often the first and only manifestation of hyperkalaemia. The pulse becomes irregular and heart block of variable degree occurs. Typical electrocardiographic changes include increase in the amplitude of the T wave, atrioventricular and intraventricular conduction defects and ultimately ventricular fibrillation or asystole.

Hyperkalaemia is of considerable clinical importance because of the danger of cardiac arrest with concentrations of plasma potassium above 7.5 mmol/l. The diagnosis is made more frequently by knowing the circumstances in which intoxication is likely to arise and confirming the suspicion by measuring plasma potassium than from any specific clinical feature.

Treatment. It is important to prevent the occurrence of potassium intoxication in conditions associated with oliguria and anuria. The recommendations made about diet in acute renal failure have this aim in view (p. 405). When dealing with an established case of hyperkalaemia, the following measures are advised:

1. Identify and, if possible, remove the cause.

2. Migration of potassium into cells should be encouraged by giving glucose and insulin and alkali. 5 to 10 units of soluble insulin and 50 ml of a 50% solution of glucose should be given intravenously and repeated if hyperkalaemia recurs. Alternatively 20% glucose solution containing 6–12 units of insulin is infused slowly over 6–12 hours. Provided there is no evidence of circulatory overload, isotonic sodium bicarbonate solution should be infused slowly until the plasma bicarbonate is in the upper reference range.

3. When severe electrocardiographic changes are present, 10 ml of 10% calcium gluconate should be injected slowly intravenously to reduce the cardiotoxic effects of the potassium ion. The ECG is monitored throughout the procedure.

4. Any deficit of sodium or water should be replaced in order to restore normal circulation. Metabolic and respiratory acidosis should be corrected (pp. 96 and 99).

Measures to prevent recurrence of hyperkalaemia include (1) dietary restriction of foods rich in potassium, and (2) administration of sodium or calcium loaded resins which adsorb potassium in the intestine. 30 g suspended in a small volume of water is given by mouth or by retention enema as required, usually 3 or 4 times a day.

If these methods fail or if the rise of concentration of potassium is rapid, removal of potassium by peritoneal dialysis or by haemodialysis is indicated.

Magnesium deficiency and excess

Disorders of magnesium metabolism are occasionally responsible for otherwise puzzling clinical features and are susceptible to therapeutic control.

Magnesium deficiency is most commonly due to prolonged acute diarrhoea, vomiting or aspiration of gastrointestinal secretions which has been treated with parenteral fluid without magnesium supplements. It is also associated with chronic diarrhoea and severe undernutrition, such as occurs in protein-energy malnutrition and the malabsorption syndrome. Uncontrolled diabetes mellitus, aldosteronism, hyperparathyroidism, the diuretic phase of acute renal failure and chronic alcoholism lead to magnesium deficiency from excessive urinary loss. It occasionally follows long continued treatment with loop diuretics or occurs after relief of acute obstruction of the urinary tract.

Clinical features are predominantly neuromuscular, with tremor and choreiform movements. Depression, confusion, agitation, epileptic fits and hallucinations also occur. The diagnosis can be confirmed by finding the concentration of magnesium in the plasma to be less than 0.75 mmol/l.

Magnesium deficiency is best treated parenterally; 30–50 mmol of magnesium chloride may be added to 1 litre of 5% glucose or other isotonic solution and given over a period of 12 to 24 hours. Thereafter 15–25 mmol of magnesium chloride should be infused daily until the plasma concentration remains within the normal range. When renal function is impaired the amount of magnesium chloride must be reduced by half.

Magnesium excess mainly occurs in acute and chronic renal disease and contributes to the central nervous features associated with uraemia. Its treatment is that of the primary disorder.

Water excess

Healthy individuals can safely drink very large volumes of water and respond to this by a vigorous water diuresis. The capacity of the kidney to excrete water without electrolytes (solute-free water) depends upon a number of physiological processes: (1) Sufficient solute must be delivered to the ascending limb and early distal convoluted tubule where urinary dilution occurs. This is determined by the glomerular filtration rate and the fractional reabsorption of solute and water in the proximal tubule. (2) The capacity to reabsorb sodium and chloride without water at the diluting sites must be unimpaired. (3) There must be an absence of ADH and ADH-like substances and the nephron distal to the diluting sites must be largely impermeable to water. Many patients who are ill have a restricted ability to dilute the urine because of disturbance of one or more of these processes, e.g. in acute and chronic renal disease, severe heart failure, hypopituitarism, adrenocortical insufficiency, severe hypothyroidism and hepatic cirrhosis or liver failure.

A variety of malignant tumours, including carcinoma of the lung (p. 253) and lymphoma may secrete a polypeptide with antidiuretic properties which induces water intoxication. Continued *inappropriate secretion of ADH* from the posterior pituitary in the absence of osmotic or haemodynamic stimuli may occur in head injury, cerebral tumours, meningitis and encephalitis and in some pulmonary diseases, notably tuberculosis and severe pneumonias. Postoperative patients are incapable of water diuresis because of liberation of ADH by the pain and stress of operation. In addition a number of drugs induce release of pituitary vasopressin and can thus cause water intoxication. These include morphine, phenothiazines, tricyclic antidepressants, vincristine and cyclophosphamide. Chlorpropamide and many non-steroidal anti-inflammatory agents exert a similar effect by enhancing the action of ADH on the distal nephron. Urinary dilution is impaired by frusemide and bumetanide which inhibit sodium chloride resorption in the ascending limb and by the thiazide diuretics which have a similar effect on the cortical diluting segment.

In all these circumstances even a modest water intake reduces the plasma osmolality and the concentration of sodium and produces symptoms which are primarily those of disordered cerebral function; these are partly due to cerebral oedema and include dizziness, headache, nausea and mental confusion. Severe water intoxication can produce convulsions, coma and death. Diagnosis depends upon being aware of the circumstances in which water intoxication is likely to occur and the demonstration of a plasma sodium concentration below 130 mmol/l. The urinary osmolality, which in these circumstances should be less than 100 mOsm/kg, is inappropriately high.

Treatment consists of dealing with the underlying cause and meanwhile restricting water intake. In severe cases 100 ml 5% sodium chloride solution should be given intravenously and repeated in a few hours if there is little or no clinical improvement. Patients who have irremediable tumours producing ADH or ADH-like peptide are sometimes treated with demeclocycline, a tetracycline derivative which inhibits the action of the ADH on the collecting duct. The drug is nephrotoxic and its use is best confined to such patients. Alternatively in these cases the plasma sodium concentration may be kept within the reference range by increasing the daily intake of sodium to about 200 mmol and giving frusemide, 40 mg per day, by mouth.

Sodium and water excess

In health, the total amount of sodium in the body is kept within narrow limits in spite of great day-to-day variations in the amount ingested. Positive sodium balance with consequent accumulation of sodium results when renal excretion fails to keep pace with the amount ingested. Sodium accumulation is accompanied by retention of water so that the concentration of sodium in the extracellular space is usually not materially altered. When the distribution of the retained fluid is generalised, the expansion in the volume of the extracellular space does not become clinically detectable until the increase is of the order of 15%.

The disturbances which initiate the accumulation of water and salt which lead to oedema, vary with the nature of the disease and are discussed in the appropriate sections of this book. They include (1) a reduction in the colloid osmotic pressure from hypoproteinaemia as occurs in the nephrotic syndrome; (2) an increase in venous hydrostatic pressure as in heart failure and (3) primary inability to eliminate salt and water in the urine as in acute glomerulonephritis. In addition several compensatory reactions occur which promote further retention of water and salt. These include an increased secretion of aldosterone mediated by the renin-angiotensin system and a rise in the level of circulating ADH.

The therapeutic use of corticosteroids, androgens or oral contraceptives with a high oestrogen content may also give rise to sodium and water retention by virtue of their action on the kidney. Other drugs which do so include carbenoxolone vasodilators and non-steroidal anti-inflammatory agents.

Some oedema is not uncommon in normal women during the premenstrual stage of the menstrual cycle. Oedema is commonly present in normal pregnancy but is more severe and is associated with proteinuria when renal disease or pregnancy hypertension is present. Other disorders associated with generalised oedema include nutritional oedema and thiamin deficiency. In some diseases several mechanisms appear to be operating simultaneously. This is exemplified particularly in the oedema and ascites of hepatic cirrhosis in which portal hypertension, hypoproteinaemia and possibly salt retaining and antidiuretic hormones all contribute.

The clinical features of water and salt accumulation depend to some extent upon the distribution of the retained fluid. These are described under the various diseases.

Principles of treatment. These are:

1. The use of measures designed to remedy specific factors leading to the oedema, e.g. digitalis and vasodilators in heart failure, corticosteroids in some forms of glomerulonephritis, intravenous administration of plasma proteins or salt-free albumin in conditions associated with hypoproteinaemia, and a high protein diet in oedema of nutritional origin, hepatic cirrhosis and the

nephrotic syndrome.

2. The restriction by dietary means of the raw materials necessary for the formation of extracellular fluid, i.e. sodium and water.

3. Increasing the excretion of sodium and water by the use of effective diuretics.

Diuretic therapy. Drugs which block reabsorption of sodium by the renal tubules also increase the urinary volume because reabsorption of water in the nephron is a passive process dependent on sodium reabsorption. The following are the most important diuretics discussed in order of their potency.

HIGH POTENCY DIURETICS (LOOP DIURETICS). The diuresis induced by these agents, which include frusemide and bumetanide, is rapid, intense and of short duration. They reduce reabsorption of sodium and chloride in the ascending limb of Henle's loop and since the most distal segment has a large capacity to reabsorb sodium chloride they induce a larger diuresis than drugs acting at other sites. Because they deliver an increased amount of sodium and water to the distal tubule they increase potassium loss in the urine. *Frusemide* may be given orally (40–80 mg) or i.v. (20–40 mg). On a weight basis *bumetanide* is more potent than frusemide, comparable oral doses being 1–2 mg, but is otherwise similar in action. These drugs are of great value in the treatment of generalised oedema and severe pulmonary oedema. They have few adverse effects but occasionally a precipitate diuresis may cause postural hypotension or acute retention of urine may develop in elderly men with prostatic enlargement. Their continued use in susceptible subjects may lead to a rise in blood sugar or plasma urate with the possible development of diabetes mellitus or an attack of gout. When frusemide is given in large doses to patients with impaired renal function (p. 412) it occasionally causes transient or permanent hearing loss. Large doses of bumetanide may cause severe myalgia in patients with renal failure. Adverse effects on electrolytes are discussed below.

MEDIUM POTENCY DIURETICS. Thiazide (benzothiadiazine) diuretics have a variable influence on the activity of carbonic anhydrase and so upon sodium bicarbonate reabsorption in the proximal tubules but their main action is to depress reabsorption of sodium and chloride in the early distal convoluted tubule. Potassium depletion results from reduced H^+ secretion and increased delivery of sodium and water to the distal tubules. Chlorthiazide was the prototype drug but those most commonly used now are *bendrofluazide* (10 mg) and *hydrochorothiazide* (100 mg). *Chlorthalidone* (100–200 mg) is similar in action but produces a slower and more prolonged diuresis extending over 48 hours. Adverse effects include impotence, postural hypertension, allergic rashes and rarely marrow depression. Hyperuricaemia and diabetes may be produced in susceptible patients. Adverse effects on electrolytes are discussed below.

LOW POTENCY DIURETICS. These agents are not sufficiently potent by themselves but, because of other properties, are sometimes valuable when combined with more potent diuretics. *Spironolactone* (100–400 mg daily) is a specific aldosterone antagonist and reverses the renal effects of this hormone. Its important clinical effect is reduction of the capacity of the kidney to excrete potassium. This it shares with other low potency diuretics.

Amiloride (20 mg) and triamterene (200 mg) are non-steroidal diuretics which reduce reabsorption of sodium in the collecting tubules by directly inhibiting sodium transport across the luminal membrane. They thereby induce a small sodium diuresis and by reducing the transepithelial P.D. inhibit potassium secretion. They are not aldosterone antagonists and are effective when the circulating aldosterone levels are low. Rarely triamterene has been shown to cause interstitial nephritis and to induce formation of calculi containing the drug. When given with indomethacin it may cause acute renal failure, therefore the combination of these drugs should be avoided. None of the low potency diuretics should be given in the presence of renal failure or with potassium supplements lest dangerous hyperkalaemia develop.

ADVERSE EFFECTS OF DIURETIC THERAPY ON ELECTROLYTES. *Potassium depletion*. High and medium potency diuretics produce potassium depletion, especially when given repeatedly over long periods and when combined with diets low in sodium. Symptoms of potassium deficit may arise before satisfactory loss of oedema has been achieved and are then superimposed upon the clinical features of water and sodium accumulation. This state of affairs is especially prone to develop in the treatment of severe cardiac failure (p. 152) and is particularly serious since it may be responsible for increased sensitivity to digitalis, with development of toxic manifestations to this drug before control of the heart failure has been attained.

In hepatic disease with oedema and ascites potassium depletion may seriously aggravate or precipitate the neurological features of hepatic insufficiency. Prophylactic administration of potassium is therefore essential when diuretics are being given frequently, e.g. on alternate days. Between 3 and 4 g potassium chloride is required daily given either as slow release or effervescent tablets.

Sodium depletion and oligaemia. Overtreatment with diuretics is likely to occur when high potency diuretics are given over prolonged periods without adequate supervision. These patients exhibit the features of sodium depletion although paradoxically some, in whom the plasma albumin is low, may still be oedematous.

The circulatory characteristics of sodium depletion, due to oligaemia, are present, namely hypotension with an increase in the pulse rate. The blood urea is increased and the plasma sodium may be reduced to 130 mmol/l or less. Such patients usually suffer from advanced cardiac or hepatic disease associated with hypoproteinaemia. In these circumstances persistent attempts to reduce the oedema lead to further deterioration. Relief may sometimes be achieved by infusion of 25–100 g plasma protein fraction to increase the blood volume. Diuretics should be withheld temporarily and a diet unrestricted in its salt content permitted.

Hyponatraemia. In cardiac and hepatic diseases associated with severe oedema hyponatraemia sometimes develops without oligaemia. This is due to inability to excrete water normally because of poor renal perfusion and increased circulating ADH. It is exacerbated by thiazide diuretics. In these circumstances the water intake should be restricted to a volume equal to, or less than, the output and a loop diuretic substituted. Occasionally, when symptoms of water intoxication are present and the plasma sodium is less than 125 mmol/l, slow infusion of 100–200 ml of 5% saline may be needed to relieve symptoms.

DIAGNOSIS OF DISTURBANCES IN WATER AND ELECTROLYTE BALANCE

It is apparent from this summary of the principal disorders of water and electrolyte balance that these disturbances present considerable diagnostic difficulty and are not characterised by pathognomonic signs or symptoms. The neuromuscular abnormalities of potassium depletion are clinically indistinguishable from those of hyperkalaemia; severe sodium depletion is attended by considerable water deficit and is not readily distinguishable on clinical grounds from severe degrees of pure water deficit. Furthermore, it is common for multiple electrolyte deficits to develop simultaneously. For example, in diabetic ketoacidosis, potassium and magnesium depletion may occur in conjunction with sodium and water depletion. In addition the symptoms of lethargy, apathy and mental confusion which are common accompaniments of major electrolyte disorders occur in many diseases in which no significant body fluid disturbance exists. Moreover, the results obtained from biochemical analysis of blood and urine are of limited diagnostic value. Potassium or magnesium deficit may occur without significant change in their plasma concentrations, and serious sodium depletion commonly develops with plasma sodium concentrations within the reference range. A low plasma sodium may not even indicate salt depletion since hyponatraemia is seen in conditions of water excess.

The measurement of electrolytes in the urine without knowledge of the dietary intake is also obviously of limited value. In the majority of conditions in which there is a reduced blood or ECF volume the urinary loss of sodium is less than 10–20 mmol/day and the presence of larger amounts in the urine of patients who are volume-depleted strongly suggests a renal salt wasting disorder. Urinary potassium determination is also of limited value but is sometimes helpful in patients who are found unexpectedly to have hypokalaemia. Then the finding of a urinary K^+ of more than 20 mmol/day indicates that the kidney is responsible unless extrarenal losses are of recent and sudden onset. In contrast the finding of a urinary K^+ of < 10 mmol/l in the presence of hypokalaemia indicates that the route of the loss is extrarenal and is usually gastrointestinal.

Accurate diagnosis largely depends upon a careful history and knowledge of the conditions and diseases which may give rise to abnormalities in water and electrolyte balance. In patients with such diseases, the suspicion that these abnormalities may exist is strengthened by the presence of the clinical features known to occur with them and possibly by the results of appropriate biochemical and electrocardiographic examinations.

By understanding the mechanism by which the economy of the fluids of the body becomes disturbed and by the intelligent use of the reparative fluids which have been described, much can be done to restore the distortions of body fluid balance wrought by disease.

HYDROGEN ION CONCENTRATION

Life is possible only if the hydrogen ion concentration, $[H^+]$, of body fluids is kept within a narrow range. In health a blood $[H^+]$ of 36–44 nmol/l (pH 7.37–7.45) is maintained by several closely integrated but widely differing mechanisms. Some understanding of these mechanisms is necessary to appreciate the clinical implications of acidosis and alkalosis.

Since $[H^+] = K[HA]/[A^-]$ the $[H^+]$ in any body fluid is determined by the ratio of the conjugate acids to the conjugate bases of the different buffer systems present in that fluid. Thus in the extracellular fluid the $[H^+]$ depends mainly upon the ratio of carbonic acid to bicarbonate. The concentration of carbonic acid in the plasma is determined by the partial pressure of carbon dioxide (PCO_2) in the alveoli. The latter is normally about 5.3 kPa (p. 199) which gives rise to little over 1 mmol/l of carbonic acid in physical solution in the plasma. The alveolar partial pressure of carbon dioxide is itself maintained steady by the equality between its rate of production by the tissues and the rate at which ventilation eliminates it from the body. On the other hand, the concentration of bicarbonate is regulated by the tubular epithelium of the kidneys and in health

is kept at about 22–27 mmol/l by the mechanism described on page 372.

A great many metabolic processes result in the production of acids which must be eliminated from the body if the reaction of the body fluids is to remain within the normal range. The route of disposal of acids depends upon whether or not they are capable of being oxidised completely to carbon dioxide and water. Carbon dioxide forms carbonic acid within the body and is eliminated as carbon dioxide by ventilation. Other acids such as phosphoric and sulphuric acids which are derived from the oxidation of phospholipids or sulphur-containing proteins respectively are excreted by the kidneys. At the site of their production in the tissues and during their carriage in the blood all acids increase the $[H^+]$. The extent of this increase is minimised by the physiologically important buffers.

Carbonic acid is produced by metabolic reactions in far greater amounts than any other acid. A small part of the carbon dioxide is transported in the blood reversibly bound to haemoglobin as a carbamino compound. A greater part is converted to carbonic acid in the red blood cells which are rich in carbonic anhydrase. The hydrogen ions of the carbonic acid are taken up by the haemoglobin in the red cells after it has given up its oxygen to tissues while the bicarbonate ions move out from the red cells to the plasma in exchange for chloride ions (chloride shift, Fig. 5.1). Most of the carbonic acid added to the blood therefore appears not as acid but as bicarbonate ion. When the blood passes through the lungs and

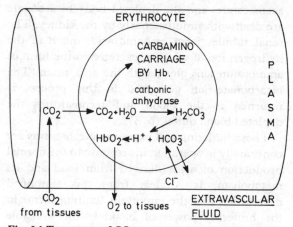

Fig. 5.1 Transport of CO_2.

the haemoglobin is reoxygenated this process is reversed and the carbon dioxide formed is exhaled.

In health, on a normal diet, 40–80 mmol of non-volatile acids are excreted in the urine daily. However in some disorders, notably diabetic ketoacidosis, a large amount of keto acids are formed. The tissues and blood are buffered against these acids by a different mechanism which involves in particular the sodium bicarbonate and carbonic acid buffer system in the plasma.

The addition of acid to the plasma results in a movement of the reactions in the direction indicated by the broad arrow (Fig. 5.2). As a result of this and of a similar reaction on the part of the other buffer systems, many of the hydrogen ions which would otherwise increase the acidity of the plasma are removed to form increased amounts of poorly dissociated acids such as carbonic acid. There is a corresponding diminution in the concentration of conjugate bases including bicarbonate ions. By this means the $[H^+]$ of the plasma rises far less than it would do if the buffers were not present.

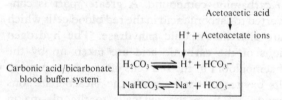

Acetoacetic acid

H^+ + Acetoacetate ions

Carbonic acid/bicarbonate blood buffer system

$H_2CO_3 \rightleftharpoons H^+ + HCO_3^-$

$NaHCO_3 \rightleftharpoons Na^+ + HCO_3^-$

Fig. 5.2 Effect of acid on the blood buffer system.

The rise in $[H^+]$ stimulates ventilation and the excess carbonic acid is removed from the body as carbon dioxide. The anion of the acid (e.g. acetoacetate) and the depleted body bicarbonate are dealt with simultaneously by the kidney. The renal tubules form carbonic acid, much of the hydrogen ion of which is excreted in the form of ammonium ions along with the acid anion. The bicarbonate ion generated in this process is returned to the blood and reconstitutes the depleted blood buffer (p. 372).

These buffering and excreting mechanisms are continually in operation in response to the normal production of acids derived from food and its metabolism. It is clear from this simplified description that the important limiting factor in the buffering power of blood is the available haemoglobin and bicarbonate. The excretory power of the kidneys is the limiting factor in the body's ability to rid itself of the hydrogen ions and anions derived from inorganic and organic acids other than carbonic acid.

DISTURBANCES IN HYDROGEN ION CONCENTRATION

Abnormalities in the reaction of the body fluids are reflected in changes in the $[H^+]$ and concentrations of carbonic acid (i.e. $PaCO_2$) and bicarbonate in the blood. The estimation of $PaCO_2$ is of particular value in respiratory disorders and its use in these conditions is described on page 208.

As there is no entirely satisfactory method available for the determination of $[HCO_3^-]$, it is usually calculated from a knowledge either of $PaCO_2$ or total CO_2 and pH using the Henderson Hasselbach equation or a nomogram based upon it. Since the concentration of bicarbonate is itself influenced by $PaCO_2$ it is common practice to express the $[HCO_3^-]$ as the concentration which would exist at a standard value of $PaCO_2$ of 5.3 kPa. It is then known as standard bicarbonate and normally ranges between 22 and 26 mmol/l.

Metabolic acidosis

Metabolic acidosis arises as a result of the production or ingestion of acids other than carbonic acid, or as a consequence of body depletion of the base bicarbonate. The condition is characterised by a rise in $[H^+]$ and a marked reduction in the concentration of bicarbonate in the plasma. The $PaCO_2$ is reduced secondarily by the hyperventilation produced by stimulation of respiration; this mitigates to some extent the increased $[H^+]$ which arises from the fall in $[HCO_3^-]$.

The production of large amounts of lactic acid in vigorous exercise is probably the most common cause of acidosis and is to be regarded as physiological. Shock from any cause, notably severe myocardial infarction or cardiac arrest, causes metabolic acidosis because of hypoxia of the tissues and the accumulation of organic acids, particularly lactic acid. Lactic acid acidosis is a recognised complication of treatment with oral hypoglycaemic biguanides such as phenformin; it is also seen in acute alcoholic intoxication and severe liver failure. In diabetic ketoacidosis β-

hydroxybutyric acid and acetoacetic acid are produced in abnormally large amounts, and at a rate which is greater than the capacity of the body to oxidise them. Salicylate intoxication produces metabolic acidosis as well as respiratory alkalosis (p. 99).

In patients with acute or chronic renal failure or renal tubular acidosis, the ability of the kidneys to conserve and generate bicarbonate ions and to produce and secrete hydrogen and ammonium ions is impaired. Depletion of body bicarbonate also occurs from direct loss of sodium bicarbonate in the stools in chronic or severe acute diarrhoea or from loss of intestinal contents from fistulae or by intestinal aspiration.

Consequences of metabolic acidosis. The most obvious consequence of acidosis is the stimulation of respiration by the abnormally high blood $[H^+]$. In severe cases the respirations become deep and rapid (Kussmaul's respiration).

It is clear, however, from the list of causes given above that the clinical picture in the individual case is largely determined by the underlying condition and by the presence of concomitant disturbances of water and salt balance. In diabetic ketoacidosis, by the time acidosis is severe, considerable water, salt and potassium depletion has usually occurred. The acidosis of chronic diarrhoea is similarly associated with salt loss and especially with potassium deficit.

As in the case of disturbances in water and electrolyte balance, the diagnosis of metabolic acidosis is facilitated by an awareness of those pathological conditions in which it is likely to arise. The diagnosis should be confirmed by the determination of $[H^+]$, $PaCO_2$ and bicarbonate concentration in the blood. In acidosis of moderate degree plasma bicarbonate is reduced to 15 mmol/l, while concentrations below 10 mmol/l represent severe degrees of acidosis.

Some information about the likely cause of metabolic acidosis can be obtained by calculating delta (Δ), the concentration of 'unmeasured anions' (albumin, sulphate, phosphate) in plasma using the equation:

$$\Delta = [Na^+] - ([Cl^-] + [HCO_3^+]).$$

In health Δ is less than 14. When metabolic acidosis is due to diarrhoea or renal tubular acidosis plasma bicarbonate is replaced by chloride and Δ is normal. In other forms of metabolic acidosis Δ is increased.

Treatment. The cause of the acidosis should be identified and where possible corrected. Treatment of diabetic ketoacidosis and lactic acidosis results in metabolism of the accumulated acids to CO_2 and water, a process which regenerates bicarbonate. Metabolic acidosis is commonly associated with some degree of sodium depletion and water deficiency and it is reasonable to correct these disturbances by the administration of isotonic NaCl solution (p. 86); this is a neutral solution and by itself might be expected to have only a little influence on the reaction of the blood and tissues. In fact, provided the kidneys are healthy and provided the degree of sodium and water depletion is not such as to impair renal function seriously, its intravenous administration is usually effective in correcting metabolic acidosis of moderate severity. Its success depends upon the capacity of the kidneys to generate bicarbonate from carbon dioxide and water and to retain this with the infused sodium, rejecting the chloride in the urine. When the blood $[H^+]$ exceeds 70 nmol/l, myocardial function and maintenance of blood pressure are compromised. It is therefore advisable in such cases to give sufficient 1.26% sodium bicarbonate solution at the start of treatment to lower the $[H^+]$ below this value. Thereafter administration of saline is usually sufficient.

In the presence of renal disease, and severe sodium depletion giving rise to uraemia, it is unwise to depend upon renal regeneration of bicarbonate. In these circumstances, isotonic sodium bicarbonate should be given by intravenous infusion in addition to isotonic sodium chloride. The two solutions should be given in a ratio of 1 to 2 and need not be mixed. The total volume of the combined solutions required varies with the severity of the sodium depletion and with the degree of acidosis. Blood $[H^+]$ and plasma bicarbonate concentration should be monitored and infusion of sodium bicarbonate stopped when the $[H^+]$ is normal. If there is still evidence of sodium and water depletion infusion of sodium chloride solution should be continued.

In severe shock or cardiac arrest, acidosis

develops without sodium depletion. In these circumstances it is best to give sodium bicarbonate in a small volume of hypertonic concentration, i.e. 50–100 ml 8.4% solution intravenously as a bolus.

The treatment of lactic acid acidosis in diabetes is given on page 480.

Metabolic alkalosis

Metabolic alkalosis, which is less common than metabolic acidosis, is characterised by an increased concentration of bicarbonate ion in plasma and a fall in the blood $[H^+]$. There may be a small compensatory increase in $PaCO_2$. In health when the plasma bicarbonate rises above normal, urinary excretion of this ion increases immediately. It is therefore extremely difficult to produce alkalosis in subjects with normal renal function by giving sodium bicarbonate and metabolic alkalosis, however induced, can be sustained only if the proportion of filtered sodium reabsorbed with bicarbonate (i.e. reabsorbed in exchange for hydrogen ion) is increased. This occurs (1) when filtered chloride is reduced and there is a strong stimulus to reabsorb sodium due to hypovolaemia and (2) when distal tubular secretion of hydrogen ion is increased directly by cellular potassium depletion, or by excess circulating mineralocorticoid or by increased delivery of sodium to the distal tubule such as occurs with potent diuretics.

Commonly several different factors contribute to the development of metabolic alkalosis. It is convenient to consider development of the commoner forms of the disorder in two phases: an initiation and maintenance phase. When hydrogen ions are secreted into the gastric lumen, bicarbonate ions from the parietal cells are added to the blood. The effect of this is normally neutralised by reabsorption of the secreted hydrogen ions in the small bowel. Loss of hydrogen ions in gastric secretions in the course of prolonged or severe vomiting therefore initiates metabolic alkalosis. The disturbance is maintained because loss of sodium, chloride, water and potassium in vomitus gives rise to hypochloraemia, extracellular fluid depletion and a potassium deficit all of which enhance renal reabsorption of sodium in exchange for protons.

In potassium deficiency, alkalosis is thought to be initiated by transfer of hydrogen ions into cells and maintained by the increased rate of secretion of protons by potassium-depleted renal tubular cells.

Prolonged use of high potency diuretics in the treatment of very oedematous patients induces metabolic alkalosis. Selective loss of sodium, chloride and water leads to contraction of the extracellular fluid and consequently induces hyperbicarbonataemia. This is sustained by increased distal tubular hydrogen ion secretion due mainly to increased delivery of sodium to this zone of the nephron in a patient with a strong stimulus to conserve sodium. Development of metabolic alkalosis in such cases is facilitated by restriction of dietary sodium and chloride.

Patients with severely impaired renal function who are given large amounts of sodium bicarbonate may develop alkalosis.

Consequences of alkalosis. The fall in $[H^+]$ suppresses ventilation and carbon dioxide is retained. This partially restores the extracellular $[H^+]$ but further stimulates $[H^+]$ secretion and thus bicarbonate reabsorption by the kidney. Because of increased secretion of hydrogen ions by distal tubular cells the urine often remains acid.

Alkalosis is commonly unattended by specific clinical disturbances. Acute alkalosis produces tetany which occurs spontaneously or may be induced by the Trousseau manoeuvre (p. 448) and which is due to reduction in the concentration of plasma ionised calcium. Another cause of increased neuromuscular excitability in alkalosis is enhanced release of acetylcholine. Apathy, personality changes, delirium and stupor may occur in severe cases. An important cause of these symptoms is cerebral vasoconstriction consequent upon the low CO_2, but since patients frequently suffer from associated sodium, water, potassium and magnesium depletion it is probably wrong to attribute such features solely to the effects of the alkalosis. Severe alkalosis of some duration is often associated with depression of renal function and uraemia. Protein and casts are found in the urine and the error of attributing vomiting due to pyloric stenosis to primary renal disease must be avoided.

Treatment. Patients with pyloric obstruction will show evidence of sodium and water depletion and this deficit should be corrected using isotonic saline of which usually 2–4 litres are required in the course of 24 hours. Sufficient potassium chloride should be added to the infusion to repair the associated potassium deficit. Restoration of extracellular fluid volume, plasma chloride concentration and cell potassium is associated with renal retention of chloride and excretion of the excess bicarbonate in urine. Patients who are being prepared for operation for relief of gastric outlet obstruction and in whom continuous gastric aspiration is needed should have the volume of fluid removed by aspiration replaced by an equal volume of isotonic saline containing potassium chloride or by an equal volume of 'gastric solution'. The latter contains 63 mmol/l of sodium chloride, 17 mmol/l of potassium chloride and 70 mmol/l of ammonium chloride. 1 litre may be given in 4–6 hours.

Alkalosis associated with primary potassium deficiency is corrected when sufficient potassium chloride is given to restore body potassium to normal. Diuretic-induced alkalosis is difficult to correct. If possible the diuretic should be stopped temporarily and the intake of sodium chloride increased for a few days. Failing this the diuretic should be stopped for one or two days during which time 500–1000 mg of the carbonic anhydrase inhibitor acetazolamide are given daily to induce a sodium bicarbonate diuresis. Any deficit of potassium should be corrected. Treatment of metabolic alkalosis must always be monitored by regular estimations of the blood [H$^+$], Paco$_2$ and plasma bicarbonate concentration.

Respiratory acidosis and alkalosis

Respiratory acidosis arises when the effective alveolar ventilation does not keep pace with the rate of production of carbon dioxide (p. 204). As a result the Paco$_2$ and carbonic acid concentration of the blood increases, and the [H$^+$] rises. The distinction between respiratory acidosis and metabolic alkalosis is usually easily made from a knowledge of the cause of the disturbance. The reaction of the arterial blood is decisive; in both the Paco$_2$ is increased, but in respiratory acidosis [H$^+$] is increased, whereas in metabolic alkalosis the [H$^+$] is reduced.

The kidney responds to an increase in Paco$_2$ by excreting an acid urine and conserving sodium bicarbonate. The causes and consequences of respiratory acidosis are given on page 000.

Respiratory alkalosis occurs when there is excessive loss of carbonic acid by overventilation of the lungs. Most commonly this occurs in hysterical overbreathing or in overventilation during the course of assisted respiration, though it may arise also in the course of lobar pneumonia, pulmonary embolism, meningitis, encephalitis, salicylate intoxication and liver failure. As a result the Paco$_2$ of the blood falls. Renal compensatory mechanisms result in the excretion of sodium bicarbonate which mitigates the fall in blood [H$^+$].

The distinction between respiratory alkalosis and metabolic acidosis is usually clear from the clinical circumstances. In both, the concentration of plasma bicarbonate is reduced and the reaction of the blood is again decisive. In respiratory alkalosis the plasma [H$^+$] falls while in metabolic acidosis it rises.

Electrolyte repair solutions play no part in the treatment of respiratory acidosis or alkalosis, and therapy should be directed to the underlying disorder. The treatment of hypercapnia is described on page 211 and that of respiratory alkalosis due to hysterical overbreathing on page 449. Tetany may be treated by an intravenous injection of 10 ml of 10% calcium gluconate if necessary. The underlying causative factors should receive appropriate attention.

ANNE T. LAMBIE

FURTHER READING:

Robinson J R 1975 Fundamentals of acid-base regulation, 5th edn. Blackwell Scientific Publications, Oxford. A straightforward account of this difficult subject.
Forrester J M 1986 Companion to medical studies, 4th edn. vol 1. Blackwell Scientific Publications, Oxford. For further information about acid-base metabolism and renal physiology
Arieff A I, DeFronzo R A 1985 Fluid, electrolyte and acid-base disorders, vols 1 & 2. Churchill Livingstone, Edinburgh. A detailed account of the physiology and pathophysiology of water and electrolyte balance. Useful accounts of the electrolyte disturbances occurring in clinical situations
The New England Journal of Medicine frequently contains reviews of the physiological basis of medical progress

6

Introduction to oncology

Oncology is the study of tumours. *Neoplasia* means abnormal new growth, which may be benign or malignant. *Cancer* is a term that is used to describe a wide variety of malignant diseases, the management of which requires several medical disciplines. Traditionally physicians have played a lesser role than surgeons or radiotherapists in the treatment of these diseases but the development of cytotoxic drugs has resulted in the greater involvement of physicians in the overall management of malignancy. The use of cytotoxic drugs requires specialised knowledge and experience but since cancer impinges on every medical discipline, it is necessary for all doctors to be aware of the basic principles of investigating and managing malignant diseases. This chapter reviews these basic principles and outlines some aspects of the aetiology and pathology of tumours, the assessment of tumour burden, the use of radiotherapy, chemotherapy and hormone therapy, and possible approaches to the prevention of these diseases, many of which may be associated with avoidable causes.

EPIDEMIOLOGY AND AETIOLOGY

Cancer is second only to coronary artery disease as being the commonest cause of death in the Western world. The age standardised mortality in England and Wales for the years 1976–1978 was 283.7 and 178.4 per 100 000 population for men and women respectively, with even higher figures for Scotland (373.5 and 274.2 per 100 000). There is considerable geographical variation in

the incidence of malignant diseases around the world but as Figure 6.1 shows, British countries are amongst the highest for mortality rates, with Scotland actually leading the world tables for its incidence of cancer in men. In many developed countries the incidence is steadily increasing (Fig. 6.2).

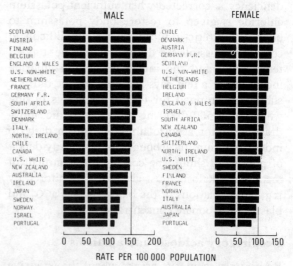

Fig. 6.1 Age-adjusted mortality rates for all cancers in various countries 1966–67.

Throughout the Western world the commonest sites of malignant disease are the lung, large bowel and breast. Over the past 25 years the incidence of lung cancer in men has increased by 125%, and even more significantly in women concomitant with their increased consumption of cigarettes. The incidence of colonic, prostatic and bladder cancer has also shown an increase but during the past decade there has been a decrease in the incidence of carcinomas arising in the stomach, uterus, rectum and oesophagus.

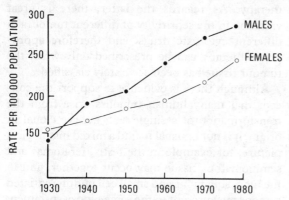

Fig. 6.2 Death rates from cancer in Scotland 1930–80.

Age has a bearing on the incidence of specific cancers. In children, cancer is the leading cause of death between the ages of 3–13 years, about half of these being due to acute lymphoblastic leukaemia. For the age group in the third and fourth decades, cancer is three times as common in women as in men but men are at greater risk than women between the ages of 60–80.

The aetiology of many malignant diseases remains unknown but studies of the geographical distribution of their incidence gives some leads as to the possible influence of particular environmental or social factors in causation. The best documented aetiological factor is cigarette tobacco which is unquestionably associated with the considerable increase in lung cancer in countries where cigarette smoking has increased over the past 30 years.

The incidence of carcinoma of the oesophagus varies greatly from country to country (over a 200-fold range) with a particularly high incidence in a geographical band covering eastern and southern Africa, Iran, Afghanistan, Soviet and central Asia, Mongolia and northern China. Suggestions that diet or cooking practices are involved are as yet unconfirmed.

The incidence of carcinoma of the pancreas is increasing in most of the developed countries but is relatively rare in Japan, whereas the reverse is true for stomach cancer which is particularly prevalent in Japan.

It has been known for a long time that the incidence of breast cancer varies appreciably in different parts of the world, being high in the USA and low in the Orient but increasing over two generations of orientals who emigrate to the USA. Population migration represents a natural experiment where the assumption of incidence levels of the host country strongly suggests an environmental rather than a genetic aetiology.

The incidence of carcinoma of the uterine cervix has increased in recent years particularly amongst younger women. This has coincided with changing social patterns of greater sexual freedom and the use of oral contraception, suggesting that a sexually transmissable agent may be the aetiological factor responsible.

There is evidence that both environmental and genetic factors are important in the pathogenesis of malignant melanoma. In the USA, figures for 1975 show an incidence of 4.2 cases per 100 000 population, but of great concern is the fact that the incidence is rising rapidly, doubling every 10–15 years. Melanoma is rare in black and oriental people suggesting that skin pigment plays a genetic role in protecting against the development of melanoma. Although not proven, there is support for the fact that sunlight is environmentally involved in the aetiology of this disease. Although the incidence between the sexes is equal, women tend to develop melanoma in the legs and exposed parts of the limbs more frequently than men who have a higher incidence of lesions on the trunk. Furthermore, studies from Norway, Canada, the USA and Australia show that the incidence of melanoma increases as one approaches the equator, consistent with greater exposure to ultraviolet light.

It has long been suspected that viruses may be involved in the pathogenesis of human neoplasms, but there is as yet no conclusive evidence of a direct aetiological relationship. There is however indirect evidence to suggest the hypothesis that viruses may act as cofactors in the development of some malignant diseases. This evidence includes the fact that viral particles can be demonstrated in the cells of certain malignancies, the enzyme reverse transcriptase (of oncornavirus-type) has been demonstrated in human cancer cells, and the nuclei of some malignant cells have been shown to contain DNA base sequences complementary to the base sequences of known tumour viruses.

The integration of viral information into the genome of the human cell that subsequently becomes malignant has led to the concept of 'oncogenes', whereby cancer results from the de-repression of these viral oncogenes to permit malignant transformation. De-repression may be caused by exposure to an external carcinogen, or by spontaneous mutation. This hypothesis is the subject of intensive research at the present time.

PATHOLOGY

A fundamental principle of oncology is to establish the pathological nature of any lesion suspected of being neoplastic before making decisions about management. This usually entails biopsy of the tumour for histological examination.

The first distinction to be made is between benign and malignant lesions. Benign tumours represent the accumulation of cells which have been transformed to reproduce in abnormal numbers but under circumstances where they remain within the tissue of origin. Malignant tumours are comprised of cells which are capable of invading adjacent tissues and leaving the tissue of origin to disseminate and form metastases. The histological distinction between benign and malignant lesions will depend, amongst other factors, on the pleomorphism of the cells, the presence of aberrations in the nucleus, increased numbers of mitoses and whether or not there is evidence of invasion into surrounding tissues.

Cancers are classified into three major groups: the *carcinomas* which arise in endodermal or ectodermal tissue, the *sarcomas* of mesodermal origin, and the *leukaemias and lymphomas* which are derived from the white blood cells and the monocyte–macrophage system. Within a given tissue there may be major differences in the cell type from which the tumour has arisen. Thus for example bronchogenic carcinomas are classified histologically into four major groups: squamous carcinomas, adenocarcinomas, small cell and large cell undifferentiated carcinomas.

Such distinctions are essential to clinical management since the choice between surgery, radiotherapy and chemotherapy will depend on whether or not the lesion is benign or malignant, and whether or not the particular histological subtype is sensitive to radiotherapy or chemotherapy. As regards the latter, there is great variation in the sensitivity of different tumours to different cytotoxic drugs, and therefore appropriate therapy can be prescribed only when the tumour tissue has been accurately classified.

Although there is evidence to support the concept that many human tumours arise from the transformation of a single cell, i.e. are clonal in origin, it is not unusual to find a mixed histological picture; for example in the testis, teratomas and seminomatous tissue may occur together, and in the lung, squamous and small cell undifferentiated tumour may present in the same biopsy specimen.

In addition to defining whether the tumour is benign or malignant and from which cell type it arises, it is useful to define the degree of differentiation or anaplasia of the cancer cell since for many tumour types this has been shown to correlate with prognosis and response to treatment of differing forms.

Whilst most histology is performed on tissue that is obtained by surgical biopsy, in certain circumstances it is possible to achieve excellent classification from cytology alone. Thus for example sputum may be examined for malignant bronchogenic cells, pleural or peritoneal effusions may provide suitable cells for diagnostic purposes and smears can be prepared from the uterine cervix. Increasing use is being made of needle aspiration for cytological diagnosis. A fine gauge needle can be inserted into breast lumps, subcutaneous deposits, intrathoracic or hepatic lesions, and a smear for cytological evaluation can be made from the aspirated material. In experienced hands, this technique has many advantages over the more conventional surgical biopsy technique, mainly because of speed and simplicity.

TUMOUR MARKERS

Malignant cells appear different histologically and vary biochemically from their normal counterparts but attempts to identify biochemical abnormalities unique to the cancer cell have proved unrewarding. Nevertheless it is now appreciated that the presence of viable tumour tissue in the body may be detectable by the presence in the blood of biochemical products known as 'tumour markers'. These are normal metabolic constituents that are found either in abnormal amounts or at an inappropriate time of life, for example fetal proteins being re-expressed in adult life.

Tumour markers of this type can be useful in a number of different clinical situations. In theory tumour markers might be useful for screening whole populations for undetected cancers but in practice this has not proved useful for the following reasons. The predictive value of a screening test depends on the sensitivity of the test, its specificity and the prevalence of the particular disease. Sensitivity refers to the number of times a test is positive for patients known to have the disease, i.e. true positives, and specificity refers to the incidence of true negatives, i.e. that the test should prove negative in people known to be free of the disease. Unfortunately sensitivity is inversely related to specificity. For example it is known that some gastrointestinal tumours contain carcinoembryonic antigen (CEA), a substance that is present in the gut during fetal life but which is not found in normal adult gastrointestinal tissues. Radio-immunoassays of CEA in blood have shown an overall 67% positivity in patients with colorectal carcinoma but the test is also positive in alcoholic cirrhosis (70%), emphysema (57%) and diabetes mellitus (38%) amongst many other diseases. Screening the population at large for subclinical carcinomas of the colon would therefore fail because of lack of specificity.

However the presence of a tumour marker can be of clinical value in monitoring the progress of individual patients known to have a given malignancy. For example testicular teratomas not infrequently secrete another oncofetal protein — alpha-fetoprotein (AFP). Figure 6.3 illustrates a typical case where during the months following surgical resection of the primary tumour, a rising level of AFP was associated with (and preceded) the clinical appearance of metastases. The successful use of chemotherapy was associated with a disappearance of the abnormal tumour marker.

Human chorionic gonadotrophin (normally produced only by placental tissue) is another tumour marker seen in testicular teratoma while the production of placental alkaline phosphatase

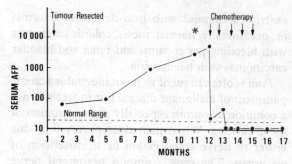

Fig. 6.3 Serum alpha-fetoprotein (AFP) levels in a young man with testicular teratoma. The levels of AFP fluctuate with disease state and can be used to monitor the effects of the treatment.

is associated with approximately 40% of testicular seminomas.

A variety of hormones can be produced ectopically by small cell anaplastic lung tumours including antidiuretic hormone (ADH) and ACTH. The levels of these hormones, or the biochemical consequences of their production — such as hyponatraemia resulting from inappropriate ADH secretion — can be useful markers of the viability of residual tumour following treatment, therefore indicating whether or not further therapy is required.

CLINICAL FEATURES

Malignant diseases manifest themselves in a variety of ways. The presence of an abnormal accumulation of cells may, by virtue of its physical bulk alone, produce clinical symptoms and signs. Thus for example painless swellings in the breast or in muscle may indicate an underlying carcinoma or sarcoma respectively. Lymphomas usually present as painless enlargements of lymph nodes or spleen. Intracranial space-occupying lesions may cause focal manifestations, fits, headaches, vomiting and papilloedema. Tumours in the distal colon may partially obstruct the lumen of the bowel with a resulting change in bowel habit. Bronchogenic tumours may cause cough or shortness of breath resulting from partial or complete occlusion of an airway.

Haemorrhage. Malignant tumours not infrequently present as haemorrhage from an eroded epithelial surface. For example bronchogenic carcinomas may present with haemoptysis, gastric carcinomas with iron deficiency anaemia or, occasionally, haematemesis, colonic carcinoma with bleeding per rectum, and renal and bladder carcinomas with haematuria.

Pain is often thought to be an inevitable accompaniment of malignant disease but in fact it is not a common symptom especially at presentation of most cancers. When pain does occur, it is due either to nerve compression or to distension of an organ. The most common peripheral nerve compressions are due to involvement of the brachial plexus (carcinomas of the lung or breast), the sacral plexus (carcinomas of the rectum or cervix) or the paraspinal nerves (carcinoma of the pancreas). Metastatic tumours in the liver may cause pain as a result of distension and stretching of its capsule. Bone pain resulting from primary, or more commonly, secondary deposits usually occurs in the weight bearing bones, and results from compression secondary to weakening of the structural component of the bone. Pathological fractures may arise as a consequence. Patients may present with referred pain, most frequently in the shoulder, hip or knee, as when a nerve root is involved directly or by metastases.

Cachexia is a clinical feature of many malignant diseases presenting at an advanced stage, especially carcinomas of the gastro-intestinal tract, lung, ovary and testis. It is, however, not a universal phenomenon and is rare in breast cancer and in tumours of the central nervous system, and uncommon in leukaemia and lymphomas.

Cachexia may arise as a direct result of malnutrition from a tumour in the gastrointestinal tract. Malabsorption may arise rarely as a consequence of tumour replacing the absorptive epithelia but more commonly from reduced exocrine function (from carcinomas of the pancreas), or loss of bile from carcinomas of the upper gastrointestinal tract that obstruct biliary outflow. Loss of taste and the malaise that accompanies many malignant diseases may contribute to poor food intake but all of these factors in promoting malnutrition do not of themselves fully explain the cachexia of malignancy. Although many patients will have a negative nitrogen balance, others who are in positive balance may show a caloric deficit. It has been shown that in the cachexia accompanying malignant disease, caloric expenditure remains high with an elevated basal metabolic rate despite reduced dietary intake (the reverse of the situation that follows starvation) which indicates that this phenomenon results from a profound systemic derangement of host metabolism, the pathogenesis of which remains unclear.

Paraneoplastic features. In addition to generalised clinical features that are commonly associated with the presentation of a malignant disease, there are a variety of syndromes for which the term 'paraneoplastic' has been used. These syndromes include many that arise as a result of the secretion into the blood of tumour products (usually polypeptide hormones) which produce clinical signs as a consequence of their action on target organs remote from the primary tumour. Although relatively rare, these syndromes are important since they may precede the clinical presentation of the primary tumour, facilitating early detection. In addition they may mimic metastatic disease and thus confuse management decisions. They may also serve as tumour markers to monitor therapy. The ectopic production of ADH and ACTH (p. 253) are most commonly associated with an underlying small cell anaplastic carcinoma of the bronchus. Squamous cell lung cancers may produce parathyroid hormone manifesting as hypercalcaemia.

A number of neurological paraneoplastic syndromes (p. 668) have been described for which the tumour product remains unknown. These include peripheral neuropathies, a myasthenia-like syndrome and subacute cerebellar degeneration. Whilst all of these syndromes may improve with successful treatment of the primary tumour, complete resolution is rare.

Dermatomyositis and polymyositis present as gradually progressive muscle weakness predominantly affecting the proximal musculature, coming on over a period of months. Whilst these disorders are not universally associated with malignancy, patients suffering from them have a greatly increased risk of an underlying neoplasm compared with the general public, and malignancies of the breast, lung, and gastrointestinal and genito-urinary tract should be considered.

Acanthosis nigricans is a rare condition characterised by the appearance of black velvety verrucose lesions in the flexures around the neck, axillae and groin. It is particularly seen in patients with carcinomas of the stomach.

PRINCIPLES OF TREATMENT

In order to plan the optimal management for an individual patient, it is necessary to consider two essential questions: (1) Is the tumour still localised to its site of origin? and (2) Is it a realistic aim to 'cure' the patient, or should treatment be focussed on palliation of symptoms? Tumours that have not metastasised are amenable to local forms of treatment, surgery or radiotherapy, whilst tumours that have already disseminated require systemic treatment with chemotherapy or hormonal therapy. Not infrequently it is necessary to use a combination of these measures, particularly if it is appropriate to aim for complete eradication of the tumour. Surgery, radiotherapy and chemotherapy all cause some degree of host toxicity and this may be enhanced by combining the treatments.

For this reason it is important to decide whether or not cure is feasible and desirable in order to minimise any treatment-related toxicity in circumstances where an aggressive therapeutic approach would be inappropriate. Thus for example lymphoma arising in a young person may require a protracted course of combination chemotherapy and radiotherapy but cure is attained in a significant proportion of patients and will be the initial intention in planning management. If the same disease presents in an 80-year-old then management should be planned to relieve symptoms as effectively as possible but to minimise hospital attendances and any treatment-related toxicity. Such an example may appear obvious but more subtle decisions are frequently required in planning management for patients with carcinomas of breast, stomach or ovary.

The patient's history and physical examination provide a starting point for planning treatment but it is usually necessary to perform specialised investigations to determine the extent of dissemination of the tumour prior to selecting treatment — the process of 'staging' the tumour. Staging investigations take time and inevitably the delay in announcing a decision about treatment causes anxiety for the patient. For this reason it cannot be overemphasised that the first interview with a patient suspected of having a malignant disease is of particular importance. It is essential to perform this interview in a quiet and unhurried manner. In addition to a routine history of symptoms and previous illnesses, it is important to ascertain whether patients already know that they have malignant disease and what this means to them. For many patients the word 'cancer' is automatically associated with an incurable disease and very distressing death. This myth of universal hopelessness is slowly being destroyed, helped by greater public interest in health and medical progress generally but the patient who holds such beliefs will be helped very considerably by positive assurance that symptoms can almost always be improved, if not completely resolved, even if the underlying disease cannot be eradicated. At the first interview the physician may not have sufficient facts to know the likelihood of cure but at this stage it is important to explain to the patient that the first aim of treatment will be to control the disease, whether or not cure can ultimately be achieved.

Whether or not to tell patients that they have malignant disease is a matter of individual circumstances but as a general rule it is recommended that patients should be informed of this, whilst it is not necessarily appropriate to inform them of the exact prognosis which in any case may be uncertain. The first interview may not be the time to discuss these matters but it is recommended that they should always be discussed prior to starting treatment. If it is necessary to arrange a series of staging investigations, patients should be informed of the purpose of these so that their natural anxiety is not accentuated. Time should be taken to counsel the patient at the earliest opportunity about these matters so that they can have confidence in those who are going to be responsible for therapy and follow-up which by the nature of these diseases need to be continued for a long period.

Staging

The concept of staging arose from the fact that survival rates were better for malignancies that were localised than for those which had metastasised at the time of clinical presentation. This was associated with the concept of 'early' and 'late' presentation, implying a regular progression with time. It is now known that the stage of disease at diagnosis is much more complex than this, and is a reflection not only of the degree of malignancy of the particular tumour but also of the tumour-host relationship. However, staging is still an essential part of oncological management since in addition to its contribution towards selecting appropriate treatment, it may give an indication of prognosis and assist in the monitoring and evaluation of treatment.

The internationally recognised staging system is known as the TNM classification in which T defines the extent of the primary tumour, N defines the extent of regional lymph node involvement and M defines the presence or absence of metastases. To T, N or M, the addition of numbers indicates the extent of the disease, thus for example T0 refers to an excised tumour, T1, 2 or 3 to (defined) increases in primary tumour size. N1, N2 and N3 apply similarly to increasing involvement of nodes, and the suffix 1 indicates the presence of metastases where M0 indicates that metastases are not present. For T and N the exact criteria of size and regions of nodal involvement have been defined for each anatomical site, for example for lung cancers:

T1	< 3cm with no invasion
T2	> 3cm ± extension to hilar region
T3	Gross extension/effusion/atelectasis
N1	Hilar nodes
N2	Mediastinal nodes
M0	Metastases absent
M1	Metastases present

The TNM system is a clinical staging system but if supplemented by the pathological examin-

Table 6.1 Performance status scale (ECOG).

0	Fully active, able to carry on all usual activities without restriction and without the aid of analgesics
1	Restricted in strenuous activity but ambulatory and able to carry out light work or pursue a sedentary occupation This group also contains patients who are fully active, as in grade 0, but only with the aid of analgesics
2	Ambulatory and capable of all self-care but unable to work. Up and about more than 50% of waking hours
3	Capable of only limited self-care, confined to bed or chair more than 50% of waking hours
4	Completely disabled, unable to carry out any self-care and confined totally to bed or chair

ation of biopsied or resected specimens the suffix p is added. Having defined the T, N and M status of the tumour, it is then possible to group patients into different stages. Thus for example in lung cancers the stage groupings are as follows:

Occult cancer	Tx*	N0	M0
Stage Ia	T1	N0	M0
	T2	N0	M0
Stage Ib	T1	N1	M0
Stage II	T2	N1	M0
Stage III	T3	N0,N1	M0
	Any T	N2	M0
Stage IV	Any T	Any N	M1

*Tx refers to tumour proven by the presence of malignant cells in bronchopulmonary secretions but not visualised by radiography or bronchoscopy.

For certain diseases it has proved useful to define specific staging systems which differ from the TNM classification, as for example the Ann Arbor staging for Hodgkin's lymphoma (p. 534), and Dukes' classification for carcinomas of the rectum. Nevertheless increasing use of the TNM system for the majority of malignant diseases is being encouraged particularly in order to facilitate comparisons of the results of treatments in different centres internationally.

The investigations required to define the T, N or M status of a tumour vary for different diseases. Primary tumours may be assessed by palpation or inspection (fibreoptic bronchoscopy, cystoscopy, etc.) or by radiography (conventional or computed tomography [CT]); nodes are assessed by palpation, excision, lymphangiography or CT scanning; and metastases are evaluated by a variety of techniques such as biochemical screening of liver function, radionuclide scans of bone, liver or brain, ultrasound of the liver, peritoneoscopy or laparotomy.

Performance status

In addition to the anatomical assessment of tumour extent evaluated by staging procedures, it is important to assess the overall degree of functional impairment that the disease is causing the patient at the time of diagnosis. A variety of 'performance status' scales have been devised such as the Eastern Cooperative Oncology Group (ECOG) scale shown in Table 6.1. The complications of disease which impinge on a patient's life and therefore affect his or her performance status are multiple and variable but these simple divisions into major groups have been found useful in prognosis in assessing the efficacy and toxicity of treatment, and in research studies comparing different forms of treatment.

Evaluation of response

With presently available therapies most methods of cancer treatment are associated with significant morbidity. For this reason alone, it is essential to evaluate the response to therapy as accurately as possible but since research into new methods of treatment is so widespread, properly defined criteria for evaluating response are necessary in order to make valid comparisons between different treatments. The concept of 'survival time', particularly the long hallowed 'five year survival' concept, places too much emphasis on cure as the only objective of treatment. Since palliation is a much commoner objective in management planning, more subtle criteria are required than crude survival figures.

The terms universally accepted for evaluating treatment are those of 'objective response', 'complete response', 'partial response', 'no response' and 'progressive disease'. These are defined as follows:

Objective response:	any response that fulfils the criteria of complete or partial response.
Complete response:	complete disappearance of all known disease in the absence of any new lesions appearing.
Partial response:	a reduction in size by at least 50% of the tumour in the absence of any new lesions appearing.
No response:	no change, or an increase or decrease of 25% in the size of the tumour in the absence of new lesions.
Progressive disease:	increase in the size of the tumour by 25% or the development of any new lesions.

The term 'complete response' may or may not indicate true eradication of the tumour and for any given disease these terms can only reflect the ability to detect viable tumour.

Principles of radiotherapy

Whilst it is outside the scope of this chapter to consider details of the radiobiological aspects of radiotherapy, it is important that physicians should be familiar with an outline of the procedures involved when their patients are referred for this form of treatment.

Radiotherapy involves the exposure of a defined area of the body to a source of ionising radiation under carefully controlled conditions. Treatment planning involves accurate localisation of the tumour and prescription of multiple daily fractions of irradiation for a specified period of time. The biological effect of radiation depends on the amount of energy absorbed per unit mass. The unit of absorbed dose is the gray and is equivalent to 1 joule per kilogram.

Ionising radiation damages cells by interaction with nuclear DNA thus preventing the normal reproduction of that cell. As with cytotoxic drugs there is only a relative selectivity in this process, and normal (non-malignant) cells are readily damaged by radiation. For this reason radiotherapy planning must take into account the exact anatomical distribution of the tumour in order to minimise the exposure of normal tissues whilst at the same time ensuring that all of the diseased tissues are included in the treated area. Great care is taken to ensure that the patient can be accurately and reproducibly repositioned whilst radiotherapy is being undertaken.

Patients are usually treated in the supine position although the prone position may be more suitable for some abdominal and pelvic tumours, and in certain situations patients may be treated seated or standing with horizontal beams rather than supine with vertical or oblique beams. In order to immobilise the area to be treated, moulds, casts and shells are constructed for the individual patient.

With the patient comfortably positioned and the treatment area immobilised, the tumour is localised by a variety of techniques such as the placement of radio-opaque seeds in the tumour or the use of contrast media as in conventional radiography. Increasingly computed tomography is being used to assist in planning radiotherapeutic treatment, especially since CT can provide information about tumour margins in the transverse plane in which most radiotherapy is administered.

Radiotherapy localisation is usually carried out on specialised equipment known as a simulator which is designed to allow isocentric rotation and thus to simulate the exact axis distance of the treatment machine. In most centres computers are now available to integrate the information obtained from simulators in order to select the optimum configuration, energy and variable loading of different treatment beams. This ensures that the least possible dose of radiation will be given to critical normal tissues and that a homogeneous high level of dose will be given to the tumour.

To maximise the absorbed dose within the tumour area and minimise the dose to normal tissues, treatment is given through multiple portals, for example as a four-field box technique for the pelvis, or through fields at right angles to each other with compensating wedge filters to even the dose distribution where the beams overlap. Compensating filters are used to overcome variations in thickness of the areas to be treated through multiple ports. Since the human body is not a symmetrical cube, the routine use of these filters compensates for the lack of consistent tissue thickness and ensures a more homogeneous dose distribution throughout the target.

Most radiotherapy is performed with 'teletherapy' techniques, i.e. where a beam of photons is used to irradiate the tumour from outside the patient. Alternatively for specific sites, 'brachytherapy' is used whereby a source of radiation is implanted in a body cavity or within the tumour itself. Teletherapy techniques include the use of low energy ortho- or kilovoltage sources and the more widely used megavoltage sources. Low energy radiation (50–100 kVp range) is useful for treating carcinomas of the skin and lip, and orthovoltage (250–300 kVp) machines are sometimes used for the palliative treatment of bone metastases and lesions of the chest wall. However, orthovoltage machines are unsuitable for the treatment of more deep seated tumours.

^{60}Cobalt machines and linear accelerators are the most widely used teletherapy equipment. Both of these types can be used isocentrically, i.e. the radiation source can be mounted in a gantry which can be rotated around the axis of the patient thus allowing direction of multiple beams to the centre of the target volume with great accuracy. ^{60}Cobalt machines which give radiation of a quality similar to that from a 4 MV linear accelerator are less expensive to operate and easier to maintain but provide a less well defined beam of radiation, lower dose rates and poorer depth doses. In general, ^{60}cobalt or 4 MV linear accelerators are used for treating carcinomas of the head and neck and breast, 6 MV linear accelerators for lymphomas and lung cancers, and higher energy accelerators for some deep seated abdominal and pelvic tumours. In addition to producing X-rays, the higher energy linear accelerators can be used to produce accelerated electrons. The latter are charged particles which are absorbed within a finite range of tissue and can be useful in the treatment of superficial lesions where it is desirable to spare underlying tissues. Thus, for example, electrons may be employed (with advantage) for the treatment of some lesions of the head and neck, lymph nodes near the spinal cord, and lesions of the chest wall such as occur in breast carcinoma.

Brachytherapy is performed with sealed sources of radioactivity introduced for a few days into a body cavity or tumour, for example the insertion of ^{137}caesium into the uterus for treating carcinoma of the cervix, or the use of ^{192}iridium wire placed within breast tumours. The advantages of brachytherapy are that a relatively high dose of radiation can be administered to a very limited volume of tissue thereby sparing any adverse effects on normal adjacent tissues. Brachytherapy is applicable only when the tumour is accessible and when its size can be accurately defined. Such treatments are often supplemented by teletherapy to treat the larger volume where microscopic disease may be present.

Radiotherapy is most frequently prescribed in daily fractions of 200 centigray (cGy) for 5 days a week where, depending on the tumour type and management plan, treatment may continue for 3–6 weeks. During and after this time a number of side-effects may occur. Many patients, particularly those treated with target volumes greater than 500 cm^3, will experience some malaise and fatigue. Nausea and anorexia are common and vomiting is a frequent problem if it is necessary to irradiate very large volumes, particularly in the upper abdomen. Acute skin reaction usually consists of mild erythema best treated by keeping the skin dry. Oral and pharyngeal mucosal reactions are common if the area receives high radiation doses. Particular attention to oral hygiene is required and close inspection for candidosis essential.

Radiation effects on the bone marrow may occur if large volumes are treated. Minor decreases in lymphocyte count are common but a frequent check on the peripheral blood must be made throughout treatment to adjust this if significant marrow suppression occurs. Maintenance of adequate haemoglobin is important to the outcome of therapy since hypoxia may render the tumour less sensitive to radiation damage. Irradiation of the gastrointestinal tract may result in temporary dysphagia, diarrhoea, tenesmus or production of mucus per rectum. Management depends on the severity and duration of the symptoms but antacids and reduction of residue in the diet may be beneficial.

Principles of chemotherapy

During the Second World War, research into the action of mustard gas showed that sulphur and nitrogen mustard could destroy dividing cells in lymph nodes and the bone marrow. The potential harnessing of this effect for therapeutic benefit was explored in treating some lymphomas with nitrogen mustard which was then developed as the first clinically useful cytotoxic drug. Study of the effects of folic acid metabolism on leukaemic cells resulted in the second cytotoxic drug of therapeutic value—the antifolate, methotrexate. Thereafter many naturally occurring substances were tested for antitumour activity in experimental systems, resulting in the present availability of some 30 effective antineoplastic drugs (Fig. 6.4).

Classification. Anticancer drugs are divided into 6 main groups (Table 6.2). The site of action of each group is shown in Figure 6.5.

1. *Antimetabolites.* Methotrexate acts to inhibit folate metabolism by preventing the cell from replenishing its source of reduced folates necessary for purine and pyrimidine synthesis (p. 504). The term 'anti-metabolite' is used for this group of drugs which includes mercaptopurine, thioguanine, fluorouracil and cytosine arabinoside.

2. *Alkylating agents.* Nitrogen mustard is

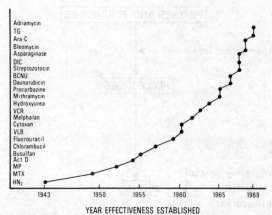

Fig. 6.4 Anticancer drugs. The year that clinical effectiveness was established for some of the commonly used anticancer drugs. TG = thioguanine, Ara C = cystosine arabinoside, DIC = dimethyl triazeno-imidazole carboxamide (DTIC), BCNU = bis-chloroethyl nitrosourea, VCR = vincristine, VLB = vinblastine, Act D = actinomycin D, MP = mercaptopurine, MTX = methotrexate, HN$_2$ = nitrogen mustard.

Table 6.2 Classification of anticancer drugs.

Antimetabolites (metabolism of substance in parenthesis is interrupted)	Methotrexate (folic acid) 6-Mercaptopurine(hypoxanthine) 6-Thioguanine (guanine) 5-Fluorouracil (uracil) Cytosine arabinoside (cytidine)
Alkylating agents	Nitrogen mustard Cyclophosphamide Chlorambucil Busulphan Melphalan Thiotepa Iphosphamide
Plant alkaloids	Vinblastine Vincristine Vindesine VP 16–213 VM 26
Antibiotics	Doxorubicin Daunorubicin Actinomycin D Bleomycin Mitomycin C
Nitrosoureas	BCNU CCNU Methyl CCNU Streptozotocin
Miscellaneous synthetic compounds	DTIC Cisplatin Procarbazine Hexamethylmelamine Hydroxyurea

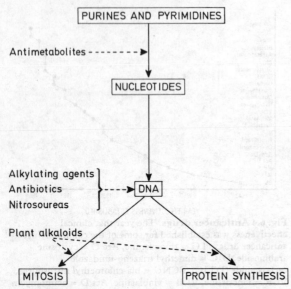

Fig. 6.5 Anticancer drugs: site of action of major groups.

curves, these factors all account for the narrow 'therapeutic index' of cytotoxic drugs. This is illustrated in Figure 6.6 which demonstrates that too low a dose is ineffective, but the dose range for optimal treatment is narrow before an increased dose produces unacceptable toxicity.

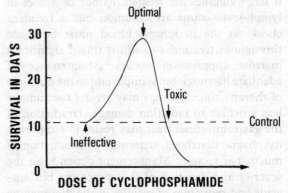

Fig. 6.6 Dose-response curve for cyclophosphamide in mice bearing the L1210 leukaemia. Too low a dose is ineffective but beyond a narrow therapeutic range too high a dose kills the animals from haematological toxicity.

thought to destroy cells by the process of alkylation — the addition of an alkyl group to constituents of DNA, thus interfering with replication and transcription of further nucleic acid. Busulphan, chlorambucil, cyclophosphamide and melphalan are other clinically useful alkylating agents.

3. *Plant alkaloids*. These inhibit cell division by binding to tubulin and disrupting the mitotic spindle.

4. *Antibiotics*. The compounds grouped altogether as antibiotics include adriamycin and actinomycin which act by intercalating between base pairs in DNA, and bleomycin which causes breaks in both single and double-stranded DNA.

5. *Nitrosoureas*. The mechanism of action of this group probably involves alkylation.

6. *Miscellaneous synthetic compounds*. Alkylation and other metabolic lesions may be involved.

Therapeutic index. Unfortunately none of these biochemical events is confined to the metabolism of malignant cells. Systemic exposure to these cellular poisons therefore must inevitably result in some damage to normal host tissues, particularly to those which rely on rapid cell division such as the bone marrow and gastrointestinal tract. In addition to their relative lack of selectivity, anticancer drugs are very potent because they act at low concentrations. Together with a tendency towards steep dose-response

The narrow therapeutic index of antineoplastic drugs is the major reason for emphasising that the greatest care is required in their administration. Certain specific toxicities are mentioned later but it is a general principle that whenever anticancer drugs are used, it is necessary to monitor the peripheral blood count and be aware of any functional disturbances such as dysphagia or diarrhoea produced by damage to the gastrointestinal tract. Since the maximum dose of any cytotoxic drug that can be prescribed on any one occasion is governed by its toxicity to normal cells, it is found that only partial tumour shrinkage results from any single treatment. It is therefore necessary to administer these drugs repeatedly, the total duration of treatment varying from a few months to several years. In order to prevent unacceptable or cumulative damage to host tissues, intermittent administration is necessary thus allowing an interval for host tissue to recover between treatments. Damage to bone marrow cells results in temporary depression of the blood counts between 10 and 14 days following drug administration. The therapeutic programme varies with different drugs but many cytotoxic drug regimens are given on 21 day cycles to preserve bone marrow integrity.

Choice of drug. In order to select the most appropriate drug for any individual clinical problem, it is necessary to know the range of activity against disease for the various drugs, and to select a drug which has the minimum toxicities in relation to the particular patient. This information is obtained through a sequence of three phases of clinical trials. Having demonstrated some antineoplastic activity in an experimental system and having been screened by conducting toxicology studies in animals, the new drug enters phase I clinical trials to establish its toxicological properties in man. For ethical reasons, phase I studies are usually performed in patients with advanced disease which has proved refractory to conventional treatment. Since the effects of the new drug are unknown, it is necessary to start phase I trials with very low doses of the drug, and increase the dose until some toxicity is observed. Pharmacokinetic studies are performed during phase I trials to establish if possible the distribution, metabolism and elimination of the compound. Then phase II trials are performed in patients with a wide variety of different malignant diseases in order to determine the range of activity of the drug. If it is effective against a particular tumour type, then phase III trials are performed. The latter are larger scale randomised trials where the new drug is compared with the best previously known treatment either alone or in combination with other drugs.

Combination chemotherapy. When in the early 1960s it was first appreciated that a variety of different types of chemical could influence the progression of malignant diseases, the concept of combining drugs in twos, threes and fours was first explored. The theory behind combination chemotherapy was to evaluate the hypothesis that simultaneous disruption of the metabolism of a tumour cell at more than one site might have far more profound effects on the cell than a single metabolic lesion. Dramatic results were produced by treating lymphomas in this way. The four-drug combination of nitrogen mustard, vincristine, procarbazine and prednisolone yielded complete remissions in more than 80% of patients with advanced Hodgkin's disease whereas these same drugs used singly rarely produced remissions in 15–20% of cases. Similarly combination

chemotherapy for acute leukaemia increased the remission rates from 20% to 90%. Over the past 20 years it has been shown that combination chemotherapy is valuable in many other malignant diseases including carcinomas of the breast, ovary, lung, testis and several of the childhood tumours. The five general principles governing the use of combination chemotherapy are:

1. Each drug in the combination should have been demonstrated to have some activity on its own against the tumour type for which the combination is being used.

2. Drugs with a similar mechanism of action should not be combined.

3. As far as is possible the major dose-limiting toxicity of each drug should differ from that of the other components of the combination.

4. Since it is rarely possible to avoid some overlap in toxicity to host tissues, it is usually necessary to reduce the dose of each of the component drugs compared with the optimal dose which would be used if the drugs were prescribed individually.

5. There should be no known adverse interaction between the drugs.

Multimodality treatment. With the development of combination chemotherapy, it became apparent that the clinical course of many different malignant diseases could be influenced by cytotoxic drugs, with cure in some and useful palliation in many others. Nevertheless, since in so many situations cytotoxic drugs are capable of shrinking only a proportion of the tumour, increasing attention has been paid to the use of chemotherapy in conjunction with surgery or radiotherapy to lessen the total tumour load. Thus chemotherapy can be used to reduce tumour bulk prior to local therapy with surgery or radiotherapy, as for example in treating head and neck tumours, or drug treatment can be introduced after primary resection or irradiation to prevent the growth of subclinical micrometastases. The latter use of chemotherapy is frequently referred to as 'adjuvant' chemotherapy, and is now widely used for treating breast carcinomas, lymphomas, and several tumours in children.

Caution must be exercised to prevent additive damage to host tissues, particularly the bone marrow if radiotherapy and chemotherapy are used together, but the principle of combining local and systemic therapy has many potential advantages since as a general principle small tumours are much more susceptible to chemotherapy than large ones. This is explained in part by the fact that drugs penetrate small tumours more effectively but also by the fact that the emergence of drug resistance may be related to the frequency of mutations in the tumour, and the potential number of such events increases with the growth of a tumour.

One major difficulty with adjuvant chemotherapy is to decide for how long it should be continued. In obvious advanced tumours, it is possible to measure tumour shrinkage and continue treatment for as long as benefit lasts. Conversely drug resistance is detectable and thus further inappropriate chemotherapy can be avoided. However, in the 'adjuvant' setting where there is no measurable tumour, it is not possible to be certain in the short term whether or not treatment is proving effective. Clinical trials have demonstrated that, for curable tumours in children, it is necessary to continue chemotherapy for 1–2 years. For lymphomas and carcinomas in adults, the optimum duration of adjuvant chemotherapy is less certain and is the subject of continuing study.

It is possible to rank many malignant diseases into groups comprising those for which chemotherapy contributes to cure, those for which effective control prolongs useful life and those for which benefit is less certain or unproven (Table 6.3). Not all patients in any of these groups prove sensitive or resistant to chemotherapy and there is considerable variation between patients in the degree of responsiveness even amongst the most favourable tumours, but such a classification gives an indication of the diseases where further research is particularly needed.

The side-effects of chemotherapy. Due to the relatively poor selectivity of presently available anticancer drugs, it is impossible to avoid some damage to normal host tissues. Nevertheless, when properly administered and monitored, many cytotoxic drugs can be given without producing side-effects which cause symptoms. For example, reversible *decreases in haemoglobin, leucocytes and platelet counts* should not cause significant symp-

Table 6.3 Contribution of chemotherapy to various malignant diseases.

Tumours for which chemotherapy can be curative:
  Acute lymphoblastic leukaemia in children
  Burkitt's lymphoma
  Hodgkin's lymphoma
  Wilms' tumour
  Rhabdomyosarcoma
  Testicular teratoma
  Choriocarcinoma
  Diffuse histiocytic lymphoma
  Ewing's sarcoma

Tumours that are highly sensitive to chemotherapy, resulting in remissions that prolong life:
  Breast carcinoma
  Ovarian carcinoma
  Small cell anaplastic lung carcinoma
  Non-Hodgkin's lymphoma
  Chronic lymphocytic leukaemia
  Acute myeloid leukaemia
  Medulloblastoma

Tumours that are sensitive to chemotherapy where life is sometimes prolonged:
  Gastric carcinoma
  Pancreatic carcinoma
  Myeloma
  Soft tissue sarcoma
  Bladder carcinoma
  Thyroid carcinoma

Tumours that are usually refractory to currently available chemotherapy:
  Squamous cell lung carcinoma
  Colorectal carcinoma
  Carcinoma of oesophagus
  Melanoma

toms provided adequate time is allowed between cycles of treatment and the blood count is monitored prior to subsequent treatment, thus preventing any cumulative effect.

Acute damage to the gastrointestinal tract may cause mouth ulceration, nausea, vomiting or diarrhoea. Mouth ulceration and diarrhoea result from necrosis of the rapidly dividing epithelial cells lining the gut. Appropriate timing of chemotherapy can prevent this but sometimes it is necessary to adjust the dose of the drug if an individual is particularly sensitive. The complex physiological events leading to nausea and vomiting almost certainly include a direct central nervous system response to many cytotoxic drugs, or their metabolites, but the nature and anatomical site of such chemoreceptors are uncertain. For the cytotoxic drugs which are known to cause nausea and vomiting, it is necessary to prescribe antiemetics, prior to and following administration of the cytotoxic drug, and skilled use of compounds such as metoclopramide (p. 280) can ameliorate these symptoms very successfully.

Alopecia. Despite the fact that it is possible to minimise many acute side-effects, there are several subacute and chronic toxicities which are less susceptible to control. Alopecia, resulting from interruption in the normal proliferation of the hair follicle, is associated with the administration of some of the cytotoxic drugs particularly adriamycin and cyclophosphamide. If such drugs are to be prescribed, it is important to warn the patient in advance and, if appropriate, to arrange for a wig to be fitted. Alopecia is almost always reversible on cessation of therapy.

The *psychological effect* of having to receive chemotherapy over a period of many months is another adverse effect of which the physician must be constantly aware. If properly counselled, many patients tolerate the impact of being informed of their diagnosis and their early treatment remarkably well, only to become anxious and depressed as treatment continues even though their tumour may be obviously responding to treatment. Awareness of this problem is essential and constant reassurance and support are necessary to help patients with the disruption in their lives occasioned by repeated visits to hospital, venepunctures and treatment.

Growth. The chronic toxicity of cancer chemotherapy is an area of increasing importance now that this form of treatment is becoming more widely available, and increasing numbers of patients are surviving for longer periods. Data from the follow-up of children cured of malignant disease have shown that physical growth can be stunted by the use of combinations of cytotoxic drugs with radiation but there is conflicting evidence as to whether or not these agents cause significant intellectual impairment.

Fertility is preserved for the majority of prepubertal children who have to be treated with cytotoxic drugs but for adults, fertility may be lost. This is particularly the case for men. For women the problem is more variable depending on their premorbid menstrual pattern and the length of time prior to the expected menopause. Many patients suffering from malignant diseases may be subfertile at the time of diagnosis and for women amenorrhoea is common for the months during which they are receiving treatment. Nevertheless, this is not a universal finding and since cytotoxic drugs are potentially teratogenic, patients of both sexes should be advised to use contraceptive measures whilst they are receiving chemotherapy.

Second malignancy. With the increasing success of chemotherapy and long-term survival, it has become apparent that cytotoxic drugs may be associated with the development of a second malignancy in a small proportion of patients. The cases described have usually been of acute myelomonocytic leukaemia developing 5–10 years following the use of alkylating agents. For example in a study of over 5000 cases of ovarian cancer treated with alkylating agents, it has been shown that the risk of developing acute leukaemia was 36 times that of the population at large. Nevertheless, it should be emphasised that only certain classes of anticancer drug are associated with this phenomenon which is rare and which has arisen only as a result of developing therapies which may cure the primary tumour.

Accumulative toxicities which are organ specific may be caused by some anticancer drugs. For example the use of adriamycin beyond a total cumulative dose of $550\,mg/m^2$ is associated with a greatly increased risk of developing cardiac failure due to the generation of free radicals that damage cardiac tissue by causing the peroxidation of cardiac lipid. This drug should therefore be prescribed only very exceptionally above this total dose.

Cisplatin causes a progressive impairment of renal function (predominantly tubular) and in addition to monitoring patients for the common side-effects mentioned above, it is necessary to assess renal function prior to subsequent doses of this drug.

Bleomycin may cause pulmonary fibrosis.

The vinca alkaloids, especially vincristine, can cause a neuropathy with cumulative effect. This manifests itself initially as peripheral sensory impairment but later involves motor function and may cause autonomic damage usually presenting as constipation or even intestinal obstruction. The neuropathy due to the vinca alkaloids is reversible on withdrawal of the drug but the cardiac effect of adriamycin, the renal toxicity of cisplatin and the pulmonary fibrosis caused by bleomycin are usually irreversible.

Principles of endocrine therapy

Tumours which develop in organs that are known to be under hormonal control sometimes retain hormonal dependency. This can be used therapeutically either by withdrawing the source of the hormone, by prescribing an anti-hormone or by the administration of another hormone. Carcinomas of the breast, prostate, endometrium and thyroid are the diseases amenable to endocrine therapy. The therapeutic use of adrenal corticosteroids is exceptional in that these compounds influence non-endocrine-related tumours, for example the lymphomas and leukaemias.

The biological effect of hormones such as oestrogen and progesterone is dependent on the hormone binding to a cytoplasmic receptor protein that transports the hormone to the nucleus where it interacts with DNA to modulate gene expression. Oestrogen-binding protein can be assayed in biopsies of breast tumours or lymph nodes containing metastases. It has been found that for about 65% of patients whose tumours possess a significant amount of this protein, removal of the source of oestrogen drive will be therapeutically useful whilst for those in whom this protein is absent, hormonal therapy is usually of no benefit. The presence of progesterone-binding protein further increases the likelihood of hormone sensitivity. The development of techniques to predict hormone sensitivity has had a major influence on the management of patients with breast carcinomas. If oestrogen receptor activity is present then premenopausal patients may benefit from oophorectomy and both pre- and postmenopausal patients may respond to the administration of tamoxifen, a compound that blocks oestrogen binding.

The use of ablative procedures such as adrenalectomy is now being superseded by the availability of compounds like aminoglutethamide which achieves the same result by 'medical' rather than surgical means. Aminoglutethamide inhibits the desmolase that catalyses the conversion of cholesterol to delta-S-pregnenolone, thus preventing the synthesis of corticosteroids, oestrogens and androgens. It also inhibits the aromatase that converts androgens to oestrogens in peripheral tissues. In order to prevent excess secretion of ACTH (as a result of the failure to produce the 11-hydroxycorticosteroids), it is necessary to prescribe hydrocortisone together with aminoglutethamide. Tumour response to tamoxifen and aminoglutethamide may not be manifest for 6–12 weeks from the start of therapy and it is therefore necessary to wait for this period before making decisions about further management. Androgen may produce responses in about 20% of patients with breast cancer, particularly in postmenopausal women with bone metastases.

Oestrogens are useful in the palliation of prostate cancer, and have a similar response rate (c. 80%) to that of orchidectomy which removes the major source of testosterone.

Progestogens are compounds related to the progesterone produced by the corpus luteum and placenta. Some women with metastatic endometrial carcinoma benefit from these drugs, particularly patients with well differentiated tumours.

Some papillary carcinomas of the thyroid remain under the influence of thyroid-stimulating hormone (TSH) and the administration of thyroid hormone may be useful as a result of its inhibiting pituitary secretion of TSH.

The major advantage of hormonal therapy over chemotherapy is that the side-effects of endocrine treatment are usually less severe than those associated with cytotoxic drugs. Tamoxifen rarely causes toxicity but aminoglutethamide can cause drowsiness, depression and transient rashes in some patients. The use of oestrogen in elderly men with prostate cancer warrants special caution in view of its known propensity to exacerbate the fluid retention that may be associated with cardiovascular disease. Research is currently in progress to evaluate compounds that inhibit pituitary gonadotrophin, thus mimicking the effects of castration but doing so in a reversible way, and in a manner that is free of important side-effects.

Terminal care

An essential component of oncological medicine is the management of patients in the terminal phase of their illness. When it becomes apparent that active measures to arrest further tumour growth are no longer proving effective, or for those patients in whom it is not appropriate to embark on such therapy, it is more important than ever to provide support and attention to the alleviation of distressing symptoms. Psychological support is the most important aspect but this can be provided only if positive measures are taken to relieve pain, to ensure adequate and appropriate nutrition and treat specific symptoms such as cough, pruritus and nausea. Successful symptomatic treatment allows patients to prepare themselves mentally for death, and the relief of physical distress in the patient will also help the patient's family to cope with impending bereavement.

An individual patient's reaction to the inevitability of death from a malignant disease depends on a host of interrelated variables including his or her cultural and religious background, age, education, the duration of the illness and the reactions of dependants. Nevertheless certain common patterns of behaviour are recognisable and an awareness of these is important in order to provide appropriate counselling and support at different stages of the patient's progression towards death. A period of initial disbelief and denial is often replaced by resentment and anger. This in turn is followed by a period of depression which is almost universal but many patients, with or without medical intervention, enter a final phase of peacefully accepting the inevitability of death.

When to tell patients that they have a terminal illness is a matter of experience and judgement that cannot easily be summarised. Death does not necessarily represent a failure of treatment and it is essential that those caring for the terminally ill do not avoid discussion of the processes of terminal illness for fear of this being seen as professional failure. Avoiding such discussions can only enhance the patient's sense of loneliness and isolation.

It is not always appropriate to present all of the facts to a patient, most especially on a single occasion, and time must be spent to determine patients' awareness of their situation, and their expectations. Non-committal, even ambiguous statements about the future may be appropriate but the patient should never be told what is known to be untrue.

Preparation for death is not the sole responsibility of the medical profession and, especially for patients dying in hospitals, it is important to make provision for the adequate access of relatives, friends and other professionals such as the clergy when patients request their support. Religious belief does not necessarily make death any easier and even for patients who hold such beliefs it should not be forgotten that fear of the unknown, most especially the unknown of death, is something shared by patients and all those who are caring for them.

The most important principle of managing terminal illness is to provide adequate time for talking with the patient. In a busy world this is difficult to find but it is sometimes easier to use the lack of time as an excuse for avoiding demanding consultations that drain the doctor's emotional resources. Nevertheless, to develop the ability to listen to patients and to learn from them how best to provide psychological support during terminal illness can be one of the most rewarding experiences in medicine.

PROSPECTS IN ONCOLOGY

In a recent survey of the trend in mortality from cancer in the USA it has been estimated that up to 90% of all such deaths could be attributed to potentially avoidable factors, namely tobacco, alcohol, diet, reproductive and sexual behaviour, occupation, pollution and geographical features.

The only cause whose effect is large, and has been reliably identified, is tobacco which is estimated to have been responsible for 130 000–140 000 deaths in the USA in 1981. The public health campaigns emphasising the indisputable association between cigarette tobacco and lung cancer are beginning to prove successful, and there are indications that cigarette consumption is at last starting to decline. There is, however, still a continuing need for such education — aimed particularly at the young to warn them of the dangers of cigarette smoking.

It appears easier to influence dietary habits but research is needed to identify the specific agents responsible for the development of tumours where diet appears to play a role such as gastrointestinal carcinomas. The increase in carcinoma of the uterine cervix appears to be related to changing patterns of sexual behaviour; the screening of women who have started sexual activity at an early age or have had multiple partners should be encouraged because early detection can be curative. As further aetiological factors are identified, it is reasonable to predict that other screening procedures will become useful for certain groups although at present there is no indication for screening the entire population.

Unfortunately, early detection does not guarantee cure for any malignant disease but generally it is easier to treat small tumours than large ones. Similarly, early detection does not necessarily guarantee that tumours have not metastasised but the treatment of localised tumours is likely to continue to yield better long-term results than those for widely disseminated lesions. Technological advances are still required to improve tumour localisation and a number of new imaging techniques are currently being investigated. Magnetic resonance imaging as an alternative to computed tomography looks promising for studying the central nervous system in particular. The development of monoclonal antibodies has lead to immunoscintigraphy, where an antibody raised to tumour tissue is 'labelled' with a radionuclide that can be detected by a camera as in other nuclear medicine procedures for scanning. This technique is limited at present by the poor specificity of available monoclonal antibodies to tumour tissue, and further research is needed before immunoscintigraphy could become generally useful.

Better tumour localisation will lead to improved selection of appropriate patients, and greater accuracy in treating localised tumours with surgery or radiotherapy. However, as regards therapy, the greatest need is to improve the systemic treatment for metastatic tumours. With the exception of endocrine therapy for hormonally-dependent tumours, the only systemic treatment of proven value is cytotoxic chemotherapy. Attempts to modify the immune response with non-specific agents such as BCG ('immunotherapy') have not proven to be successful. However, the antiviral compound interferon has been shown to have antitumour activity—particularly for low grade non-Hodgkin lymphoma and hairy cell leukaemia. Current research is evaluating the effect of combining interferons with cytotoxic drugs for the treatment of several more common malignancies.

The major problem with cytotoxic drugs is their relatively low selectivity for tumour tissues, and much investigation is being pursued to develop less toxic drugs that still maintain their antineoplastic efficacy. Such research is beginning to show results and a number of 'second generation' compounds are now available. For example, analogues of cisplatin with less nephrotoxicity and analogues of doxorubicin with less cardiotoxicity are currently entering clinical trials. Alternative approaches to overcome toxic effects on the host are also being explored, such as the harvesting of bone marrow prior to administering chemotherapy likely to damage the marrow so that unexposed marrow can be reinfused after the drug or drugs have been given. To minimise the unwanted exposure of host tissues, research is being carried out on the use of monoclonal antibodies raised against the tumour to target cytotoxic drugs exclusively to the malignant cells. The efficacy of this attractive idea awaits clinical evaluation. Further research is needed to understand the gastrointestinal side-effects of many cytotoxic drugs but increasing knowledge of the physiological mechanisms controlling nausea and emesis is being used to improve antiemetic therapy.

One of the major problems in cancer chemotherapy is the fact that patients with apparently identical diseases do not respond uniformly to treatment, with the relative predictability of many other pharmaceutical situations. One approach to this variable response is being investigated with the use of monoclonal antibodies to 'phenotype' individual tumours. It is hoped that such characterisation of individual variables will allow more exact classification of tumour subtypes with regard to chemosensitivity, leading to more precise selection of optimal treatment for individual patients.

With such a wide spectrum of clinical problems created by malignant diseases, it is unwise to make specific prediction about the future. Nevertheless it is a fact that at no time in the past has so much attention been focused on the management of these diseases. With the significant progress that has been achieved over the past 20 years, it is reasonable to be cautiously optimistic about the future. This applies most especially to the changing emphasis away from the ultimate objective of cure to the more practical issues of ameliorating symptoms, controlling further progression and relieving the anxieties so frequently created by malignant disease.

J.F. SMYTH

FURTHER READING:

Calman K C, Smyth J F, Tattersall M H N 1980 Basic principles of cancer chemotherapy. MacMillan, New York. A brief introduction to the subject

Clabner B 1982 Pharmacologic principles of cancer treatment. Saunders, Philadelphia. A detailed account both preclinical and clinical

DeVita V T, Hellman S, Rosenburg S A 1982 Cancer, principles and practice of oncology. Lippincott, Philadelphia. This is a comprehensive textbook

Doll R, Peto R 1981 The causes of cancer. Oxford Medical Publications, Oxford. This is a short resumé of the known epidemiological factors

Saunders Dame Cecily 1978 The management of terminal disease. The management of malignant disease, vol 1. Arnold, London. A summary of the theory and practice of terminal care by the Medical Director of St Christopher's Hospice, London

7

Diseases of the cardiovascular system

At all ages and in all countries, diseases of the cardiovascular system are major causes of death and disability, but the pattern of cardiovascular disease varies strikingly between different coun tries and age groups. For example, rheumatic fever, still a major cause of morbidity in young adults in many parts of the world, is now exceedingly rare in Britain. In contrast, ischaemic heart disease is an increasing problem in many countries where it was formerly uncommon, though in the United States and Australia its contribution to mortality seems to be declining. As more people live on into old age, degenerative causes of valvular disease and cardiac conduction problems become increasingly prevalent, while at the other extreme of life a reduction of infant mortality from infective and nutritional causes focuses attention on morbidity from congenital heart disease.

Patients with heart disease present not only with breathlessness, swollen ankles and chest pain, which are its cardinal symptoms, but also with other symptoms less obviously related to the heart, such as stroke resulting from thromboembolism, or fever and anaemia from endocarditis. The presentation of cardiovascular disease is thus protean.

The symptoms of heart disease

Dyspnoea. Awareness of undue breathlessness on exertion is frequently the first symptom of heart failure. From the history alone it may be hard to distinguish this from the dyspnoea which is due to lung disease (p. 203) but the differentiation is often possible if the patient is observed at the time. Typically, patients with cardiac failure take rapid, shallow breaths, and wheezing or the excessive use of accessory respiratory muscles is uncommon. There is often a repetitive cough which, initially at least, is unproductive. Occasionally, in the presence of pulmonary oedema (see below) wheezing does become prominent; this is sometimes called cardiac asthma.

Orthopnoea is the name given to breathlessness which prevents the patient lying flat. On lying down, there is a rise in right atrial pressure and hence in right ventricular output, forcing more blood into the lungs, a tendency for the redistribution of oedema fluid, and perhaps an alteration in the pattern of bloodflow within the lungs. The sensation of breathlessness is probably due partly to increased stiffness of the congested lungs and partly to direct stimulation of fine nerve endings around the alveoli.

Accumulation of excess fluid in the lungs at night may reach a critical level before the patient is wakened by breathlessness and has to sit up to gain relief. This is *paroxysmal nocturnal dyspnoea*. Usually the attack subsides within a few minutes.

The clinical syndrome of *pulmonary oedema* may develop from orthopnoea or paroxysmal nocturnal dyspnoea, or may come on without previous warning as a consequence of myocardial infarction or an arrhythmia. There is extreme breathlessness, and the patient coughs up white frothy sputum which may be tinged with blood. There is tachycardia and peripheral vasoconstriction, and the patient is usually very anxious.

Cheyne Stokes respiration (periodic breathing), in which there is waxing and waning of ventilation from hyperventilation to apnoea, is common in severe cardiac failure. It may also occur in elderly people without evidence of cardiac failure, particularly during sleep.

Peripheral oedema occurs in cardiac failure as a consequence of excessive salt and water retention (p. 92). It is found mainly in the feet and ankles in ambulant patients, as its site is largely determined by gravity. Pressure with the thumb, if sustained, will displace the fluid and leave a pit. On going to bed the oedema is redistributed, principally to the sacrum and thighs. In severe cardiac failure fluid may accumulate in the abdominal cavity (ascites) and as pleural effusions. Oedema resulting from cardiac failure needs to be distinguished from that caused by chronic venous insufficiency in the legs or the nephrotic syndrome (p. 382).

Chest pain. The cardinal symptom of cardiac ischaemia is the pain known as angina pectoris (p. 163). The pain of pericarditis is described on page 182. Precordial catch is the name given to a stabbing pain felt momentarily at the cardiac apex; it is often indicated by a finger pointing below the left breast. It is not associated with cardiac pathology but frequently causes undue concern to the anxious. Hepatic pain felt in the epigastrium is sometimes a feature of acute or worsening cardiac failure. It is due to hepatic distension resulting from a rise in central venous pressure. Pleuritic pain is a feature of pulmonary infarction, which often complicates cardiac failure. A sudden 'tearing' pain in the back, between the shoulder blades, may be due to a dissecting aneurysm of the aorta.

Palpitation is undue awareness of the heart beat; it is a common result of exercise or anxiety and occurs with increased catecholamine secretion or with sympathomimetic drugs. Patients often feel the thump of an ectopic beat or, more often, of the more powerful beat which follows a compensatory pause. Palpitation may be the only symptom of paroxysmal tachycardia; often the patient can indicate its rate, and usually is able to say whether the heart beat is regular as in supraventricular tachycardia or irregular as in atrial fibrillation.

Syncope ('fainting') is loss of consciousness resulting from a fall in blood pressure. The latter may be due to decreased cardiac output, decreased peripheral resistance, or a combination of the two. *Simple* or *vasovagal* syncope is the product of a complex reflex which causes bradycardia and peripheral vasodilatation. It usually occurs in circumstances where venous return to the heart is not adequately maintained, e.g. with prolonged standing, particularly when it is hot or when there is a loss of fluid, as from diarrhoea. Simple syncope may also occur as a result of a frightening, unpleasant or painful experience. A feeling of nausea and sometimes a failure of vision and a ringing in the ears may herald its onset. Pallor, sweating and a slow pulse are characteristic. Recovery is usually rapid when venous return is restored by raising the patient's legs. If the patient is kept upright, convulsions and occasionally brain damage may ensue.

Syncope can also occur when a rise in intrathoracic pressure reduces venous return sufficiently, as in the Valsalva manoeuvre. This may happen with prolonged vigorous coughing (*cough syncope*) or when elderly men strain to empty the bladder (*micturition syncope*). Syncope on standing, *postural syncope*, is a feature in some patients with an unusually low blood pressure as in adrenal insufficiency. More commonly it is due to antihypertensive or vasodilator drugs, and it sometimes results from a failure of the normal vasomotor reflexes as in diabetic autonomic neuropathy.

Cardiac causes of syncope should be suspected when syncope occurs on exertion (*exercise syncope*) or when it occurs in the absence of obvious precipitating circumstances. Exercise syncope may be due to cardiac arrhythmias, or to exercise-induced vasodilatation in patients unable to increase their cardiac output appropriately, perhaps because of severe coronary artery or valvular heart disease. It may be a feature of aortic stenosis, severe pulmonary stenosis or hypertrophic cardiomyopathy. Syncope which occurs without obvious precipitating circumstances needs to be distinguished from epilepsy (p. 616). It is frequently due to cardiac arrhythmias, either excessive bradycardia or tachycardia.

Other symptoms. Tiredness is a common complaint with severe heart failure and with ischaemic heart disease. Sometimes it is the consequence of treatment rather than the disease itself, e.g. beta-blockade or hypokalaemia from diuretics. In those with valvular disease without heart failure it should lead to a suspicion of infective endocarditis.

Nocturia, or a reversal of the usual diurnal rhythm of diuresis, sometimes occurs in ambulant patients with cardiac failure. It probably reflects improved renal perfusion during bed-rest rather than a simple mobilisation of oedema fluid from the ankles. Cough is a feature of pulmonary oedema. Anorexia, nausea and vomiting are all common in severe protracted heart failure; they may also be manifestations of digitalis intoxication (p. 138).

Physical examination

While taking the history and before proceeding to the examination of the heart, certain pertinent observations may be made. The presence should be noted of any anaemia, obesity, breathlessness or cyanosis.

Peripheral cyanosis is due to an excessive extraction of oxygen from the blood when the circulation is impaired from vasoconstriction, low cardiac output or stasis; it occurs in healthy people when the extremities are cold, and warmth abolishes it.

Central cyanosis is due to oxygen under-saturation of the arterial blood from poor gaseous exchange in the lungs resulting from respiratory failure or pulmonary oedema, or when there is a right-to-left shunt as in congenital heart disease. If the tongue is cyanosed it may be deduced that the cyanosis is central in origin. A combination of central and peripheral cyanosis is often seen in cardiac failure.

Other observations. The temperature of the skin varies with the skin blood flow. In cardiac failure, except in those rare forms where the cardiac output is increased, the extremities are abnormally cold, even in a warm environment. Unduly moist palms suggest anxiety if they are cold or thyrotoxicosis if they are warm. Clubbing of the fingers occurs in cyanotic congenital heart disease and in advanced infective endocarditis, as well as in a variety of respiratory and other diseases (p. 205).

Subungual or 'splinter' haemorrhages may result from trauma and occur in normal individuals, but they are also a feature of infective endocarditis.

The arterial pulse should be examined for rate, rhythm and volume, and for the character of the pulse wave. The radial pulse is traditionally used, but the carotid is more reliable for assessing the pulse wave because its form is less altered by transmission. Bradycardia (p. 129) describes a heart rate of 60 per minute or less, and tachycardia (p. 130) a heart rate of 100 or more. In health the pulse is normally regular, but a slowing of the pulse in expiration (sinus arrhythmia p. 129) is common, particularly in children. The other causes of irregularity are discussed on pages 129–135.

A pulse of small volume is a feature of reduced cardiac output, as in major haemorrhage or pulmonary embolism, or with severe obstruction to bloodflow at a cardiac valve. A pulse of large volume, sometimes called a collapsing pulse, is found where there is rapid flow of blood out of the arterial system with peripheral vasodilatation as in fever or hyperthyroidism, or with aortic regurgitation. A pulse of large volume may also accompany bradycardia, as in complete heart block.

Pulsus paradoxus is a name given to a variation of pulse volume with breathing, in which systolic pressure diminishes with inspiration. A small variation of this nature is physiological (so the 'paradox' is misnamed), but it is abnormal for there to be more than 5 mmHg difference between inspiratory and expiratory systolic blood pressures during ordinary quiet breathing, or for the difference to be readily palpable. An exaggerated fall in systolic pressure during inspiration may occur in asthma or, for a different reason, in patients with constrictive pericarditis or pericardial tamponade from a tense pericardial effusion (p. 182).

Pulsus alternans is regular but its amplitude is alternately large and small. It is best detected with the sphygmomanometer; there may be a difference of 10–40 mmHg between the strong and weak beats. It is a sign of left ventricular failure.

In aortic stenosis the pulse is characteristically slow-rising, with a shudder or vibratory feel to the upstroke. A pulse with a double peak, *pulsus bisferiens*, is suggestive of combined aortic stenosis (usually mild) and <u>regurgitation</u>.

In old age, arteries become more rigid, and this may affect the way they transmit the pulse wave. They also elongate and become more tortuous. In elderly patients, particularly hypertensive women, an arterial pulsation may be seen above the right clavicle because of 'kinking' of a tortuous carotid artery.

Arterial pulsation in the neck is increased in <u>aortic regurgitation</u> and sometimes in <u>coarctation of the aorta</u>. A bruit heard over a major artery with the stethoscope bell is an important sign of partial obstruction but needs to be distinguished from a murmur conducted from the aortic valve.

In hypertensive patients, and in children suspected of having congenital heart disease, the <u>radial and femoral pulses should be palpated simultaneously</u> in order to detect <u>coarctation of the aorta</u>. In this condition the femoral pulse is seldom absent, but it is of small volume, delayed after the radial pulse, and measurement of the arterial pressure in the legs with a suitably large cuff shows it to be lower than in the arms.

Jugular venous pulse. With the patient reclining against pillows at about <u>45°</u>, and with the neck muscles relaxed, the jugular venous pulse may be examined from movement of the skin overlying the internal jugular vein, although the vein itself is not visible. Unlike arterial pulsation, jugular venous pulsation represents the zone of transition between distended and collapsed segments of vein, and the height of this above the level of the right atrium is a measure of the right atrial, or central venous, pressure. In normal subjects, or in those with a low central venous pressure, jugular pulsation is often hidden behind the clavicle in this position, and rarely extends for more than 2 or 3 cm above the sternal angle. When venous pressure is transiently increased by pressure on the abdomen, the level of pulsation moves upwards in the neck: this is called *hepato-jugular reflux* and is one of the ways in which the jugular pulse can be distinguished from arterial pulsation.

The venous pulse varies with the patient's position and the phase of respiration; it frequently exhibits <u>two peaks</u> to every one of the arterial pulse (Fig. 7.1), and the most prominent movement is often an inward one. It is often taught that the venous pulse is <u>impalpable</u> and that it can be

abolished by pressure on the root of the neck, but these criteria are not infallible.

It is usual to express *jugular venous pressure* (which is equivalent to central venous pressure) as the vertical distance in centimetres between the zone of jugular pulsation and the sternal angle. Sometimes the jugular pressure is so high that pulsation is apparent only when the patient sits or stands upright. <u>The commonest and most</u> important cause of a raised jugular venous pressure is cardiac failure. Sometimes it is possible to find out more about the cause of the failure by analysing the wave form of the pulse.

The *wave form of the jugular venous pulse* in a patient in sinus rhythm is shown in Figure 7.1. The *a* wave is due to <u>atrial systole</u>. It is <u>absent in atrial fibrillation,</u> and may be <u>abnormally large when there is obstruction to right atrial discharge, as in tricuspid stenosis,</u> or when the <u>right ventricle is hypertrophied and stiff, as in pulmonary stenosis or pulmonary hypertension</u>. With tricus-

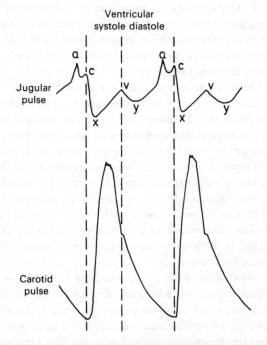

Fig. 7.1 Carotid and jugular pulses. Simultaneous central arterial and venous pulses to demonstrate carotid and jugular pulse wave form. a = atrial contraction, c = onset of ventricular contraction, v = pressure peak immediately prior to opening of tricuspid valve, c–x = x descent, v–y = y descent.

pid regurgitation there are prominent waves in the venous pulse in time with ventricular systole; these are often called *v* waves but the mechanism and timing are different from the physiological *v* waves shown in Figure 7.1.

In patients with atrioventricular dissociation (p. 140) intermittent large volume systolic waves may be seen in the venous pulse; these are called *cannon waves,* and occur when the atrium contracts against a closed tricuspid valve.

Examination of the heart. The methods employed are inspection, palpation, percussion and auscultation; at each stage the intelligent use of one of these methods often makes the deployment of the next easier.

INSPECTION. In children, enlargement of the right ventricle during the growing period may show as a prominence to the left of the sternum. The apical impulse (see below) may be visible, and its position may give a clue to cardiac enlargement. The sustained apical impulse of left ventricular hypertrophy, and the diffuse pulsation over a left ventricular aneurysm can often be seen as well as felt. Occasionally an aneurysm of the aortic arch can be seen to move the upper sternum with each systole; when the heart is very much enlarged, as with advanced valvular disease, the whole chest may move with each beat.

Systolic pulsation in the epigastrium caused by aortic pulsation is quite common in thin healthy individuals. Pulsation in the epigastrium and right hypochondrium may also be due to hepatic pulsation in tricuspid regurgitation; correct interpretation is enabled by recognising the accompanying systolic jugular venous pulsation.

PALPATION. It is best briefly to palpate the whole of the precordium with the flat of the hand before attempting to localise the apex beat, and then to return to areas of special interest for detailed analysis.

The *apex beat* is the furthest outward and downward point where the finger is lifted during systole; localisation may be impossible if there is obesity or emphysema. In health the apex beat is within the mid-clavicular line in the fifth intercostal space. Significant displacement of the apex beat to the left usually indicates cardiac enlargement, but more reliable evidence is provided by a chest radiograph. If the mediastinum is displaced by fibrosis, collapse or removal of the lung on the left side or by a large pleural effusion on the right, the apex beat may lie to the left in the absence of cardiac enlargement.

The quality of the cardiac impulse should be noted. In left ventricular hypertrophy it is forceful and sustained, while abrupt closure of the mitral valve, either with anxiety or when associated with mitral stenosis, may give it a tapping quality. When the heart is dilated, as for example in dilated cardiomyopathy or advanced ischaemic heart disease, the apex is displaced to the left but the impulse is diffuse rather than forceful.

With right ventricular hypertrophy a pulsation may be imparted to the hand on the chest to the left of the sternum. This may also result when the heart is displaced forward by a dilated left atrium. A dilated pulmonary artery under abnormally high pressure may cause a pulsation in the second left intercostal space beside the sternum. Closure of the semilunar valves under abnormal pressure may give a diastolic shock, or palpable second heart sound.

Thrills. Turbulent flow may impart a vibration to the hand; this thrill is the palpable equivalent of a murmur. Usually only loud murmurs are associated with thrills, but a low-pitched vibration is sometimes felt as readily as it is heard. A systolic thrill at the apex usually indicates mitral regurgitation, and a diastolic thrill mitral stenosis. A systolic thrill can often be felt at the lower left sternal edge with a ventricular septal defect, and at the upper sternal edge in aortic or pulmonary stenosis. An aortic diastolic thrill is very rare and usually indicates rupture of an aortic valve cusp.

PERCUSSION is seldom used except when seeking abnormal dullness to the right of the sternum in a patient with a suspected pericardial effusion. One of the physical signs of emphysema is a loss of the normal area of cardiac dullness.

AUSCULTATION. It is essential to use a satisfactory stethoscope with both diaphragm and bell. The diaphragm, firmly pressed against the chest, preferentially conveys high pitched sounds and murmurs, whereas the bell, lightly applied to the skin, favours the transmission of those that are lower pitched.

Sounds. The *first heart sound* results particularly from the closure of the mitral, and to a lesser extent of the tricuspid valve. It is loudest at the apex and may be diminished in the presence of obesity or emphysema. It is accentuated by tachycardia, as in anxiety or thyrotoxicosis, and is often abnormally loud in mitral stenosis (p. 155). The first sound may be diminished when the valve fails to close properly in mitral regurgitation, or when left ventricular function is impaired by myocarditis or cardiomyopathy. It may be obscured by the murmur of mitral regurgitation. Both mitral and tricuspid components may be audible (as a 'split' first heart sound) when contraction of one ventricle is delayed, as in bundle branch block and also in some healthy individuals.

The *second heart sound* is due to closure of the aortic and pulmonary valves. Normally, closure is synchronous in expiration, but in inspiration the pulmonary component is delayed because of increased right ventricular filling and the aortic component is advanced because of decreased left ventricular filling, so the second heart sound becomes split. This *physiological inspiratory splitting* is most prominent in children and young adults. Abnormally delayed closure of one of the semilunar valves may result from conduction or mechanical factors. An example of the former is when aortic closure is delayed by left bundle branch block. This leads to *reversed splitting* of the second heart sound, splitting being heard in expiration rather than in inspiration. Increased right ventricular stroke volume from a left to right shunt, together with equalisation of left and right atrial pressures, leads to wide, *fixed splitting* of the second heart sound throughout the respiratory cycle in atrial septal defect.

Various added sounds may also be significant. In the young a low pitched mid-diastolic *third heart sound*, at the end of the rapid phase of diastolic left ventricular filling, is often heard at the apex. In older patients this sound is associated with abnormal left ventricular filling, either from an increased stroke volume as in mitral regurgitation, or from altered left ventricular compliance, as in cardiomyopathy. In the latter case it usually implies actual or incipient cardiac failure.

A *fourth heart sound* indicates an abnormally forceful left ventricular distension as a result of atrial discharge; it occurs just before the first heart sound, and may be palpable as well as audible.

It is a feature of long-standing hypertension, hypertrophic cardiomyopathy, ischaemic heart disease and other conditions associated with left ventricular hypertrophy or reduced compliance.

The *opening snap* is a feature of mitral stenosis with a pliant mitral valve. It is best heard with the diaphragm of the stethoscope to the left of the lower sternum.

An *ejection sound* is an early systolic click which occurs at the time of opening of the relevant semilunar valve in aortic or pulmonary stenosis or when there is dilatation of the proximal aorta or pulmonary artery. A *systolic click*, or sometimes multiple clicks, may be a feature of mitral valve prolapse.

Prosthetic sounds. Mechanical replacement heart valves also produce added heart sounds; there is usually a loud click indicating valve closure and a quieter one indicating valve opening. With a mitral prosthesis the closing sound accompanies the first heart sound, and the opening click has the same timing as an opening snap.

Murmurs are associated with turbulent blood flow. When cardiac output is greatly increased, as with pregnancy or severe anaemia, the blood flow through a normal pulmonary or aortic valve may become turbulent and give rise to a systolic murmur, usually best heard in the second left intercostal space at the sternal border. Murmurs also arise when blood is projected through, or leaks back through, abnormal valves; the murmurs then usually radiate in the direction of the abnormal flow.

In coming to a decision as to the cause of a murmur it is important to note whether it occurs in systole or diastole, where it is best heard, and the direction in which the sound of the murmur is conducted. The pitch and quality of the murmur are also important. The characteristics of the main murmurs are shown in Figures 7.29, 7.30 and 7.32. As a general rule a harsh murmur, like a saw, is usually systolic; this should be confirmed by simultaneous palpation of the carotid artery or by identifying that the murmur precedes the second heart sound. The murmur of regurgitation through either of the semilunar valves is usually best heard down the left sternal edge. Because of its quality it is easily confused with a breath sound, and it is often best heard with the patient leaning forward and the breath held in expiration. The murmur of mitral stenosis, on the other hand, is low pitched and is most likely to be heard if the bell of the stethoscope is lightly pressed at or near the apex with the patient turned half towards the left side, particularly after exercise.

Blood pressure. The inflatable cuff of a sphygmomanometer is wrapped carefully round the upper arm with the bag over the brachial artery and is connected with a mercury or aneroid manometer. The bell of the stethoscope is applied over the brachial artery and the cuff is inflated to a level well above that which abolishes the Korotkov sounds. The pressure in the cuff is then allowed to fall slowly and the point of return of the sounds is taken as the systolic pressure. As the pressure falls further the sounds become louder, and then usually quite suddenly they become muffled (phase 4) and later disappear (phase 5). In some people a phase 5 endpoint cannot be reached. Although it has been traditional in Britain to use the phase 4 reading to indicate diastolic pressure, there is less observer variation with the phase 5 endpoint. It is good practice to record both, e.g. 140/90–85, where 140 mmHg is the systolic and 90 and 85 mmHg the phase 4 and 5 diastolic readings respectively.

When the blood pressure is to be recorded in the leg the patient lies prone, a special large cuff is applied to the thigh, and the stethoscope diaphragm is placed over the popliteal fossa.

The *pulse pressure* is the difference between the systolic and diastolic pressures; it tends to be abnormally high in the elderly who have rigid arteries and in patients with conditions that give rise to an increased stroke volume.

Arterial pressure is difficult to measure by the cuff method when there is severe peripheral vasoconstriction, or when there is marked beat to beat variation as in atrial fibrillation.

Blood pressure varies throughout the day, falling to low levels during sleep and rising with stress or anxiety. Isolated blood pressure records can therefore prove misleading, particularly in those who are unduly anxious. Sometimes this is manifest from tremor, sweating or tachycardia. In nervous patients repeated blood pressure estimations tend to result in progressively lower figures, but not invariably.

It would be helpful if normal blood pressure could be clearly defined, but this is not feasible because it varies according to circumstances, particularly age. In an infant, levels of 90/60 would be normal; in the 20-year-old age group, blood pressure taken at rest in most normal subjects varies between about 140/90 and 95/55, and there is a tendency for systolic, and to a lesser extent diastolic, pressures to increase with age. The problem is further discussed in the section on hypertension.

Investigation

Electrocardiography plays an essential role in the diagnosis and investigation of heart disease. Its main value lies in the elucidation of cardiac arrhythmias and conduction defects, and in the diagnosis and localisation of myocardial infarction. It also provides important information about problems such as digitalis toxicity, electrolyte disturbances and hypertrophy of the various chambers of the heart. However, difficulties with interpretation are common and the electrocardiogram (ECG) must always be viewed in the light of the clinical findings and the results of other investigations.

The normal resting cardiac cell is polarised as a result of an ionic gradient across the cell wall produced by a sodium pump which reduces the intracellular and increases the extracellular sodium concentration; the ionic balance is preserved by a high intracellular and low extracellular potassium concentration. It is the potassium gradient across the cell membrane which is mainly responsible for the electrical potential difference across it.

When the membrane is electrically stimulated, there is a sudden inrush of sodium ions, and the cell becomes depolarised. Although impermeability to sodium is rapidly restored, a slow inward flux of calcium ions is also triggered, and helps to prolong the depolarisation. Repolarisation is finally achieved by inactivation of the calcium flux and a transient increase in potassium permeability. Since cardiac cells are connected by electrically-conducting junctions, membrane depolarisation spreads as a wave through the whole myocardium.

It is principally the movement of the depolarisation wave, and the ensuing wave of repolarisation, which are detected by the surface electrocardiogram.

It is conventional to use a series of different electrode positions to record the ECG. Each pair of electrode positions is called a *lead*. Usually, 12 leads are recorded, called leads I, II, III, aVR, aVL and aVF (the limb leads) and V1 to V6 (the chest leads). Further details on the placement of the electrodes and the names of the leads are given in Figure 7.2. It is a useful simplification to imagine each lead 'looking at' electrical activity in the heart from a specific direction (Fig. 7.3). The machine is connected so that movement of the depolarisation wave towards the 'observer' causes an upward deflection and movement away from the observer a downward one. As depolarisation proceeds in many directions simultaneously, the

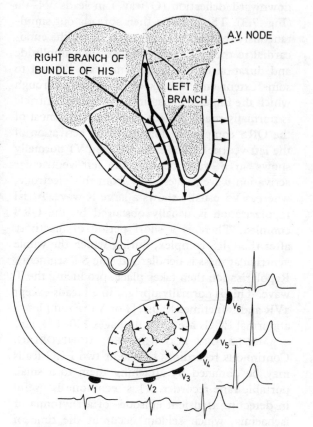

Fig. 7.3 Activation of septum and ventricles. Activation of the septum is from left to right by the left branch of the bundle of His and is followed by spread of the impulse throughout both ventricles. The lower illustration also shows the placement of the chest leads and how each 'looks at' the heart.

ECG represents the summation of these events.

Normally cardiac activation starts in the sinoatrial (SA) node, but this cannot be detected by the ECG. The impulse then flows through the atrium producing the P wave. The only point at which it can pass to ventricular tissue is at the atrioventricular (AV) node, through which conduction is relatively slow. It then goes rapidly through the right and left branches of the bundle of His to the Purkinje fibres of the ventricles. The next part of the ECG—the QRS complex— represents various components of ventricular depolarisation. The interventricular septum is first activated by the left bundle branch from left to right, producing an initial upward deflection (R wave) in leads V1 and V2, and an initial

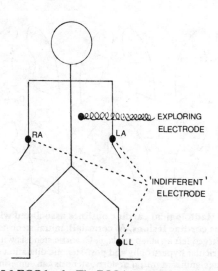

Fig. 7.2 ECG leads. The ECG is recorded using electrodes attached to each of the limbs and a mobile electrode which is moved to different positions to record the chest leads. The electrode attached to the right leg is used as an earth connection. The standard (bipolar) leads record the potential difference between the two limbs (lead I: left arm — right arm; lead II: left leg — right arm; lead III: left leg — left arm). Unipolar leads, designated by the letter V, use an exploring electrode placed on a chosen site and linked with an indifferent electrode whose potential is close to zero. The indifferent electrode is formed by connecting all three limb electrodes (i.e. both arms and left leg as shown above) in the case of the chest leads, or in the case of the augmented (a) unipolar limb leads (aVR, aVL, aVF) by connecting the two limb electrodes which are not being used as the exploring electrode.

downward deflection (Q wave) in leads V4–V6 (Fig. 7.3). The impulse then spreads out simultaneously through both ventricles from the endocardial to the epicardial surfaces. The amplitude and duration of the QRS complexes depend to some extent on the bulk of the muscle through which the impulse is passing; as the left ventricle is normally much thicker than the right, most of the QRS complex is dominated by activation of the left ventricle. For example, lead V1 normally shows an S wave because the left ventricular activation wave moves away from this electrode, whereas V5 usually shows a large R wave. Atrial repolarisation is usually obscured by the QRS complex. There is a short period of inactivity after the QRS complex, during which the whole ventricular mass is depolarised (the ST segment). Repolarisation then takes place, producing the T wave. This is normally upright in all leads except aVR and sometimes leads III or V1. Examples of abnormal ECGs are given on pages 130–134, etc.

AMBULATORY ECG (HOLTER) MONITORING. Continuous recordings of one or two ECG leads may be obtained by attaching them to a small portable tape recorder. This technique is useful in detecting transient episodes of arrhythmia or ischaemia, which seldom occur at the time of routine 12-lead ECG recordings.

Radiological examination is important for determining the size and shape of the heart, and the state of the pulmonary blood vessels. Most information is given by a postero-anterior (PA) projection taken in full inspiration. Antero-posterior (AP) projections are less useful because the heart outline is distorted owing to its distance from the film.

A rough estimate of overall heart size can be made by comparing the maximum width of the cardiac outline with the transverse diameter of the thoracic cavity at the same level. The cardiothoracic ratio so determined should be less than 0.5. Dilatation of individual cardiac chambers can be recognised by the characteristic alterations they cause to the cardiac silhouette (Figs 7.4 and 7.5 and also the sections on valvular heart disease). A barium swallow to outline the oesophagus coupled with a lateral or oblique projection sometimes helps to determine the size of the left atrium. Lateral or oblique projections are also useful in

detecting aortic or mitral valve calcification, which may be obscured by the spine on the PA view.

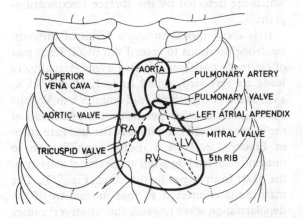

Fig. 7.4 The radiological outline of the heart and the surface projection of its valves.

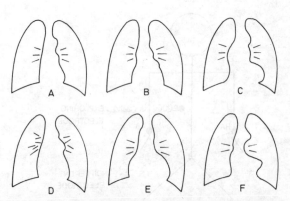

Fig. 7.5 Radiological cardiac outlines associated with different cardiac lesions. A: normal; B: mitral stenosis with enlarged left atrial appendage; C: aortic stenosis with left ventricular hypertrophy and post-stenotic dilatation of the aorta (significant mitral or aortic stenosis can sometimes occur without any visible abnormality of the postero-anterior chest radiograph); D: dilatation of the main pulmonary artery and its proximal branches in pulmonary hypertension; E: generalised cardiac enlargement (or pericardial effusion); F: tetralogy of Fallot. Note lack of prominence of pulmonary artery and its branches, and elevation of cardiac apex by enlarged right ventricle.

A rise in pulmonary venous pressure from left-sided cardiac failure first shows on the chest radiograph as an abnormal distension of the upper lobe pulmonary veins in the erect position. Subsequently, interstitial oedema causes thickened septa and dilated lymphatics which show as horizontal lines in the costophrenic angles (Kerley 'B' lines). More advanced changes are a hazy opacification spreading from the hilar region, and pleural effusion. An increased pulmonary blood flow, as in congenital heart disease with a left-to-right shunt, causes enlargement of the pulmonary artery and a generalised increase in pulmonary vascular markings. Pulmonary arterial hypertension also causes an enlargement of the main pulmonary artery and of the proximal pulmonary arteries, but the peripheral lung vascular markings tend to be diminished.

Radioscopy (screening) of the heart, using an image intensifier, may help in the detection of abnormal cardiac pulsations and of valvular calcification. Its main use, however, is during cardiac catheterisation and pacemaker implantation.

Echocardiography uses ultrasound to study the disposition and movement of valves and other structures within the heart. It depends on the reflection of ultrasound waves at interfaces between blood and more solid tissues.

In *M-mode echocardiography* the ultrasound is focused into a narrow beam, and the output is a graph against time of the movement relative to the chest wall of those structures through which the beam passes (Fig. 7.6). Characteristic patterns of movement are produced in, for example, mitral stenosis, and pericardial effusions are easily recognised. Accurate measurements can be made of cardiac dimensions.

In *two-dimensional (or cross-sectional) real-time echocardiography*, the ultrasound beam is swung rapidly back and forth over an arc or sector and the resulting information synthesised into a two-dimensional map or picture of the position of the reflecting structures on a television screen (Fig. 7.7). The picture is the equivalent of a 'slice' through the heart, and the structures shown will depend on the position and orientation of the ultrasound crystal. Because the beam oscillates very rapidly, the ultrasound image accurately reproduces the movement of structures in the living heart (hence 'real time'). This type of echocardiography is particularly good at detecting intracardiac masses, such as thrombi or tumours, or endocarditic vegetations. It is also very useful in sorting out complex structural abnormalities in congenital heart disease.

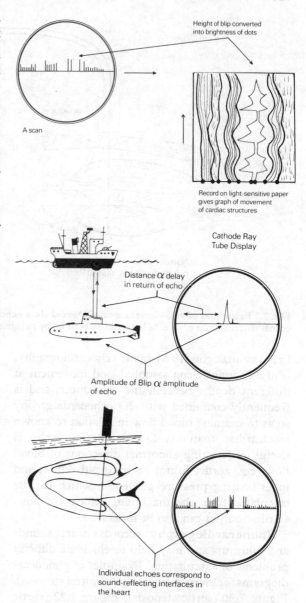

Height of blip converted into brightness of dots

A scan

Record on light-sensitive paper gives graph of movement of cardiac structures

Cathode Ray Tube Display

Distance α delay in return of echo

Amplitude of Blip α amplitude of echo

Individual echoes correspond to sound-reflecting interfaces in the heart

Fig. 7.6 Principles of M-Mode echocardiography. The reflected echoes of ultrasound are converted into blips of light on a cathode-ray tube. The blips can be used to plot a 'graph against time' of the position of cardiac structures on a moving strip of paper.

Doppler cardiography depends on the fact that sound waves reflected from moving objects, such as intracardiac red blood cells, undergo a frequency shift. This can be used to detect the speed and direction of movement of the red cells, and thus of the blood in the heart. 'Continuous wave' doppler uses a narrow beam of ultrasound

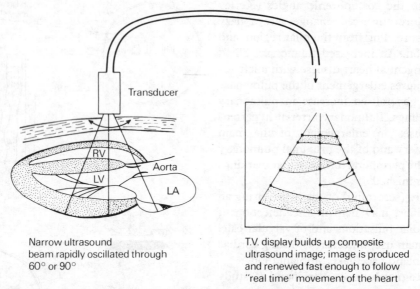

Narrow ultrasound
beam rapidly oscillated through
60° or 90°

T.V. display builds up composite
ultrasound image; image is produced
and renewed fast enough to follow
"real time" movement of the heart

Fig. 7.7 Principles of two-dimensional (2D) real time echocardiography. A moving, two-dimensional image of the echoes detected from a 'slice' of heart can be built up by swinging the ultrasound beam rapidly back and forth.

in a way analogous to M-mode echocardiography. 'Pulsed' doppler can sample blood movement at different depths beneath the transducer, and is frequently combined with 2D echocardiography so as to examine blood flow in relation to known intracardiac anatomy. Doppler cardiography is useful in detecting abnormal directions of blood flow, e.g. aortic, mitral or tricuspid reflux, and in estimating pressure gradients, which can be calculated from the maximum velocity of flow. Cardiac output can also be measured.

Phonocardiography records heart sounds and murmurs and may help to elucidate difficult problems of auscultation. Examples of phonocardiograms are given in Figure 7.29 (mitral stenosis), Figure 7.30 (aortic stenosis), Figure 7.32 (aortic regurgitation), Figure 7.39 (persistent ductus arteriosus), Figure 7.41 (atrial septal defect) and Figure 7.42 (ventricular septal defect).

Cardiac catheterisation and angiocardiography. In contrast to the preceding investigations, these are invasive techniques. A catheter inserted into a vein can be advanced into the right atrium, and then manipulated into the right ventricle and pulmonary artery. In the presence of an atrial septal defect or patent foramen ovale, venous catheters can also enter the left atrium and left ventricle. If the atrial septum is intact, access

to the left ventricle is usually by retrograde passage of a catheter across the aortic valve. Left atrial pressure can be measured directly by puncturing the interatrial septum with a special long, curved needle via a catheter passed up the femoral vein to the right atrium. For many purposes, however, a satisfactory approximation to left atrial pressure can be recorded by 'wedging' an end-hole venous catheter in a branch of the pulmonary artery.

Cardiac catheters are usually manipulated under radiographic control using an image-intensifier, but if a venous catheter is provided at its distal end with a small balloon which can be inflated when the catheter is in the right atrium then the blood stream itself will guide the catheter through the right ventricle and into the pulmonary artery. The balloon also makes it easy to 'wedge' the catheters so as to estimate left atrial pressure. These Swan-Ganz catheters (p. 145) are used in intensive and coronary care units, where they can be inserted without the need to transfer the patient to a radiology department.

Pressure measurements obtained through cardiac catheters can be used to assess the severity of valvular stenoses, and measurement of ventricular end-diastolic pressures gives an indication of ventricular compliance and indirectly of ventricular function. Measurement of oxygen saturation in samples withdrawn via the catheters at different sites in the heart allow the detection of intracardiac left to right or right to left shunts, and also allows calculation of pulmonary and systemic blood flow. Cardiac output can also be measured by dye-dilution or thermodilution techniques.

Catheters allow the injection of radio-opaque contrast medium into individual chambers of the heart, the aorta or pulmonary artery, or, using specially shaped catheters, into either coronary artery.

Radionuclide scanning. The availability of radionuclides of short half life emitting gamma rays, together with the gamma camera for detecting this radiation has made it possible to use radionuclides for studying cardiac function. Two basic types of technique are available:

1. BLOOD POOL SCANNING. The isotope is injected into the blood stream and mixes with the circulating blood. The gamma camera detects the amount of isotope-emitting blood in the heart at different phases of the cardiac cycle, and also the size and 'shape' of the cardiac chambers. By linking the gamma camera to the ECG it is possible to collect information over several cardiac cycles. The principal use of blood pool scanning is as an accurate and reproducible measure of left ventricular function, and for detecting left ventricular aneurysms.

2. MYOCARDIAL SCANNING. Although this uses the same gamma camera, both the radionuclides used and the concepts involved differ from blood pool scanning. The object is usually to distinguish between ischaemic and non-ischaemic myocardium (using radioactive thallium) or between normal and damaged myocardium (using radio-active pyrophosphate).

Radionuclide scanning is also of great value in detecting pulmonary embolism, particularly if the injection of an isotope into the blood stream is combined with a study of the distribution of an inhaled radioactive gas (ventilation-perfusion scanning).

DISORDERS OF CARDIAC RATE, RHYTHM AND CONDUCTION

The control of cardiac rate. Some cardiac cells have the faculty of self excitation. The pacemaking of the heart is due to this activity, and it is normally controlled by the cells with the fastest natural rate. These are usually in the sinoatrial node. The SA node has its own intrinsic rate but it is also under nervous control; vagal activity slows it and sympathetic activity accelerates it. If the sinus rate becomes unduly slow, lower centres may take over the pacemaking, e.g. either the AV node (junctional rhythm), or sometimes an ectopic ventricular focus. At other times the natural rate of lower centres may be increased as a result of disturbances of cellular metabolism, such as occur with electrolyte disorders, digitalis excess, or as a result of cellular damage from myocardial disease.

Sometimes, as a consequence of congenital abnormality or acquired disease, there are alternative pathways for the conduction of the impulse. A premature, ectopic impulse may find the normal pathway refractory, and then has to take a different course. As shown in Figure 7.8, this can sometimes lead to an abnormal re-entry movement of electrical activity and is one of the causes of paroxysmal tachycardia.

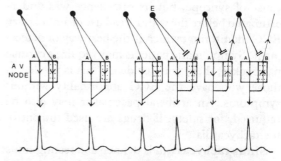

Fig. 7.8 Mechanism of re-entry tachycardia. In this example there are two alternative pathways, A and B, through the AV node. B has a longer refractory period than A. The atrial ectopic beat E finds pathway B refractory, but travels through A. On reaching the end of A, the impulse finds that B has now completed its refractory period, so the impulse can now travel retrogradely to give a further premature atrial beat, which repeats the process. The result is a re-entry or reciprocating tachycardia.

Sinus rhythms

Sinus arrhythmia is a phasic alteration in heart rate in time with breathing; the rate increases in inspiration. It is a manifestation of normal autonomic nervous activity, and is often particularly pronounced in children. A complete absence of variation in heart rate with breathing or with changes in posture may be a feature of autonomic neuropathy.

Sinus bradycardia is arbitrarily defined as a sinus rate of less than 60 per minute. This may occur in normal people during sleep, and is a common finding in athletes. It can be caused by several drugs, e.g. beta-adrenoceptor antagonists. It may also be a feature of myxoedema, jaundice or raised intracranial pressure, and occurs in some patients after myocardial infarction.

Sinoatrial disease (the sick sinus syndrome) is characterised by inappropriate bradycardia, episodes of sinus arrest (with absent P waves on the ECG), an increased liability to paroxysmal tachyarrhythmias, and a tendency to delayed or absent return of sinus node activity following termination of a tachyarrhythmia. The underlying pathology is uncertain but SA node fibrosis or degeneration may occur. There may be associated AV node dysfunction.

Sinoatrial disease may occur at any age, but is most common in the elderly. It is an important cause of syncope, but its prevalence was underestimated before the widespread use of ambulatory ECG monitoring, which is the best way of detecting it. Symptomatic patients may require a cardiac pacemaker; there is no evidence this is needed in those who have the ECG abnormality without symptoms. An artificial pacemaker may also be required, for safety, if drugs are used to control the tachycardia.

Sinus tachycardia is defined as a resting sinus rate of more than 100 per minute. It is a feature of anxiety, fever, hyperthyroidism and acute circulatory or cardiac failure. Except in infants, the rate seldom exceeds 160 per minute. Apart from the rapid rate, the ECG is normal.

Ectopic rhythms

When the impulses arise elsewhere than in the SA node the rhythm is called ectopic; it may be regular or irregular. Ectopic rhythms arise either because of increased automaticity of pacemaker cells, or because of re-entry circuits (Fig. 7.8).

They can broadly be classified into supraventricular (arising in the atria, AV node or other AV junctional tissue) and ventricular.

Supraventricular ectopic rhythms

Ectopic beats (*extrasystoles, premature beats*). These usually cause no symptoms but can give the sensation of an extra or thumping beat. The rhythm is basically regular, but premature beats may occur either at regular intervals or apparently randomly. If sufficiently premature they may produce no pulse, but their presence can usually be detected with the stethoscope. The ECG (Fig. 7.9) shows a premature beat with a normal QRS complex; the conformation of the P wave is often different because the impulse starts at an abnormal site.

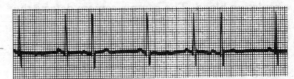

Fig. 7.9 Atrial ectopic beats. The QRS complexes of the two ectopic beats are similar to those of the normal beats and are preceded by a P wave.

Supraventricular tachycardia (Fig. 7.10). Paroxysmal tachycardia may occur with a rate of between 140 and 220 as a result of re-entry or a rapidly firing ectopic focus in the atria or AV node. This usually occurs in hearts which are otherwise normal and may last from a few seconds to a day or two when untreated. The patient is usually aware that the heart has suddenly started to beat fast, and may feel faint or breathless. With prolonged attacks polyuria is sometimes a feature. Particularly if the heart is otherwise abnormal, cardiac pain or left ventricular failure may occur.

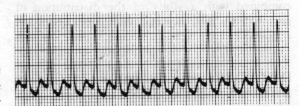

Fig. 7.10 Atrial tachycardia. The rate is 190 per minute. The QRS complexes are normal.

Coffee, alcohol, tobacco, anxiety or hyperthyroidism may be precipitating factors.

The ECG confirms the tachycardia and shows a QRST of normal configuration; occasionally, bundle branch block develops at rapid rates. Massage of the carotid sinus on one side for a few seconds may terminate an attack. If it does not do so, a sedative and retiring to bed may be all that is required; many patients then awake to find that the attack is over. If the attack is causing severe symptoms it can usually be terminated by intravenous verapamil, by a beta-adrenoceptor antagonist or disopyramide, or in an emergency by cardioversion (p. 142). Digoxin is also effective but takes longer to work. If attacks are frequent or otherwise disabling, oral therapy with any of the above drugs may help to reduce their frequency. In resistant cases amiodarone is helpful. Further information about antiarrhythmic drugs is given on pages 136-139.

The Wolff-Parkinson-White (WPW) syndrome results from the presence of an abnormal band of atrioventricular conducting tissue which can bypass the AV node. In normal sinus rhythm conduction takes place partly through the AV node and partly through the more rapidly conducting bypass, which produces a shortening of the PR interval and a slurring of the QRS complex called a delta wave (Fig. 7.11). Because the AV node and the bypass pathway have different conduction speeds and refractory periods, a re- entry circuit

can develop causing paroxysms of tachycardia. Because the bypass pathway lacks the rate-limiting properties of the normal AV node, patients are at risk from very rapid ventricular rates, and sometimes ventricular fibrillation and death, should they develop atrial fibrillation or a rapid atrial tachycardia.

Treatment is aimed at reducing conduction rate and increasing the refractory period of the bypass, using disopyramide, quinidine or amiodarone (pp. 136-137).

Atrial tachycardia with atrioventricular block. In this condition there is an atrial tachycardia of 140–220 per minute accompanied by atrioventricular block, usually either 2:1 or variable (p. 139). Carotid sinus massage may slow the pulse by increasing the degree of block (Fig. 7.12), but seldom terminates the attack. Atrial

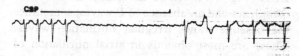

Fig. 7.12 Atrial tachycardia with atrioventricular block induced by carotid sinus pressure (CSP).

tachycardia with block seldom occurs in otherwise normal hearts, and it is sometimes a manifestation of digitalis toxicity. If the latter is suspected, digitalis should be stopped, potassium supplements given (the intracellular potassium is often low even if plasma potassium is normal) and the heart rate controlled if necessary, with a beta-adrenoceptor antagonist. If this arrhythmia develops in a patient not already taking a digitalis preparation, then digoxin is, paradoxically, the drug of choice for controlling the ventricular rate.

Atrial flutter. This is also a condition in which a rapid atrial rate is associated with 2:1, 3:1, or 4:1 atrioventricular block. The atrial rate however tends to be more rapid, usually about 300 per minute, and the aetiology resembles that of the commoner atrial fibrillation. The ECG shows characteristic saw-toothed flutter waves (Fig. 7.13). With a regular 2:1 AV block it may be difficult to distinguish atrial flutter from supraventricular or even sinus tachycardia, but carotid sinus pressure may help by temporarily increasing the degree of block.

Digoxin is traditionally used to control the

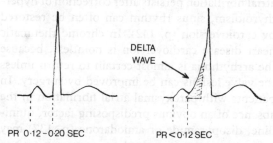

PR 0·12 – 0·20 SEC   PR < 0·12 SEC

Fig. 7.11 A normal ECG complex (left) compared with one from a patient with the **Wolff-Parkinson-White syndrome** (right). In this syndrome, premature excitation of part of the ventricles through an accessory atrioventricular conduction pathway produces the delta wave, which gives the appearance of a short PR interval and a broad QRS complex. These patients are prone to re-entry tachycardias — during such a tachycardia the QRS usually becomes normal, since ventricular activation is taking place only through the AV node, and the accessory pathway is conducting the impulses back to the atria.

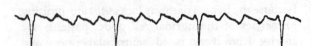

Fig. 7.13 Atrial flutter. ECG showing saw-toothed atrial flutter waves and 4:1 atrioventricular block.

ventricular rate, and as prophylaxis in patients with paroxysmal atrial flutter. In some patients atrial flutter is difficult to control without inducing digitalis toxicity, and cardioversion may be preferable (p. 142). If digoxin alone does not give adequate prophylaxis, quinidine or disopyramide may be added (p. 136).

Atrial fibrillation. In this arrhythmia the atria beat rapidly, chaotically and ineffectively; the ventricles respond at irregular intervals giving the characteristic 'irregularly irregular' pulse. The ECG (Fig. 7.14) shows no change in the QRS complexes and an absence of P waves; sometimes the baseline shows irregular fibrillation waves. These are most obvious in atrial fibrillation of recent onset.

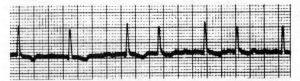

Fig. 7.14 Atrial fibrillation. The ventricular complexes are irregular, there are no P waves and irregular oscillations (f waves) disturb the baseline.

Atrial fibrillation may result from any stimulus which produces atrial dilatation. Mitral valve disease is the commonest cause in young and middle aged patients; in older patients the reason is often obscure, though many have hypertension or ischaemic heart disease. Atrial fibrillation may occur temporarily with myocardial infarction, with pericarditis, or after thoracic operations. It is rare in congenital or pulmonary heart disease, and it is a late complication of isolated aortic valve disease. Thyrotoxicosis, which increases atrial excitability, is an important and often undetected cause, particularly in the elderly.

'Lone' atrial fibrillation may be found in the absence of any other evidence of heart disease, and then may be intermittent at first, but later is often permanent; it is frequently a component of the sick sinus syndrome. Episodes of atrial fibrillation can be provoked, in those who are prone to it, by alcohol or infections.

Atrial fibrillation may be asymptomatic, more commonly in the elderly. Patients with paroxysmal atrial fibrillation are more aware of the arrhythmia than those in whom it is established. Atrial fibrillation frequently precipitates or aggravates cardiac failure in those with an abnormal heart, particularly with mitral stenosis. The ventricular rate at the onset of atrial fibrillation is usually rapid, diastole is shortened, and the left atrial pressure rises, sometimes leading to pulmonary oedema. The absence of the contribution of atrial systole to ventricular filling is another adverse factor.

Ineffective atrial contraction coupled with left atrial dilatation predisposes to stasis, thrombosis, and a risk of systemic thromboembolism. The risk is greatest when atrial fibrillation coexists with mitral valve disease, in patients with paroxysmal atrial fibrillation, and in the weeks immediately following the onset of fibrillation; however there is some risk of systemic embolism in all patients with atrial fibrillation.

Treatment. Digoxin is used to reduce the ventricular rate by increasing the degree of AV block, and this alone may result in a striking improvement, particularly in patients with mitral stenosis. In atrial fibrillation due to thyrotoxicosis, beta-blockade may be better than digoxin. When atrial fibrillation persists after correction of hyperthyroidism, sinus rhythm can often be restored by cardioversion (p. 142). In chronic rheumatic heart disease cardioversion is pointless, because the arrhythmia is almost certain to return unless the valve lesions can be improved by surgery. In patients with paroxysmal atrial fibrillation in the absence of an obvious predisposing factor, quinidine, disopyramide or amiodarone (p. 137) may help to preserve sinus rhythm.

Long-term anticoagulant therapy with warfarin reduces the risk of systemic embolism in patients with mitral valve disease, and is probably also indicated in patients with paroxysmal atrial fibrillation and to cover elective cardioversion. The potential benefits have to be weighed against the risks of anticoagulant therapy in each case. Although patients with lone atrial fibrillation have an increased risk of stroke, there is no evidence that this is reduced by anticoagulation.

Refractory atrial and junctional arrhythmias may be treated by high-energy shocks to the conduction pathway via a trans-venous pacing catheter. Heart block which is usually complete and persistent is induced, and a permanent pacemaker is required.

Ventricular ectopic rhythms

Ectopic beats. The symptoms and signs are the same as those of atrial ectopic beats, from which they can be distinguished by their abnormally widened QRS complex on the ECG (Fig. 7.15). They are fairly frequent in normal people, and their prevalence increases with age. They are sometimes precipitated by excessive tea, coffee or alcohol consumption. Ectopic beats in patients with otherwise normal hearts are often more prominent at rest, and tend to disappear with exercise. Ventricular ectopic beats often occur at a fixed interval after a sinus beat, and together with the compensatory pause after the ectopic beats produce a coupled or bigeminal pulse rhythm.

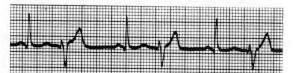

Fig. 7.15 Ventricular ectopic beats. Alternate beats have an abnormally wide QRS complex with no preceding P waves, i.e. coupling of the pulse results.

Ventricular ectopic beats are sometimes a manifestation of underlying heart disease, particularly disease of ventricular muscle which enhances ventricular excitability and increases the scope for ventricular re-entry circuits. Examples include acute myocardial infarction and myocarditis. Under these conditions an unusually premature ectopic beat falling on the T wave of a normal beat ('R on T') may initiate ventricular tachycardia or ventricular fibrillation.

Frequent ventricular ectopic beats, often against a background of bradycardia, are a feature of digitalis intoxication, and here too they may be a herald of more serious arrhythmias. Hypokal-

aemia may cause ventricular ectopic beats on its own, and will potentiate other causes. Ventricular ectopic beats are sometimes a feature of mitral valve prolapse, and occasionally they occur as 'escape beats' in the presence of an underlying bradycardia.

Treatment should be directed at the underlying causes. The use of lignocaine to suppress ventricular ectopic beats after myocardial infarction has not been shown to improve survival. If frequent ectopic beats are causing annoyance in an otherwise healthy patient, beta-adrenoceptor antagonists, quinidine, disopyramide or mexiletine may help to suppress them (pp. 136–137)

Ventricular tachycardia (Fig. 7.16) is a grave arrhythmia because it is nearly always associated with serious heart disease, because the ventricular rate may be very rapid, and because it may degenerate into ventricular fibrillation. Patients sometimes complain of palpitation, but more often the symptoms are those of a low cardiac output — dizziness and dyspnoea, or even loss of consciousness. The ventricular rate is usually between 140 and 220 per minute, and carotid sinus pressure is ineffective. The ECG shows broad, abnormal QRS complexes; P waves are difficult to see, and when visible they may bear no regular relationship to the QRS complex. Ventricular tachycardia is sometimes difficult to distinguish from supraventricular tachycardia with bundle branch block; when there is doubt, it is safer to treat for ventricular tachycardia.

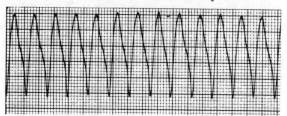

Fig. 7.16 Ventricular tachycardia. The rate is 220 per minute. The complexes are broad and abnormal.

The commonest cause of ventricular tachycardia is acute myocardial infarction. It may also be due to myocarditis, cardiomyopathy, or chronic ischaemic heart disease, especially when the last is associated with a ventricular aneurysm. In a few individuals a predisposition to ventricular arrhythmia is associated with abnormal prolongation of the QT interval of the ECG, a trait which is sometimes hereditary. Hypokalaemia, hypomagnesaemia or digitalis excess are also predisposing factors.

Patients recovering from myocardial infarction sometimes have periods of idioventricular rhythm ('slow' ventricular tachycardia) at a rate only slightly above the preceding sinus rate. These episodes are usually self limiting, asymptomatic, and do not require treatment. Most other instances of ventricular tachycardia, if they last for more than a few beats, will require treatment, often as an emergency.

Treatment of choice in urgent cases is intravenous lignocaine given as a bolus (1.5 mg per kg) followed by an infusion of 4 mg per minute reducing to 2 mg per minute over a period of 2 to 4 hours. The dose may need to be reduced in the elderly, the frail and those with liver disease. Lignocaine toxicity is manifested by confusion, paraesthesiae and twitching; if these are observed the dose should be curtailed. Mexiletine or disopyramide may be effective, either as alternatives to lignocaine or when lignocaine has failed, but if the patient is gravely ill then cardioversion is preferable to polypharmacy. Hypokalaemia, hypomagnesaemia and acidosis must be corrected. Cardioversion should be avoided if digitalis toxicity is likely; if it is considered necessary in these circumstances the first attempts should be made at low energy settings.

Urgent treatment of ventricular tachycardia should be followed by oral prophylaxis with mexiletine, disopyramide, procainamide or quinidine (p. 136). Slow release preparations may help in maintaining adequate plasma concentrations. Treatment can usually be stopped after 6 weeks in patients who develop ventricular tachycardia as a complication of acute infarction, but it may need to be continued indefinitely in patients with recurrent attacks. Procainamide should be avoided for long-term treatment (p. 136). Amiodarone (p. 137) may be helpful in difficult cases.

Ventricular fibrillation is the commonest immediate cause of sudden death. It results from critical anoxia or ischaemia of ventricular muscle, most commonly as a result of coronary artery disease, or from inappropriate electrical stimulation, as in electrocution. Susceptibility to ventricular fibrillation can be enhanced by underlying heart disease, by hypokalaemia or by drugs such as the catecholamines. The ventricles have a rapid, ineffective uncoordinated movement which produces no pulse, and the ECG (Fig. 7.17) has broad, bizarre, irregular complexes.

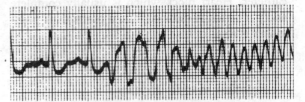

Fig. 7.17 Ventricular fibrillation. The change from sinus rhythm to ventricular fibrillation occurs when a ventricular ectopic beat falls on the T of the previous complex.

Within seconds of the onset of the attack the patient loses consciousness. Respiration ceases and the pupils begin to dilate. Death is virtually inevitable unless treatment is started promptly. If a defibrillator is available, the immediate application of a direct current shock may restore sinus rhythm within seconds. Under other circumstances the circulation has to be maintained by the resuscitation procedures described on page 135. Failure of circulation causes acidosis, and sodium bicarbonate should be given intravenously (p. 97). If sinus rhythm is restored, lignocaine should be given to reduce the likelihood of recurrence, followed by oral prophylaxis as described for ventricular tachycardia.

Ventricular asystole is another arrhythmia which can cause sudden death. It may be due either to a localised failure of impulse-conducting tissue, with delay in the emergence of a ventricular escape rhythm, or to massive ventricular damage complicating myocardial infarction. With the former, cardiac massage or a blow to the chest will often restore cardiac activity, although an artificial pacemaker may be needed to prevent recurrent attacks. When asystole occurs as a consequence of massive myocardial damage, it is nearly always resistant to treatment. Sometimes, electrical activity returns but is not accompanied by effective ventricular contraction.

Cardiac arrest

Cardiac arrest is the sudden and complete loss of cardiac function. It is usually due to ventricular fibrillation, less often to asystole. These can usually be distinguished only by an ECG, or during cardiac surgery when the heart is visible. Most attempts at resuscitation have to be commenced before an ECG is available. The development of the technique of closed-chest cardiac massage together with mouth-to-mouth ventilation, has improved the outlook immeasurably, and all doctors, nurses, ambulance drivers and attendants should receive instruction in this vitally important form of first aid.

The indication for resuscitation is clearest when the arrest has occurred as a result of an accident, such as electrocution or drowning, or when it occurs during an investigation such as cardiac catheterisation. One of the problems in hospital practice is to determine when it is inappropriate to attempt resuscitation because the nature of the patient's illness is such that recovery would be unprecedented. Inevitably it is sometimes necessary to institute resuscitation until someone familiar with the patient can make the decision as to whether the attempt should continue.

Treatment. The brain suffers irreversible damage unless some circulation of oxygenated blood can be achieved within 2 or 3 minutes. A smart blow should be given to the left of the sternum with the hand or fist, and both legs should be elevated to 90 degrees. If the heart does not start immediately, as indicated by the return of the carotid or femoral pulse, closed-chest cardiac massage (external cardiac compression) and mouth-to-mouth ventilation (expired air resuscitation) should be commenced.

TECHNIQUE OF CARDIOPULMONARY RESUSCITATION. The patient is laid on the back on the floor or some other firm surface. The operator places the hands one on top of the other (Fig. 7.18) on the patient's lower sternum and commences forceful, rhythmic compressions at the rate of 60–100 per minute. The danger of fracturing ribs is reduced if the pressure is transmitted through the ball of the hand on to the sternum. Previous practice with a dummy or mannikin is very helpful. At the same time, ventilation must be ensured. The head is extended, and the jaw pulled forward. Mouth-to-mouth, mouth-to-nose or mouth-to-airway ventilation is employed until a face mask and bag are available. When there are two oper-

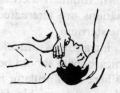

1. Head hyperextended and chin raised

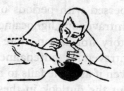

2. Direct mouth-to-mouth breathing

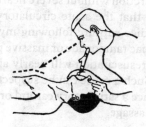

3. Indirect mouth-to-mouth breathing

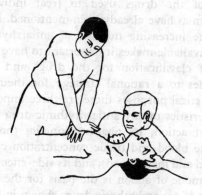

4. Cardiac massage

Fig. 7.18 Emergency resuscitation.

ators the lungs should be inflated after every fifth compression of the sternum. If there is only one operator, two inflations are alternated with 15 compressions of the sternum.

Meanwhile an intravenous infusion of 50 mmol of sodium bicarbonate should be set up to combat acidosis. Where a defibrillator is available it should be used as soon as possible, for no harm is done if the patient proves to have asystole rather than ventricular fibrillation. 200 joules (watt-seconds) is an adequate energy level for all but the largest adults. Repeated attempts at defibrillation should be interspersed with periods of massage and ventilation. Intravenous lignocaine (100 mg) may make refractory fibrillation more amenable to correction. Intravenous adrenaline (1 ml of 1:1000) can be given if asystole fails to respond to massage alone, but the outlook in these cases is poor.

Resuscitation is most likely to be successful in cardiac arrest resulting from accidents, or from myocardial infarction without severe heart failure. If it transpires that the acute circulatory failure was due to cardiac rupture following myocardial infarction, cardiac tamponade or massive pulmonary embolism, resuscitation will nearly always be unsuccessful. Such a cause can be suspected from failure to produce a satisfactory carotid or femoral pulse during massage.

Antiarrhythmic drugs

Some of the drugs used to treat individual arrhythmias have already been mentioned. However, the increasing number of antiarrhythmic agents available makes it important to have some form of classification for the drugs and some guidelines to a rational strategy for their use. For practical purposes there are three important characteristics of any antiarrhythmic drug — its mode of action, its pharmacokinetics (how an adequate blood and tissue concentration can be achieved and maintained), and its side-effects.

The mode of action is the basis for the classification of antiarrhythmic drugs shown in Table 7.1.

Class I drugs act principally by depressing excitability and slowing conduction in atrial or ventricular muscle. Lignocaine and mexiletine are

Table 7.1 Classification of antiarrhythmic drugs. (Adapted from Singh B, Vaughan Williams E M 1972 Cardiovascular Research 6:109.)

Class	Action	Examples
I	Slow fast-rising phase of ventricular action potential (by inhibiting 'fast sodium current')	Quinidine Lignocaine Mexiletine
II	Beta-adrenoceptor antagonists	Propranolol
III	Delay repolarisation; prolong 'plateau' of ventricular action potential	Amiodarone
IV	Calcium-channel antagonists	Verapamil

used mainly for ventricular arrhythmias; procainamide, quinidine and disopyramide can be used for both atrial and ventricular arrhythmias. Phenytoin is claimed to be particularly useful in digitalis induced arrhythmias.

Lignocaine has to be given parenterally, and has a very short plasma half-life, so its concentration will depend on the rate of infusion. It is mainly used for the urgent treatment or prophylaxis of ventricular tachycardia or fibrillation (p. 133).

Procainamide can also be given intravenously, but tends to cause hypotension. It is effective orally, and has been used in the prophylaxis of ventricular arrhythmias. The plasma half-life is short, and it is best given as a sustained-release preparation. With prolonged usage there is a risk of a systemic lupus erythematosus-like syndrome (p. 575), which is usually reversible on withdrawal of the drug.

Mexiletine can be given intravenously or orally in the treatment or prophylaxis of ventricular arrhythmias. It is tending to supersede procainamide as it seems to have fewer side-effects. These mainly take the form of nausea and vomiting but ataxia can also be troublesome. The usual oral dose is 200 to 250 mg 8-hourly; the manufacturer's literature should be consulted for the parenteral dosage schedule. Metabolism is mainly hepatic, and can be impaired in liver disease.

Disopyramide can be used for the treatment or prophylaxis of both atrial and ventricular tachyarrhythmias. It can be given intravenously or orally. If it is used in patients with atrial flutter and AV block, there is a risk of a paradoxical increase in heart rate as the atria slow and 2:1 block changes to 1:1 conduction; this can be prevented by previous administration of digoxin.

Disopyramide and mexiletine are of similar efficacy in treating ventricular arrhythmias, but differ in their side effects and metabolism. Disopyramide has weak atropine-like effects and may cause urinary retention or precipitate glaucoma. It has a depressant effect on ventricular function and should be avoided in cardiac failure. Metabolism is renal as well as hepatic. The plasma half-life is quite short, and the oral dose is 100 to 150 mg every 6 hours, or as slow-release disopyramide 250 mg twice a day. The manufacturer's instructions should be consulted for the intravenous dose schedule.

Quinidine gained a bad reputation when it used to be given in large doses to convert atrial fibrillation to sinus rhythm. In more modest doses (e.g. oral slow-release quinidine 500 mg b.d.) it is of similar efficacy and safety to disopyramide in the prophylaxis of atrial arrhythmias and to disopyramide or mexiletine in the prevention of ventricular arrhythmias. In practical terms, a choice between these drugs will often be determined by personal experience, patient tolerance and availability. Quinidine tends to cause abdominal discomfort and diarrhoea; rarely an auto-immune thrombocytopenia or haemolytic anaemia may occur. It is a myocardial depressant, and should be avoided in patients with poor left ventricular function. Excretion is almost entirely renal, and the drug will accumulate in renal failure.

Phenytoin can be given by slow intravenous injection (up to 5 mg per kg) to patients with a refractory ventricular tachycardia, particularly if this is due to digitalis toxicity. It is seldom used for the long-term treatment of arrhythmias.

Class II drugs comprise the beta-adrenoceptor antagonists. They are useful in treating supraventricular arrhythmias, and as an adjunct to digoxin in controlling the ventricular rate in atrial fibrillation. They can be useful in treating ventricular arrhythmias, but are seldom the drugs of first choice for this purpose. Their tendency to depress ventricular function is a disadvantage. Choice is determined by availability, duration of action, and side-effects.

Propranolol is an effective drug but needs to be taken three times a day, or as a sustained release preparation, in order to maintain adequate plasma concentrations. Because it is extensively metabolised the effective dose is unpredictable; 10 mg is a safe starting dose, but some patients need up to 320 mg daily, or more in thyrotoxicosis. Intravenous propranolol is very potent, and an initial dose should not exceed 1 mg. Intravenous metoprolol, atenolol or sotalol are preferable.

Metoprolol is a cardioselective β_1-antagonist (p. 177), which may have fewer side-effects than propranolol. Oral metoprolol needs to be given twice or thrice daily, or as a slow-release preparation. The usual oral starting dose is 50 mg b.d. Intravenous metoprolol (or atenolol or sotalol) may be used to treat supraventricular tachycardia. The intravenous dose of metoprolol is up to 5 mg initially given at 1–2 mg per minute, repeated at 5 minute intervals to a maximum of 15 mg.

Atenolol is a cardioselective beta-adrenoceptor antagonist with a long duration of action. It is usually given once daily. The oral dose is usually 100 mg daily, but 50 mg is a safer starting dose in the elderly. The intravenous dose of atenolol is 2.5 mg initially, repeated at 5 minute intervals to a maximum of 10 mg.

Sotalol is not cardioselective, but has a long half-life and also has some class III antiarrhythmic activity. The oral dose is usually 80 mg twice daily, increasing to 320 mg daily or more if necessary. The intravenous dose is 10-20 mg given slowly.

Other adverse effects of these beta-blockers are discussed on page 177.

Class III drugs act by prolonging the plateau phase of the action potential, thus lengthening the refractory period. *Amiodarone* is the principal drug in this class although both disopyramide and sotalol have class III activity. Amiodarone also has unusual pharmacokinetics, and it is unclear whether these or its mode of action contribute more to its undoubted efficacy as an antiarrhythmic agent. It is effective against a wide variety of atrial arrhythmias, and is probably the most potent drug in controlling paroxysmal atrial fibrillation and the arrhythmias of the Wolff-Parkinson-White syndrome. It is also useful in preventing recurrent ventricular tachycardia.

Tissue levels are built up slowly, and with oral therapy it may take 2 weeks or longer to achieve therapeutic concentrations. Conversely, amiodarone is a very persistent drug, and traces can still be detected weeks or months after treatment has ceased. The oral dosage is 200 mg thrice daily for 1 or 2 weeks, reducing thereafter to 200 or 400 mg daily. After several months it may be possible to reduce the dosage further.

Side-effects are numerous, and have to be balanced against the advantages of therapy. Corneal deposits are virtually universal, but do not affect vision and seem to regress after withdrawal of the drug. Photosensitisation of the skin is also very common. Gastrointestinal problems tend to get better when the dose is reduced. Amiodarone is an iodine-containing compound, and both hypo- and hyperthyroidism have been reported. Hepatitis and allergic alveolitis are other potentially serious complications. Drug interac tions may be a problem, particularly with digoxinand with warfarin. Patients taking amiodarone should be kept under review and have regular examination of the eyes, thyroid, liver and lung function.

Class IV drugs block the 'slow calcium channel' (p. 166) which is particularly important for impulse generation and conduction in atrial and nodal tissue, although it is also present in ventricular muscle.

Verapamil is the only widely used antiarrhythmic drug in this class; nifedipine (p. 166) has no significant antiarrhythmic effect in man. Verapamil may be given intravenously, in 5 mg aliquots to a maximum of 20 mg, to patients with supraventricular tachycardia. Although very effective, bradycardia and hypotension may occur and this treatment is not recommended outside hospital. Intravenous verapamil must not be combined with a beta-adrenoceptor antagonist, or given to patients who have taken such drugs within 48 hours. Oral verapamil (40–120 mg t.i.d.) can be used to control recurrent atrial arrhythmias, or as an adjunct to digoxin in treating atrial fibrillation. It is not used for ventricular arrhythmias. Side-effects include dizziness, constipation, and sometimes myocardial depression.

Digoxin. This is an important antiarrhythmic drug which does not feature in the above classification. Its principal value lies in its ability to slow conduction and prolong the refractory period in the AV node. This effect helps to control the ventricular rate in atrial fibrillation or paroxysmal atrial tachycardia, and will often interrupt re-entry tachycardias involving the AV node. On the other hand the effect of digoxin on sodium and potassium pumping tends to enhance excitability and conduction, and shorten the refractory period, in other parts of the heart; therefore atrial or ventricular tachycardias may be features of digoxin toxicity.

Digoxin is a purified glycoside from the European foxglove, *Digitalis lanata*. Digitalis is a less precise term sometimes used for the powdered leaves of *D. lanata*, sometimes as a generic term for the whole family of cardiac glycosides.

Digoxin is widely distributed in body tissues, and to achieve a rapid therapeutic effect it is best to give a loading dose of approximately 0.02 mg per kg over the first 48 hours, followed by a maintenance dose of 0.25 mg daily. Digoxin is largely excreted by the kidneys, and the maintenance dose should be reduced in children, the elderly and those with renal impairment. In an emergency, digoxin can be given intravenously as an infusion of 0.5 mg in 100 ml saline over 30 minutes, repeated every 6 hours until the required loading dose has been given. Digoxin has a long plasma half-life, and effects may persist 24–36 hours after the last dose. Measurements of plasma digoxin concentrations (p. 818) are useful, (1) in determining that the dose being used is inadequate and (2) in confirming a clinical impression of toxicity. Treatment of suspected toxicity should not be delayed pending concentration measurements, particularly as a fall in plasma potassium concentration may induce digoxin toxicity without a change in plasma digoxin concentration.

Digoxin toxicity. Extracardiac manifestations include anorexia, nausea, vomiting, diarrhoea and altered colour vision (xanthopsia). Cardiac manifestations include bradycardia, ventricular ectopic beats, often multiple or coupled, paroxysmal atrial tachycardia and ventricular tachycardia or fibrillation. Digoxin administration should be stopped, and blood taken for plasma digoxin levels, urea and electrolyte estimation. Fluid loss should be replaced, intravenously if necessary, and potassium supplements given as required. Symptomatic bradycardia should be treated with atropine and if necessary an artificial pacemaker.

Symptomatic atrial tachycardia can be controlled with a beta-adrenoceptor antagonist. Ventricular tachycardia is treated with lignocaine, or if this fails with phenytoin. Cardioversion carries an increased risk of provoking ventricular fibrillation, but will be required for refractory ventricular tachycardia or for ventricular fibrillation. Treatment with antibodies to digoxin has been used with success for digoxin overdosage in self-poisoning.

Strategy in antiarrhythmic therapy. The availability of many agents is an invitation to overtreatment. Many arrhythmias are benign, asymptomatic or self limited, and best left alone. Simple measures such as rest, reassurance, analgesia and sedation must not be forgotten. Any causative factor must be dealt with, notably alcohol, caffeine or hyperthyroidism. Acidosis, hypokalaemia and hypomagnesaemia need to be corrected. If treatment is needed it is best to use as few drugs as possible, and to give them in the maximum possible dose before discarding them as ineffective.

If a patient's condition is deteriorating because of a tachyarrhythmia then cardioversion should not be delayed; even if the relief is only temporary it will buy time for a review of drug therapy and correction of adverse factors. Perseverance is often rewarded, particularly after myocardial infarction where arrhythmias tend to settle with time. When it is considered necessary to use a combination of drugs, it would seem sensible to combine drugs with different modes of action, though objective evidence for this is scanty. In refractory cases the ability to induce the arrhythmia in the laboratory using programmed stimulation via a pacing electrode may be useful in deciding the best drug combination. Patients on long-term anti-arrhythmic drugs should be reviewed regularly, and attempts made to withdraw therapy if it appears that the factors which precipitated the arrhythmias are no longer operative.

If the patient has recurrent supraventricular arrhythmias in spite of drug therapy, or if side-effects, idiosyncrasy or personal preference make drug therapy undesirable, either His bundle ablation or an antitachycardia pacemaker should be considered. These pacemakers are able to detect the onset of an abnormal rhythm, and respond by emitting appropriately timed impulses which block the re-entry circuit (Fig. 7.8). Their use for ventricular arrhythmias is controversial.

HEART BLOCK

Sinoatrial (SA) block

In this condition a complete cardiac cycle is missed so that a gap appears in the pulse. The electrocardiogram shows that both atrial and ventricular complexes are absent. Sinoatrial block is one of the features of the sick sinus syndrome.

Sinoatrial block does not require treatment if it is asymptomatic. Sinoatrial disorders causing symptoms may require the implantation of an artificial pacemaker.

Atrioventricular (AV) block

In this condition conduction between the atria and ventricles is impaired.

1. In *first degree heart block* (delayed AV conduction) the PR interval is prolonged beyond the upper limit of normal (0.20 second) (Fig. 7.19).

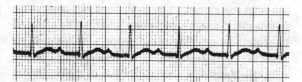

Fig. 7.19 First degree heart block. The PR interval is 0.26 sec.

2. In *second degree heart block* (partial heart block) some impulses from the atria fail to get through to the ventricles, i.e. dropped beats occur. Sometimes there is progressive lengthening of successive PR intervals followed by a dropped

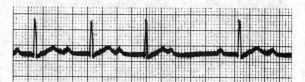

Fig. 7.20 Second degree heart block (Wenckebach's phenomenon). The first beat in the cycle has a PR of 0.28 sec; it lengthens with the next two beats and the fourth P wave is not followed by a QRS — the dropped beat.

beat. This is known as *Wenckebach's phenomenon* (Fig. 7.20) and is due to progressive fatigue of the AV bundle with recovery following the rest period when the dropped beat occurs. Second degree heart block sometimes occurs with atrial tachyarrhythmias.

3. In *complete heart block* no impulses from the atria reach the ventricles. Cardiac action is maintained by an escape rhythm arising in the bundle of His or in the ventricles (Fig. 7.21).

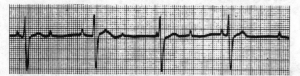

Fig. 7.21 Complete heart block. There is complete dissociation of atrial and ventricular complexes. The atrial rate is 90 and the ventricular rate 40 per minute.

Aetiology. Depression of atrioventricular conduction may be due to ischaemia, fibrosis or inflammation of the atrioventricular node or proximal part of the bundle of His, to vagal stimulation or to drugs. Myocardial infarction is the most frequent cause of heart block which develops suddenly. Idiopathic fibrosis of the bundle of His is a common cause of chronic heart block in the elderly. The bundle of His runs close to the aortic and mitral valves and may be affected by calcification extending from a valve, by an abscess cavity resulting from endocarditis, or by surgical trauma. Other causes of complete heart block include congenital maldevelopment of the bundle of His, digitalis poisoning, sarcoidosis and Chagas' disease (p. 781).

Clinical features. *First degree heart block* can be diagnosed only by ECG.

Second degree heart block. When the atrial and ventricular contractions bear a simple ratio to one another such as in 2:1 and 3:1 block, the pulse is slow and regular. Change in the degree of partial heart block may give rise to sudden changes in the pulse rate. More complex ratios such as 3:2 or 4:3 block give rise to dropped beats. Partial heart block is usually transient and may occur during an acute infection, from digitalis overdose, or after myocardial infarction. It is sometimes observed at rest or during sleep in athletic young adults with a high vagal tone.

Complete heart block may be chronic or intermittent. Chronic complete heart block should be suspected when the pulse is slow (30 to 40 per minute) and regular, and does not vary with exercise. It may be possible to see dissociation between jugular venous pulsation, reflecting atrial activity, and the carotid pulse. Venous cannon waves may occur (p. 122). The arterial pulse volume is large, and the increased stroke volume may produce a systolic murmur.

Intermittent complete heart block may cause fairly prolonged ventricular asystole because of a delay in establishing a ventricular escape rhythm. It is one of the causes of cardiac syncope. Temporary ventricular asystole, resulting from prolonged sinoatrial block in the sick sinus syndrome or from transient failure of the ventricular escape rhythm in chronic complete heart block, produces the same clinical picture, called the *Adams-Stokes syndrome*. Attacks frequently occur without warning, although some patients describe a prodrome. Consciousness is rapidly lost and the patient may fall. Convulsions may occur if the heart does not begin to beat again within about 10 seconds, and death will result if the arrest is prolonged. The skin blanches at the beginning of the attack, but when the heart starts beating again there is a characteristic flush as the emptied vessels are filled with blood.

Treatment. *First degree heart block* does not require treatment, but may be an indication of underlying heart disease, a warning of drug toxicity, or a contraindication to the use of drugs which might further impair conduction.

Asymptomatic *second degree heart block* does not require treatment, but the patient should be observed in case it progresses to complete heart block. 24-hour ECG monitoring may be helpful. Symptomatic second degree block following inferior myocardial infarction usually responds to atropine (0.3 mg i.v., repeated to a maximum of 1.2 mg). If it does not, a temporary pacemaker may be needed. Chronic symptomatic second degree block may be an indication for a permanent artificial pacemaker.

Complete heart block complicating acute inferior myocardial infarction is often accompanied by an escape rhythm at a satisfactory rate; it may need no treatment, or it may respond to atropine. If the latter is unsuccessful a temporary pacemaker may be needed. Complete heart block following acute anterior infarction requires a temporary pacemaker. If the patient presents with asystole, atropine and isoprenaline (1–5 mg in 500 ml glucose, infused intravenously at the minimum rate needed to produce a satisfactory heart rhythm) may help to maintain the circulation until a temporary pacing electrode can be inserted.

Most cases of chronic complete heart block, or of intermittent complete heart block unrelated to myocardial infarction or to drug administration, require a permanent artificial pacemaker. An exception may be made in young asymptomatic patients with congenital complete heart block or in frail and asymptomatic elderly patients. Sustained release isoprenaline (30 mg or more four times daily) may help to relieve heart failure and reduce the frequency of Adams-Stokes attacks in patients for whom pacemaker implantation is impracticable or unacceptable.

Bundle branch block and hemiblock

Interruption of the left or right branches of the bundle of His causes delay in the activation of the appropriate ventricle, broadening of the QRS complex on the ECG to 0.12 seconds or more, and characteristic alterations to QRS morphology shown in Figures 7.22 and 7.23.

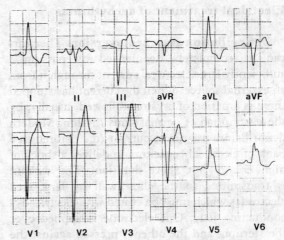

Fig. 7.23 Left bundle branch block from a patient with ischaemic heart disease. The QRS complexes are broad, with a large broad S wave in V2 and V3, and an 'M'-shaped QRS in V5 and V6. The normal septal Q wave is absent in V5 and V6. The T wave in bundle branch block usually goes in the opposite direction to the terminal part of the QRS complex, i.e. upright in V1, 2, 3, inverted in V5 and V6.

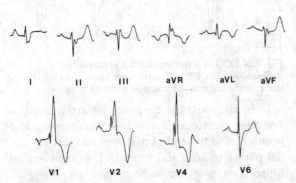

Fig. 7.22 Right bundle branch block from a child who had undergone surgical correction of the tetralogy of Fallot. Note the wide QRS complexes with 'M'-shaped complexes in leads V1 and V2, and an S wave in lead V6.

Right bundle branch block is occasionally congenital, sometimes results from gross hypertrophy or dilatation of the right ventricle or from surgical damage, and is usually (in adults) a manifestation of ischaemic heart disease.

Left bundle branch block is most commonly due to ischaemic heart disease; it is sometimes a feature of cardiomyopathy or of calcific infiltration of the bundle of His from a calcified aortic valve. The left branch of the bundle of His rapidly divides into a fan-like array of conducting tissue on the left side of the interventricular septum. Partial interruption of the bundle at this point (hemiblock) does not broaden the QRS complex, but alters the mean direction of ventricular depolarisation (cardiac axis). Damage to the anterior part of the system (*left anterior hemiblock*) shifts the axis to the left (large R in leads I and aVL, large S in II, III, aVF). Damage to the posterior part (*left posterior hemiblock*) shifts the axis to the right (S in I, aVL, large R in III, aVF).

The treatment and prognosis of bundle branch block are in general those of the underlying disease. The development of left bundle branch block, or of right bundle branch block plus anterior or posterior hemiblock after myocardial infarction indicates extensive myocardial damage, and often a poor prognosis.

Electrical treatment of arrhythmias

Defibrillation and cardioversion. The heart can be completely depolarised by passing a sufficiently large electrical current through it from an external source. When the current has stopped there is a period of asystole followed, usually, by the resumption of normal sinus rhythm. Modern defibrillators use direct current (d.c.) stored in a bank of electrical capacitors to deliver a shock of high energy but short duration. The current is transmitted to the chest wall by large-area electrodes which must be coated with electrically-conducting jelly. One electrode is applied over the sternum and the other is pressed against the chest wall beneath the left scapula or in the left axilla.

The precise timing of the discharge is unimportant in ventricular fibrillation, but when the technique is used to treat supraventricular or ventricular tachycardia or atrial fibrillation discharge should be synchronised with the R wave of the ECG. The reason for this is that if a current, not large enough to cause total depolarisation, is applied during a critical period at the end of the T wave it may provoke ventricular fibrillation.

In *ventricular fibrillation* neither preparation, anaesthesia nor synchronisation are required. Discharge energy should be set at 200 Joules (Watt-seconds) and the sooner the shock is applied the more likely it is to succeed. For other arrhythmias there is less urgency, a synchronised discharge should be used, and the patient should be anaesthetised. *Atrial fibrillation* often requires energies of 150 to 200 J to restore sinus rhythm. In *atrial flutter* or *supraventricular tachycardia* lower energies of 50 J or less may suffice.

Digitalis intoxication increases the risk of untoward arrhythmias after cardioversion, and ideally digitalis therapy should be withdrawn 36 hours before elective cardioversion. Patients with long-standing atrial arrhythmias are at risk of systemic embolism after cardioversion, unless this is preceded by a period of anticoagulation.

Artificial pacemakers. *Temporary procedures.* In an emergency it is sometimes possible to stimulate the heart by passing an electric current through electrodes placed on the chest wall, or passed down the oesophagus, or inserted directly through the chest wall into the myocardium. None of these methods is satisfactory for longer than a few minutes, if at all, and the most effective technique for temporary artificial pacemaking is to insert a bipolar pacing electrode via an antecubital, subclavian or femoral vein and position it under radioscopic control in the apex of the right ventricle. The electrode is connected to an external pulse generator. The threshold for reliable ventricular stimulation should be less than 1 volt, and the pulse generator should be set to deliver at least three times this figure — usually 3 to 4 volts.

The ECG of a patient whose rhythm is controlled by an artificial ventricular pacemaker shows regular broad QRS complexes with a left bundle branch block pattern and left axis deviation. Each complex is immediately preceded by a 'pacing spike' (Fig. 7.24). Nearly all pulse generators are used in a 'demand' or 'ventricular-inhibited' mode whereby a spontaneously generated QRS complex can inhibit the artificial impulse. In other words, if the patient's spontaneous rhythm recovers and its rate exceeds that at which the artificial pacemaker is set, the latter is inhibited, but if the patient's spontaneous rate drops below that set on the pulse generator then artificial pacing will be resumed.

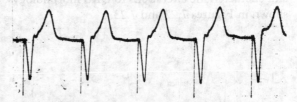

Fig. 7.24 ECG of a patient with a ventricular pacemaker. The QRS complexes are broad and each is immediately preceded by a narrow pacemaker 'spike'.

It is also possible to pace the atria, using a J-shaped electrode inserted percutaneously and positioned in the right atrial appendage. Sequential pacing of atria and ventricles, using a special pulse generator, reproduces the physiological sequence of atrial and ventricular contraction, and gives a better cardiac output than ventricular pacing alone. This may be important when there is impaired left ventricular function, e.g. after myocardial infarction.

Temporary pacemakers are invaluable where

heart block is transient, as is usually the case after myocardial infarction, but their long term use is inconvenient and the insertion site is prone to infection. Only in very exceptional circumstances should one be used for longer than 2 weeks.

Permanent artificial pacemakers utilise the same principles, but the pulse generator is smaller, completely enclosed, and can be implanted under the skin. The electrode passed to the heart is usually unipolar, the body of the pulse generator providing the other terminal for the current. The battery capacity of the pulse generator will usually sustain it for 5 to 10 years, after which it needs to be replaced. A longer lifespan can be achieved either by using a larger and bulkier battery, or by providing a facility for 'programming' the pacemaker, i.e. controlling its rate, output etc. by external radio frequency or magnetic stimuli so as to minimise the drain on its resources. Programming can also be used to increase output in the face of an unexpected increase in threshold, or to alter sensitivity if the pacemaker is inappropriately inhibited by electrical potentials generated in the pectoral muscles.

Atrial electrodes can also be used with permanent pacemakers. They can detect the atrial P wave and use it to initiate the impulse delivered to the ventricle. This has the dual advantage that atrioventricular synchrony is preserved and that the ventricular rate can increase together with the atrial rate during exercise. Atrial-triggered permanent pacemakers are the treatment of choice in physically active patients with complete heart block but normal atrial rhythm. Conversion to an atrial triggered pacing system may cure 'pacemaker syncope'—a fall in blood pressure and dizziness precipitated by the start of ventricular pacing. Other 'rate responsive' pacemakers are sensitive to QT interval (as an index of sympathetic tone), pH, or physical movement, and may be helpful if an atrial triggered system is impracticable.

ACUTE CIRCULATORY FAILURE

Acute circulatory failure, *shock* and *low output state* are terms used to describe a clinical syndrome of hypotension, peripheral vasoconstriction, oliguria, and often impairment of consciousness. The

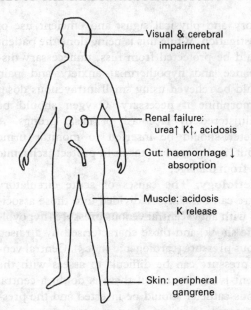

Fig. 7.25 Systemic consequences of acute circulatory failure.

Labels:
- Visual & cerebral impairment
- Renal failure: urea↑ K↑, acidosis
- Gut: haemorrhage ↓ absorption
- Muscle: acidosis K release
- Skin: peripheral gangrene

basic cause is an inadequate cardiac output with compensatory vasoconstriction and renal and cerebral hypoperfusion.

Onset may be sudden or gradual. The skin is·cold, pale and sweaty and in advanced cases there may be peripheral cyanosis or gangrene. The systolic blood pressure is usually low, often under 100 mmHg. With peripheral constriction the blood pressure, measured by cuff, is often an underestimate of central pressure. There is usually tachycardia, and the heart sounds may be difficult to analyse. Urine output is often less than 30 ml per hour. There may be Cheyne-Stokes breathing. Consciousness may be superficially preserved, but frequently there is confusion and irritability.

If treatment is not prompt and effective, systemic consequences may ensue (Fig. 7.25). Oliguria may progress to acute tubular necrosis (p.403). A rising plasma potassium concentration and progressive acidosis both from renal failure and ischaemic necrosis of skeletal muscle cause cardiac arrhythmias which may eventually be intractable. Even if recovery occurs, permanent cerebral damage or loss of peripheral tissues may be inevitable.

Successful treatment of acute circulatory failure is absolutely dependent on identification of the cause; this requires meticulous assessment of the history and physical signs, and efficient use of investigation. While this is being done the patient should be protected from fuss, unnecessary disturbance and hypothermia; anxiety and pain should be relieved using small intravenous doses of morphine if necessary. Oxygen should be administered by facemask or nasal prongs. A catheter should be inserted to monitor urine output, and great care taken to protect ischaemic skin from damage.

Aetiology. The causes of acute circulatory failure can basically be divided into those associated with a low central venous pressure (hypovolaemic shock) and those characterised by a raised venous pressure (cardiogenic shock). Central venous pressure can be difficult to assess with the patient lying flat, and if there is doubt a central venous catheter should be inserted and the pressure measured with a saline manometer.

HYPOVOLAEMIC SHOCK. The commonest cause of hypovolaemia is haemorrhage—external, into the bowel, or into a body cavity. Gastrointestinal haemorrhage can often be diagnosed on the basis of history and rectal examination; its further assessment is considered on page 289. Intra-abdominal haemorrhage, from a leaking aortic aneurysm in the elderly or a ruptured spleen or ectopic gestation sac in younger patient, is often insidious in its presentation, and atypical in its physical signs.

Less common causes of hypovolaemia include plasma loss in severe burns, or into the abdominal cavity in acute pancreatitis, inappropriate vasodilatation in bacteraemic shock (p. 48) and anaphylactic shock (p. 25), and excess urinary fluid loss as in diabetic ketoacidosis.

CARDIOGENIC SHOCK. Acute circulatory failure with a raised central venous pressure is caused by problems affecting the left or right side of the heart or the pulmonary circulation. The two most common causes are acute myocardial infarction and acute massive pulmonary embolism. When the diagnosis is not immediately apparent, it is useful to consider possible causes in a methodical order (Fig. 7.26).

Dissecting aneurysm of the aorta (p. 192) presents with severe pain, often between the shoulders. There may be an inappropriate bradycardia and an early diastolic murmur may be heard. Chest

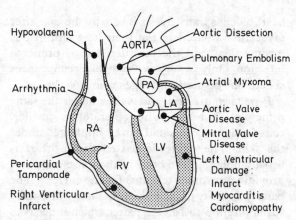

Fig. 7.26 Some possible cardiac causes of acute circulatory failure.

radiography and echocardiography are helpful.

Pericardial tamponade (p. 182) is an important cause of acute circulatory failure because it carries a high mortality if neglected and because it usually responds dramatically to treatment. Characteristically there is severe circulatory failure with oliguria, a grossly elevated venous pressure, and pulsus paradoxus. The chest radiograph shows an enlarged cardiac shadow. Echocardiography, which may be done at the bedside, is the best way of confirming the diagnosis, and helps to indicate the best site for paracentesis.

Aortic valve disease may precipitate acute circulatory failure by causing left ventricular failure and pulmonary oedema. The signs of *aortic stenosis* (p. 157) may be masked by a low cardiac output, the characteristic murmur becoming quiet. Acute severe *aortic regurgitation*, from cusp rupture or endocarditis, may also be atypical, with an unimpressive murmur and little cardiac enlargement on the chest radiograph. Echocardiography is helpful.

Myocardial infarction extensive enough to cause acute circulatory failure is usually obvious from the ECG, but occasionally ECG changes of ischaemia are a secondary result of circulatory failure from some other catastrophe such as pulmonary embolism. Usually, circulatory failure from myocardial infarction is associated with pulmonary oedema, but if the infarct predominantly affects the right ventricle (see below) this is not always the case.

Progressive *myocarditis*, including that of rheumatic fever, sometimes presents as acute circulatory failure; the chest radiograph usually shows an enlarged heart and echocardiography reveals severely impaired left ventricular function.

Tachyarrhythmias are usually obvious clinically and from the ECG. The onset of atrial fibrillation may precipitate acute circulatory failure, often with severe pulmonary oedema, in patients with impaired left ventricular function or *mitral stenosis*. The murmur of mitral stenosis (p. 155) is difficult to hear in the presence of tachycardia, but the history, chest radiograph and echocardiogram will confirm the diagnosis.

Acute massive pulmonary embolism (p. 179) is a sequel to leg or pelvic vein thrombosis. Collapse is sudden, often with extreme breathlessness. A tachycardia and elevated jugular venous pressure are invariable; other physical signs such as a parasternal lift, wide splitting of the second heart sound and a third sound over the right ventricle are helpful supportive findings. The ECG may show signs of acute right ventricular strain (Fig. 7.27) or may be normal apart from a tachycardia. The chest radiograph is of value mainly in excluding other diagnoses. Echocardiography shows a dilated right ventricle and, often, a small vigorously contracting left ventricle. Radionuclide perfusion lung scanning is helpful provided it can be done quickly enough. Pulmonary angiography is the definitive diagnostic procedure, but is not without risks—including those of moving a severely ill patient and of delay in instituting treatment.

Pure 'right sided' causes of acute circulatory failure are rare apart from pulmonary embolism. Probably the most common is the combination of a right ventricular infarct with excessive diuretic therapy; this can be suspected if cardiac output and urine production decline after an inferior infarct in the absence of pulmonary congestion, and confirmed by demonstrating a high central venous pressure but a low pulmonary artery wedge pressure (measured with a Swan-Ganz catheter, see below). Other causes include right atrial or right ventricular tumours, or right atrial tamponade from a localised pericardial effusion.

Treatment. The immediate objective is to restore and maintain cardiac output at a satisfactory level until the cause of the circulatory failure can be identified and specifically treated or allowed to resolve.

FLUID REPLACEMENT. In hypovolaemic circulatory failure the most important step is to replace fluid lost from the vascular compartment. Initially, it matters little whether isotonic saline, plasma or plasma substitutes are used, but when large quantities are required the nature of the fluid lost should determine the nature of its replacement. The rate of fluid replacement is judged according to estimates of the fluid lost, the clinical state of the patient, observation of the jugular venous pressure, and in severely ill patients by manometer measurement of the central venous pressure. Where large transfusions are needed rapidly it is important to warm the fluid used to body temperature.

Hypovolaemic shock sometimes occurs in patients with pre-existing cardiac disease. Under these conditions central venous or right atrial pressure may be an unreliable guide to fluid replacement, and it is better to obtain an estimate of pulmonary venous or left atrial pressure by *bedside haemodynamic monitoring*. This can be done using a Swan-Ganz catheter, which is a flexible double-lumen tube with a small balloon at the distal end. The catheter is introduced into a vein and advanced to the right atrium. One lumen is then used to inflate the balloon with about 1 cm^3 of air; the force of the bloodstream carries the balloon and attached catheter through the right ventricle to the pulmonary artery, the changing pressures measured through the other lumen indicating its progress. Ideally the tip of the catheter is positioned in a peripheral branch of the pulmonary artery. When the balloon is deflated it records pulmonary artery pressure, but when the balloon is inflated the tip is isolated from the main pulmonary artery and instead registers left atrial pressure. The mean left atrial pressure is normally between 5 and 10 mmHg; in left sided cardiac failure it may rise as high as 30 mmHg. In managing patients with acute circulatory failure a left atrial pressure of about 15 mmHg is usually aimed at; this is high enough to give good left ventricular filling but carries a low risk of pulmonary oedema.

ACUTE PULMONARY OEDEMA. This is usually a feature of circulatory failure caused by left sided

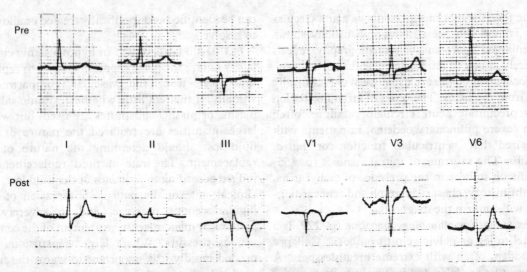

Fig. 7.27 ECGs from a patient before and immediately after a massive pulmonary embolism (the embolus was successfully removed surgically shortly after this record was taken). Right ventricular dilatation and strain are manifested by the development of an S wave in lead I and a Q wave plus T inversion in lead III (the 'S₁Q₃T₃' pattern). There is also acute T wave inversion in V1 and a shift from a left ventricular to a right ventricular pattern in V3. Note that many of these features can be seen in ECGs from normal subjects, and it is only by taking the pattern as a whole, and particularly by comparison with a previous ECG, that the full significance is appreciated.

cardiac problems. The three initial steps in its management are the administration of (1) morphine, to alleviate breathlessness and reverse reflex peripheral vasoconstriction, (2) a powerful diuretic such as frusemide (40–80 mg i.v.) both for its diuretic effect and also as a vasodilator, and (3) a high concentration of oxygen.

If these immediate measures are inadequate, one may try to stimulate the heart using inotropic agents, or to reduce left ventricular load by using more powerful vasodilators.

CONTROLLED VASODILATATION. This is an important concept in the management of pulmonary oedema and of left sided cardiac failure in general. *Venodilatation* reduces central venous pressure and right ventricular output, and slows the accumulation of pulmonary oedema, while *arteriolar dilatation* improves left ventricular function by reducing the afterload against which it has to work.

Glyceryl trinitrate and isosorbide dinitrate are predominantly venodilators, hydralazine, nifedipine and salbutamol predominantly arteriolar dilators, and sodium nitroprusside does both very powerfully. These distinctions become blurred in patients with severe circulatory failure. Small doses of vasodilating drugs improve cardiac output and reduce pulmonary oedema but have little effect on blood pressure — the increased efficiency of left ventricular contraction more than compensating for the fall in peripheral resistance. Larger doses may however cause dangerous hypotension. It is therefore essential, if vasodilators are used in treating acute circulatory failure, that their administration should be carefully controlled (e.g. by slow intravenous infusion using a paediatric burette or infusion pump) and their effects carefully monitored, if possible by measurement of left atrial as well as systemic arterial pressure.

INOTROPIC AGENTS. These increase ventricular output for a given filling pressure, but at the cost of increased oxygen consumption. Digoxin, though an inotrope, is of little immediate value because of the time taken to achieve a therapeutic level; it may have a role in persistent circulatory failure.

Noradrenaline, adrenaline and isoprenaline all have effects on peripheral resistance as well as inotropic properties. These range from vasoconstriction for noradrenaline to vasodilatation for isoprenaline. They all cause a tachycardia and increase the risk of arrhythmias. For this reason they are tending to be superseded by dobutamine and dopamine. Dobutamine is an inotropic agent with little effect on peripheral resistance, and less tendency to produce tachycardia than isoprenaline. It may be given by continuous intravenous infusion. Dopamine has an inotropic action and complex effects on peripheral resistance. In low doses (2–4 micrograms per kg per minute) it has a selective renal vasodilating effect, in larger doses it produces more widespread vasodilatation, while in very large doses it causes vasoconstriction.

There is no hard and fast rule about the order in which inotropic agents and vasodilators should be used. Dopamine is useful because at low doses it combines the benefits of both, and in severely ill patients inotropes and vasodilators are frequently used in combination.

In pure right sided cardiac failure it is important to maintain an adequate filling pressure for the right side of the heart, and the left atrial pressure may be a better guide to this than the central venous pressure. Inotropic agents may be helpful, but diuretics should be used with care and venodilators are contraindicated.

CARE OF OTHER SYSTEMS. Renal failure (p. 403) is a common complication of acute circulatory failure. The kidney responds to a severe fall in blood pressure by vasoconstriction and by redistribution of blood flow between medulla and cortex. If this vasoconstriction persists, tubular necrosis may ensue. Inducing a diuresis with frusemide or the osmotic diuretic mannitol may help protect the kidney from vasoconstriction, but perhaps the most effective antidote to renal vasoconstriction is low-dose dopamine. Once tubular necrosis has occurred it is important to restrict fluid intake, or pulmonary oedema will follow. Correction of the acidosis which often accompanies circulatory failure presents a dilemma in the presence of tubular necrosis, because of the sodium and fluid load involved. Peritoneal or haemodialysis are sometimes needed.

Hypoxaemia is common in acute circulatory failure, particularly when there is pulmonary oedema. If it does not respond rapidly to oxygen and diuretic therapy, early consideration should be given to endotracheal intubation and positive-pressure ventilation. This often has a strikingly beneficial effect on pulmonary oedema, by reducing right ventricular output.

Prognosis of acute circulatory failure is determined by the underlying cause. No amount of medication can compensate for massive and irretrievable myocardial damage, and the prognosis for circulatory failure complicating extensive myocardial infarction is poor. In contrast the prognosis after drainage of a pericardial effusion, replacement of a diseased valve, or dissolution of a pulmonary embolus may be exellent.

CARDIAC FAILURE

Acute circulatory failure is at one end of the range of possible manifestations of cardiac failure. The other manifestations are less dramatic, but can be responsible for a great deal of ill health. The common factor in all forms of cardiac failure is the inability of the heart to produce an output sufficient for the needs of the patient. In the mildest forms of cardiac failure, cardiac output is adequate at rest and becomes inadequate only during exercise. In more severe forms, even when the patient is examined at rest, it is possible to detect at least some features of cardiac failure and of the complex haemodynamic, endocrine and renal compensatory mechanisms it evokes. The successful management of cardiac failure depends both on an understanding of its pathophysiology and on an accurate diagnosis of its cause.

Pathophysiology. It is convenient to consider separately the consequences of impaired function of the left and the right sides of the heart. The left side of the heart is a term for the functional unit of the left atrium and left ventricle together with the mitral and aortic valves, and the right side stands for the right atrium and ventricle and the tricuspid and pulmonary valves.

Left sided cardiac failure is characterised by a reduction in effective left ventricular output for a given pulmonary venous or left atrial pressure, or conversely, an increase in the left atrial pressure needed to sustain a given cardiac output. An acute increase in left atrial pressure may cause pulmonary congestion or pulmonary oedema; with a more gradual increase in left atrial pressure there tends to be, for reasons at present poorly understood, reflex pulmonary vasoconstriction which protects the patient from pulmonary oedema at the cost of increasing pulmonary hypertension. This is one reason why right sided and left sided failure often occur together, another is that the same disease process (e.g. ischaemic heart disease) frequently affects both ventricles.

In *right sided cardiac failure* there is similarly a reduction of right ventricular output for a given right atrial pressure, or a need for an increased right atrial pressure to maintain a given output. The increased right atrial pressure is manifested as an increase in jugular venous pressure and as hepatic engorgement.

In both left and right sided cardiac failure the body attempts to compensate for the drop in cardiac output by activation of the sympathetic nervous system, causing tachycardia and vaso-constriction, and retention of salt and water by the kidneys. Fluid retention is accompanied by the development of oedema; in pure left sided failure this is principally pulmonary, and a small accumulation may cause prominent symptoms. In right sided failure, or in a combination of right and left sided failure, most of the oedema is peripheral and its site is determined mainly by gravity. It affects the ankles in ambulant patients, and the thighs or sacrum in the bed-bound. Considerable quantities of peripheral oedema may accumulate without causing distress. Massive accumulation of fluid may cause ascites or pleural effusions (p. 261).

CAUSES OF LEFT OR RIGHT SIDED CARDIAC FAILURE. Nearly all causes of these can be accounted for under four headings: (1) ventricular outflow obstruction, (2) ventricular inflow obstruction, (3) impaired ventricular function and (4) volume overload.

1. *Ventricular outflow obstruction.* Obstruction to the outflow of blood from either ventricle causes an increase in ventricular afterload. It may occur as a result of systemic or pulmonary hypertension or of aortic or pulmonary valve stenosis. The initial response is ventricular hypertrophy, the size of the ventricular cavity remaining the same. The increased muscle bulk makes the ventricle stiffer, and higher atrial pressures are needed for diastolic filling. This leads to atrial hypertrophy, and on the left side may precipitate pulmonary oedema. Eventually the increase in afterload may reach a point where the muscle fibres are no longer able to contract fully with each systole. The

ventricle then begins to dilate, and as a result, a higher wall tension is needed to maintain the same systolic pressure. (Laplace's law states that the wall tension required to counteract a given pressure in a spherical cavity is proportional to the radius of the cavity.) At the same time, it becomes increasingly difficult for the coronary vessels to supply the hypertrophied muscle, and fibres begin to die and to be replaced by fibrous tissue. It is characteristic of this cause of cardiac failure that it is initially well tolerated, but that once deterioration begins it progresses rapidly.

2. *Ventricular inflow obstruction.* The commonest cause is mitral or tricuspid valve stenosis; rarer causes include cardiac tumours, external pressure or constriction as in constrictive pericarditis, and occasionally endomyocardial fibrosis. The ventricle itself remains small and usually contracts vigorously; however, the chamber upstream, the atrium, often becomes dilated. With obstructed ventricular inflow, atrial contraction becomes increasingly important, and the onset of the atrial fibrillation may cause a striking deterioration.

3. *Impaired ventricular function.* This can be divided into two subgroups: (a) cases where ventricular muscle is diffusely affected, as in myocarditis, and (b) cases where part of the ventricle is virtually normal and part has been damaged, usually by myocardial infarction and subsequent fibrosis.

a. In the first group cardiac enlargement is usually observed as a result of ventricular dilatation. The damaged muscle fibres require to be stretched more in diastole (i.e. they need an increased preload) to enable them to exert the same contractile effort. Unfortunately, in accordance with Laplace's law, the dilated ventricle requires an even greater tension to be developed, so a vicious circle may be set up. The pericardium initially tends to limit the amount of ventricular dilatation, but it stretches in response to prolonged pressure. The stroke volume divided by the ventricular end-diastolic volume is called the *ejection fraction*; it is less than 0.5 in patients with impaired ventricular function. A global reduction in ventricular function of this type may result not only from primary disease of the ventricular muscle, but as the end stage in ventricular outflow obstruction or volume overload.

b. Areas of ventricular muscle which have been damaged or converted to scar tissue contract less well than adjacent normal muscle, and are called *akinetic areas or segments*. They may impede the function of the normal segments by distorting their contraction pattern. An extensive area of scar tissue may actually bulge outward while the rest of the ventricle is contracting; this is called dyskinetic movement. A circumscribed dyskinetic segment constitutes a ventricular aneurysm.

4. *Volume overload* occurs as a consequence of a chronically increased cardiac output, as in patients with an arteriovenous fistula, because of leakage of the mitral or aortic valves (or their right sided equivalents), or as a result of left-to-right intracardiac shunting, as in atrial septal defect. In all cases there is an increase in diastolic filling or preload, which in turn causes an increase in the diastolic volume of the ventricle. Healthy muscle responds by contracting vigorously, causing the large stroke volume and hyperdynamic cardiac impulse characteristic of these conditions. Eventually however progressive ventricular dilatation occurs, together with a reduction in ejection fraction and impairment of ventricular function.

Clinical features. The symptoms of cardiac failure have been considered (p. 118), as have the clinical features of acute circulatory failure, pulmonary oedema and massive pulmonary embolism. This section considers the ways in which the pathophysiological mechanisms involved in a particular patient can be deduced from the clinical examination and investigation.

The first priority is to decide whether the patient has left sided or right sided failure, or a combination of the two. Symptoms of orthopnoea or paroxysmal nocturnal dyspnoea, or the crepitations heard during inspiration over the lung bases in pulmonary oedema, indicate a left sided problem. They may however not occur in the presence of pulmonary vasoconstriction (p. 178). The chest radiograph is often a more sensitive indicator of pulmonary venous congestion than the clinical signs, and shows characteristic abnormalities (p. 126) even in the presence of pulmonary vasoconstriction. The most characteristic features of right sided cardiac failure are a raised jugular venous pressure and the presence of peripheral oedema.

Palpation of the precordium often gives a clue to the presence of left or right ventricular hypertrophy or dilatation, and this can be confirmed by the ECG, chest radiograph, and echocardiography. The detection of ventricular hypertrophy demands a search for signs of systemic or pulmonary hypertension, or a murmur indicating aortic or pulmonary stenosis. Ventricular hypertrophy in the absence of hypertension may be due to hypertrophic cardiomyopathy. A hyperdynamic, rather than a hypertrophic, character to the cardiac impulse should concentrate attention on causes of volume overload.

The detection of a murmur or murmurs suggests the possibility of a valvular lesion, or less probably, an intracardiac shunt. It is sometimes difficult to be sure whether a valve lesion is the cause of the cardiac failure, a minor incidental finding, or the consequence of some other mechanism of cardiac failure; for example, dilatation of the left or right ventricle may cause mitral or tricuspid regurgitation respectively. Echocardiography is often of great value in assessing valve lesions.

Cardiac failure in the absence of murmurs or ventricular hypertrophy is most commonly due to impaired ventricular function, and if necessary this can be confirmed by echocardiography or by radionuclide ventriculography. The ECG may provide clues to the aetiology, for example evidence of previous infarction. Other less common causes include pericardial effusion or a peripheral cause for volume overload.

High output cardiac failure is a term applied to situations where signs of cardiac failure coexist with peripheral vasodilatation and an increased cardiac output, as in severe anaemia, beri-beri and thyrotoxicosis. In many of these cases there are other reasons for the cardiac failure, and the high output requirements may be a precipitating rather than a causative factor.

HEPATIC IMPAIRMENT. Liver function is disturbed by a combination of increased hepatic venous pressure and reduced hepatic artery perfusion. Both the synthesis of coagulation factors and the metabolism of warfarin are affected early, leading to a potentiation of anticoagulant therapy. Later, there may be a rise in plasma bilirubin, alkaline phosphatase and alanine aminotransferase, but severe jaundice or hepatic failure are very unusual.

URAEMIA, HYPOKALAEMIA, AND HYPONATRAEMIA are discussed on page 152.

Treatment. There are three aspects to the treatment of chronic cardiac failure, the eradication of the precipitating cause, the improvement of cardiac output and efficiency, and the treatment of consequences such as pulmonary oedema. The cause of the failure can be tackled only in a selected group of patients by eliminating arrhythmia, correcting structural defects and repairing or replacing damaged valves. The other two aspects are interrelated, and the principles of treatment involved are common to different causes and varieties of cardiac failure.

As discussed under acute circulatory failure (p. 143), the main ways in which cardiac function can be improved are by increasing ventricular contractility, by optimising preload and by decreasing afterload. It is more convenient however to discuss the treatment of chronic cardiac failure under the headings of the principal classes of therapeutic agents which may be employed: digoxin, diuretics, and vasodilator drugs.

DIGOXIN. There is general agreement that digoxin is the agent of choice for controlling the ventricular rate in patients with atrial fibrillation and that it is a useful drug for treating certain supraventricular arrhythmias (p. 138). There is less certainty concerning its use as an inotropic agent, and in particular its value for the long-term treatment of patients with cardiac failure who remain in sinus rhythm. Digoxin and other digitalis glycosides seem to exert their inotropic action by increasing intracellular calcium availability, and it has been suggested that with long-continued use some form of adaptation occurs to lessen the effect.

Some clinical trials support, and others deny, the long-term efficacy of digoxin as an inotrope. The most likely explanation is that the effect is selective, but there are no well-validated rules for deciding whether an individual patient will benefit or not from long-term digoxin therapy. In general, digoxin is often particularly effective when myocardial function is depressed by drug therapy, e.g. with beta-adrenoceptor antagonists or quinidine, and largely ineffective in the presence of extensive ventricular damage from ischaemic heart disease. In practice, digoxin therapy should be given a trial in patients whose heart failure can be attributed to impaired ventricular function, but discontinued if there is no evidence of benefit. Because of the possibility of digoxin toxicity, the long-term use of digoxin in patients who remain in sinus rhythm should be subject to periodic review. Digoxin dosage and toxicity are discussed on page 138. Attempts have been made to produce other inotropic drugs suitable for long-term use, but such agents are not at present generally available.

DIURETICS. This therapy is extensively used in cardiac failure. All diuretics cause an increased urinary output of sodium, chloride and water, by inhibiting the reabsorption of these substances from the glomerular filtrate. The main effects are:

1. A reduction in oedema, both pulmonary and peripheral. This relieves breathlessness and improves the patient's comfort.

2. A reduction in blood, and especially plasma, volume. This reduces right and left ventricular preload, lowers jugular and pulmonary venous pressure, and relieves hepatic congestion. Although a reduction in ventricular filling pressure will tend to reduce cardiac output (Starling's law), the curve relating output to filling pressure is 'flat' in cardiac failure, so unless excessive doses of diuretics are used, the reduction in output will be minimal (Fig. 7.28). At the same time, ventricular size tends to diminish and the ventricles contract more effectively.

3. There is also often a small but significant reduction in left ventricular afterload as a result of peripheral arteriolar dilatation, which also helps to improve cardiac function.

Commonly used diuretics have been classified in three groups (p. 93), (a) high potency, loop diuretics, e.g. frusemide and bumetanide; (b) medium potency thiazide diuretics, e.g. bendrofluazide and hydrochlorothiazide. Chlorthalidone, though not chemically a thiazide is similar; and (c) low potency, potassium sparing diuretics, e.g. amiloride, triamterene and spironolactone. Dosage, mode of action and adverse effects are described on pages 93-94.

It is logical to combine diuretics from different classes if an increased effect is desired, but the

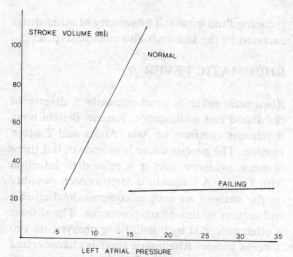

Fig. 7.28 Starling curves relating stroke volume to filling pressure in a normal subject and one with a failing ventricle. The curves shown are for the left ventricle; right ventricular curves show a similar relationship but at lower filling pressures. Because the 'curve' for the failing ventricle is very flat, preload reduction (lowering the filling pressure) makes little difference to output, but enables left atrial pressure to be lowered so that pulmonary oedema does not accumulate.

use of multiple agents increases the responsibility of the prescriber for monitoring potentially dangerous upsets of fluid or electrolyte imbalance. Combining a thiazide or a loop diuretic with a potassium sparing diuretic will give an increased diuresis while helping to conserve potassium. Even though thiazides are less potent than loop diuretics, the addition of a thiazide to a combination of loop diuretic and potassium sparing diuretic will often produce a further increase in diuretic effect.

Several diuretic combinations are commercially available. They tend to be expensive, and the use of a theoretically balanced combination is no substitute for electrolyte monitoring. Occasionally however they may help by reducing the number of pills the patient is expected to take.

VASODILATORS. The availability of angiotensin converting enzyme (ACE) inhibitors has revolutionised vasodilator therapy in chronic cardiac failure. Captopril and enalapril are powerful arteriolar and venodilators which also inhibit aldosterone release. Unlike other classes of vasodilator, therapeutic efficiency is usually maintained for prolonged periods. Most patients will require a moderate dose of diuretic in conjunction

with an ACE inhibitor, but large doses of diuretics can often be markedly reduced. Before starting an ACE inhibitor it is prudent to reduce diuretic doses until the jugular venous pressure is slightly elevated; this helps to prevent initial hypotension. Therapy should be started with a small dose (6.25 mg of captopril; 2.5 mg of enalapril) and gradually increased until the desired effect is achieved or postural hypotension prevents further increase. Because of the aldosterone antagonism, potassium supplements are not usually needed, and plasma potassium should be monitored. Apart from postural hypotension, the main side-effects are 'indigestion' and rashes. A rising plasma urea usually results from over-diuresis, and is reversible. Blood dyscrasias and a true nephropathy have been reported but are rare. Patients should be warned to stop the drug if severe diarrhoea develops, as serious fluid depletion may occur.

OTHER TREATMENT. Physical rest is a valuable aid to the management of cardiac failure. Bed-rest increases renal blood flow and will often initiate a diuresis in an oedematous patient without any adjustment of diuretic therapy. Conversely, patients often need a larger dose of diuretic when they are up and about than when in bed. Patients with left ventricular failure may be unable to lie flat, and prefer to rest and sleep in a chair or raised on pillows.

Patients should be discouraged from adding extra salt to food, or consuming salty foods or drugs containing or retaining sodium (p. 357), but there is little place for special low salt diets. Fluid restriction is necessary only when oedema is present with a low plasma sodium concentration.

Obesity seriously impairs effort tolerance, and should be vigorously treated. In contrast, patients with severe cardiac failure become cachectic, and it is difficult to reverse this unless the cardiac failure can be controlled. Anaemia must also be corrected.

Complications of cardiac failure and their treatment. Patients with advanced cardiac failure often exhibit complex metabolic and endocrine upsets which are partly the consequence of the cardiac failure and partly the result of therapy.

URAEMIA. Renal function is impaired by a reduction in renal blood flow. This may be caused by reflex vasoconstriction, by severe damage to cardiac function, or most commonly by excessive use of potent diuretics. A rising plasma urea concentration is an indication for reviewing the patient's state of hydration, and perhaps reducing the dose of diuretic. When renal function is deteriorating in spite of adequate hydration a renal vasodilator such as dopamine may help, but the possibility of acute tubular necrosis should also be considered (p. 403).

HYPOKALAEMIA. Under conditions of reduced renal blood flow, renin production is increased and leads in turn to increased aldosterone production. Renin output is further enhanced by the salt-depleting effects of diuretics, and aldosterone metabolism is hindered by hepatic congestion. The resulting *secondary hyperaldosteronism* may in itself cause hypokalaemia and alkalosis, and it potentiates the potassium depleting properties of diuretics. Most of the body's potassium is intracellular, and there may be substantial depletion of potassium stores even when the plasma concentration is in the normal range. Potassium depletion should be treated by replacement therapy with potassium chloride and/or a potassium sparing diuretic. If cardiac failure is so severe as to cause renal failure, hyperkalaemia may become a problem, and potassium supplements must be stopped.

HYPONATRAEMIA. A falling plasma sodium concentration may sometimes be encountered in severely ill patients on large doses of diuretics. If the patient is oedematous and has a high venous pressure this usually represents inappropriate water retention and responds to a moderate restriction of water intake (p. 92). On the other hand if there is no oedema and the venous pressure is low it is more likely to reflect severe sodium depletion, and oligaemia. This calls for diuretic withdrawal and perhaps fluid replacement (p. 94). In very ill patients the ion pump of the cell membrane may fail to function normally, leading to a falling plasma sodium and a rising potassium concentration.

DRUG TOXICITY. Digoxin toxicity is often a feature of worsening cardiac failure, as renal function becomes impaired. It is potentiated by hypokalaemia. The characteristic vomiting makes things worse by increasing potassium loss and reducing fluid intake. The toxicity of other drugs excreted by the kidney is also enhanced (p. 412).

RHEUMATIC FEVER

Rheumatic fever is predominantly a disease of childhood and adolescence. Rare in Britain now, it remains common in Asia, Africa and Eastern Europe. The precise cause is unknown, but there is much evidence that it is related to infection with Group A haemolytic streptococci, possibly on the basis of an antigen common to the heart and certain strains of streptococcus. The disease is often preceded by tonsillitis or pharyngitis 1 to 3 weeks before. Rheumatic fever is characterised by acute arthritis and/or carditis, sometimes with involvement of the nervous system. Recurrences are frequent unless prophylactic treatment is given. After the acute attack, which may sometimes be mild or subclinical, progressive damage to the heart valves may occur, often not manifesting itself until several years later. This is called chronic rheumatic heart disease.

Pathology. In the acute attack the connective tissues of the myocardium, pericardium, synovial membranes and tendons are affected by inflammation, with oedema, hyperaemia and leucocyte infiltration. The hallmark of rheumatic fever is the Aschoff nodule, a central area of necrosis surrounded by small round cells, histiocytes and giant cells. The mitral, and to a lesser extent the aortic valves, have pinhead-size warty vegetations. In some aggressive forms of rheumatic fever, valve tissue is rapidly destroyed. Subsequent scarring leads to the valve changes of chronic rheumatic heart disease.

Clinical features. The onset may be sudden with pain, swelling and stiffness in one or more joints, fever, sweating and tachycardia, or it may be insidious with fatigue, and loss of weight. The large joints are principally affected. Characteristically there is a migrating polyarthritis, one joint improving as another becomes worse. In severe cases the joints become hot, swollen, red and very tender; effusions may develop. The joints return to normal when the attack is over. Tachycardia tends to be out of proportion to the degree of fever, and may persist after the latter has settled. Although pancarditis probably occurs to some extent in all cases of rheumatic fever, only about half of them have later evidence of chronic rheumatic heart disease. In the early stages, endocarditis may be suspected from the diminished intensity of the first heart sound or from the development of a systolic murmur. A transient mitral diastolic murmur may be heard (Carey Coombs murmur). Aortic regurgitation can also occur. Myocarditis may be assumed to be present if there is endocarditis or pericarditis. Its presence is also suggested by undue tachycardia, increasing enlargement of the heart, evidence of cardiac failure and abnormalities in the ECG (see below).

Pericarditis is characterised by retrosternal pain and pericardial friction may be heard. An effusion may develop. Pericarditis is not in itself a serious manifestation of rheumatic fever.

Rheumatic nodules occur most often in childhood, and their significance lies in the almost invariable association with active carditis. They are painless, subcutaneous, not attached to skin and tend to occur over bony prominences such as elbows, knees, scapulae, occiput and vertebrae, or on tendons.

Erythema marginatum (erythema annulare) consists of transient pink patches which appear mainly on the trunk and rapidly enlarge to form irregular crescents which join to form larger areas with a pale centre. The margins are slightly elevated.

Sydenham's chorea is described on page 652. The majority of children with chorea subsequently develop evidence of chronic rheumatic valvular disease.

A raised ESR is usually present and may persist as evidence of the activity of the rheumatic process when all other manifestations have subsided. In about a quarter, a group A streptococcus can be grown from the throat. A high ASO (antistreptolysin 'O') titre rising or raised to above 300 units provides evidence of recent streptococcal infection. The chest radiograph often shows cardiac enlargement. Echocardiography may confirm ventricular dilatation or demonstrate a pericardial effusion. The commoner ECG changes are prolongation of the PR interval and abnormalities of the ST segments and T waves.

Diagnosis. Since there is no single diagnostic test, diagnosis depends on an assessment of the whole clinical picture together with the laboratory findings. The Duckett Jones criteria have been proposed as an aid to diagnosis. They classify the clinical manifestations into major criteria (carditis, arthritis, nodules, erythema marginatum and chorea) and minor criteria (fever, arthralgia and a previous history of rheumatic fever). A raised ESR and a prolonged PR interval also qualify as minor criteria. It is suggested that a diagnosis should be based on two major criteria or one major and two minor criteria plus in each case evidence of previous streptococcal infections.

Treatment. Rest in bed is indicated until symptoms and fever have subsided, the sleeping pulse rate, white count and haemoglobin level have returned to normal, and weight is being regained. Thereafter the return to activity should be gradual. The ESR is a useful guide to progress. Phenoxymethylpenicillin should be given, routinely for 7 to 10 days, to kill any remaining haemolytic streptococci in the nose or throat. Erythromycin is an alternative in patients allergic to penicillin.

Aspirin is effective in combating pain and fever. The daily dose is 50 mg per kg body weight divided into 4-hourly doses, with a double dose at night to avoid waking the patient. This dose should be continued until fever and symptoms have been controlled for at least 10 days and then gradually reduced. Should rheumatic manifestations return, larger quantities will have to be resumed. If toxic symptoms develop the dose must be reduced to a level which can be tolerated. Nausea, headache, dizziness, tinnitus and deafness are the early toxic symptoms, followed by vomiting, hyperventilation and confusion. Aspirin relieves symptoms but probably does not shorten the course of the disease or reduce the incidence of cardiac complications.

Corticosteroids such as prednisolone (60–80 mg per day, or 3 mg per kg in children, tailing off after 10 days) may help to relieve severe symptoms, but there is little convincing evidence they affect long-term results.

Convalescence in a suitable environment will be required when the acute attack is over and before return to school or work. Its length will depend on the duration of the preceding illness and the severity of any complications.

Prevention. Children who have had rheumatic fever should have continuous antibiotic prophylaxis until about 20 years of age. Intramuscular benzathine penicillin 1.2 mega units per month is more effective, though less convenient, than phenoxymethylpenicillin (125 mg b.d.) or sulphadimidine (550 mg b.d.).

DISEASES OF THE HEART VALVES

A diseased valve may be narrowed (stenosed) or it may fail to close adequately and thus permit regurgitation of blood. The term incompetence may be used synonymously with regurgitation but the latter is preferable as a stenosed valve is obviously not 'competent'. Regurgitation may be present without structural change in the cusps, e.g. from dilatation of the mitral valve ring in left ventricular failure, the tricuspid valve ring in right ventricular failure, the pulmonary valve ring in pulmonary hypertension or the aortic valve ring in aortic aneurysm.

The principal worldwide cause of symptomatic valvular disease is rheumatic endocarditis, but in many countries it is being overtaken by congenital and degenerative causes. Chronic rheumatic disease most commonly affects the mitral valve, next the aortic, comparatively infrequently the tricuspid and very rarely the pulmonary valve.

Mitral valve prolapse is possibly the most common valvular abnormality; it has been claimed to be present in about 5% of the young adult population. About one child in 80 is born with a bicuspid aortic valve; initially this is asymptomatic, but it may become the seat of infective endocarditis, and in middle or old age degeneration and calcification may result in aortic stenosis or regurgitation. Congenital aortic stenosis may occur, but is much less common. Congenital lesions are responsible for most cases of pulmonary valve disease.

Infective endocarditis may transform a trivial valve lesion into a major one; it usually affects valves deformed by congenital abnormality or rheumatic disease. Syphilis may cause aortic regurgitation from dilatation of the aorta. Exceptionally, a cusp may rupture spontaneously or as a result of external trauma.

Mitral stenosis

In about half the patients there is a history of rheumatic fever or chorea. The gradual scarring process in the heart takes many years to develop fully. The commissures of the mitral valve become adherent and the chordae are often short and deformed. The mitral valve orifice is about 5 cm^2 in diastole in health, and is reduced in severe mitral stenosis to about 1cm^2. With the reduction in the size of the valve orifice, cardiac output can be maintained only by a rise in left atrial, pulmonary venous and pulmonary capillary pressures with a resultant loss of lung compliance. A sudden increase in pulmonary venous pressure, caused perhaps by the onset of atrial fibrillation, may precipitate pulmonary oedema. With a more gradual rise in pressure, there tends to be an increase in pulmonary vascular resistance which provides some protection against pulmonary oedema.

In about 80% of cases left atrial dilatation is prominent, and may be accompanied by atrial fibrillation. In a minority, the left atrium remains small but becomes hypertrophied and sinus rhythm tends to persist in spite of severe stenosis. All cases may develop pulmonary hypertension and right ventricular hypertrophy, but this is often more severe in those who remain in sinus rhythm. All patients with mitral stenosis are at risk from left atrial thrombosis and systemic thromboembolism, particularly those with atrial fibrillation. Mitral stenosis is frequently associated with mitral regurgitation or disease of the aortic or tricuspid valves.

Clinical features. The gradual reduction in the mitral valve orifice usually produces breathlessness in about the third decade. The extra demands of pregnancy, or the impairment of function brought about by tachycardia or atrial fibrillation may precipitate a deterioration, and may bring on breathlessness even at rest. Pulmonary congestion may cause a cough, and pulmonary hypertension lead to haemoptysis. Systemic embolism is sometimes the presenting feature.

In some patients with mitral stenosis the face may have a malar flush but this is not specific. The major signs are those which are due to the abnormal valve (p. 124). It closes with an unusually loud sound which may be palpable—

the tapping apex beat. The turbulent flow, which is heralded by the opening snap, causes the characteristic diastolic murmur, and often a thrill (Fig. 7.29). The murmur may be accentuated during atrial systole, and in early or asymptomatic patients this presystolic murmur may be the only auscultatory abnormality. In patients with symptoms the murmur usually extends from the opening snap to the first heart sound. The opening snap may be inaudible if the valve is heavily calcified. Accompanying mitral regurgitation may cause a pansystolic murmur.

An abnormal pulsation is often felt to the left of the sternum; this may be due either to right ventricular hypertrophy or to forward displacement of the heart by a dilated left atrium. Pulmonary hypertension may cause a loud pulmonary component of the second heart sound, and right atrial hypertrophy may produce a prominent *a* wave in the jugular venous pulse. Tricuspid regurgitation secondary to right ventricular dilatation causes a systolic murmur and systolic waves in the venous pulse.

The physical signs of mitral stenosis are often found before symptoms develop, and their recognition is of particular importance in the obstetric department, since the identification of mitral disease allows appropriate decisions to be made about its management.

Investigation. The ECG may show either the bifid P waves associated with left atrial hypertrophy or atrial fibrillation. There may be evidence of right ventricular hypertrophy; one of the earliest signs is a reduction in the size of the usual QS complex in lead V1. Enlargement of the left atrium and its appendage and of the main pulmonary artery may be seen on the chest radiograph (Fig. 7.29). There may be enlargement of the upper pulmonary veins and horizontal linear shadows in the costophrenic angles as indications of a high left atrial and pulmonary venous pressure. In the lateral and right anterior oblique position an enlarged left atrium causes a backward displacement of the barium-filled oesophagus.

Echocardiography is very useful in the evaluation of mitral stenosis; apart from confirming the diagnosis it allows an estimate to be made of its severity and it also provides information on the rigidity and state of calcification of the valve cusps, the size of the left atrium, and the state of left ventricular function. Cardiac catheterisation has been extensively used to confirm the severity of mitral stenosis by measurement of the gradient across the mitral valve from recording pressures simultaneously in the left ventricle and left atrium (or pulmonary arterial wedge position). Increasing confidence in echocardiography has considerably reduced the need for this, although catheterisation

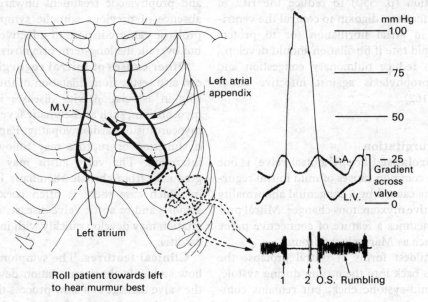

Fig. 7.29 Mitral stenosis. O.S. = opening snap.

may still have a role in assessing mitral regurgitation and associated coronary disease.

Treatment. The definitive treatment of mitral stenosis is surgical, in the form either of mitral valvotomy or mitral valve replacement, but since surgery is not without risk and its long-term results somewhat unpredictable, patients with minor symptoms should be treated medically. Management in relation to pregnancy is discussed on page 189.

Mitral valvotomy remains the surgical treatment of choice in patients with significant symptoms, pure mitral stenosis, no mitral regurgitation, and a thin, mobile and non-calcified mitral valve. It may be done with a dilator introduced into the mitral valve through the left ventricle under guidance from a finger inserted into the left atrium, or under direct vision using cardiopulmonary by pass. The results are dependent on the expertise of the surgeon, but when the operation is successful patients can expect 5 to 20 years of benefit before the stenosis recurs. In some patients traumatic mitral regurgitation is produced which is usually slight but may require subsequent mitral valve replacement.

Mitral valve replacement is indicated if there is substantial mitral regurgitation, or if the valve is rigid or heavily calcified.

Medical treatment of mitral stenosis consists of anticoagulation (p. 550) to reduce the risk of systemic embolism, digoxin to control the ventricular rate in atrial fibrillation (or to protect against a rapid rate if fibrillation should develop), diuretics to reduce pulmonary congestion and antibiotic prophylaxis against infective endocarditis (p. 162).

Mitral regurgitation

Mitral prolapse ('floppy' mitral valve) is one of the more common causes of mild mitral regurgitation. It is caused by a congenital abnormality or degenerative myxomatous changes. Mitral prolapse is sometimes a feature of connective tissue disorders such as Marfan's syndrome.

In the mildest forms of mitral prolapse the valve bulges back into the atrium during systole, causing a mid-systolic click, but remains competent and so produces no murmur. Frequently however the click is followed by a late systolic murmur, and the combination of mid-systolic click and late systolic murmur is the clinical hallmark of mitral prolapse. Sometimes multiple clicks are heard, while in other cases prolapse occurs at the start of systole, the click is obscured by the first heart sound, and the pansystolic murmur is indistinguishable from other causes of mitral regurgitation. The physical signs may vary with posture or respiration.The diagnosis can be confirmed by echo- or angiocardiography.

Progressive elongation of the chordae tendineae may lead to increasing mitral regurgitation, while if chordal rupture occurs, regurgitation may suddenly become severe. These complications are rare before the fifth or sixth decade.

Mitral prolapse is associated with an increased incidence of arrhythmias; these are usually benign but a small minority of patients have frequent and bizarre arrhythmias and perhaps an increased risk of sudden death. Many patients found to have mitral prolapse present with atypical chest pain but the specificity of this association is uncertain. Telling a patient there is an abnormal valve sometimes exacerbates or perpetuates a cardiac neurosis. Mitral prolapse is more common than would be expected in young people with embolic stroke or transient cerebral ischaemic attacks, but the overall risk of the complication is very small and prophylactic treatment unwarranted in the absence of previous embolic symptoms. Mitral prolapse can predispose to infective endocarditis but overall, the long-term prognosis is good.

Other causes of mitral regurgitation. This can also result from dilatation of the mitral valve ring in association with diseases involving the myocardium, such as rheumatic fever, diphtheria, myocarditis or cardiomyopathy. Papillary muscle dysfunction or rupture may follow myocardial infarction. The valve cusps may be damaged gradually from chronic rheumatic heart disease, in which case there is often coexisting mitral stenosis and/or aortic valve disease. Mitral regurgitation may develop quickly with infective endocarditis.

Clinical features. The symptoms depend on how suddenly the regurgitation develops. When the valve damage is a slow process the symptoms are similar to those in mitral stenosis. In myocardial disease, the mitral regurgitation exacerbates an already serious situation.

The physical signs arise from the regurgitant jet which causes an apical systolic murmur. This often radiates into the axilla, and may be accompanied by a thrill. The apex beat is usually displaced to the left as a result of dilatation of the left ventricle. The abnormal valve closure is often associated with a quiet first heart sound, and the increased forward flow through the mitral valve may give rise to a loud third heart sound or a short mid-diastolic murmur.

Investigation. The radiograph and ECG often give evidence of left atrial or left ventricular hypertrophy. Atrial fibrillation is common as a consequence of atrial dilatation. Echocardiography provides information about the state of the mitral valve, but Doppler cardiography gives a better estimate of the extent of regurgitation. At cardiac catheterisation the severity of mitral regurgitation may be indicated by the size of the v waves in the left atrial or pulmonary artery wedge trace, or by left ventricular angiography. In practice, the usual problem lies in deciding the extent to which cardiac failure is due to mitral regurgitation and the extent to which it reflects impaired left ventricular function.

Treatment. If mitral regurgitation is due to myocardial disease, treatment, when available, is directed to the latter. When the valve disease is predominant and the symptoms severe, mitral valve replacement is indicated. Infective endocarditis should be treated, if possible, prior to surgery. Mitral regurgitation of moderate severity can often be managed medically, using a diuretic, digoxin and perhaps a vasodilator. Anticoagulation should be considered if there is atrial fibrillation.

Aortic stenosis

This may be a congenital fault, may arise from fusion of the valve cusps from rheumatic damage, or it may be a late development from premature calcification in a congenital bicuspid aortic valve. Rarely congenital aortic stenosis may be due to a subvalvar diaphragm or more rarely still to a supravalvar stenosis. Except in the congenital forms, aortic stenosis develops slowly; the cardiac output is maintained at the cost of a steadily increasing gradient across the aortic valve. The left ventricle becomes increasingly hypertrophied and fibrotic changes may follow. The coronary blood flow may become inadequate, particularly if there is concomitant coronary atheroma. There is often accompanying aortic regurgitation.

Clinical features. Symptoms arise from restriction of the cardiac output on exercise, which may cause syncope. Breathlessness does not develop until left ventricular hypertrophy fails to compensate for the obstruction and is therefore a late feature of the disease. Inadequate coronary blood flow may cause angina or arrhythmias. Sudden death is common with severe aortic stenosis.

The physical signs arise from the jet through the aortic valve (Fig. 7.30) which causes a systolic murmur and often a thrill which may be transmitted to the carotid pulse as the 'carotid shudder'. There is sometimes an ejection sound (ejection click) from movement of the stenotic aortic valve prior to the onset of the murmur; this is absent when the valve is rigid and calcified.

The sustained, thrusting, apical impulse is characteristic of left ventricular hypertrophy. The combination of a stiff left ventricle and hypertrophied left atrium may cause a fourth heart sound. The restricted cardiac output is often reflected in a small volume, slow-rising arterial pulse. The physical signs are usually diagnostic, the slow-rising pulse helping to distinguish aortic stenosis from hypertrophic cardiomyopathy (p. 181) or mitral regurgitation.

Investigation. The radiographic changes are shown in Figure 7.30. Under the image intensifier calcification of the aortic valve can often be seen. The ECG may show left atrial and left ventricular hypertrophy, and in advanced cases changes of the latter are gross (Fig. 7.31). Echocardiography may demonstrate a disorganised aortic valve, left ventricular hypertrophy or left ventricular dilatation. Doppler cardiography or cardiac catheterisation can be used to determine the gradient across the aortic valve which together with a measurement of cardiac output can be used to calculate the aortic valve area. As with mitral stenosis, echocardiography has tended to reduce the need for catheterisation, but it is still valuable

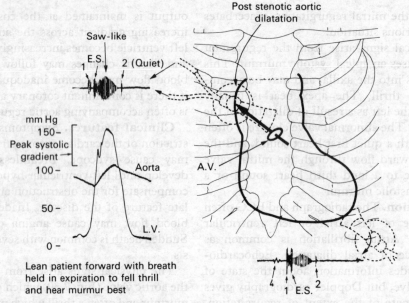

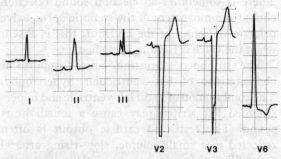

Fig. 7.30 Aortic stenosis. E.S. = ejection sound (p. 123).

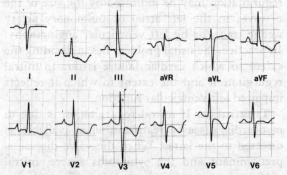

Fig. 7.31 Left ventricular hypertrophy from a 75-year-old woman with aortic stenosis. The QRS complexes in the limb leads I, II and III are slightly widened to 0.10 seconds, but of normal amplitude in this case. However, there is a very large S wave in V2 and a large R wave in V6, with T wave inversion in V6.

for assessing the state of the coronary arteries.

Treatment. Unlike patients with mitral stenosis, it is often necessary to recommend surgical replacement of the valve when symptoms are slight or even absent if the aortic stenosis is severe. To wait too long may result in irreversible damage to the left ventricle. The valve is replaced, under cardiopulmonary bypass, with a prosthetic or heterograft valve. Postoperatively there is usually ECG and other evidence of reduction in the left ventricular hypertrophy. In some cases of severe congenital aortic stenosis, valvotomy may be required as an intermediate measure until an

Figure 7.32 Right ventricular hypertrophy and right atrial hypertrophy. ECG from a 38-year-old woman with primary pulmonary hypertension. There is a tall (3 mm) peaked P wave in leads II and aVF; there is a tall R wave with T wave inversion in the right sided chest leads V1–V3 and a deep S wave in the left sided chest leads V4–V6.

adult-size valve can be inserted. Long-term medical treatment of symptomatic aortic stenosis is justified only if extreme age or intercurrent illness preclude surgery.

Aortic regurgitation

This results from abnormal aortic cusps as in congenital bicuspid valves, or when valves have been damaged by rheumatic heart disease or infective endocarditis. Aortic regurgitation may also be due to dilatation of the first part of the aorta in cystic medial necrosis, Marfan's syndrome, ankylosing spondylitis, late syphilis or atheroma. When the leak is large the stroke output of the left ventricle may be doubled or trebled. The major arteries are then conspicuously pulsatile; the left ventricle dilates and hypertrophies and initially compensates for the fault in the valve. The left ventricular diastolic pressure rises, at first only with exercise; the pulmonary vascular pressures then also increase and breathlessness develops.

Clinical features. Until the onset of breathlessness the only symptom may be an awareness of the heartbeat, particularly when lying on the left side. Paroxysmal nocturnal dyspnoea may be the first symptom. Peripheral oedema may follow. Angina may occur particularly when there is coexisting coronary atheroma or when the coronary ostia are involved in syphilitic aortitis.

The characteristic murmur is illustrated in Figure 7.33; although it is usually best heard to the left of the sternum it is sometimes louder to the right, particularly with syphilitic aortitis. A thrill is uncommon. When the leak is small the murmur will be heard only if the steps shown in Figure 7.33 are followed; this is of crucial importance in the early detection of infective endocarditis affecting the aortic valve. A systolic murmur due to the increased stroke volume is

common and should not be regarded as due to accompanying stenosis without other evidence of the latter. When the leak is large the diagnosis is usually easy, with gross pulsation in the large arteries, a collapsing pulse, a low diastolic and an increased pulse pressure. There is usually a thrusting apical impulse and often a presystolic impulse and a fourth heart sound as evidence of left atrial hypertrophy.

Investigation. The change in the radiographic outline is illustrated in Figure 7.5. The ECG usually shows left ventricular hypertrophy (Fig. 7.31). Echocardiography in aortic regurgitation often shows fluttering of the anterior mitral leaflet in the regurgitant jet and the jet is usually readily detected by Doppler cardiography. In severe aortic regurgitation the mitral valve may close completely before the onset of ventricular systole. The echocardiogram may reveal vegetations in infective endocarditis, and gives information about left ventricular function. Cardiac catheterisation and aortography are also helpful in assessing severity.

Treatment. Aortic valve replacement under cardiopulmonary bypass is indicated when aortic regurgitation is beginning to cause symptoms or when an enlarging heart or progressive ECG changes give evidence of increasing left ventricular overload.

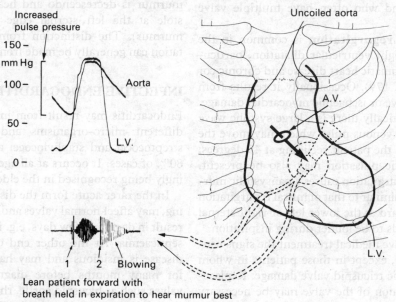

Fig. 7.33 Aortic regurgitation.

Tricuspid and pulmonary valve disease

Tricuspid stenosis is usually due to chronic rheumatic heart disease and is almost always accompanied by mitral stenosis and often also by aortic valve disease. Very rarely, tricuspid valve disease may be associated with the carcinoid syndrome (p. 312). The symptoms tend to be those of accompanying mitral disease, but if tricuspid stenosis is severe there is an increased likelihood of the development of ascites and peripheral oedema.

With sinus rhythm the *a* wave in the jugular venous pulse is conspicuous and often easily palpable. There may be presystolic hepatic pulsation. Mid-diastolic and presystolic murmurs may be heard, similar in timing to those in mitral stenosis but lacking the rumbling quality and increased in inspiration. Tricuspid murmurs are best heard at the lower left or right sternal edge rather than at the apex. The radiograph may show disproportionate enlargement of the right atrium, but this is unreliable; in the ECG there may be the peaked P waves of right atrial hypertrophy. The echocardiogram is often helpful.

Occasionally tricuspid valve replacement is required, but the operation is often less satisfactory than those for mitral and aortic valve disease, partly because tricuspid stenosis tends to occur in those patients who have had severe rheumatic pancarditis and who often have multiple valve lesions.

Tricuspid regurgitation is common in the presence of right ventricular dilatation, particularly with rheumatic heart disease and chronic cor pulmonale (p. 179). Occasionally it results from rheumatic valve or ischaemic myocardial damage.

Characteristically there is a large systolic wave in the jugular venous pulse which may move the ear lobes with the patient reclining at 45 degrees; systolic hepatic pulsation may also be present. Tricuspid regurgitation causes a pansystolic murmur which is similar to that of mitral regurgitation but is best heard at the lower left or right sternal edge, and tends to be louder during inspiration.

With effective medical treatment the signs usually disappear, except in those patients in whom there is organic tricuspid valve damage. Replacement or plication of the valve may be necessary in a few of these patients.

Pulmonary stenosis is usually congenital and may be isolated or part of Fallot's tetralogy (p. 188). It is recognisable from an ejection systolic murmur to the left of the upper sternum, radiating towards the left shoulder, often accompanied by a thrill which is best appreciated when the patient leans forward and breathes out. The murmur is often preceded by an ejection sound. Delay in right ventricular ejection may cause wide splitting of the second heart sound, but pulmonary valve closure is often abnormally quiet and the splitting may be recognised only on phonocardiography. Mild pulmonary stenosis is fairly common and does not require treatment.

Severe pulmonary stenosis is characterised clinically by a loud, harsh murmur, an increased right ventricular thrust, prominent *a* waves in the jugular pulse, ECG evidence of right ventricular and right atrial hypertrophy, and post-stenotic pulmonary artery dilatation on the chest radiograph. The severity of stenosis can be further assessed by cardiac catheterization. Pulmonary valvotomy is indicated for patients with severe stenosis; it is carried out under cardiopulmonary bypass. Percutaneous balloon pulmonary valvuloplasty is an alternative to valvotomy, and may supersede it.

Pulmonary regurgitation is rare and is usually a feature of pulmonary hypertension. The murmur is decrescendo and heard in early diastole at the left sternal edge (Graham Steell murmur). The distinction from aortic regurgitation can generally be made from other evidence.

INFECTIVE ENDOCARDITIS

Endocarditis may result from infection by many different micro-organisms and by fungi but streptococci and staphylococci account for over 80% of cases. It occurs at all ages and is increasingly being recognised in the elderly.

In the rarer acute form the disease is fulminating, may affect normal valves and if untreated may result in death in a few days, e.g. in staphylococcal septicaemia. At the other end of the range the disease is insidious and may have been present for many months before diagnosis. Abnormal valves such as bicuspid aortic, rheumatic or prosthetic valves, or various forms of congenital heart disease, e.g. ventricular septal defect or persistent ductus arteriosus, are the usual underlying lesions. Regurgitant mitral and aortic valves are the commonest to be affected. Normal valves, particularly the tricuspid, are liable to become infected in 'main line' drug addicts.

Pathology. Damage to the delicate endothelial covering of the heart valves leads to the deposition of platelets and fibrin. The process is exaggerated with abnormal valves, or where an abnormal jet impinges on the endocardium. Colonisation of such deposits by blood borne organisms may occur and cause infective endocarditis. The structure of the valve cusps, and the presence of fibrin aggregates may serve to protect the organisms from the usual defence mechanisms of the host.

Streptococcus sanguis, a common cause of periodontal infections, is liable to enter the bloodstream at the time of a dental extraction. Staphylococci (p. 742) and *Streptococcus faecalis* are other common causative organisms; with the latter there may be a history of urethral or pelvic surgery. *Coxiella burnetii* (Q fever) endocarditis is more common in, but not confined to, those who work with sheep or with carcasses.

Affected valves develop vegetations, composed of organisms, fibrin and platelets, which may be a source of embolism. Regurgitation may develop or increase owing to the perforation of a cusp. Weeks or months after the onset, mycotic aneurysms may develop in systemic arteries, and rupture. At post mortem it is common to find infarction of the spleen and kidneys as well as other organs. Glomerulonephritis is also found, possibly associated with an immune complex reaction.

Clinical features. Infective endocarditis should be suspected when a patient known to have congenital or valvular heart disease develops a fever or complains of unusual tiredness. Often, however, infective endocarditis occurs in patients whose heart disease has been hitherto unsuspected and the diagnosis may be dangerously delayed because it has not been considered. Persistent fever, often recognisable from a history of sweating at night, unexplained arterial occlusion, or the discovery of anaemia or splenomegaly may be presenting features. The disease is almost invariably fatal if untreated, and even if the infection is controlled there is a high mortality. Delay in diagnosis may result in an embolic stroke, progressive valve damage, heart failure and death.

In the early stages the patient looks well but later pallor may be obvious. Other features commonly listed should nowadays be regarded as evidence of delay in diagnosis; these include purpura and petechial haemorrhages in the skin and mucous membranes and splinter haemorrhages under the finger nails. Osler's nodes consist of painful tender swellings at the fingertips; they probably result from vasculitis rather than embolism, and are rare. Finger clubbing is a late sign. The spleen is frequently just palpable, but in coxiella infections both it and the liver may be considerably enlarged. Microscopic haematuria is common. The finding of any of these features in a patient with fever or malaise is an indication for re-examination for hitherto unrecognised heart disease such as trivial aortic regurgitation.

Investigation. Elevation of the ESR is usual; a normocytic, normochromic anaemia and a leucocytosis are common but not invariable. Blood culture is the crucial investigation; it should identify the infection and give guidance about therapy. Three specimens taken at intervals of 2–3 hours should be sufficient.

Echocardiography is of value for detecting and following the progress of vegetations. It is, however, possible for these to be too small for echocardiographic detection.

Treatment. The basic objective is to give a suitable antibiotic in adequate dosage for a long enough period. The treatment of streptococcal and staphylococcal infections has been studied by a working party whose report (p. 196) should be consulted for details. Their main recommendations are: (1) for penicillin sensitive streptococci give benzylpenicillin i.v. and gentamicin for 2 weeks; then amoxycillin for 2 weeks; (2) for less sensitive streptococci continue gentamicin for 4 weeks; (3) for elderly patients or those with impaired renal function netilmicin is an alternative to gentamicin; (4) for staphylococcal infections give flucloxacillin plus fusidic acid; (5) for patients allergic to penicillin, vancomycin is recommended. Further information about these antibiotics is available in Chapter 3. Metronidazole is of value in endocarditis caused by anaerobes. Coxiella endocarditis responds to tetracycline combined with clindamycin.

Any source of infection should be removed if possible, for example a tooth with an apical abscess should be extracted. Cardiac surgery is indicated if valve damage causes progressive cardiac failure, if the endocarditis involves a prosthetic valve, or if active infection persists in spite of adequate treatment, as evidenced by continuing fever, raised ESR and changing murmurs. Antimicrobial therapy should be started before surgery.

Prevention. Every patient with heart disease susceptible to infective endocarditis should be warned of the absolute necessity of taking special care of the teeth, and of having antibiotic cover for dental extractions or other dental procedures which go below the gum margin. For outpatient dental procedures, oral amoxycillin (3 g as a single dose one hour before) is effective and practical. Erythromycin is an alternative for those allergic to penicillin. Patients undergoing operations on the gastrointestinal or urinary tracts should be given ampicillin (1 g i.m. pre-operatively and 500 mg t.d.s. for 48 hours afterwards). Prolonged antibiotic therapy prior to the procedure may encourage the overgrowth of resistant organisms.

ISCHAEMIC (CORONARY) HEART DISEASE

Atheromatous disease of the coronary arteries is the most important single cause of death in the Western world. Although its global incidence is still increasing there has been a recent marked fall in the United States and elsewhere. Atheroma is the commonest cause of angina pectoris, and leads also to myocardial infarction and its complications, to cardiac failure and to sudden death.

The coronary circulation. The right coronary artery arises from the right sinus of Valsalva and passes in the right atrioventricular groove to supply the right ventricle, part of the interventricular septum and the inferior part of the left ventricle; a branch supplies the AV node. The left coronary artery arises from the left sinus and divides into (1) an anterior descending branch, which supplies part of the septum and the anterior and apical parts of the heart and (2) the circumflex branch, which passes in the left atrioventricular groove and supplies the lateral and posterior surfaces of the heart. In health there are small anastomoses between the coronary arteries; these enlarge under the influence of ischaemia if the flow through a neighbouring coronary artery is compromised. With advancing years an extensive network of anastomotic vessels may develop.

Aetiology. The aetiology of ischaemic heart disease is complex, and much of our understanding of it is based on epidemiological evidence. For a more detailed review and references to the original data the reader should consult the review by Oliver (p. 196). Although there are broad similarities between the prevalence of coronary atheroma at autopsy, the clinical prevalence of angina, and the incidences of myocardial infarction and sudden cardiac death, there are also striking differences. Thus the incidence of sudden cardiac death may vary threefold between areas with a similar prevalence of coronary atheroma.

Geography. There are large differences between countries in the manifestations of all aspects of ischaemic heart disease. In some countries ischaemic heart disease mortality is increasing, in others (e.g. USA, Finland, Australia) it has been high and is now falling. Immigration studies suggest that cultural factors such as smoking and diet outweigh genetic and environmental factors in their effects.

Smoking. There is evidence of a strong, consistent and dose-linked relationship between cigarette smoking and ischaemic heart disease. The relative risk of death from ischaemic heart disease for smokers compared to non-smokers is highest in young patients and declines in older age groups.

Diet. Population studies show a good, though non-linear, correlation between mean population plasma cholesterol and prevalence of atheroma, and between an individual's plasma cholesterol and the risk of a coronary event. However, the relationship between dietary and plasma cholesterol is indirect (much of the body's cholesterol is synthesised *de novo*) and it is possible that plasma cholesterol is simply a marker for something more fundamentally relevant. Much interest has centred on diets rich in certain polyunsaturated fatty acids which appear to protect against coronary heart disease, but by mechanisms perhaps independent of their cholesterol content. Studies which have attempted to alter plasma cholesterol by diet or drugs have produced positive results in those with the highest initial cholesterol concentrations, but non-significant results in other groups.

Arterial hypertension. There is evidence, particularly from the Framingham study in the USA, that even mild hypertension is a risk factor for ischaemic heart disease. However, prospective studies have failed to show a reduction in the mortality of ischaemic heart disease in treated hypertensives, even though mortality from stroke and cardiac failure are markedly diminished.

Stress. Occupations and events of a stressful nature, and particular ways of dealing with stress have all been linked epidemiologically with increased morbidity from ischaemic heart disease. The efficacy of 'stress prevention strategies' in reducing such morbidity is unproven.

Pathology. Reduction in the lumen of a coronary artery may be due to atheroma affecting the intima, fibrin and platelet deposition on the intima, haemorrhage under the intima, thrombosis or a combination of these factors. When angina develops one or more coronary arteries is usually already critically reduced in lumen or even occluded. The anterior descending coronary artery is especially vulnerable to atheroma and sudden occlusion of this vessel is particularly dangerous.

In myocardial infarction there is usually complete, but sometimes temporary, occlusion of a coronary artery. There is usually an atheromatous plaque at the site of occlusion, but the final obliteration of the lumen may be due to vascular spasm, thrombosis, or haemorrhage into the plaque. This may result in subendocardial or transmural infarction. Following acute infarction there is an inflammatory reaction, and if the epicardial surface is involved there is usually overlying pericarditis; if the endocardium is affected there may be intraventricular thrombosis. Over a period of 1 to 2 months the area damaged by infarction is replaced by fibrosis; it may ultimately become difficult to find which area was involved even at post mortem.

Angina pectoris

Angina pectoris is the name for a clinical syndrome rather than a disease. The term is used to describe a discomfort due to transient myocardial ischaemia. It is likely to occur when the coronary bloodflow is less than is required. Coronary atheroma is the commonest cause. Factors which increase myocardial oxygen requirement include any which add to the ventricular preload such as exercise, anaemia or hyperthyroidism, and those which increase afterload such as hypertension, aortic stenosis or obstructive cardiomyopathy. Increased tension of the ventricular wall, as occurs in dilatation or hypertrophy, may also reduce coronary flow. Tachycardia increases cardiac work and often brings on pain. A rapid arterial run-off during diastole reduces coronary arterial pressure and flow in aortic regurgitation. Coronary artery spasm can cause or exacerbate angina pectoris.

Clinical features. The history is by far the most important factor in making the diagnosis. Angina pectoris is usually experienced as a sense of oppression or tightness in the middle of the chest — 'like a band round the chest'; when describing it the patient commonly places the hand or clenched fist on the sternum, or both hands on the lower chest with the fingers touching at the sternum. It is usually induced by exertion and relieved by rest, lasting only a few minutes. Angina is likely to be worse when walking against a wind, uphill, on a cold day, and particularly after meals. Some patients find that the pain comes when they start walking and that later it does not return despite greater effort. Others can 'walk it off'. Some experience the pain when lying flat (*angina decubitus*), and some are awakened by it (*nocturnal angina*) particularly with 'energetic' or alarming dreams. Rarely, pain may come capriciously as a result of coronary arterial spasm, and be accompanied by transient ST elevation in the ECG (*Prinzmetal's or variant angina*).

The pain is often accompanied by discomfort in the arms, more commonly the left, the wrists and sometimes the hands; the patient may describe a feeling of uselessness in the limbs. Angina may more rarely be epigastric or interscapular or may radiate to the neck and jaw, or occur at any of these places of reference without chest discomfort. The precipitation by effort or anxiety, and the relief by rest or with the use of glyceryl trinitrate, should allow the pain to be recognised. There may be accompanying breathlessness. Pain may sometimes be induced by a cardiac arrhythmia.

Physical examination is frequently negative, but evidence of contributory or concomitant disease should be sought. The presence of tendon xanthomas, thickening of the achilles tendons and an arcus lipidus in a young patient may indicate a hereditary hyperlipidaemia. Aortic valve disease, particularly aortic stenosis, may cause angina. The patient should be examined for anaemia, obesity, diabetes, thyroid and peripheral vascular disease.

Investigation. *Electrocardiography*. The ECG is normal in most patients at rest between attacks. Occasionally T wave flattening or inversion may be seen in some leads; this is non-specific evidence of myocardial ischaemia or damage. A few patients may show ECG signs of established infarction (p. 169). The most convincing ECG evidence is the demonstration of reversible ST segment depression or elevation, with or without T wave inversion, at the time the patient is experiencing symptoms — whether spontaneous or induced by exercise testing. Formal exercise testing is usually done using a treadmill or bicycle ergometer and a standard procedure which ensures a progressive and reproducible increase in work load. Exercise testing should be done only where resuscitation facilities are available and the test should be stopped if the patient develops significant chest pain or discomfort or suffers arrhythmias or a fall in blood pressure. The amount of exercise which can be tolerated under these conditions is a useful guide to the extent of coronary disease.

Scanning. Myocardial perfusion scanning using radioactive thallium may be helpful, in conjunction with exercise testing, in evaluating the minority of patients with an atypical history, or the small group who have severe symptoms but no significant ECG abnormality on exercise testing. Echocardiography or radionuclide bloodpool scanning provide information about ventricular function, which may be relevant in making a decision about coronary arteriography.

Coronary arteriography provides detailed information about the extent and site of coronary artery stenosis. It is usually performed with a view to subsequent coronary bypass grafting or angioplasty (p. 167). In a small minority it may be indicated when a full range of non-invasive tests have failed to elucidate the cause of atypical chest pain.

Differential diagnosis. This includes musculoskeletal, pericardial and oesophageal pain. Musculoskeletal pains are provoked by specific movement rather than by walking, and background pain often persists at rest. There may be marked tenderness over the costal cartilages and manubriosternal angle. The pain of pericarditis is occasionally provoked by exercise, but its other characteristics (p. 182) should help to make the distinction. Angina occurring at rest may be confused with oesophagitis, with or without a hiatus hernia, but pain due to oesophagitis usually has a burning quality and is relieved by alkalis. Oesophageal spasm however causes a different type of pain which may be difficult to distinguish from variant angina.

Treatment of angina pectoris involves three phases: a proper assessment of the severity of the symptoms and the likely extent of the disease; the use of measures to control symptoms; and treatment which will improve life expectancy. The first phase has been discussed under diagnosis, and a suggested sequence of investigation is shown as a flow chart in Figure 7.34.

Control of symptoms should start with an explanation of how they are caused. Patients usually respond to a careful presentation of the problem as what it is — a mismatch between coronary supply and cardiac needs. The natural process of repair by development of anastomoses should be stressed. Patients can then learn how to help themselves, e.g. by avoiding walking after meals, particularly in the cold or against a wind, and by avoiding severe unaccustomed exertion. They may need encouragement and support in their endeavours to stop smoking and to lose weight. In a few patients hyperlipidaemia requires treatment by diet and other measures (p. 489).

DRUG TREATMENT. There are three principal groups of drugs which help to relieve or prevent the symptoms of angina: nitrates, beta-adrenoceptor antagonists (beta-blockers) and calcium antagonists.

Nitrates. Fresh glyceryl trinitrate (GTN 500 micrograms), allowed to dissolve under the tongue or crunched for more rapid effect and retained in the mouth, usually relieves the pain in 2 to 3

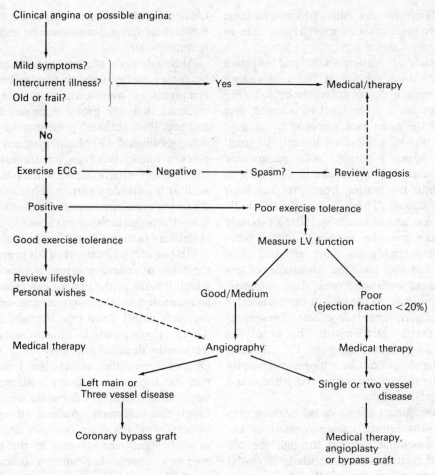

Clinical angina or possible angina:

Mild symptoms?
Intercurrent illness? } ——————→ Yes ——————→ Medical/therapy
Old or frail?

No

Exercise ECG ——————→ Negative ——————→ Spasm? ——————→ Review diagosis

Positive ——————————————————→ Poor exercise tolerance

Good exercise tolerance   Measure LV function

Review lifestyle
Personal wishes   Good/Medium   Poor
                                                     (ejection fraction <20%)

Medical therapy   Angiography   Medical therapy

Left main or   Single or two vessel
Three vessel disease   disease

Coronary bypass graft   Medical therapy,
                                      angioplasty
                                      or bypass graft

Fig. 7.34 Angina pectoris — sequence of investigation and treatment.

minutes, and about the same time it often produces a slight headache. The headache may become severe in some patients if the tablet is left in the mouth, so the patient should be instructed to spit it out or swallow it once the angina is relieved. The best use of GTN is prophylactically before exercise known as liable to produce pain. The good effect comes from venous and arteriolar dilatation, which lowers the blood pressure and also dilates the coronary vessels provided their disease does not prevent this. Patients can be reassured that GTN is not dangerous or habit forming, and that it does not lose its effect. The tablets themselves have a limited shelf life, particularly if kept in a warm place. Not more than about two tablets per hour should be used; if the requirement for it increases significantly the patient should seek medical advice. The appro-

priate use of GTN (or other drugs) allows more exercise to be taken; this should be encouraged because physical activity promotes the formation of collateral vessels. As sublingual GTN has a short duration of action, there has been much interest in ways of giving more prolonged nitrate therapy. GTN can be given percutaneously as a paste or plasters, or as a slow-release buccal tablet. Some patients find these helpful, but they are much more expensive than sublingual tablets. GTN is virtually ineffective when swallowed, but other nitrates such as isosorbide dinitrate (10 mg or more, 3–6 per day) can be given by mouth. Headache is common when patients are started on oral nitrates, but tends to improve on persevering with the therapy. Tolerance frequently occurs, and the dose needs to be increased to maintain efficacy. The use of slow-release preparations may make it possible for the patient to accept large doses. Intravenous nitrates may have a role in treating unstable angina.

Beta-blockade is an important and effective way of preventing angina. It helps to reduce myocardial oxygen demand, largely by reducing the heart rate for a given level of exercise, and by reducing the heart rate response to anxiety. *Propranolol* can be prescribed initially in small doses (e.g. 20 mg 6-hourly) with progressive increments until benefit is obtained, which is often not until the resting heart rate has been significantly slowed. There is considerable individual variation and as much as 160 mg 6-hourly or even more may be required. Other beta-blockers are probably no more effective than propranolol but may have the advantages of less individual dose variation, once daily administration and possibly, in the case of cardioselective agents, fewer peripheral side-effects. These matters are discussed, together with other properties of beta-blocking drugs, on page 177. A beta-blocking drug should not be withdrawn abruptly because of the risks of dangerous arrhythmias and myocardial infarction.

Calcium antagonists are so called because they inhibit the slow inward current caused by the entry of extracellular calcium through the cell membrane of excited cells, particularly arteriolar smooth muscle and cardiac atrial cells. In arterioles, the result is vasodilatation and hence a fall in blood presure. In cardiac muscle, the principal effects are a reduction in excitability and conductivity, with large doses causing reduced contractility. Different calcium antagonists vary greatly in their pharmacological range of action. *Nifedipine* is a powerful coronary and systemic arteriolar dilator, and most of its antianginal effects can be explained by these actions. The initial dosage is one 10 mg capsule t.i.d. with food. For rapid effect, a capsule may be bitten before swallowing it. Side-effects are headache, dizziness, flushing, itching skin and mild fluid retention. It is often given in combination with a beta-blocker. *Verapamil* is enjoying a resurgence of popularity as an antianginal agent, at doses considerably higher than originally used (120–240 mg t.i.d.). It seems less likely to cause side-effects related to vasodilatation than nifedipine, but should be used cautiously in a patient suspected of a cardiac conduction defect. Its commonest unwanted effect is constipation.

Although each of these groups of drugs can be shown to be superior to placebo in treating symptoms of angina, there is little convincing evidence that one group is more effective than another. The authors' present policy is to start with sublingual GTN, to progress to a beta-blocker unless there are contraindications and then to add nifedipine or a long-acting nitrate such as isosorbide dinitrate. The ultimate aim of achieving excellent control of angina with minimal side-effects and the simplest possible tablet regime is unlikely to be reached without trial and error.

SURGICAL TREATMENT. This principally takes the form of coronary artery bypass grafting, in which lengths of the patient's saphenous vein are anastomosed to the aorta at one end and to a coronary vessel distal to a stenosis at the other. There is symptomatic improvement, which is frequently dramatic, in over 80% of patients. Operative mortality is between 1 and 2%, but may be higher in patients with impaired left ventricular function. Controlled trials have indicated that coronary grafting in symptomatic patients with left main coronary artery stenosis, or with significant stenosis in the three major coronary vessels (left anterior descending, left circumflex and right coronary arteries) gives a better chance of survival over a 5-year period than medical treatment. There is as yet no clearcut evidence of improved survival in patients with less extensive disease, although they may benefit symptomatically, nor is there definite evidence of improved survival after surgery in asymptomatic patients.

Coronary arteriography is a necessary preliminary to coronary artery surgery, and should be considered in those patients whose severe symptoms or poor performance on exercise testing suggest extensive disease, as well as in those who continue to have unacceptable symptoms in spite of adequate medical treatment. Poor left ventricular function (which may be assessed by echocardiography or radionuclide scanning) or intercurrent illness are relative contraindications.

Coronary angioplasty is the dilatation of coronary artery stenoses by a small balloon introduced percutaneously via an arterial catheter. Most experience has been with single vessel coronary disease but patients with multiple lesions are being treated in increasing numbers. In experienced hands the initial success rate is of the order of 90% with an operative mortality similar to that of coronary artery grafting. Recurrence of symptoms within 3 months occurs in about 20% of patients, but the dilatation can be repeated. Overall, it is probably a less definitive procedure than coronary artery grafting for stable angina, but it involves a shorter hospital stay and may be more acceptable to the patient. It is the treatment of choice for unstable angina when rest pain recurs despite full medical treatment. Its role as an adjunct to acute coronary thrombolysis is being investigated.

Prognosis. Overall, more than half of a group of patients with angina will live for 5 years, and a third for 10 years from the time of diagnosis. Spontaneous recovery, which may prove temporary, may occur in as many as a third, a fact which is useful to remember in talking to patients about their disease. Prognosis is worse in the patient who has had multiple cardiac infarcts or who has cardiac failure.

Unstable angina

The term 'unstable' is used to describe angina which has become abruptly more severe or more prolonged in the absence of evidence of infarction. Many different factors may be responsible, including the natural progression of coronary atherosclerosis, thrombus formation or the development of coronary artery spasm. Affected patients are often admitted to hospital under suspicion of myocardial infarction.

Most patients will respond to rest, mild sedation, nitrates and beta-adrenergic blocking drugs. Aspirin (approximately 300 mg/d) has been shown to reduce the risk of progression to myocardial infarction presumably because of an antiplatelet effect (p. 542) Calcium antagonists such as nifedipine may also be useful. The persistence of symptoms in spite of these measures should lead to consideration of coronary arteriography and the possibility of surgical treatment.

Myocardial infarction

This is myocardial necrosis occurring as a result of a critical imbalance between coronary blood supply and myocardial demand. The infarct may be confined to the subendocardial region, or may affect the full thickness of the myocardium (transmural infarction). The latter is usually associated with the total, but sometimes transient, occlusion of the coronary artery supplying the area and mainly occurs at the site of a pre-existing atheromatous plaque. It is difficult to be certain of the precise factors causing occlusion in individual cases, but fissuring and dissection of the plaque, coronary spasm, and thrombosis probably all play a part.

In its mildest form the infarct may be unrecognised ('silent') and be disclosed subsequently only by ECG evidence; at the other end of the range there is permanent severe disability or death. At the onset of the illness, sudden death, presumably from ventricular fibrillation or asystole, may occur immediately, and many of the patients who die do so within the first hour. If the patient survives this most critical stage, the liability to dangerous arrhythmias remains, but diminishes as each hour goes by. The development of cardiac failure reflects the extent of myocardial damage; its severity may range from slight reduction in skin perfusion and basal lung crepitations at one end to acute circulatory failure at the other. Cardiac failure is the major cause of death in those who survive the first few hours of infarction.

Clinical features. The cardinal symptom is pain, but breathlessness, syncope, vomiting and extreme tiredness are common. The pain occurs in the same sites as for angina but is usually more severe and lasts longer. It is most often described as a tightness, heaviness or constriction in the chest. At its worst the pain is one of the most severe which can be experienced and the patient's expression and pallor may vividly convey the seriousness of the situation.

Many patients are breathless and in some this is the only symptom; a few develop pulmonary oedema at the onset. Syncope may occur and the blood pressure falls particularly if the patient is upright, or from the development of a serious arrhythmia or heart block. Vomiting is common, particularly in the more severe cases. It may also result from morphine given for pain relief. In rare cases the infarct may go unnoticed until endocardial thrombosis resulting from it leads to systemic embolism.

At any time after the first 12 hours or so the patient may recognise that a different pain has developed, even though it is at the same site. It is worse, or only appears, on inspiration and may be altered by a change of position. It is due to pericarditis consequent on the infarct, and the diagnosis is confirmed if a pericardial rub is heard.

The *physical signs* may be few in a mild attack but in severe cases there is usually pallor, sweating and breathlessness. The heart rate is usually increased, and with circulatory failure the pulse volume may be much reduced and the skin perfusion poor. Most patients seen early after myocardial infarction have a normal initial blood pressure, but transiently it may be high as a result of pain or anxiety. The blood pressure gradually falls over the first 3 or 4 days. It is low in the minority who develop circulatory failure. The jugular venous pressure is often elevated when the patient is first seen; this may be due to cardiac failure but vasoconstriction and anxiety may contribute. Later, the JVP may remain high in patients with inferior infarction even when there is no evidence of fluid overload; this is because inferior infarcts often involve the right ventricle and make it less compliant than usual.

The first heart sound is often quiet and a third or a fourth sound may develop. Extensive anterior myocardial damage may be manifest in a diffuse apical pulsation. Pericardial friction is most often heard on the second or third day, and is usually transitory. Crepitations, particularly if widespread and persistent after coughing, suggest pulmonary oedema. Oliguria is common if the blood pressure is low. It is not an indication for diuretic therapy unless there are other signs of fluid overload. In many cases there is a fever, reaching a maximum on the third or fourth day, and not much higher than 38°C.

Complications. ARRHYTHMIAS. Nearly all patients with myocardial infarction have some form of arrhythmia, but in most cases this is mild and of no haemodynamic or prognostic significance. Various degrees of heart block (p. 139) are also frequent.

Sinus tachycardia is the commonest arrhythmia; anxiety may contribute to it. If persistent, it may warn of incipient cardiac failure. Sinus bradycardia is more common after inferior infarction; it does not usually need treatment unless it is associated with hypotension. Severe bradycardia may lead to ventricular escape and the development of more dangerous rhythms. Atrial tachycardia or fibrillation occur in about 15% of patients; these arrhythmias may exacerbate hypotension or cardiac failure and require prompt treatment if the ventricular rate is excessively fast.

Ventricular ectopic beats are almost invariable, and are frequently numerous. They are usually of little consequence but may indicate an increased liability to ventricular fibrillation if they fall on the T wave of the preceding beat ('R on T'). Ventricular tachycardia is also common. If it persists at a fast rate for more than a few seconds it may have serious haemodynamic effects.

Ventricular fibrillation occurs in about 5–10% of patients in hospital. The risk is much higher in the first hour after infarction, and ventricular fibrillation is thought to be the major cause of death before reaching hospital. Its potential reversibility in those patients who do not have extensive myocardial damage is one of the main foundations on which the policy of acute coronary care is built.

ACUTE CIRCULATORY FAILURE. If there is a reversible arrhythmia as an important contributory factor its correction may bring about considerable improvement. In a few cases excessive diuretic therapy leading to hypovolaemia may be the cause. If neither of these is responsible, acute circulatory failure usually reflects extensive myocardial damage and indicates a bad prognosis. In its presence, all the other complications of myocardial infarction are more likely.

OTHER COMPLICATIONS. *Cardiac failure* may occur, and pulmonary oedema is its commonest form. Regular examination for basal lung crepitations and chest radiography should lead to its early detection.

Rarer complications include *infarction of a mitral papillary muscle*, which leads to mitral regurgitation and may precipitate pulmonary oedema. *Rupture of the interventricular septum* is diagnosed by the development of the characteristic murmur of a ventricular septal defect (p. 186) and may cause severe hypotension and venous hypertension. Rupture of the ventricle into the pericardial space may lead to *cardiac tamponade* (p. 182).

Embolism, cerebral or peripheral, can occur when a thrombus forms on the endocardium of the left ventricle. *Venous thrombosis* is less common now than when patients were routinely kept in bed for 6 weeks; it often first announces its presence by pulmonary embolism.

The *post-myocardial infarction syndrome* (Dressler's syndrome), which is probably an auto-immune reaction to necrotic myocardium, is characterised by persistent fever, pericarditis and pleurisy. It occurs a few weeks or even months after the infarct and often subsides after a few days but may require aspirin, other anti-inflammatory drugs or corticosteroids for its control if symptoms are prolonged.

Ventricular aneurysm and dyskinetic or akinetic segments (p. 149) can develop later.

Investigation. ELECTROCARDIOGRAPHY. The ECG is usually a sensitive and specific way of confirming the diagnosis, but the typical changes may take some hours to develop. The ECG may also be difficult to interpret after previous infarction and occasionally it will not be significantly altered in spite of clinical and biochemical evidence of re-infarction. The earliest ECG change is usually ST elevation, which reflects acute myocardial injury. At the same time or slightly later there is diminution in the size of the R wave, and a Q wave begins to develop. One explanation for the Q wave is that the myocardial infarct acts as an 'electrical window' transmitting the changes of potential from within the ventricular cavity, and allowing the ECG to 'see' the reciprocal R wave from the other wall of the ventricle. Subsequently the T wave becomes inverted because of a change in ventricular repolarisation, and this change persists after the ST segment has returned to normal. These features are shown diagrammatically in Figure 7.35 and their sequence is sufficiently reliable for the approximate age of the infarct to be deduced. In contrast to transmural lesions, with subendocardial infarction there is usually no Q wave or ST elevation, but symmetrical T wave inversion

develops.

The ECG changes are best seen in the leads which 'face' the infarcted areas (Fig. 7.2). When there has been anteroseptal infarction abnormalities are found in one or more leads from V1 to V4 (Fig. 7.36) while anterolateral infarction produces changes from V4 to V6, in aVL and hence also in lead I. In strict anterior infarction the changes may be confined to V3 and V4. Inferior infarction is best shown in leads II, III and aVF, while leads I, aVL and the lateral chest leads show 'reciprocal' changes of ST depression (Fig. 7.37). Infarction of the posterior wall of the left ventricle is not recorded in the standard leads by ST elevation or Q waves, but the reciprocal changes of ST depression and a tall R wave may be seen in leads V1-V4.

PLASMA ENZYMES. Myocardial infarction leads to a detectable rise in the plasma concentration of enzymes normally confined within cardiac cells. The enzymes most widely used in the detection of myocardial infarction are creatine kinase (CK), aspartate aminotransferase (AST) and lactate dehydrogenase (LD). CK starts to rise at 4–6 hours, peaks about 12 hours and falls to normal in 48–72 hours. CK is also present in skeletal muscle, and a rise in CK may be due to an intramuscular injection or vigorous physical exercise. Measurement of the myocardial iso-enzyme of CK (CK-MB) is more specific for myocardial damage (p. 815). AST starts to rise about 12 hours after infarction, and reaches a peak on the first or second day. LD is also liberated from haemolysed red cells and is therefore less specific. It starts to rise after 12 hours, reaches a peak after 2 or 3 days and may be elevated for about a week. LD estimation may be useful when the diagnosis is uncertain several days after a possible infarct. Serial estimations are necessary in doubtful cases, for it is the change in enzyme levels which is of diagnostic value.

OTHER BLOOD TESTS. A leucocytosis is usual, reaching a peak on the first day. The ESR becomes raised and may remain so for several days.

CHEST RADIOGRAPHY may demonstrate pulmonary oedema which has been undetected clinically. The heart size is usually normal. Enlargement of the cardiac shadow may indicate previous myocardial damage or a developing pericardial

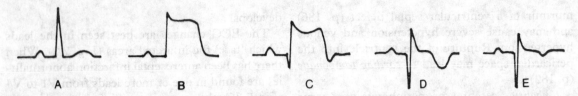

Fig. 7.35 The serial evolution of ECG changes in myocardial infarction. A: pre-infarct; B: ST elevation owing to a myocardial 'injury current', also some reduction in R wave size; C: developing Q wave and terminal T wave inversion; D: established Q wave and T inversion; E: 'old infarct' pattern — the Q wave tends to persist but T wave changes become less marked. The rate of evolution is very variable. In general stage C is usually reached in hours, stage D in days and stage E after some months. This diagrammatic representation should be compared with the actual ECGs in Figures 7.36 and 7.37.

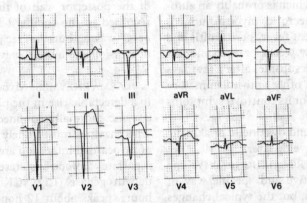

Fig. 7.36 Established anterior myocardial infarct, from a 43-year-old man with chest pain starting 6 hours previously. There are Q waves in leads V2, V3 and V4, ST elevation in the same leads, and loss of the normal R wave pattern in all the chest leads. Anterior infarcts with Q waves most prominent in leads V2, V3 and V4 are sometimes called 'anteroseptal' infarcts to distinguish them from 'anterolateral' infarcts with Q waves most prominent in leads V4, V5 and V6.

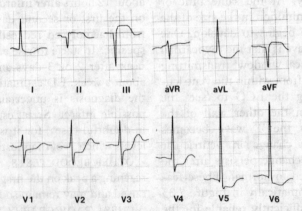

Fig. 7.37 Established inferior myocardial infarction with Q waves and ST elevation in leads II, III and aVF, from a 55-year-old man with a severe episode of chest pain 24 hours before. In this patient there is also 'reciprocal' ST depression in the chest leads V2 to V6.

effusion.

RADIONUCLIDE SCANNING (p. 129). A pyrophosphate scan may show the site of myocardial necrosis. A radionuclide ventriculogram indicates the extent of impairment of ventricular function and may give useful prognostic information.

Treatment. The main immediate needs are for the relief of pain and the prevention or treatment of arrhythmias and other complications. Later, efforts are concentrated on rehabilitation of the patient and the attempted prevention of further infarction.

In the first 3 or 4 hours when the risk of fatal arrhythmia is highest it is best for patients to be cared for where there is immediate access to resuscitation facilities; this will usually be in a coronary care unit. Patients seen and diagnosed after the first few hours may be cared for at home if they are free of cardiac failure or other complications and are adequately supported domestically.

ACUTE CORONARY THROMBOLYSIS with intravenous streptokinase (1 500 000 units over 1 hour) has been shown to improve survival in myocardial infarction, and helps to preserve left ventricular function if instituted within 3 hours from the onset of symptoms. Subsequent anticoagulation for 3 to 6 months reduces the risk of re-occlusion, but many patients are left with a more or less severe coronary stenosis which may require subsequent angioplasty or coronary grafting.

RELIEF OF PAIN. The patient with a severe attack is in pain and is frightened. An effective remedy is morphine given intravenously in 5 or 10 mg aliquots titrated against the patient's response. Diamorphine (2.5–5 mg) is slightly more potent on a weight for weight basis, and produces analgesia slightly more rapidly, but has no other advantages to compensate for its expense, instability and addiction potential. Either drug may be given subcutaneously or intramuscularly (morphine 10–20 mg, diamorphine 5–10 mg) but this is less satisfactory because peripheral vasoconstriction initially delays absorption, while later vasodilation leads to rapid absorption and possible respiratory depression. Opiates should be supplemented with an antiemetic such as cyclizine (50 mg i.v.) or a phenothiazine. The anxiety must be

recognised even if it is not overt; it is essential to reassure the patient that recovery is the most likely outcome and that the most dangerous phase of the illness is already over.

ARRHYTHMIAS. Pain relief, rest, reassurance and the correction of hypokalaemia all play a major role in preventing arrhythmias. Lignocaine (p. 136) is given after resuscitation from ventricular fibrillation or to treat ventricular tachycardia with a rapid rate. In some units lignocaine is also given if multiple ectopic beats, or the potentially dangerous 'R on T' ectopics are observed during the acute phase of the illness. If lignocaine is ineffective, mexiletine (p. 136) may be used instead; sometimes an intravenous beta-blocker (e.g. atenolol 5–10 mg or sotalol 10 mg) may be helpful.

Ventricular fibrillation should be treated with an immediate d.c. shock (p. 142). Failing this, the cardiac resuscitation procedure (p. 135) should be used until the defibrillator is available. Atrial tachycardia, flutter or fibrillation are best treated with digoxin if the ventricular rate is rapid, and spontaneous reversion to sinus rhythm is common. If the arrhythmia causes severe hypotension, synchronised d.c. shock treatment should be considered.

Sinus bradycardia does not usually require treatment, but if there is hypotension or ventricular escape, atropine may be given (0.3 mg i.v. every 5 min to a maximum of 1.5 mg). Heart block complicating inferior infarction often responds to atropine and a temporary pacemaker is needed only if this drug is ineffective in preventing hypotension. Heart block complicating anterior infarction is an indication for the prophylactic insertion of a temporary pacemaker, as asystole may suddenly supervene. Asystole sometimes responds to cardiac massage, and following this a pacemaker electrode should be inserted.

ACUTE CIRCULATORY and CARDIAC FAILURE are treated as described on pages 143 and 147.

ANTICOAGULANTS (p. 550) are indicated in the treatment of venous thrombosis and pulmonary embolism and may be used prophylactically if the patient is at risk because of prolonged immobilisation. Whether or not the long-term use of anticoagulants protects against further infarction has been controversial for many years, and is presently undergoing further evaluation.

REHABILITATION. There is histological evidence that an infarct takes 4–6 weeks to become replaced with fibrous tissue. Accordingly it is generally thought reasonable to restrict physical activities during this period. When there are no complications the patient can sit in a chair within a few days, be ambulant within a week, return home in 7–10 days and gradually increase activity with the prospect of a return to work after 6 weeks. When there are complications the regime has to be adjusted accordingly. Reassurance is essential at every stage because many patients are severely and even permanently incapacitated as a result of psychological rather than physical effects of myocardial infarction. The success of restoring a patient to normal life depends very much on the attitudes of the physician. The naturally vigorous person may require restraint in the early stages but more often the anxious will need encouragement. In general, patients can be reassured that exercise within the limits set by angina and tiredness will do no harm and much good. The same limits apply to sexual activity. The spouse has often to learn to stop reminding the patient of former disability. Formal rehabilitation programmes based on graded exercise and counselling may be of great psychological benefit, although it has not been possible to show convincing effects on eventual exercise ability or survival.

Post-infarct angina is associated with a worse prognosis, and provided ventricular function is adequate some of these patients may be helped by coronary bypass grafting.

Secondary prevention. Primary prevention is the term used for measures which are applied in the absence of clinical manifestations of disease. It is discussed on page 173. Secondary prevention refers to measures put into practice after the disease has become apparent, usually as a result of the development of angina or following myocardial infarction.

Much advice given to patients after myocardial infarction is based on common sense rather than on objective demonstration of benefit, but control of obesity, regular exercise and the adoption of a less frenetic way of life are unlikely to do harm. Stopping smoking improves survival, more so in younger than in older patients. There is no overall evidence that control of plasma lipids, by dietary or other means, affects survival in patients who have had an infarct, but lipid control may still be worthwhile in young patients with familial hyperlipidaemias.

The beta-adrenoceptor blocking drugs, propranolol, metoprolol and timolol have all been shown in prospective controlled trials to reduce cardiovascular mortality in patients taking them on a long-term basis following myocardial infarction. Contraindications to the use of these drugs include persistent cardiac failure or heart block, and some patients are unable to tolerate them because of side-effects such as breathlessness, hypotension or cold extremities. The reduction in mortality from the use of these drugs is of the order of 25% over a 1–2 year period: although this might have a considerable impact on community mortality, the improvement in survival for the individual patient is in the order of only 2–5%, so patients reluctant to take this medication should not be subjected to undue pressure to do so.

Prognosis. In about a quarter of all cases of myocardial infarction death occurs within a few minutes without medical care. Half the deaths from myocardial infarction occur within 2 hours of the onset of symptoms and three quarters within 24 hours. About 40% of all affected patients die within the first month. Unfavourable features are poor left ventricular function, heart block and persistent ventricular arrhythmias. The prognosis is worse for anterior than for inferior infarcts. Bundle branch block and high enzyme levels both indicate extensive myocardial damage. Old age, stress and social isolation are also associated with a higher mortality. In the absence of unfavourable features, the outlook is as good for those who survive ventricular fibrillation as for the others. Of those who survive an acute attack, more than 80% live for a further year, about 75% for 5 years, 50% for 10 years and 25% for 20 years. It is therefore appropriate to be reassuring to patients about their prospects.

Sudden death

This term can be applied when a person previously in apparent good health falls ill and dies within minutes or at most a few hours. Some of these patients have an identifiable non-cardiac cause of death such as cerebral haemorrhage or a ruptured aortic aneurysm. Many have extensive coronary atherosclerosis; the proportion of these who have thrombotic occlusion of a coronary vessel is small when death is virtually instantaneous but higher in those who survive for a few hours. The explanation for this is uncertain but possibly coronary spasm may occlude a vessel for long enough to produce fatal consequences without a thrombus developing. Alternatively, death might be due to an arrhythmia in the absence of coronary occlusion. Arrhythmias are probably the immediate cause of sudden death in patients with other cardiac abnormalities such as severe aortic or pulmonary stenosis or hypertrophic cardiomyopathy.

A small group of patients who die suddenly have no obvious pathological cause of death on post-mortem examination; cardiac arrhythmia seems the most likely cause in this group also, and in some cases a previous ECG has been found to be abnormal. There is evidence both from patients who have died during ambulatory ECG monitoring and from acute resuscitation services that ventricular fibrillation is the commonest arrhythmia causing sudden death, and resuscitation, if promptly applied, may restore effective cardiac action.

Relatives of patients who have died suddenly often seek reassurance, and should be examined, if appropriate, for evidence of hypertrophic cardiomyopathy, Marfan's syndrome and hyperlipidaemia. A family history of sudden death in childhood or young adult life is sometimes associated with prolongation of the QT interval on the ECG, and beta-blockade may improve prognosis in this group.

Primary prevention of ischaemic heart disease

Persisting uncertainty about the basic cause of ischaemic heart disease (p. 162) makes definitive advice about primary prevention difficult. Even when a risk factor is clearly identified, prospective trials are needed to show that correction of the risk factor improves prognosis. Stopping cigarette smoking has been shown to reduce both the risk

of an initial ischaemic event and to be effective in secondary prevention. Lowering plasma cholesterol by diet, and/or medication, reduces risk in patients with initial plasma total cholesterol concentrations above about 7 mmol/l. Obesity in itself is a weak risk factor for ischaemic heart disease, but in Britain obesity is closely linked to the most common form of hypercholesterolaemia. There is suggestive evidence, short of proof, that a diet with a higher proportion of polyunsaturated to saturated fats and a lower proportion of total energy derived from fat, may reduce the risk of ischaemic heart disease. In sedentary sections of the community ischaemic heart disease is more prevalent than in those who take regular physical exercise, and, although direct proof of a beneficial effect is lacking, regular daily exercise to the point of breathlessness is recommended.

SYSTEMIC HYPERTENSION

In Western societies the average systolic and diastolic blood pressures gradually rise with age. Hypertension is defined arbitrarily at levels above generally accepted 'normals', for example 140/90 at the age of 20, 160/95 at the age of 50 and 170/105 at the age of 75. It is recommended that the phase 5 diastolic pressure (p. 124) be used in defining hypertension. Exercise, anxiety, discomfort and unfamiliar surroundings can all lead to a transient rise in blood pressure, and measurements should be repeated under conditions with the patient resting and relaxed until consistent readings are obtained. Patients who have a high blood pressure on first examination which subsequently settles with rest may not require treatment but should be kept under review because they are more likely to develop sustained hypertension. According to these criteria, some 15% of the population can be regarded as hypertensive, though only a proportion of these will be diagnosed or receive treatment.

Aetiology. In about 10–15% of cases, hypertension can be shown to be a consequence of a specific disease or abnormality. The most important of these are:

1. Coarctation of the aorta.
2. Renal disease: (a) Parenchymatous, e.g. acute

and chronic glomerulonephritis, pyelo-nephritis, analgesic-induced nephropathy, systemic lupus erythematosus and poly-arteritis nodosa; (b) Polycystic kidneys; (c) Renal artery stenosis.

3. Endocrine disorders and hormone therapy: (a) Phaeochromocytoma; (b) Cushing's syn-drome, spontaneous and drug induced; (c) Primary aldosteronism (Conn's syndrome); (d) Oral contraception and oestrogen therapy.

4. Pregnancy.

These conditions give an insight into the possible mechanisms by which hypertension may be caused. In phaeochromocytoma, it results from an increased cardiac output and/or a raised peripheral resistance due to excessive catecholamines. Cush-ing's syndrome and Conn's syndrome are associ-ated with increased sodium retention, and prob-ably an alteration in the reactivity of vascular smooth muscle. Renal causes of hypertension are also often associated with sodium retention, and in many cases with high plasma concentrations of renin, which causes the production of the potent vasoconstrictor agent angiotensin II. The latter stimulates aldosterone release and thus also encourages sodium retention. In sustained hyper-tension it is often found that the carotid sinus baroreceptors, which help to smooth out fluctu-ations in blood pressure, become 'reset' to a higher level.

In the majority of patients with hypertension, although some of these mechanisms may be oper-ating, it is not possible to define a specific under-lying cause, and they are said to have *essential hypertension*. In 70% of such patients another member of the family is affected. Essential hyper-tension is especially frequent in some races, par-ticularly American Blacks and Japanese. It is commoner where there is a high salt intake.

Clinical features. In the majority of patients there are no specific symptoms attributable to hypertension, which is detected on routine exami-nation or because of one of its complications. Acute hypertension occasionally causes headache or polyuria, but these are transient. Similarly, there are few specific physical signs unless the hypertension is severe. Long-standing hyperten-sion leads to left ventricular hypertrophy and may

be indicated by a forceful and sustained apical impulse. Left atrial hypertrophy may accompany that of the left ventricle, and a fourth heart sound may be heard. The aortic second sound may be increased, and there is sometimes a very short aortic early diastolic murmur. Paroxysmal noctur-nal dyspnoea and/or crepitations at the lung bases may give evidence of left ventricular failure. The optic fundi provide valuable evidence about the severity of the hypertension (see below).

The three main objectives of clinical examina-tion in a hypertensive patient are to identify any underlying cause, to recognise risk factors for the development of complications and to detect any complications already present.

Patients with phaeochromocytoma sometimes give a history of panic attacks, paroxysmal head-aches, or palpitation. A history of recurrent back-ache or undiagnosed fever is sometimes a clue to chronic pyelonephritis, and specific enquiry should be made about analgesic intake. Apart from oral contraceptives and other steroids, drugs which may cause hypertension include liquorice and carbenoxolone used for peptic ulcer and non-steroidal anti-inflammatory drugs. Physical examination should detect the delay between rad-ial and femoral pulses characteristic of coarctation of the aorta, and the enlarged kidneys in polycystic disease. The characteristic facies and habitus of Cushing's syndrome may be recognised, and a bruit is sometimes audible over the abdomen in renal artery stenosis.

It is important to identify risk factors such as smoking, obesity and hyperlipidaemia which may interact with hypertension, particularly in the genesis of ischaemic heart disease.

Complications. The adverse effects of hyper-tension principally involve the central nervous system, the retina, the heart and the kidneys.

CENTRAL NERVOUS SYSTEM. *Stroke* resulting from cerebral haemorrhage or from cerebral ischaemia is a common complication of hyperten-sion and a major cause of death in hypertensive patients. Carotid atheroma and transient cerebral ischaemic attacks are more common in hyperten-sive patients.

Hypertensive encephalopathy is a rare condition characterised by a very high blood pressure and neurological symptoms including transient disturbances of speech or vision, paraesthesiae, disorientation, fits and loss of consciousness. Papilloedema is common. The neurological deficit is usually reversible if the hypertension is properly controlled.

Subarachnoid haemorrhage is more common in hypertensive patients.

RETINA. *Hypertensive retinopathy* (Plate I). In long-standing hypertension of moderate severity the major change is a thickening of the walls of retinal arterioles, causing diffuse or segmental narrowing of the blood columns, varying width of the light reflex from the vessel wall and often some arteriovenous nipping. With more severe hypertension, retinal haemorrhages are seen, and are usually flame shaped. Soft (cotton wool) exudates are associated with retinal ischaemia or infarction and fade in a few weeks Hard exudates are small white dense deposits of lipid which may persist for years. Papilloedema indicates the most advanced stage of hypertension. In early retinopathy there is little effect on visual acuity, but extensive exudates or haemorrhages can cause visual field defects, or blindness if the macula is affected.

HEART. Hypertension is a major risk factor for ischaemic heart disease, and myocardial infarction is a common cause of death. The heart initially responds to hypertension with left ventricular hypertrophy (Fig. 7.31), and angina may be precipitated if there is concomitant coronary disease. Subsequently, the persistently high afterload may lead to left ventricular failure. Hypertension also contributes to the pathogenesis of aortic aneurysm and acute aortic dissection (p. 192).

KIDNEYS. In addition to being a cause, renal disease may also be a result of hypertensive damage to the renal vessels. Long-standing hypertension may cause proteinuria and progressive renal failure. Sometimes, renal damage resulting from hypertension produces an increased release of renin, and a vicious circle may be set up with worsening renal failure and very severe hypertension. This *accelerated phase* or *malignant hypertension* has a bad prognosis unless the cycle is interrupted. There is fibrinoid necrosis in the small arterioles of the kidney and also in those of the heart, brain and retina where the presence of soft exudates is evidence of accelerated phase

hypertension, and later, papilloedema is indicative of malignant hypertension.

Investigation of the hypertensive patient has the same basic objectives as the clinical examination, but because hypertension is so common it is prudent to be selective in the use of resources. Some investigations need to be done on all patients, while others can be reserved for those with specific features of a particular condition or who are refractory to the initial treatment.

The most basic investigations are urine analysis for protein (which may indicate renal disease) and sugar (diabetes mellitus may coexist with hypertension and is another important risk factor for vascular disease), and estimation of plasma urea and electrolyte concentrations. The urea or creatinine estimation is a measure of renal excretory function, and the plasma electrolytes may give a clue to the cause of the hypertension. In particular, hypokalaemia and a metabolic alkalosis may indicate hyperaldosteronism, provided diuretic therapy can be excluded as a cause. Plasma cholesterol concentration should be measured in younger patients, and plasma urate concentration is worth estimating because hyperuricaemia is associated with hypertension and gout is liable to be precipitated if diuretics are used for treatment.

A chest radiograph and ECG are not essential but are useful as a baseline in the event of subsequent complications. Screening for phaeochromocytoma is indicated in patients with clinical features of the disease (p. 458) and in other patients whose hypertension is severe or refractory to treatment.

Further investigation of the urinary tract by excretion urography or radionuclide renography is indicated: (1) in patients under the age of 40, (2) in those whose history, clinical examination or baseline investigation suggests renal pathology, and (3) in older patients where difficulty in the control of hypertension or a sudden increase in severity may indicate a renal artery stenosis. Excretion urography provides more information about urinary tract anatomy whereas radionuclide studies give a more direct estimate of renal haemodynamics. Measurement of plasma renin activity is a useful test in suspected renovascular hypertension but care is needed to ensure that samples are taken under proper basal conditions and are not affected by diuretic therapy or salt restriction. Renal arteriography provides the most detailed information about the renal vessels, and it can sometimes be combined with percutaneous balloon dilatation of a renal artery stenosis.

Treatment. The object of treating systemic arterial hypertension is to reduce the risk of complications and to improve patient survival. The benefits of treatment have to be weighed against its inconvenience and the possibility that the agents used may themselves have potentially harmful effects. In most instances, the discovery of hypertension commits the patient to a lifetime of supervision and treatment. It is important to treat the whole patient, and not just the blood pressure. Because of these considerations it is not particularly helpful to set up arbitrary levels of blood pressure at which treatment should be commenced. Decisions about treatment should also take into account the fact that the natural history of hypertension tends to be more benign in women than in men, and that black people and diabetics are more prone to hypertensive complications.

There is general agreement that hypertension should be treated with antihypertensive drugs if it is severe (e.g. over 160/100 at age 20, 170/110 in men aged 50) or if it is associated with retinal, cardiac or renal damage. There is less certainty concerning the benefits of such treatment in mild or 'borderline' hypertensives, e.g. 140/90 at age 20, 160/95 at age 50. A large-scale trial conducted in Britain by the Medical Research Council tested the effects of treating mild hypertension with a beta-blocker (propranolol), a thiazide diuretic or a placebo. There was no significant overall reduction in mortality in the treated patients, though the trial confirmed an increased mortality risk in hypertensive patients who continued to smoke, and showed some benefit in the subgroup of smoking patients who received active treatment. It remains to be seen whether further trials will be conducted on this scale with other antihypertensive agents.

The trials which have shown the most consistent benefits of treatment have tended to be those in which the 'treated' group has been subject to close medical supervision, and attention has been paid to the correction of other risk factors. Perhaps it is best to regard borderline hypertensives as an 'at risk' population which requires continuing supervision, redoubled efforts at health education, and judicious intervention as determined by individual circumstances.

There is also controversy concerning the drug treatment of hypertension in the elderly. On one hand, hypertension sometimes develops quite rapidly in an elderly person, and responds to treatment with gratifying clinical results. On the other hand, elderly patients with long-standing hypertension often respond badly to ill-judged attempts at lowering the pressure. A recent large-scale European trial showed that there was a reduction in cardiovascular mortality in elderly hypertensive patients treated with a thiazide/triamterene combination, but there was no significant reduction in overall mortality. Rather than attempting to define 'thresholds' of blood pressure requiring treatment in the elderly, it is sensible to rely more on evidence of end-organ damage, or of a recent rise in pressure above previously recorded levels.

GENERAL MEASURES. *Diet*. Very low sodium diets may reduce blood pressure, but there is little evidence that more socially-acceptable diets will do this consistently. Patients may be advised a 'prudent' mixed diet, and encouraged not to add excess salt at table or eat foods with a high sodium content (p. 357). The blood pressure of obese, hypertensive patients often falls in response to weight reduction. There is evidence that excessive alcohol consumption may cause or exacerbate hypertension, and this should be moderated.

Smoking. The effects of cigarette smoking and hypertension on cardiovascular morbidity are additive, and smoking should be discouraged.

Exercise. Regular exercise improves physical fitness and is to be encouraged. Vigorous 'isometric' exercise, e.g. weight lifting, may cause a considerable rise in blood pressure and should be avoided.

Relaxation. It is customary to advise patients to 'avoid stress' but this is usually a pious hope. Spouses should be dissuaded from perpetually reminding patients of their hypertension. Formal relaxation classes, meditation and biofeedback have all been shown to reduce blood pressure in small groups of patients; their efficacy is usually proportional to the enthusiasm of the teacher and the commitment of the participant.

ANTIHYPERTENSIVE DRUG THERAPY. Many patients can be satisfactorily treated with a single antihypertensive drug, the choice of which will be determined by safety, convenience and freedom from side-effects. Another large group will require a combination of two or three antihypertensive agents to give good control with a low level of side-effects. A small minority will have severe hypertension refractory to conventional treatment and requiring intensive investigation and special treatment.

The principal agents used in single drug treatment of hypertension are thiazide diuretics, beta-adrenoceptor antagonists and ACE inhibitors; calcium antagonists and some other vasodilators are also effective.

Thiazide diuretics and their adverse effects have been discussed on page 93. The mechanism of their hypotensive action is incompletely understood, and it may take up to a month for the maximum effect to be observed. More potent diuretics such as frusemide have few advantages over thiazides in the treatment of hypertension unless there is substantial renal impairment, when their greater ability to cause sodium excretion may be useful.

Beta-adrenoceptor antagonists are the most widely used of the sympatholytic agents. In addition to an antihypertensive effect thay may also relieve anxiety, palpitation and angina pectoris. *Propranolol* (p. 137) is effective and reliable, but its dose has to be adjusted to the individual's needs because a large and variable proportion of the drug is destroyed in its first passage through the liver; even with equivalent blood concentrations there is some variation in response. Often twice daily dosage will suffice, but in others high doses may be required, so that treatment initiated in a dose of 40 mg b.d. may have to be increased to as much as 160 mg 6-hourly or more. The slow-release form has the advantage that the patient has to remember only a single daily dose. Many patients have no side-effects but minor gastric disturbance, bradycardia, cardiac failure, bronchospasm, tiredness, bad dreams, hallucinations, cold hands and, occasionally, muscle weakness are all recognised complications.

Metoprolol and *atenolol* are appropriate if a cardioselective drug is indicated, as in patients who have airways obstruction, peripheral vascular disease or insulin dependent diabetes. Cardioselective drugs have a greater effect on the cardiac (β_1) receptors than on the β_2 receptors which subserve bronchodilatation and vasodilatation. They also delay less the return of the blood sugar to normal after hypoglycaemia.

Metabolic side effects of beta-blocking drugs include a tendency to increase plasma concentrations of cholesterol in low density lipoproteins, which could in theory have a deleterious effect on the progression of atheroma, and a tendency for nonselective beta-blockers to cause a rise in plasma potassium concentration, particularly after exercise.

Labetalol is a combined alpha and beta adrenoceptor antagonist which is sometimes more effective than pure beta-blockers. The usual dose is 100–200 mg twice daily.

Angiotensin converting enzyme (ACE) inhibitors (p. 151) have been a major advance in the treatment of moderate to severe hypertension. Apart from causing postural hypotension, they are largely free from unpleasant side-effects and compliance tends to be good. They should be used with care in patients with impaired renal function or renal artery stenosis, as a sudden reduction in renal perfusion may precipitate renal failure. As in the treatment of cardiac failure, it is best to start with a small dose and increase it gradually.

Calcium antagonists such as verapamil or nifedipine are effective and usually well tolerated antihypertensive drugs. They are particularly useful when hypertension coexists with angina.

Drug combinations. Another approach to the problem of side-effects is to use drug combinations—most commonly a thiazide diuretic together with a beta-blocker. This may allow control of hypertension refractory to either drug alone at doses insufficient to cause serious side-effects. In some respects the drugs have complementary actions; thiazides increase renin production while beta-blockers depress it, and the hypokalaemic effect of thiazides may be countered by the hyperkalaemic effect of a nonselective beta-blocker. On the other hand the complexity of combination therapy may discourage compliance and the risk of side-effects unrelated to the dose of drug is increased. A number of beta-blocker/thiazide combination tablets have been marketed, but the proportion of the two drugs is not necessarily optimal for every patient.

If satisfactory hypertensive control (usually defined as a phase 5 diastolic pressure of 90 or less) cannot be achieved with a beta-blocker and thiazide combination, a third drug may be added—usually a peripheral vasodilator such as hydralazine. This drug is rarely used alone as it tends to cause a tachycardia. The usual dose of hydralazine is 50–200 mg daily in divided doses. It is sometimes the cause of an allergic vasculitis or a syndrome resembling SLE (p. 575).

The emergency treatment of hypertension. It is virtually never necessary or desirable to cause an instantaneous fall in blood pressure. Even in the presence of cardiac failure or hypertensive encephalopathy a controlled reduction over a period of 30–60 minutes to a level of about 150/90 is adequate, and there is often less urgency. Too rapid a fall in pressure may cause permanent cerebral ischaemic damage, including blindness, and may sometimes precipitate coronary or renal insufficiency.

The most effective agent for blood pressure reduction in an emergency is a controlled intravenous infusion of sodium nitroprusside, but this requires very careful supervision, preferably in an intensive care unit. Alternatives are intravenous or intramuscular labetalol (2 mg/min to a maximum of 200 mg) or intramuscular hydralazine (5 or 10 mg aliquots repeated at half-hourly intervals and titrated against the blood pressure response). Bed-rest, sedation and a diuretic are also helpful. Urinary output and plasma electrolytes should be monitored, and urgent enquiry made into the cause of the hypertension.

Hypertensive emergencies in young patients may result from acute glomerulonephritis or from an acute exacerbation of chronic renal failure. The latter is also an important cause in older patients, but these are also likely to suffer from acute renal ischaemia caused by atheroma or embolism. The possibility of phaeochromocytoma should also be considered.

Refractory hypertension. The common causes of treatment failure in hypertension are non-compliance with drug therapy, inadequate therapy, and failure to recognise an underlying cause such as renal artery stenosis or phaeochromocytoma; of these the first is by far the most prevalent. There is no easy solution to compliance problems, but a simple treatment regime, attempts to improve rapport with the patient, and careful supervision may all help.

DISEASES OF THE PULMONARY CIRCULATION

Pulmonary arterial hypertension

Aetiology. The principal cause of severe pulmonary hypertension in adults is an increase in pulmonary vascular resistance. In infancy another important cause is an increased pulmonary blood flow resulting from left to right shunting, as in atrial and ventricular septal defects and in persistent ductus arteriosus. While this is initially reversible when the shunt is corrected, prolonged exposure of a child's lungs to pulmonary hypertension causes irreversible vascular damage, and a rise in pulmonary vascular resistance perpetuates the hypertension.

Pulmonary hypertension developing in adult life may be due to: (1) reflex increase in pulmonary vascular resistance in response to a rise in pulmonary capillary pressure; (2) pulmonary vasoconstriction as a response to alveolar hypoxia or arterial hypoxaemia (p. 154); (3) thromboembolic obliteration of the pulmonary vascular bed, or (4) a variety of disease processes directly affecting the pulmonary vessels. Any cause of left sided cardiac failure may produce pulmonary hypertension, but it is most prominent when there has been a very gradual rise in left atrial pressure, as in some cases of mitral stenosis. The combined burden of a raised left atrial pressure and an increased pulmonary vascular resistance may produce secondary right heart failure. Provided the left sided failure is relieved, e.g. by mitral valvotomy, the pulmonary hypertension will usually regress.

Pulmonary vasoconstriction in response to hypoxia is to some extent a protective reflex, which will divert blood flow away from poorly ventilated alveoli. It may be responsible however for the chronic pulmonary hypertension seen in some people who live at high altitude, and for the pulmonary hypertension and right heart failure associated with chronic alveolar hypoventilation. Another important cause of right heart failure in association with chronic lung disease (*cor pulmonale*) is a rise in pulmonary vascular resistance as the result of loss of pulmonary vessels in destructive lung diseases such as emphysema (p. 246). Pulmonary thromboembolism is particularly important and is considered in the next section. Pulmonary vessels can be affected by connective tissue diseases such as systemic sclerosis, by drugs such as fenfluramine and by schistosomiasis (p. 783).

In primary pulmonary hypertension the underlying cause is obscure. This is a rare disease most common in young women, and there is sometimes a family history.

Clinical features. There may be a left parasternal impulse either from right ventricular hypertrophy, or from an enlarged pulmonary artery, or both. If there is accompanying right atrial hypertrophy a large *a* wave is to be expected in the jugular venous pulse. There may be an ejection sound and a loud second heart sound over the pulmonary valve, and pulmonary regurgitation may produce a soft early diastolic murmur. Associated conditions such as left sided cardiac failure or chronic lung disease may also produce their own clinical features.

Investigation. The ECG usually shows evidence of right atrial and right ventricular hypertrophy (Fig. 7.32). The chest radiograph may show enlargement of the pulmonary artery and its main branches. Echocardiography is important to exclude left sided obstructive lesions such as 'silent' mitral stenosis, and radionuclide lung scanning may suggest pulmonary embolism. Pulmonary arteriography and lung biopsy have a role in a few selected cases.

Treatment is basically that of the underlying cause. Prognosis is fairly good if the hypertension is due to correctable left heart failure, treatable hypoxia or to drugs which can be withdrawn; the outlook is poor if the cause is advanced lung disease or thromboembolism. Primary pulmonary hypertension generally has a poor prognosis; vasodilators have been tried but with inconsistent results. Continuous intravenous infusion of prostacyclin has been successful in some patients. Very occasionally, spontaneous recovery has been reported. Patients with irreversible pulmonary hypertension may be candidates for heart-lung transplantation, but this is still largely experimental.

Pulmonary embolism and infarction

Pulmonary embolism occurs when a portion of thrombus in a systemic vein, or less commonly the right side of the heart, is discharged into the circulation. It may lodge in the main pulmonary artery and cause sudden death, or in a smaller pulmonary artery and result in pulmonary infarction. Recurrent 'silent' pulmonary embolism may come to light only when pulmonary hypertension and chronic right heart failure develop.

Aetiology. Thrombosis in a pelvic vein or a deep vein of the legs (p. 194) is the most frequent source. As this is usually the result of stasis, pulmonary embolism most often affects people who have been confined to bed. It is particularly liable to occur within 10 days after a surgical operation or after childbirth. A long journey in an aircraft or car can cause thrombosis in a leg vein. The presence of phlebothrombosis is frequently not recognised until after the embolism.

In less than 10% of cases thrombi responsible for pulmonary embolism form in the right atrium in patients with atrial fibrillation, especially if cardiac failure is present.

Clinical features. Massive pulmonary embolism has been described on page 145. In cases of lesser severity, symptoms and signs may be absent or there may be transient dyspnoea, tachycardia or syncope. In *pulmonary infarction*, which is usually due to a small peripheral embolus, the signs are pleural pain which may be severe, and haemoptysis which may be profuse and repetitive. There may be dyspnoea, tachycardia, central cyanosis, pyrexia and polymorphonuclear leucocytosis. Secondary infection may occur. Often, pulmonary infarction produces no symptoms.

Investigation. RADIOLOGICAL EXAMINATION. In massive pulmonary embolism the lung fields often appear normal but sometimes there is a hilar opacity from the blocked vessel and ischaemia distal to the embolus causes a reduction in the usual vascular markings of a lung or lobe. Pulmonary angiography is the most reliable method of diagnosis, but should not be allowed to delay urgent treatment.

In pulmonary infarction there may be a pulmonary opacity due to a recent infarct or a linear scar from an earlier one. A small pleural effusion is common. The ipsilateral hemidiaphragm may be elevated. These radiological abnormalities are usually most marked at the base of one lung but are often bilateral.

Venous thrombosis can be demonstrated by bilateral ascending phlebography.

RADIONUCLIDE SCANNING. The intravenous injection of radionuclide-labelled macroaggregated albumin can be used to delineate underperfused areas of lung not detected on a plain radiograph. This technique is of value in the diagnosis of pulmonary embolism, especially if combined with ventilation scanning following the inhalation of a radionuclide-labelled gas. Radionuclide lung scans may be difficult to interpret if the chest radiograph is abnormal.

ELECTROCARDIOGRAPHY may show evidence of right ventricular dilatation and strain in cases of massive pulmonary embolism (right axis deviation, T wave inversion in the right ventricular leads and displacement of the interventricular septum to the left), or the pattern of incomplete right bundle branch block (Fig. 7.27). In cases of lesser severity the ECG is usually normal, except for a sinus tachycardia.

Course and prognosis. Massive pulmonary embolism is frequently fatal. Minor and medium sized emboli are much less dangerous, but may herald subsequent massive embolism. Recurrent emboli may cause pulmonary hypertension and right ventricular failure. The vast majority of pulmonary infarcts resolve completely. Occasionally an infarct may become secondarily infected and result in a lung abscess.

Treatment. Intravenous heparin should be injected immediately and a heparin infusion continued for 3 days (p. 550). Thereafter oral anticoagulants should be given to prevent further venous thrombosis (p. 551). Depending on the circumstances such treatment should be continued for 6 weeks to 6 months. Pain and apprehension should be allayed but morphine must be avoided if there is severe hypotension. Oxygen should be administered if central cyanosis is present.

Massive pulmonary embolism is best managed in an area where intensive care can be provided. If there is no detectable cardiac output, cardiac massage may sometimes help by fragmenting a thrombus in the pulmonary artery. Vasodilators are contraindicated and a high venous pressure should be maintained. Pulmonary embolectomy under cardiopulmonary bypass may be life-saving, but often takes too long to organise. Thrombolytic therapy with streptokinase or urokinase produces more rapid angiographic resolution of thrombus, but its ability to improve survival has been less convincing. Heparin and oxygen therapy should not be neglected while these measures are being considered.

Prevention of pulmonary embolism and infarction consists of those measures directed at prophylaxis against venous thrombosis in the legs (p. 194). In cases of recurrent pulmonary embolism despite anticoagulation, venous interruption may be necessary either by inserting a filter into, or plicating, the inferior vena cava.

DISEASES OF THE MYOCARDIUM

The myocardium is involved in most types of heart disease, but the terms myocarditis and cardiomyopathy tend to be used, not always consistently, for diseases which primarily affect the heart muscle rather than the heart valves or coronary arteries. Myocarditis implies an inflammatory process; this is true of rheumatic myocarditis and many types of viral myocarditis, but diphtheritic myocarditis is due to a toxin, and sarcoid heart disease and that associated with systemic lupus erythematosus have in the past been classed as cardiomyopathies. An international commission has now recommended that the term cardiomyopathy should be confined to forms of chronic myocardial disease without a known cause, and that where a cause is known the term (specific) heart disease, e.g. sarcoid heart disease, should be used instead. In practice, myocarditis usually means an acute and potentially reversible illness affecting heart muscle, and it is convenient to consider together the chronic diseases, namely the cardiomyopathies and the specific conditions which often closely resemble them in their clinical presentation.

Acute myocarditis

Acute myocarditis may occur as a complication of infections such as diphtheria, chickenpox, pneumonia, typhoid fever, scrub typhus fever and meningitis. Chagas' disease (American trypanosomiasis, p. 781) is the commonest cause in South America. Myocarditis may also be due to viral infection such as in influenza, poliomyelitis, infectious mononucleosis and, particularly, Coxsackie B infections. Rheumatic myocarditis is described on page 152.

Often the only evidence of myocarditis is a sinus tachycardia which is out of proportion to the severity of the infection. In more severe cases there may be a third heart sound, arrhythmias, conduction defects or acute cardiac failure. Prognosis in most types of acute myocarditis is usually good, but it may cause death in diphtheria. In Chagas' disease, the patient usually recovers from the acute phase and after a latent period of 10 or 20 years a chronic cardiomyopathy develops which is eventually fatal.

There is no specific therapy for acute myocarditis; the usual forms of treatment for cardiac failure and arrhythmias should be undertaken. Corticosteroids have been tried, but are of no proven value. Prolonged rest is sometimes necessary.

Specific diseases of heart muscle and cardiomyopathy

Damage to cardiac muscle is part of a number of systemic disorders such as haemochromatosis, sarcoidosis, amyloidosis, systemic lupus erythematosus, systemic sclerosis and polyarteritis nodosa. There are often, but not invariably, extracardiac clues to the diagnosis in these conditions. Heart muscle damage may also be associated with a variety of toxins, of which the most important is alcohol.

In the cardiomyopathies there is no generalised disorder and frequently no aetiological agent can be found, although in a proportion of such cases there is a family history. Sometimes there is a definite or suspected history of myocarditis. Cardiomyopathies are classified into three groups: dilated; hypertrophic; and restrictive or obliterative. Clinically, most cases of heart muscle disease for which a specific cause is known resemble one or other of these varieties.

Dilated cardiomyopathy is characterised by left and right ventricular dilatation, impaired ventricular contraction with a reduced ventricular ejection fraction (p. 148) and often mitral and/or tricuspid regurgitation. The ventricular end-diastolic pressure is elevated, and the clinical picture is one of progressive left sided and, later, right sided cardiac failure. The ECG is usually nonspecific, but may show evidence of left ventricular hypertrophy. Arrhythmias are common. Echocardiography is useful in making the diagnosis. It is this form of cardiomyopathy which specific heart muscle disease (e.g. that due to alcohol) most often resembles. A similar picture is sometimes seen in advanced ischaemic heart disease.

The treatment of dilated cardiomyopathy is directed at the associated cardiac failure; specific treatment is possible only when there is a recognisable cause. The prognosis is usually poor, particularly when there is no known aetiology.

Hypertrophic cardiomyopathy is often familial. A similar condition is associated with the hereditary disorder Friedreich's ataxia.

Hypertrophic cardiomyopathy is characterised by increased thickness of the ventricular wall; this may be generalised or may principally affect the interventricular septum. If asymmetrical septal hypertrophy is present, it may cause left ventricular outflow obstruction, but this is not essential to the diagnosis. In many cases the diagnosis is made only at autopsy following sudden death in a young person. In others, the condition may present with syncopal episodes or with angina.

On examination, there is usually palpable left ventricular hypertrophy, and there may be an apical double impulse reflecting also atrial hypertrophy. On auscultation there is commonly a midsystolic murmur over the left ventricular outflow, and there may be associated mitral regurgitation. The pulse is characteristically 'jerky' and not slow-rising. The ECG usually shows left ventricular hypertrophy; there may be bizarre T wave abnormalities and an inferior myocardial infarct may be mimicked. Echocardiography is usually diagnostic.

The natural history is variable. Sometimes patients who present with hypertrophic cardiomyopathy gradually develop features of a dilated cardiomyopathy over the course of some years. The prognosis may be better in those who have the condition discovered incidentally in adult life than in those who present with symptoms in childhood or adolescence.

No treatment is definitely known to improve prognosis, but propranolol helps to relieve angina and sometimes prevents syncopal attacks, particularly in those with ventricular outflow obstruction. Arrhythmias are common, and amiodarone is useful in their control. Digoxin and vasodilators may increase outflow obstruction and should be used with caution.

Restrictive or obliterative cardiomyopathy is characterised by an increased ventricular 'stiffness' effectively causing ventricular inflow obstruction. It is found with endomyocardial fibrosis in the tropics (p. 716) and with endocardial eosinophilia. Amyloidosis of the heart can produce a similar picture. Diagnosis can be very difficult, especially where the condition is uncommon. The combination of severe left or right heart failure with a normal heart size and no murmurs is suggestive. Endocardial biopsy may be diagnostic. Treatment is usually symptomatic, but successful excision of fibrotic endocardium has been reported.

DISEASES OF THE PERICARDIUM

Acute pericarditis

The most common identifiable causes of acute pericarditis in Britain are myocardial infarction and viral infections, e.g. with Coxsackie B viruses. Rheumatic fever and tuberculosis are also important, but are now rare in Britain. Pericarditis may occur as a complication of bacterial infection and of malignant disease. Other causes include uraemia, trauma and connective tissue disorders such as systemic lupus erythematosus. In many cases of pericarditis it is not possible to identify a cause, and these are referred to as 'idiopathic'.

Pathology. Pericarditis may be fibrinous, serous, haemorrhagic or purulent. In the first there is a fibrinous exudate on the surface which may eventually lead to varying degrees of adhesion formation. In serous pericarditis there is in addition an exudate of anything from a few millilitres to a litre or more. The effusion is straw-coloured and often slightly turbid with a high protein content. A haemorrhagic effusion suggests a malignant origin. Purulent pericarditis is due to a pyogenic infection.

Clinical features. The characteristic pain of pericarditis is retrosternal and often radiates to the shoulders and neck. It may be present on, or made worse by, a deep breath, movement, change of position, exercise or swallowing.

A friction rub is the diagnostic sign of pericarditis. It consists of a superficial scratching sound, best heard to the left of the lower sternum; it is usually systolic but may be audible also in diastole. It frequently has a 'to and fro' quality. Friction is often better heard when the stethoscope diaphragm is pressed firmly upon the chest, the patient's breath being held for a time in inspiration and then in expiration. If a pericardial effusion develops there is sometimes a sensation of retrosternal oppression. An effusion may be difficult to detect clinically — the heart sounds may become quieter, but pericardial friction is not always abolished.

CARDIAC TAMPONADE refers to compression of the heart by a large or rapidly developing effusion which interferes with diastolic filling. The amount of fluid which is needed to produce tamponade depends in part on the compliance of the pericardium, and is variable. In the presence of tamponade, jugular venous pressure rises and cardiac output falls. Pulsus paradoxus (p. 120) may be found, and urine output is suppressed. The clinical picture of acute circulatory failure may develop. Pulmonary oedema is unusual but not unknown. Atypical presentations may occur when the effusion is loculated as a result of previous pericarditis or cardiac surgery.

Investigation. The ECG shows ST elevation with upward concavity over the affected area, which may be widespread. Later, there may be T wave inversion. QRS voltage is often reduced in the presence of an effusion. Serial radiographs may show a rapid increase in the size of the cardiac shadow over days or even hours, and with a large effusion the heart may have a pear shaped appearance. Echocardiography is particularly useful in detecting pericardial effusion.

Treatment. The pain can usually be relieved by aspirin, but a more potent anti-inflammatory agent such as indomethacin may be required.

PARACENTESIS of a pericardial effusion may be indicated for diagnostic purposes or to relieve symptoms from cardiac tamponade. Either of two approaches may be used depending on the experience of the operator and the configuration of the patient: (1) the needle is inserted to the left of the xiphoid process, insinuated deep to the left costal margin, and then directed towards the left shoulder; (2) the needle is inserted medial to the cardiac apex at a point where echocardiography reveals the presence of a layer of fluid lying in front of the heart.

For diagnostic purposes it is usually enough to withdraw a few millilitres of fluid. If therapeutic drainage is needed it may be safer to use a plastic cannula inserted over a needle or guidewire than to attempt aspiration of the whole effusion through a rigid needle. A viscous or loculated effusion may require surgical drainage. The main dangers of pericardiocentesis are arrhythmia, damage to a coronary artery, and exacerbation of tamponade as a result of injury to the right ventricle. It is however life saving in the presence of severe tamponade.

Viral, tuberculous and purulent pericarditis

Viral pericarditis may follow an upper respiratory infection, and in about 10% of cases a Coxsackie infection can be established. Recovery usually occurs within a few days or weeks, but there may be recurrences. There is no specific treatment; corticosteroids may help suppress symptoms but there is little evidence they accelerate cure.

Tuberculous pericarditis may be secondary to manifest pulmonary tuberculosis, or the primary source may not be detectable. The disease is commonly insidious in onset and the subsequent course is chronic. An effusion usually develops and the pericardium may become thick and unyielding so that the heart is compressed. Pleural effusions are often associated.

The diagnosis may be confirmed by aspiration of the fluid and direct examination or culture for tubercle bacilli. Antituberculous chemotherapy is prescribed (p. 230). Corticosteroids may help to prevent the development of constrictive pericarditis. Pericardial aspiration may be carried out as required to relieve symptoms. In the inactive stage surgical relief may be necessary.

Purulent pericarditis is rare. It occurs as a complication of septicaemia, by direct spread from an intrathoracic infection, or from a penetrating injury. Treatment is by antimicrobial therapy and if necessary surgical drainage.

Chronic pericardial constriction

Tuberculosis was formerly a frequent cause. Some cases accompany rheumatoid arthritis and others follow a haemopericardium or, rarely, acute pericarditis. Often the cause is obscure. A slowly progressive fibrosis of the pericardium develops and constricts the movement of the heart, so that it cannot expand in diastole. The fibrous tissue is dense and inelastic and calcification is common. The inflow to the heart is impeded, so that cardiac output is diminished and systemic venous pressure raised.

Clinical features. Breathlessness is not a prominent symptom as the lungs are seldom congested. A raised jugular venous pressure is present, with a rapid and transitory y descent (Fig. 7.1). The arterial pulse tends to be rapid, of small volume, and pulsus paradoxus may be present. Hepatomegaly and ascites occur relatively early compared with peripheral oedema. The heart is usually not enlarged but chest radiography may show pericardial calcification. The main differential diagnosis is from restrictive cardiomyopathy.

Treatment. The problem is primarily a mechanical one, and rapid improvement is usual if surgical resection of the pericardium is performed.

CONGENITAL HEART DISEASE

The incidence of haemodynamically significant congenital cardiac abnormalities is about 1% of live births. In most cases the cause of the abnormality is unknown, but some fetal defects are due to maternal infections in the early weeks of pregnancy, e.g. rubella. All degrees of severity occur. Many defects are not compatible with extrauterine life, or only for a short time. Early diagnosis is important because most types are amenable to surgical treatment, but this opportunity may be lost if secondary changes, for example pulmonary vascular damage, occur.

Symptoms may be absent, or the child may be noticed to be breathless, or may fail to thrive and grow normally. Local signs vary with the 8anatomical lesion.

Central cyanosis occurs when desaturated blood enters the systemic circulation without passing through the lungs (i.e. there is a right to left shunt). In the neonate the commonest cause of this is transposition of the great arteries, in which the aorta derives from the right ventricle and the pulmonary artery from the left. In older children cyanosis is usually the consequence of a ventricular septal defect combined with severe pulmonary stenosis (tetralogy of Fallot, p. 188) or with pulmonary vascular disease (Eisenmenger's syndrome, p. 187).

Persistent ductus arteriosus

During fetal life, before the lungs begin to function, most of the blood from the pulmonary artery passes through the ductus arteriosus into the aorta just below the origin of the left subclavian artery. Normally the ductus closes soon after birth but sometimes it fails to do so. Since the pressure in the aorta is higher than that in the pulmonary artery there will be a continuous arteriovenous shunt, the volume of which depends on the size of the ductus. As much as 50% of the left ventricular output may be recirculated through the lungs, with a consequent increase in the work of the heart. The condition, which may be associated with other abnormalities, is much commoner in females.

With small shunts there may be no symptoms for years but, if the ductus is large, growth and development are retarded. There is usually no disability, but cardiac failure may eventually ensue, dyspnoea being the first symptom. A continuous 'machinery' murmur is heard with late systolic accentuation, maximal at the second left rib near the sternum (Fig. 7.38). It is frequently accompanied by a thrill. Enlargement of the pulmonary artery may be detected radiologically.

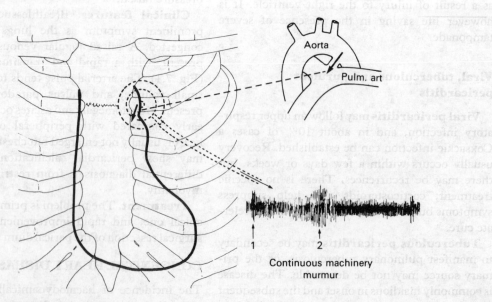

Fig. 7.38 Persistent ductus arteriosus.

The ECG is usually normal.

A large left to right shunt in infancy may cause a considerable rise in pulmonary artery pressure, and sometimes this leads to progressive pulmonary vascular damage. With the resulting rise in pulmonary vascular resistance, pulmonary artery pressure rises further until it equals or exceeds aortic pressure. The shunt through the defect may then reverse, causing central cyanosis; with a persistent ductus arteriosus this cyanosis may be more apparent in the feet and toes than in the upper part of the body. The murmur becomes quieter, may be confined to systole, or may disappear. The ECG shows evidence of right ventricular hypertrophy.

In uncomplicated cases the ductus can be divided with little risk, especially in children, and there is general agreement that this should be advised in all cases to remove the risks of infective endocarditis or of cardiac failure in adult life. Operation is contraindicated when the pulmonary vascular resistance is elevated and the shunt has become reversed.

Coarctation of the aorta

Narrowing of the aorta most commonly occurs in the region where the ductus arteriosus joins the aorta, i.e. just below the origin of the left subclavian artery (Fig. 7.39). The condition is more common in males, and is sometimes associated with other abnormalities, of which the most frequent is a bicuspid aortic valve. Acquired coarctation of the aorta is rare; it may follow trauma, or be a complication of a progressive arteritis (Takayasu disease, p. 193).

Aortic coarctation is an important cause of cardiac failure in the newborn, but symptoms are often absent in older children or adults. Headaches may occur from hypertension in the upper part of the body, and occasionally weakness or cramps in the legs may result from decreased circulation in the lower part of the body. The blood pressure is raised in the arms but normal or low in the legs. Unduly large arterial pulsations may be seen in the neck. The femoral pulses are weak, and delayed after the radial. A systolic murmur may sometimes be heard over the coarctation posteriorly. There may also be an ejection systolic

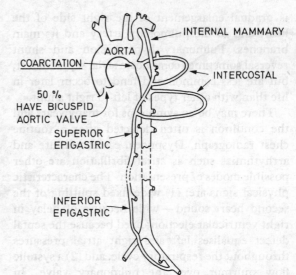

Fig. 7.39 Coarctation of the aorta.

murmur in the aortic area. Evidence of a collateral circulation may be detectable in older children and adults in the form of visible or palpable dilated and tortuous arteries around the scapulae and below the ribs posteriorly.

Radiological examination in early childhood is often normal but at a later age may show changes in the contour of the aorta and notching of the undersurfaces of the ribs from tortuous loops of enlarged intercostal arteries. The ECG may show left ventricular hypertrophy.

In untreated severe cases, death may occur from left ventricular failure, dissection of the aorta or cerebral haemorrhage. Surgical correction is advisable in all but the mildest cases. If this is done early enough in childhood the risk of persistent hypertension may be avoided, but patients operated on in late childhood or adult life often remain hypertensive or become hypertensive again. Coexistent aortic valve disease is another reason for long-term follow-up.

Atrial septal defect

Atrial septal defect is more common in females. Since the normal right ventricle is much more compliant than the left, a large volume of blood shunts through the defect from the left to right atrium and thence to the right ventricle and pulmonary arteries (Fig. 7.40). As a result there is gradual enlargement of the right side of the heart and of the pulmonary artery and its main branches. Pulmonary hypertension and shunt reversal sometimes complicate atrial septal defect, but are less common and tend to occur later in life than with other types of left to right shunt.

There may be no symptoms for many years and the condition is often detected after a routine chest radiograph. Dyspnoea, cardiac failure and arrhythmias such as atrial fibrillation are other possible modes of presentation. The characteristic physical signs are: (1) wide fixed splitting of the second heart sound—wide because of delay in right ventricular ejection, fixed because the septal defect equalises left and right atrial pressures throughout the respiratory cycle; and (2) a systolic flow murmur over the pulmonary valve. In children with a large shunt there may be a diastolic flow murmur over the tricuspid valve; unlike a mitral flow murmur, this is usually high-pitched.

The chest radiograph shows enlargement of the heart and of the pulmonary artery; increased pulsation of these vessels can be seen on screening. The ECG usually shows incomplete right bundle branch block because right ventricular depolarisation is delayed as a result of ventricular dilatation. Echocardiography is very useful, and cross-sectional echocardiography may directly demonstrate the defect.

Atrial septal defects large enough to be clinically recognisable should be closed surgically, and the long-term prognosis thereafter is excellent. Pul-monary hypertension and shunt reversal are contraindications to surgery.

Ventricular septal defect

The clinical features of ventricular septal defect depend on the size of the defect and the age of the patient. At birth, there may be little shunting through a large defect because fetal pulmonary vascular resistance and right ventricular pressure are high and may fall only gradually in the first few days of life. As right ventricular pressure falls, the left to right shunt increases, and children with a large ventricular septal defect commonly develop heart failure between 3 and 6 weeks of age. Following this, the defect may spontaneously diminish in size, or the pulmonary vascular resistance may increase, reducing the shunt at the price of progressive pulmonary vascular damage and eventually shunt reversal. Most patients seen with a congenital ventricular septal defect in late childhood or adult life therefore have either a small defect with a small or moderate left to right shunt or a large defect with shunt reversal. The latter is sometimes called Eisenmenger's syndrome (p. 187).

Small ventricular septal defects are characterised clinically by a harsh pansystolic murmur, often accompanied by a thrill, best heard in the fourth intercostal space to the left of the sternum. Symptoms are absent, and the chest radiograph and ECG are normal. The loudness of the murmur

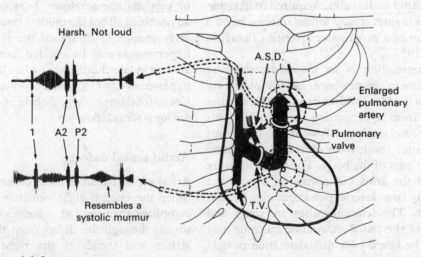

Fig. 7.40 Atrial septal defect.

often seems out of keeping with the absence of other signs (Fig. 7.41). The natural history of this type of defect is usually benign, but there is a risk of infective endocarditis. Surgical closure is rarely justified unless there are complications, and many defects probably close spontaneously.

Large ventricular septal defects with left to right shunt. For reasons already given, this combination is usually seen in infants, or in adults as a complication of myocardial infarction with secondary rupture of the ventricular septum. A systolic murmur is usual, but its loudness is not a good indicator of the size of the shunt. There is often a mid-diastolic mitral flow murmur.

The chest radiograph shows an enlarged heart and dilatation of the pulmonary vessels. The ECG may show both right and left ventricular hypertrophy. Cardiac catheterisation is often required to confirm the diagnosis and measure the pulmonary vascular resistance.

Cardiac failure is treated in the usual way with digoxin and diuretics, but inability to control the failure or evidence of increasing pulmonary vascular resistance are indications for early surgery. In adults with post-infarction septal defects the prognosis is poor but early investigation and surgery may be life saving.

Eisenmenger's syndrome. This term is used for patients with pulmonary hypertension and a reversed (right to left) shunt associated with a ventricular or atrial septal defect or with a persistent ductus arteriosus. For practical purposes the management and prognosis of patients with a raised pulmonary vascular resistance, pulmonary hypertension and reversed shunting is the same whatever the site of the shunt. By this stage the time for surgery is past, and closure of the defect simply hastens death from right heart failure.

These patients usually present in childhood or early adolescence with effort intolerance or failure to thrive. Frequent respiratory infections are a common cause of complaint. The patient is centrally cyanosed with finger and toe clubbing. There is usually clinical evidence of right ventricular hypertrophy. Shunt murmurs are usually absent; there may be an early diastolic murmur of pulmonary regurgitation. The chest radiograph may show an enlarged pulmonary artery, but the heart shadow is often not enlarged. Polycythaemia is usual, and if extreme may lead to neurological symptoms. The natural history is one of slow and inexorable decline; in the later stages pulmonary infarction and haemoptysis may occur.

There is no specific treatment. Periodic venesection helps symptomatically but iron deficiency is to be avoided. With the aid of venesection,

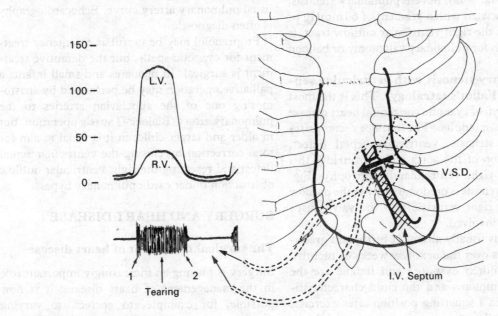

Fig. 7.41 Ventricular septal defect.

diuretics and antibiotics more of these patients are reaching early adulthood, but few survive beyond the fourth decade. The prevention of Eisenmengers' syndrome by the detection and correction of large left to right shunts in infancy is an important reason for regular cardiac examination in infants and young children.

Pulmonary stenosis

Pulmonary stenosis may occur as an isolated anomaly, in which case there is no cyanosis, or in association with an atrial or ventricular septal defect, in which case there may or may not be cyanosis depending on the relative pressures on the two sides of the defect. Stenosis may occur at the level of the pulmonary valve or in the infundibular region of the right ventricle.

Pulmonary stenosis with intact interventricular septum. Mild congenital pulmonary stenosis is fairly common, asymptomatic and rarely deteriorates. In severe pulmonary stenosis there may be dyspnoea, fatigue, or exertional syncope. The physical signs are discussed on page 160. Guides to the severity of the stenosis include the loudness of the murmur, the width of splitting of the second heart sound, and most importantly the presence of right ventricular hypertrophy on the ECG (Fig. 7.32). Severe pulmonary stenosis, usually associated with a gradient of 60 mmHg or more across the right ventricular outflow tract, is an indication for pulmonary valvotomy or balloon dilatation.

Pulmonary stenosis with ventricular septal defect (Fallot's tetralogy). This is the most common form of cyanotic congenital heart disease in children or adults. The tetralogy comprises pulmonary stenosis, ventricular septal defect, dextroposition of the aorta which overrides this defect, and right ventricular hypertrophy (Fig. 7.42). The stenosis is predominantly in the outflow tract of the right ventricle, but the valve cusps may also be involved.

Cyanosis is usually absent at birth, and gradually develops over the next few weeks or months. In older children dyspnoea and fatigue are the principal symptoms and the child characteristically assumes a squatting position after exercise. Cyanotic spells may occur in infants or children

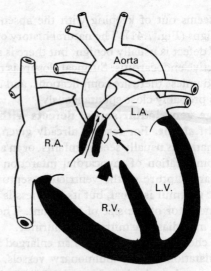

Fig. 7.42 Fallot's tetralogy. The stenosis is in the infundibulum of the right ventricle.

after feeds or exertion; the child becomes deeply cyanosed and flaccid for several seconds, with gradual recovery. The principal signs are central cyanosis with a systolic murmur maximal to the left of the upper sternum. The pulmonary component of the second heart sound is soft and may be inaudible. The ECG shows right ventricular hypertrophy, and the chest radiograph has a characteristic cardiac contour with absence of the usual pulmonary artery curve. Echocardiography is often diagnostic.

Propranolol may be useful as emergency treatment for cyanotic spells, but the definitive treatment is surgical. In neonates and small infants a palliative operation may be performed by anastomosing one of the subclavian arteries to the pulmonary artery (Blalock-Taussig operation) but in older and larger children it is usual to aim for total correction by closing the ventricular septal defect and resecting the right ventricular outflow obstruction under cardiopulmonary bypass.

SURGERY AND HEART DISEASE

The surgical treatment of heart disease

Surgery is playing an increasingly important role in the management of heart disease; it is now possible, for example, to correct, to varying degrees, most types of congenital heart disease and to alleviate many cases of rheumatic and ischaemic heart disease. It is not possible, short of cardiac transplantation, to replace cardiac muscle which has been lost or irretrievably damaged.

Some operations such as mitral valvotomy and the correction of coarctation can be performed under normal circulatory conditions with blood continuing to flow through the heart. Most procedures however require an open or immobile heart, so cardiac function must be taken over by an extracorporeal circulation (cardiopulmonary bypass). With this technique, venous blood is drained from the great veins into a reservoir and is then passed through an oxygenator before being pumped back into the aorta. The heart can then be stopped for some hours though an adequate circulation is maintained to the other vital organs. The mortality of cardiopulmonary bypass should be less than 1%, but patients are nevertheless at risk from several hazards, including air embolism, trauma to the blood from the pump and oxygenator, and electrolyte and acid-base disturbances.

Some surgical procedures require the use of prosthetic material such as a patch to close an atrial or ventricular septal defect, a tube graft for aortic repair, or an artificial heart valve. To a greater or lesser extent this material is a substrate for the ingrowth of host tissue, and with the exception of mechanical valve prostheses is eventually completely covered with host endothelium. Temporary anticoagulation may help to prevent thrombosis and embolism while this process is taking place. The choice between mechanical valves and heterograft 'tissue' valves is still controversial.

Heart transplantation has recently become a practicable procedure. The principal indication is otherwise intractable cardiac failure usually due to cardiomyopathy in a patient under 50 years of age with a normal pulmonary vascular resistance. The overall 2 year survival is approximately 70%.

It is often necessary to devote considerable effort to the physical and psychological rehabilitation of patients after cardiac surgery, particularly in those who have had a prolonged spell of disability. In contrast, patients who have had coronary artery vein grafts sometimes need reminding that their new freedom from symptoms is unlikely to be maintained unless they make efforts to correct risk factors such as cigarette smoking.

Surgery in patients with heart disease

Patients with heart disease undergoing surgery are at risk from the anaesthetic and from the surgery itself. Skilled anaesthesia is particularly important. Continuous monitoring of the ECG, systemic arterial pressure, central venous pressure or pulmonary artery and pulmonary artery wedge pressure may be advisable in appropriate cases, both during surgery and in the early postoperative period.

On the whole, patients with heart disease tolerate surgery remarkably well. Exceptions to this rule are patients with recent myocardial infarction and those who have cardiac or respiratory failure. Only in exceptional circumstances should patients be operated on within 3 months of myocardial infarction; cardiac and respiratory failure should be brought under control before operation if possible. If heart block is present, a pacemaker should be inserted prior to surgery. Surgical diathermy should be avoided if possible in patients with pacemakers; if it is essential, the diathermy electrodes should be kept as far from the pacemaker as possible.

Hypertension is not usually a contraindication to surgery, but it is necessary for the anaesthetist to be aware of what antihypertensive therapy is being used, as excessive hypotension may result from interactions between antihypertensive drugs and anaesthetic agents.

In some patients it is better to defer surgery until the heart disease has been corrected or ameliorated. Thus, elective general surgery should be deferred until after mitral valvotomy, if this is indicated. On the other hand if the cardiac surgery will necessitate long-term anticoagulant therapy it may be better to undertake general surgery first.

HEART DISEASE IN PREGNANCY

Pregnancy leads to increases of blood volume and cardiac output of up to 50%. These changes produce characteristic physical signs. The extremities feel warm and the pulse is of large volume. Tachycardia is present and there may be a rise in venous pressure. The arterial diastolic pressure is lower than in the nonpregnant state because of vasodilatation. The heart may be slightly enlarged and may be displaced outwards because of the high diaphragm. A pulmonary systolic murmur from increased blood flow is common and there may be a physiological third heart sound. Following delivery there is often a transient rise in venous pressure as a consequence of uterine contraction. There is also a period of blood hypercoagulability following delivery.

The increased load on the heart often provokes or worsens symptoms in patients with heart disease. These do not usually occur before about the 12th week, and tend to become maximal from the 24th week onwards. The main symptom of heart disease in pregnancy is breathlessness, but oedema may also occur. It is unusual for angina to present during pregnancy, though patients with pre-existing ischaemic heart disease tend to tolerate pregnancy badly. Symptoms are a poor guide to the severity of the heart disease as some patients are totally asymptomatic until they develop acute pulmonary oedema in late pregnancy or shortly after delivery.

The commonest major form of heart disease encountered in pregnancy is mitral stenosis. Pregnancy should be deferred in patients with severe mitral stenosis, but is usually safe after valvotomy has been performed. If a patient with advanced mitral stenosis does become pregnant either valvotomy or termination should be carried out before the 16th week. With less serious degrees of mitral stenosis and with other forms of heart disease, pregnancy can be allowed to continue and in most cases is uncomplicated. However, if objective evidence of deterioration is apparent, bed-rest must be enforced, combined if necessary with digoxin and diuretics. With careful management, even those with advanced heart disease can be carried successfully through pregnancy and delivery.

Patients with mechanical heart valves who require continuous anticoagulation pose a particular problem during pregnancy because warfarin is capable of causing fetal abnormalities. With care and cooperation it is sometimes possible to maintain heparin anticoagulation throughout pregnancy, but a more satisfactory alternative may be to avoid this type of operation in patients likely to become pregnant.

Patients with congenital heart disease are being seen with increasing frequency during pregnancy, but usually the lesion has been corrected beforehand. In most cases no problems arise but pregnancy is a formidable hazard in those who have pulmonary vascular disease in association with congenital heart disease, and maternal mortality approaches 33% in this group if pregnancy is allowed to go to term.

DISEASES OF ARTERIES AND VEINS

For clinical purposes it is convenient to classify arterial disease under the general headings of degenerative, inflammatory and vasospastic causes.

DEGENERATIVE ARTERIAL DISEASE

Arteriosclerosis is a term which in the past has been applied rather indiscriminately to various unrelated forms of arterial disease. Its retention is justified only if it is confined to the degenerative changes which are part of the usual ageing process and which affect the whole arterial tree.

Medial or Mönckeberg's sclerosis is the name given to degenerative changes which occur in old age in the muscular coats of medium sized arteries such as the radial. Calcification of the media is the characteristic change and accounts for the 'pipe stem' arteries so commonly palpable in the elderly. Arteries become elongated and tortuous and the lumina enlarges; clinical features, other than some rise in systolic pressure, are absent.

Atherosclerosis is a condition which principally affects the aorta and large and medium-sized vessels. It becomes increasingly common as age advances, but it is not an inevitable concomitant of ageing, and there is a great variation in its extent and severity. Although often associated with and accelerated by hypertension, atherosclerosis may be advanced even in the presence of a normal blood pressure. It may also occur in response to a persistent elevation of pressure in the pulmonary arteries.

The basic atheromatous lesion is the plaque, the most important constituents of which are cholesterol and other lipids which may be free in the intimal tissues or intracellular. At a later stage the plaque becomes sclerosed and calcified. Thrombosis is liable to occur on the surface of the plaque, particularly if it ulcerates. Embolism is frequent. Narrowing or obliteration of the lumen leads to symptoms due to ischaemia particularly in the coronary, cerebral, carotid and lower limb vessels.

Atherosclerosis obliterans

This condition is usually confined to the lower limbs. It affects males more commonly than females and usually after the age of 50. It is particularly common in diabetics and is rare in non-smokers.

Clinical features. The principal symptoms which follow impairment of blood supply to the extremities are (1) pain, which occurs on exercise (intermittent claudication) and (2) cold extremities. Although the pathological changes are usually bilateral, symptoms commonly present first in one leg.

Intermittent claudication appears on walking and is rapidly relieved by rest. It most commonly occurs in the calf and causes the patient to limp or stop. Pain occurs at rest with severe ischaemia and relief by dependency suggests gross arterial obstruction. Pain which is relieved by elevation of the part suggests venous obstruction.

Ischaemia may lead to dryness, scaling and inelasticity of the skin, loss of hair, brittle nails, ulceration or gangrene. There may be a change of colour of the skin and delay in the return of colour after blanching with light finger pressure. Where gross lesions are present in one limb, the lower temperature is appreciable to the touch but in chronic ischaemia the affected part may feel warmer on palpation because of a superficial collateral circulation. If the ischaemic limb is first raised 75 degrees above the horizontal, it will blanch more quickly than normal. If then placed in the dependent position, there will be delay in flushing and in venous filling.

Loss of pulsation of one or more peripheral arteries is a common and important feature of arterial disease; bruits may be heard over the larger arteries if they are partially obstructed.

Patients frequently die from myocardial infarction.

Investigation. A radiograph may show calcification. This is especially common in Mönckeberg's sclerosis but does not necessarily indicate that the arterial lumen is significantly narrowed. Ultrasound (Doppler) flow probes are a useful adjunct to clinical examination. Angiography will show the site of vascular occlusion and the extent of any collateral circulation.

Treatment. Until the pathogenesis of atherosclerosis has been clearly established and until specific therapy is discovered the treatment of peripheral vascular disease must continue to be unsatisfactory. Diabetes or obesity may require attention. The patient may need help in getting rid of the tobacco habit.

Cold should be avoided and suitable woollen clothing worn, especially on the limbs. The application of heat to the affected limb is harmful because it increases local metabolism in the ischaemic area without improving blood flow. Pain at rest may be reduced by raising the head of the bed or by lowering the limb below the horizontal and keeping it cool.

Protection against trauma and the early treatment of sepsis are most important. Fungal infection between the toes should be treated. Detailed instructions on the care of the feet and nails must be given. The feet should be kept scrupulously clean, carefully dried after washing, especially between the toes, and dusting powder containing zinc oxide and salicylic acid applied. Nails should be cut carefully and corns pared with caution. It is wise to employ the services of a chiropodist. Socks and shoes should be well fitting. Even the slightest abrasion should be taken seriously and medical advice sought. Dressings to keep the part dry are required for any breach of the surface.

Regular exercise encourages the development of collateral vessels. Patients should not be alarmed by the development of pain and they should be encouraged to believe that with exercise and the stopping of smoking improvement is expected and that the occurrence of gangrene is improbable. Vasodilators are not recommended as they act by dilating normal vessels elsewhere and may divert blood from the affected site.

Areas of gangrene should be kept clean and

dry until a clear line of demarcation appears. Thereafter surgical treatment may be required. Sympathectomy may be of value when the limb is cold or rest pain is present but it seldom helps claudication. Direct arterial surgery is indicated for disabling claudication, rest pain or gangrene provided the vessels are shown by arteriography to be suitable. Balloon angioplasty, which can often be done at the same time as angiography, is an effective treatment for short stenosed segments and may avoid the need for major surgery.

Atherosclerosis and aneurysm formation

Atherosclerosis is frequently present in the aorta but seldom affects its function. It may, however, be responsible for aneurysms of any part of this vessel. An aneurysm of the arch of the aorta may produce hoarseness from pressure on the left recurrent laryngeal nerve. Aneurysms of the abdominal aorta cause abdominal pain, backache and a pulsatile mass; their rupture leads usually to sudden death. The results of elective resection and replacement with a prosthesis are improving.

Dissecting aneurysm of the aorta. In this condition a tear occurs through the intima secondary to degeneration of the media. As a result blood makes its way in a split in the media to form a new channel. Death usually occurs from rupture through the adventitia into the pericardium, pleural cavity or elsewhere. Most patients have been hypertensive. There is an increased risk of aortic dissection in pregnancy and in patients with *Marfan's syndrome*, a connective tissue disorder characterised by long, thin extremities, a high arched palate and subluxation of the lens.

The onset of dissection is sudden with severe, tearing, chest pain which often radiates into the neck, abdomen, legs or back of the chest. It may be precipitated by exertion and may simulate or include myocardial infarction. Neurological features may result from occlusion of branches of the aorta supplying the spinal cord. One or more of the peripheral pulses may be obliterated.

Diagnosis is suggested by the sudden onset of the characteristic pain and the absence of the ECG and enzyme abnormalities of myocardial infarction unless the dissection includes a coronary artery. The chest radiograph may be helpful in showing a broadened mediastinum due to widening of the aorta. CT scanning or aortography is required for precise assessment.

In the initial stages the blood pressure, if high, should be lowered by antihypertensive drugs to normal levels. Surgical treatment is usually necessary for dissecting aneurysms affecting the ascending aorta or aortic arch. Dissecting aneurysms confined to the descending aorta can often be managed medically.

Sudden occlusion of a major artery

This is usually due to embolism from the heart as a result of rheumatic heart disease, myocardial infarction or, rarely, an atrial myxoma. Emboli lodge commonly at the aortic, iliac or popliteal bifurcations. The limb becomes painful, cold, numb and pale, and pulses distal to the block are absent. Surgical embolectomy should be considered without delay. A Fogarty balloon catheter is used to extract the embolus through a small arteriotomy, and the procedure is often performed under local anaesthesia. While preparations for surgery are being made, pain should be relieved and the limb kept at rest and at room temperature.

INFLAMMATORY ARTERIAL DISEASE

The principal types of inflammatory arterial disease are syphilitic aortitis, polyarteritis nodosa, thromboangiitis obliterans, cranial (giant cell) arteritis and Takayasu disease (pulseless disease). Arteritis may involve the kidneys (p. 391), connective tissues (p. 558) or brain (p. 631).

Syphilitic aortitis is now very rare in Britain. There is often a latent period of 15 to 20 years following an infection before clinical manifestations are evident in the cardiovascular system. Neurosyphilis sometimes coexists.

The disease begins just above the aortic valve cusps. Elastic tissue is gradually replaced by fibrous tissue and this leads to dilatation and aneurysm of the aorta. Proliferation of the intima occurs and may involve the mouths of the coronary arteries leading to myocardial ischaemia, or spread along the valve cusps which become thickened, everted and incompetent.

The diagnosis is difficult in the early uncomplicated stages. Suspicion may be aroused by an aortic systolic murmur, together with accentuation of the second sound. Later there is the characteristic diastolic murmur of aortic regurgitation. Dilatation and calcification of the ascending aorta may be demonstrated by radiological examination. The diagnosis is confirmed by serological tests (p. 416).

If adequate antisyphilitic therapy is given in the early stages of the infection cardiovascular manifestations in later life are prevented. Treatment of syphilitic aortitis consists of a course of procaine penicillin (p. 417). If cardiac failure is present this should first be controlled. Surgical treatment may be indicated for aortic regurgitation or aneurysm.

Thromboangiitis obliterans (*Buerger's disease*) is an uncommon condition of obscure origin. It usually begins before the age of 40 and is almost confined to males who smoke cigarettes heavily. The wall of the artery is infiltrated with polymorphs and the lumen may be obstructed by thrombus. The adjacent vein is often involved.

The symptoms and signs are essentially those of diminished blood supply to the limbs, especially the legs; persistent pain in a cold, cyanosed toe is often the presenting complaint. This is followed by intermittent claudication and rest pain and finally gangrene may develop. Involvement of the veins may cause recurrent thrombophlebitis.

There is no specific treatment but it is essential that cigarette smoking is stopped.

Polyarteritis nodosa is an uncommon condition most often seen in men between the ages of 20 and 50 and thought to have an immunological basis. The characteristic lesions consist of multiple nodules on the smaller arteries. The vessel wall is infiltrated by polymorphs and necrosis follows with resultant aneurysmal dilatation. Thrombosis may occur.

Clinical features such as fever, tachycardia, wasting, sweating and generalised pain are accompanied by local manifestations of ischaemia in various parts of the body. The vessels of the kidney, gastrointestinal tract, heart, peripheral nerves and skin are particularly affected giving rise to such varied manifestations as haematuria, abdominal pain, angina, myocardial infarction, pericarditis, peripheral neuropathy, subcutaneous nodules or ulcers. Involvement of the lungs may cause asthma. There may be leucocytosis or eosinophilia. Hypertension is common.

The course is usually progressive although mild cases may recover. There is no curative treatment, but corticosteroids, administered before vascular damage is extensive, may produce a remission.

Cranial or giant cell arteritis is a panarteritis of medium-sized vessels affecting elderly persons. The disease may be immunologically determined; it is related to polymyalgia rheumatica (p. 578).

The vessel wall is infiltrated by mononuclear cells, plasma cells and giant cells. Thrombosis may occur. The temporal arteries are usually affected and may be thickened and tender. Other arteries may also be involved, notably the ophthalmic and cerebral.

Intense headache is usual and blindness may occur. Other manifestations include fever, pain and stiffness of hips and shoulders, weakness and loss of weight. Spontaneous recovery usually occurs after several months but cranial arteritis responds promptly to prednisolone; at least 50 mg daily should be given initially because of the risk of blindness; the dose is then reduced to the minimum for control of symptoms.

Takayasu disease, known also as *pulseless disease* and the *aortic arch syndrome*, is rare except in some communities, e.g. Japan. It predominantly affects young females. An arteritis, probably of immunological origin, involves the aortic arch with narrowing of its major branches. The pulses are diminished or absent in the upper extremities, neck and head. Headache, syncope, visual disturbance and muscular wasting may occur. The prognosis is poor but corticosteroids are sometimes of value.

VASOSPASTIC DISORDERS

Raynaud's disease is the name given to a peripheral vascular disturbance consisting of spasmodic contraction of the digital arteries, which is precipitated by cold, emotion and by other causative factors mentioned below. Primary Raynaud's disease is commonest in young women and is an exaggerated physiological response to cold. Secondary Raynaud's disease or phenomenon occurs in (1) disorders of connective tissue, especially systemic sclerosis, (2) obliterative arterial disease, (3) occupations in which the hands are exposed to vibration, e.g. from pneumatic drills, or (4) occasionally from cold agglutinins and cryoglobulins. In the early, uncomplicated stages there are no pathological changes. Later, obliterative endarteritis may occur and result in thrombosis, ischaemic changes in the skin of the digits and nails, superficial necrosis and finally gangrene.

The disorder is usually bilateral and fingers are more affected than toes. Numbness, tingling and burning are more prominent than pain. Sensitivity to cold may be extreme and disabling. Colour changes usually consist of three phases: pallor, cyanosis and redness. If the limb is bloodless it will be pale. If blood flow is sluggish, excessive deoxygenation results in cyanosis. Redness is in some cases due to reactive hyperaemia which may follow the vasospasm.

Any primary disease should be treated and protection from cold is obviously indicated. Cigarette smoking should be stopped. Nifedipine (p. 166) may be helpful.

VENOUS THROMBOSIS

A distinction may be made between *thrombophlebitis* when the endothelium is injured by inflammation, and *phlebothrombosis* when thrombosis is the primary disturbance. The latter is the more common condition and carries a much greater risk of pulmonary embolism.

Aetiology. The following factors are of importance:

1. *Slowing or obstruction of the blood stream.* This may result from rest in bed, particularly if a pillow is placed under the knees, especially in the elderly or from unduly prolonged sitting, e.g. in journeys by air. Cardiac failure also leads to slowing of the circulation.

2. *Injury to the vein.* This may be due to trauma and may follow accidents, operations, childbirth, intravenous infusions or injections.

3. *Increased coagulability of the blood.* Many factors may disturb the dynamic equilibrium which normally exists between coagulation and fibrinolysis, notably an increase in platelet adhesiveness. This may occur for example in malignant disease or with the use of oral contraceptives. An increased liability to thrombosis also occurs in dehydration and polycythaemia due to an increase in the blood viscosity.

Pathology. At first the thrombus consists mainly of dense layers of platelets and fibrin; later it is a loose, friable, jelly-like mass of fibrin and red cells which readily becomes detached to form an embolus. After a few days inflammatory changes occur in the wall of the vein. The thrombus may undergo lysis or organisation.

Venous thrombosis is most common in the lower limbs, particularly in the venous sinuses of the soleus muscle in the calf and in the femoral and iliac veins. It is much less frequent in the upper limb but the axillary vein may be involved as a complication of trauma, neoplasm or radiotherapy. Superficial thrombophlebitis most commonly occurs in the saphenous vein, particularly if there are associated varicosities.

Suppurative thrombophlebitis is a rare but very serious condition usually involving the veins of the pelvis following sepsis.

Tropical phlebitis is described on page 718.

Clinical features. The patient may complain of pain in the calf but the process is often silent and undiagnosed. An unexplained slight pyrexia may be the only warning. If the lumen of a main vein is occluded, there is dilatation of the superficial veins, the skin may be warm and pink and there may be oedema at the ankle. In extensive occlusive iliofemoral thrombosis the whole lower limb is swollen and white if the collateral channels remain patent. If the collaterals are also occluded, the leg is blue—a pregangrenous condition. In contrast there are frequently no signs in the presence of an extensive non-occlusive, potentially lethal thrombus. Pulmonary embolism is often the first clinical manifestation of venous thrombosis.

Investigation. The veins from the ankle to the inguinal ligament can be demonstrated by ascending lower limb phlebography. Percutaneous iliofemoral phlebography may also be required. Phlebography may precipitate venous thrombosis, and heparin should be given before it is undertaken. Ultrasound is used to assess the patency of deep veins in patients who present with a swollen leg or with pulmonary embolism. The uptake of ^{123}I-labelled fibrinogen is used for the early detection of thrombosis, for example postoperatively; it has the advantage of being non-invasive but is less reliable than phlebography, particularly for the detection of thrombosis in the pelvic and common femoral veins.

Treatment aims at preventing the propagation of thrombus and pulmonary embolism, damage to the valves of the vein and chronic venous insufficiency. Unless there is an obvious contraindication, such as active peptic ulceration or a bleeding surface as after prostatectomy, treatment is initiated with heparin and continued with warfarin (p. 550). Thrombolysis with streptokinase (p. 171) can be considered for iliofemoral thrombosis. Thrombectomy may occasionally be required for a recent non-occlusive thrombosis at this site.

The legs should be elevated to 15 degrees and physiotherapy commenced after 48 hours. Straining at stool often causes separation of venous thrombi and should be avoided. The venous flow is accelerated by the support of graduated elastic hose but care must be taken to avoid a constricting effect by the hose rolling up. The ambulant woman should wear elastic support tights and for men knee-length elastic hose is best. Support of this kind will probably be necessary permanently after a severe thrombosis to control chronic venous insufficiency. Superficial thrombophlebitis usually responds to an elastic support and a non-steroidal anti-inflammatory drug (p. 560).

Prevention. Efforts must chiefly be directed to the avoidance of venous stasis. This is easiest in surgical patients when the period of risk can be defined. Almost all postoperative thromboses begin during, or within 72 hours of, operation. Early ambulation should be encouraged after surgery and medical illnesses. This means more than simply transferring the patient from lying in bed to sitting in a chair. Active exercises should be prescribed and at other times the leg should be elevated. A graduated elastic support should be worn if the patient is at particular risk. If confinement to bed is unavoidable, the patient should be encouraged to move the lower limbs frequently. In hospital, exercises can be organised under the supervision of a physiotherapist. Faulty posture in bed must be corrected, constricting bandages avoided and cardiac failure and dehy-

dration should receive attention.

For patients at particular risk other prophylactic measures include low dose subcutaneous heparin or intravenous dextran 70.

PROSPECTS IN CARDIOLOGY

One of the fascinations of medicine is the way in which new ideas and techniques suddenly bear fruit in fields which have remained relatively fallow for some years. There has been a striking expansion of interest in coronary thrombolysis, and a number of new thrombolytic agents such as human tissue type plasminogen activator, acylated plasminogen streptokinase complex and pro-urokinase are now under investigation. Angiotensin converting enzyme inhibitors have been a major advance in the treatment of both hypertension and cardiac failure, and orally-effective dopamine analogues may hold similar promise in cardiac failure. Better understanding of renal physiology may be bringing nearer a fundamental understanding of hypertension. Advances in molecular genetics may elucidate the heredity and mechanism of atheroma and cardiomyopathy, and will have implications for genetic counselling and possible antenatal diagnosis.

It is salutary also to consider some retreats and reverses. We still do not have an ideal artificial heart valve, we are still arguing over the primary prevention of ischaemic heart disease, mortality from infective endocarditis is too high, and trials of platelet anti-aggregant drugs have, with a couple of striking exceptions, been disappointing. A major trial of antihypertensive therapy in mild to moderate hypertension has shown less benefit than some of us had hoped, and the increasing cost of mounting large-scale clinical trials is a worrying feature.

D.G. JULIAN

D.P. DE BONO

FURTHER READING:

De Bono D 1986 Examination of the cardiovascular system. In: Macleod J, Munro J (eds) Clinical examination, 7th edn. Churchill Livingstone, Edinburgh
Julian D G 1987 Cardiology, 5th edn. Baillière Tindall, London. An introduction to cardiology for the non-specialist

Braunwald E 1984 Heart disease: a textbook of cardiovascular medicine. Saunders, Philadelphia. A detailed and comprehensive textbook

Bradley R D 1977 Studies in acute heart failure. Arnold, London. An elegant discussion of the application of physiological principles to the management of heart failure

Levy R I 1985 Cholesterol and cardiovascular disease. Circulation 72: 686–691. See next paper

Oliver M F 1986 Prevention of coronary heart disease. Circulation 73: 1–9. This and the preceding paper provide up-to-date perspectives, from very different points of view, on the prevention of ischaemic heart disease

Report of a Working Party of the British Society for Antimicrobial Chemotherapy 1985 Antibiotic treatment of streptococcal and staphylococcal endocarditis. Lancet 2: 815–817

Many advances in cardiology are well described in original articles or editorials in general medical journals such as the Lancet or New England Journal of Medicine. More specialised journals include the British Heart Journal and Circulation

8

Diseases of the respiratory system

Knowledge of the normal anatomy and processes of respiration is essential in the understanding of the effects of disease on the airways and lungs, and is of great importance in the comprehension of investigation and treatment.

ANATOMY

The *upper respiratory tract*, which includes the nose, nasopharynx and larynx, is lined by vascular mucous membrane. The rich blood supply ensures that the inspired air enters the lungs at body temperature and fully saturated with water vapour. The whole respiratory epithelium down to the terminal bronchioles is ciliated. The cilia, and the thin film of mucus covering them, have the important function of trapping foreign particles including bacteria, and propelling them towards the pharynx. They contribute to the prevention of respiratory infection, as do the alveolar macrophages by means of their secretory, phagocytic and bactericidal activity.

The *nasal sinuses* (maxillary, frontal, ethmoidal and sphenoidal) drain into the nose by narrow openings which are frequently blocked in upper respiratory infections.

The *larynx*, in addition to being the organ of voice production, has the function of preventing nasal secretions, food, vomitus, foreign bodies, etc. from reaching the lower respiratory tract. The larynx, like the large bronchi, is supplied with vagal receptors, which form the sensory side of the cough reflex and perhaps also of reflexes concerned with bronchoconstriction.

The *trachea* begins at the cricoid cartilage and ends at the level of the sternal angle by bifurcation into the two main bronchi. The trachea is usually palpable in the suprasternal notch, where in normal subjects it is in the midline. Deviation of the trachea to either side, in the absence of a local lesion in the neck, is a valuable indication of displacement of the upper mediastinum.

Of the *main bronchi*, the right is more vertical than the left, with the result that a foreign body entering the trachea is more likely to lodge in that bronchus or one of its divisions than the left.

The lobar bronchi (Fig. 8.1) divide and subdivide like the branches of a tree (the term 'bronchial tree' is in common use) until the terminal bronchioles are reached. The portion of lung supplied by a terminal bronchiole is called an acinus, which is the basic functional unit of lung tissue. Each acinus contains branching respiratory bronchioles communicating with clusters of alveoli. The alveoli are lined by a single layer of flattened epithelial cells (Type I pneumocytes) which are in direct contact with the pulmonary capillaries. Exchange of the respiratory gases, oxygen and carbon dioxide, takes place between the air in the alveoli and the blood in the pulmonary capillaries. Pulmonary surfactant, a phospholipid which by reducing surface tension prevents alveolar collapse, is secreted by Type II granular pneumocytes.

The fissures, lobes and segments of the lung are shown in Figure 8.1.

In many diseases, e.g. pneumococcal pneumonia, collapse and lung abscess, the lesion is

MAJOR BRONCHIAL SUBDIVISIONS

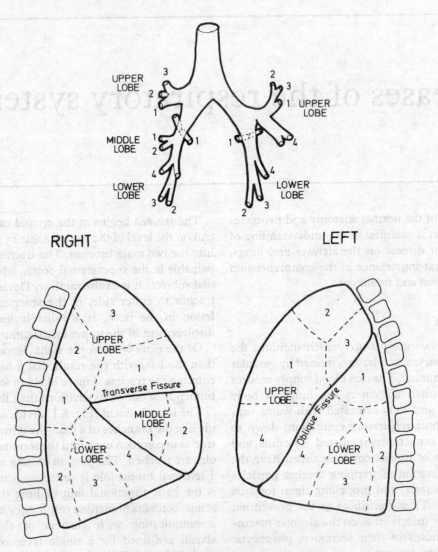

LATERAL ASPECTS OF LUNGS

Fig. 8.1 The major bronchial divisions and the fissures, lobes and segments of the lungs. The position of the oblique fissure is such that the left upper lobe is largely anterior to the lower lobe. On the right side the transverse fissure separates the upper from the anteriorly placed middle lobe which is matched by the lingular segment on the left side. The site of the lobe determines whether physical signs are mainly anterior or posterior. Each lobe is composed of two or more bronchopulmonary segments, i.e. the lung tissue supplied by the main branches of each lobar bronchus.
BRONCHOPULMONARY SEGMENTS: Right *Upper lobe* 1. Anterior 2. Posterior 3. Apical. *Middle lobe* 1. Lateral 2. Medial. *Lower lobe* 1. Apical 2. Posterior basal 3. Lateral basal 4. Anterior basal 5. Medial basal. **Left** *Upper lobe* 1. Anterior 2. Apical 3. Posterior 4. Lingular. *Lower lobe* 1. Apical 2. Posterior basal 3. Lateral basal 4. Anterior basal.

typically confined to a single lobe or segment. A knowledge of pulmonary anatomy, when applied to the interpretation of radiographs, is thus of value in determining the nature of the lesion as well as its situation.

Pleura. Each lung is closely invested with visceral pleura. Parietal pleura lines the chest wall, mediastinum and diaphragm, and is continuous with the visceral pleura at the pulmonary hilum. In health the two pleural layers are separated only by a thin film of liquid, and are kept in apposition by negative (subatmospheric) pressure. This results from the natural tendency of the lung to recoil towards the hilum, because of its inherent elastic properties.

If a communication develops with the atmosphere as, for example, with a penetrating wound of the chest wall or from spontaneous rupture of an emphysematous bulla, the negative pressure draws air between the pleural layers and the potential space becomes a real one. There is then said to be a *pneumothorax*. When the space is created by the presence of serous fluid there is said to be a pleural effusion or a hydrothorax — by pus, an empyema; by blood, a haemothorax; by both serous fluid and air, a hydropneumothorax; by both pus and air, a pyopneumothorax; and by both blood and air, a haemopneumothorax.

When the pleural space contains large amounts of air or fluid the elastic recoil of the underlying lung causes the lung to shrink towards the hilum. Impairment of function is dependent upon the degree of pulmonary collapse. If the quantity of air or fluid is very large it causes displacement of the mediastinum towards the opposite side, with the result that function of the opposite lung is also impaired. A gross degree of mediastinal displacement may, in addition, embarrass the action of the heart. Mediastinal displacement is recognised clinically by alteration in position of the trachea and of the cardiac apex beat.

Collapse of the lung, referred to as absorption collapse, also occurs, without air or fluid in the pleural space, as a result of bronchial obstruction.

The anatomy of the *mediastinum* has an important bearing on the diagnosis of intrathoracic disease, particularly tumours which often involve mediastinal structures, producing readily recognisable symptoms, physical signs and radiological abnormalities (p. 255).

PHYSIOLOGY

The aspects of the physiology of respiration which merit special attention are:

1. *Ventilation*, which includes (a) the mechanical processes of inspiration and expiration and (b) the control of ventilation at a level appropriate to metabolic needs.

2. *Perfusion* of the lungs by the output of the right ventricle.

3. *Distribution* of ventilation and perfusion within the lungs.

4. *Diffusion* of oxygen and carbon dioxide, which occurs both within the terminal airways and alveoli, and also between the alveoli and the pulmonary capillary blood.

In a typical adult at rest the pulmonary blood flow of about 5 l/min carries 11 mmol/min (250 ml/min) of oxygen from the lungs to the tissues and ventilation of about 6 l/min carries 9 mmol/min (200 ml/min) of carbon dioxide out of the body. The pressures of oxygen and carbon dioxide in the arterial blood are closely controlled. The normal range of PaO_2 is 11–13 kPa (83–98 mmHg) and of $PaCO_2$ 4.8–6.0 kPa (36–45 mmHg). Observation of changes in these pressures in disease is of importance in assessing the nature and severity of any disturbance of lung function (p. 204).

Ventilation

The respiratory muscles, in ventilating the lungs, work against resistance of two kinds, elastic and non-elastic. The first is performed against elastic forces in the lungs and chest wall which together tend to bring the chest to the position it occupies at the end of a normal expiration. Work resulting in chest expansion from this position of equilibrium results in the storage of kinetic energy which is then used to return the chest to the resting position. This second kind of work is largely expended in overcoming the resistance of the airways to the inspiratory and expiratory flow of air and to a smaller extent in displacing soft and inelastic tissues. Most of the resistance in normal subjects lies in the large central airways. The peripheral airways, though individually smaller in calibre, contribute less to total resistance because of their large combined cross-sectional area.

During quiet breathing inspiration is 'active' and expiration 'passive'. Inspiration against abnormal resistance (whether elastic or non-elastic) may bring accessory muscles such as the sternomastoids and scaleni into play; expiration, if forced or performed against abnormal resistance, is accomplished with the aid of the accessory muscles of expiration, chiefly those of the abdominal wall.

Elastic work is increased when the lungs are made more rigid (less compliant) by pulmonary oedema or fibrosis or when the chest wall is made more unyielding, e.g. by ankylosing spondylitis. Rapid shallow breathing is often observed in these conditions. Work against non-elastic resistance is increased by rapid breathing and by conditions causing airflow obstruction such as asthma, chronic bronchitis, emphysema and tumours of major bronchi.

The metabolic cost of breathing is normally low: an increase in ventilation of 1 l/min raises oxygen uptake by about 45 μmol/min (1 ml/min) at most. In disease, this figure may rise to as much as 450 μmol (10 ml) oxygen per min per l/min increase in ventilation. Under such circumstances breathing accounts for an important fraction of the total metabolic oxygen uptake.

Not all of the inspired air takes part in gas exchange in the lungs. Some of each breath ventilates the conducting airways (down to the respiratory bronchioles), which constitute the 'anatomical' dead space; also because of maldistribution (see below) some of each breath is wasted in ventilating underperfused parts of the lungs. The proportion of wasted ventilation in each breath (physiological dead space : tidal volume ratio, Vd/Vt) is normally one-fifth to one-third, but may be much increased, sometimes to as much as two-thirds, in disease. The volume which remains takes part in gas exchange and provides *alveolar ventilation*, which is normally about 5 l/min at rest. It follows that if the proportion of wasted ventilation is greater than normal a greater total ventilation is needed to achieve normal alveolar ventilation.

Normally, alveolar ventilation is closely matched to the excretion of carbon dioxide and this matching is reflected in a normal level of arterial PCO_2. If alveolar ventilation is reduced in proportion to carbon dioxide excretion, the arterial PCO_2 rises (hypercapnia), and if alveolar ventilation becomes excessive, the arterial PCO_2

falls (hypocapnia). Indeed, the arterial PCO_2 reflects alveolar ventilation and the production of carbon dioxide just as the blood urea concentration reflects renal urea clearance and the metabolic production of urea.

Generalised alveolar underventilation is most commonly found as a late result of chronic bronchitis and emphysema. It also occurs if respiration is centrally depressed by narcotics, anaesthetics or intracranial disease. It may ensue when the respiratory muscles are paralysed, when gross deformity of the chest wall limits thoracic or diaphragmatic movement or in some cases of gross obesity. Lowering of the arterial PO_2 (hypoxaemia) is an inevitable result of alveolar underventilation when air is breathed. Giving oxygen will correct this, but hypercapnia is corrected only when alveolar ventilation is improved.

Alveolar overventilation occurs in asthma of mild or moderate severity, in interstitial lung disease, in pulmonary vascular disease (e.g. pulmonary thromboembolic disease), in salicylate overdosage, as a result of upper brain stem lesions, or from anxiety or hysteria. It is also a prominent manifestation of metabolic acidosis.

Control of breathing. Rhythmical discharges originating in the reticular substance of the brain stem provide the basis for co-ordinated respiratory movements; it is convenient to use the term 'respiratory centre' for the neurones involved in breathing, but the distribution and organisation of these neurones is highly complex. From the respiratory centre, impulses reach the spinal motor neurones by the reticulospinal tracts, in contrast to impulses mediating conscious changes in breathing, which travel via the corticospinal tracts. Normal breathing is modified by afferent impulses from many sources, which are best considered in two groups:

1. Those arising within the central nervous system and from receptors other than chemoreceptors ('neural stimuli').

2. Those arising from chemoreceptors sensitive to the composition of blood or cerebrospinal fluid ('chemical stimuli').

Afferent impulses of the first group mediate (a) the changes in rate and depth of breathing which may be consciously maintained for short periods, (b) the central neurogenic overventilation which occurs in certain lesions of the upper brain stem, (c) the respiratory depression associated with medullary compression and (d) the respiratory stimulation which originates in limb receptors, as in exercise. These impulses may also arise from receptors in muscles and joints in the chest wall, and from pulmonary receptors sensitive to stretch, bronchial irritation or pulmonary capillary distension. Pulmonary inflation and deflation (Hering-Breuer) reflexes are present in the newborn, but are weak in adults except under general anaesthesia.

The second group of afferent impulses arises in chemosensitive cells located in the carotid and aortic bodies (peripheral chemoreceptors) and intracranially (central chemoreceptors). In animals central chemosensitive areas are located on the ventrolateral surface of the medulla, but in man their situation is uncertain.

Ventilation is increased when the peripheral chemoreceptors are stimulated by arterial hypoxia; at rest, the stimulus is not strong unless arterial PO_2 is below 8 kPa (60 mmHg), and becomes powerful at about 4 kPa (30 mmHg). The peripheral chemoreceptors are also stimulated by an increase in the hydrogen ion concentration of arterial blood. Central chemoreceptors are stimulated by an increase in the hydrogen ion concentration of cerebrospinal fluid (CSF). A rise in PCO_2 of the arterial blood is accompanied by increasing acidity of both blood and CSF and therefore stimulates both central and peripheral chemoreceptors. For this reason, inhalation of carbon dioxide is one of the strongest known respiratory stimulants. In the presence of mild or moderate hypoxia its effect is increased, but severe hypoxia acts as a central depressant. Pyrexia increases the sensitivity of the respiratory centre; all sedatives, particularly opiates, depress it.

In some patients with chronic bronchitis the normal sensitivity to increased arterial PCO_2 is greatly reduced. In such patients chronic alveolar underventilation may occur and relief of the concurrent hypoxaemia may, by removing one of the remaining stimuli to breathing, be followed by worsening of the hypercapnia.

Distribution of gas and blood in the lungs

Gas exchange in the lungs is inefficient unless alveolar ventilation is distributed uniformly to different parts of the lungs and is matched by uniform distribution of blood flow. The composition of blood leaving an individual alveolus depends on the composition of the mixed venous blood entering the pulmonary capillaries and the ratio between the ventilation of and blood flow around the alveolus. The possible values of this ventilation:perfusion ratio ($\dot{V}A/\dot{Q}$) lie between infinity (ventilation but no perfusion) and zero (perfusion but no ventilation). Thus areas of lung with $\dot{V}A/\dot{Q} = \infty$ behave as dead space, giving rise to wasted ventilation, while areas with $\dot{V}A/\dot{Q} = 0$ behave as a physiological right-to-left shunt or venous admixture effect, giving rise to wasted perfusion.

The possible range of alveolar ventilation:perfusion ratios is so large that it has become conventional to treat the lungs as if they were made up of three compartments:

1. A compartment ventilated and perfused normally.

2. Physiological dead space, contributed to by all alveoli whose $\dot{V}A/\dot{Q}$ exceeds unity, and including the anatomical dead space.

3. Physiological shunt, contributed to by all alveoli with $\dot{V}A/\dot{Q}$ less than unity, and including the small anatomical or 'true' right-to-left shunts through such pathways as bronchial-pulmonary venous anastomoses.

It follows that if the range of ventilation:perfusion ratios found in the lungs is wider than normal the physiological dead space and physiological shunt will be larger than normal and gas exchange will become less efficient.

Even in the normal lung, distribution of ventilation and perfusion is imperfect. In the erect posture, gravity affects distribution of both ventilation and blood flow, causing $\dot{V}A/\dot{Q}$ to be increased at the apices and reduced at the bases of the lungs. In most forms of lung disease, distribution of ventilation and perfusion is further impaired, and it is easy to visualise how pathological mechanisms may have this effect. For example, distribution of ventilation may be impaired by

1. Bronchial or bronchiolar obstruction (tumour, secretions, mucosal oedema, bronchoconstriction).

2. Destruction of elastic tissue (as in emphysema).

3. Pulmonary collapse, consolidation, fibrosis or oedema.

4. Chest wall deformities.

Blood flow is reduced or abolished by pulmonary embolism or thrombosis or by obliteration of areas of the pulmonary capillary bed by necrosis or fibrosis.

Maldistribution, with areas of low $\dot{V}A/\dot{Q}$ ratio, is the most important single cause of hypoxaemia in disease, and is found in a wide variety of conditions. Fortunately, administration of oxygen raises the alveolar PO_2, even in poorly ventilated alveoli, and corrects the hypoxaemia, but oxygen therapy has some dangers (p. 210).

Diffusion of gases in the lungs

Oxygen and carbon dioxide move by molecular diffusion in the gas phase along the terminal airways and alveoli, and are also exchanged across the alveolar membrane by diffusion in the liquid phase from a site of higher to one of lower partial pressure. It might be expected that if the alveolar wall became thickened, as in interstitial lung disease, diffusion of gases, particularly of oxygen, would be impaired. However, most conditions which might be expected to have this effect can also give rise to maldistribution of ventilation and perfusion, and analysis suggests that this is usually the chief cause of hypoxaemia in these conditions.

If the area available for gas exchange is reduced (e.g. in emphysema) or if, because of maldistribution, the effective area is reduced, the ability of the lung to transfer gases will also diminish. Such a reduction may not be significant at rest, but may limit the amount of oxygen which can be taken up during exercise and may become a cause of hypoxaemia under these circumstances.

The overall ability of the lung to transfer gases can be readily measured by relating the uptake of carbon monoxide to the alveolar CO pressure when a low concentration of the gas is breathed. By this method, values for *gas transfer factor* or *diffusing capacity* are obtained.

COMMON MANIFESTATIONS OF RESPIRATORY DISEASE

Cough. This is the most frequent of all respiratory symptoms. It may be short, painful and half-suppressed, as when pleurisy accompanies pneumonia, loose and readily productive of sputum, as in bronchiectasis, or paroxysmal, ineffectual and exhausting, as in some cases of chronic bronchitis and asthma. In bronchial carcinoma it is usually an early symptom but may be relatively late in pulmonary tuberculosis. Generally it is worse at night or on waking and often is aggravated by changes in temperature or humidity. The explosive character of a normal cough is lost when laryngeal paralysis is present ('bovine cough'). It is accompanied by stridor (p. 204) in whooping cough and in the presence of partial obstruction of the larynx or trachea.

Sputum. Purulent sputum is usually due to bacterial infection in the respiratory tract and is typically seen in acute bronchitis, infective exacerbations of chronic bronchitis, bacterial pneumonia and lung abscess. In the last condition the sputum may be copious and is sometimes fetid. Sputum containing large numbers of eosinophils has the same macroscopic appearance as sputum in which there are many polymorphonuclear leucocytes. Mucoid sputum is due to oversecretion of bronchial mucus. It is frequently present in chronic bronchitis and bronchial asthma. In early cases of pulmonary tuberculosis the sputum is mucoid but in advanced cases it is usually purulent.

Haemoptysis. All grades of severity may occur, from slight streaking of sputum with blood to a massive haemorrhage. Although it is a common symptom in acute and chronic bronchitis, bleeding from the lower respiratory tract, however slight, must be regarded as of potentially serious significance demanding full investigation. Bronchial carcinoma, pulmonary infarction, bronchiectasis, pulmonary tuberculosis and mitral stenosis are its main causes.

Chest pain. There are four types of chest pain associated with respiratory disease:

1. Central retrosternal pain of a tearing character made worse by coughing, usually caused by inflammation of the trachea.

2. Central chest discomfort caused by rapidly enlarging mediastinal tumours.

3. Constant pain, unrelated to breathing, resulting from direct invasion of the chest wall by a malignant tumour, metastatic deposits in ribs

or vertebral metastatic deposits compressing or invading intercostal nerve roots.

4. Unilateral chest pain of a sharp stabbing character, made worse by deep breathing and coughing, and caused by inflammation of the pleura—pleural pain. Rib fracture causes a similar pain.

Pleural pain is thought to be due to stretching of the inflamed parietal pleura (the visceral pleura is insensitive to painful stimuli) and is maximal towards the end of inspiration. Patients try to minimise pleural pain by taking shallow breaths and by suppressing cough as much as possible.

The pain is referred to the area of skin supplied by the same spinal nerves as those from the inflamed area of pleura. Usually it is referred to the chest wall, but, when the pleura lining the diaphragm is affected, pain may be felt in the cutaneous distribution of the supraclavicular nerves which have the same spinal roots (C 3 and 4) as the phrenic nerve. Pain in the front and top of the shoulder is thus often a feature of diaphragmatic pleurisy. Pleural pain may also be referred to the anterior abdominal wall, where it may be difficult to distinguish from the pain of an abdominal emergency.

Pleural friction, which is a common physical sign in pleurisy, is due to the rubbing together of pleural surfaces roughened by fibrinous exudate. The effusion of fluid between the layers of the pleura diminishes pain and abolishes the pleural rub by separating the pleural surfaces.

Dyspnoea. It has been said that breathing is the only involuntary act which is carried out by voluntary muscle, and this is normally so. Dyspnoea is a subjective sensation in which the effort of breathing reaches consciousness, usually under circumstances in which a normal person would not be aware of it. Dyspnoea should be distinguished from *hyperpnoea*, where the volume of ventilation is increased, but no abnormal sensation is felt, and *tachypnoea*, an excessive respiratory rate.

Dyspnoea is a symptom of a wide variety of diseases, and no single theory can adequately explain why it occurs. In conditions where resistance to airflow is high, such as asthma or chronic bronchitis, the increased mechanical work needed to achieve a given volume of ventilation may account for it. A similar explanation may be given for dyspnoea in diseases causing lung stiffness, such as fibrosing alveolitis, with the added factor that the hypoxaemia which occurs readily during exercise in such diseases may still further increase the drive to breathe. This explanation is less satisfactory for the dyspnoea of heart disease, and still less so for the dyspnoea found in anaemia, where both the lungs and the arterial oxygen pressure are normal. Stimulation of certain receptors in the lungs (e.g. J receptors) may play a role in the generation of dyspnoea in many conditions.

In mild heart or lung disease, dyspnoea is noticeable only on effort, and the presence of dyspnoea at rest is an indication that the disease is severe or advanced. In conditions such as chronic bronchitis, much of the respiratory reserve may have been lost before a sedentary patient complains of dyspnoea, but measurements of ventilatory capacity will confirm that severe airflow obstruction is already established. Complaints of dyspnoea should therefore be taken seriously, for although the symptom is commonly found in anxiety states, it also may occur early in diseases such as pulmonary thromboembolism or allergic alveolitis at a stage when abnormalities may not be apparent clinically or radiologically. Tests of pulmonary function and objective assessment of exercise capacity are then of value.

Apnoea and sleep apnoea. Apnoea (cessation of breathing) can be voluntary (breath-holding) or a manifestation of disease. Recurring periods of apnoea are a feature of *Cheyne-Stokes respiration* (p. 119) which is seen in severe cardiac failure and certain neurological disorders involving the brain stem. Occasional periods of cessation of breathing, lasting for 10 seconds or more, can occur during sleep in healthy individuals. The term *sleep apnoea syndrome* is used when patients have frequent episodes of apnoea during sleep. These can be of two types: *obstructive sleep apnoea*, the more common, associated with loud snoring, and caused by transient total obstruction to ubreathing in the upper air passages, and *central sleep apnoea* due to transient failure of respiratory drive.

In severe chronic bronchitis periods of disordered breathing during sleep, with associated falls in arterial oxygen saturation, usually are due to profound hypoventilation rather than true apnoea.

Wheeze. In all diseases causing airflow obstruction, particularly bronchial asthma, wheeze is usually a conspicuous symptom. It is a musical sound heard best during expiration, and is associated with numerous rhonchi on auscultation. *Stridor*, on the other hand, occurs when one of the major airways (larynx, trachea or main bronchus) is almost completely obstructed. It is a crowing sound heard best during inspiration, especially after coughing, and is associated with a persistent low-pitched rhonchus audible all over the chest.

Hypoxaemia is present if either the pressure or content of oxygen in arterial blood is reduced, and if severe enough may result in visible central cyanosis. The normal arterial PO_2 is over 12 kPa (90 mmHg) at the age of 20, and falls to around 11 kPa (82 mmHg) at 60. Above this age a further fall in PO_2 of up to 1.3 kPa (10 mmHg) may occur on recumbency because of closure of airways in the dependent regions of the lungs.

The most frequent and important cause of hypoxaemia in respiratory disease is the presence in the lungs of areas where the distribution of ventilation and perfusion is disturbed and where ventilation is low in relation to perfusion. Hypoxaemia also inevitably results from alveolar underventilation (because alveolar and arterial PCO_2 are increased and a rise in the partial pressure of one gas inevitably results in a fall of the others) or if an atmosphere poor in oxygen is breathed, as at high altitudes. Impairment of diffusion across the alveolar wall may cause hypoxaemia during exercise, but is hardly ever an important factor at rest. The hypoxaemia due to all these causes is reversed by giving oxygen.

Hypoxaemia due to congenital heart disease or vascular anomalies, with shunting of blood from the right to the left of the circulation past the lungs, cannot be entirely reversed by oxygen. Hypoxaemia also occurs if the oxygen capacity of the blood is reduced, as in anaemia or carbon monoxide poisoning.

Hypercapnia is present if the pressure of carbon dioxide in the arterial blood ($PaCO_2$) is above the upper limit of normal of 6.0 kPa or 45 mmHg at rest, but values of up to 6.5 kPa (50 mmHg) are seldom of clinical importance. As has been explained, the finding of a raised $PaCO_2$ implies that alveolar ventilation is inadequate in relation to the carbon dioxide production of the body; the causes of hypercapnia are therefore those of alveolar underventilation. Alveoli in which the ventilation:perfusion ratio is low also contribute to hypercapnia.

The finding of hypercapnia implies either that the normal sensitivity of the respiratory centre to carbon dioxide has been reduced, or that mechanical limitation or failure of neuromuscular transmission prevents a normally responsive centre from maintaining adequate alveolar ventilation.

Clinical features suggestive of hypercapnia include peripheral vasodilatation, with warm extremities and bounding pulses, sweating, muscle twitching, flapping tremor, headache, drowsiness, coma, retinal venous distension and, rarely, papilloedema. Unfortunately, none of these signs is specific and the diagnosis must be made by measurement of the pressure of carbon dioxide in arterial blood.

Hypercapnia has three consequences of clinical importance: (1) it aggravates hypoxaemia by lowering the pressure of oxygen in the alveolar gas, (2) when acute, it increases the arterial hydrogen ion concentration (respiratory acidosis), although renal retention of bicarbonate tends to compensate for this over a period of hours or days (p. 372), and (3) when of a severe degree, it induces drowsiness, which may proceed to coma.

Respiratory failure is said to occur when the normal pressures of oxygen and carbon dioxide in the arterial blood are no longer maintained. For practical purposes, this means the finding of either a PaO_2 of less than 8 kPa (60 mmHg) or a $PaCO_2$ of more than 6.5 kPa (50 mmHg).

It follows that two varieties of respiratory failure can be recognised. In Type I respiratory failure the $PaCO_2$ is normal or low, but PaO_2 is reduced. Type II respiratory failure, in which the $PaCO_2$ is elevated and the PaO_2 is reduced, is often termed 'ventilatory failure'. The mechanisms responsible for the hypoxaemia in each type have been discussed above.

The causes of Type I respiratory failure are many, and include any of the pathological causes of maldistribution of ventilation and perfusion in the lungs (p. 200). Among the most important are bronchial asthma, pneumonia, pulmonary oedema, allergic and fibrosing alveolitis and pulmonary thromboembolism.

Adult respiratory distress syndrome (ARDS) is a severe form of Type I respiratory failure caused by non-cardiogenic pulmonary oedema (p. 213).

The most common pulmonary cause of Type II respiratory failure is chronic bronchitis, particularly when complicated by acute respiratory infection. Other causes include respiratory paralysis (p. 644), deformities of the chest such as severe kyphoscoliosis, depression of the respiratory centre, particularly by narcotic or sedative drugs and, in a few patients, gross obesity.

Clubbing of the fingers and toes. The cause of clubbing, which is most readily recognised in the fingers, is not known but it is frequently found in patients with certain types of respiratory disease, notably bronchial carcinoma, chronic intrathoracic suppuration and fibrosing alveolitis.

Clubbing also occurs in certain other conditions. It is present in cyanotic congenital heart disease, sometimes in infective endocarditis, occasionally in Crohn's disease, malabsorption syndrome and cirrhosis of the liver, and rarely in healthy subjects as a familial trait.

The earliest indication of finger clubbing is an abnormal degree of fluctuation at the bases of the nails. With more advanced clubbing there is, in addition, an increase in the curvature of the nails and bulbous swelling of the fingertips.

THE INVESTIGATION OF RESPIRATORY DISEASE

In most respiratory diseases a reasonably accurate diagnosis can be made from the history and physical examination alone, but in several important conditions, notably pulmonary tuberculosis and bronchial carcinoma, these methods are inadequate and the diagnosis can be confirmed or excluded only by more specialised procedures such as radiological, bacteriological or endoscopic examination.

The patient must always be asked about symptoms such as cough, sputum, haemoptysis, pain,

breathlessness, wheeze and nasal discharge. Since some respiratory diseases are related to present or past occupational hazards (p. 257), contact with animals, particularly birds (pp. 219 and 242), or drug treatment (p. 241), a thorough enquiry must be made into these potential causes of respiratory illness.

Physical examination

Before the chest itself is examined a note should be made of the rate and character of breathing, the type and severity of cough and the amount and nature of any sputum. In addition, particular care must be taken to determine whether or not there is cyanosis, clubbing of the fingers or enlargement of the supraclavicular lymph nodes, these features being of special significance in respiratory disease.

The upper respiratory tract should be examined next, with particular regard to nasal discharge or obstruction, postnasal discharge, oral sepsis, and infection of the tonsils.

The chest wall should then be carefully inspected for soft tissue abnormalities such as cutaneous lesions, subcutaneous swellings (including lumps in the breast) and bulging or indrawing of intercostal spaces, and for skeletal abnormalities such as an increase in the anteroposterior diameter of the chest relative to its lateral diameter.

The position of the trachea and of the apex beat should be noted and the chest expansion measured. Chest wall movement, vocal fremitus and the percussion note should be compared in equivalent positions on the two sides. The terms used to describe the various types of percussion note are: hyperresonant, normal, impaired, dull and stony dull.

At auscultation, attention should be directed in turn to the breath sounds, added sounds and vocal resonance.

BREATH SOUNDS. The following terms are used: vesicular, vesicular with prolonged expiration, diminished vesicular, absent breath sounds, and high-pitched and low-pitched bronchial breath sounds.

ADDED SOUNDS. *Rhonchi* (sometimes called

'wheezes') seem to be related to narrowing of the lumen of the bronchi caused by spasm of bronchial muscle, swelling of bronchial mucosa or tenacious mucus adherent to bronchial walls. Rhonchi may be high-pitched, medium-pitched or low-pitched, according to the size of the bronchi in which they originate.

Crepitations ('crackles') usually indicate the presence of secretions within alveoli, bronchi or pulmonary cavities. Loud end-inspiratory crackles, unaltered by coughing, are a feature of interstitial lung disease (p. 256).

Pleural rub is a diagnostic sign of pleurisy. It is a grating or creaking sound, unaltered by coughing, audible during both inspiration and expiration.

VOCAL RESONANCE. The following terms are used: normal, increased, diminished or absent vocal resonance, and whispering pectoriloquy.

The interpretation of physical signs. Certain groups of physical signs are typically associated with various pathological changes in the lungs and pleura. Such changes are not necessarily specific for one particular disease. For example, consolidation may occur in pneumonia or tuberculosis, and fluid may be present in the pleural space in tuberculous pleurisy, empyema, malignant disease or cardiac failure. Each group of physical signs should therefore be interpreted in terms of a physical state rather than any specific disease, the diagnosis of which depends on an analysis of all the clinical and other evidence.

The physical signs of the more common lesions are shown in Table 8.1 (p. 207).

Special methods of investigation

Radiological examination of the chest. Many pulmonary diseases, including bronchial carcinoma and pulmonary tuberculosis, cannot be detected at an early stage without radiological examination of the chest. Facilities for this investigation are now readily available to most doctors, and it should always be undertaken whenever any serious form of intrathoracic disease is suspected. A lateral film may provide additional information about the nature and situation of a pulmonary, pleural or mediastinal abnormality.

Specialised techniques, such as bronchography, fluoroscopy (screening), conventional and computed tomography, radionuclide ventilation and perfusion scanning and pulmonary angiography may be of considerable diagnostic value in selected cases.

It may be very useful to obtain chest radiographs taken previously for comparison with a current film, since this may show whether a radiographic opacity is 'new' or progressive, and thus potentially serious, or 'old' and probably of no importance.

Some respiratory diseases, such as bronchial asthma and chronic bronchitis, and occasionally bronchial carcinoma, may not be associated with any radiographic abnormality, and a normal chest radiograph in these circumstances does not necessarily exclude serious intrathoracic disease.

Microbiological and cytological examination. *Sputum* can be examined for bacteria, fungi and viruses. Microbiological examination seldom provides conclusive diagnostic information except when *Mycobacterium tuberculosis* is isolated. The findings in other circumstances must be interpreted in conjunction with the results of clinical and, if necessary, radiological examination. The demonstration of malignant cells in the sputum confirms a diagnosis of bronchial carcinoma in the absence of malignant disease in the mouth or nasopharynx. Sputum cytology may also identify excessive numbers of eosinophil leucocytes, as in asthma and bronchopulmonary eosinophilia.

Pleural fluid. This should always be examined cytologically and bacteriologically. A special search should be made for *Myco. tuberculosis* and also for pyogenic organisms if the fluid is purulent. The fluid should also be examined cytologically, particularly if malignant disease is suspected.

Blood examination. Serological examination may be of value in the diagnosis of viral infections and allergic disorders.

Estimation of the total and differential leucocyte count may help to distinguish pyogenic infection from tuberculous or viral infection. An increase in the eosinophil count may occur for a variety of reasons (p. 241).

Skin tests. The tuberculin test (p. 227) and Kveim test (p. 261) may be of value in the diagnosis of tuberculosis and sarcoidosis respectively. Skin sensitivity tests (p. 237) are useful in

Table 8.1 Summary of typical physical signs in the more common respiratory diseases.

Pathological process	Movement of chest wall	Mediastinal displacement	Percussion note	Breath sounds	Vocal resonance	Added sounds
Consolidation as in lobar pneumonia	Reduction on affected side	None	Dull	High-pitched bronchial	Increased Whispering pectoriloquy	Fine crepitations early Coarse crepitations later
Collapse due to obstruction of major bronchus	Reduced on side affected	Towards lesion	Dull	Diminished or absent	Reduced or absent	None
Collapse due to peripheral bronchial obstruction	Reduced on side affected	Towards lesion	Dull	High-pitched bronchial	Increased Whispering pectoriloquy	None early—coarse crepitations later
Localised fibrosis and/or bronchiectasis	Slightly reduced on side affected	Towards lesion	Impaired	Low-pitched bronchial	Increased	Coarse crepitations
Cavitation (usually associated with consolidation or fibrosis)	Slightly reduced on side affected	None, or towards lesion	Impaired	'Amphoric' bronchial	Increased Whispering pectoriloquy	Coarse crepitations
Pleural effusion Empyema	Reduced or absent (depending on size) on side affected	Towards opposite side	Stony dull	Diminished or absent (occasionally bronchial)	Reduced or absent (occasionally increased)	Pleural rub in some cases (above effusion)
Pneumothorax	Reduced or absent (depending on size) on side affected	Towards opposite side	Normal or hyper-resonant	Diminished or absent (occasionally faint bronchial)	Reduced or absent	Tinkling crepitations when fluid present
Bronchitis: Acute Chronic	Normal or symmetrically diminished	None	Normal	Vesicular with prolonged expiration	Normal	Rhonchi, usually with some coarse crepitations
Bronchial asthma	Symmetrically diminished	None	Normal	Vesicular with prolonged expiration	Normal or reduced	Rhonchi, mainly expiratory and high-pitched
Bronchopneumonia	Symmetrically diminished	None	May be impaired	Usually harsh vesicular with prolonged expiration	Normal	Rhonchi and coarse crepitations
Diffuse pulmonary emphysema	Symmetrically diminished	None	Normal	Diminished vesicular with prolonged expiration	Normal or reduced	Expiratory rhonchi
Interstitial lung disease	Symmetrically diminished	None	Normal	Harsh vesicular with prolonged expiration	Usually increased	End-inspiratory crepitations uninfluenced by coughing

the investigation of allergic diseases.

Laryngoscopy and bronchoscopy. The larynx is inspected either by means of a mirror placed in front of the uvula (indirect laryngoscopy) or with a laryngoscope (direct laryngoscopy).

The trachea and larger bronchi are inspected by a bronchoscope of either rigid or flexible fibreoptic type. Abnormal tissue can be removed for histological examination (bronchial biopsy), and bronchial brushings and washings can be taken for cytological and bacteriological examination. The range of vision with the rigid instrument extends to the origins of all segmental bronchi but the fibreoptic bronchoscope is more useful for the inspection and biopsy of lesions situated more peripherally, particularly in the upper lobes.

Biopsy. Histological examination of an enlarged lymph node removed from the neck or axilla, or cytological examination of a needle aspirate, may provide a diagnosis in conditions such as bronchial carcinoma, tuberculosis, lymphoma and sarcoidosis. A lymph node can also be obtained for histological examination from the mediastinum by the technique of *mediastinoscopy*.

In patients with pleural effusion it is possible to obtain a specimen of parietal pleura suitable for histological examination. This procedure is simple and safe and may be of considerable value in determining the cause of a pleural effusion. If it is unsuccessful, the pleural surfaces can be inspected with a thoracoscope inserted through an intercostal space under general anaesthesia, and if a pleural lesion is seen, a biopsy can be performed under telescopic vision.

When a diagnosis cannot be made in any other way it may be necessary to obtain a specimen of lung tissue for histological examination by needle biopsy through the chest wall, by transbronchial lung biopsy via a fibreoptic bronchoscope or by thoracotomy.

Tests of pulmonary function. Many of the procedures mentioned above are of great assistance in arriving at a pathological diagnosis, but investigations of a different type are necessary to determine the effects of disease on pulmonary function and to assess the response to therapy. Disturbances of the mechanical properties of the lungs, of ventilation, of control of breathing, of the distribution of ventilation and perfusion within the lungs and of diffusing capacity can all be measured (Fig. 8.2). Some of the tests require a high degree of skill and elaborate apparatus, but others are simple routine procedures which can be undertaken by any doctor without special training.

1. ESTIMATION OF VENTILATORY CAPACITY. The patient is asked to take in as deep a breath as possible and then expel it as hard and as fast as possible. If the forced expiration is made into a recording spirometer of low resistance and low inertia, the *forced expiratory volume* in the standard time of 1 second (FEV_1) can be measured; if the forced expiration is continued till no more gas can be expelled, the *forced vital capacity* (FVC) is measured. In some diseases, especially emphysema, measurement of vital capacity (VC) during a relaxed rather than a forced expiration may be more appropriate in order to avoid 'air trapping'. The ratio of these two volumes may be expressed as a percentage (FEV/VC%); normal people can expel between 65 and 80% of the VC in 1 second, depending on age and sex.

In diseases which cause narrowing of the airways during expiration, such as asthma and chronic bronchitis, the FEV/VC% is reduced, sometimes to 40% or less. This is due to a greater reduction in FEV than in VC, and this type of ventilatory defect is called *obstructive*. In diseases such as interstitial lung disease or ankylosing spondylitis, which make the lungs or chest wall more rigid, FEV and VC are reduced in the same proportion and FEV/VC% is normal, as the airflow is relatively unaffected. This is called a *restrictive* ventilatory defect. Discovery of airflow obstruction is an indication to repeat the spirometric measurements after a bronchodilator drug has been given; reversibility of airflow obstruction is found in asthma and in some patients with chronic bronchitis.

During forced expiration, *peak expiratory flow* (PEF) can be measured by a gauge or meter which is simpler and cheaper than a spirometer. PEF is reduced in conditions causing airflow obstruction, and is a good indicator of the severity of the obstruction. The measurement has therefore become popular in clinical practice because of its speed and simplicity and the ease with which serial measurements can be made. PEF is less affected by conditions causing a restrictive type of ventilatory defect, and is therefore of little value in diagnosing or assessing them.

Even if no apparatus other than a watch and stethoscope is available, forced expiration can still be used to assess ventilatory capacity. Normal people can empty their chests from full inspiration in 4 seconds or less. Prolongation of the *forced expiratory time* (FET) to more than 6 seconds indicates airflow obstruction and a reduction in FEV/VC% to less than 50%. The end-point of FET is detected by listening through a stethoscope placed over the trachea in the suprasternal notch.

2. ANALYSIS OF ARTERIAL BLOOD. Apparatus for arterial blood-gas analysis is now available in most hospitals. Knowledge of the $PaCO_2$ provides the answer to the question, 'Is the patient breathing enough?', and is of particular value in the management of Type II respiratory failure (p. 204). If the arterial hydrogen ion concentration (or pH) is known, it is often possible to deduce the type of disturbance of acid:base balance (p. 99) which may be present. Knowledge of the PaO_2, or arterial oxygen saturation (which can be measured non-invasively with an oximeter) allows accurate assessment of hypoxaemia and of the effects of oxygen therapy.

These simple measurements are thus of value in distinguishing between some types of respiratory disorder, as well as in providing an index of their severity. Serial measurements are valuable in following changes in pulmonary function, whether occurring spontaneously or in response to treatment.

THE TREATMENT OF RESPIRATORY DISEASE

Infection

The antimicrobial therapy of infection of the bronchi, lungs and pleura will be described in the

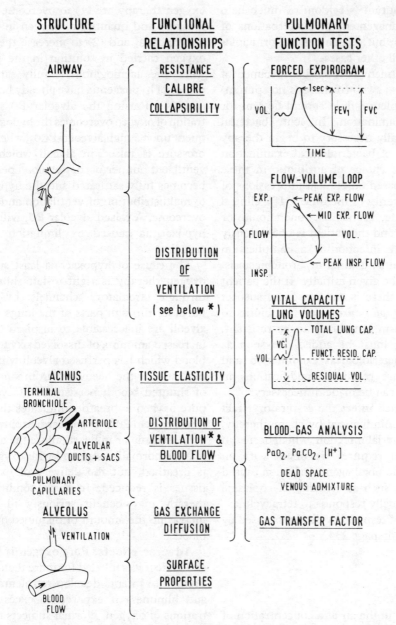

Fig. 8.2 Relationships between structure and function of lungs and pulmonary function tests. The forced expirogram gives information about airway resistance and calibre. The maximal flow-volume loop supplements this with information about inspiratory resistance, airway collapsibility and behaviour of small peripheral airways. In this test the rates at which air flows out of and into the lungs during forced maximum expiration and inspiration are measured and plotted against lung volume. Expiratory flow rates are decreased with airways collapse (e.g. emphysema) and the expiratory limb of the loop is scooped out compared with the almost straight line seen in health. Vital capacity and lung volume measurements are influenced by tissue elasticity and airway resistance. Distribution of ventilation and blood flow may be assessed by blood-gas analysis and by measurement of dead space and venous admixture. Overall gas exchange is assessed by arterial P_{O_2} and P_{CO_2} and by gas transfer factor.

sections on individual diseases. Bacteriological examination of sputum is seldom of much help in the clinical management of exacerbations of chronic bronchitis, but certain general principles are applicable to all other cases.

Before any treatment is started a specimen of sputum, a laryngeal swab (if there is no sputum) or a specimen of pleural fluid should be sent for bacteriological examination. In acute bacterial infection it is usually necessary to begin therapy before the results of bacteriological examination are available. The choice of antibiotic in these circumstances is based on clinical impressions of the nature and severity of the illness. If a clinical diagnosis of acute bronchitis, pneumonia or empyema is made and the patient is not seriously ill or if the acute infection is a complication of chronic bronchitis, asthma or bronchiectasis, ampicillin should be given initially. If the patient is gravely ill and there is any reason to suspect infection with *Staph. aureus*, an antibiotic to which that organism is unlikely to be resistant, e.g. flucloxacillin, must be added. As soon as the results of bacteriological examination and sensitivity tests are received, modifications in antibiotic therapy can be made, if necessary.

The viruses which infect the respiratory tract are, in the main, uninfluenced by chemotherapy, but secondary bacterial infection, which occurs in many cases, often requires treatment with an appropriate antimicrobial agent. Infection caused by small bacteria, such as coxiella, mycoplasma and chlamydia, usually responds to tetracycline.

The treatment of respiratory diseases caused by fungi is described on page 234.

Oxygen therapy

Oxygen is present in the air at a concentration of 21% and at sea level the pressure of oxygen in inspired tracheal air is almost 20 kPa (150 mmHg). Arterial blood of normal haemoglobin concentration contains about 9 mmol oxygen per litre (20 ml/100 ml); at a PaO_2 of 13.5 kPa (100 mmHg) 135 μmol oxygen per litre (0.3 ml/100 ml) are dissolved in the plasma (i.e. a solubility of 10 μmol/l/kPa) and the rest is bound to haemoglobin.

Therapeutic indications. The objectives of oxygen therapy are (1) to overcome the reduced pressure and quantity of oxygen in the blood in hypoxaemia, and (2) to increase the quantity of oxygen carried in solution in the plasma even when the haemoglobin is fully saturated. The causes of hypoxaemia have already been discussed (p. 204). Raising the alveolar PO_2 by administration of oxygen overcomes the hypoxaemia consequent upon a high alveolar PCO_2; when the oxygen pressure is raised in alveoli which are poorly ventilated but perfused, the blood perfusing them becomes fully saturated and the hypoxaemia due to maldistribution of ventilation and perfusion is overcome. A raised alveolar PO_2 will also correct hypoxaemia caused by limitation of diffusing capacity.

The cause of hypoxaemia least susceptible to oxygen therapy is right-to-left shunting, either through circulatory channels by-passing the lungs, or through parts of the lungs in which the alveoli are inaccessible to inspired oxygen. The increased amounts of dissolved oxygen carried by blood which has perfused alveoli with a high PO_2 can saturate the haemoglobin in small quantities of shunted blood; persistence of cyanosis when pure oxygen is breathed indicates that the shunt is larger than 20% of the cardiac output.

In anaemia or in heart failure the arterial blood may be normally saturated with oxygen when air is breathed, but the delivery of oxygen to the tissues is reduced. In these conditions oxygen therapy may benefit seriously ill patients by increasing the amount of dissolved oxygen in the blood.

Adverse effects. Pure oxygen is both irritant and toxic if it is inhaled for more than a few hours. Premature infants develop retrolental fibroplasia and blindness if exposed to excessive concentrations of oxygen. Normal subjects notice cough and bronchial irritation, and in patients ventilated with high concentrations of oxygen for several days pulmonary oedema and consolidation may occur. Pulmonary damage by oxygen is one of the possible causes of ARDS (p. 213) and poses a therapeutic dilemma because hypoxaemia is a consequence of that syndrome and treatment may make it worse. If such patients require oxygen it is important to give, whenever possible, an inspired concentration which corrects hypoxaemia but does not exceed 60 to 70%.

Technique of oxygen administration. Hypoxaemia is such a common consequence of respiratory diseases that oxygen may well be the most frequently prescribed 'drug' used in their treatment. It is important that prescriptions for oxygen should be in writing, and that flow rates or concentrations should be clearly specified. Administration of oxygen should be continuous though this may prove difficult in confused or restless patients. The risk of fire should never be forgotten when any patient is treated with oxygen.

Oxygen masks are of two types: 1. Those which are designed to produce a high concentration of O_2 in the inspired air. An example of this type of mask is the MC mask which delivers about 60% O_2 when the flow rate is 4–6 l per minute.

2. Those which are designed to produce slight O_2 enrichment of the inspired air and do not permit the rebreathing of expired CO_2. A suitable mask of this type is the Ventimask available in models delivering 24, 28, 35, 45 and 60% O_2 respectively. The last two require very high oxygen flow rates.

Nasal cannulae. Double nasal cannulae fit comfortably into the nostrils. Their main advantages are that they do not permit rebreathing of CO_2 and do not interfere with eating, drinking and the wearing of spectacles. The inspired O_2 concentration they provide is somewhat unpredictable, but an O_2 flow rate of 2 l/min. will usually raise it to about 30%. They are of particular value if oxygen is administered for long periods.

Humidification. When MC masks are used, the oxygen must be humidified, either by passing it over the surface of warm water in an electrically heated canister (East-Radcliffe humidifier) or through a nebuliser. This is not necessary with Ventimasks or nasal cannulae, as a high proportion of atmospheric air is mixed with the oxygen when these devices are used.

Treatment of respiratory failure

Acute Type I respiratory failure. Severe hypoxaemia associated with a normal or low $PaCO_2$ can develop rapidly in many respiratory and cardiac disorders. Treatment is that of the underlying cause (e.g. pulmonary oedema, pneumonia, adult respiratory distress syndrome) and correction of the hypoxaemia by administration of oxygen in high concentration by oronasal mask. Young children may have to be treated in oxygen tents since few of them tolerate masks. Very ill patients may require artificial ventilation with oxygen-enriched air through a cuffed endotracheal tube.

Chronic Type I respiratory failure. Chronic hypoxaemia without carbon dioxide retention has many causes, mainly respiratory, which include fibrosing alveolitis and other types of interstitial lung disease (p. 256). Treatment is that of the underlying disorder, combined with high concentration oxygen therapy. Patients with chronic respiratory failure of this type are rarely treated with artificial ventilation, since the prognosis is generally poor and aggressive therapy is usually considered to be ethically unjustified.

Acute Type II respiratory failure. Acute Type II respiratory failure (asphyxia) may be produced by: (1) obstruction of the upper airways, (2) severe acute asthma, (3) major chest injuries, particularly those associated with tension pneumothorax, massive haemothorax or multiple rib fractures (flail chest), (4) acute brain stem and cervical cord lesions resulting from trauma to the head and neck, viral infection or ischaemia of the brain stem, (5) paralysis of respiratory muscles and (6) poisoning with narcotic and other drugs.

Acute retention of carbon dioxide in this form of Type II respiratory failure causes severe respiratory acidosis (p. 99). This may also supervene when carbon dioxide retention increases rapidly in patients with chronic Type II respiratory failure who develop a respiratory infection.

The treatment of the various causes of acute Type II respiratory failure is summarised in Table 8.2.

Chronic Type II respiratory failure. The most important cause of chronic retention of carbon dioxide (hypercapnia) and associated hypoxaemia is chronic bronchitis, but Type II respiratory failure also occurs preterminally in other progressive respiratory diseases. Chronic hypercapnia leads to renal conservation of bicarbonate which usually corrects the resultant respir-

Table 8.2 Treatment of acute Type II respiratory failure.

Cause	Treatment
1. *Upper airways obstruction* (a) Inhaled foreign body	Try to dislodge it by turning child upside down and forcibly compressing the thoracic cage or by Heimlich manoeuvre (p. 000) in adult. If ineffective, extract foreign body by laryngoscopy or bronchoscopy
(b) Acute epiglottitis laryngeal oedema, bilateral vocal cord paralysis	Treatment of cause. If medical treatment ineffective, tracheal intubation or tracheostomy
2. *Severe acute asthma*	Medical treatment (p. 000). If not rapidly effective, tracheal intubation and intermittent positive-pressure ventilation.
3. *Chest injuries* (a) Tension pneumothorax	Pleural decompression by intercostal tube
(b) Massive haemothorax	Drainage of blood through intercostal tube. Thoracotomy if necessary for evacuation of clot and ligation of bleeding points
(c) Flail chest	Tracheal intubation and intermittent positive-pressure ventilation. Fixation of rib and sternal fractures
4. *Brain stem and cervical cord lesions. Paralysis of respiratory muscles*	Tracheal intubation and intermittent positive-pressure ventilation. Treatment of cause where possible
5. *Poisoning with narcotic and other drugs*	Measures to eliminate poison. Specific antidote (e.g. naloxone for opium alkaloids). Tracheal intubation and intermittent positive-pressure ventilation.

atory acidosis. In these circumstances the arterial hydrogen ion concentration may be normal, but acidaemia recurs whenever a further reduction in alveolar ventilation again increases the degree of hypercapnia. High concentrations of oxygen can cause deterioration because they reduce the hypoxic drive to breathing in patients whose central (brain stem) response to carbon dioxide is diminished or absent.

Associated right ventricular failure is almost invariably made worse by hypoxaemia, which aggravates pulmonary hypertension.

Respiratory infection and retained bronchial secretions are the main factors responsible for exacerbations of Type II respiratory failure in patients with chronic lung disease. Efforts to encourage efficient expectoration, which may be difficult in patients made drowsy by carbon dioxide retention, must be pursued with the utmost vigour and appropriate antimicrobial therapy prescribed. If there is evidence of bronchospasm, bronchodilators and, if necessary, corticosteroids should be given in an attempt to reduce airflow obstruction. Analeptic drugs have a limited but useful place in drowsy and comatose patients. Nikethamide (0.5–2 g 1–2 hourly) or doxapram (infusions of up to 3 mg/min) given intravenously for 24 hours, may successfully tide the patient over a period of hypoventilation during which time bronchopulmonary infection, bronchospasm and right ventricular failure can be treated, the last with a powerful diuretic. The main reason for giving analeptic drugs is to improve the level of consciousness so that effective expectoration can be encouraged. If these measures fail patients who were able to lead a fairly active life before the onset of the acute episode may be considered for artificial ventilation.

Mechanical ventilation — intermittent positive-pressure ventilation (IPPV). Patients with both types of respiratory failure may have to be treated by IPPV through a cuffed endotracheal tube introduced through the mouth or nose under general anaesthesia. Positive end-expiratory pressure (PEEP) may be useful in some cases with Type I respiratory failure to correct ventilation-perfusion imbalance. Powerful ventilators delivering a fixed volume are required for the treatment of patients with Type II respiratory failure associated with airflow obstruction, e.g. asthma and chronic bronchitis. Whenever IPPV is likely to be necessary for more than a few days, for example in patients with respiratory muscle paralysis, the patient should have a tracheostomy and the endotracheal tube should be replaced by a cuffed tracheostomy tube.

Endotracheal intubation and tracheostomy allow tracheo-bronchial suction to be performed as often as necessary to clear the airways of secretions. This can be done more efficiently by fibreoptic bronchoscopy which is of particular value if lobar collapse has occurred because of retained secretions.

Most adults require a ventilatory volume of about 10 l/min to maintain a normal $PaCO_2$ and sufficient oxygen is added to the 'inspired' air in order to achieve a satisfactory PaO_2. Attempts to discontinue ventilation can be started as soon as the underlying cause of respiratory failure has been successfully treated. It is usual for the patient to be allowed to breathe humidified air spontaneously through the tracheostomy tube for longer periods each day until assisted ventilation is no longer required. At this stage the tracheostomy tube can be removed, providing it is not still necessary to prevent aspiration of secretions into the trachea in patients who cannot swallow normally because of brain stem lesions.

Adult respiratory distress syndrome (ARDS). ARDS may not be a single disease entity but it is convenient to think of it as such. In this syndrome there is damage to the alveolar epithelium and capillary endothelium which allows the alveolar spaces to become flooded with oedema of high protein content (non-cardiogenic pulmonary oedema). There are many disorders which may be complicated by the development of this serious condition (Table 8.3).

ARDS is characterised by dyspnoea, hypoxaemia and hypotension. It usually affects both lungs and crepitations are audible over all areas, especially the bases. The chest X-ray shows rapidly progressive widespread 'fluffy or soft' and sometimes homogeneous shadowing. Often the costophrenic angles remain clear in the early stages.

Treatment is of the underlying cause together with correction of the hypoxaemia, keeping in mind possible adverse effects of oxygen therapy (p. 210). Many patients require assisted ventilation with PEEP to maintain an adequate arterial oxygen pressure. There is a high mortality in patients who require to be treated by ventilation.

Symptomatic treatment in respiratory disease

Cough, when productive of sputum, should be encouraged and not suppressed. Those who are physically weak should be exhorted at regular intervals to clear their bronchi of secretion. Those with bronchiectasis or lung abscess should practise postural drainage, and those with tenacious sputum should be given hot drinks and inhalations of either steam or nebulised normal saline to help them to bring up sputum more easily.

Unproductive, distressing cough should be suppressed. The two most effective preparations, suitable for use in acute bronchitis, pneumonia, bronchial carcinoma and pulmonary tuberculosis, are pholcodine and methadone.

Haemoptysis. A sedative may be given to allay anxiety, e.g. diazepam. Morphine, which depresses the cough reflex, may have the effect of allowing blood clot to accumulate in the bronchi and should not be prescribed. Haemoptysis nearly always stops spontaneously and reassurance to this effect lessens the strain of what, to patient and relatives, is a most alarming experience.

If the haemorrhage is very severe blood volume should be restored by transfusion and, if respiratory obstruction develops, the blood must be removed from the bronchi by aspiration through a bronchoscope. Control of the bleeding by surgical measures is occasionally required.

Airflow obstruction in bronchitis and asthma is treated by bronchodilators (p. 238) and in some cases by corticosteroids given by inhalation or as tablets (p. 238).

Table 8.3 Causes of adult respiratory distress syndrome.

Pneumonias	Viral, bacterial, tuberculous, fungal, *Pneumocystis carinii*, *Mycoplasma pneumoniae*
Inhaled toxic substances	Corrosive chemicals (ammonia, chlorine, nitrogen dioxide), oxygen in high concentration, smoke
Aspiration of irritant substances	Vomitus, water (fresh and salt), hydrocarbons
Systemic disorders	Shock of any cause, septicaemia, eclampsia, uraemia
Blood disorders	Disseminated intravascular coagulation, blood product transfusion, thrombocytopenic purpura
Lung emboli	Fat, air, amniotic fluid, X-ray contrast media
Lung trauma	Contusion, irradiation
Drugs	Diamorphine, methadone, thiazides, barbiturates
Miscellaneous	Acute pancreatitis, high altitude, increased intracranial pressure, cardiopulmonary bypass

Chest pain. For pleural pain mild analgesics are rarely adequate and most patients require pethidine, 50–100 mg by mouth or intramuscular injection, or even morphine, 10–15 mg i.m. Opiates must, however, be used with caution in patients with poor respiratory function.

The pain of acute tracheitis usually responds to mild analgesics such as acetylsalicylic acid or paracetamol, combined with inhalations of steam. Pain due to invasion of the chest wall by a malignant tumour, if not relieved by radiotherapy, usually demands a powerful analgesic such as pethidine or morphine, given by injection or constant infusion. In advanced cases these drugs may become ineffective and neurosurgical measures may be required for the relief of intractable pain.

INFECTIONS OF THE RESPIRATORY SYSTEM

Infections of the respiratory tract may be caused by viruses, bacteria or fungi. Viruses are frequently responsible for upper respiratory illnesses. Although viral infection is a relatively uncommon specific cause of pneumonia, it is often complicated by bacterial infection of the bronchi and lungs as, for example, in influenza. The bacteria most frequently responsible for respiratory infection, including pneumonia, are *Streptococcus pneumoniae*, often in association with *Haemophilus influenzae*, *Staphylococcus aureus* and various species of Gram-negative bacilli. The so-called small bacteria, such as mycoplasma, coxiella and chlamydia, and also legionnella, are other, but much less common, causes of acute pneumonia. Pulmonary infection by *Mycobacterium tuberculosis*, atypical mycobacteria and fungi results in diseases of a more chronic type, which are described in separate sections.

Upper respiratory tract infections

The vast majority of these illnesses, of which acute coryza is by far the most common, are caused by viruses (Table 8.4). Immunity is short-lived, and specific for each virus. The average person can, therefore, expect to have at least two or three attacks of coryza every year. Other viral infections include acute laryngitis and acute laryngotracheobronchitis. Bacterial infection is the cause of acute tonsillitis, otitis media and epiglottitis.

Acute coryza (common cold). The onset is usually sudden with a burning and tickling sensation in the nose accompanied by sneezing. The throat often feels dry and sore, the head feels

Table 8.4 Respiratory infections caused by viruses.

Clinical syndrome	Usual cause (other causes in parentheses)
Epidemic influenza	Influenza A and B
'Flu-like' illness	Adenoviruses rhinoviruses. (Enteroviruses)
Sore throat	Adenoviruses. (Enteroviruses, parainfluenza viruses, influenza A and B in partially immune)
Common cold (Coryza)	Rhinoviruses. (Coronaviruses, enteroviruses, adenoviruses, respiratory syncytial virus)
'Feverish' cold	Rhinoviruses, enteroviruses. (Influenza A and B, para-influenza viruses, respiratory syncytial virus)
Croup	Parainfluenza 1, 2, 3. (Rhinoviruses, enteroviruses)
Bronchitis	Rhinoviruses, adenoviruses. (Influenza A and B)
Bronchiolitis	Respiratory syncytial virus. (Parainfluenza 3)
Pneumonia	Influenza A and B. (Respiratory syncytial virus and parainfluenza viruses in adults)

'stuffed' and there is a profuse watery nasal discharge (rhinorrhoea). These symptoms last for 1 to 2 days, after which, with secondary infection, the secretion becomes thick and purulent, and impedes nasal breathing.

Coryza may be complicated by sinusitis which can become chronic, particularly in the maxillary sinuses, causing persistent purulent discharge from the front and back of the nose, often accompanied by nasal obstruction and headaches. Other complications are infections of the lower respiratory tract, occlusion of the auditory tubes causing deafness, and otitis media.

Frequent attacks of sneezing and watery rhinorrhoea, without systemic upset, suggest nasal allergy rather than viral infection.

Acute laryngitis. This usually occurs either as a complication of coryza or as a manifestation of one of the infectious fevers, for example, measles. The laryngeal mucous membrane is swollen, congested and coated with mucus.

The throat is dry and sore. The voice is at first hoarse and then reduced to a whisper. Speaking may be painful. There is an irritating non-productive cough, but the general upset is usually mild. In children the small laryngeal opening may be almost completely obstructed by oedema and viscid secretion, giving rise to stridor.

Acute laryngitis usually clears up in a few days, but frequently recurring episodes may predispose to chronic laryngitis. Downward spread of the infection may cause tracheitis, bronchitis or even pneumonia.

Acute laryngotracheobronchitis (croup). This illness, which is particularly serious in very young children because of the small calibre of their airways, may be caused by several viruses (Table 8.4). Superinfection with bacteria, especially *Strep. pneumoniae* and *Staph. aureus*, may occur. The mucosa is intensely inflamed, the secretions are extremely tenacious and fibrinous casts of the bronchi may form.

The initial symptoms may be those of the common cold. These are followed by severe and sometimes violent cough which may be paroxysmal, accompanied by dyspnoea and stridor (croup), contraction of accessory muscles and indrawing of intercostal spaces. The child may be cyanosed, and asphyxia may occur if appropriate treatment is not given.

Acute epiglottitis. This is a rare, but serious disease of young children. Bacterial infection, almost always with *Haemophilus influenzae*, is the cause of this condition which presents with fever and sore throat. Stridor develops rapidly because of inflammatory swelling of the epiglottis and surrounding submucosa, and death may occur from asphyxia. In acute epiglottitis, stridor and cough in the absence of hoarseness help to distinguish it from laryngeal causes of stridor. When epiglottitis is suspected, attempts to examine the throat using a tongue depressor or any instrument should be avoided, unless facilities for tracheal intubation or tracheostomy are immediately available, since this may cause complete respiratory obstruction.

Investigation and treatment of upper respiratory tract infections

Most patients with these infections recover rapidly and specific investigation is indicated only in the more severe cases. Viruses can be isolated from throat swabs, and viral infections may be identified retrospectively by serological tests. Exfoliated cells colonised by certain viruses (e.g. influenza A and B) can be identified by the fluorescent antibody technique, allowing the pathogen to be rapidly defined. Throat swabs may also be helpful if streptococcal sore throat is suspected, and examination of the blood will identify infectious mononucleosis. Radiographic examination may be required to confirm the presence of chronic sinus infection.

The spread of viral infections can be reduced by voluntary isolation of patients for 2–3 days during the early highly infectious stage. Excessive nasal secretions can be reduced by periodic use of decongestants either sprayed or dropped into the nose. Lozenges containing local anaesthetic, for example benzocaine, are helpful when the throat is painful. A mild analgesic, such as aspirin or paracetamol, relieves systemic symptoms. Antibiotics are unnecessary except in the treatment of acute epiglottitis, streptococcal sore throat and bacterial complications of viral infection, such as acute sinusitis or otitis media. Ampicillin is normally the drug of choice in these conditions. In acute epiglottitis, however, either ampicillin in high dosage, or chloramphenicol, should be given intravenously. Ampicillin should be avoided whenever a diagnosis of infectious mononucleosis is suspected (p. 522).

Inhalations of steam are helpful in laryngitis. In acute laryngotracheobronchitis clearing of secretions is of utmost importance. Bronchoscopy, endotracheal intubation or tracheostomy may be required as life-saving measures in patients with severe respiratory obstruction. Oxygen therapy is necessary in some patients and adequate hydration should be maintained.

INFLUENZA

Influenza is a specific acute illness caused by a group of myxoviruses. It occurs in epidemics, and occasionally pandemics, often explosive in nature.

Aetiology. There are two common types of virus, A and B. At least four strains of influenza A, which is responsible for the pandemics, have been identified. The H3N2 strain (Hong Kong) has been implicated in most recent epidemics. Influenza B is usually associated with smaller and less virulent outbreaks. The immunity which follows infection is type-specific and of relatively short duration. This causes problems in providing effective immunisation.

Clinical features. The incubation period is 24 to 48 hours. The illness starts suddenly with headache, pain in the back and limbs, anorexia and sometimes nausea and vomiting. Pyrexia to 39°C remits for 2 to 3 days, with shivering but seldom rigors. The fauces are hyperaemic with prominent lymphoid follicles. There may be a harsh unproductive cough, without physical signs over the lungs. Leucopenia is common.

The disease may spread rapidly throughout a household or institution. During epidemics, the diagnosis is usually easy. Most sporadic cases are identifiable only as respiratory viral infections unless the virus is isolated, or demonstrated by the fluorescent antibody technique, or if serological tests for specific antibodies are positive.

Course and complications. In many cases, no further symptoms develop and recovery ensues within 3 to 5 days. The disease may, however, be complicated by tracheitis, bronchitis, bronchiolitis and bronchopneumonia. Secondary bacterial invasion by *Strep. pneumoniae*, *H. influenzae* and occasionally *Staph. aureus* causes these complications.

Toxic cardiomyopathy may cause sudden death, especially when there is pre-existing cardiac disease. Encephalitis and post-influenzal demyelinating encephalopathy are rare complications. Post-influenzal asthenia and depression are common, often marked, and may last for a few weeks.

Treatment and prevention. The patient should be kept in bed until the fever has subsided. A mild analgesic usually relieves the headache and generalised pains. Aspirin should not be given to children under 12 years, with this or other febrile illnesses, because of the risk of Reye's syndrome (p. 347). Pholcodine or methadone may be used to suppress unproductive cough. The treatment of complications such as bronchitis and pneumonia is dealt with later.

Immunity is type-specific and if the antigenic constitution of a new strain can be detected early, a specific vaccine may give about 70% protection. Annual winter vaccination is recommended for patients suffering from chronic pulmonary, cardiac or renal disease.

ACUTE BRONCHITIS

Aetiology. This condition is an acute inflammation of the trachea and bronchi caused by viruses and pyogenic organisms such as *Strep. pneumoniae*, *H. influenzae* and, rarely, *Staph. aureus*. Bacterial infection is a common sequel of coryza, influenza, measles and whooping-cough. Other factors predisposing to bacterial infection include cold, damp, foggy and dusty atmospheres and cigarette smoking.

Clinical features. The first symptom is an irritating, unproductive cough accompanied by upper retrosternal discomfort or pain caused by tracheitis. When the bronchi become involved there is also a sensation of tightness in the chest, and dyspnoea with wheeze may be present. Respiratory distress may be particularly severe when acute bronchitis complicates chronic bronchitis and emphysema.

The sputum is at first scanty, mucoid, viscid and difficult to bring up, and occasionally may be streaked with blood. A day or two later it becomes mucopurulent and more copious. As the infection extends down the bronchial tree there may be a rise in temperature to 38–39°C and a neutrophil leucocytosis. In the vast majority of cases recovery takes place gradually over the next 4 to 8 days without the patient ever becoming seriously ill. Occasionally the dyspnoea and cough increase, cyanosis appears, and if the infection reaches the smaller bronchi and bronchioles ('bronchiolitis') the condition becomes indistinguishable from bronchopneumonia.

Tracheitis without bronchitis produces no abnormal physical signs. In bronchitis there may be prolonged expiration accompanied by rhonchi and, in bronchiolitis, crepitations.

Treatment. The patient should be confined to bed and oxytetracycline or ampicillin, 250–500 mg 4 times daily, given by mouth. Cotrimoxazole is equally effective in a dose of 2 tablets twice daily. In the early stages, when cough is painful and unproductive, the tough viscid secretion should be loosened by steam inhalation 3 or 4 times a day. Cough should be controlled at night by pholcodine. If symptoms or signs of airflow obstruction are present a bronchodilator drug should be given. Oxygen is seldom required in uncomplicated acute bronchitis.

THE PNEUMONIAS

Pneumonia is the term used to describe inflammation of the lung. There are many different kinds of pneumonia, some common, others rare. Aetiologically, they can be divided into the *primary pneumonias*, in which the disease is caused by a specific pathogenic organism, and the *secondary pneumonias*, in which some abnormality of the respiratory system predisposes to the invasion of the lung by organisms of relatively low virulence, and infection generally reaches the alveoli by aspiration from other parts of the respiratory tract.

In the secondary pneumonias, *H. influenzae*, some types of *Strep. pneumoniae* and certain of the bacteria forming the flora of the upper respiratory tract and mouth are the organisms most frequently cultured from the sputum.

Occasionally in some types of both primary and secondary pneumonia, prominent features are destruction of lung tissue by the inflammatory process, a high incidence of abscess formation and the subsequent development of pulmonary fibrosis and bronchiectasis. The term 'suppurative pneumonia' has been applied to this group of cases and this condition merits separate description (p. 221).

THE PRIMARY PNEUMONIAS

Pneumococcal pneumonia, caused by *Strep. pneumoniae*, is the most common type of primary pneumonia. Other bacteria which may cause primary pneumonia include *Staph. aureus*, *Strep. pyogenes*, *Klebsiella pneumoniae*, *H. influenzae*, *Legionella pneumophila* and so-called small bacteria such as *Mycoplasma pneumoniae*, *Coxiella burnetii* and *Chlamydia psittaci* (psittacosis and ornithosis). Anaerobic organisms, including *Actinomyces israeli*, are rare causes of primary pneumonia. Primary viral pneumonia is most frequently due to influenza viruses in adults.

Pneumococcal pneumonia

Pneumococcal pneumonia is characterised by homogeneous consolidation of one or more lobes or segments. The disease occurs at all ages but most frequently in early and middle adult life. The highest incidence is in winter. It is usually a sporadic disease, the mode of spread being by droplet infection.

Clinical features. The onset is sudden, often with rigors, or with vomiting or a convulsion in children. The temperature rises in a few hours to 39–40°C. Loss of appetite, headache, and aching pains in the body and limbs accompany the pyrexia. Localised pain of pleural type in the chest wall often develops at an early stage in the illness. Occasionally it may be referred to the shoulder or to the abdominal wall. There is a short, painful cough, dry at first but later productive of tenacious sputum which is often rust-coloured and occasionally frankly blood-stained. Respiration is rapid (30–40 per minute in adults, 50–60 in children), and shallow when pleural pain is present. The pulse is rapid, the skin is hot and dry, the face is flushed, and central cyanosis may be observed in severe cases. Herpes labialis is often present. A marked neutrophil leucocytosis is characteristic. *Strep. pneumoniae* can usually be isolated from the sputum, and a positive blood culture may be obtained.

Physical signs in the chest. In the first 24 to 48 hours of the illness, there is diminution of respiratory movement, slight impairment of the percussion note and often a pleural rub on the affected side. At a variable time after the onset, generally within 2 days, signs of consolidation appear (p. 207), the breath sounds being of high-pitched bronchial type. When resolution begins, numerous coarse crepitations are heard, indicating liquefaction of the alveolar exudate. If a pleural effusion develops, the physical signs of fluid in the pleural space are usually found, but bronchial breath sounds can persist and the presence of an effusion may be suspected only from stony dullness on percussion.

Radiological examination shows a homogeneous opacity localised to the affected lobe or segment, appearing within 12 to 18 hours of the onset of the illness. Radiological examination is particularly helpful if a complication such as pleural effusion or empyema is suspected.

Course. Most cases respond promptly to chemotherapy (p. 223) and within a week the patient is well again. Delayed recovery suggests either that some complication such as empyema has developed or that the diagnosis is incorrect.

Other types of primary pneumonia

Staphylococcal pneumonia. Pneumonia due to *Staph. aureus* may occur either as a primary respiratory infection or as a blood-borne infection from a staphylococcal lesion elsewhere in the body, for example, osteomyelitis. The second condition is essentially one of pyaemic abscess formation in the lungs. Unless an empyema is produced by rupture of an abscess into the pleura, the pulmonary lesions may pass unnoticed, overshadowed by the severe general illness.

Primary staphylococcal pneumonia, although it occurs much less frequently than pneumococcal pneumonia, is a relatively common illness, especially as a complication of influenza. It may present as a lobar or segmental pneumonia, which may be difficult to distinguish clinically from a severe pneumococcal infection, or as a suppurative pneumonia (p. 221) with multiple lung abscesses which may persist as thin-walled cysts after the acute infection has subsided.

Treatment of this and other forms of primary pneumonia is discussed on page 223.

Klebsiella pneumonia. Pneumonia due to *Kl. pneumoniae* is a rare disease with a high mortality. There is usually massive consolidation and excavation of one or more lobes, the upper lobes being most often involved, with profound systemic disturbance and the expectoration of large amounts of purulent sputum, sometimes chocolate-coloured. The diagnosis is made by the radiological appearances and the isolation of the causative organism from the sputum.

Legionella pneumonia (legionnaires' disease) is caused by a bacillus (*L. pneumophila*) which appears to be transmitted in water droplets often originating in infected humidifier cooling towers and perhaps from stagnant water in cisterns and shower heads. Epidemics traced to institutions such as hospitals receive much publicity but sporadic cases infected from unknown sources are not uncommon. It can be a serious and fatal illness, but most patients survive. Gastro-intestinal symptoms, mental confusion, hyponatraemia and proteinuria often accompany the pneumonia.

Actinomycosis. Formerly included amongst the fungal diseases, this is now regarded as a bacterial infection. It is caused by *A. israeli*, an anaerobic organism, which exists as a commensal in the mouth. When local defences are impaired, actinomycosis can cause cervicofacial, abdominal or, occasionally, pulmonary infection such as a widespread suppurative pneumonia (p. 221). Empyema, often bilateral and associated with persistent chest wall sinuses, may develop. The pus may contain 'sulphur grains' (p. 767). Sinuses are also a feature of cervicofacial and abdominal infections.

Pneumonia caused by viruses and small bacteria. A distinctive form of pneumonia may be produced by certain viruses, and also by small bacteria which affect lung tissue in a similar way. The clinical picture differs from that of the bacterial pneumonias in that fever and toxaemia usually precede the respiratory symptoms by several days. Severe headache, malaise and anorexia are characteristic features in the early stages. The physical signs in the chest, if there are any, appear later and are seldom gross. The existence of a pulmonary lesion may not be recognised without a radiograph. The spleen may be palpable in the first week. The white blood count is generally normal and the pyrexia does not respond to penicillins. The diagnosis can often be confirmed by isolation of the causal organism or by serological tests.

The disease is usually self-limiting. The pyrexia subsides by lysis after 5 to 10 days, and complete recovery and radiographic resolution follow, the latter sometimes being slow. Very rarely, death takes place from widespread extension of the pneumonia or from viral encephalitis.

The *influenza, parainfluenza* and *measles* viruses rarely produce a specific pneumonia. In adults pneumonia caused by *chickenpox* virus, however, is usually characteristic. The radiograph shows numerous miliary nodular shadows which may eventually calcify. The *adenoviruses* cause occasional mild epidemics of primary pneumonia.

Respiratory syncytial virus is the most important respiratory pathogen of early childhood, especially in the first 2 months of life. This is because it causes bronchiolitis and occasionally pneumonia, and carries a risk of mortality. The infant is fevered, and cough, wheezy respiration and occasionally an erythematous rash are prominent features. The virus is not susceptible to any known therapy, and immunisation is ineffective.

Chlamydia psittaci causes psittacosis (ornithosis), a systemic illness contracted from infected birds. The pneumonia associated with it may be extensive, with severe toxaemia. Headache is a prominent early symptom.

Mycoplasma pneumoniae is a pleomorphic bacterium which is susceptible to tetracyclines though a few strains are sensitive only to erythromycin. Cold agglutinins (p. 517) can be demonstrated in a high proportion of cases. Antibodies can be detected, and haemagglutination and complement-fixation tests are available for diagnosis. Outbreaks of pneumonia caused by this organism are common in barracks and institutions. Most cases occur in children and young adults. Maculopapular rashes, haemolytic anaemia and meningoencephalitis occur rarely.

Coxiella (Rickettsia) burnetii is the organism responsible for *Q-fever*. Endocarditis may occur, as well as pneumonia, in this disease (p. 741).

Pneumonia due to opportunistic infections. Patients whose immunological defences have been compromised by disease (e.g. lymphomas and monocyte-macrophage system disorders) or by immunosuppressive and corticosteroid therapy, and in particular patients who have developed the acquired immune deficiency syndrome (AIDS) (p. 726), are prone to opportunistic pulmonary infections. The commonest causes are Gram-negative bacilli (coliforms and *Ps. aeruginosa*), fungi (*Cryptococcus neoformans, Candida albicans* and *Aspergillus fumigatus*), viruses (cytomegaloviruses, herpes viruses) and a protozoon (*Pneumocystis carinii*). Cytomegaloviral and *Pneumocystis carinii* infections are especially common in AIDS patients and a definitive diagnosis may require bronchial washings, brushings and/or trans-bronchial biopsy to identify the pathogen.

THE SECONDARY PNEUMONIAS

This group, sometimes described as 'non-specific' or aspiration pneumonias, comprises a large number of different conditions. Their common features are the absence of any specific pathogenic organism in the sputum and the existence of some abnormality of the respiratory system. This predisposes to the invasion of the lung by organisms of relatively low virulence derived from the upper respiratory tract or from the mouth, for example, streptococci, certain types of pneumococci, *H. influenzae* and various species of anaerobic bacteria.

Infection may reach the lungs in various ways. Pus may be aspirated from an infected nasal sinus, or septic matter may be inhaled during tonsillectomy or dental extraction under general anaesthesia. Vomitus or the contents of a dilated oesophagus may enter the larynx during general anaesthesia, coma or even sleep, and aspiration may also occur in patients with gastro-oesophageal reflux (p. 279). Infected secretion in the bronchi and pus from acute bronchitis, dilated bronchi or a lung abscess may also be carried into the alveoli by the air stream or by gravity.

Ineffective coughing caused by postoperative or post-traumatic thoracic or abdominal pain, by debility or immobility, or by laryngeal paralysis may also predispose to the development of secondary (aspiration) pneumonia.

Partial bronchial obstruction, as for example by a carcinoma, is another potential cause of secondary pneumonia, as it allows infection derived from the upper air passages to become established in the inadequately drained portion of lung beyond the obstruction.

Acute bronchopneumonia

This type of secondary pneumonia is invariably preceded by bronchial infection, which accounts for the widespread patchy distribution of the lesions. It occurs most frequently at the extremes of life, and may be described as 'hypostatic pneumonia' when it occurs in elderly or debilitated patients. In children, it is often a complication of measles or whooping cough, and in adults, of acute bronchitis or influenza. It is particularly common in patients with chronic bronchitis.

Pathology. There is acute inflammation of the bronchi, especially the terminal bronchioles, which are filled with pus. Collapse and consoli-

dation of the associated groups of alveoli follow. The lesions are distributed bilaterally in small patches which tend to become larger by confluence and are often more extensive in the lower lobes. There is interstitial oedema and compensatory emphysema around the collapsed alveoli.

Clinical features. After 2 or 3 days of acute bronchitis, as bronchopneumonia develops, the temperature rises to a higher level, the pulse and respiration rates increase, and dyspnoea and central cyanosis appear. There is generally a severe cough with purulent sputum. Pleural pain is uncommon, in contrast to pneumococcal pneumonia.

During the early stages the physical signs are those of acute bronchitis but crepitations later become more numerous. In many cases, no signs of consolidation can be detected. Radiological examination shows mottled opacities in both lung fields, chiefly in the lower zones. A neutrophil leucocytosis is present.

Course and complications. The disease is of more insidious onset and tends to run a more protracted course (up to 10 days) than pneumococcal pneumonia. Incomplete resolution may lead to bronchiectasis and replacement fibrosis (p. 255). The mortality is higher at the extremes of life, especially if the disease supervenes on chronic bronchitis and emphysema or any debilitating illness.

Prevention. The incidence of bronchopneumonia can be reduced by careful attention to apparently benign upper respiratory infections and acute bronchitis, especially when they occur in children or elderly subjects and in patients with chronic bronchitis.

Benign aspiration pneumonia

This type of secondary pneumonia is due to the aspiration of infected secretion into the lungs during the course of an upper respiratory infection such as coryza or sinusitis. The organisms causing the pneumonia, being derived from the upper respiratory tract, are generally of low virulence and the degree of systemic disturbance is usually slight. In fact, the symptoms are often no more severe than would be expected with an uncomplicated upper respiratory infection and the existence of pneumonia may be discovered only by radiological examination.

As a rule, however, the condition manifests itself by cough, purulent sputum, low-grade pyrexia and sometimes pleural pain, in association with a frank upper respiratory infection. Localised crepitations are often the only abnormal physical finding. A neutrophil leucocytosis is usually present. The radiological lesions are typically unilateral, the characteristic appearance being a mottled opacity involving a single lobe or segment, which in some cases may be partially collapsed.

The condition is liable to be confused with viral pneumonia, but the coexistent upper respiratory infection and the minimal systemic upset are useful distinguishing features. Pulmonary tuberculosis may be erroneously diagnosed on the basis of a single radiograph. Re-examination 10 to 14 days later, following treatment with an antibiotic, will clarify the diagnosis as resolution is generally rapid in aspiration pneumonia.

Suppurative pneumonia (including pulmonary abscess)

Suppurative pneumonia is the term used to describe a form of pneumonic consolidation in which there is destruction of lung parenchyma by the inflammatory process. Although microabscess formation is a characteristic histological feature of suppurative pneumonia, it is usual to restrict the term 'pulmonary abscess' to lesions in which there is a fairly large localised collection of pus, or a cavity lined by chronic inflammatory tissue, from which pus has ruptured into a bronchus.

Suppurative pneumonia and pulmonary abscess may be produced by infection of previously healthy lung tissue with Staph. aureus or Kl. pneumoniae. These are, in effect, primary bacterial pneumonias associated with pulmonary suppuration. More frequently, suppurative pneumonia and pulmonary abscess are forms of secondary pneumonia. They may develop after the inhalation of septic material during operations on the nose, mouth or throat under general anaesthesia, or of vomitus during anaesthesia or coma.

In such circumstances gross oral sepsis may be an important predisposing factor. Bacterial infection of a pulmonary infarct or of a collapsed lobe, may also produce a suppurative pneumonia or a pulmonary abscess. The organisms isolated from the sputum may include Strep. pneumoniae, Staph. aureus, Strep. pyogenes, H. influenzae, and in some cases, anaerobic bacteria. In many cases, however, no pathogens can be isolated, particularly when antibiotics have been given.

Clinical features. These depend to a large extent on the pathogenesis of the lesion. The onset of the illness may be either insidious or acute, but cough with purulent sputum, usually large in amount, sometimes fetid and occasionally bloodstained, is present from an early stage. There is high, remittent pyrexia with shivering and sweating, and a neutrophil leucocytosis. Pleural pain is common and clubbing of the fingers may develop as early as 10 to 14 days after the onset of the illness. Progressive deterioration in general health with marked loss of weight ensues if the patient remains untreated. The rupture of a large abscess into a bronchus can be assumed when a large quantity of pus is suddenly expectorated. Such an incident is often preceded by bloodstaining of the sputum and followed by remission of the pyrexia and systemic symptoms.

Physical signs in the chest also depend on the nature of the primary pathological process. Signs of consolidation (p. 207) are the most frequent; signs of cavitation are rarely found. A pleural rub is often present.

Radiological examination. There is a homogeneous lobar or segmental opacity consistent with consolidation or collapse. A large, dense opacity, which may later cavitate and show a fluid level within it, is the characteristic finding when a frank pulmonary abscess is present.

Course and prognosis. In most cases, there is a good response to antibacterial therapy (p. 223), and although residual fibrosis and bronchiectasis are common sequelae, these seldom give rise to serious morbidity. Empyema (p. 263) may complicate the acute phase of the disease.

Prevention. Every precaution should be taken during operations on the mouth, nose and throat to prevent the inhalation of blood, tonsillar fragments, etc. Oral sepsis should be eradicated, especially if a general anaesthetic is contemplated.

Investigation of pneumonia

An attempt should always be made to establish a positive microbiological diagnosis, though this is not always possible, particularly if antibiotics have been given before specimens are submitted for examination. Direct smear examination of *sputum* by Gram and Ziehl-Neelsen stains may give an immediate indication of possible pathogens, and indicate what treatment should be prescribed. Culture (including anaerobic culture where indicated) and sensitivity testing should be carried out.

Where a microbiological diagnosis is essential, as in severely ill immunosuppressed patients, and a specimen of sputum cannot be obtained, an attempt should be made to aspirate secretions or washings from the trachea or bronchi either by bronchoscopy or by inserting a needle through the cricothyroid membrane. Transthoracic lung puncture has been advocated if the other techniques are unsuccessful, but carries the risk of pneumothorax, which may have lethal consequences in dangerously ill patients.

Blood culture should be performed in patients with severe pneumonia, and may yield a positive result when sputum examination is negative, particularly in pneumococcal pneumonia. Pneumococcal antigen may also be detected in serum.

Serological tests may be helpful, specimens being examined at 10-day intervals for viral titres. A four-fold rise suggests recent infection. Nose and throat swabs, and post-nasal and bronchial aspirates, can be cultured for viruses or examined by immunofluorescence or electron microscopy.

The *total and differential white blood count* is often below $5.0 \times 10^9/l$ in patients with viral infection, and a high neutrophil polymorph leucocytosis favours bacterial infection. The ESR is usually elevated, but is of no help in diagnosis.

Arterial blood-gas studies are of vital importance in all patients who are seriously ill and in those with a previous history of chronic respiratory disease. It is impossible to make any rational decisions on oxygen therapy unless the PO_2 and PCO_2 and the hydrogen ion concentration or pH of arterial blood are known.

Radiological examination is essential for confirmation of the diagnosis and for the early detection of complications such as pleural effusion and empyema. Follow-up radiological examination is important, because if a pneumonia fails to resolve, it may be secondary to bronchial obstruction by a carcinoma.

Complications of pneumonia

Pulmonary. In most cases, the abnormal physical signs disappear within 2 weeks and the radiographic opacity within 4 weeks. Although resolution is occasionally delayed for longer periods, and may be incomplete, particularly in patients with suppurative pneumonia, such delay is always an indication for further investigation, including bronchoscopic examination. Bronchiectasis is a common complication of suppurative pneumonia.

Pleural. Spread of the infection to the pleura may occur, with the development of a sterile pleural effusion or empyema. Staphylococcal lung abscess may be complicated by pyopneumothorax.

Cardiovascular. These are acute circulatory failure (due to septicaemia), acute pericarditis and rarely endocarditis.

Neurological. Meningism is not uncommon in children and lumbar puncture may be required to distinguish it from meningitis. Mental confusion may be a prominent feature of legionnaires' disease.

Differential diagnosis of pneumonia

The following conditions may be difficult to distinguish from pneumonia:

Pulmonary infarction, in which pyrexia is less marked and is uninfluenced by antibiotics, frank haemoptysis is common, cough is inconspicuous and the source of an embolus can be identified in a few cases.

Tuberculous pleurisy with effusion, in which the correct diagnosis can usually be suspected from the insidious onset, the virtual absence of cough and sputum, the physical signs of pleural effusion, the absence of leucocytosis, the failure of the pyrexia to respond to antibiotics, the radiological findings and the aspiration of serous fluid, in which lymphocytes predominate, from the pleural space.

Pulmonary tuberculosis, acute cases of which

may simulate pneumonia. The patient is, however, seldom as acutely ill as in other primary pneumonias, it is uncommon for the respiratory rate to be markedly increased and the white blood count is seldom above $12.0 \times 10^9/l$. The diagnosis can usually be made by radiological examination, and the demonstration of tubercle bacilli puts it beyond doubt.

Pulmonary oedema, which may be difficult to distinguish from pneumonia. If fever is present, pneumonia is the more likely diagnosis, but where there is any doubt, both an antibiotic and a diuretic should be given.

Inflammatory conditions below the diaphragm, such as cholecystitis, perforated duodenal ulcer, acute appendicitis, subphrenic abscess, generalised peritonitis, acute pancreatitis and hepatic amoebiasis, which may occasionally be mistaken for pneumonia. A carefully taken history is one of the most valuable means of determining the site and nature of the primary disease. A high temperature and a rapid respiratory rate favour a diagnosis of pneumonia, whereas tenderness of the abdominal wall suggests that the primary lesion is below the diaphragm. Sometimes radiological examination of the chest is necessary before the presence of pneumonia can be confirmed or excluded.

Treatment of pneumonia

Antimicrobial therapy. When a clinical diagnosis of pneumonia is made, provided the patient is not seriously ill, the initial treatment should consist of ampicillin, 500 mg four times daily, or co-trimoxazole, 2 tablets twice daily. Patients who are gravely ill and in whom a staphylococcal or a Gram-negative infection is suspected, should receive, in addition to ampicillin by intravenous injection, antibiotics to which the causative organism is unlikely to be resistant, for example, flucloxacillin, 250 mg 6-hourly by intravenous injection, and gentamicin, 2–5 mg/kg daily in divided doses 8-hourly by intramuscular or intravenous injection.

1. If *Strep. pneumoniae, Strep. pyogenes* or *H. influenzae* is isolated, or no pathogenic organisms are reported on culture, and the patient appears to be making satisfactory clinical progress, treatment with ampicillin or co-trimoxazole should be continued, but the dose of ampicillin can be reduced to 250 mg 6-hourly.

2. If *Staph. aureus* is isolated, treatment must be modified in accordance with the results of sensitivity tests. Alternative therapy for organisms resistant to penicillin, which is usually the case, and for patients allergic to penicillin is given on page 743.

3. *Pneumocystis carinii* pneumonia is best treated with intravenous high-dose co-trimoxazole (20 mg trimethoprim and 100 mg sulphamethoxazole per kg per day in two divided doses) with substitution of oral therapy as soon as possible.

4. *Legionella pneumophilia* is sensitive to erythromycin, but in very ill patients rifampicin 450–600 mg daily should be added.

5. *Antimicrobial therapy for other organisms* causing pneumonia is:
Actinomyces israelii—benzylpenicillin,
Klebsiella pneumoniae—chloramphenicol, mezlocillin, cefotaxime or gentamicin,
Proteus mirabilis—ampicillin, co-trimoxazole or gentamicin,
Pseudomonas aeruginosa—ticarcillin, azlocillin or ceftazidime.

6. *If bacteriological examination is uninformative* and there is no neutrophil leucocytosis in the blood, the pneumonia may be due to *Coxiella burnetii, Mycoplasma pneumoniae* or *Chlamydia psittaci*. In these circumstances, tetracycline, 500 mg four times daily is recommended. Pneumonia caused by viruses does not respond to antibiotic therapy.

7. *If an anaerobic bacterial infection* is suspected from fetor of the sputum, a combination of benzylpenicillin and metronidazole should be given.

8. *If recovery is progressing satisfactorily,* the isolation of an organism showing in vitro resistance to the antibiotic in use is not necessarily an indication for a change in treatment. If, however, the patient is not improving and is still febrile when such an organism is isolated, an appropriate change in antibiotic is imperative.

9. *Duration of therapy*. No definite rule can be laid down for the duration of chemotherapy. In most cases of uncomplicated pneumococcal pneumonia, a 7-day course of treatment is usually adequate but this may have to be extended if the

response to treatment is slow. In staphylococcal and klebsiella pneumonia, and in other forms of suppurative pneumonia, chemotherapy should be continued for a minimum of 2 weeks and should not be stopped until the causative organism has been eliminated from the sputum.

10. *Bacteraemic shock* carries a high mortality and admission to an intensive therapy unit affords the best prospect of survival. Appropriate antibiotics must be continued in high dosage and oxygenation maintained, if necessary by tracheal intubation and intermittent positive-pressure ventilation. Additional measures are described on page 48.

11. *Abscess formation.* Suppurative pneumonia is not in itself a reason for any departure from standard antibiotic policy. When an abscess cavity is present, however, it must be kept empty by regular postural drainage. Medical treatment is almost invariably successful and surgical measures nowadays are seldom required. In occasional instances, however, a large abscess may have to be drained externally or residual bronchiectasis resected.

General measures. The usual regimen of treatment for an acute infection should be instituted and attention paid to hydration, oral hygiene and care of the skin. If respiratory distress is marked the patient should be propped up comfortably with pillows or a backrest.

Cough, when distressing and unproductive, should be controlled by the measures described on page 213. When secretions are present in the bronchi the patient should be firmly encouraged to cough up sputum, even if the effort to do so causes pleural pain. In these circumstances an analgesic and the support of a hand on the painful side of the chest may ease the distress of coughing. Postural drainage is of value if the sputum is difficult to bring up, particularly if it is copious, as in suppurative pneumonia, or when pneumonia complicates bronchiectasis. Skilled physiotherapy may be invaluable.

Pleural pain should be treated with analgesics (p. 214). It can, however, be dangerous to use opiates if even a mild degree of ventilatory insufficiency is present.

Hypoxia demands oxygen therapy (p. 210).

Delirium, which in the early stages is caused mainly by the high temperature, and later by cerebral hypoxia, may have to be controlled by sedation. The safest drug to use is diazepam (5–10 mg i.m. or i.v.).

TUBERCULOSIS

Although tuberculosis is a problem of rapidly diminishing proportions in Western Europe and North America, it remains, in the words of a WHO report: 'the most important specific communicable disease in the world'. As the disease decreases in frequency there is a tendency for tuberculosis to be overlooked.

Aetiology. Three types of mycobacteria are responsible for disease in man: (1) *Myco. tuberculosis* (human type) — now the cause of almost all infections in man; (2) *Myco. bovis* — endemic in cattle, but now rarely responsible for disease in man, and (3) the *atypical* or *opportunistic* mycobacteria. The clinical importance of the last group of organisms lies in their ability to cause infection in cervical lymph nodes in children and, rarely, pulmonary disease in adults, when treatment may be a problem because the mycobacteria are primarily resistant to many drugs.

Entry of the tubercle bacillus into the body by the alimentary or respiratory tract is not necessarily followed by a clinical illness, the development of which is dependent on several other factors. Those of most practical importance are:

Age and sex. In Europe and America, tuberculosis used to affect predominantly the young people in the community, especially females, but there has been a radical change in the age and sex incidence. Thirty years ago, 80% of notifications were of patients under 45 years of age, but nowadays most patients are over that age, males predominating.

Natural resistance. Susceptibility to tuberculosis is not inherited in the strict sense of the word, but the fact that certain races, and even certain regional groups, are more prone to develop the disease suggests that natural resistance varies from race to race and from region to region. The natural resistance of a community tends to rise as the period of exposure increases. Immigrants to Britain from Asia are more prone to have the disease than the indigenous population, and tend to have more florid types of tuberculosis.

Standard of living. The prevalence of tuberculosis diminishes as social and economic conditions improve. Poor housing with associated overcrowding increases the risk of massive infection or reinfection.

Conditions affecting individual patients. Diabetes mellitus, gastrectomy and silicosis all predispose to the development of tuberculosis, as does treatment with corticosteroids or immunosuppressive drugs.

Pathology. The initial '*primary*' tuberculous *infection* usually occurs in the lung but occasionally in the tonsil or alimentary tract, especially the ileocaecal region. The primary infection differs from subsequent infections in that the primary focus in lung, tonsil or bowel is almost invariably accompanied by caseous lesions in the regional lymph nodes, i.e. in the mediastinal, cervical or mesenteric groups respectively.

In most people the primary infection and the associated lymph node lesions heal and calcify. In a few, healing, particularly in lymph nodes, is incomplete and viable tubercle bacilli may enter the blood-stream. In consequence tuberculous lesions may develop elsewhere. '*Haematogenous*' *lesions* of this kind are most common in the lungs, bones, joints and kidneys. Such lesions may develop months or even years after the primary infection.

The primary infection may in some cases fail to heal. A primary pulmonary lesion, particularly when it occurs during adolescence or early adult life, may lead to progressive pulmonary tuberculosis. A tuberculous mediastinal lymph node, in children especially, may compress a lobar or segmental bronchus (rarely a main bronchus) and produce pulmonary collapse. Occasionally the node may ulcerate through the bronchial wall and discharge caseous material into the lumen, with the production of acute tuberculous lesions in the related lobe or segment. Infection may also be carried by lymphatics from tuberculous mediastinal lymph nodes to the pleura or pericardium with the production of tuberculous pleurisy or pericarditis. Comparable complications may occur when the primary lesion is in the tonsil or gut, e.g. 'cold abscess' of the neck or tuberculous peritonitis.

Rarely, a caseous tuberculous focus ruptures into a vein and produces acute dissemination throughout the body, a condition known as *acute miliary tuberculosis*. Meningitis often complicates this condition.

Progressive pulmonary tuberculosis may develop directly from a primary lesion or it may occur later, following reactivation of an incompletely healed primary focus. Alternatively it may be the result of reinfection.

Postprimary pulmonary tuberculosis is the term used to describe lung disease, the characteristic pathological feature of which is the tuberculous cavity, formed when the caseated and liquefied centre of a tuberculous pulmonary lesion is discharged into a bronchus. Extension of infection to the pleura causes tuberculous pleurisy, which is sometimes accompanied by effusion and is occasionally followed by the development of a tuberculous empyema. Blood-borne dissemination to other organs is uncommon in post-primary pulmonary tuberculosis.

Clinical features. There are two groups of clinical features in tuberculosis:

1. Those due to the systemic effects of the disease, which include lassitude, impairment of appetite, loss of weight, anaemia, sweating especially during sleep, tachycardia and pyrexia. The last is usually most marked in the evening and sometimes occurs only at this time. Absence of symptoms does not mean that the disease is inactive.

2. Those caused by the local effects of the tuberculous lesions, which are summarised below according to anatomical site:

Lungs and bronchi: cough, sputum, haemoptysis, dyspnoea.

Pleura: pleural pain, dyspnoea due to pleural effusion.

Larynx: hoarseness, stridor.

Tongue: ulceration (rare).

Intestine: diarrhoea, malabsorption or intestinal obstruction.

Peritoneum: ascites, intestinal obstruction.

Pericardium: pericardial effusion, constrictive pericarditis later.

Kidneys and bladder: haematuria, increased frequency of micturition. These are relatively late developments, early renal lesions being symptomless.

Epididymis: painless craggy swelling, sinus formation later.

Fallopian tubes: salpingitis, tubal abscess, infertility.

Brain: tuberculoma with or without focal neurological signs.

Meninges: headache, neck stiffness, vomiting, coma.

Lymph nodes: enlargement of nodes, often with 'cold' abscess and sinus formation later.

Adrenal glands: Addison's disease.

Bones and joints: arthritis, osteomyelitis, 'cold' abscesses.

Skin: erythema nodosum, lupus vulgaris.

Eyes: phlyctenular keratoconjunctivitis, iritis, choroiditis.

In the sections which follow an account is given of those manifestations of tuberculosis which involve the lungs, namely primary pulmonary tuberculosis, acute miliary tuberculosis and postprimary pulmonary tuberculosis. In some cases the pleura is also involved. For information regarding other manifestations of tuberculosis the reader should refer to appropriate sections of the book. The treatment and prevention of tuberculosis are dealt with on pages 230–233.

Primary pulmonary tuberculosis

The pathological features of this type of tuberculosis have been described on page 225. The primary infection usually occurs in childhood. A history of contact with a case of active pulmonary tuberculosis is obtained in many instances.

Clinical features. In the vast majority of patients the primary infection produces no symptoms or signs and passes unnoticed unless routine radiological examination of the chest happens to be carried out at the appropriate time or serial tuberculin tests show conversion from negative to positive.

In a few patients the primary infection produces a febrile illness which is generally mild and lasts for no more than 7 to 14 days. It is unusual for gross focal symptoms or signs to develop but a slight dry cough is occasionally present. The

leucocyte count is usually normal but the ESR is raised.

The primary infection may be accompanied by *erythema nodosum*. This condition is characterised by bluish-red, raised, tender cutaneous lesions on the shins and, less commonly, on the thighs, and is associated in some cases with pyrexia and polyarthralgia. Erythema nodosum may be the first clinical indication of a tuberculous infection. In such cases the tuberculin reaction (below) is always strongly positive and evidence of primary tuberculosis can usually be detected on the chest radiograph. Erythema nodosum is, however, seen in conditions other than primary tuberculosis, e.g. sarcoidosis, streptococcal infections and drug reactions.

Occasionally the primary pulmonary infection pursues a progressive course (p. 225). Symptoms and signs due to its complications may appear either during the course of the initial illness or after a latent interval of weeks or months. Such complications include pleurisy or pleural effusion (p. 263), lobar or segmental collapse (p. 251), acute miliary tuberculosis (p. 227), tuberculous meningitis (p. 639), and postprimary pulmonary tuberculosis (p. 228).

Investigation. The three most valuable diagnostic investigations in primary pulmonary tuberculosis are:

1. *Radiological examination of the chest*. In children this usually shows unilateral enlargement of the hilar lymph nodes and demonstrates the primary intrapulmonary lesion if it is large enough. In adolescents and young adults the lymph node component of the primary complex is usually less conspicuous than in children and the pulmonary lesion more prominent. Complications such as pleural effusion, lobar or segmental collapse and acute progressive pulmonary tuberculosis may be superimposed.

2. *Tuberculin test*. With the Mantoux technique a solution of Old Tuberculin or purified protein derivative (PPD) tuberculin is injected intradermally on the flexor aspect of the forearm. The test is regarded as positive if, 2 to 4 days after injection, there is a reaction consisting of a raised area of inflammatory oedema not less than 5 mm in diameter, with surrounding erythema.

The test should first be carried out with 1

tuberculin unit (TU) in 0.1 ml of normal saline. If there is no reaction it should be repeated with 10 TU in the same volume of saline. In order to obtain accurate results it is essential to use freshly prepared dilutions of tuberculin. Differential tuberculin testing with antigens prepared from other mycobacteria, e.g. PPD-A (*Myco. avium*) or PPD-Y (*Myco. kansasii*) is often a satisfactory method of distinguishing atypical mycobacterial infection from tuberculosis.

The younger the patient the greater is the diagnostic significance of a positive tuberculin test. A repeatedly negative test over a period of 6 weeks from the onset of symptoms practically rules out tuberculosis except in the elderly, after acute exanthemata, in the later stages of miliary tuberculosis and tuberculous meningitis and in patients taking immunosuppressive drugs. The tuberculin test is almost invariably negative in patients with sarcoidosis.

Tuberculin testing is an essential part of the examination of family contacts. Apart from its value as a diagnostic measure it indicates which of the contacts should be vaccinated with BCG. When large numbers are being tested, particularly children, a *multiple puncture technique*, which is quick and almost painless, is preferable to the Mantoux test. A disposable tine test unit should be used for this purpose. It has four prongs ('tines') 2 mm in length mounted on a disc and coated with Old Tuberculin. If firmly pressed on the skin of the forearm, it yields results as reliable as those obtained with the Heaf unit which, being difficult to sterilise, may carry some risk of transmitting viral infections such as hepatitis or AIDS.

The test should be read after 3 days and the following four grades of positivity are recognised:

Grade I: One or two faint papules
       II: Four discrete papules
       III: The area encircled by the papules is completely indurated.
       IV: Any reaction which is greater than III, including central necrosis.

Reaction in grades III and IV indicates infection with mammalian tubercle bacilli and a grade I reaction may indicate infection with atypical mycobacteria. The significance of a grade II reaction is uncertain.

3. *Bacteriological examination.* Sputum is seldom available in cases of primary pulmonary tuberculosis, but tubercle bacilli can sometimes be isolated by culture of fasting gastric washings or of secretion obtained by swabbing the larynx. At least three specimens should be examined. The isolation of tubercle bacilli is absolute proof of the diagnosis, but a negative result does not exclude it.

Prognosis. Since primary pulmonary tuberculosis and its complications respond satisfactorily to antituberculosis chemotherapy (p. 230), which should be given in every case, the prognosis is excellent.

Miliary tuberculosis

The pathogenesis of this condition has already been discussed. Hitherto it has occurred chiefly in children and young adults. With the changing age-structure of tuberculosis in many countries it is now affecting persons in older age groups in whom it tends to take the form of an insidious illness — the so-called 'cryptic' type — which is often difficult to diagnose. Before the introduction of chemotherapy the disease was invariably fatal but most treated patients now recover completely.

Clinical features. The disease may start suddenly or may be preceded by a few weeks of vague ill-health. In children and young adults the systemic disturbance rapidly becomes profound. In particular there is a high pyrexia with drenching sweats during sleep, marked tachycardia, loss of weight and usually progressive anaemia. Cough and dyspnoea are only occasionally present. There may be no abnormal physical signs in the lungs, although widespread crepitations may be heard late in the disease. The liver is often enlarged and the spleen may be palpable. Choroidal tubercles may be visible on ophthalmoscopy but are rarely present in the elderly. Leucocytosis is usually absent or slight. If chemotherapy is not given death takes place within days or weeks.

'Cryptic' miliary tuberculosis occurs in older age groups, particularly females. Lassitude and exhaustion, loss of weight, and anaemia are common presenting features. Respiratory symptoms are rare, and the characteristic miliary shadows are absent. A variety of blood disorders — neutropenia, pancytopenia and leukaemoid reaction—may be found. The clinical features are often non-specific and diagnosis is made at autopsy.

Investigation. The diagnosis of acute miliary tuberculosis can be made with confidence only when radiological examination of the chest shows the characteristic 'miliary' mottling symmetrically distributed throughout both lung fields or when choroidal tubercles are seen. The diagnosis can often be suspected at an earlier stage by the symptoms, progressive clinical deterioration, persistent pyrexia and splenomegaly.

Bacteriological confirmation should be sought by culture of sputum, urine or bone-marrow. In difficult cases, liver biopsy may be diagnostic. Although the tuberculin reaction is usually positive in young patients, a negative result does not always exclude acute miliary tuberculosis, as tuberculin sensitivity is occasionally depressed in the later stages of the illness.

In patients suspected to have the cryptic form of miliary tuberculosis a therapeutic trial of chemotherapy with ethambutol and isoniazid (p. 230) is indicated; if the diagnosis is correct, clinical improvement is usually evident within 10 days.

Prognosis. Antituberculosis chemotherapy (p. 230) has reduced the mortality of miliary tuberculosis from 100% to virtually zero, providing the diagnosis is made at an early stage.

Postprimary pulmonary tuberculosis

Most of the morbidity and mortality from tuberculosis is caused by this form of the disease. Although in developing countries it is most prevalent in adolescence and early adult life, the majority of cases in Western Europe and North America now occur in middle-aged and elderly subjects.

The lesions are most frequently situated in the upper lobes. The disease is often bilateral. Occasionally, a whole lobe may be consolidated in acute pneumonic tuberculosis.

Clinical features. The onset of postprimary pulmonary tuberculosis is usually insidious, with the gradual development of general symptoms or of cough and sputum. Sometimes a dramatic incident such as haemoptysis, pleural pain or a spontaneous pneumothorax marks the onset, but

the diagnosis is now frequently made by radiography before any symptoms have appeared.

The following respiratory symptoms may occur during the course of postprimary tuberculosis:

Cough may be one of the earliest symptoms or may not be troublesome until a late stage.

Sputum, like cough, may not become a prominent feature until the disease has reached an advanced stage. It is usually mucoid at first but later becomes purulent.

Haemoptysis, in the early stages, is due to the erosion of a small vessel in a caseating lesion and the bleeding is usually slight. In the late stages it can originate from a large vessel in the wall of a cavity and haemorrhage may be large, occasionally fatal.

Dyspnoea on exertion is usually a late symptom, but may develop acutely when due to a spontaneous pneumothorax or to a rapidly developing pleural effusion.

Pleural pain is usually due to pleurisy but occasionally to spontaneous pneumothorax.

At first, no abnormal physical signs may be present, but despite this an extensive lesion may be visible radiologically. The earliest physical signs consist of a few crepitations, usually situated over one or other lung apex posteriorly. Ultimately, physical signs of consolidation, cavitation and fibrosis may develop, and occasionally those of pleurisy, with or without effusion, or spontaneous pneumothorax (Table 8.1).

Radiological examination. This is of paramount importance for diagnosis in the early stages before physical signs appear and for assessment of the extent and progress of the disease.

The earliest radiological change is an ill-defined opacity or opacities, usually situated in one of the upper lobes. In more advanced cases opacities are larger and more widespread, and may be bilateral. Occasionally there is a dense, homogeneous shadow involving a whole lobe ('pneumonic tuberculosis'). An area or areas of translucency within the opacities indicates cavitation. Very large cavities may be visible in some cases. The presence of cavitation in an untreated case usually indicates that the disease is active. When fibrosis is marked the trachea and heart shadow are displaced towards the side of the lesion.

The radiological appearances of pleural effusion

and pneumothorax, which may accompany those of pulmonary tuberculosis, are described on pages 262 and 265.

Diagnosis. The symptoms and signs suggesting a diagnosis of tuberculosis have already been stated. The grounds on which pulmonary tuberculosis should be suspected are: (1) unexplained cough persisting for more than a few weeks; (2) haemoptysis; (3) pleural pain not associated with an acute illness; (4) spontaneous pneumothorax (although most cases are not caused by tuberculosis); (5) unexplained tiredness or loss of weight, even in the absence of respiratory symptoms.

The presence of any of these symptoms demands immediate radiological examination of the lungs and, if an abnormality is found, the examination of at least three specimens of sputum for tubercle bacilli. When bacilli are numerous, the diagnosis can readily be made by microscopical examination of sputum smears stained by the Ziehl-Neelsen method. Culture of sputum (or fasting gastric washings or laryngeal swabs, if no sputum can be obtained) is necessary when smears are negative and essential for the detection of drug resistance (p. 231). Cultural methods are thus of great practical value and should be used in the examination of every specimen, if facilities permit.

In the vast majority of cases the diagnosis of pulmonary tuberculosis can be made with confidence by radiological examination of the chest and examination of the sputum. In some cases it is necessary to carry out further radiological examination after a course of treatment with an antibiotic, such as ampicillin, in order to exclude an acute inflammatory cause for an abnormal X-ray shadow.

Complications

Pleurisy with or without effusion (p. 261).

Spontaneous pneumothorax may be due to rupture of a tuberculous lesion into the pleural space (p. 265).

Tuberculous empyema or pyopneumothorax (p. 265) may complicate spontaneous pneumothorax.

Tuberculous laryngitis (p. 226) usually occurs as a complication of advanced pulmonary disease.

Tuberculous enteritis is practically confined to advanced cases. It is due to the swallowing of heavily infected sputum which causes ulceration of the ileum and diarrhoea.

Ischiorectal abscess and fistula-in-ano. The abscess forms as a result of tubercle bacilli passing through the rectal mucosa. Secondary pyogenic infection invariably occurs.

Dissemination of tuberculosis via the bloodstream is very unusual in postprimary pulmonary tuberculosis, but may occur in advanced cases.

Respiratory failure (p. 204) and *right ventricular failure* (p. 148) are important late complications of extensive pulmonary destruction and fibrosis. Although the infection itself can be controlled, the residual pulmonary damage may leave the patient seriously disabled.

Secondary infection of a healed cavity with fungi such as *Aspergillus fumigatus* may lead to the development of an aspergilloma (p. 233). This can be a cause of haemoptysis, as can post-tuberculous bronchiectasis.

Prognosis. With the advent of effective chemotherapy there has been a remarkable decline in the mortality from pulmonary tuberculosis. Provided the tubercle bacilli are not initially drug-resistant and chemotherapy is used correctly, a fatal outcome is extremely uncommon, even if the disease has reached an advanced stage when it is first recognised. Late complications of respiratory failure and secondary infection with pyogenic bacteria or fungi can be prevented if pulmonary tuberculosis is diagnosed at a reasonably early stage and is efficiently treated.

THE TREATMENT OF TUBERCULOSIS

General principles

Antituberculosis chemotherapy is by far the most important measure in the treatment of all forms of tuberculosis and should be given to every patient with active disease.

Rest is unimportant except in a few specific circumstances. The majority of patients are ambulant throughout treatment, many of them remaining at work. Immobilisation is of course necessary in certain forms of skeletal tuberculosis.

Isolation of patients who are excreting tubercle bacilli and who are therefore potentially infectious has previously been an important principle. The observation made in Madras that the frequency of disease amongst contacts was no greater when the patient was treated at home than in a sanatorium has led to the adoption of a policy whereby the majority of patients are treated wholly as outpatients. However, many authorities still prefer to isolate patients from contact with young children. An initial period of treatment in hospital, as distinct from isolation, may be recommended for patients who cannot be relied upon to take their drugs regularly and for those who present difficult therapeutic problems.

Surgical treatment such as pulmonary resection, nephrectomy or removal of superficial lymph nodes is now rarely required. However, drainage of an abscess from tuberculous lymph nodes or of an empyema may be necessary. Surgical treatment of tuberculosis of the spine may be essential to prevent paraplegia.

Chemotherapy

Effective treatment of tuberculosis demands not only a detailed knowledge of the drugs available but also of the most appropriate regimen for the individual patient.

In Britain, five drugs—rifampicin, isoniazid, ethambutol, streptomycin and pyrazinamide— are normally considered in the initial treatment of tuberculosis. Thiacetazone, which is cheap, is widely used in developing countries. Pyrazinamide is particularly useful in the treatment of tuberculous meningitis because it diffuses well into the cerebrospinal fluid. Apart from a few minor variations in dose and duration of treatment (see below and p. 231) the policy governing the use of antituberculosis drugs is the same for all forms of the disease.

The drugs should be used in the following once daily doses:

Rifampicin †	Children	10–20 mg/kg
	Adults weighing less than 50 kg and in the elderly	450 mg
	Adults weighing more than 50 kg	600 mg
Isoniazid	Children	3 mg/kg
	Adults	200–300 mg
	Intermittent regimen	15 mg/kg*
	Miliary/meningitis	10–12 mg/kg*

Ethambutol	Children and adults:	
	initial 8 weeks	25 mg/kg
	subsequently	15 mg/kg
	In renal failure	According to serum levels
Strepto-mycin sulphate	Children	30 mg/kg
	Adults under 40 years and weighing more than 45 kg	1 g
	Adults 40–60 years or weighing less than 45 kg	0.75 g
	Adults over 60 years or in patients with renal failure	According to serum levels
	Intermittent regimens	0.75–1 g
Pyrazin-amide	Children and adults	35 mg/kg (max 2.5 g)

† Taken at least 30 minutes before breakfast.
* Plus pyridoxine 10 mg to prevent peripheral neuropathy (p. 74).

ADVERSE EFFECTS. In choosing a suitable drug regimen for individual patients it is important to bear in mind those side-effects which are particularly liable to cause serious chronic disability, such as vestibular disturbance due to streptomycin which accordingly must be prescribed with caution. Even in the relatively low dose recommended for ethambutol, a few patients develop optic neuritis and some are left with a permanent visual defect. This potential hazard must be taken into consideration whenever ethambutol is prescribed, particularly in children.

Streptomycin and occasionally isoniazid, ethambutol and rifampicin may produce a hypersensitivity reaction, consisting of pyrexia and an erythematous skin eruption, which usually develops 2 to 4 weeks after treatment is started.

Rifampicin, which colours the urine orange-pink, is a potent liver enzyme inducer (p. 330) and should be used with appropriate caution when the following drugs are prescribed: oestrogens (e.g. oral contraceptives), warfarin, corticosteroids, oral hypoglycaemic drugs, phenytoin and digoxin. It should, if possible, be avoided in patients with liver disease.

The principal adverse effects of the most commonly prescribed drugs are:

Rifampicin: drug interaction (see above); hypersensitivity (occasionally, see above); hepatitis (rare); vasculitis (rare); fever, skin flushing, nausea and abdominal pain, breathlessness and wheeze (intermittent regimens only). Rifampicin should not be given again to any patient in whom it has caused vasculitis.

Isoniazid: hypersensitivity (occasionally, see above); polyneuropathy (rare); lack of mental concentration (rare).

Ethambutol: optic neuritis (see above); hypersensitivity (rare, see above).

Streptomycin: vestibular disturbance (see above); hypersensitivity (see above); deafness (rare).

Pyrazinamide: hepatitis; gout; hypersensitivity (rare).

REGIMENS. The following regimens are virtually 100% effective in the treatment of tuberculosis:

1. *Duration 9 months*

Initial phase (2 months): ethambutol or streptomycin plus isoniazid plus rifampicin.

Continuation phase (7 months): isoniazid plus rifampicin.

2. *Duration 6 months*

Initial phase (2 months): ethambutol or streptomycin plus isoniazid plus rifampicin plus pyrazinamide.

Continuation phase (4 months): isoniazid plus rifampicin.

Any patient who cannot be trusted to take oral antituberculosis drugs regularly without supervision should be kept in hospital for the initial (2-month) phase of treatment. Thereafter, for 10 months, the following should be given at home twice weekly (at 3 and 4 day intervals): streptomycin sulphate (1 g i.m.), and isoniazid (15 mg/kg by mouth), with pyridoxine (10 mg), to prevent peripheral neuropathy. This type of chemotherapy should be wholly supervised, the tablets being administered at the same time as the injections.

Inexpensive treatment regimens. In developing countries it will usually be impossible for economic reasons to adhere to ideal chemotherapeutic regimens. The following inexpensive forms of treatment are reasonably effective if administered for 12 months: (1) Streptomycin (1g) by intramuscular injection *plus* isoniazid (15 mg/kg) by mouth with pyridoxine (10 mg) on 2 days per week. This is 90 to 95% effective: if daily treatment with standard doses of streptomycin and isoniazid can be afforded for the initial phase of 2–3 months, the effectiveness of this regimen is nearly 100% in the absence of primary drug resistance. (2) Isoniazid (300 mg) *plus* thiacetazone (150 mg) given in a single daily dose by mouth is extremely cheap, and is about 80 to 95% effective.

RESPONSE TO TREATMENT. If the bacilli at the start of treatment are fully sensitive to the drugs it is most unusual, even in advanced cases, for cultures to remain positive for longer than 6 months. Where facilities for sensitivity testing do not exist, reliance must be placed on smear examination.

DRUG-RESISTANT TUBERCLE BACILLI. The treatment of patients infected with drug-resistant tubercle bacilli presents a problem requiring specialised knowledge. Additional drugs available for the treatment of such cases are: Sodium aminosalicylate (PAS–5 g b.d. by mouth), ethionamide or prothionamide (0.75–1 g once daily by mouth), capreomycin (0.75–1 g once daily i.m.) and cycloserine (0.75–1 g once daily by mouth).

Corticosteroid drugs

These agents suppress the cell-mediated reaction induced by the tubercle bacillus and by interfering with tissue defence mechanisms may promote a rapid dissemination of infection. If, however, a corticosteroid drug is given in conjunction with effective antituberculous chemotherapy, it may exert a favourable influence on the course of the disease by reducing the severity both of the local inflammatory reaction and of the associated systemic disturbance. In acute pulmonary tuberculosis such treatment will rapidly relieve pyrexia and will often produce a dramatic improvement in the radiological appearances. The effect is temporary and ceases when the corticosteroid drug is withdrawn, but it may save the lives of patients with fulminating infection by enabling them to survive until antituberculous chemotherapy has had time to exert its influence. Prednisolone is given in a dose of 20 mg daily for about 3 months.

Corticosteroid drugs in combination with chemotherapy may also be of value in tuberculosis affecting the pleura, pericardium, intrathoracic or superficial lymph nodes, the eye and meninges. Whenever there is evidence of ureteric obstruction, corticosteroids should be administered in addition to chemotherapy, for such treatment significantly reduces the need for surgery.

Symptomatic treatment

Pleural pain due to pleurisy or spontaneous pneumothorax, *cough* and *haemoptysis* are treated as described on page 213. *Fever and sweating* usually subside soon after chemotherapy is started. *Hoarseness* is usually due to tuberculous laryngitis, which responds rapidly to specific chemotherapy. *Diarrhoea*, when persistent in a patient with pulmonary tuberculosis, is usually due to tuberculous enteritis which in most cases is rapidly controlled by chemotherapy.

The prevention of tuberculosis

Mortality rates are no longer considered so important in the assessment of the success of control measures because of the very low rates now existing in some countries and the inaccuracy of certification in the many countries where tuberculosis remains a major problem. Notification rates are of limited value because of the adoption of varying standards, but the annual recording of the number of smear-positive patients with pulmonary tuberculosis is a useful indication of the efficiency of preventive measures.

The *tuberculin index* is another useful parameter. It is the percentage of positive reactors to tuberculin at a standard age, e.g. 5 or 13 years. It is important to assess the possible influence of the prevalence of atypical mycobacteria in the community and of BCG vaccination policy on the tuberculin index.

The following control measures are important in the achievement of the goal of eradication of the disease.

Improvement in socio-economic conditions mainly in respect of adequate housing, ventilation and nutrition may still be the most important control measure of all.

Case-finding. Mass radiography is an expensive method of case-finding and should now be used in a selective manner concentrating on certain specific groups. The highest yield by far is from patients referred by general practitioners because of symptoms. Open access to chest radiography for general practitioners and minimum waiting time for patients are essential for success.

Sputum-smear examination is an important and inexpensive method of case-finding in developing countries.

Contact examination achieves a high yield in case-finding. Efforts should be concentrated on the immediate examination of household contacts of sputum smear-positive patients especially amongst contacts under 25 years of age.

Chemotherapy. The proper use of modern highly-effective chemotherapy, by rendering patients non-infectious rapidly, makes a very important contribution to the control of the disease.

Isolation of patients is rarely considered necessary nowadays even in smear-positive patients except where very young children are at risk, provided the source case is being properly treated by chemotherapy.

BCG vaccination. This is carried out by the administration of freeze-dried vaccine, reconstituted at the time of use, by the intradermal route (0.1ml) injected at the junction of the upper and middle thirds of the upper arm. Complications such as local abscess formation and enlargement of regional lymph nodes are very rare. BCG vaccine should not be given in the presence of immunodeficiency. The duration of protection is up to 7 years. Vaccination reduces the incidence of pulmonary tuberculosis in young adults by 80% and minimises the risk of serious disseminated disease — miliary tuberculosis and tuberculous meningitis.

Policy in relation to BCG vaccination in a community depends upon the size of the problem locally. If the infection rate is very low (1% or less) vaccination is inappropriate on the grounds of cost and the fact that BCG interferes with the diagnostic value of the tuberculin test in such a situation. Where there are many positive tuberculin reactors, as occurs in communities with low living standards, vaccination of the newborn is usually indicated. Where infection rates are falling to low levels, vaccination at puberty is practical.

Chemoprophylaxis. The concept of administering chemotherapy to individuals in order to try to prevent the development of tuberculosis is adopted in different communities with varying degrees of enthusiasm. Chemoprophylaxis, using isoniazid (5 mg/kg by mouth) daily for 1 year, can be employed in: (1) non-BCG vaccinated tuberculin positive children under 3 years of age, as this is a vulnerable group in respect of miliary tuberculosis and tuberculous meningitis; (2) unvaccinated individuals who have recently become tuberculin-positive; (3) patients on immunosuppressive drugs.

Chemoprophylaxis may also be considered in: (1) tuberculin-positive adolescents with a high level of tuberculin sensitivity; (2) infants of highly infectious parents, when isoniazid-resistant BCG vaccine may be administered, isoniazid chemoprophylaxis being given for 6 weeks thereafter.

Elimination of bovine infection. Although such infection is now extremely rare in Western countries constant vigilance will be required to ensure that it remains so.

RESPIRATORY DISEASES CAUSED BY FUNGI

Most fungi encountered by man are harmless saprophytes, but some species may in certain circumstances infect human tissue or promote damaging allergic reactions.

The term *mycosis* is applied to disease caused by fungal infection. Predisposing factors include metabolic disorders such as diabetes mellitus, toxic states such as chronic alcoholism, diseases in which immunological responses are disturbed such as AIDS, treatment with corticosteroids and immunosuppressive drugs, and radiotherapy. Local factors, such as tissue damage by suppuration or necrosis and the elimination of the competitive influence of a normal bacterial flora by antibiotics, may also facilitate fungal infection.

Allergic reactions to fungi may cause bronchial asthma (*Aspergillus fumigatus* and *Cladosporium herbarum*), bronchopulmonary eosinophilia (*A. fumigatus*) or extrinsic allergic alveolitis (*Micropolyspora faeni, Thermoactinomyces vulgaris, Coniosporium corticale* and *A. clavatus*). These conditions are described in the following section on allergic diseases of the respiratory tract.

The diagnosis of fungal diseases is usually made by mycological examination of the sputum, supported by serological tests for precipitating antibodies, and in some instances by skin sensitivity tests.

Aspergillosis. This is the most common res-piratory mycosis in Britain. Inhaled air-borne spores of *Aspergillus fumigatus* lodge and germinate in damaged pulmonary tissue. In some cases the fungal infection remains localised to the site of the original lesion, but, particularly in immuno-deficient or immunosuppressed patients, it may spread rapidly, with the production of consolidation, necrosis and cavitation and grave systemic disturbance (*invasive pulmonary aspergillosis*).

When a pre-existing pulmonary cavity or cyst is infected by *A. fumigatus,* a large spherical mass of fungal mycelium may form within the cavity, producing on radiological examination a tumour-like opacity to which the term *aspergilloma* is applied. This type of lesion can readily be distinguished from a peripheral bronchial carcinoma by the presence of a crescent of air between the mycelial mass and the cavity wall. An aspergilloma often produces no specific symptoms, but may be responsible for recurrent haemoptysis, often severe.

Whenever a large amount of mycelium is present in a pulmonary cavity, or in any other lesion, precipitating antibodies can be detected in the serum by means of a gel diffusion test, using an antigen derived from *A. fumigatus*. This test is of considerable diagnostic value.

Candidosis. Occasionally, in debilitated subjects oral thrush (p. 277) extends into the respiratory tract to involve the bronchi or lungs.

Other pulmonary mycoses. These, all of which are rare, include nocardiosis, cryptococcosis (p. 770), mucormycosis, blastomycosis (p. 770) and sporotrichosis (p. 768). Only the first three of these conditions have been encountered in Britain. In a somewhat different category are histoplasmosis (p. 768) and coccidioidomycosis (p. 770), which are endemic in certain areas of North America and Africa, and produce local or systemic granulomatous lesions resembling tuberculosis.

Treatment of the pulmonary mycoses is difficult and unsatisfactory. The administration of antibacterial drugs should be stopped, and antifungal agents substituted. Nystatin or natamycin by inhalation may control the more superficial respiratory mycoses involving the trachea and bronchi. For grave pulmonary infections amphotericin (p. 46), a potent but highly toxic antifungal agent, may have to be given intravenously. Flucytosine and the antifungal imidazoles (p. 46) may be useful in the treatment of less severe infections. The effective dose of amphotericin, and thus its toxic effects on the kidney, can be reduced by combining it with flucytosine. Surgical treatment for an aspergilloma may have to be considered if severe haemoptysis occurs.

ALLERGIC DISEASES

Three types of allergic response are concerned in the production of respiratory disease. The anaphylactic response (p. 25), mediated by immunoglobulin IgE, is associated with an immediate hypersensitivity reaction, the clinical manifestations of which include allergic rhinitis and bronchial asthma. The tuberculin test is the classical example of delayed hypersensitivity. The immune complex response, possibly associated with a delayed hypersensitivity reaction may contribute to the production of allergic alveolitis. Both anaphylactic and immune complex reactions may be concerned in the production of some forms of bronchopulmonary eosinophilia, such as allergic aspergillosis.

ALLERGIC RHINITIS

This is a disorder in which there are episodes of nasal congestion, watery nasal discharge and sneezing. It may be *seasonal* or *perennial*.

Aetiology. Allergic rhinitis is due to an immediate hypersensitivity reaction in the nasal mucosa (p. 25). The antigens concerned in the seasonal form of the disorder are pollens from grasses, flowers, weeds or trees. Grass pollen is responsible for *hay fever (pollenosis)*, the most common type of seasonal allergic rhinitis in Britain, and this disorder is at its peak between May and July.

Perennial allergic rhinitis may be a specific reaction to antigens derived from house dust, fungal spores or animal dander, but similar symptoms can be caused by physical or chemical irritants, such as pungent odours or fumes, including strong perfumes, cold air and dry atmospheres. In this context the term 'allergic' is a misnomer.

Clinical features. In the seasonal type there are frequent sudden attacks of sneezing, with profuse watery nasal discharge and nasal obstruction. These attacks last for a few hours, and are often accompanied by smarting and watering of the eyes and conjunctival injection. In the perennial type the symptoms are similar, but more continuous and generally less severe.

In seasonal allergic rhinitis, skin sensitivity tests with the relevant antigen are usually positive, and are thus of diagnostic value, but these tests are less useful in perennial rhinitis, and may all be negative.

Treatment. The following symptomatic measures, singly or in combination, are usually effective in both seasonal and perennial allergic rhinitis: (1) an antihistamine drug, such as terfenadine (60 mg b.d.); (2) sodium cromoglycate nasal spray, one metered dose of a 2% solution, into each nostril 4 to 6 times daily; (3) beclomethasone dipropionate or budesonide nasal spray, one or two metered doses of 50 μg into each nostril twice daily.

Patients failing to respond to these measures may obtain symptomatic relief from intramuscular injection of a long-acting corticosteroid preparation, but this form of treatment should be reserved for occasional use in patients whose symptoms are very severe and interfere seriously with school, business or social activities.

Prevention. In the seasonal type an attempt should be made to reduce exposure to pollen, for example by avoiding country districts and keeping indoors as much as possible, with the windows closed, during the pollen season. Some patients with hay fever may benefit from pre-seasonal hyposensitisation (p. 238) with a grass pollen extract. The prevention of perennial rhinitis consists of avoiding, as far as possible, exposure to any identifiable aetiological factors. Specific hyposensitisation is of little value.

BRONCHIAL ASTHMA

Bronchial asthma is characterised by paroxysms of dyspnoea accompanied by wheezing, resulting from narrowing of the bronchial airways by muscle spasm, mucosal swelling or viscid secretion. The airflow obstruction, which characteristically fluctuates markedly, causes mismatching of alveolar ventilation and perfusion and increases the work of breathing. Being more marked during expiration it also causes air to be 'trapped' in the lungs. The narrowed bronchi can no longer be effectively cleared of mucus by the act of coughing, and in patients with severe acute asthma many of the smaller bronchi become obstructed by mucus. This is usually the most conspicuous finding at autopsy. Death can occur from alveolar hypoventilation and severe arterial hypoxaemia, culminating in cardiac arrest.

Aetiology. Asthma in most cases starts either in childhood or in middle age. 'Early onset' asthma is slightly more common in males, and 'late onset' asthma in females.

Early onset asthma generally occurs in atopic individuals, i.e. those who readily form IgE antibodies to commonly encountered allergens (p. 236). Such individuals can be identified by skin sensitivity tests (p. 237), which produce positive reactions to a wide range of common allergens. They often suffer from other allergic disorders, such as allergic rhinitis and eczema, and a family history of these disorders and of 'early onset' asthma is common. It is unusual for a single allergen to be the sole cause of asthma, and clinical experience indicates that many different allergens are implicated in almost every case, although the importance of each of them may vary from time to time.

Late onset asthma generally occurs in non-atopic individuals, and it would appear that external allergens play no part in the production of this form of the disease, to which the term 'intrinsic asthma' is sometimes applied (Fig. 8.3).

The allergens responsible for asthma in atopic individuals generally enter the bronchi with the inspired air, and are derived from organic material, such as pollen, mite-containing house dust, feathers, animal dander and fungal spores. Previous exposure to these agents will have stimulated the formation of IgE and an anaphylactic antigen-antibody reaction in the bronchi may follow further exposure to specific allergen. This causes the release, from mast cells, of pharmacologically active substances which provoke bronchial constriction and an inflammatory reaction of

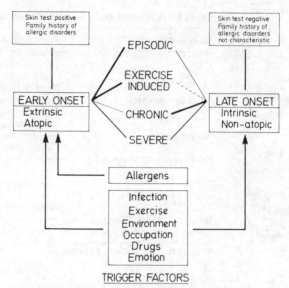

Fig. 8.3 Aetiology and types of asthma.

allergic type in the bronchial wall. Much less frequently, similar effects may be produced by ingested allergens derived from certain foods, such as fish, eggs, milk, yeasts and wheat, which presumably reach the bronchi via the bloodstream.

An immune complex allergic reaction may also be implicated in the pathogenesis of bronchial asthma, particularly where antigens derived from fungi, such as *A. fumigatus*, are implicated. Acute attacks of asthma may be caused by drugs such as aspirin and by exposure to chemical substances in the electronics, plastics and other industries (Tables 8.5 and 8.11).

Asthma is often aggravated by non-specific factors, such as bronchial irritation caused by tobacco smoke, dust and acrid fumes, respiratory infection, and emotional stress. In children and young adults, usually atopic subjects, an attack of asthma may follow strenuous exertion (*exercise-induced asthma*) or exposure to cold air.

Clinical features. Bronchial asthma may be either *episodic* or *chronic*, and although there is a good deal of overlap between these two syndromes, the distinction is clinically useful, particularly in terms of prognosis and management. In general, atopic individuals tend to develop episodic asthma, and non-atopic individuals chronic asthma.

In *episodic asthma* paroxysms of wheeze and dyspnoea occur at any hour of the day or night,

Table 8.5 Allergens and other substances liable to provoke attacks of asthma.

Causative agent	Preventive measures	Efficacy
Pollens	Try to avoid exposure to flowering vegetation	Low
	Keep bedroom windows closed	
Mites in house dust	Vacuum-clean mattress daily	Doubtful
	Shake out blankets daily	
	Dust bedroom thoroughly	
Animal dander	Avoid contact with dogs, cats, horses or other animals	High
Feathers in pillows or quilts	Substitute latex foam pillows and terylene quilts.	High
Drugs (e.g. beta-blockers)	Avoid all preparations of relevant drugs	High
Foods	Identify and eliminate from diet	Low*
Industrial chemicals (e.g. isocyanates, epoxy resins)	Avoid exposure to chemical, or change occupation	High

*More effective in control of eczema.

are of sudden onset, and may be preceded by a feeling of tightness in the chest. Breathing is exhausting and initially expiration is difficult and prolonged compared with inspiration. The patient adopts an upright position, fixing the shoulder-girdle to assist the accessory muscles of respiration. Wheeze is chiefly expiratory and there is often an unproductive cough which aggravates the dyspnoea. In severe attacks there is tachycardia, pulsus paradoxus (p. 120) and central cyanosis.

An attack may end abruptly within an hour or two, sometimes with the coughing up of viscid sputum, or may persist for many hours or even for several days. Sputum, usually scanty, may contain numerous eosinophil leucocytes and, occasionally, gelatinous casts of small bronchi. In most cases there is an increase in the number of eosinophil leucocytes in the blood.

The term, *severe acute asthma*, has replaced 'status asthmaticus' for the description of life-threatening attacks associated with extreme respiratory distress and arterial hypoxaemia.

In *chronic asthma* the paroxysmal character of the symptoms is usually less conspicuous, the chief clinical features being wheeze and breathlessness on exertion and spontaneous cough and wheeze during the night. Cough and mucoid sputum, with recurrent episodes of frank respiratory infection, are common in this type of asthma, which may be difficult to distinguish from chronic bronchitis.

The various types of asthma are contrasted in Figure 8.3.

Physical signs in the chest. 1. During an attack the chest is held near the position of full inspiration. The percussion note may be hyper-resonant. The breath sounds, which are obscured by numerous high pitched rhonchi, are vesicular in character with prolonged expiration. In very severe asthma airflow may be insufficient to produce rhonchi, and a 'silent chest' in such patients is an ominous sign.

2. Between paroxysms there are usually no abnormal physical signs except in patients with chronic asthma, who are seldom without expiratory rhonchi. Severe asthma persisting from childhood may cause a 'pigeon chest' deformity.

Investigation. *Radiological examination.* In an acute attack of asthma the lungs appear hyper-inflated. In long-standing cases the appearances may be indistinguishable from emphysema, and the lateral view may demonstrate a 'pigeon chest' deformity. Occasionally, when a bronchus is obstructed by tenacious mucus, there is an opacity caused by lobar or segmental collapse.

Pulmonary function tests. Measurements of the forced expiratory volume in 1 second (FEV_1) and vital capacity (VC) or of peak expiratory flow (PEF) provide a fairly reliable indication of the degree of airflow obstruction (p. 207), and can also be used to determine whether and to what extent it can be relieved by bronchodilator drugs or corticosteroids, or to confirm that it is provoked by exercise (Fig. 8.4) or hyperventilation. Such

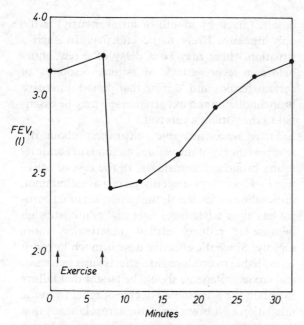

Fig. 8.4 Exercise-induced asthma: serial recordings of forced expiratory volume in one second (FEV_1) in patient with bronchial asthma before, during and after 6 minutes of strenuous exercise. Note initial slight rise on completion of exercise, followed by sudden fall and gradual recovery.

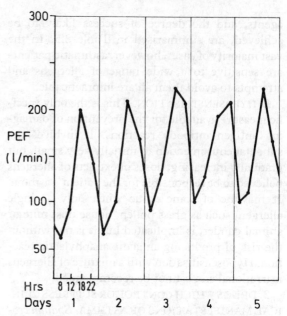

Fig. 8.5 'Morning dipping': serial recordings of peak expiratory flow (PEF) in patient with chronic asthma showing marked diurnal variations. Note sharp overnight fall and subsequent rise during the day.

tests thus have an important place in the diagnosis and treatment of bronchial asthma. Serial recordings of PEF are useful in the assessment of those patients ('morning dippers') whose asthma shows marked diurnal variations in severity (Fig. 8.5). Measurements of arterial blood-gas pressures (PaO_2 and $PaCO_2$) are indispensable in the management of patients with severe acute asthma.

Skin sensitivity tests. A prick is made in the skin with a fine needle through a drop of an aqueous extract of the substance to be tested, and a positive reaction is indicated by the development of a wheal and flare, which begin to appear within a few minutes. Tests are usually performed with a group of common allergens known to cause bronchial asthma. It is seldom possible with these tests to identify one particular allergen as the cause of asthma in an individual case, and their chief value is to distinguish atopic from non-atopic subjects.

Course and prognosis. The prognosis of the individual attack is good, except in severe acute asthma where there is occasionally a fatal outcome, especially if treatment is inadequate or delayed. Spontaneous remission is fairly common in epi-

sodic asthma, particularly in children, but rare in chronic asthma, which can lead to irreversible airflow obstruction. Seasonal fluctuations occur in both types of asthma. Atopic subjects with episodic asthma are usually worse in the summer, when they are more heavily exposed to antigens, while chronic asthmatics are usually worse in the winter months because of their increased liability to viral infections.

Treatment. The following measures may be of value in the management of patients with bronchial asthma: (1) Avoidance of relevant allergens. (2) Hyposensitisation (rarely of great benefit). (3) Drugs, such as sodium cromoglycate, bronchodilators, or corticosteroids to control or suppress the clinical manifestations of asthma. (4) Measures to counter the effects of aggravating factors such as exercise, infection and emotional stress.

1. AVOIDANCE OF ALLERGENS. There are a few instances in which a single agent can be identified as the cause of attacks of asthma. These allergens include grass pollens, mites, animal dander, drugs, industrial chemicals such as isocyanates and certain articles of diet. The measures which can be taken to prevent or reduce exposure to these

agents, and the degree of success likely to be achieved, are summarised in Table 8.5. In the vast majority of cases, however, asthmatic patients are sensitive to a wide range of allergens and attempts to avoid them all are impracticable.

2. HYPOSENSITISATION. This is the only specific measure available for the prevention of damaging antigen-antibody reactions. It involves the subcutaneous injection of initially very small, but gradually increasing, doses of extracts of allergens believed to be responsible for the patient's asthma. It may be of some value when only a single allergen, such as grass pollen, house dust mite or animal dander, is implicated but it is not without the risk of producing an acute anaphylactic reaction. Hyposensitisation with a mixture of allergens is irrational and cannot be recommended.

3. DRUGS WHICH CONTROL OR SUPPRESS CLINICAL MANIFESTATIONS OF ASTHMA. *Sodium cromoglycate* administered by inhalation has actions which include prevention of mediator release from mast cells. It seems to be of particular value in children with extrinsic (atopic) asthma, and should be given a trial of at least 4 weeks' duration in all such patients. If it is found to be effective, regular inhalation of 20 mg in a dry powder by 'Spinhaler' or of 2–10 mg from a metered dose inhaler 4 times daily may completely prevent recurrence of asthma in this group of patients. It may also be of value in some cases of intrinsic (non-atopic) asthma, but has no place in the management of severe asthma.

Ketotifen by mouth has a similar mode of action, but that drug is less effective than sodium cromoglycate and has the serious disadvantage in some patients of causing drowsiness which may be a dangerous side-effect in patients driving cars or operating machinery.

Bronchodilators and corticosteroids. It is important to distinguish between bronchodilators, which have a direct and immediate effect on airflow obstruction, and corticosteroids, which relieve or prevent airflow obstruction indirectly by their less rapid anti-inflammatory action. Thus a corticosteroid aerosol cannot be expected to relieve an acute episode of asthma. On the other hand, if a patient with severe acute asthma does not respond rapidly to a bronchodilator aerosol, systemic treatment with corticosteroids in high dosage (given by mouth or intravenously) is the only measure likely to be effective. In such a situation, there may be a delay of a few hours before a severe attack of asthma responds to corticosteroids and, during that period, intensive bronchodilator and oxygen therapy may be essential to the patient's survival.

There is considerable controversy about the relative efficacy of the various methods of administering bronchodilator drugs. In the case of selective β_2-adrenoceptor agonists, such as salbutamol, terbutaline or fenoterol, the inhalation of an aerosol has clear advantages over oral administration because it reduces airflow obstruction more rapidly. Since the effective dose is much lower, it is less liable to produce side-effects such as tremor and anxiety. Patients should be taught that failure to obtain the accustomed degree of relief from the inhalation of a bronchodilator aerosol means that the asthma is in a refractory phase, and that a more potent form of treatment, such as a course of prednisolone by mouth, is urgently required.

Methylxanthine derivatives, such as theophylline or aminophylline, can be given by intravenous injection, mouth or suppository. Intravenous aminophylline (5 mg/kg) is often an effective form of treatment for severe acute asthma, although it is probably not superior to salbutamol (4 μg/kg) administered by the same route. There has been a revival of interest in the oral methylxanthines since the introduction of sustained-release formulations. This is based chiefly on the claim that these preparations can maintain serum concentrations of theophylline at therapeutically effective but subtoxic levels. It is, however, still open to doubt whether oral methylxanthines, even when the dose is monitored by serum concentrations, have any real advantage in terms of efficacy and safety over the regular inhalation of β_2-adrenoceptor agonist aerosols, except possibly for the prevention of nocturnal asthma.

The above measures can be applied to the management of the different types of asthma as follows:

1. *Episodic asthma.* Where episodes of asthma are mild and infrequent, they can be controlled by inhalation of a bronchodilator aerosol, for example, 2 metered doses of salbutamol (200 μg) as required. When the episodes are more frequent,

this should be supplemented by a regular prophylactic measure, such as sodium cromoglycate or a corticosteroid by inhalation. Sodium cromoglycate has virtually no side-effects, but corticosteroid aerosols are apt to cause oropharyngeal candidiasis and a husky voice.

2. *Exercise-induced asthma.* This common phenomenon, which occurs particularly in children and young adults, can often be prevented by the inhalation of two metered doses of salbutamol a few minutes before exercise. Regular treatment with sodium cromoglycate may also be effective and if these measures fail an inhaled corticosteroid preparation should be tried.

3. *Chronic asthma.* Some form of suppressive treatment is necessary in all patients with chronic asthma. Sodium cromoglycate is always worth a trial, but there is usually a better response to the regular inhalation of a corticosteroid aerosol — beclomethasone dipropionate ($200\,\mu$g) or budesonide ($200\,\mu$g) twice daily. In severe cases higher doses may be necessary, occasionally supplemented by a small maintenance dose of prednisolone given by mouth (5–7.5 mg/day) and/or by occasional short courses of prednisolone in higher dosage (20 mg/day or more for a week).

There is evidence that supplementary treatment with oral prednisolone is required less frequently if the dose of inhaled corticosteroid aerosol is increased, e.g. beclomethasone dipropionate to $1500\,\mu$g per day, budesonide to $2000\,\mu$g per day. These doses should, however, not be exceeded because systemic absorption may then cause impairment of pituitary-adrenal function. Most patients with chronic asthma also require to inhale a bronchodilator aerosol either regularly or periodically to control recurrences of wheeze. When regular treatment is needed, it is best given a few minutes before the inhalation of sodium cromoglycate or a corticosteroid aerosol to ensure that the largest possible amounts of these drugs enter the bronchi. Oral bronchodilator drugs are seldom as effective as aerosols in the treatment of chronic asthma, but slow-release oral preparations of β_2-adrenoceptor agonists and methylxanthines taken at bedtime can be useful in preventing nocturnal symptoms.

4. *Severe acute asthma.* When an acute attack of asthma becomes severe and life-threatening, the patient will have ceased to show any response to bronchodilator inhalers. All such patients should be admitted to hospital as quickly as possible and emergency admission schemes, which eliminate the delays inherent in normal hospital admission procedures, can do much to reduce the number of unnecessary deaths from severe acute asthma. It is equally important that, before the ambulance arrives, the general practitioner should start effective treatment (Table 8.6).

Table 8.6 Treatment of severe acute asthma in the home.

1. Administer oxygen from portable cylinder (preferably by MC mask)
2. Give bronchodilator intravenously: aminophylline (5 mg/kg) *or* salbutamol (4 µg/kg) *or* terbutaline (0.5 mg in 20 ml of saline). Alternatively, give salbutamol (5 mg) or terbutaline (10 mg) by inhalation
3. Give hydrocortisone sodium succinate 200 mg intravenously
4. Arrange for emergency admission to hospital in ambulance equipped for oxygen and nebulised β_2 agonist therapy
5. Give prednisolone 60 mg by mouth

N.B. The above doses are for adults — those for children should be proportionately smaller.

Since all bronchodilator drugs have the potential to increase arterial hypoxaemia, which may have grave consequences in patients with severe acute asthma, it is strongly advisable for oxygen to be given from a portable cylinder before and after these drugs are administered at home. High concentration oxygen therapy should be continued in the ambulance conveying the patient to hospital.

In hospital most patients respond to treatment with high doses of corticosteroid, supplemented by bronchodilator drugs administered in the form of an aqueous aerosol delivered in oxygen from a nebuliser or by intravenous injection or infusion. Only occasionally is it necessary to employ major resuscitative measures, such as tracheal intubation and mechanical ventilation.

Recently there has been an increase in the use of electric nebulisers for the self-administration of bronchodilators by patients in their homes, but those who are hypoxaemic and do not have access to oxygen may be at some risk from this form of treatment. Furthermore, overconfidence in the efficacy of this treatment can lead to delay in seeking medical advice during an episode of severe asthma when prompt admission to hospital may be vital to survival. Doctors must, therefore, ensure that patients who are provided with nebulisers fully understand their potential dangers and how these can be avoided. This is just one illustration of the place of the education of patients in the management of their disease. Such involvement and understanding is as necessary in asthma as it is in diabetes mellitus and many other diseases.

BRONCHOPULMONARY EOSINOPHILIA

This term is applied to a group of allergic disorders of different aetiology in which lesions of the bronchi and/or the lungs are associated with an increase in the number of eosinophil leucocytes in the blood. In some of these diseases the bronchi appear to be primarily affected, although there may be secondary effects on lung tissue, while in others the pathological changes are confined to the lungs. It is therefore appropriate to subdivide the syndrome into bronchial and pulmonary eosinophilia.

Bronchial eosinophilia

Although bronchial asthma could logically be included in this category, it is not customary to do so, and the term is normally restricted to patients with a severe allergic reaction in the bronchi which gives rise to the production of inspissated mucus heavily infiltrated with eosinophils (asthmatic pulmonary eosinophilia). These casts frequently obstruct bronchi and produce lobar or segmental collapse. In some cases, the allergic reaction extends into the collapsed lung tissue, but because lung biopsy is seldom indicated in patients with bronchopulmonary eosinophilia, the frequency of this complication is uncertain.

There is evidence that eosinophilic bronchitis is the result of dual anaphylactic and immune complex reactions in the bronchial wall, and that an antigen derived from a fungus, usually Aspergillus fumigatus, is often the causal agent. In many cases the fungus can be isolated from the sputum or from a bronchial cast, skin tests with an A. fumigatus antigen are positive and precipitating antibodies can be detected in the serum. The term, allergic bronchopulmonary aspergillosis can be used to describe such cases. Occasionally all investigations are negative and a causal antigen cannot be identified.

Clinical features. Chronic asthma is the dominant clinical manifestation of bronchial eosinophilia, but at irregular intervals bronchi, usually in the upper lobes, are obstructed by casts, with the production of lobar or segmental collapse, which may cause a mild febrile illness. When these episodes recur over a period of years, as they usually do, they result in permanent damage to the bronchi and lungs. Cast formation first produces dilatation of the larger bronchi (proximal bronchiectasis), and at a later stage bacterial and possibly fungal infection in lung tissue beyond the bronchial obstruction causes extensive pulmonary fibrosis and distal bronchiectasis. These changes, together with the associated chronic asthma, which seldom responds well to treatment, eventually cause respiratory failure, pulmonary hypertension and right ventricular failure.

Investigation. In early cases, the diagnosis is made by observing recurrent transient radiographic opacities, usually of lobar or segmental distribution, in young adults (seldom children) with chronic asthma and an increased eosinophil count in the blood. Often the investigations already described will identify A. fumigatus as the cause of the allergic reaction. In advanced cases, however, chronic respiratory failure overshadows the earlier and more specific features, and radiological examination shows extensive bilateral fibrosis and bronchiectasis predominantly affecting the upper lobes.

Treatment. Initially, a short course of prednisolone (40 mg/d for 7–10 days), presumably by relieving airflow obstruction, may be followed by the expectoration of bronchial casts and clearing of the pulmonary opacities. If not, it may be necessary to extract the cast or casts by bronchoscopy in an attempt to avert permanent bronchopulmonary damage. Further cast formation can in some cases be prevented by a maintenance dose of prednisolone (5–10 mg per day), but in many cases this does not halt the development of bronchiectasis and progressive pulmonary fibrosis, particularly when bronchial eosinophilia is a manifestation of allergic aspergillosis.

Pulmonary eosinophilia

This condition predominantly involves lung tissues although in a few cases it may be associated with chronic bronchial asthma. There is a cellular infiltrate, chiefly consisting of eosinophil leucocytes, in the alveoli and alveolar walls, to which the term, *eosinophilic pneumonia*, is applied. This may be localised or diffuse, and appears to be an immunological reaction in the lung to a variety of antigens (Table 8.7). In some cases eosinophilic pneumonia, which may be severe and extensive, develops in the absence of any identifiable cause. The term, *cryptogenic pulmonary eosinophilia*, is applied to this form of the disease, for which an autoimmune mechanism may be responsible.

Table 8.7 Causes of pulmonary eosinophilia.

*Helminths	Filariae—*Dirofilaria* or *Brugia pahangi* unable to mature in man
	Microfilaria—*Wuchereria bancrofti* or *Brugia malayi*
	Ancylostomiasis
	Ascaris lumbricoides
Fungi	*Aspergillus fumigatus*
Drugs	Nitrofurantoin, para-aminosalicyclic acid, sulphasalazine, imipramine, chlorpropamide, phenylbutazone, aspirin
Chemicals	Isocyanates

*Tropical pulmonary eosinophilia is found in India, Sri Lanka, Malaysia, China, Philippines, Australia, South America and other tropical regions but uncommonly in Africa.

Clinical features vary widely in severity, depending on the aetiology and on the extent of pulmonary involvement. Many patients have only a trivial febrile illness, the nature of which would have passed unrecognised in the absence of radiological and haematological investigation. Others, particularly those in whom the illness is an allergic reaction to worms (*tropical pulmonary eosinophilia*, Table 8.7) or to drugs, may become gravely ill with high fever and severe dyspnoea. In such patients, the absolute eosinophil count in the blood is high, often exceeding $5.0 \times 10^9/l$. After the diagnosis is established, an attempt should be made to discover the aetiological factor. If all such causes are excluded, and tests for fungal allergy are negative, a diagnosis of cryptogenic pulmonary eosinophilia has to be accepted.

Treatment. If a cause is found or suspected it must be treated or removed. Helminthic infections should be eradicated and any drug likely to be responsible should be withdrawn. When the condition is due to filariae the patient should be given diethylcarbamazine (10 mg/kg/d for 10 days) and rapid clinical and radiographic improvement will follow. Cryptogenic pulmonary eosinophilia usually responds dramatically to prednisolone (5 mg 6 hourly by mouth) but because it is apt to recur after corticosteroid therapy is withdrawn, a small maintenance dose may have to be continued for some months, or even for a few years.

EXTRINSIC ALLERGIC ALVEOLITIS

In this condition the inhalation of certain types of organic dust produces a diffuse immune complex reaction (p. 26) in the walls of the alveoli and bronchioles. The finding of small pulmonary granulomata suggests that cell-mediated hypersensitivity may also be implicated.

Some of the agents which produce extrinsic allergic alveolitis, the source of these agents, and the names applied to the resulting diseases are shown in Table 8.8. If patients with this disorder continue to be exposed to the relevant antigen for long periods, they may eventually develop permanent pulmonary damage with severe respiratory disability.

Table 8.8 Examples of extrinsic allergic alveolitis.

Agent	Source	Disease
Avian protein from pigeons and budgerigars	Pigeon loft or bird cage	Bird fancier's lung
Micropolyspora faeni	Mouldy hay	Farmer's lung
Thermophilic actinomycetes	Compost	Mushroom worker's lung
	Mouldy sugar cane fibre	Bagassosis
Aspergillus clavatus	Malting barley	Maltworker's lung
Coniosporium corticale	Bark of maple trees	Maple bark disease

Clinical features. Extrinsic allergic alveolitis should be suspected when a person regularly exposed to a heavy concentration of organic dust complains, a few hours after re-exposure to the same dust, of malaise, pyrexia, dry cough and dyspnoea without wheeze, or insidiously develops similar symptoms after constant exposure to antigen, as in some cases of bird fancier's lung.

Soon after exposure the patient may be febrile, cyanosed and dyspnoeic at rest, end-inspiratory crepitations (crackles) but no rhonchi can be heard over both lungs and a chest radiograph may show diffuse micronodular shadowing. The FEV_1 and VC are both reduced, but the FEV_1/VC ratio is normal, indicating a restrictive ventilatory defect without airflow obstruction. The PaO_2 is reduced, and the $PaCO_2$ is often below normal as a result of overventilation. Gas transfer is impaired.

The diagnosis of extrinsic allergic alveolitis is confirmed serologically by a positive precipitin test and, if necessary, by a positive provocation test, in which the inhalation of the relevant antigen is followed after 3 to 6 hours by pyrexia and a reduction in VC, often associated with a recurrence of symptoms.

Treatment. Mild forms of extrinsic allergic alveolitis rapidly subside when exposure to the antigen ceases. In acute cases a corticosteroid preparation should be given for 3 to 4 weeks, starting with 40–60 mg of prednisolone per day, and severely hypoxic patients may require oxygen in high concentration. Most of these patients recover completely, but when there has been prolonged exposure to the relevant antigen, the development of interstitial fibrosis causes permanent disability.

DISEASES OF THE LARYNX, TRACHEA AND BRONCHI

Acute infections have already been described (p. 215). Other disorders of the larynx include chronic laryngitis, laryngeal tuberculosis (p. 226), laryngeal paralysis and laryngeal obstruction. Tumours of the larynx are relatively common, but for information on these conditions the reader should refer to a textbook of diseases of the ear, nose and throat.

Chronic laryngitis

Chronic laryngitis occurs as a result of (1) repeated attacks of acute laryngitis, (2) excessive use of the voice, especially in dusty atmospheres, e.g. in auctioneers, (3) heavy tobacco smoking, (4) mouth-breathing from nasal obstruction and (5) chronic infection of the nasal sinuses. The chief symptom is hoarseness and the voice may be lost. There is irritation of the throat and spasmodic cough. The disease pursues a chronic course frequently uninfluenced by treatment, and in long-standing cases the voice is often permanently impaired.

As chronic and progressive hoarseness may also be caused by tuberculosis and tumours of the larynx and by laryngeal paralysis, these conditions must be considered in the differential diagnosis if the hoarseness does not improve within a few weeks. In some cases a chest radiograph may bring to light unsuspected pulmonary tuberculosis or a bronchial carcinoma. If no such abnormality is found the patient should be referred to a specialist for laryngoscopic examination.

The voice must be rested completely. This is particularly important in the case of public speakers. Smoking should be prohibited. Some benefit may be obtained from frequent inhalations of medicated steam.

Laryngeal paralysis

Aetiology. Paralysis is due to interference with the motor nerve supply of the larynx. It is nearly always unilateral and, by reason of the intrathoracic course of the left recurrent laryngeal nerve, usually left-sided. One or both recurrent laryngeal nerves may be damaged at thyroidectomy or by carcinoma of the thyroid. Rarely the vagal trunk itself is involved by tumour, aneurysm or trauma.

Hoarseness or complete loss of voice (aphonia) may occur as a manifestation of hysteria.

Clinical features. *Hoarseness* always accompanies laryngeal paralysis whatever its cause. Paralysis of organic origin is seldom reversible, but when only one vocal cord is affected the hoarseness may improve or even disappear after a few weeks as a result of a compensatory adjustment whereby the unparalysed cord crosses the midline and approximates with the paralysed cord on phonation.

'Bovine' cough, which is a characteristic feature of organic laryngeal paralysis, results from the loss of the explosive phase of normal coughing consequent upon the failure of the cords to close

the glottis. The difficulty in bringing up sputum which some of these patients experience can be explained on the same basis. A normal cough in patients with partial loss of voice or aphonia virtually excludes laryngeal paralysis.

Dyspnoea and *stridor* are occasionally present but are seldom severe except with bilateral laryngeal paralysis.

Laryngoscopy is necessary to establish the diagnosis of laryngeal paralysis with certainty. The paralysed cord lies in the so-called 'cadaveric' position, midway between abduction and adduction. In hysteria only adduction of the cords, a voluntary movement, is affected.

Treatment. The cause of the laryngeal paralysis should be treated if that is possible. In unilateral paralysis the voice can be improved by the injection of teflon into the affected vocal cord. In bilateral organic paralysis, tracheal intubation, tracheostomy or a plastic operation on the larynx may be necessary. Psychiatric treatment is indicated for hysterical aphonia.

Laryngeal obstruction

Aetiology. The laryngeal opening (glottis) may be obstructed by (1) inflammatory or allergic oedema or exudate, (2) spasm of the laryngeal muscles, (3) inhaled foreign body, (4) inhaled vomitus in an unconscious patient, (5) tumours of the larynx, (6) bilateral vocal cord paralysis and (7) fixation of both cords in advanced rheumatoid arthritis. Laryngeal obstruction is more liable to occur in children than in adults because of the smaller size of the glottis.

Clinical features. Sudden complete laryngeal obstruction by a foreign body produces the clinical picture of acute asphyxia — violent but ineffective inspiratory efforts with indrawing of the intercostal spaces and the unsupported lower ribs, accompanied by deep cyanosis. Unrelieved, the condition progresses rapidly to coma, and death ensues within 5 to 10 minutes. When, as in most cases, the obstruction is incomplete at first, the main clinical features are progressive dyspnoea and cyanosis, stridor and indrawing of the intercostal spaces and lower ribs on both sides. The great danger in these cases is that the obstruction may at any time become complete and result in sudden death.

Treatment. Transient attacks of laryngeal obstruction due to exudate and spasm, which may occur with acute laryngitis in children (p. 215) and with whooping cough, are potentially dangerous but can usually be relieved by the inhalation of steam.

Laryngeal obstruction from all other causes carries a high mortality and demands prompt treatment. The following measures may have to be employed:

1. *The relief of obstruction by mechanical means.* When a foreign body is known to be the cause of the obstruction in children it can often be dislodged by turning the patient head downwards and thumping the back vigorously. In adults this is often impossible, but sudden forceful compression of the upper abdomen (Heimlich manoeuvre) may be effective. In other circumstances the cause of the obstruction should be investigated by direct laryngoscopy, which may also permit the removal of an unsuspected foreign body or the insertion of a tube past the obstruction into the trachea. Tracheostomy must be performed without delay if these procedures fail to relieve the obstruction, but except in dire emergencies the operation should be performed in the operating theatre by a surgeon.

2. *Treatment of the cause.* In cases of diphtheria, antitoxin should be administered and for other infections the appropriate antibiotic should be given. In angio-oedema the patient should receive adrenaline (0.5–1.0 ml of 1:1000 solution s.c.), chlorpheniramine maleate (10–20 mg i.v.) and hydrocortisone hemisuccinate (100 mg i.v.). These remedies take time to act and tracheostomy may be required in the intervening period.

Diseases of the trachea

Acute tracheitis is a common complication of viral and bacterial infection of the upper respiratory tract (p. 215), and is usually associated with acute bronchitis (p. 217). Other primary disorders of the trachea are rare.

Tracheal obstruction. External compression by enlarged mediastinal lymph nodes containing metastatic deposits from a bronchial carcinoma causes tracheal obstruction more often than intrinsic benign or malignant tumours. Rarely, the trachea may be compressed by an aneurysm of the aortic arch, or in children by tuberculous mediastinal lymph nodes. Tracheal stricture is an occasional complication of tracheostomy.

Stridor can be detected in every patient with severe tracheal narrowing. Endoscopic examination of the trachea should be undertaken without delay in these patients to determine the degree of obstruction and its nature.

Localised tumours of the trachea can be resected, but reconstruction of the resected segment may present complex technical problems. Radiotherapy or the administration of cytotoxic drugs may temporarily relieve compression by malignant lymph nodes. Tracheal strictures can sometimes be dilated, but may have to be resected.

Tracheo-oesophageal fistula. This may be present in newborn infants as a congenital abnormality. In adults, it is usually due to malignant lesions in the mediastinum, such as carcinoma or lymphoma, eroding both the trachea and oesophagus, to produce a communication between them. Swallowed liquids enter the trachea and bronchi through the fistula, and provoke a 'spluttering' cough. Surgical closure of a congenital fistula, if undertaken promptly, is usually successful, but malignant fistulae are incurable, and death from overwhelming pulmonary infection rapidly supervenes.

CHRONIC OBSTRUCTIVE AIRWAYS DISEASE

Although chronic bronchitis and emphysema are pathologically distinct, they frequently coexist, and it may then be difficult or impossible to determine the relative importance of each condition in the individual case. Generalised airflow obstruction is the dominant feature of both diseases.

Chronic bronchitis and emphysema are often grouped together under the heading of 'chronic obstructive airways disease', and can be regarded as forming a spectrum, with 'pure' chronic bronchitis at one end and 'pure' emphysema at the other. For descriptive purposes, however, it is convenient to deal with them separately, with emphasis on their similarities and differences, and on the relationships which frequently exist between them.

Chronic bronchitis

Aetiology. Chronic bronchitis is the name given to the clinical syndrome which many individuals develop in response to the long-continued action of various types of irritant on the bronchial mucosa. The most important of these is tobacco smoke, but they also include dust, smoke and fumes occurring as specific occupational hazards or as part of a general atmospheric pollution in industrial cities and towns. Infection is sometimes a precipitating factor in the onset of chronic bronchitis, but its main role is in aggravating the established condition. Exposure to dampness, to sudden changes in temperature and to fog may also be responsible for exacerbations of chronic bronchitis.

The disorder occurs most commonly in middle and late adult life and more males are affected than females. It is much more common in smokers than in non-smokers, and in urban than in rural dwellers.

On culture of the sputum, *Strep. pneumoniae* and/or *H. influenzae* are isolated in most cases. These organisms become more numerous during acute exacerbations.

Pathology. In all cases there is overactivity of the mucus-secreting glands and goblet cells in the bronchi and bronchioles. The vast excess of mucus so produced coats the bronchial walls and clogs the bronchioles. Mucosal oedema further reduces the calibre of the air passages and as the degree of obstruction is greater during expiration air is 'trapped' in the alveoli. With the passage of time the alveoli become permanently overdistended and there is extensive rupture of their walls. These changes, which constitute one form of 'emphysema', are also discussed on page 246.

Clinical features. The disease usually starts with repeated attacks of 'winter cough', which show a steady increase in severity and duration with successive years, until cough is present all the year round. Wheeze, dyspnoea and tightness in the chest are common complaints, especially in the morning before the bronchial secretions are cleared, often with difficulty, by coughing. The sputum may be scanty, tenacious mucoid, and occasionally streaked with blood. A frankly purulent sputum is indicative of bacterial infection, which supervenes from time to time in most cases of bronchitis.

Dyspnoea in chronic bronchitis is chiefly caused by airflow obstruction, and is aggravated by infection, excessive cigarette smoking and adverse atmospheric conditions.

Variable numbers of inspiratory and expiratory rhonchi, mainly low and medium pitched, are present in most cases of chronic bronchitis and there may also be some crepitations. Physical signs attributable to emphysema may coexist.

Investigation. *Radiological examination.* Chronic bronchitis produces no characteristic abnormality in the radiograph, but the features of emphysema (p. 246) may be prominent in some cases. Bronchography shows various irregularities of bronchial outline, calibre and branching, but is not a routine investigation in chronic bronchitis.

Pulmonary function tests. 1. The forced expiratory volume in 1 second (FEV_1) is reduced, and the ratio of FEV_1 to vital capacity (VC) is also subnormal. In advanced cases the FEV_1 may be less than 1 litre, and the FEV/VC ratio may be as low as 30%.

2. With 'air trapping' and alveolar distension the residual volume of the lungs is increased at the expense of vital capacity.

3. As the distribution of ventilation and perfusion within the lungs becomes disturbed (p. 199), the PaO_2 falls below normal.

4. Impairment of gas transfer occurs in a proportion of patients and marked reduction may provide an indication of the presence of emphysema.

5. In the later stages, when generalised alveolar underventilation supervenes, there is a further fall in PaO_2 and a sustained rise in $PaCO_2$ (chronic Type II respiratory failure p. 205). Hypoxaemia becomes more severe during sleep, and some patients have periods of marked hypoventilation and 'sleep apnoea' (p. 203) which cause profound falls in PaO_2. These may be factors in the production of pulmonary hypertension (p. 178).

Course and prognosis. Chronic bronchitis is usually a progressive disease, punctuated by acute exacerbations and remissions, and eventually causing respiratory and cardiac failure. Some patients die within a few years of the onset of symptoms, while others survive for many years, with gradually diminishing respiratory reserve.

Treatment. *Bronchial irritation* must be reduced to a minimum. If a smoker, the patient should be urged to give up the habit completely and permanently. Dusty and smoke-laden atmospheres should be avoided, which may involve a change of occupation.

Respiratory infection must be promptly controlled, as it aggravates dyspnoea and may precipitate Type II respiratory failure. The patient should be instructed to observe the colour of the sputum every morning, and, if it becomes purulent, should be given oxytetracycline or ampicillin in a dose of 250 mg four times daily or co-trimoxazole, 2 tablets twice daily, for 5 to 7 days. Intelligent patients can be given a supply and permitted to start a course of treatment on their own initiative when the need arises.

As the vast majority of bacterial infections in chronic bronchitis are caused by *Strep. pneumoniae* or *H. influenzae*, bacteriological examination of sputum is essential only when the response to standard treatment is unsatisfactory, and the sputum remains purulent. In that event a change of antibiotic, guided by the results of bacterial sensitivity tests, will be indicated. Continuous suppressive treatment with a tetracycline or ampicillin is not advised, since it is apt to promote the emergence of a drug-resistant respiratory tract flora.

Symptomatic measures may be required to control unproductive cough during the night, to enable sputum to be coughed up more easily and to relieve breathlessness and wheeze. Nocturnal unproductive cough will often be less troublesome if the patient sleeps in a heated bedroom, but pholcodine may be required to control it. A hot drink or the inhalation of steam helps to liquefy sputum and make it easier to bring up. So-called expectorant cough mixtures and drugs claimed to reduce sputum viscosity are of little or no value. Bronchodilators are much less effective in chronic bronchitis than in asthma, but are of value in those patients with demonstrable reversibility of airflow obstruction.

Respiratory failure must be promptly treated (p. 211).

Prevention. The abandonment of smoking is the most important preventive measure. The control of atmospheric pollution in urban areas and the increased use of measures to prevent the inhalation of dust by industrial workers will also help to reduce the prevalence of chronic bronchitis. Respiratory infection should be promptly and efficiently treated.

Emphysema

The word 'emphysema' means 'inflation' in the sense of unnatural distension with air, and, although normally confined to the lungs (*pulmonary emphysema*), can occur elsewhere. Air may, for example, enter the mediastinum (*mediastinal emphysema*) following the rupture of over-distended alveoli into the interstitial tissues of the lung in patients with severe bronchial asthma, or following rupture of the oesophagus. If a very large amount of air escapes rapidly into the mediastinum, it may produce cardiac tamponade (p. 182), but in most cases it tracks harmlessly upwards into the soft tissues of the neck, where it imparts a characteristic crackling sensation to the palpating fingers (*subcutaneous emphysema*). Penetrating wounds of the chest wall may also cause subcutaneous emphysema, and when a spontaneous pneumothorax is treated by pleural decompression with an intercostal tube (p. 266), widespread subcutaneous emphysema is an occasional complication, which is alarming but not serious.

Pulmonary emphysema. This term covers a wide variety of pathological processes, ranging from overdistension of otherwise normal alveoli in conditions such as bronchial asthma, to the widespread disruption of the alveolar walls which occurs in the more serious forms of pulmonary emphysema. There is a close association between the latter and chronic bronchitis, but the physical signs and radiological changes attributable to 'emphysema' may be more conspicuous in some cases of chronic bronchitis than in others.

In 'pure' emphysema generalised destruction of the alveolar walls ('panacinar' emphysema) is the dominant lesion. Where emphysema occurs along with a major component of chronic bronchitis, it is usually 'centrilobular' or 'centriacinar', and principally affects those alveoli which are most closely related to the respiratory bronchioles.

Although these two types of emphysema develop in different ways, factors such as bacterial infection, alveolar overdistension and distortion of the airways may eventually blur their distinctive features. The predominance of either chronic bronchitis or emphysema may, however, be sufficiently clear-cut to produce two separately identifiable syndromes. In the chronic bronchitis syndrome severe hypoxia and hypercapnia, pulmonary hypertension and right ventricular failure with peripheral oedema occur at an early stage (the *'blue bloater'*). In the emphysema syndrome, on the other hand, disabling exertional dyspnoea may antedate by many years the manifestations of respiratory and cardiac failure (the *'pink puffer'*). A mixed syndrome of chronic bronchitis and emphysema is, however, much more commonly seen than either of the two individual syndromes.

Emphysema in young adults may be associated with genetically determined α_1-antitrypsin deficiency (p. 336). It is believed that connective tissue in the lung is digested by proteolytic enzymes normally inhibited by α_1-antitrypsin. Cigarette smoking may promote emphysema by releasing proteases from cells within the alveoli and bronchioles.

Clinical features. Most patients with pulmonary emphysema complain of exertional dyspnoea, but since other causes of airflow obstruction, such as chronic bronchitis and bronchial asthma, often coexist, it is seldom possible to assess the contribution of emphysema *per se* to the production of this symptom. There is a progressive increase in respiratory disability, but the tempo of deterioration varies widely from one patient to another.

The physical signs which may be observed in emphysema and other forms of chronic airflow obstruction are summarised in Table 8.1. Other clinical abnormalities include (1) a reduction in the length of the trachea palpable above the sternal notch, (2) tracheal descent during inspiration, (3) contraction of the sternomastoid and scalene muscles on inspiration, (4) excavation of the suprasternal and supraclavicular fossae during inspiration, (5) jugular venous filling during expiration, (6) indrawing of the costal margins during inspiration, and (7) an increase in the antero-posterior diameter of the chest relative to the lateral diameter.

Investigation. *Radiological examination.* A diagnosis of emphysema can be made with reasonable confidence if the following abnormalities are present: (1) Unusually translucent lung fields, with loss of peripheral vascular markings. (2) Bullae. (3) A low flat diaphragm. (4) Prominence of the pulmonary arterial shadows at both hila.

It is often difficult radiographically to distinguish emphysema from pulmonary hyperinflation, unless bullae are visible. Computed tomography can detect emphysema with greater certainty, but is not yet routinely used for this purpose. X-ray abnormalities caused by pulmonary infection ('inflammatory shadowing') may also be present. In the late stages, when pulmonary hypertension and right ventricular failure supervene, there is enlargement of the main pulmonary artery, the right ventricle and the right atrium.

Pulmonary function tests. See page 207.

Complications. 1. *Type I and II respiratory failure.* The latter may be associated with *secondary polycythaemia* as a consequence of prolonged hypoxaemia.

2. *Pulmonary hypertension and right ventricular failure.* The increase in pulmonary arterial pressure is due to vasoconstriction mediated by the effect of hypoxia on pulmonary arterioles and ultimately to destruction of the pulmonary vascular bed. As hypoxia is aggravated by any increase in the degree of airflow obstruction, bacterial infection in the respiratory tract, oedema of the bronchial mucosa, oversecretion of bronchial mucus and spasm of the bronchial muscles are all liable to increase the pulmonary arterial pressure and precipitate right ventricular failure. Similarly, falls in arterial oxygen saturation occurring during sleep (p. 203) may also contribute. Conversely, effective treatment of these causes of hypoxia, combined with oxygen therapy and diuretics, may relieve pulmonary hypertension and cardiac failure, at least for a time.

3. *Pulmonary bullae*, single or multiple, large or small, may develop in emphysematous lung tissue, regardless of the primary pathology. Bullae are inflated thin-walled spaces created by rupture of the alveolar walls. They are usually situated subpleurally, and are commonly found along the anterior borders of the lungs. A bulla may rupture, causing spontaneous pneumothorax. In other circumstances bullae may increase progressively in size, and eventually become so large that they interfere seriously with pulmonary ventilation.

Treatment. There is no specific remedy for emphysema, but the patient may benefit considerably from the treatment of associated chronic bronchitis, and of respiratory failure, which is a common complication. Obesity must be prevented or corrected, as excess weight is an intolerable burden on the reduced cardiorespiratory reserve. The purpose of physiotherapy should be to induce relaxation of the cervical muscles and to show the patient how to exhale slowly and steadily through pursed lips. It should also be used to encourage expectoration. Regular mild exercise has also been shown to increase mobility, even in severely disabled patients. The surgical ablation of giant bullae, where this is feasible, may allow relatively normal lung tissue compressed by the bullae to re-expand and may bring about a dramatic improvement in pulmonary function.

BRONCHIECTASIS

Aetiology and pathogenesis. Bronchiectasis, which is the term used to describe abnormal dilatation of the bronchi, may be produced in different ways. It may be acquired or, less commonly, congenital (Table 8.9). In most cases bronchiectasis is secondary to severe bacterial infection in childhood often as a complication of whooping cough or measles.

Table 8.9 Causes of bronchiectasis.

Congenital	Ciliary dysfunction syndromes, cystic fibrosis, primary hypogammaglobulinaemia
Acquired	
Children	Pneumonia (whooping cough and measles), primary tuberculosis, foreign body
Adults	Suppurative pneumonia, pulmonary tuberculosis, bronchial eosinophilia, bronchial tumours

Bronchiectasis may be due to bronchial distension resulting from the accumulation of pus beyond a lesion obstructing a major bronchus, such as a tuberculous hilar lymph node, an inhaled foreign body or a bronchial carcinoma. In cystic fibrosis (p. 300) recurrent infection and chronic obstruction by viscid mucus are both factors in causing bronchiectasis. Rarely, it may be the result of congenital dysfunction of the cilia, which is a feature of, for example, Kartagener's syndrome (bronchiectasis, sinusitis and transposition of the viscera). Because of the many different causes of bronchiectasis no precise age incidence can be stated.

Pathology. Although bronchiectasis may involve any part of the lungs the more efficient drainage by gravity of the upper lobes renders bronchiectasis there less liable to produce serious symptoms than when it involves the lower lobes. The bronchiectatic cavities may be lined by granulation tissue, squamous epithelium or normal ciliated epithelium. There may also be inflammatory changes in the deeper layers of the bronchial walls and chronic inflammatory and fibrotic changes in the surrounding lung tissue.

Clinical features. In many patients, symptoms are slight. In more severe cases three groups of clinical features occur:

1. *Those due to the accumulation of pus in the dilated bronchi* are chronic cough, usually worse in the mornings and often induced by changes in posture, and purulent sputum which in advanced cases is copious and sometimes fetid.

2. *Those due to inflammatory changes in the surrounding lung tissue and pleura.* Febrile episodes usually last for a few days but occasionally for weeks. Malaise, shivering and sleep sweating accompany the pyrexia; there is an increase in the amount of cough and sputum, a neutrophil leucocytosis is usually present and there may be radiological evidence of pneumonia. Pleurisy frequently accompanies the febrile episodes and empyema is an occasional complication.

When chronic suppuration is a marked feature it causes a decline in the patient's general health, with lassitude, anorexia, loss of weight, sleep sweating and clubbing of the fingers and toes.

3. *Haemoptysis* is caused by bleeding from thin-walled vessels situated in the walls of the dilated bronchi. It ranges in amount from blood-stained sputum to massive haemorrhage. It may be present in association with the first two groups of symptoms, but recurrent haemoptysis may also occur as an isolated symptom in the absence of cough and sputum ('dry' bronchiectasis).

Physical signs may be unilateral or bilateral and are usually basal. If, however, the bronchiectatic cavities are dry and there is no lobar collapse, there may be no abnormal physical signs. If a large amount of secretion is present, numerous coarse crepitations are heard over the affected areas. When collapse is present the character of the physical signs depends on whether or not the proximal bronchi in the collapsed lobe are patent (Table 8.1).

Investigation. Bacteriological examination of the sputum is necessary in every case. In ordinary radiographs changes may be produced by associated pulmonary inflammation or collapse. A diagnosis of bronchiectasis can be made with certainty only by bronchography.

Treatment. *Postural drainage.* The purpose of this measure is to keep the dilated bronchi emptied of secretion. Efficiently performed it is of great value both in reducing the amount of cough and sputum and in preventing the 'toxaemia' caused by associated bronchopulmonary infection. In its simplest form, postural drainage consists of adopting a position in which the lobe to be drained is uppermost, so as to allow secretions in the dilated bronchi to gravitate towards the trachea, from which they can readily be cleared by vigorous coughing. The optimum duration and frequency of postural drainage depends on the amount of sputum, but 5 to 10 minutes once or twice daily is adequate in most cases.

Chemotherapy. The policy governing the use of antibiotics in bronchiectasis is the same as that in chronic bronchitis. Some patients, including those with cystic fibrosis, present difficult therapeutic problems because of secondary infection with bacteria such as staphylococci and Gram-negative bacilli, especially pseudomonas species.

Surgical treatment. If this is being considered, it is essential to obtain bronchograms demonstrating exactly the extent of the bronchiectasis. For this purpose the bronchi of all segments of both lungs must be outlined. Pulmonary function should also be assessed. Unfortunately many of the cases in which medical treatment proves unsuccessful are also unsuitable for resection either because the bronchiectasis is too extensive or because most of the symptoms are due to coexisting chronic bronchitis. Emphysema of even moderate severity is a contraindication to surgical treatment. The most favourable cases for surgery are children and young adults in whom the bronchiectasis is confined to a single lobe or part of a lobe.

Prevention. As bronchiectasis commonly starts in childhood following measles, whooping cough or a primary tuberculous infection, it is essential that these conditions receive adequate prophylaxis and treatment. The early recognition and treatment of bronchial obstruction is particularly important in this respect.

Prognosis. The disease is progressive when associated with ciliary dysfunction and cystic fibrosis. In other cases the prognosis is relatively good if postural drainage is performed regularly and antibiotics are used judiciously.

BRONCHIAL OBSTRUCTION

Aetiology. The lesions most likely to obstruct a large bronchus are: (1) tumours, e.g. bronchial carcinoma or adenoma; (2) enlarged tracheobronchial lymph nodes, malignant or tuberculous; (3) inhaled foreign bodies; (4) bronchial casts or plugs, consisting of inspissated mucus or blood clot; (5) collections of mucus or mucopus retained in the bronchi as a result of ineffective expectoration.

Rare causes of bronchial obstruction include congenital bronchial atresia, fibrous bronchial stricture (often post-tuberculous), aortic aneurysm, giant left atrium and pericardial effusion.

Clinical features. The manifestations of obstruction of a large bronchus depend on whether the obstruction is complete or partial, on secondary infection and on the effect on pulmonary function. The clinical features also vary with the cause of the obstruction.

1. COMPLETE OBSTRUCTION. When a large bronchus is completely obstructed, the air in the lung, lobe or segment it supplies is absorbed, the alveolar spaces close, and the affected portion of lung tissue becomes collapsed and solid. The percussion note over the collapsed lung or lobe is dull, and the breath sounds are absent or diminished. Radiological examination shows displacement of the trachea and/or heart shadow towards the side of the lesion, elevation of the diaphragm on the same side and a dense pulmonary opacity of characteristic size, shape and position (Figs 8.6 and 8.7).

If the collapse involves a smaller portion of lung (e.g. the right middle lobe or a bronchopulmonary segment), displacement of the mediastinum may not occur, and abnormal physical signs may be difficult to detect, but a characteristic radiographic opacity will be present.

2. PARTIAL OBSTRUCTION. If a large bronchus is partially obstructed, a situation occasionally arises in which there is less resistance to airflow through the narrowed bronchus during inspiration than during expiration, when the obstruction may become temporarily complete. This differential between inspiratory and expiratory airflow, which is increased by coughing, results in overdistension of the lung, lobe or segment supplied by the partially obstructed bronchus (*obstructive emphysema*). The percussion note over such a lesion is resonant or hyperresonant, and the breath sounds are diminished. A chest radiograph shows hypertranslucency of the affected part of lung, and on fluoroscopic examination the mediastinum can be seen to move towards the opposite side of the chest during expiration, because the volume of the affected lung then exceeds that of the contralateral lung.

3. SECONDARY INFECTION. Whenever a bronchus is narrowed, bacterial infection of the lung tissue it supplies is virtually inevitable, and this may occur even when the degree of obstruction is insufficient to cause collapse. This explains why pneumonia may be the first clinical manifestation of bronchial carcinoma. The infection is usually of low virulence, but in some cases severe pulmonary suppuration may occur.

4. IMPAIRED PULMONARY FUNCTION. This is unlikely to produce symptoms unless a main or lobar bronchus is involved, or the patient's overall pulmonary function is so poor that obstruction of a smaller bronchus critically diminishes the respiratory reserve. Sudden occlusion of a main or lobar bronchus by mucus or mucopus occurring as a postoperative complication may cause severe dyspnoea and hypoxaemia.

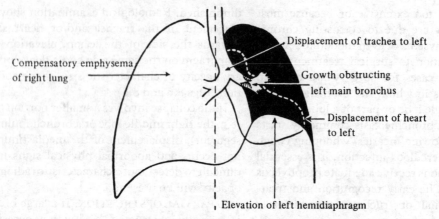

Compensatory emphysema of right lung

Displacement of trachea to left

Growth obstructing left main bronchus

Displacement of heart to left

Elevation of left hemidiaphragm

Fig. 8.6 Collapse of the left lung—effects on neighbouring structures.

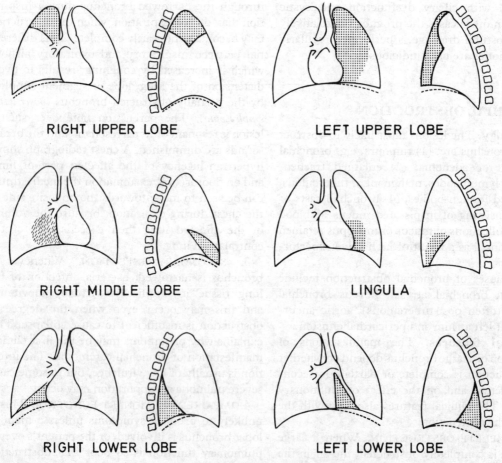

RIGHT UPPER LOBE

LEFT UPPER LOBE

RIGHT MIDDLE LOBE

LINGULA

RIGHT LOWER LOBE

LEFT LOWER LOBE

Fig. 8.7 Radiological features of lobar collapse caused by bronchial obstruction. The dotted line represents the normal position of the diaphragm.

5. CLINICAL FEATURES RELATED TO THE CAUSE OF THE OBSTRUCTION.

a. *Tumours.* Bronchial obstruction by a carcinoma usually produces pulmonary collapse at an early stage and seldom causes obstructive emphysema. Pulmonary infection is common, and this may be complicated by empyema. The degree of exertional dyspnoea produced by a bronchial carcinoma is directly related to the size of the obstructed bronchus. The rate of growth of a bronchial adenoma (p. 254) is much less rapid than that of a carcinoma. Complete bronchial obstruction and pulmonary collapse are therefore later developments in the presence of an adenoma, and obstructive emphysema, caused by partial bronchial obstruction, may be observed during the intervening period.

b. *Enlarged tracheobronchial lymph nodes.* By compressing or invading the bronchial wall, enlarged lymph nodes may produce the same clinical manifestations of bronchial obstruction as a tumour within the lumen, and in bronchial carcinoma both types of lesion may co-exist. Bronchial obstruction by enlarged lymph nodes in Hodgkin's disease and other forms of lymphoma is less common than in bronchial carcinoma, presumably because these are less invasive types of tumour.

In some children with primary tuberculous infection, large caseous tracheobronchial lymph nodes may compress and erode lobar or segmental bronchi, occasionally even a main bronchus. Caseous material and granulation tissue from the lymph node may be extruded into the bronchial lumen and increase the degree of bronchial obstruction. Tuberculous infection may develop in the collapsed lobe or segment, and later complications include bronchial stricture and bronchiectasis.

In all these conditions the supraclavicular lymph nodes may also be involved, and biopsy of one of these nodes may provide a positive histological diagnosis of tumour, lymphoma or tuberculosis.

c. *Foreign bodies.* An inhaled foreign body generally lodges in the right main, intermediate or lower bronchus, as these bronchi are almost directly in line with the trachea. Children, more often than adults, inhale foreign bodies such as nuts (usually peanuts), peas, beans and small pieces of pens or toys. Adults, on the other hand, are more likely to inhale fragments of tooth during extractions under general anaesthesia, and pieces of mutton or chicken bone.

When a foreign body becomes impacted in a bronchus, it first produces, after an initial episode of choking, either obstructive emphysema or lobar collapse. A persistent low-pitched rhonchus may be audible all over the chest if the bronchial lumen is not totally occluded. Within a few days pathogenic bacteria, carried into the respiratory tract with the foreign body, give rise to a suppurative pneumonia in the collapsed lobe. The patient at this stage often has a high temperature, cough productive of purulent sputum, and pleural pain. On clinical examination there may be a pleural rub and physical signs of either collapse or consolidation. Radiological examination shows either obstructive emphysema or collapse and/or pneumonic consolidation. It may also detect and locate a radio-opaque foreign body.

d. *Bronchial casts or plugs.* These may consist of either inspissated mucus or blood clot. Plugs of mucus may cause bronchial obstruction in patients with asthma or bronchial eosinophilia (p. 240). Secondary bacterial infection of the collapsed lung may occur, but is seldom severe. Bronchial obstruction by blood clot frequently follows severe haemoptysis, but as this complication is usually recognised and treated at an early stage, secondary bacterial infection of collapsed lung tissue seldom occurs.

e. *Retained secretions.* A main, lobar or segmental bronchus may be obstructed by retained mucus or mucopus when a patient is unable to cough effectively because of chest pain, muscular weakness or debility, e.g. following an upper abdominal or thoracic operation, or an injury to the chest wall. Secondary bacterial infection of the collapsed lung tissue supervenes at an early stage.

Investigation and treatment of bronchial obstruction. The cause of the bronchial obstruction can be discovered by bronchoscopic examination, and in the case of tumour and tuberculosis histological confirmation of the diagnosis can usually be obtained by biopsy. Foreign bodies can be extracted by bronchoscopy or bronchotomy. If bronchial casts, plugs or secretions cannot be dislodged by postural coughing, they should be removed through a bronchoscope. In other forms of bronchial obstruction the treatment is that of the primary condition.

Measures which may help to prevent postoperative pulmonary collapse include forbidding patients to smoke for 3 weeks prior to operation, vigorous pre- and postoperative breathing exercises, and regularly supervised coughing during the immediate postoperative period.

INTRATHORACIC TUMOURS

TUMOURS OF BRONCHUS AND LUNG

Bronchial carcinoma is by far the most common malignant pulmonary tumour. Benign tumours are rare. A primary carcinoma in any organ, but particularly in breast, kidney, uterus, ovary, testis, thyroid or in lung itself, may give rise to pulmonary metastatic deposits, as may an osteogenic or other sarcoma.

Bronchial carcinoma

Bronchial carcinoma accounts for more than 50% of all male deaths from malignant disease. It is more common in men than in women (although the gap is now narrowing), and occurs most frequently between the ages of 50 and 75. Cigarette smoking is responsible for most cases of bronchial carcinoma, and the increased risk is directly proportional to the amount smoked and to the tar content of the cigarettes. For example, the death rate from the disease in heavy cigarette smokers is 40 times that in non-smokers. It is slightly higher in urban than in rural dwellers, presumably because of atmospheric pollution. There is also a higher incidence of bronchial carcinoma in asbestosis.

Pathology. The tumour may be a squamous carcinoma (55%), a small cell carcinoma (25%), a large cell carcinoma (10%) or an adenocarcinoma (10%). It arises from bronchial epithelium or mucous glands and at an early stage may occlude the bronchial lumen. It also invades the deeper layers of the bronchial wall and the surrounding lung tissue. When the tumour obstructs a major bronchus it causes collapse and infection. A tumour arising from a peripheral bronchus may attain a very large size without producing a significant degree of collapse. Such a tumour, which is usually of the squamous type, may undergo central necrosis and cavitation.

The tumour may involve the pleura either directly or by lymphatic spread, causing a pleural effusion which is often blood-stained. It may also extend into the chest wall and cause severe pain by invading intercostal nerves or the brachial plexus. The tumour or its lymph node metastases may extend into the mediastinum, involving the left recurrent laryngeal and phrenic nerves, the sympathetic trunk, the superior vena cava, the pericardium and myocardium, the trachea and the oesophagus.

Lymphatic spread may occur to the supraclavicular ('scalene') as well as to the mediastinal lymph nodes. Blood-borne metastases occur most commonly in liver, bone, brain, suprarenals, skin and kidneys. Even a small primary tumour may cause widespread metastatic deposits. A carcinoma of the small cell type has often spread beyond the lung by the time it is diagnosed.

Clinical features. Cough is the most common early symptom. Sputum is purulent if there is secondary bacterial infection. Repeated slight haemoptysis is a common and characteristic feature. Dyspnoea may occur early when a lobe or lung is collapsed, or if there is a large pleural effusion, but in other circumstances is a late symptom unless the patient is coincidentally suffering from chronic bronchitis and emphysema. Pleural pain is a frequent symptom and may be due either to infective pleurisy or to malignant invasion of the pleura. Pain in the chest wall or in an upper limb with a nerve root distribution may be present if the tumour involves intercostal nerves or the brachial plexus. An apical bronchial carcinoma may cause Horner's syndrome (p. 616). The symptoms and signs which may occur if the tumour invades the mediastinum are described in the section on mediastinal tumours (p. 254).

Occasionally the presenting feature is the result of metastases, e.g. focal neurological signs, fits or personality change, jaundice, bone pain or skin nodules which may be tender. Lassitude, anorexia and loss of weight are late symptoms, usually indicative of extensive metastatic spread.

Clubbing of the fingers is often seen and a few patients present with the features of hypertrophic pulmonary osteoarthropathy. These are examples of non-metastatic extra-pulmonary manifestations of bronchial carcinoma; other paraneoplastic syndromes are listed in Table 8.10. Two of the endocrine syndromes, inappropriate ADH secretion (p. 90) and ectopic ACTH secretion (p. 451) are associated with small cell carcinoma, and a third, hypercalcaemia, usually with squamous carcinoma. The neurological syndromes (p. 668) may occur with any type of bronchial carcinoma, but perhaps more often with small cell tumours.

Table 8.10 Non-metastatic extra-pulmonary manifestations of bronchial carcinoma.

Endocrine	Inappropriate secretion of antidiuretic hormone (ADH)
	Ectopic ACTH secretion
	Hypercalcaemia
	Carcinoid syndrome
	Gynaecomastia
Neurological	Polyneuropathy
	Myelopathy
	Cerebellar degeneration
Other	Digital clubbing
	Hypertrophic pulmonary osteoarthropathy
	Nephrotic syndrome
	Myasthenia
	Polymyositis and dermatomyositis

Physical signs in the chest depend on the size of the tumour, but even more on the nature and extent of its secondary effects on lung and pleura. In the early stages a tumour may cause no abnormal physical signs. A tumour obstructing a large bronchus produces the physical signs of collapse or obstructive emphysema. Pulmonary infection beyond an obstructing tumour gives rise to pneumonia which is unusually slow to respond to treatment. A massive tumour may give rise to signs resembling those of a pleural effusion. Involvement of the pleura either by infection or by tumour may produce signs of pleurisy or of a pleural effusion.

Investigation. *Radiological examination.* A bronchial carcinoma may produce (1) a dense, irregular, hilar opacity, (2) a dense, fairly well circumscribed, peripheral pulmonary opacity, often large when first discovered, sometimes irregularly cavitated or (3) an opacity consistent with collapse of a whole lung, a lobe or a segment which may be associated with a hilar opacity due to the tumour itself.

In some cases radiological examination may show a pleural effusion (usually due to malignant spread but occasionally to bacterial infection), broadening of the mediastinal shadow (due to lymph node metastases), osteolytic lesions of the ribs (indicating either direct invasion by tumour or blood-borne metastases) or unilateral diaphragmatic paralysis (indicating involvement of the phrenic nerve). A paralysed hemidiaphragm is usually raised and on fluoroscopic examination moves 'paradoxically' upwards when the patient sniffs.

Bronchoscopy. Inspection of the intrabronchial portion of the tumour and removal of tissue for histological examination is possible in over 70% of cases.

Cytological examination of sputum or bronchial brushings for malignant cells is a valuable diagnostic measure when practised by a pathologist with special expertise in this technique. Percutaneous needle aspiration biopsy is a useful method of obtaining a positive cytological diagnosis in peripheral tumours, and when metastatic spread has occurred to lymph nodes, skin or liver.

Other investigations, such as transbronchial lung biopsy, scalene node biopsy or mediastinoscopy may be required to confirm the diagnosis.

Staging of the tumour (p. 105) is defined from the information obtained from the foregoing procedures.

Treatment and prognosis. Unless surgical treatment is practicable, the average period of survival, after the diagnosis is made, is less than a year. Resection of the lung (pneumonectomy) or, in some cases, of the lobe containing the tumour (lobectomy) offers the best prospect of survival. The operation can be performed only on the small number of cases (about 20%) in which the tumour is discovered at an early and relatively localised stage and pulmonary function is adequate. The tumour is liable to recur even after an apparently successful operation, and only 30% of such patients survive for more than 5 years. Early diagnosis provides slightly better results, but the prognosis depends to an even greater extent on the histological type of tumour and on the presence or absence of metastatic deposits in the hilar lymph nodes. The outlook is particularly unfavourable when the tumour is a small cell carcinoma.

Small tumours can occasionally be eradicated by radiotherapy, but this form of treatment is of greatest value in the palliation of distressing complications such as superior vena caval obstruction, recurrent haemoptysis and pain caused by chest wall invasion or by skeletal metastatic deposits. Obstruction of the trachea and main bronchi can also be relieved temporarily by radiotherapy, but as the latter may initially produce tumour swelling and a dangerous increase in the degree of obstruction, prednisolone should be given for 24–48 hours before treatment is started.

The treatment of small cell carcinoma with combinations of cytotoxic drugs can increase the median survival of patients with this highly malignant type of bronchial carcinoma from 3 months to over a year. This form of treatment is, however, still in the experimental stage and because of problems arising from the toxicity of the drugs it should for the present be undertaken only in specialised centres. Chemotherapy is of little value in the treatment of other histological types of bronchial carcinoma.

Bronchial adenoma

This is an uncommon tumour occurring in a younger age group than carcinoma, and affecting females as often as males. Although classified as a benign tumour it possesses some of the properties of a malignant growth and may eventually give rise to metastases. There are two histological types of bronchial adenoma, the relatively more common bronchial carcinoid and the rare cylindroma, or 'adenoid cystic carcinoma', which often arises at the tracheal bifurcation.

The clinical features, which may have a duration of several years, are recurrent haemoptysis, due to the vascularity of the tumour, recurrent pulmonary infection resulting from bronchial obstruction and, in rare cases, usually when metastatic spread has occurred, the carcinoid syndrome (p. 312). The physical signs most frequently found are those of collapse. The diagnosis from bronchial carcinoma can be made only by bronchoscopy and histological examination of a portion of the tumour.

Treatment consists of resection of the pulmonary lobe or segment containing the tumour along with the bronchus from which it arises.

Secondary tumours of the lung

Blood-borne metastatic deposits in the lungs may be derived from many primary tumours (p. 252). The secondary deposits are usually multiple and bilateral. Haemoptysis occurs in a few cases but often there are no respiratory symptoms and the diagnosis is made by radiological examination.

Lymphatic infiltration may develop in patients with carcinoma of breast, stomach, pancreas or bronchus. This grave condition, *pulmonary lymphatic carcinomatosis*, causes severe and rapidly progressive dyspnoea.

TUMOURS OF THE MEDIASTINUM

Classification. *Tumours of the lymph nodes*, e.g. secondary carcinoma, usually from bronchus or breast; lymphomas; leukaemia.

Oesophageal tumours, e.g. carcinoma (p. 282).

Thymic tumours, e.g. benign or malignant thymoma.

Connective tissue tumours, e.g. fibroma, lipoma (benign); sarcoma (malignant).

Neural tumours, e.g. neurofibroma.

Developmental tumours and cysts, e.g. teratoma; dermoid, bronchogenic and pleuro-pericardial cysts.

Other lesions may present as mediastinal tumours, e.g. aortic aneurysm, aneurysmal dilatation of left atrium, intrathoracic goitre, sarcoidosis involving lymph nodes.

Pathology and clinical features

BENIGN TUMOURS AND CYSTS. The conditions in this category, which are all rare, include neural tumours, teratoma, developmental cysts and intrathoracic goitre. They may compress, but do not invade, vital structures. The diagnosis of benign tumour or cyst is usually made by chance, when radiological examination of the chest is undertaken for some other reason. If a tumour becomes very large it may cause dyspnoea by compression of lung tissue, or occasionally by narrowing the trachea. A benign tumour in the upper part of the thorax occasionally compresses the superior vena cava (below). A dermoid cyst occasionally ruptures into a bronchus.

MALIGNANT TUMOURS. Included in this category are mediastinal lymph node metastases, lymphomas, leukaemia, malignant thymic tumours and mediastinal sarcoma. Aortic and innominate aneurysms have destructive features resembling those of malignant mediastinal tumours. All these conditions, except lymph node metastases, are uncommon.

The distinguishing feature of this group of tumours is their power to invade as well as to compress mediastinal structures, bronchi and lungs. As a result of this property even a small malignant tumour can produce symptoms, although as a rule the tumour has attained a considerable size before this happens. The structures which may be invaded or compressed and the symptoms and signs produced in each case are:

Trachea: dyspnoea, stridor, paroxysmal cough.

Main bronchus: dyspnoea, stridor, pulmonary collapse.

Oesophagus: dysphagia, oesophageal displacement or obstruction on barium swallow examination.

Phrenic nerve: diaphragmatic paralysis.

Left recurrent laryngeal nerve: paralysis of left vocal cord, hoarseness, bovine cough.

Sympathetic trunk: Horner's syndrome.

Superior vena cava: oedema and cyanosis of head and neck, and sometimes of upper limbs also, with distension of external jugular veins and dilated anastomotic veins on anterior chest wall and in axillary regions.

Pericardium: pericarditis, either dry with pericardial rub, or with effusion.

Investigation. *Radiological examination.* A benign mediastinal tumour generally appears as a large, round, sharply circumscribed opacity, situated mainly in the mediastinum but often encroaching on one or both lung fields. A malignant mediastinal tumour seldom has a clearly defined margin and often presents as a general broadening of the mediastinal shadow. Fluoroscopic examination of the diaphragm and oeso-

phagus should be undertaken in all suspected cases of mediastinal tumour.

As bronchial carcinoma is such a common primary cause of mediastinal tumour, *bronchoscopy* should be carried out in all cases. If enlarged mediastinal lymph nodes are suspected one of these can be removed for histological examination by the technique of *mediastinoscopy* (p. 207). In some cases, however, an exact diagnosis cannot be made without *surgical exploration* of the chest and removal of the tumour or a portion of it for histological examination.

Treatment. Benign mediastinal tumours should be removed surgically as soon as they are discovered because (1) they tend to produce symptoms sooner or later and (2) some of them, particularly cysts, may become infected while others, especially neural tumours, may become malignant. The operative mortality is low.

The treatment of lymphoma and leukaemia is described on pages 534 and 525 respectively. A malignant thymoma usually responds dramatically to radiotherapy. Lymph node metastases from bronchial carcinoma may respond well temporarily to radiotherapy or to cytotoxic chemotherapy, especially if the tumour is of the small cell type; complications such as superior vena caval and tracheal obstruction can often be relieved in this way.

PULMONARY FIBROSIS AND RELATED DISEASES

There are three main types of pulmonary fibrosis:

1. *Replacement fibrosis,* in which the fibrous tissue replaces lung parenchyma damaged by infection or by some other destructive process (e.g. infarction). Fibrosis of this type is a common feature of pulmonary tuberculosis and of all types of pulmonary suppuration (p. 221), and is often associated with bronchiectasis.

2. *Focal fibrosis,* which is a common manifestation of pneumoconiosis.

3. *Interstitial fibrosis,* which is the end-result of interstitial lung disease.

If pulmonary fibrosis is extensive, it will cause exertional dyspnoea and hypoxaemia, and this is more likely to be the case in focal and interstitial fibrosis than in replacement fibrosis. On the other hand, the physical signs and radiological changes will usually be more conspicuous in replacement fibrosis, which generally produces gross localised abnormalities.

INTERSTITIAL LUNG DISEASE

This term is applied to a group of pulmonary diseases which have the following features in common: (1) thickening of the alveolar walls by oedema, cellular exudate or fibrosis; (2) increased stiffness of the lungs (reduced compliance), associated with exertional dyspnoea; (3) maldistribution of pulmonary ventilation and perfusion, and a gas transfer defect leading to hypoxaemia, hyperventilation and hypocapnia.

Aetiology. Interstitial lung disease is caused by several different pathological processes, but these all give rise to similar symptoms, physical signs, radiological changes and disturbances of pulmonary function. They are thus worthy of collective consideration. Causes of interstitial lung disease are:

1. Chronic pulmonary oedema e.g. secondary to mitral valve disease.

2. Extrinsic allergic alveolitis.

3. Fibrosing alveolitis associated with the connective tissue disorders.

4. Pulmonary damage following radiotherapy to the thorax.

5. Drugs, e.g. bleomycin (p. 113), busulphan (p. 528), methotrexate (p. 109), amiodarone (p. 137) and gold (p. 562).

6. Sarcoidosis (p. 260), asbestosis (p. 259), and idiopathic pulmonary haemosiderosis (see below).

Fibrosing alveolitis exemplifies many of the typical features of interstitial lung disease. It may be a manifestation of one of the connective tissue disorders, such as rheumatoid disease, systemic lupus erythematosus or systemic sclerosis, or it may occur as an isolated pulmonary abnormality (cryptogenic fibrosing alveolitis).

Progressive exertional dyspnoea is usually the presenting symptom, often accompanied by a persistent dry cough. In most cases there is gross clubbing of the fingers and toes. Chest expansion is poor, but hyperventilation is always a striking feature. Numerous bilateral end-inspiratory crepitations (crackles) are audible on auscultation.

Radiologically, there are diffuse pulmonary opacities, the diaphragm is high and the lungs appear small. There is a restrictive ventilatory defect, with proportionate reduction of FEV_1 and VC. The carbon monoxide transfer factor is low, and there is arterial hypoxaemia and hypocapnia. Broncho-alveolar lavage fluid usually contains an increase in the numbers of neutrophils and eosinophils. The diagnosis can usually be made with confidence from these findings. Serological tests for antinuclear and rheumatoid factors may be positive, even in cases without evidence of a connective tissue disorder.

The rate of progression of the pulmonary changes varies considerably, from death within a few months to survival with minimal symptoms for many years.

Treatment with corticosteroids is effective in perhaps 30% of the acute cases, but is of little or no value in the others, few of whom survive for more than 5 years.

Honeycomb lung. The radiological phenomenon of 'honeycomb lung' in which diffuse pulmonary shadowing is interspersed with small cystic translucencies, may be observed in some cases of interstitial lung disease, but it may also be a characteristic feature of certain rare diseases, such as histiocytosis X and tuberous sclerosis. Honeycomb lung, whatever its cause, is associated with an increased incidence of spontaneous pneumothorax, and eventually produces respiratory failure, pulmonary hypertension and right ventricular failure.

Idiopathic pulmonary haemosiderosis is a rare disease of unknown cause, in which spontaneous haemorrhage into the lungs causes recurrent episodes of pyrexia, haemoptysis and iron-deficiency anaemia. If the patient survives the acute haemorrhagic episodes, interstitial fibrosis may eventually cause respiratory failure and pulmonary hypertension. Pulmonary haemosiderosis may also be associated with acute glomerulonephritis (Goodpasture's syndrome, p. 388).

OCCUPATIONAL LUNG DISEASES

In certain occupations the inhalation of dusts, fumes or other noxious substances may give rise to specific pathological changes in the lungs. The nature of each substance, the occupation in which the hazard occurs, the description of each disease and the pathological changes produced in the lungs are summarised in Table 8.11.

Since a diagnosis of occupational lung disease can easily be overlooked and the victims of it may be eligible for compensation, it is most important to take a detailed occupational history, past as well as present. It must also be emphasised that in many types of pneumoconiosis a long period of exposure to dust is required before radiological changes appear and these may precede symptoms by several years. Notes on diagnosis and claims for benefits in pneumoconiosis, occupational asthma and other related occupational diseases in Britain are contained in government pamphlets (p. 268). New industrial processes are constantly being introduced and it is necessary to remain alert to the possibility that they may be associated with new occupational lung diseases.

DISEASES CAUSED BY MINERAL DUSTS (PNEUMOCONIOSIS)

The dust particles, after inhalation, are conveyed by macrophages from the bronchial mucosa to minute foci of lymphoid tissue throughout the lungs. There the irritation produced by solution of the particles in tissue fluid may initiate widespread pulmonary fibrosis. The fibrogenic capacities of mineral dusts vary, silica being markedly fibrogenic whereas iron is almost inert. The most important types of pneumoconiosis are coal-worker's pneumoconiosis, silicosis and asbestosis.

Coal-worker's pneumoconiosis

The disease results from prolonged inhalation of coal dust. For clinical purposes (and for certification) the condition is subdivided into simple pneumoconiosis and progressive massive fibrosis. It must be emphasised that for certification purposes in Britain the diagnosis rests at present on radiological, and not clinical, features.

Simple coal-worker's pneumoconiosis. This is categorised radiologically into 3 grades, depending on the size and extent of the nodulation present. It does not progress if the miner leaves the industry.

Progressive massive fibrosis. In this form of the disease, large dense masses, single or multiple, occur mainly in the upper lobes. These may be irregular in shape and may cavitate. This type of disease may be complicated by tuberculosis. It may be disabling, may shorten life expectancy and may progress even after the miner leaves the industry.

Cough and sputum due to associated chronic bronchitis are frequently present. The sputum may be black. Progressive breathlessness on exertion occurs in the later stages, and ventilatory and right ventricular failure supervene as terminal events. There may be no abnormal physical signs in the chest, but where present they are those of chronic obstructive airways disease.

Antinuclear factor is present in the serum of about 15% of patients with coal-worker's pneumoconiosis. Rheumatoid factor is present in some patients, as in *Caplan's syndrome*, in which rheumatoid arthritis coexists with rounded fibrotic nodules 0.5 to 5 cm in diameter, mainly in the periphery of the lung fields. This syndrome may also occur in other types of pneumoconiosis.

Silicosis

This disease is becoming much more rare as the standards of industrial hygiene improve. It is caused by the inhalation of fine free crystalline silicon dioxide (silica) dust or quartz particles. It occurs in the following occupations: mining of coal, tin, gold and other minerals; quarrying, mining and dressing of sandstone and granite; the pottery and ceramics industry; the manufacture of silica bricks and abrasive soaps; iron and steel industries; sand blasting, metal grinding and boiler scaling.

Silica is a very fibrogenic dust and causes the development of hard nodules which coalesce as the disease progresses. Tuberculosis may modify the silicotic process, and caseation and calcification may occur. The radiological features are similar to those seen in coal-worker's pneumoconiosis though the changes tend to be more marked in the upper zones. The hilar shadows may be enlarged and 'egg-shell' calcification in the hilar lymph nodes is a distinctive feature. The

Table 8.11 Causes and effects of occupational lung disease.

Cause	Occupation	Description of disease	Characteristic features
Mineral dusts:			
Coal dust	Coal mining	Coal-worker's pneumoconiosis	
Silica	Gold mining Iron and steel industries Metal grinding Stone dressing Pottery	Silicosis	Focal and interstitial fibrosis Centrilobular emphysema Progressive massive fibrosis
Asbestos	Manufacture of fireproof and insulating materials Shipbreaking	Asbestos-related disease	Asbestos bodies Interstitial fibrosis Pleural plaques and effusion Bronchial carcinoma Pleural mesothelioma
Iron oxide Tin dioxide	Arc welding Tin ore mining	Siderosis Stannosis	Mineral deposition only
Beryllium	Aircraft and atomic energy industries	Berylliosis	Granulomata Interstitial fibrosis
Organic dusts:			
Cotton, flax or hemp dust	Textile industries	Byssinosis	Acute bronchiolitis Bronchoconstriction
Fungal spores from mouldy hay, straw or grain, mushroom compost, bagasse, etc.	Agriculture and related industries	Farmer's lung Maltworker's lung Mushroom worker's lung Bagassosis	Extrinsic allergic alveolitis
Gases and fumes:			
Irritant gases (ammonia, chlorine, phosgene, sulphur and nitrogen dioxide)	Various industries (accidental exposure)		Acute pulmonary oedema
Cadmium	Welding and electroplating		Chronic bronchitis and emphysema
Isocyanates, e.g. toluene di-isocyanate	Manufacture of plastic foam, paints and adhesives Paint-spraying of vehicles in motor industry		Bronchial asthma Eosinophilic pneumonia Alveolitis
Platinum salts	Platinum refining Laboratory work involving platinum compounds		Bronchial asthma
Acid anhydride and amine hardening agents (including epoxy resin curing agents)	Manufacture of epoxy resins Manufacture of adhesives Moulding of resins and plastics		Bronchial asthma
Rosin (colophony) used in soldering fluxes	Electronics industry		Bronchial asthma
Biological substances:			
Proteolytic enzymes, e.g. *Bacillus subtilis*, pancreatic extracts, papain	Detergent manufacturing Pharmaceutical industry Food processing		Bronchial asthma
Animal and insect excreta	Animal laboratories Farming Flour milling		Bronchial asthma
Grain dust contaminated by mites and fungal spores	Combine harvesting Handling of stored grain		Bronchial asthma

disease tends to progress even when exposure to dust ceases. The sufferer should therefore be removed from the offending environment as soon as possible.

Clinical features are similar to those described in coal-worker's pneumoconiosis.

Asbestos-related diseases of the lungs and pleura

The main types of asbestos are chrysotile, which accounts for 90% of the world's production, and crocidolite (blue asbestos). Exposure occurs in the following occupations: mining and milling of the mineral; manufacturing processes involving asbestos; pipe lagging and spraying of limpet asbestos. Demolition workers, including those who may work alongside them, e.g. joiners, painters and electricians are also at risk.

Four forms of disease related to inhalation of asbestos are recognised — benign pleural plaques, benign pleural effusion, progressive pulmonary fibrosis (pulmonary asbestosis) and malignant disease of pleura (mesothelioma). Of these, only two qualify for industrial injury benefit in Britain.

1. *Benign pleural plaques*, which are often calcified, are best seen in the early stages on oblique films. They are most commonly found on the diaphragm and anterolaterally.

2. *Benign pleural effusion* is considered to be a specific asbestos-related entity and may be associated with pleural pain, fever and leucocytosis. The pleural liquid may be blood-stained and differentiation of this benign condition from a malignant effusion caused by mesothelioma can be difficult.

3. *Pulmonary asbestosis* is characterised by increasing shortness of breath on exertion and cough, by the presence of clubbing of the fingers and end-inspiratory crepitations at the bases and anterolaterally, and by typical radiological and physiological abnormalities.

The radiological abnormalities are usually confined to the lower two-thirds of the lung fields and consist of mottled shadows with some streaky opacities and sometimes 'honeycombing'. The cardiac silhouette becomes 'shaggy'.

The most important physiological abnormalities are a reduced carbon monoxide transfer factor and a restrictive ventilatory defect. Respiratory and right ventricular failure eventually supervene. The incidence of bronchial carcinoma is much increased, about ten-fold, in persons suffering from asbestosis.

Lung biopsy may be required to confirm the diagnosis, but is not without risk and should not be carried out solely for the purpose of allowing patients to claim benefits.

4. *Mesothelioma of the pleura* is usually linked with exposure, often relatively trivial, to blue asbestos. The patient frequently presents with chest pain. A pleural effusion, often blood-stained, may develop, and cause breathlessness. In some cases the diagnosis can be confirmed histologically by pleural biopsy, but tumour masses may later develop in the chest wall at the site of biopsy. Thoracotomy is seldom justified as a diagnostic procedure in patients with suspected mesothelioma.

Treatment and prevention of pneumoconiosis

No specific treatment is available. In the later stages treatment is required for associated conditions such as chronic bronchitis and respiratory failure, pulmonary tuberculosis or malignant pleural effusion.

Improvement of standards of industrial hygiene are now enforced by law in many countries; such measures as wearing respirators, damping dust and efficient ventilation systems are already proving effective in a number of industries.

DISEASES CAUSED BY ORGANIC DUSTS

In *byssinosis* the initial lesion is an acute bronchiolitis, associated with symptoms and signs of generalised airflow obstruction which tend to be worse after weekend breaks, but eventually become continuous. There is no radiological abnormality. Recovery usually follows removal from exposure to the dust hazard.

Humidifier fever is a disease with a similar pattern of symptoms during the working week. It is thought to be caused by water-borne microorganisms from contaminated humidifiers in forced air ventilation systems.

Other diseases caused by organic dusts are forms of asthma or extrinsic allergic alveolitis, described on pages 241 and 242.

SARCOIDOSIS

Sarcoidosis is a multisystem granulomatous disease. It is associated with imbalance between subsets of T lymphocytes and other disturbances of cell-mediated immunity, but the relationship between these phenomena and sarcoidosis has not so far been explained. Apart from absence of caseation and tubercle bacilli, the lesions are histologically similar to tuberculous follicles, but there is no convincing evidence to support the view that the disease is caused by any of the mycobacteria. Chronic beryllium poisoning produces a disease which mimics sarcoidosis both pathologically and clinically, but exposure to beryllium is extremely uncommon and such cases are rare. Histological changes resembling those of sarcoidosis are occasionally seen in individual organs, such as lymph nodes, in conditions such as carcinoma, and fungal infections, but these localised 'sarcoid reactions' are not associated with systemic sarcoidosis.

Pathology. The mediastinal and superficial lymph nodes, lungs, liver, spleen, skin, eyes, parotid glands and phalangeal bones are most frequently involved. The characteristic histological feature consists of non-caseating epithelioid follicles. These lesions usually resolve spontaneously but in some cases they stimulate the production of fibrous tissue, which may have grave effects on local structure and function. The disease is seldom fatal, and then only when it affects vital organs such as the lungs, the heart or the central nervous system. Calcium metabolism may be disturbed causing hypercalcaemia and, rarely, nephrocalcinosis and renal failure.

Clinical features. Sarcoidosis may present in a subacute or a chronic form. The pulmonary changes are described in three stages.

SUBACUTE SARCOIDOSIS is usually a benign and self-limiting disorder, spontaneous resolution occurring within a year in most cases. One of its most common manifestations is bilateral and often symmetrical enlargement of the hilar lymph nodes (*Stage* 1). The paratracheal lymph nodes may also be involved. Erythema nodosum, pyrexia and polyarthralgia (p. 573) may be present at the outset. Later, transient pulmonary changes may be seen on radiological examination in addition to the lymph node enlargement (*Stage* 2).

CHRONIC SARCOIDOSIS is a more serious condition, which is less likely to resolve spontaneously and is more liable to cause permanent damage to the structures it involves. Chronic pulmonary sarcoidosis (*Stage* 3) may lead to the development of interstitial fibrosis, pulmonary hypertension and cor pulmonale. The vital capacity and carbon monoxide transfer factor are the most useful indices of impairment of lung function in this form of the disease.

EXTRA-PULMONARY MANIFESTATIONS. Sarcoidosis is a multisystem disease of which the following are examples:

Eyes. Bilateral chronic iritis which, if untreated, may cause blindness. Lachrimal gland involvement.

Skin. Erythema nodosum (see above). Cutaneous 'sarcoids' (reddish-brown papules). Lupus pernio (raised purple plaques usually on nose and cheeks). Infiltration of scars.

Salivary glands. Parotid gland enlargement.

Heart. Myocarditis.

Kidneys. Nephrocalcinosis.

Liver and spleen. Granulomas.

Nervous system. Cerebral, meningeal and cranial or peripheral nerve lesions.

Bones and joints. Phalangeal cysts and arthritis (p. 573).

Investigation. In most cases skin sensitivity to tuberculin is depressed or absent, and the Mantoux reaction is therefore a useful 'screening' test, a strongly positive reaction to 1 TU virtually excluding sarcoidosis. Although the diagnosis can often be made with a fair measure of confidence from the clinical and radiological features and the tuberculin test, it should, if possible, be confirmed histologically by biopsy of a superficial lymph node or of a skin lesion, when these are present. Transbronchial lung biopsy almost always confirms the diagnosis.

The Kveim test is also a useful diagnostic procedure, provided a potent antigen can be obtained from human sarcoid tissue. The antigen (0.1 ml) is injected intradermally and when the test is positive a small nodule develops about 4 weeks later, biopsy of which reveals typical sarcoid follicles.

Bronchoalveolar lavage usually yields fluid with an increased proportion of lymphocytes and ^{67}gallium scanning shows increased pulmonary uptake of this isotope when the disease is active. There is also an elevation of the plasma level of the angiotensin-converting enzyme from the endothelium of the pulmonary capillaries. Although these investigations are not specific for sarcoidosis they may be of value in the assessment of disease activity and response to treatment.

Treatment. As subacute sarcoidosis usually resolves spontaneously treatment is seldom required, but occasionally patients with persistent erythema nodosum, pyrexia, parotid swelling or iridocyclitis may have to be given oral corticosteroid therapy for a short period.

Chronic sarcoidosis, particularly if it involves the lungs, eyes or other vital organs, is much more likely to require treatment with corticosteroids, which may have to be continued for several years. The dose should be kept to the minimum required to suppress the manifestations of the disease.

DISEASES OF THE PLEURA AND CHEST WALL

FIBRINOUS PLEURISY

This term is used to describe cases of pleurisy at the stage of fibrinous exudation when there is no significant degree of effusion. It is usually secondary to bacterial infection in the underlying lung, but may also occur in association with a viral infection (Coxsackie B), which primarily involves the intercostal muscles and is known as 'Bornholm disease'. Pleurisy is a common feature of pulmonary infarction, and may be an early manifestation of pleural invasion by a pulmonary tumour or of pulmonary tuberculosis.

Clinical features. Pleural pain is the characteristic symptom. On examination, rib movement is restricted and the breath sounds may be diminished on the affected side. A pleural rub is present in many cases, particularly when the patient is asked to take a deep breath. It is not heard when the breath is held, except near the pericardium where a so-called pleuropericardial rub may be present.

The other clinical features depend on the nature of the lesion causing the pleurisy. Depending on the cause, complete clinical recovery may ensue or an effusion may develop, either serous or purulent.

Radiological examination must be performed in every case but a negative radiograph does not necessarily exclude a pulmonary cause for the pleurisy. A preceding history of a few days of cough, purulent sputum, and pyrexia is presumptive evidence of a pulmonary infection which may not have been severe enough to produce a radiographic abnormality or which may have resolved before the film was taken.

Treatment. The primary cause of the pleurisy must be treated. The symptomatic treatment of pleural pain is described on page 214.

PLEURAL EFFUSION

This term is applied only to serous effusions. The condition of purulent effusion or empyema is described on page 263. The passive transudation of fluid into the pleural cavity (*hydrothorax*) occurs in cardiac failure, nephrotic syndrome, advanced cirrhosis of the liver and severe malnutrition.

The most common causes of pleural effusion are pneumonia, tuberculosis, malignant disease and pulmonary infarction. Pleural effusion, often bilateral, may also be a manifestation of rheumatoid disease, systemic lupus erythematosus and lymphoma. Inflammatory lesions below the diaphragm, such as subphrenic abscess, amoebic liver abscess and pancreatitis, occasionally produce a pleural effusion. The cause of the majority of pleural effusions can be identified if a careful history is taken and comprehensive clinical examination performed.

Where the cause is obscure a lead may be given by enquiry regarding travel abroad, occupation (for example exposure to asbestos), contact with tuberculosis, or causes of thromboembolism (oral contraception; recent operation). Detailed investigations as described below may, however, be necessary.

Clinical features. The symptoms and signs of pleurisy often precede the development of effusion, but the onset in other cases may be insidious. Dyspnoea is the only symptom related to the effusion itself. Its severity depends on the size of the effusion and the rate at which it accumulates. The physical signs in the chest are those of fluid in the pleural space (p. 207).

Investigation. *Radiological examination* shows a dense uniform opacity in the lower and lateral parts of the hemithorax shading off above and medially into translucent lung. Occasionally the fluid is localised below the lower lobe, the appearances simulating an elevated hemidiaphragm. When the effusion is loculated, for example, in an interlobar fissure, a localised opacity is seen.

Ultrasonography is of value in detecting and localising an effusion.

Pleural aspiration. Absolute proof that an effusion is present can be obtained only by the aspiration of fluid. A needle should be inserted through an intercostal space over the area of maximum dullness on percussion, at the site of maximum radiological opacity as shown by postero-anterior and lateral films or at a site determined by ultrasound. At least 50 ml of fluid should be withdrawn, 20 ml or more being placed in a sterile container for bacteriological examination, 20 ml in a citrated container for cytological examination and 10 ml in a chemically clean container for biochemical examination. Pleural biopsy is always indicated whenever a diagnostic aspiration of pleural fluid is performed.

The appearance of the fluid should be noted — straw-coloured, blood-stained, purulent or chylous. The protein content will give an indication as to whether the effusion is an exudate ($>30\,g/l$) or a transudate ($<30\,g/l$). The predominant cell type (polymorph, lymphocyte, red blood cell) gives useful information, and the fluid should be examined for malignant cells.

There is a high amylase level in effusions secondary to acute pancreatitis and a high concentration of cholesterol in most chronic rheumatoid effusions. Microbiological investigation, including culture for *Myco. tuberculosis* should be performed where appropriate.

Other investigations may be required to determine the primary cause of a pleural effusion. Estimation of the total and differential leucocyte count in the peripheral blood, a tuberculin test, and examination of the sputum for tubercle bacilli should never be omitted. Radiological examination of the chest may disclose underlying pulmonary disease and indicate its nature. If the lung is obscured by a massive effusion, this examination should be repeated after a large volume of fluid has been aspirated. Other investigations which may help to determine the cause of a pleural effusion include bronchoscopy, biopsy or aspiration of a scalene lymph node, thoracoscopy and serological tests for antinuclear and rheumatoid factors.

The main features of the more important causes of pleural effusion are shown in Table 8.12.

Treatment. Aspiration of pleural fluid may be necessary to relieve breathlessness. It is inadvisable to remove more than 1 litre on the first occasion, since pulmonary oedema occasionally follows the aspiration of larger amounts. Even a careful operator may accidentally produce a pneumothorax (hydropneumothorax) and a radiograph of the chest should be taken after the procedure.

Treatment of the underlying cause, for example heart failure, pneumonia, pulmonary embolism and subphrenic abscess, will often be followed by resolution of the effusion, but certain conditions require special measures.

Postpneumonic pleural effusion may require aspiration, as necessary, to ensure that an empyema has not developed and to prevent pleural thickening.

Tuberculous pleural effusion should always be treated with antituberculous chemotherapy (p. 230). Aspiration is required initially if the effusion is large and causing dyspnoea, but the addition of prednisolone by mouth will promote rapid absorption of the fluid and obviate the need for further aspiration.

Malignant effusions reaccumulate and to avoid the distress of repeated aspirations, an attempt should be made to obliterate the pleural space (pleurodesis) by injecting substances which produce an inflammatory reaction and extensive pleural adhesions. The agents most frequently

Table 8.12 Pleural effusion: main causes and features.

	Appearance of fluid	Type of fluid	Predominant cells in fluid	Other diagnostic features
Tuberculous	Serous, usually amber coloured	Exudate	Lymphocytes (occas. polymorphs)	Positive tuberculin test. Isolation of *Myco. tuberculosis* Positive pleural biopsy (80%)
Malignant disease	Serous, often blood-stained	Exudate	Serosal cells and lymphocytes Often clumps of malignant cells	Positive pleural biopsy (40%) Evidence of malignant disease elsewhere
*Cardiac failure	Serous, straw-coloured	Transudate	Few serosal cells	Other evidence of left heart failure Response to diuretics
*Pulmonary infarction	Serous or blood-stained	Exudate	Red blood cells Eosinophils	Contralateral evidence of infarction Source of embolism. Factors predisposing to venous thrombosis
*Rheumatoid disease	Serous Turbid if chronic	Exudate	Lymphocytes (occas. polymorphs)	Rheumatoid arthritis Rheumatoid factor in serum. Cholesterol in chronic effusion. Low glucose
*Systemic lupus erythematosus	Serous	Exudate	Lymphocytes and serosal cells	Other manifestations of SLE. ANF or anti-DNA in serum
Obstruction of thoracic duct	Milky	Chyle	None	Chylomicrons

*Effusion often bilateral.

used for this purpose are, inactivated *Corynebacterium parvum*, tetracycline and mustine hydrochloride.

EMPYEMA THORACIS

This is the term used to describe the presence of pus in the pleural space. The pus may be as thin as serous fluid, or so thick that it is difficult to aspirate even through a wide-bore needle. Microscopically, neutrophil leucocytes are present in large numbers. The causative organism may or may not be isolated from the pus. An empyema may involve the whole pleural space ('total' empyema) or only part of it ('loculated' or 'encysted' empyema). It is almost invariably unilateral.

Aetiology. Empyema is always secondary to infection in a neighbouring structure, usually the lung. The principal infections liable to produce empyema are the bacterial pneumonias and tuberculosis. Other causes of empyema are infection of a

haemothorax and rupture of a subphrenic abscess through the diaphragm. Empyema has become a relatively rare disease because pulmonary infection can now be so readily controlled by antibacterial therapy.

Pathology. Both layers of pleura are covered with a thick, shaggy, inflammatory exudate. The pus in the pleural space is often under considerable pressure and if the condition is not adequately treated it may rupture into a bronchus, from which it is expectorated, or through an intercostal space with the formation of a subcutaneous abscess or sinus. When an empyema ruptures into a bronchus, a bronchopleural fistula is produced and a pyopneumothorax is formed.

The only way in which an empyema can heal is by apposition of the visceral and parietal layers of the pleura with obliteration of the empyema space by organisation of the intervening exudate. This cannot occur unless re-expansion of the collapsed lung is secured at an early stage by removal of all the pus from the pleural space. Re-expansion of the lung cannot take place if, (1) through delay in treatment or inadequate drainage, the visceral pleura becomes grossly thickened and rigid, (2) if the pleural layers are kept apart by air entering the pleura through a bronchopleural fistula, or (3) if disease in the lung itself, such as bronchiectasis, bronchial carcinoma or pulmonary tuberculosis, renders it incapable of re-expansion. In all these circumstances an empyema tends to become chronic and healing may not take place without recourse to major thoracic surgery.

Clinical features. Empyema should be suspected in patients with pulmonary infection if there is a recurrence of pyrexia in spite of the continued administration of a suitable antibiotic. In other cases the illness produced by the primary infective lesion may be so slight that it passes unrecognised and the first definite clinical features are due to the empyema itself.

In the fully developed case two separate groups of clinical features are found:

Systemic features: (1) Pyrexia, usually high and remittent but sometimes slight. (2) Rigors, sweating, malaise, anorexia and loss of weight. (3) Neutrophil leucocytosis.

Local features: (1) Dyspnoea, when the empyema is large. (2) Pleural pain, usually confined to the initial stage of the illness. (3) Cough and purulent sputum, usually related to the primary lung disease, but occasionally caused by the rupture of an empyema into a bronchus. An empyema usually produces the typical signs of fluid in the pleural space (p. 207), unless it is small or localised.

Investigation. *Radiological examination.* The appearances are indistinguishable from those of pleural effusion. When air is present in addition to pus (pyopneumothorax), a horizontal 'fluid level' marks the interface of liquid and air if the film is taken in the erect position.

Aspiration of pus confirms the presence of an empyema. A wide-bore needle should be inserted through an intercostal space over the area of maximal dullness on percussion. Whenever possible the position of the empyema should have previously been confirmed by posteroanterior and lateral radiographs or by ultrasonography.

Bacteriological examination of the pus may help to determine the cause of the empyema. In post-pneumonic cases where intensive treatment with antibiotics has been given the pus is frequently sterile. The distinction between tuberculous and non-tuberculous cases can usually be made from the radiological changes in the lungs or by the isolation of tubercle bacilli from pus or sputum.

Treatment

NON-TUBERCULOUS EMPYEMA

1. *Acute.* When the patient is acutely ill, and the pus is thin in consistency:

a. An intercostal tube should be inserted into the most dependent part of the empyema space and connected to a water seal drainage system.

b. An antibiotic to which the organism causing the empyema is sensitive should be given.

If treatment is started early enough, and the organisms are drug-sensitive, an empyema can often be aborted by these measures. If, however, the intercostal tube is not providing adequate drainage, which is apt to happen when the pus thickens and clots, a short segment of rib should be resected, the empyema cavity cleared of pus and clot, and a wide-bore tube inserted.

2. *Chronic.* If the diagnosis is made before any drainage procedure is carried out, it may be feasible to resect the empyema sac *in toto*, provided the patient is fairly fit and the underlying lung is healthy. If open drainage has been performed, and re-expansion of the lung is prevented by gross thickening of the visceral pleura, 'decortication' may be required. This procedure will allow the lung to re-expand and obliterate the pleural space.

TUBERCULOUS EMPYEMA. Antituberculous chemotherapy should be started immediately, and the pus in the pleural space should be aspirated through a wide-bore needle until it ceases to reaccumulate. In many cases no other treatment is necessary, but surgery is occasionally required to ablate the residual empyema space.

SPONTANEOUS PNEUMOTHORAX

Aetiology. The two chief causes of spontaneous pneumothorax are: (1) rupture of a subpleural emphysematous bulla or of the pulmonary end of a pleural adhesion; (2) rupture of a subpleural tuberculous focus into the pleural space. In Britain the first cause is very much more common. Other conditions such as staphylococcal lung abscess, pulmonary infarction and bronchial carcinoma may, in rare instances, give rise to spontaneous pneumothorax.

Pathology. There are three types of spontaneous pneumothorax (Fig. 8.8):

1. *Closed*. The communication between pleura and lung seals off as the lung collapses, and does not reopen. In this type of case the air is gradually absorbed and the lung re-expands.

2. *Open*. The communication is generally with a bronchus (bronchopleural fistula) and does not seal off when the lung collapses. The air pressure in the pleural space thus approximates to atmospheric pressure on both inspiration and expiration and the lung cannot re-expand. Moreover, the large bronchial communication facilitates the transmission of infection from the air passages into the pleural space and empyema is a common complication. The term 'open' is also applied to a pneumothorax resulting from a penetrating wound of the chest wall.

3. *Tension (valvular)*. The communication between pleura and lung persists but is small and acts as a one-way valve which allows air to enter the pleura during inspiration but prevents it from escaping during expiration. Very large amounts of air may be trapped in the pleural space during bouts of coughing and the intrapleural pressure may rise to well above atmospheric level. This results not only in complete collapse of the underlying lung but also in mediastinal displacement towards the opposite side with compression of the opposite lung.

Clinical features. The onset is usually sudden, with pain or a feeling of tightness on the affected side of the chest, which may be aggravated by deep inspiration. The patient then becomes increasingly breathless and, in severe cases, cyanosed. The physical signs in the chest are those of air in the pleural space (p. 207). When the pneumothorax is small and localised there may be no abnormal signs, and the condition may be revealed only by radiological examination.

Closed spontaneous pneumothorax. Dyspnoea, which is seldom severe, gradually abates over the course of a few days. Progressive spontaneous absorption of the air takes place and re-expansion of the lung is complete between 2 and 4 weeks later, depending on the initial size of the pneumo-

thorax. Pleural infection is uncommon in this type of pneumothorax.

Open spontaneous pneumothorax is usually due to rupture of an emphysematous bulla, a tuberculous cavity or a lung abscess into the pleural space. The onset is similar to that of the closed type, but the dyspnoea does not improve and, when tuberculosis or lung abscess has been the cause, pyrexia and systemic disturbance soon ensue. There are physical and radiological signs of air and fluid in the pleural space. In tuberculous cases acid-fast bacilli can be isolated from the pleural fluid.

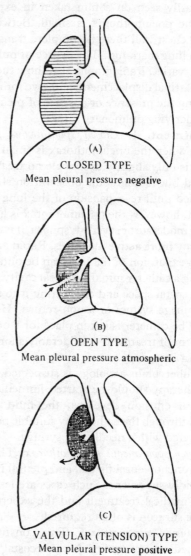

(A)
CLOSED TYPE
Mean pleural pressure **negative**

(B)
OPEN TYPE
Mean pleural pressure **atmospheric**

(C)
VALVULAR (TENSION) TYPE
Mean pleural pressure **positive**

Fig. 8.8 Types of spontaneous pneumothorax.

Tension pneumothorax produces the most dramatic clinical picture. The dyspnoea is rapidly progressive and is accompanied by central cyanosis. The patient may die from asphyxia within a few minutes, but usually the course of events is less rapid and medical attention can be obtained in time to avert a fatal outcome.

Recurrent spontaneous pneumothorax is not uncommon, especially in patients with emphysematous bullae. Subsequent incidents are usually on the same side.

Radiological examination shows the sharply defined edge of the collapsed lung which may be more easily seen on a film taken in expiration, when the pneumothorax is small. Between this and the chest wall there is complete translucency with no lung markings. The degree of pulmonary collapse varies. Radiographs also show the degree of mediastinal displacement, and give information regarding the presence or absence of pleural fluid and underlying pulmonary disease.

Treatment. 1. *Closed spontaneous pneumothorax.* When the pneumothorax is small and the patient is only slightly dyspnoeic no treatment is required but radiographic observation should be continued until re-expansion of the lung is complete. If, however, the pneumothorax is large and causing moderate or severe dyspnoea, it is essential to employ more active measures. Rapid and complete re-expansion of the lung can be obtained by inserting a catheter into the pleural cavity through an intercostal space and connecting it to a water-seal drainage system or a non-return (Heimlich) valve. The catheter is left in place for 5 or 6 days. This form of treatment considerably shortens the period of incapacity.

If a tuberculous aetiology is suspected, specific chemotherapy should be started immediately. If a pleural effusion develops, the fluid may be drained through the catheter by suitable posturing or aspirated with a needle and syringe.

2. *Open spontaneous pneumothorax.* There is a large bronchopleural fistula, and pleural infection can rapidly supervene. Such cases are less amenable to medical treatment and the expertise of a thoracic surgeon is often required.

3. *Tension pneumothorax.* This constitutes an acute medical emergency. An intercostal catheter should be inserted at once and connected to a water-seal drainage system. Symptomatic relief is immediate and dramatic. If suitable equipment for this procedure is not at hand a wide-bore plastic cannula should be used instead. This should be attached to a length of tubing, the end of which should be placed under water in a bottle or basin.

4. *Recurrent spontaneous pneumothorax*, unilateral or bilateral, is first treated by the introduction of an irritant substance, such as kaolin, into the pleural space. This procedure (artificial pleurodesis) produces an aseptic pleurisy, which results in the formation of extensive adhesions between the parietal and visceral surfaces, and usually prevents further episodes of spontaneous pneumothorax. In a few cases thoracotomy and abrasion of the parietal pleura, or parietal pleurectomy, may be required to obliterate the pleural space.

DEFORMITIES OF THE CHEST WALL

Thoracic kyphoscoliosis, if severe, restricts and distorts expansion of the chest wall causing maldistribution of ventilation and blood flow in the lungs. Such patients may later develop Type II respiratory failure, pulmonary hypertension and right ventricular failure, and few survive beyond middle age. The tempo of deterioration is often accelerated by bacterial infection in the bronchi and lungs. The prognosis in these cases can be improved only by early surgical correction of the spinal deformity. Respiratory failure may also occur in ankylosing spondylitis, particularly if there is any interference with the function of the diaphragm.

Pectus carinatum ('pigeon chest') is seen in patients who have suffered from chronic asthma since early childhood.

Pectus excavatum ('funnel chest') is a condition in which the body of the sternum, often only its lower end, is curved backwards. The heart is displaced to the left, and may be compressed between the sternum and vertebral column, but only very rarely is this associated with disturbance of cardiac function. It may, however, restrict chest expansion and reduce the vital capacity. The impairment of cardiac or pulmonary function is seldom sufficiently severe to warrant surgical correction, but this may be indicated for cosmetic reasons.

PROSPECTS IN RESPIRATORY MEDICINE

Because the lungs are open to the external environment, the microcosm of changes within the lungs themselves—whether structural, functional, immunological, or microbiological—is closely related to the macrocosm of epidemiological, environmental, occupational, personal and social factors, so that the study of respiratory medicine has wider horizons than the lung or even the whole body. At the local level, advances in immunology, immunopathology and immunopharmacology have led to clearer understanding of bronchial asthma, bronchopulmonary eosinophilia and extrinsic allergic alveolitis, and may in time help to elucidate the pathogenesis of cryptogenic fibrosing alveolitis, some types of occupational lung disease and even bronchial carcinoma. Cytological, microbiological and biochemical examination of material obtained by bronchoalveolar lavage is proving to be a useful diagnostic and research technique. Diagnosis of peripheral lung tumours, rapid identification of opportunistic organisms in the increasing number of immunocompromised patients and assessment of the activity of interstitial lung disease are examples of its value. Immunology also plays a part in the study of the mechanisms which protect the lungs against acute and chronic infection by bacteria, viruses and fungi, and cell biology throws light on the ways in which enzymatic attack on alveolar elastic tissue takes place in emphysema. At subcellular level, DNA gene probes raise hopes of clarifying the genetic defects in cystic fibrosis and α_1-antitrypsin deficiency.

New non-invasive techniques have simplified the assessment of exercise tolerance and demonstrated changes in breathing and gas exchange taking place in sleep. New methods are becoming available for the diagnosis of localised pulmonary lesions and of diseases which cause abnormalities of ventilation and perfusion, such as emphysema and pulmonary thromboembolism. Such techniques as nuclear magnetic imaging and new methods of radionuclide scanning are certain, when fully exploited, to have a major impact on the investigation of respiratory disease. Further improvements can be expected in the techniques of bronchoscopy, and of bronchial and pulmonary biopsy.

Effective and safe antiviral agents are now becoming available and should soon allow us to combat many conditions with variable degrees of mortality and morbidity, which affect all age groups and carry particular risks for adults with lung disease and for children. In those in whom lung damage is far advanced, the benefits of long-term oxygen therapy are being clarified, and the oxygen concentrator provides a less costly way of providing treatment for those patients in whom it is indicated.

Epidemiologists and occupational health specialists can bring precise measures to bear on a widening field; for example the hazards to the individual inhaling platinum fumes, to workers in a large building supplied by a contaminated humidifier system or to the mass victims of toxic fumes from an industrial plant. If the role of the cardiothoracic surgeon seems to have diminished during recent decades, this is a reflection of the greater efficacy of the treatment of tuberculosis and of the pleuro-pulmonary infections which were a frequent cause of empyema, lung abscess and bronchiectasis. The treatment of 'operable' bronchial carcinoma remains today the chief link between the thoracic physician and surgeon. However, the results of organ transplantation are encouraging enough to suggest that cardiopulmonary transplantation will be used more often in future in managing end-stage pulmonary disease, or even for bronchial tumours now considered inoperable because of their central site.

The chief burden of respiratory disease in the community lies not only in acute infections but in bronchial carcinoma, with its appalling mortality and prognosis, and in the long progress of the morbidity of chronic bronchitis and emphysema. Therapeutic advances resulting from the greater understanding of the pathogenesis of chronic bronchitis and emphysema may merely delay the onset of severe disability; effective chemotherapy for bronchial carcinoma—especially for small-cell tumours—is also likely to be developed long before the incidence of the disease falls as cigarette smoking decreases. Reduction in cigarette smoking remains the chief measure to reduce these burdens, and the struggle to influence personal habits and commercial interests in the community will long remain the chief social task of all doctors.

G. K. CROMPTON
G. J. R. McHARDY

FURTHER READING:

Crompton G K 1986 In: Macleod J and Munro J (eds) Clinical examination, 7th edn. Churchill Livingstone, Edinburgh. For information about examination of the respiratory system
Crofton J W, Douglas A C 1981 Respiratory diseases, 3rd edn. Blackwell Scientific Publications, Oxford. A detailed reference work
James D G, Studdy P R 1981 A colour atlas of respiratory diseases. Wolfe, London. Fine illustrations of a somewhat limited range of conditions

Cotes J E 1979 Lung function: assessment and application in medicine, 4th edn. Blackwell Scientific Publications, Oxford. A comprehensive review of methods and an excellent source of normal values
Ross J D, Horne N W 1983 Modern drug treatment in tuberculosis, 6th edn. Chest, Heart and Stroke Association, London. All the essential information in concise form
Parkes W R 1982 Occupational lung disorders, 2nd edn. Butterworth, London. A detailed account which has become a classic
Department of Health and Social Security NI 226 1979 Pneumoconiosis and related occupational diseases: notes on diagnosis and claims for industrial injuries scheme benefits. DHSS, London
Department of Health and Social Security NI 238 1982 Clinical notes on occupational asthma: a disease prescribed under the industrial injuries scheme. DHSS, London

Periodicals
Thorax. British Medical Association, London. A wide-ranging medical and surgical journal with valuable editorial reviews
American Review of Respiratory Disease. American Thoracic Society, New York. A prestigious journal with excellent 'state of the art' reviews

9

Diseases of the alimentary tract and pancreas

PHYSIOLOGY OF THE ALIMENTARY TRACT

The alimentary tract is a co-ordinated structure with the function of ingesting and absorbing nutrients and excreting unabsorbed and waste products. It should not be regarded as a series of separate organs, since the role of each component is closely related to that of other parts of the tract. Its operation may be considered under the following headings:

1. *Controlling and co-ordinating mechanisms.* The autonomic nervous system, hormones and paracrine substances control and co-ordinate motility and secretion.

2. *Motility.* The carefully controlled motility of the tract is responsible for the orderly progression of nutrients through the system at a rate appropriate to the stage of digestion and absorption in a given region of the tract.

3. *Secretion.* The secretion of enzymes and detergents enables protein, carbohydrate and fat to be digested prior to absorption. The secretion of electrolytes provides the correct pH for each stage of digestion.

4. *Absorption.* The absorptive system consists of specialised cells, together with the portal venous system and lymphatics.

5. *Defence mechanisms.* These are necessary to protect the mucosa from its own digestive enzymes and from the bacterial population to which it is exposed. These mechanisms include a rapid turnover of the epithelial cells, the production of mucus and a specialised immunological system.

1. The controlling and co-ordinating mechanisms

Cellular function of the gastrointestinal tract is controlled by chemical messengers which may be hormones, or amino acids or their derivatives, amines or peptides. The transmission of the message is called neurocrine when it is across a synapse, paracrine when it is through an intercellular space, and endocrine when it is via the blood. Hormones or paracrine substances are produced by a distinctive cell type in the gastrointestinal mucosa or pancreas released in response to food in the stomach and intestine. Their role is to control the progression of nutrients by modifying nervous stimuli, and to stimulate or inhibit secretions. Gastrointestinal function is influenced by a multitude of nervous and hormonal stimuli. For example, the secretion of acid by the stomach is stimulated mainly by the release of gastrin and by the vagus nerves, but many other enteric hormones probably have smaller roles to play.

A peptide system is now recognised as an important component of the autonomic nervous system. The nerves contain mediators such as vasoactive intestinal peptide, substance P and encephalins. The autonomic nervous system exerts an effect on the contraction of the smooth muscle cells and on the secretion of enzymes, electrolytes and hormones by the mucosa and the pancreas. It is influenced by sensory nerves in the mucosa and gut wall which respond to chemical stimuli and to stretch, by the enteric hormones and by the release of paracrine substances.

2. Motility

Apart from the striated muscle in the upper oesophagus, smooth muscle is responsible for the motility of the gastrointestinal tract. The smooth muscle produces 'slow waves' which are conducted over long distances. These do not result in contraction but they enable contractions in different areas to be co-ordinated.

Oesophagus. The upper oesophageal sphincter is formed by the striated cricopharyngeus muscle which exerts constant tone to keep the sphincter closed except during swallowing. Once the upper oesophageal sphincter relaxes, peristalsis sweeps along the length of the body of the oesophagus, but occasionally, even in the normal oesophagus, the contractions are not co-ordinated. In the disorder of diffuse spasm these unco-ordinated contractions predominate. The lowest few centimetres of the oesophagus form the lower oesophageal sphincter. This has a high resting tension which prevents reflux of gastric contents into the oesophagus. Normally the sphincter relaxes when the peristaltic wave arrives but the characteristic feature in achalasia is that it fails to do so. The sphincter is controlled by nervous and hormonal mechanisms.

Stomach. The normal tonic contraction of the stomach is inhibited by the arrival of food probably by means of a centrally mediated vagal reflex. This is termed receptive relaxation so that a large increase in volume is accompanied by only a small rise in pressure within the lumen. The gastric slow wave controls the frequency and direction of antral peristalsis which is responsible for the thorough mixing of the gastric contents and their progressive emptying into the duodenum.

Several mechanisms exist to prevent the duodenum receiving more nutrient that it can deal with. Chemoreceptors for fat and acid and osmoreceptors in the duodenal mucosa control gastric emptying by means of local reflexes and the release of secretin, cholecystokinin and other enteric hormones. Approximately half of a semi-solid meal has left the stomach in about 30 minutes.

Small intestine. Here the co-ordination is due to the slow wave in the longitudinal muscle fibres. It is the pacemaker which dictates the times at which any given segment of the gut can contract. The frequency of the slow wave in the duodenum is greater than in the ileum, thus enabling the proximal bowel to override more distal areas. By this means contractions are co-ordinated both to mix and propel the small bowel content so that all nutrients can be exposed to the absorptive cells. It is thought that the myenteric plexus and the enteric hormones determine the local response to the slow wave so that contraction may or may not occur depending on the state of affairs in the lumen at any one time.

Colon. Motility here is poorly understood. There is probably a slow wave but it is not known how it co-ordinates contractions. Observation of the colon suggests two main types of contraction occur which may be associated with two different functions. First, there is segmentation which consists of contraction rings forming and disappearing over long periods: these produce a slow mixing of faeces but no propulsion, thus facilitating the absorption of water and electrolytes. Second, propulsion occurs through 'mass movement,' a peristaltic wave which occurs several times a day. This action carries out the second function of the colon, namely the elimination of faeces.

All activity in the colon is increased after eating, and defecation is more likely to occur postprandially. The enteric hormones may be responsible for this activity. The main activity in the colon, segmentation, causes mixing only and is responsible for the resistance to flow along the lumen. In constipation, segmentation is increased and there is resistance to flow along the lumen whereas in diarrhoea there is a reduction in segmentation so that the semi-formed contents of the right colon have an unimpeded transit through the colon.

3. Secretion

The production of secretions for the digestion of nutrients is under nervous and hormonal control.

Gastric secretion. In response to the sight or smell of food, the vagus stimulates acid and pepsin secretion by a direct effect on the parietal and peptic cells. It also initiates the release of gastrin from the antrum. More sustained output of this hormone is produced by a rise in pH and by ingested protein. Gastrin then enters the bloodstream and acts on the body of the stomach to produce acid and pepsin to digest the protein. The parietal cell has receptors for gastrin, acetylcholine (vagal stimulation) and for histamine (the H_2 receptor). Each receptor has a secondary messenger system within the parietal cell, but the proton pump $H^+ K^+$ adenosine triphosphatase is the final common pathway for acid secretion. Mechanisms are also required to turn off gastric secretion once digestion within the stomach is complete. These are largely the same as those which slow gastric emptying, i.e. the release of secretin and other enteric hormones and also the presence of a low pH in the gastric antrum which inhibits the further release of gastrin.

Pancreatic secretion, bile and intestinal secretions. Acid and fat in the duodenum release the hormones secretin and cholecystokinin from the duodenal mucosa into the bloodstream. Secretin stimulates the entire duct system of the pancreas to produce bicarbonate which neutralises the gastric acid and provides a neutral pH for the activity of the pancreatic enzymes, lipase, amylase and trypsin. These are produced in response to cholecystokinin, which also causes contraction of the gall bladder so that an adequate supply of bile acids reaches the intestine at a time when fat has to be digested. The acinar cells have cholecystokinin, secretin and cholinergic receptors. The enteric hormones are also responsible for the secretion, by the mucosa of the small intestine, of succus entericus which contains bicarbonate and additional enzymes.

4. The absorptive system

The area for absorption in the small intestine is increased several hundredfold by the presence of villi and microvilli. The surface of the individual cell is formed of microvilli which possess a multitude of enzyme systems for the final stages of digestion of nutrients followed by their absorption. In coeliac disease and tropical sprue the surface area of the small intestine is reduced because of the atrophy or loss of villi, and malabsorption results.

Under normal circumstances nutrients are transported from the absorptive cell by the lymphatic system (e.g. fat and fat-soluble vitamins) or by the portal venous system (e.g. amino acids and hexoses).

The absorptive system is discussed in more detail on page 301.

5. Defence mechanisms

Cell turnover. The epithelial cells of the gastrointestinal tract are constantly renewed so that, for example, the epithelial surface of the small intestine is replaced every 48 hours. The desquamated cells are digested and their products reabsorbed. In the intestine, cellular turnover has been shown to be slower than normal in germ-free animals and it can be argued that this turnover is to some extent a protective mechanism.

Production of mucus. Mucus producing cells are present throughout the gastrointestinal tract and mucus has a protective function. In the stomach, the mucous layer on the surface of the epithelium contains bicarbonate ions which form part of the barrier to gastric acid.

Immunological system. The lamina propria of the stomach and intestines contains many lymphocytes and plasma cells. Some of these cells synthesise secretory IgA which is resistant to digestion by intestinal enzymes and has a role in protecting mucosal surfaces from bacterial invasion. It is thus of particular importance in the small intestine where bacterial colonisation is deleterious.

THE SYMPTOMS OF ALIMENTARY DISEASE

Pain is often the most important symptom of gastrointestinal disease. It must be analysed in relation to its main site, radiation, character, severity, duration, frequency, times of occurrence, aggravating and relieving factors and any associated phenomena. The characteristics of abdominal pain are sometimes diagnostic, for example in acute appendicitis or helpful as in peptic ulceration.

Loss of appetite (anorexia) may have a local cause such as carcinoma of the stomach but may also be a feature of any debilitating disease or of a psychological disturbance.

Waterbrash is the sudden filling of the mouth with saliva which is produced as a reflex response to a variety of symptoms from the upper gastrointestinal tract, e.g. peptic ulcer pain.

Vomiting may occur in any acute disorder of the alimentary tract, including intestinal obstruction. Numerous other conditions may also be responsible, for example meningitis, uraemia, migraine, drugs such as digoxin or morphine and, in the child, infection. The type, timing and related features of the vomiting are important diagnostically. Sudden vomiting without preceding nausea may be due to direct stimulation of the vomiting centre in the medulla and thus be an indication of intracranial disease. Vomiting in the morning may be due to pregnancy, alcoholism or anxiety. Vomiting of large quantities of food and secretions late in the day or night indicates gastric outlet obstruction. Vomiting which relieves pain is often due to a peptic ulcer. The complaint of persistent vomiting without loss of weight is nearly always indicative of psychological disturbance.

Heartburn is a burning retrosternal sensation usually due to inflammation of the oesophagus as in reflux oesophagitis. Sometimes dysmotility of the oesophagus produces a similar sensation.

Regurgitation is the appearance of previously swallowed food in the mouth without vomiting. It usually has an acid or bitter taste because of the presence of gastric juice or bile but not in patients with obstruction in the oesophagus.

Dysphagia, i.e. difficulty in swallowing, is discussed on page 278.

Flatulence is often due to excessive swallowing of air (aerophagy) which in turn may be due to anxiety. Under normal circumstances a small amount of air is swallowed with food, drink and saliva. Some of this gas may be expelled as a belch. The remainder passes into the intestine. Some will be absorbed but most, particularly the nitrogen, will be expelled per rectum. A plain radiograph of the abdomen shows that gas is normally present in the stomach and colon but that very little is seen in the small intestine.

Constipation and diarrhoea are sometimes difficult to define. In Britain fewer than 10% of people have less than one bowel motion per day and only 1% have a bowel movement less frequently than 3 times a week. These latter should be regarded as constipated. In addition, if the stool is hard and difficult to pass the patient should be regarded as constipated whatever the frequency of bowel movement. In contrast, less than 1% of the population have more than three bowel movements daily and this should be regarded as abnormal, particularly if the stool is not formed. When the stool is liquid or semiformed it must be regarded as abnormal whatever the frequency of bowel movement. The diet in Western countries is low in roughage; where a high residue diet is usual, more than three bowel movements daily may be normal. An explanation must be found for any change in bowel habit.

Loss of weight may be due to a reduced intake of food because of anorexia, nausea or vomiting, to malabsorption of nutrients or to the loss of protein from a diseased bowel as in ulcerative colitis. Carcinoma is the most important alimentary cause of loss of weight.

INVESTIGATION OF THE ALIMENTARY TRACT

In addition to systematic examination of the abdomen by inspection, palpation, percussion and auscultation and of the rectum by digital examination along the lines described in *Clinical examination* (p. 324), further investigation is frequently required.

Radiological examination

Plain radiographs show the normal soft tissue shadows due to the liver, spleen and kidneys and also abnormal shadows. Gas in the intestine acts as a contrast medium so that the distribution of the bowel within the abdomen can be assessed. In obstruction there may be an excessive amount of gas and fluid in the bowel above the obstruction and films with the patient erect will demonstrate fluid levels. Finally, areas of opacification due to stones or to calcification in the liver, pancreas, cysts or blood vessels may provide important diagnostic information.

A chest radiograph will show the diaphragms. Free gas may be seen under the diaphragm and may indicate a perforation. Gas with a fluid level may be associated with a subphrenic abscess. Pulmonary lesions, from which pain may be referred to the abdomen, can also be identified.

Barium studies. These will demonstrate a break in the continuity of the outline of the organ, abnormalities in the appearance of the mucosa and disorders of motility. Preparation of the patient for each examination should always be undertaken so that mucosal details will not be obscured by contents. For studies of the upper gastrointestinal tract, the patient is fasted and for barium enema examination the colon should be cleared of faeces by means of laxatives and colonic lavage.

The barium swallow and meal examination. Since pharyngeal swallowing is rapid, video recording or rapid sequence films are often necessary. The oesophagus is studied while barium is being swallowed so that it is seen distended with barium. Mucosal films are taken immediately after the barium has passed through the area. The procedure may demonstrate a disorder of motility, a filling defect caused by a tumour or varices, a stricture, a diverticulum or a hiatus hernia (Fig. 9.1).

The mucosa of the stomach is usually examined by a double contrast study in which a small amount of barium is used together with the introduction of gas to distend the stomach. An ulcer is usually seen face on as a small collection of barium with radiating folds of mucosa (Figs. 9.4 and 9.5). An ulcer may also appear as a projection beyond the normal outline while tumours cause filling defects. Small cancers can be detected by irregularity in the mucosal pattern. Observation of the motility of the stomach may indicate an inert area caused by infiltrating carcinoma. The duodenal cap is examined by studying its contours when it is completely filled with barium, and its mucosal pattern when it is distended with gas and the mucosa coated with barium.

The follow-through examination. When disease of the small intestine is suspected, barium is observed during its passage through the small intestine and radiographs are taken at intervals. The outline of the barium may indicate structural abnormalities such as diverticula or strictures. When there is malabsorption, excess secretions may cause the barium to clump and flocculate (Fig. 9.8). As variations in this procedure, a tube can be passed into the duodenum for the direct introduction of barium in order to obtain more precise films. Duodenal atony is induced by glucagon to obtain films of the duodenum (hypotonic duodenography) and for films of the small intestine, the introduction of barium is followed by a large volume of water (small bowel enteroclysis).

Barium enema. This procedure is uncomfortable and sometimes exhausting, particularly in the elderly or in those with cardiac disease in whom arrhythmia may be induced. Barium enema must always have been preceded by digital examination of the rectum and preferably also by sigmoidoscopy a few days earlier. The colon must be meticulously cleared of faeces by means of laxatives followed by a cleansing enema just before the barium enema. Barium alone or, for double contrast examination, barium and air, is run into the bowel through a self-retaining catheter. Radiographs are taken with the colonic mucosa coated with barium and the lumen distended with air. In this way the colonic mucosa can be studied in detail and polyps or small tumours identified (Fig. 9.13). In inflammatory bowel disease mucosal abnormalities are readily recognised (Figs 9.9 and 9.11). In some patients there will be a reflux of barium into the terminal ileum which can be outlined.

Cautionary note. Exposure to X-rays in the early months of pregnancy may upset normal development of the fetus and be responsible for deformity or still birth. These risks apply not only to radiographic examination of the abdomen such as barium enema but also to procedures such as excretion urography and radiographs of the lumbar spine and pelvis. Inadvertent irradiation in the first few weeks of pregnancy can be avoided by restricting radiological examination of the lower abdomen in women at risk to the 10 days immediately following the onset of the last menstrual period — 'the 10 day rule'.

Imaging studies

CT and magnetic resonance imaging. CT is an important technique for defining certain intra-abdominal diseases particularly those involving inaccessible organs or regions. Thus it is used in the diagnosis and management of acute pancreatitis and pancreatic cancer, and in diagnosing diseases of the retroperitoneal space and lymph nodes. It is also of importance in assessing the spread of tumour, e.g. gastric cancer so that decisions can be made on whether surgery should be palliative or curative. Magnetic resonance imaging has not yet proven to be superior to CT for any intra-abdominal diagnostic problem.

Ultrasonography. This non-invasive technique is of value in detecting cysts, particularly of the pancreas, and abscesses and can show the size of the pancreatic duct.

Radionuclide scanning is used for examining the liver and spleen (p. 337) and for detecting the approximate site of gastrointestinal haemorrhage.

Endoscopy

With fibreoptic instruments it is not difficult to examine the whole of the oesophagus, stomach, duodenum and colon. Two bundles of many thousands of fine glass fibres are contained in the instrument's shaft. One bundle carries light to the tip of the instrument in order to illuminate the organ being examined whilst the other can transmit an image back to the observer. The fibre bundles are flexible so that the whole shaft can be bent and easily passed into the upper gastrointestinal tract or colon. The shaft of the instrument also carries controls so that the tip of the instrument can be moved, and channels through which air or forceps can be passed to insufflate the organ or to take a biopsy from the mucosa. Endoscopic instruments can also be used for the therapeutic procedures which would otherwise require laparotomy such as removal of a polyp.

Rigid instruments are used to examine the rectum and lower pelvic colon (sigmoidoscope) and occasionally the oesophagus (oesophagoscope).

Upper alimentary tract. It is usual to carry out the procedure with the patient under sedation, often as an out-patient. After a 12-hour fast the pharynx is anaesthetised with a spray or gargle. The instrument is passed with the assistance of the patient in swallowing, and the procedure, whilst uncomfortable, should be no more so than any other intubation. Possible complications are perforation of the oesophagus or stomach whilst passing the instrument or during biopsy, the inhalation of secretions, cardiac arrhythmias or arrest, and the transmission of infections. All these are rare when appropriate precautions are used but resuscitation and after-care facilities must be available in endoscopy units.

Where possible, the oesophagus, stomach and duodenum are all inspected at the same examination (*panendoscopy*), because the presence of one lesion does not exclude another and double lesions are not uncommon, e.g. oesophagitis and duodenal ulcer. This is particularly important when endoscopy is carried out in patients with haematemesis or melaena, since there may be more than one source of bleeding.

Oesophagoscopy should be carried out when there is dysphagia or when barium examination suggests a tumour or stricture. Other indications include suspected oesophagitis, varices or a motility disorder. Therapeutic procedures that can be carried out include dilatation of a stricture and injection of sclerosing material into oesophageal varices to control bleeding.

Gastroscopy is always indicated when a gastric ulcer has been demonstrated on barium studies so that biopsies can be taken to exclude malignancy; subsequent healing of the ulcer should also be confirmed. Gastroscopy is nearly always necessary in the investigation of patients with symptoms after gastric surgery because the appearances are difficult to define radiologically.

Duodenoscopy is indicated in cases of duodenal ulceration and when cancer of the head of the pancreas or ampulla is suspected.

Endoscopic retrograde cholangio-pancreatography (ERCP) is a special application of fibreoptic endoscopy. At duodenoscopy the ampulla of Vater is cannulated with a fine bore catheter passed through the shaft of the instrument and radio-opaque dye is injected into the biliary and pancreatic ducts. The procedure is of great value in patients suspected of having pancreatic disease since distortion or obstruction of the ductal system may indicate a diagnosis of chronic pancreatitis or pancreatic carcinoma. It is of value in the diagnosis of pancreas divisum (p. 297). Obstruction or distortion of the common bile duct by a stone or a tumour can also be demonstrated and sphincterotomy can be performed to allow removal of stones.

Lower alimentary tract. *Proctoscopy and sigmoidoscopy.* These are simple procedures which should always be carried out in patients with symptoms referable to the lower bowel or anus. Both terms are inaccurate since proctoscopy visualises the anal canal and only 2–3 cm of the rectum, and sigmoidoscopy examines the rectum and the lower few centimetres of the pelvic colon. It is usual to carry out the procedures without preparation but if the rectum contains faeces, then endoscopy is repeated after the bowel has been emptied. The examination is carried out with the patient in the knee-elbow position, or on the left side with the knees drawn up. Digital examination of the rectum should always precede endoscopy and the instruments should be warmed and well lubricated. Proctoscopy is used for the demonstration and injection of haemorrhoids. Sigmoidoscopy is necessary for the diagnosis of polyps, cancer of the rectum, ulcerative proctitis or colitis and Crohn's disease of the large bowel. Biopsy of the mucosa or lesion may also be taken. Sigmoidoscopy is carried out under anaesthesia when there is a painful condition of the anus such as a fissure; it should be performed only with extreme care in fulminating ulcerative colitis because of the danger of perforation.

Colonoscopy. The fibreoptic colonoscope permits inspection of the entire colon but the procedure is time-consuming and occasionally difficult. More often a short colonoscope is used to examine the sigmoid and left colon where most lesions will be found. The bowel must be carefully prepared over several days, first with laxatives and then by lavage so that no faecal material remains. During colonoscopy it is possible to take a biopsy of suspicious lesions and polyps can be removed using a diathermy snare.

Other investigations

Biopsy of lesions is an essential part of each endoscopic procedure but the small size of the specimen may make interpretation by the pathologist difficult.

Biopsy of the small intestine is indicated if malabsorption is suspected and is carried out by means of the Crosby capsule. After an overnight fast the capsule is passed into the jejunum attached to a stiff radio-opaque catheter and the biopsy is taken just distal to the duodeno-jejunal flexure. Suction via the catheter draws mucosa into a small port on the side of the instrument. The negative pressure which develops within the capsule also fires the knife which severs the mucosa. The intubation and biopsy are completed in about one hour. Bleeding occurs occasionally and for this reason biopsies should not be carried out unless the platelet count and prothrombin time are normal. Another rare complication is perforation of the intestine. The biopsy specimens are inspected under the dissecting microscope immediately after removal from the capsule prior to fixation and histological examination (p. 303).

Secretory studies. *The pentagastrin test.* The acid output is measured in response to pentagastrin, a synthetic pentapeptide which exerts the biological effects of gastrin. Preparation consists of an overnight fast and H_2-receptor antagonist drugs must be stopped for at least 48 hours before the test. The fasting contents of the stomach are aspirated and their volume measured; then the secretions are collected continuously for one hour. This is termed the 'basal acid output'. Then pentagastrin is given subcutaneously and the secretions are collected for a further hour. The acid output in this hour is termed the 'maximum acid output'.

The pentagastrin test is helpful because: (1) a large volume of fasting juice indicates obstruction of the gastric outlet; (2) a very high basal acid output suggests that the patient has the Zollinger-Ellison syndrome (p. 291); (3) in patients with peptic ulcer it provides a pre-operative base line; (4) achlorhydria can be demonstrated.

The insulin test is used after gastric surgery to indicate the completeness of vagotomy. The preparation and procedure are similar to those described above but the gastric stimulant is unmodified insulin which is given intravenously. The resulting hypoglycaemia stimulates the vagal centres and gastric acid is secreted if the vagal innervation of the stomach has not been completely divided.

Bacteriological studies. The malabsorption syndrome may be due occasionally to bacterial colonisation of the small intestine. When this is suspected, secretion can be obtained for bacteriological studies by passing a fine sterile tube into the upper small intestine. A mercury bag attached to the tip of the tube ensures that the tube moves rapidly to the correct site. The patient should not be receiving antibiotics.

Motility studies. Barium examination gives a poor demonstration of the motility of the oesophagus, stomach and small intestine. The isotope ^{99m}Technetium sulphur colloid incorporated into a solid or liquid bolus can be used to measure transit down the oesophagus. This is often delayed in dysphagia and in most motility disorders. Radioactive markers incorporated into solid food and liquids are also used to measure emptying of the stomach. Small intestinal motility can be estimated by giving a non-absorbable carbohydrate. When this reaches the caecum it is metabolised by bacteria and hydrogen is excreted in the breath, where it is detected.

Motility can be studied more accurately by measuring the pressure changes in the lumen of the organ but only in the case of the oesophagus is this manometry of diagnostic value. Fine open ended tubes are passed into the stomach and pressures are transmitted to transducers and measured at intervals whilst the tube is gradually withdrawn with the patient swallowing. The procedure may be of value in establishing the relationship between chest pain and abnormal oesophageal contractions, for the diagnosis of motility disorders of the oesophagus and in determining the position and competence of the lower oesophageal sphincter.

Examination of the stool. In malabsorption the stool may be pale and frothy; in the irritable bowel syndrome it may be like pellets or ribbon with or without mucus. In mild ulcerative disease of the colon there may be flecks of blood in the mucus. Inspection of the stool is sufficient to diagnose fresh bleeding from the lower alimentary tract while the loss of over 60 ml of blood from a site proximal to the ascending colon will produce a black tarry stool.

Tests for occult blood (e.g. Hemoccult) detect small amounts in the stool and are performed for several successive days because bleeding from the gastrointestinal tract is often intermittent. Specimens obtained on the fingerstall at rectal examination can be readily examined.

Microscopic examination is of value particularly in distinguishing amoebic dysentry and other parasitic diseases.

DISEASES OF THE MOUTH

The mouth acts as a receptacle in which food can be broken down into small particles during mastication. Into the mouth flows the saliva which is secreted in response to the act of chewing and to the sight, taste and smell of food. Saliva facilitates speech, moistens the food and lubricates the process of swallowing. By its solvent action on the foodstuffs, it enables tasting to take place. Saliva also contains an enzyme ptyalin which is concerned in the digestion of polysaccharides to disaccharides and bicarbonate which helps to neutralise acid reflux into the oesophagus.

Disorders of the teeth

Mastication of food to a soft pulp is a prerequisite for good digestion. The teeth should be inspected to determine if they are healthy, present in adequate numbers and in correct apposition in the upper and lower jaws to allow efficient mastication. If dentures are worn it should be ascertained if they are comfortable and efficient. Bacteraemia may have its source in gingivitis or an apical abscess. It is particularly liable to occur after dental manipulation and may cause endocarditis in patients with valvular disease of the heart. All patients should be advised to consult a dentist regularly in order to conserve the teeth and to prevent or treat foci of infection in the mouth.

Stomatitis

The mouth harbours a population of commensal micro-organisms which normally is controlled by a reasonable standard of oral hygiene; if this is neglected the bacterial population may proliferate and cause stomatitis. This may also occur when resistance to the commensal population is lowered by disease especially in the compromised host. Stomatitis may also be due to nutritional deficiencies or other factors.

Ulcerative stomatitis (Vincent's infection) occurs mainly in adults with malnutrition and poor dental hygiene. Ulcers with ragged necrotic margins occur especially on the gums, but may involve the palate, the lips, or the inner aspects of the cheeks; the ulcers are covered by a grey slough surrounded by an erythematous margin. A stained smear shows many spirochaetes and fusiform bacilli; these organisms are present in small numbers in the normal commensal population of the mouth and the condition may be regarded as an endogenous infection due to impairment of host resistance. The condition is infectious, so that the patient's food vessels and cutlery should be sterilised.

The acute phase responds to local treatment with metronidazole (200 mg t.i.d. for 4 d), or to penicillin. Necrosis of the gums may occur, so that when the acute phase has been controlled it is important that proper dental treatment is undertaken.

Candidosis. The fungus *Candida albicans* (p. 767) is a normal commensal in the mouth but it may proliferate to cause *thrush* in babies, in the aged and particularly in debilitated or compromised patients. Thrush is also common in those receiving prolonged treatment with oral antibiotics. White patches appear on the tongue and buccal mucosa and may enlarge and coalesce to form an easily detached membrane; there is little surrounding inflammation. In severe infection, the lower pharynx and oesophagus may be affected, causing dysphagia, or the fungus may spread to the lungs.

Thrush may be treated by gentian violet mouth wash three times a day for 4 days or by nystatin tablets (500 000 units) retained in the mouth for as long as possible, and given four times daily for at least 4 days.

Stomatitis due to deficiency of nutritional factors may arise directly from an insufficient intake or indirectly as a result of impaired absorption of vitamins, especially niacin, riboflavin, folate, and vitamin B_{12}. When the deficiency is acute and severe, the tongue is red, raw and painful. When the deficiency is chronic and less severe the tongue appears moist and unduly clean because of atrophy of the papillae. Angular stomatitis often accompanies glossitis, especially in the case of

gross iron deficiency. In severe vitamin C deficiency the gums become swollen and spongy and bleed readily.

Aphthous ulceration is a common recurrent condition characterised by painful superficial ulceration in the mouth. The lesion beings as an indurated erythematous area followed in a day or so by ulceration. The ulcers are often multiple and may recur over several weeks. The aetiology is unknown and the patient is usually healthy otherwise. Emotional stress may precipitate an attack, and in some women ulcers tend to recur in cyclical fashion during the premenstrual phase. Severe chronic aphthous ulceration may be found in association with Crohn's disease, ulcerative colitis or coeliac disease.

Hydrocortisone hemisuccinate lozenges (2.5 mg t.i.d.) may be effective in the early phase of lesions. Pain can be reduced with topical anaesthetics and secondary infection controlled with tetracycline mouth washes.

Other forms of stomatitis. An allergic reaction to chemicals in toothpaste, dentures, foodstuffs and many drugs, especially antibiotics, can cause stomatitis. A characteristic blue-black punctate line may be seen where the gum margins adjoin the teeth in lead poisoning. Skin diseases such as lichen planus, pemphigus and erythema multiforme involve the mouth, sometimes before being seen on the skin.

Diseases of the tongue

In health the tongue is moist with only a slight white fur on the dorsum. The papillae are readily seen. Mouth breathing causes a dry tongue, but otherwise dryness of the tongue is an indication of dehydration. The tongue may be coated with whitish-yellow fur in persons who smoke excessively but in general, the presence of fur on the tongue has little clinical significance.

Glossitis may be a prominent feature of stomatitis resulting from nutritional deficiency.

Geographical tongue is the name given to a chronic migrating superficial glossitis; it looks odd but has no clinical significance.

Glossodynia is a persistently painful tongue which appears normal on inspection and, unlike true glossitis, is not exacerbated by hot liquids;

the symptom is usually psychogenic. A bad taste in the mouth may be caused by local disease in the oropharynx and by some drugs; when these causes can be excluded the symptom is usually neurotic in origin.

Syphilis may occur as a primary chancre, in the secondary stage as 'mucous patches', or in the tertiary stage as painless gummatous ulcers.

Leukoplakia is a chronic condition characterised by white, firm, smooth patches beginning at the side of the tongue and later spreading over the dorsum. In the early stages the tongue is not painful but later the patches are split by fissures with resultant tenderness. The significance of leukoplakia is that it may precede the development of carcinoma, and a biopsy of such lesions should always be undertaken.

Carcinoma of the mouth and tongue is often related to excessive consumption of tobacco and alcohol and poor oral hygiene. It must be considered in all cases of chronic ulcer of the tongue; if any doubt exists biopsy should be carried out.

Diseases of the salivary glands

Xerostomia (dryness of the mouth) may be due to dehydration or may be caused by anticholinergic or antidepressant drugs; commonly it is due to anxiety. Xerostomia is one of the features of Sjögren's syndrome (p. 557). Excessive salivary secretion may be a response to irritation or inflammation in the mouth, e.g. oral sepsis.

Parotitis may be due to the virus of mumps or to bacterial infection of the gland. The latter tends to develop during severe febrile illnesses and after major abdominal operations if adequate attention is not given to oral hygiene and to the prevention of dehydration and infection. Its treatment consists of the parenteral administration of penicillin and surgical drainage if abscess formation has occurred.

Sarcoidosis is another cause of enlargement of the parotid glands.

Salivary calculi occur occasionally in the submandibular gland or its duct. They cause pain and swelling brought on by eating. Infection of the gland is a complication. Stones in the duct can be felt in the floor of the mouth and can be removed by incision over the duct. Stones in the

gland may require excision of the gland.

A *'mixed' salivary tumour* presents as a slow, painless enlargement of one salivary gland. The tumour is essentially of epithelial origin but may contain stromal elements and shows a variable degree of malignancy. It is treated either by excision or excision and radiotherapy.

DISEASES OF THE OESOPHAGUS

Dysphagia

Since its only function is the transmission of food from mouth to stomach most diseases of the oesophagus and its adjacent structures cause difficulty in swallowing (dysphagia).

Causes of dysphagia. 1. PAINFUL DISEASES of the mouth and pharynx, e.g. stomatitis, tonsillitis, tuberculous laryngitis or retropharyngeal abscess, produce dysphagia, the cause of which is usually apparent.

2. NEUROMUSCULAR DISORDERS. Pharyngeal causes of dysphagia include bulbar and pseudobulbar paralysis and myasthenia gravis. Motility disorders of the oesophagus, e.g. achalasia, diffuse spasm, Chagas' disease and systemic sclerosis also cause dysphagia.

3. EXTRINSIC COMPRESSION — goitre or a mediastinal mass, e.g. malignant lymph nodes or aneurysm of the aorta.

4. INTRINSIC DISEASE OF THE OESOPHAGUS

a. *Congenital abnormalities.* Atresia, the upper oesophagus ending blindly at about the level of the tracheal bifurcation, occurs occasionally requiring urgent surgery in the newborn.

b. *Oesophagitis, ulceration and stricture.* Oesophagitis is most commonly due to reflux of gastric contents. There is acid-pepsin digestion of the oesophageal mucosa immediately above the hernia, with ulceration, spasm and eventual stricture formation. Oesophagitis and stricture are occasionally caused by the ingestion, accidental or otherwise, of corrosives such as bleach and caustic soda. More unusual causes of oesophagitis are herpes viral infections and candidosis in the immunocompromised. A variety of drugs given as tablets or capsules may lodge in the oesophagus, particularly in the elderly, to cause local ulceration.

c. *Sideropenic dysphagia (Plummer-Vinson syndrome)*. This rare form of dysphagia is associated with iron deficiency anaemia, glossitis, and perhaps koilonychia and splenic enlargement. There is degeneration and atrophy of the epithelium of the tongue, pharynx, oesophagus and stomach. A fold of atrophic epithelial cells — the 'postcricoid web' — may be demonstrable radiographically or endoscopically. The dysphagia is to solids rather than to liquids, is intermittent, and may therefore mistakenly be thought to be hysterical. The dilatation associated with diagnostic endoscopy is often sufficient to relieve the dysphagia. Treatment is with iron.

d. *Carcinoma* of the oesophagus or of the cardia of the stomach is the usual cause in elderly patients with no previous history of dysphagia.

Investigation. The exclusion of malignant disease is essential in any patient who complains of dysphagia. Barium swallow and oesophagoscopy are required. Where the disorder appears to be one of function rather than structure, as for example in achalasia or systemic sclerosis, then manometry can give additional information.

Oesophageal hiatus hernia and reflux oesophagitis

Several mechanisms operate to prevent reflux of food and fluid from the stomach into the lower oesophagus. The most important is the lower oesophageal sphincter just above the oesophagogastric junction. Because this sphincter is situated below the diaphragm it is reinforced by intra-abdominal pressure and, furthermore, the oblique entry of the oesophagus into the stomach leads to closure of the intra-abdominal oesophagus when the stomach is distended. The latter two mechanisms are lost when the oesophagogastric junction 'slides' though the oesophageal hiatus in the diaphragm. Some degree of reflux occurs in all individuals and there are mechanisms to clear the refluxed acid from the oesophagus by secondary peristaltic waves and the swallowing of saliva. If reflux persists the continued exposure of the lower oesophageal mucosa to the effects of gastric juice or bile results in oesophagitis.

Hiatus hernia and reflux oesophagitis are most frequent in middle-aged and elderly women. An increase in intra-abdominal pressure, as a result of obesity, and hormonal changes in pregnancy promote their development in earlier years.

Clinical features. Heartburn is the characteristic symptom of reflux oesophagitis. It is a deeply placed 'burning' pain, felt retrosternally and brought on by bending, or by the exertion of lifting or straining with consequent increase in intra-abdominal pressure. It may also occur on lying down at night and keep the patient awake; relief is obtained by sitting up, or by taking food or alkali. No other pain produced in the alimentary tract is so closely linked to change of posture as that of reflux oesophagitis. Chest pain indistinguishable from angina may occur, with radiation to neck, jaws and arms, but it is not related to exercise.

Transient dysphagia for solids is usually caused by spasm while persistent dysphagia indicates the development of stricture. Regurgitation of gastric contents may occur during bending or at night when it can result in aspiration and coughing. Many patients with hiatus hernia have no symptoms as these are related to the presence of oesophagitis. Occasionally the latter is itself symptomless and it may present with severe iron deficiency anaemia due to blood loss. Bleeding may also occur from a gastric ulcer situated in the herniated gastric mucosa.

In patients with long standing oesophagitis, the inflamed mucosa may change from squamous to columnar mucosa. This is termed a Barrett's oesophagus and when an ulcer develops in the columnar mucosa it is called a Barrett's ulcer. It is suspected that an increased incidence of oesophageal adenocarcinoma may occur in these patients.

The diagnosis of oesophagitis and the presence of stricture or Barrett's mucosa is made on the visual and biopsy findings at endoscopy. The presence of a hiatus hernia is shown by a barium meal (Fig. 9.1) and ulcer in the hiatus hernia can be revealed by endoscopy or barium studies. Some patients have symptoms of oesophagitis, yet have minimal or no endoscopic or biopsy evidence. In them, the perfusion of acid into the oesophagus may be useful diagnostically by reproducing the symptoms. In those patients with chest pain which might be either cardiac or oesophageal, a resting ECG and exercise stress testing is indicated. If these are negative a search for abnormal oesophageal motility should be investigated with barium swallow followed by oesophageal motility studies. When a patient with gastro-oesophageal reflux develops angina-like chest pain, it is often because the refluxed material initiates abnormal motility in the oesophagus.

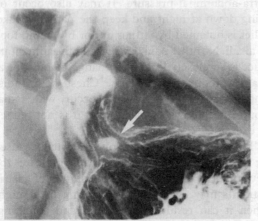

Fig. 9.1 **Hiatus hernia** with an ulcer (arrow) in the herniated portion of the stomach. (Courtesy of Dr G.M. Fraser.)

Treatment. There are several practical dietary and postural measures which the patient can take to minimise reflux and these should be explained. Meals should be of small volume and fatty foods should be avoided as they tend to promote reflux and delay gastric emptying. Weight reduction is essential in obese subjects and may be all that is required to relieve symptoms. Stooping from the waist should be avoided as far as possible. To reduce reflux at night, the patient should sleep with the head of the bed elevated. Smoking reduces lower oesophageal sphincter pressure and should be stopped.

All medications consumed by the patient should be reviewed. Non steroidal anti-inflammatory drugs should be reduced or stopped if possible and the patient should be instructed to take all tablets with a large volume of water when sitting or standing in order to ensure complete swallowing.

Heartburn can be effectively relieved by antacids which, when symptoms are severe, should be taken one and three hours after meals, before sleep, and whenever heartburn occurs. The antiemetic metoclopramide (10 mg t.i.d.) may be helpful; it increases the contraction of the lower oesophageal sphincter and promotes emptying of the stomach. Cimetidine or ranitidine (p. 286) relieve symptoms and a prolonged course may induce healing of oesophagitis. Patients with strictures will require a liquid or semi-liquid diet, pending dilatation. Anaemia will usually respond to oral iron, but transfusion may be required if blood loss has been severe.

Surgery is indicated if severe symptoms persist despite adequate medical therapy. The aim of surgery is to return the lower oesophageal sphincter to the abdomen and to construct an additional valve mechanism. Most oesophageal strictures can be treated by dilatation at endoscopy followed by further dilatation as necessary. However, a small proportion cannot be helped in this way and surgical resection of the stricture is necessary.

Paraoesophageal hernia

Here a knuckle of the greater curvature of the stomach passes alongside the oesophagus through the hiatus. The lower oesophageal sphincter remains below the diaphragm and competent even in the extreme cases when most of the stomach rotates to follow the herniated knuckle into the chest. There may be epigastric fullness, and intermittent mild dysphagia; a large hernia in the posterior mediastinum may cause cardiac arrhythmias and breathlessness but often there are no symptoms and the hernia is found incidentally on chest radiography. Occasionally symptoms become acute because of obstruction, distension and even gangrene of the herniated portion of stomach and then surgery may be required urgently. In a few patients, and as a planned procedure, surgical repair of the hernia is indicated if the disability is severe.

Diverticulum of the oesophagus

A traction diverticulum is most commonly situated in the anterior wall of the oesophagus just below the level of the tracheal bifurcation. It is due to chronic inflammation, usually tuberculous, in adjacent lymph nodes. By the time the diverticulum is discovered, often accidentally during barium swallow, the disease in the lymph nodes has healed. It is seldom that diverticulum itself causes symptoms and surgical treatment is rarely necessary.

A pharyngeal pouch develops at the site of the inferior constrictor of the pharynx probably as a result of muscle inco-ordination. It begins as a posterior bulge of mucosa which enlarges to form a sac that extends downwards between oesophagus and cervical spine. The fully-formed pouch causes dysphagia due to forward displacement of the oesophagus. There is swelling and gurgling in the neck on swallowing. The patient may present with recurrent attacks of stridor, or inhalation of contents of the sac may lead to pneumonia.

Treatment is surgical. In Edinburgh, pharyngeal pouch is remembered as the affliction of Lord Jeffrey (1773–1850), a Scottish judge and wit who, in those days before surgery, emptied his pouch with a specially designed silver spoon.

Achalasia of the cardia

Although apparently confined to the lower end where there is failure of the sphincter to relax, this is in fact a motility disorder of the whole oesophagus which shows progressive atony and dilatation. The cause is probably a failure of nerve conduction due to diminution in the number of ganglion cells. Chagas' disease (American trypanosomiasis, p. 781) produces similar changes. Achalasia is also known, less appropriately, as *cardiospasm*.

Clinical features. Dysphagia may at first be intermittent but later is always present. It is caused both by solids and liquids and may be localised behind the lower end of the sternum. Retrosternal pain occurs in some patients. In the initial stages, the patient continues to eat a normal diet but food accumulates in the capacious non-contractile oesophagus. Later the retained food cannot be expelled into the stomach and weight loss ensues. Inhalation of food and secretions may occur at night and cause recurrent pulmonary infection.

Investigation. A chest radiograph may be sufficient to show a dilated oesophageal outline, perhaps with a fluid level behind the heart shadow. A barium swallow shows the dilated atonic

oesophagus coming to a smooth pointed termination (Fig. 9.2). There is absence of the usual gas shadow in the fundus of the stomach. While the appearances are typical, they are not diagnostic because they can be mimicked by a carcinoma at the lower end of the oesophagus or in the cardiac portion of the stomach. Treated or untreated, patients with achalasia have an increased liability to carcinoma of the oesophagus which makes initial endoscopy essential and periodic review after treatment desirable.

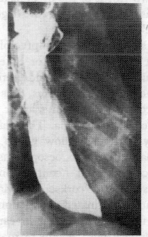

Fig. 9.2 Achalasia of cardia (Courtesy of Dr D.H. Cummack.)

Oesophagoscopy should always be carried out. Usually cleansing of the oesophagus is required with mechanical removal of the larger retained food fragments, and this may involve repeated lavage, aspiration and oesophagoscopy. Once the oesophagus is clean it can be inspected and biopsies taken if necessary. Motility studies (p. 276) are of value in establishing the diagnosis and in determining the severity of the lesion.

Treatment may be by dilatation or cardiomyotomy. In the first a hydrostatic or pneumatic bag is positioned at the level of the diaphragm and then distended forcibly so as to weaken the lower oesophageal sphincter. One or more dilatations may be required to bring about adequate swallowing.

Failure of hydrostatic dilatation or inability to introduce the dilator are indications for operation, which takes the form of cardiomyotomy (Heller's operation). Here the muscle at the lower end of the oesophagus, and for some distance above and below, is slit to expose but not to penetrate the mucosa. The operation is relatively effective and safe, even in the elderly, but both dilatation and cardiomyotomy may be complicated by reflux oesophagitis, or occasionally by oesophageal perforation.

Diffuse spasm of the oesophagus

In this condition there is muscular hypertrophy of the lower two-thirds of the oesophagus; Auerbach's plexus is normal, but there are degenerative changes in the vagus nerves.

The main symptom is pain precipitated by eating, by hot and cold liquids or by emotional stress. The pain is retrosternal and there may be radiation to the back, neck or arms, thus mimicking angina pectoris. The pain may or may not be accompanied by dysphagia. The diagnosis is established by barium swallow which shows a hold-up of barium in the oesophagus due to multiple unco-ordinated contractions. The appearance resembles a 'corkscrew'. Manometry shows strong unco-ordinated contractions.

Treatment involves education in eating in a relaxed atmosphere with adequate mastication. Any emotional stress should receive attention. Nitroglycerine, hydralazine or nifedipine may all relieve pain in some patients. Since most patients are over the age of 60, the physician has to persist with medical management but in the occasional younger patient, an extended cardiomyotomy may be required.

Carcinoma of the oesophagus

There are wide geographical variations in the incidence of this tumour; it is very common around the Caspian Sea and some parts of Southern Africa (p. 101). In Europe and the USA, alcohol and tobacco are important aetiological factors. In other parts of the world, chewing various noxious substances contributes.

In Western communities, the average age of patients with carcinoma of the oesophagus is between 60 and 70 years. The most frequent site is the lower third of the oesophagus; it is less common in the middle third and least common in the upper third. The lesion is usually ulcerative and it extends circumferentially and longitudinally in the wall of the oesophagus, often producing stenosis. Direct invasion of surrounding structures and involvement of related lymph nodes is common by the time of diagnosis. Squamous carcinoma is most frequent. Of the 10–20% of adenocarcinomas, the majority probably arises in Barrett's columnar epithelium, the remainder invading the lower oesophagus from the stomach.

Clinical features. Progressive dysphagia is typical. It starts with the 'sticking' of solid food, at first intermittently and then regularly and proceeds to difficulty with semisolids and eventually with liquids. There is discomfort, not amounting to pain, at the site of the obstruction which is usually well localised by the patient. The development of symptoms occupies some months so that by the time the patient first attends, weight loss is already a feature and there may be metastases in lymph nodes, liver and the mediastinum.

Investigation. Obstruction and an irregular narrowing of the oesophagus, seen at barium swallow, are highly suggestive of the diagnosis (Fig. 9.3). At the lower end it may not be possible to distinguish between carcinoma of the oesophagus and achalasia of the cardia. Oesophagitis and a benign stricture may also simulate carcinoma.

Oesophagoscopy and biopsy should always be carried out. Repeated biopsy may be required to obtain positive confirmation of the diagnosis, and this is particularly so when stricture formation prevents further insertion of the oesophagoscope or the biopsy forceps. In these circumstances, the passage of a brush through the narrowed area dislodges cells which can be examined for malignancy.

Treatment. The choice lies between palliation and radical measures. The chances of cure seldom exceed 10%. In squamous carcinoma, particularly of the upper and middle thirds, high voltage radiotherapy is the treatment of choice in those centres possessing the necessary facilities. Otherwise, and with tumours of the lower third, oesophagogastrectomy offers the best hope. There is the possibility that a combined approach of sur-

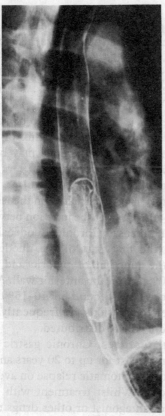

Fig. 9.3 Carcinoma of the oesophagus. (Courtesy of Dr G. M. Fraser.)

gery with pre-operative radiotherapy may lead to enhanced survival.

Extensive tumours that are unsuitable for radical surgery or for intensive radiotherapy are treated palliatively, occasionally by bypass surgery, but more often by endoscopic insertion of a permanent tube into the oesophagus. This allows liquids to be taken and is effective in relieving the patient of that most distressing problem — the inability to swallow saliva.

Gastrostomy as a palliative measure offers no relief to the patient, fails to prolong survival and is therefore not advisable.

DISEASES OF THE STOMACH AND DUODENUM

PEPTIC ULCER

The term 'peptic ulcer' refers to an ulcer in the lower oesophagus, stomach or duodenum, in the jejunum after surgical anastomosis to the stomach, or rarely in the ileum adjacent to a Meckel's diverticulum. Ulcers in the stomach or duodenum may be acute or chronic; both penetrate the muscularis mucosae but the acute ulcer shows no evidence of fibrosis. Erosions do not penetrate the muscularis mucosae.

Although the incidence of peptic ulcer is decreasing in many Western communities, it still affects, at some time, approximately 10% of all adult males. The male to female ratio for duodenal ulcer varies from 4:1 to 2:1 in different communities whilst that for gastric ulcer is 2:1 or less. Variations in the incidence of gastric and duodenal ulcer occur between different countries and between different parts of the same country; the incidence of peptic ulcer is higher in Scotland than in Southern England due to a preponderance of duodenal ulcers in Scotland. Peptic ulcer is becoming more common in many developing countries. There is growing evidence that cigarette smoking prevents healing of gastric and duodenal ulcers and may be a factor contributing to their development.

Aetiology of chronic ulceration. HEREDITY. Patients with peptic ulcer often have a family history of the disease; this is particularly the case with duodenal ulcers which develop below the age of 20 years. Gastric and duodenal ulcers are inherited as separate disorders; thus, the relatives of gastric ulcer patients have three times the expected number of gastric ulcers but duodenal ulcer occurs with the same frequency amongst relatives as in the general population.

ACID-PEPSIN VERSUS MUCOSAL RESISTANCE. The immediate cause of peptic ulceration is digestion of the mucosa by acid and pepsin of the gastric juice, but the sequence of events leading to this is unknown. Digestion by acid and pepsin cannot be the only factor involved, since the normal stomach is obviously capable of resisting digestion by its own secretions. The concept of ulcer aetiology may be written as 'acid plus pepsin versus mucosal resistance'. Some factors which affect this balance can be identified.

Gastric hypersecretion. Ulcers occur only in the presence of acid and pepsin; they are never found in achlorhydric patients such as those with pernicious anaemia. On the other hand, severe intractable peptic ulceration nearly always occurs in patients with the Zollinger-Ellison syndrome which is characterised by very high acid secretion. Acid secretion is more important in the aetiology of duodenal than gastric ulcer, because patients with duodenal ulcer, as a group, secrete more hydrochloric acid than normal individuals.

Mucosal resistance. Several mechanisms protect the gastric mucosa from hydrogen ions secreted into the lumen of the stomach. The surface epithelial cells secrete bicarbonate which creates an alkaline milieu at the surface of the mucosa; this bicarbonate secretion is under the influence of mucosal prostaglandins. The tight junctions between the epithelial cells, and their surface lipoprotein layer provide a mechanical barrier. The normal turnover of epithelial cells and gastric mucus also has a protective function. Collectively, all these mechanisms can be described as the 'gastric mucosal barrier'. Its integrity is important in preventing gastric ulcer and some of these mechanisms may also operate in the duodenum.

Factors reducing mucosal resistance. Several drugs, particularly those used in rheumatoid arthritis, will disrupt the gastric mucosal barrier. When aspirin is in solution at a pH below 3.5 it is undissociated and fat-soluble, so that it is absorbed through the lipoprotein membrane of the surface epithelial cells; during absorption it damages the membrane and the tight junctions. It also inhibits prostaglandin synthesis thus reducing bicarbonate secretion by the surface epithelial cells. Aspirin has been shown to be an important aetiological factor in gastric ulcer in Australia, and this may also be so in other countries where there is a high consumption of aspirin. There is also a relationship between aspirin ingestion and acute bleeding from the upper gastrointestinal tract.

Reflux of bile and intestinal secretions into the stomach occurs more frequently in patients with gastric ulcers than in normal individuals or patients with duodenal ulcer, due presumably to a poorly functioning pyloric sphincter. Bile damages the gastric mucosal barrier, predisposing the mucosa to ulceration. Chronic gastritis is more common in patients with gastric ulcer and it may be caused by damage from regurgitated bile and intestinal secretions or by *Campylobacter pyloridis*

(p. 293).

Aetiology of acute and stress ulcers. Many of the factors described above also contribute to the development of acute ulcers. Aspirin is particularly important. Acute peptic ulcers developing after head injury, burns, severe sepsis, surgery or trauma are termed *stress ulcers*. Gastric hypersecretion is the usual cause of acute ulcer after head injury, while the reflux of duodenal contents and mucosal ischaemia may be responsible factors after burns or shock.

Pathology. Chronic gastric ulcer is nearly always single; 90% are situated on the lesser curve within the antrum or at the junction between body and antral mucosa. Chronic duodenal ulcer is usually in the first part of the duodenum just distal to the junction of pyloric and duodenal mucosa; 50% are on the anterior wall. More than one peptic ulcer is found in 10–15% of cases. Acute ulcers or erosions are frequently multiple, and are more widely distributed.

Clinical features. Chronic gastric and duodenal ulcers persist for up to 20 years and perhaps for life with symptomatic relapse on average once every 2 years. Whilst treatment with histamine H_2-receptor antagonist or other drugs may effect prompt healing, there is no evidence that the natural history of the ulcer is affected. While there are good grounds for believing that gastric and duodenal ulcers are different diseases it is convenient to describe the general features of 'peptic ulcer' as inclusive of both, noting differences where they occur.

Peptic ulcer may present in different ways. The commonest is chronic, episodic pain extending over months or years. However, the ulcer may come to attention as an acute episode with bleeding or perforation, with little or no previous history. Occasionally the patient presents with the symptoms of gastric outlet obstruction, having had negligible trouble previously.

Pain is the characteristic symptom of peptic ulcer, and it has three notable features—localisation to the epigastrium, relationship to food, and periodicity. Ulcer pain is typically referred to the epigastrium, in the midline or to the right; it is usually localised so that the patient can indicate the site with one finger, 'the pointing sign'. Occasionally ulcer pain is not clearly localised; it may be referred diffusely in the epigastrium, the lower chest or to the back in the interscapular region in the fifth to eighth thoracic segments. Pain referred to the interscapular area suggests duodenal or post-bulbar ulceration. The description of the pain is not especially helpful, although patients commonly describe it as gnawing or burning. Pain varies considerably in severity, and it is sometimes helpful to ask the patient to qualify the symptom as 'pain' or as 'discomfort' as a measure of its intensity.

Most patients recognise a relationship of the pain to food, although the relationship varies between patients, and in the same patient from time to time. Duodenal ulcer pain tends to occur between meal times, so that the patient may describe it as 'hunger' pain, which is characteristically relieved by food. A notable feature of duodenal ulcer is pain awakening the patient from sleep 2 to 3 hours after retiring. The pain of gastric ulcer occurs less regularly; it frequently occurs within an hour of eating, is less often relieved by food and it rarely occurs at night. Besides the characteristic relief obtained after eating, ulcer pain is almost invariably relieved by antacids or vomiting.

Ulcer pain is characteristically episodic occurring regularly each day for days or weeks at a time, then disappearing, to recur weeks or months later. Between attacks, the patient feels perfectly well, and may eat and drink with impunity. Bouts of pain may at first last only a day or so at a time, and occur only once or twice a year. As the natural history evolves, however, episodes begin to last longer and occur more frequently, so that in severe cases remissions of pain may be short lived and pain or discomfort becomes more or less persistent. The cause for these relapses is difficult to establish. Seasonal factors may be operative, sometimes psychological stress may be blamed, sometimes dietary indiscretion, and sometimes alcoholic excess. Most commonly, no reason can be found for the relapse.

Pain is sometimes absent or so slight as to be dismissed by the patient. Such individuals may complain of other symptoms such as a feeling of 'distension' in the epigastrium or a poorly defined sense of unease after eating. Other complaints include episodic nausea and sometimes anorexia,

as well as heartburn or waterbrash. Vomiting in ulcer patients almost always relieves pain and when it is persistent may result in weight loss. This helps to distinguish it from vomiting of psychological origin, in which weight is usually maintained. Persistent vomiting in an ulcer subject usually indicates some degree of gastric outflow obstruction, whether due to spasm or organic narrowing. In such patients, vomiting is usually copious, so that the patient is 'surprised' at the volume; the patient often recognises food eaten 12 or more hours previously. Although there is no constant change in bowel rhythm during an ulcer relapse, some patients are aware of constipation or diarrhoea when dyspepsia reappears.

Physical signs. The only physical sign that may be present is 'the pointing sign' which, when accompanied by localised tenderness, is practically diagnostic of an ulcer. However, tenderness may be completely absent. In patients with gastric outlet obstruction, the stomach may be visibly distended, a succussion splash may be present and gastric peristalsis may be seen.

Investigation. At double contrast barium meal the ulcer is seen *en face* as a small collection of barium with mucosal folds radiating to the edge of the crater (Figs 9.4 and 9.5). Even when an ulcer cannot be seen, deformity of the duodenal cap can be important evidence of duodenal ulcer disease. Endoscopy is preferred by most physicians particularly when the ulcer is gastric, because a biopsy can be carried out to exclude carcinoma. Endoscopy will also locate some duodenal ulcers which are difficult to detect radiologically. In addition it will diagnose *duodenitis*, a generalised inflammation of the first part of the duodenum. This may be regarded as a variant of duodenal ulcer disease in which no ulcer crater is present.

Treatment. While various measures are available to alleviate symptoms and heal the ulcer, there is no evidence that the long-term course of the disease is affected.

INJURIOUS DRUGS, TOBACCO, ALCOHOL AND DIET. It is particularly important that aspirin and other anti-inflammatory drugs are not used in peptic ulceration. Their injurious action should be explained to the patient. Stopping smoking accelerates the healing of ulcers and patients must

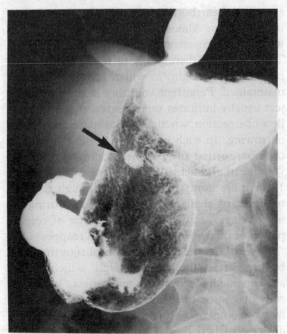

Fig. 9.4 Gastric ulcer. (Courtesy of Dr G. M. Fraser.)

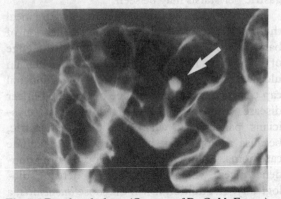

Fig. 9.5 Duodenal ulcer. (Courtesy of Dr G. M. Fraser.)

therefore be advised to give up cigarettes. Most patients cannot consume alcohol during exacerbations of ulcer disease because it aggravates their symptoms. It seems reasonable to encourage moderation in drinking habits in all patients with peptic ulceration. There is no evidence that dietary manipulation affects symptoms or ulcer healing, and strict diets are not indicated.

DRUGS. *Antacids* provide symptomatic relief in peptic ulcer disease; in large doses, given for 4 to 6 weeks they will induce healing but side-effects usually preclude this usage. Many preparations are available, varying in neutralising capacity, side-effects, palatability and cost. Sodium bicarbonate is the quickest acting and is widely used for self-medication. However, it is very readily absorbed with the risk of alkalosis, so that its use should be discouraged and it should not be prescribed. The majority of antacids are based on combinations of calcium, aluminium and magnesium salts, all of which may cause side-effects. Frequently calcium and aluminium cause constipation and magnesium causes diarrhoea. Calcium compounds may lead to hypercalcaemia if dosage is high and prolonged. Aluminium compounds block the absorption of phosphate and may cause phosphate depletion, an effect which is utilised in the management of renal failure. They may also bind other drugs whose absorption will be reduced if given at the same time as the antacid. Magnesium compounds may cause toxic hypermagnesaemia when renal function is impaired. Almost all antacids contain appreciable amounts of sodium which may exacerbate fluid retention in patients with cardiac or liver disease.

For relief of minor discomfort, antacid preparations in tablet form are convenient; they may be carried in the pocket and chewed or sucked whenever pain occurs. For relief of more severe pain during exacerbations, 15–30 ml of liquid antacid are usually required. To heal duodenal ulcer, it is necessary to give 30 ml of liquid antacid one and three hours after food and at bedtime. Patient acceptance of this form of therapy is low because of poor palatability and the frequent occurrence of constipation or diarrhoea.

Histamine H_2-receptor antagonist drugs. The fact that the stimulating effect of histamine on gastric secretion could not be blocked by the standard antihistamines led to the idea that there was a second type of histamine receptor situated on, or near, the parietal cells, blocking of which would reduce gastric secretion. This led to the development of the histamine H_2-receptor antagonists which are now the treatment of choice for all forms of peptic ulcer. Two of these drugs, cimetidine and ranitidine, when given for 4 weeks will heal over 80% of duodenal ulcers and 70% of gastric ulcers. Cimetidine is used in a dose of 200 mg three times a day with meals and 400 mg at night, or 400 mg with breakfast and 400 mg at night, or in a single dose of 800 mg at night. Ranitidine is given in a dose of 150 mg with breakfast and 150 mg at night or in a single dose of 300 mg at night.

The use of cimetidine in large numbers of patients suggests that it is a very safe drug. Gynaecomastia occurs in a few patients; confusion in the elderly and diarrhoea are other occasional side-effects. Cimetidine also impairs the metabolism of some drugs and this is particularly important in the case of warfarin and phenytoin Ranitidine does not cause any of the above side-effects.

Treatment with either drug usually renders nearly all patients asymptomatic within a week of the commencement of therapy, and most are asymptomatic within 48 hours. Failure to relieve symptoms should lead to a reconsideration of the diagnosis. Most patients with peptic ulceration will have one or two exacerbations per year and each can be treated with a 4-week course of cimetidine or ranitidine. However, for those patients with more frequent relapses or who have contraindications to elective surgery, such as age, respiratory or cardiac disease, the frequency of further relapses can be reduced by giving maintenance therapy of cimetidine (400 mg) or ranitidine (150 mg) at night for several years or permanently.

Tri-potassium di-citrato bismuthate is an ammoniacal suspension of a complex colloidal bismuth salt which precipitates in acid conditions and binds to proteins in the ulcer base. One tablet is chewed four times daily 30 minutes before each meal and 2 hours after the evening meal for 4 weeks. Because of the risk of bismuth toxicity, it should not be used for maintenance treatment.

Sucralfate is the aluminium salt of sucrose octasulphate. It acts by binding to the ulcer crater and has the same efficacy as cimetidine for healing duodenal ulcer. It is given in a dose of 1 g three times a day before meals and 1 g at bedtime for 4 weeks.

Other drugs used for healing ulcers. Carbenoxolone sodium accelerates the healing of both gastric and duodenal ulcers. However, because of its aldosterone-like effects, it may cause sodium retention with oedema, hypokalaemia and hypertension, so it is little used now. Pirenzepine is a tricyclic compound which preferentially blocks the subclass of muscarinic receptors in the stomach. Its efficacy in healing ulcers is less than

that of cimetidine and some patients complain of a dry mouth or blurred vision. Prostaglandin analogues heal both gastric and duodenal ulcers with approximately the same efficacy as cimetidine.

Choice of drug. The H_2-receptor antagonist drugs are favoured as the treatment of choice by the majority of physicians because they are effective and have a demonstrated record of safety over the short and long term. Sucralfate and tripotassium di-citrato bismuthate are acceptable alternatives for short-term therapy. Carbenoxolone and pirenzepine are not recommended because of side-effects. Prostaglandin analogues are likely to gain acceptance because they may act partly by strengthening the gastric mucosal barrier.

SURGICAL TREATMENT. This has much to offer the patient with intractable peptic ulceration. It can relieve severe or persistent symptoms and prevent complications. While in many cases the assessment of the disability is straightforward, in patients in whom anxiety or depression is present, the decision becomes difficult. Elective surgery should be considered in the following circumstances:

1. When the ulcer relapses promptly after several courses of cimetidine or other ulcer-healing drugs, when relapse occurs during maintenance therapy, or more rarely when the ulcer fails to heal at all, particularly when symptoms interfere with the enjoyment of life or reduce the capacity to work. The indications for surgery are strengthened if the ulcer has developed in adolescence or young adult life, if there is a strong family history, or if there has been a previous complication such as haemorrhage or perforation. Finally, some patients fail to comply with medical therapy or express reservations about prolonged therapy, both points being in favour of elective surgical treatment.

2. When there is an ulcer which has produced gastric outlet obstruction, or an hour-glass stomach because of fibrosis.

3. In a recurrent ulcer following previous gastric surgery.

There is no single, ideal operation suitable for all ulcers and all patients. For a gastric ulcer, the operation of choice is partial gastrectomy preferably with a Billroth I anastomosis, in which the ulcer itself and the ulcer-bearing area of the stomach is resected (Fig. 9.6). For duodenal ulcer the acid secretory capacity of the stomach may be reduced by vagotomy which eliminates nervous stimulation (Fig. 9.6). At truncal vagotomy the main nerves are divided and thereafter gastric emptying may be retarded so that a drainage operation such as pyloroplasty or gastroenterostomy has to be added. A drainage procedure is also required in selective vagotomy in which vagal innervation to the small intestine, pancreas and biliary tree is preserved.

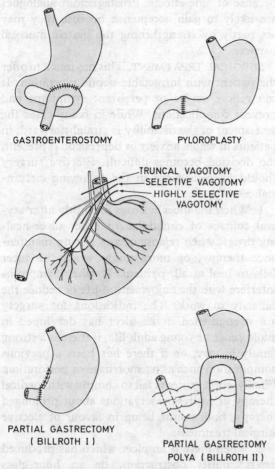

GASTROENTEROSTOMY

PYLOROPLASTY

TRUNCAL VAGOTOMY
SELECTIVE VAGOTOMY
HIGHLY SELECTIVE VAGOTOMY

PARTIAL GASTRECTOMY
(BILLROTH I)

PARTIAL GASTRECTOMY
POLYA (BILLROTH II)

Fig. 9.6 Operations for peptic ulcer.

The aim of highly selective vagotomy is to denervate only the acid-producing area of the stomach while leaving intact the vagal supply of the antrum and pylorus. Gastric emptying is thus not impaired and a drainage procedure is not required unless there is stenosis from ulcer scarring. The avoidance of a drainage procedure markedly reduces the incidence of post-cibal syndromes and in particular dumping (p. 292). Vagotomy is preferred to partial gastrectomy because of the lesser mortality and lower incidence of long-term complications.

Complications of peptic ulcer are haemorrhage, perforation and gastric outlet obstruction. Ulcer-cancer is discussed on page 294.

Gastroduodenal haemorrhage

Gastroduodenal haemorrhage is recognised by *haematemesis* (vomiting of blood) and/or *melaena* (passage of blood in the stools), and usually there are symptoms of hypovolaemia. Gastroduodenal haemorrhage carries a mortality that may reach 30% in elderly and shocked patients. A history of significant blood loss within the previous 48 hours should lead to immediate admission to hospital.

Aetiology. The common causes of bleeding are chronic gastric and duodenal ulcers (50%), erosions (15–30%), oesophageal varices (10%) and mucosal lacerations at the cardia due to vomiting (Mallory-Weiss syndrome — 7%). Less frequent causes are cancer of the stomach and other tumours such as leiomyoma, oesophagitis, stress ulcers and bleeding disorders.

Erosions are usually caused by the ingestion of aspirin either alone or in combination with alcohol or by non-steroidal anti-inflammatory drugs. In some patients the stomach shows petechiae, multiple erosions and areas of confluent mucosal bleeding; this appearance is called *acute haemorrhagic gastritis*. The usual presentation of stress ulcer, caused by burns or head injury, is with haematemesis and melaena.

Clinical features. In severe bleeding from whatever cause, the patient complains of weakness, faintness, nausea, and sweating: these symptoms are followed by haematemesis or melaena. Haematemesis and melaena occur together with a sudden large bleed whereas melaena alone indicates that bleeding is slower and less in amount. If blood remains in the stomach it becomes partially digested and appears brown and granular in the vomit or gastric aspirate, like 'coffee grounds'. Blood passing through the intestinal canal is also altered in appearance, so that the faeces become black and sticky, (a 'tarry' stool) but in severe bleeding, transit may be so rapid that the blood in the rectum is bright red.

The patient may be shocked or restless and disorientated because of cerebral anoxia. These signs may be absent in the young patient in whom compensatory mechanisms are more effective. The haemoglobin level will not alter until haemodilution occurs and this may not take place for some hours, nor be complete for some days. A reduced haematocrit on admission to hospital often indicates chronic bleeding prior to the acute episode. A raised urea with a normal serum creatinine indicates a blood loss of at least one litre. There is no simple laboratory procedure which will give a reliable estimate of the amount of blood loss until haemodilution is complete, so that in ordinary circumstances the assessment of the degree or rate of bleeding depends on clinical judgement. Serial recordings of the pulse rate and blood pressure give some indication, but for a more accurate assessment in patients who continue to bleed, measurement of central venous pressure is necessary. In patients with severe bleeding a record of urinary output by catheterisation is helpful.

Investigation. On admission there should be joint assessment by physician and surgeon and in large centres the management of gastroduodenal bleeding can with advantage be centralised in a single unit. The diagnosis and bleeding status should be established at the outset. Emergency endoscopy will show the source of the bleeding, whether it is continuing or whether it is likely to recur. Endoscopy is preferable to emergency barium studies in that it can demonstrate erosions and in the event of more than one lesion being present it can confirm which is bleeding.

The bleeding status is ascertained by passage of a nasogastric tube which should be aspirated at half-hourly intervals and the quantity and type of aspirate recorded.

Treatment. Urgent treatment of hypovolaemic shock requires rapid and adequate blood replacement. Whole blood should be given as soon as it is available; until then, a colloidal solution such as dextran can be used. A blood transfusion is also indicated if the pulse rate is faster than 100 per minute or the systolic pressure lower than 100 mmHg. Transfusion must keep pace with the estimated loss. This may be difficult in the elderly patient who is liable to develop cardiac or renal failure or cerebral anoxia and in whom coronary blood supply may also be impaired leading to angina or even myocardial infarction.

To control restlessness and anxiety, the injection of drugs such as diazepam is to be preferred to morphine which may itself cause vomiting.

Subsequent management depends on the initial response and on the site and cause of bleeding. In general, emergency surgery should be advised in patients over the age of 50 in whom there is continued or recurrent bleeding from a gastric or duodenal ulcer. Conversely operation is unlikely to be necessary in such patients under the age of 30 or in patients with erosions in whom conservative management, including cimetidine or ranitidine, will usually suffice. The greatest risks are in the shocked and elderly with continued severe bleeding and when operation is delayed too long.

The need for surgery does not disappear once the crisis is over. Early elective operation may still be indicated in patients with chronic ulcers which have bled, in those requiring continued treatment with salicylates, non-steroidal analgesics or corticosteroids, and in patients whose occupation or residence makes supervision difficult. In general, excision of the bleeding gastric ulcer, or exposure and suture of the duodenal ulcer coupled in either case with vagotomy is safer than partial gastrectomy which should be reserved for the complicated case in expert hands.

Bleeding from oesophageal varices secondary to portal hypertension can be extremely severe and demands special management (p. 357).

Acute perforation of a peptic ulcer

When free perforation occurs, the contents of the stomach escape into the peritoneal cavity. If perforation occurs without loss of contents, as in the accidental perforation of the empty stomach at gastroscopy, few symptoms are produced and the accident may even pass unnoticed. It follows that the symptoms of perforation are those of peritonitis, and they are in proportion to the extent of peritoneal soiling. Occasionally the symptoms of perforation appear and rapidly subside; presumably the perforation has then closed spontaneously, or more commonly the ulcer has perforated locally into an area confined by adhesions to adjacent structures. Perforation occurs more commonly in duodenal than in gastric ulcers, and usually in ulcers on the anterior wall. About one-quarter of all perforations occur in acute ulcers.

Clinical features. Although perforation may be the first sign of ulcer, usually there is a history of recurrent epigastric pain. The most striking symptom is sudden, severe pain; its distribution follows the spread of the gastric contents over the peritoneum. Thus, initially the pain may be referred to the upper abdomen, but very quickly it becomes generalised; shoulder tip pain may occur as a result of irritation of the diaphragm. The pain is accompanied by shallow respiration due to limitation of diaphragmatic movements and by shock. The abdomen is held immobile, and there is generalised board-like rigidity. Intestinal sounds are absent, and liver dullness to percussion may decrease due to the presence of gas under the diaphragm. Vomiting is common. After some hours, the symptoms improve, though the abdominal rigidity remains. This period of improvement may deceive the clinician examining the patient for the first time; after this temporary improvement, manifestations of general peritonitis follow the initial peritoneal irritation and the patient's condition deteriorates.

A radiograph of the upper abdomen in the erect position may help to establish the diagnosis since free gas within the peritoneal cavity, if in sufficient amount, will show as a translucent crescent between the liver and diaphragm. Where doubt remains, an emergency gastrografin meal may confirm that perforation has occurred.

Treatment and prognosis. After initial treatment of the patient for shock, the acute perforation should be treated surgically either by simple closure, or occasionally in the case of perforation of a chronic ulcer by closure combined with vagotomy and drainage. More than half the patients who have a simple closure will eventually require a further elective operation for recurrence of ulcer symptoms, and for this reason some surgeons recommend a definitive procedure for the ulcer at the time of operation.

Acute perforation carries a mortality of about 5%. The outlook is poorest in elderly patients, when a large perforation results in extensive peritonitis or when operation is delayed.

Gastric outlet obstruction

An ulcer in the region of the pylorus may lead to gastric outlet obstruction. This may be due to fibrous stricture or to oedema or spasm produced by the ulcer; frequently it is a combination of all three. Gastric outlet obstruction may also be caused by carcinoma of the antrum and by a rare condition, adult hypertrophic pyloric stenosis. The syndrome of gastric outlet obstruction is loosely described as 'pyloric stenosis', even when the cause is chronic duodenal ulcer; here the stenosis is distal to the pylorus which itself may be seen radiologically to be greatly dilated.

Clinical features. Symptoms of obstruction are usually preceded by a long history of duodenal ulceration. Without such symptoms, a patient with gastric outlet obstruction is likely to have a pyloric carcinoma. When there has been an ulcer, the symptoms change, so that vomiting becomes a prominent feature, and nausea replaces normal appetite. Vomiting produces such striking relief that a patient may start to eat immediately after the stomach has been emptied. If the obstruction progresses, the stomach dilates so that, eventually, surprisingly large amounts of gastric content may be vomited. Articles of food which have been eaten 24 hours or more previously may be recognised in the vomit. The loss of gastric contents results in water and electrolyte depletion. The blood urea may be raised because of dehydration. Alkalosis develops if large amounts of hydrochloric acid are lost, as occurs particularly in obstruction due to duodenal ulcer.

Physical examination shows evidence of wasting and dehydration, and there may be signs of tetany (p. 448). A succussion splash may be elicited four hours or more after the last meal or drink. In normal persons splashing occurs for less than an hour after meals because gastric emptying is rapid.

Visible gastric peristalsis is diagnostic of gastric outlet obstruction and the abdomen should be inspected for its presence.

Investigation. *Aspiration of the stomach contents* will confirm the diagnosis if the volume is in excess of 100 ml after fasting overnight or if the aspirate contains food residue, or is foul.

Barium meal shows: (1) an increase in the fasting residue of the stomach, (2) dilatation of the stomach with or without excessive peristalsis, (3) a lesion at or near the pylorus, and (4) delayed gastric emptying.

Endoscopy may demonstrate the cause of the obstruction and its degree.

Treatment. The stomach is washed out to remove all food debris and then aspirated 2 to 4 hourly for 3 to 4 days at which point, if the volume of aspirate has decreased, it may be possible to allow fluids by mouth. Dehydration and metabolic alkalosis must be treated (p. 98). A multivitamin preparation should be given by injection to all but the mildest cases. The majority of patients will be greatly improved by these methods; the volume of the gastric aspirate steadily declines, and the size of the stomach returns to near normal. Relief of obstruction by conservative measures provides an opportunity to complete investigation and to render the patient as fit as possible for subsequent elective surgery.

Zollinger-Ellison syndrome

This is a rare disorder in which severe peptic ulceration occurs due usually to an adenoma or hyperplasia of the islets of the pancreas secreting large amounts of gastrin which stimulates the parietal cells of the stomach excessively. The acid output may be so great that the 'acid tide' may reach the upper small intestine, reducing the luminal pH to 2 or less; at this pH, pancreatic lipase is inactivated and bile acids may be precipitated, causing diarrhoea and steatorrhoea. Excessive gastric secretion results in large volumes on aspiration under 'basal' conditions. Pentagastrin does not increase the secretory rate much above 'basal' values, since the stomach is already continuously secreting at or near maximal rates.

The ulcers are often multiple and severe and may occur in unusual sites such as the jejunum or the oesophagus. The history is usually short and bleeding and perforation are common. The syndrome may present in the form of severe recurrent ulceration following a standard operation for peptic ulcer, the underlying cause not having been recognised.

The diagnosis should be suspected in all patients with unusual or severe peptic ulceration, especially if the barium meal examination shows abnormally coarse gastric mucosal folds. It may be confirmed by finding very high levels of gastrin in the circulation.

Theoretically the condition should be cured by removing the pancreatic tumour, but this may not be possible because of its diffuse nature. In these circumstances it is necessary to eliminate, or very greatly reduce, acid secretion so that the ulcers may heal. In most patients continuous therapy with cimetidine or ranitidine is effective, but larger doses than those used to treat duodenal ulcer are required. In unresponsive patients, total gastrectomy is necessary.

Late complications following gastric surgery

Although most operations carried out for the relief of peptic ulcer are successful, 10% of patients will develop complications months or years afterwards. Some of these, such as anaemia and nutritional impairment, develop insidiously, so that patients who have had an operation on the stomach should be reviewed at least once a year.

Recurrent ulcer, after surgery for duodenal ulcer, is usually due to insufficient reduction of the secretory capacity of the stomach because of incomplete vagotomy or inadequate gastrectomy. A *jejunal ulcer* develops just distal to the jejuno-gastric anastomosis, because the jejunal mucosa is more susceptible to acid-pepsin digestion than gastric or duodenal mucosa. About 15% of patients develop recurrent ulcer after highly selective vagotomy but the operation has the virtue of being free from the side-effects associated with resection, truncal vagotomy or drainage procedures.

After months or years of freedom following the operation, ulcer pain recurs or the patient may present with melaena or severe anaemia without any dyspeptic symptoms. Occasionally, perforation occurs. Rarely a jejunal ulcer penetrates the colon causing a *gastro-jejunal-colic fistula*; then there is bacterial contamination of the small bowel causing diarrhoea, malabsorption and wasting. The fistula can be demonstrated by barium enema.

Recurrent ulcer uncomplicated by perforation or fistula is best diagnosed by endoscopy which will also reveal the occasional ulcer due to an unabsorbed suture which can be removed endoscopically. Recurrent ulcer can be treated by H_2-receptor antagonists but if this fails, a more radical surgical procedure may be necessary.

Biliary gastritis is the result of reflux of bile into the stomach through a drainage stoma. It may be symptomless and observed only on routine postoperative endoscopy. There may be epigastric discomfort, nausea, heartburn or vomiting of bile. Reduction in fluid intake, the eating of meals dry, avoidance of alcohol and stopping smoking may bring relief. Drugs are of little value but some patients have symptoms due to delayed gastric emptying which are helped by metoclopramide (p. 280). Revisional surgery may be required if dietetic measures fail and especially when there is a mechanical cause for the reflux.

Post-cibal syndromes are mainly associated with gastrectomy and have become less frequent with the more general adoption of vagotomy.

1. *The small stomach syndrome*. Discomfort and distension with meals leads to diminished intake and weight loss or failure to regain weight. High energy small meals and, in some cases, revisional surgery are indicated.

2. *Dumping syndrome* After a meal and particularly after hot sweet foods, there is a feeling of intense drowsiness with weakness and nausea; there may also be flushing and palpitations. The syndrome usually improves with time. The ingestion of small dry meals with the avoidance of fluids at meal times is often of value. Occasionally further surgery may be necessary.

3. *Hypoglycaemia*. Rarely, one or two hours after a meal, the patient experiences attacks of weakness, tremor and faintness. The hypoglycaemia responsible for these symptoms can be relieved by glucose or barley sugar.

Diarrhoea may occur after any operation on the stomach, but especially after truncal vagotomy when most patients report some looseness of the stools. Moderate or severe diarrhoea occurs in about 10% and is characteristically episodic, several watery stools being passed daily for several days. A striking feature is the sense of urgency associated with the diarrhoea; defecation may be precipitate, and the patient becomes worried because of the fear of soiling. Loperamide or codeine should be tried.

Mild steatorrhoea is common after all ulcer operations and does not require treatment, but if severe steatorrhoea occurs the cause (p. 303) should be identified so that appropriate treatment may be undertaken.

Anaemia is a common sequel to operations on the stomach, particularly partial gastrectomy, due to inadequate absorption of iron, or to recurrent minor blood loss from gastritis or oesophagitis. Its incidence increases in the first 10 years as the stores of iron are exhausted. The occurrence of anaemia is a measure of the adequacy of postoperative supervision, because it is preventable by and responds to the administration of iron. Megaloblastic anaemia may also occur (p. 506).

Nutritional impairment and osteomalacia. In a small proportion of patients there is some nutritional impairment following gastric surgery, and this increases with the extent of any resection. Severe weight loss is its most common manifestation. There may also be malabsorption with steatorrhoea and osteomalacia which may develop for the first time 15 to 20 years after partial gastrectomy, and may present as bone pain or as a pathological fracture. Treatment is described on page 67.

GASTRITIS

Gastritis signifies an acute or chronic inflammation of the stomach. Knowledge of the changes that occur in the gastric mucosa has been obtained by direct studies of the gastric mucosa in patients with gastrostomies, by gastroscopic observation and by histological examination of specimens removed at operation, biopsy or autopsy. There is poor agreement between these three approaches, so that the classification of gastritis is difficult. If histological specimens are examined, it is very rare to find a normal stomach completely free from any signs of inflammation. In this sense 'gastritis' is almost an invariable finding in adults. However, there are gross departures from this 'normal' state of affairs, even if they do not give rise to symptoms. For these reasons the condition is best defined in histological terms as acute or chronic gastritis.

Acute gastritis

This is most commonly caused by the ingestion of aspirin, anti-inflammatory drugs and probably alcohol. It is also caused by the regurgitation of bile into the stomach, especially after gastric surgery. Macroscopically, there is engorgement of the mucosa with oedema and erosions or an acute haemorrhagic gastritis (p. 288). Microscopically there is loss of the surface epithelium, hyperaemia and some infiltration with inflammatory cells.

Acute gastritis may be asymptomatic. In some patients, there is anorexia, nausea, epigastric pain and heartburn. If gastritis persists, a slow loss of blood may lead to anaemia. The condition is diagnosed by gastroscopy.

Drug consumption should be reviewed with a view to omitting or reducing drugs which are known to cause gastric mucosal damage. Alcohol should be avoided. The treatment of biliary gastritis is discussed on page 292.

Chronic gastritis

The classification is histological; there are three stages which are progressive over many years. In *chronic superficial gastritis,* the mucosa is normal in thickness and there is patchy infiltration of lymphocytes and plasma cells. In *atrophic gastritis* there is a reduction of the specialised cells in the glands of the body and of mucous cells in the pyloric glands. There is epithelial metaplasia and an infiltrate of lymphocytes and plasma cells. In *gastric atrophy* the thickness of the mucosa is reduced, metaplasia is common but round cell infiltration is slight.

In pernicious anaemia and other autoimmune disorders, the chronic gastritis is due to an im-

munological process, and circulating antibodies to parietal cells and intrinsic factor are frequently found. Chronic gastritis is common in peptic ulcer, gastric cancer and after gastric surgery. In these instances, the gastritis is thought not to be immunological and circulating antibodies are absent. *Campylobacter pyloridis* can be demonstrated in biopsies from many patients with chronic gastritis and chronic peptic ulcer. This organism is likely to play an aetiological part in chronic gastritis but whether it has a role in peptic ulcer remains to be decided.

The condition is asymptomatic; its importance lies in its association with the disorders noted above. The diagnosis may be suspected from the absence of mucosal folds at barium meal examination or from the gastroscopic appearances. However, the diagnosis is confirmed only by gastric biopsy. No treatment is known for stimulating the mucosa to regenerate.

CARCINOMA OF THE STOMACH

The incidence of this tumour varies considerably in different parts of the world — for example, it is frequent in Japan but relatively uncommon in the USA. Its incidence is falling in many countries. Japanese immigrants to America have a lower incidence than in Japan indicating the possible importance of environmental factors such as trace elements in water, or differences in methods of food preparation. It has been suggested that nitrites, often used as preservatives in food, can be converted to the carcinogens nitrosamines in the milieu of the stomach. Patients with pernicious anaemia have an increased risk of developing gastric cancer and this may extend to gastric atrophy from other causes. In particular there is an increased incidence of cancer of the stomach after partial gastrectomy or gastroenterostomy.

Pathology. Almost 60% of all gastric cancers occur at the pylorus or in the antrum; the lesion does not spread to the duodenum. Such growths may produce symptoms of obstruction to the gastric outlet. Cancer of the body of the stomach occurs in 20–30% of cases and often produces a fungating ulcerating mass. In 5–20% of cases, the tumour is cardiac and produces dysphagia. Least common is a diffuse infiltrating scirrhous lesion spreading throughout the body of the stomach and producing the 'leather-bottle stomach'. These are the descriptions of advanced cancer.

Gastric dysplasia is the term applied to precancerous lesions of the stomach; it is recognised by cytological changes in the epithelial cells. Early gastric cancer is defined as cancer confined to the mucosa or mucosa and submucosa regardless of the presence of lymph node metastasis. The lesion may be represented only by a depressed area with obliteration or distortion of the mucosal folds, by irregular ulceration on an elevated base, or by a small polypoid lesion. Such changes can be seen and a biopsy taken during gastroscopy at a stage when the cancer is potentially curable.

The tumour is an adenocarcinoma of intestinal or diffuse type. The intestinal type has well-defined cells and a clear margin and it is this type which has shown a fall in incidence in several countries. The diffuse type consists of clusters of cells which spread widely within the mucosa. The tumour spreads by extension through the stomach wall, by lymphatic permeation and by embolism via the portal vein to the liver and thence to the systemic bloodstream.

Gastric carcinoma may present as a malignant ulcer, and whether it is then the result of malignant transformation of a benign ulcer is debatable. Most authorities believe that chronic peptic ulcer rarely becomes malignant, and that malignant ulcers, however long they have been present, have always been malignant. Whatever the truth of the matter the problem in the individual case is to decide whether a chronic gastric ulcer is benign or malignant.

Clinical features. Loss of appetite, slight nausea and discomfort after meals occurring for the first time in middle age should always arouse suspicion. If the diagnosis is to be made early, then such patients require careful investigation. Unfortunately, the majority of patients have advanced gastric carcinoma before they seek advice. In some there have been no symptoms; in others symptoms have been present for 6 months or even a year. Dyspepsia, which is at first vague, becomes troublesome with increasing anorexia and nausea, discomfort or pain, vomiting and weight loss. There may be cachexia and pallor, a mass may be palpable or peristalsis visible. The abdomen may be distended by ascites from peritoneal metastases. Sometimes it is acanthosis nigricans (p. 104) or the presence of metastases in the liver, pelvis or scalene lymph nodes which first brings the patient to the physician.

Carcinoma of the stomach should always be considered as a cause of unexplained iron deficiency anaemia in the middle-aged person or as an uncommon cause of haematemesis or melaena. Tumours at the cardia may cause dysphagia, and tumours at the gastric outlet may cause vomiting. In the infiltrating type of tumour, diarrhoea may occur because of rapid emptying from the stomach.

Investigation. Early curable cancer is usually missed by a barium meal examination unless a double contrast study is carried out to show distortion of the mucosal pattern. The only method of establishing a positive diagnosis is by gastroscopy and biopsy of suspicious areas. These procedures are also necessary to distinguish malignant from benign gastric ulceration. The commonest appearance at barium meal is a filling defect in the antrum or body of the stomach (Fig. 9.7). In the rare diffuse infiltrating carcinoma, the radiograph is that of a rigid tube through which the barium pours rapidly into the intestine. If dysphagia is the presenting symptom, a lesion in the cardia will probably be found, but symptomless lesions in this area can be easily missed. Exfoliative cytology is sometimes used for diagnosis.

Treatment and prognosis. The only curative treatment is gastrectomy, but it is usually only at laparotomy that the possibility of resection can be decided. About one-third of patients coming to operation are found to have tumours capable of removal; in the remainder it is possible to perform only a palliative procedure. This is worthwhile if pyloric obstruction is present, even if there are secondary deposits; such an operation relieves the distressing vomiting and gives the patient some comfort.

A total gastrectomy may be required for tumours involving the upper part of the stomach. Careful preoperative treatment is essential; this may require the restoration of fluid and electrolyte

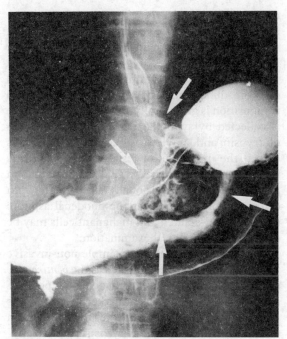

Fig. 9.7 Carcinoma of the stomach. (Courtesy of Dr G. M. Fraser.)

balance and the correction of anaemia. Every effort should be made to improve nutrition, if necessary by parenteral or enteral feeding.

A small proportion of patients with cancer of the stomach obtain worthwhile remission with cytotoxic drugs.

The prognosis in carcinoma of the stomach is very poor and has shown little improvement in the last 40 years. After an apparently successful resection, the 5-year survival rate is in the region of 20%. The overall 5-year survival rate is 5%. However for early gastric cancer, the 5-year survival rate is 85%. Thus, pending an entirely new approach to the problem, the only means currently available by which the prognosis can be improved is the detection of gastric cancer when it is at a curable stage; this requires a vigorous approach to the problem of dyspepsia in the middle-aged, including careful radiological and endoscopic examination and the critical follow-up of doubtful abnormalities.

Malignant ascites

Carcinoma of the stomach and other intra-abdominal tumours, including carcinoma of the colon and ovary, may be associated with the exudation of fluid into the peritoneal cavity. This follows the deposition of malignant cells on the peritoneal surface and is a sign of gross spread of the disease. The fluid is rich in protein and its sediment contains malignant cells which may be identifiable on microscopy.

Treatment is palliative. Relief of abdominal distension can be obtained by paracentesis, whilst instillation of an antimitotic agent such as methotrexate may slow the rate of reaccumulation.

DISEASES OF THE PANCREAS

The pancreas produces exocrine secretions which are important to digestion and also endocrine secretions concerned with the regulation of carbohydrate metabolism. The exocrine tissue, composed of acinar cells grouped in lobules and drained by a duct system, forms almost the entire mass of the gland. The exocrine secretion is discharged into the intestine through the pancreatic duct, which usually enters the duodenum together with the common bile duct at the sphincter of Oddi; in about 10% of individuals, however, the main outflow of the pancreatic juice reaches the duodenum by a separate duct.

The endocrine tissue is composed of specialised cells collected together in the small islets of Langerhans scattered throughout the gland, and accounts for only 1% of the mass of the pancreas. The endocrine secretions include insulin, which is produced by the beta cells of the islets, and glucagon from the alpha cells; both are discussed in the section on diabetes mellitus. The delta cell is one source of somatostatin (p. 425).

Pancreatic juice is an alkaline secretion which is isotonic with plasma, the main cations being sodium and potassium while the main anion is bicarbonate which is produced by the cells lining the duct system. The juice also contains enzymes which digest carbohydrate, fat and protein, the main ones being amylase, lipase and trypsin. These enzymes are synthesised by the serous cells of the pancreatic acini, and they are secreted in parallel concentrations; they all require an alkaline medium for optimal efficiency, so that theoretically digestion may be impaired if the bicarbonate content of the pancreatic juice is reduced.

Exocrine pancreatic secretion is stimulated partly through nervous and partly through hormonal mechanisms, and a maximum flow is reached between 2 and 3 hours after a meal; in all, about 1 litre is secreted daily.

Investigation of the pancreas

A plain radiograph may show evidence of duodeno-jejunal ileus in acute pancreatitis and calcification in chronic pancreatitis.

A barium meal will usually show stretching of the duodenal loop and upward displacement of the stomach when the head of the pancreas is enlarged by acute pancreatitis, cysts or tumours. Abnormalities of the mucosal folds of the duodenum, particularly on the medial wall, may be seen but these are best demonstrated by hypotonic duodenography.

The size, shape and position of the pancreas and the presence of tumours, cysts, oedema and dilated ducts can be shown by ultrasonography or by computed tomography. The former is more widely available and less expensive than CT scanning, but its value in the investigation of pancreatic disorders is greatly reduced if gas is present in overlying loops of bowel. CT scanning is more accurate in detecting pancreatic tumours especially in the tail of the gland. More specialised techniques include retrograde pancreatography of the duct system (ERCP, p. 274).

Selective arteriography of the coeliac and superior mesenteric arteries can show distortion, compression, or abnormal distribution of vessels in relation to tumours. Radionuclide studies are now little used.

Tests of exocrine pancreatic function. The exocrine function may be measured directly by passing a tube into the second part of the duodenum and collecting the secretory output of the gland in response to exogenous stimulation (secretin-cholecystokinin test) or endogenous stimulation by a meal (Lundh test). In the *secretin-cholecystokinin test* the hormones are injected intravenously and pancreatic secretions are collected for 1 hour. Measurements are made of the volume of secretion and the concentration of bicarbonate and amylase or lipase. A special double lumened tube allows gastric and pancreatic secretions to be collected separately to prevent neutralisation of pancreatic bicarbonate by gastric hydrochloric acid.

The *Lundh test* is simpler. A tube is passed into the duodenum and a liquid meal of fixed composition is given orally. The duodenal aspirate is collected by syphonage and the concentration of trypsin and amylase is recorded. Both tests detect the presence of established pancreatic insufficiency, but usually give no information as to the cause; occasionally in patients with carcinoma of the pancreas the duodenal aspirate may be blood-stained and malignant cells may be detected on cytological examination.

There is now a variety of simple non-invasive tests of pancreatic function such as the *bentiromide* and *pancreolauryl tests* which depend upon the cleavage of an orally given marker by pancreatic enzyme and its excretion in the urine, or serum trypsin-like immunoreactivity or serum isoamylase determinations. When normal values for these tests are obtained, pancreatic insufficiency is excluded but none is reliable in the presence of pancreatic insufficiency.

Tests of endocrine pancreatic function. A diabetic response to a glucose tolerance test in a patient with steatorrhoea suggests a pancreatic cause for the malabsorption of fat. When carcinoma of the pancreas is suspected, an abnormal glucose tolerance test is a frequent finding in a condition which is difficult to diagnose.

Acute pancreatitis

This acute condition, typically presenting with abdominal pain, and usually associated with raised pancreatic enzymes in blood or urine, is due to inflammatory disease of the pancreas. There is digestion of the pancreas by its own enzymes and this process may extend to adjacent organs. The passage of enzymes into the bloodstream leads to complications in distant organs, particularly the lungs. In the mildest cases the gland becomes swollen and oedematous; in more severe pancreatitis haemorrhagic necrosis occurs with the accumulation of large volumes of blood and other tissue fluids in and around the pancreas. As a result, hypovolaemic shock is common.

Aetiology. In Britain about 50% of cases are associated with biliary disease and about 20% with alcoholism while in about 20% no cause can be identified. Alcoholism accounts for a much higher proportion in some countries, especially the USA and South Africa. There are several other aetiological factors; for example pancreas divisum, when the duct systems of the dorsal and ventral pancreas fail to unite and so enter the duodenum separately, and duodenal diverticulum, which may interfere with the ampulla of Vater. Pancreatitis occurs in infections (such as mumps), with some drugs (particularly azathioprine and other antimitotic agents), with some forms of hyperlipoproteinaemia and in some vascular diseases and hypothermia. It is also associated with abdominal trauma and surgery.

The mechanisms which initiate the destruction of pancreatic tissue are not known. The frequent association with disease of the biliary tract led to the theory that obstruction of the sphincter of Oddi by a gallstone, oedema or spasm allows reflux of bile along the pancreatic duct, so activating the pancreatic enzymes and leading to autodigestion of the gland. Obstruction of the duct system by a tumour or a stone may also precipitate pancreatitis. Alcohol by itself rarely causes acute pancreatitis in a previously normal pancreas. More commonly it will cause an acute attack in a patient with chronic pancreatitis (p. 298).

Clinical features. The onset is sudden with severe pain in the epigastrium or right hypochondrium. It often occurs within 12 to 24 hours following a large meal and alcohol. The pain is usually persistent and radiates most frequently through to the back, to either shoulder or to one of the iliac fossae before spreading to involve the whole abdomen. Nausea and vomiting are frequent. In severe cases profound shock supervenes so that there is tachycardia, hypotension, cardiac arrhythmias and renal failure. An increased respiratory rate and hypoxia are common and shock lung may develop. The pancreatic inflammation may cause obstructive jaundice by direct pressure on the common bile duct or duodenal or gastric obstruction because of the inflammatory mass; inflammation may spread to cause ileus and bowel obstruction. Erosion of vessels may cause bleeding into the peritoneal cavity or into the lumen of the gastrointestinal tract.

Despite the severity of the pain, there may be little or no guarding of the abdominal muscles at first. Later the upper abdomen becomes tender and rigid as peritoneal irritation increases and the initial shock passes off. The condition may simulate acute cholecystitis (with which it may coexist), and myocardial infarction. About one-third of cases are recognised for the first time at laparotomy, having been diagnosed as perforated peptic ulcer or acute appendicitis.

Investigation. *Biochemical findings.* The serum amylase rises 2–12 hours after the onset of symptoms and activities of more than twice normal (p. 814) are almost specific for acute pancreatitis. A persistently raised serum amylase suggests the formation of a pseudocyst.

Biochemical findings may be helpful in the detection and monitoring of some complications. Hyperglycaemia is common in the first two days and hypocalcaemia may occur later because calcium is sequestered into the areas of fat necrosis which occur in severe pancreatitis.

Imaging. A wide range of abnormalities may be seen on plain radiographs of the abdomen and chest and these together with the clinical and biochemical findings are often sufficient to make the diagnosis. The plain radiograph of the abdomen may show the pancreatic region as a soft tissue mass, there may be localised or generalised dilatation of the stomach and intestines, sometimes with fluid levels, and absent psoas shadows. The plain radiograph of the chest often shows a left pleural effusion, collapse or consolidation of the lung. When the clinical findings suggest that the pancreatitis may be accompanied by cholecystitis, then the gall bladder is visualised by cholescintigraphy (p. 364). In all but the mildest cases of pancreatitis, computed tomography is carried out for it illustrates the severity of the pancreatic damage and in particular it provides an early indication of severe complications such as pancreatic abscess. Ultrasound is of value in defining biliary tract obstruction and pseudocysts (p. 299).

Laparotomy is essential if diagnostic uncertainty persists.

Treatment. The reduced mortality from acute pancreatitis in recent years is due to an understanding of the complications which may arise and the application of effective supportive therapy. Each patient must be investigated for possible remediable aetiological factors such as cholelithiasis in the hope of preventing further attacks.

The immediate requirements are the energetic treatment of shock (p. 48) and of respiratory failure (p. 211) and the relief of pain. A central venous line may be necessary to monitor the need for fluid replacement, and to guard against overloading the circulation. Serial arterial oxygen pressures should be recorded because if respiratory failure becomes a major factor, endotracheal intubation and positive-pressure assisted ventilation will be required (p. 213). The bladder should be catheterised so that urinary output can be measured. Intravenous saline, plasma, plasma expanders or whole blood may be required in large volumes as determined by the clinical response, urinary output and central venous pressure. Oral feeding should be withheld until pain, tenderness, fever and leucocytosis have resolved and parenteral alimentation is necessary in all but the milder cases. Gastric intubation and aspiration are used for symptomatic benefit.

Pain is best relieved by intravenous or intramuscular administrations of pethidine (100 mg) as required; morphine should be avoided because of its undesirable effect of causing spasm of the sphincter of Oddi.

Ileus is almost inevitable in the acute phase and nasogastric suction is continued until distension is relieved and active peristalsis has returned. When obstruction continues a barium or gastrografin meal will indicate if the duodenum is obstructed.

Haemorrhage from the upper gastrointestinal tract is investigated and treated (p. 288); bleeding into a cyst or the peritoneal cavity can be confirmed by computed tomography. Selective arteriography and therapeutic embolisation may be necessary to control haemorrhage.

Surgical treatment is necessary for pancreatic abscess and when there is cholecystitis the gall bladder should be drained or removed. Sometimes the diagnosis of acute pancreatitis is made when laparotomy is undertaken for diagnostic uncertainty. Under these circumstances no direct surgical intervention should be attempted unless there is cholecystitis.

Prognosis depends upon the severity of the attack. Overall, the mortality is 10–20%. Patients with haemorrhagic pancreatitis have a mortality of over 50% whereas when there is only oedema of the pancreas, the mortality is less than 5%. Pancreatitis secondary to gallstones is unlikely to recur provided these are removed. Alcoholic pancreatitis will recur if alcohol consumption continues.

Chronic pancreatitis

Chronic pancreatitis is defined as a continuing inflammatory disease of the pancreas, characterised by irreversible morphological change and typically causing pain and/or permanent impairment of function. In the Western world the majority of cases of chronic pancreatitis occurs as a result of high alcohol consumption. It is possible that a small number result from cholelithiasis, but a causative relationship is difficult to establish because coincidental gallstones would be expected in a significant proportion of patients. It is rare for acute attacks of pancreatitis to proceed to chronic pancreatitis. In a few patients chronic pancreatitis may be caused by stenosis or disease of the sphincter of Oddi. In some parts of the tropics, chronic pancreatitis is common and malnutrition may be an aetiological factor.

Plugs of protein and calcium carbonate crystals form in the ducts and these progress to stones, which in turn lead to duct obstruction and dilatation. On microscopy the pancreas shows fibrosis around the ducts and acinae which are gradually replaced. By contrast, there is usually preservation of the islets.

Clinical features. The disease is most common in males between the ages of 35 and 45. Nearly all patients present with abdominal pain. Recurrent attacks occur at intervals of several weeks or months often within a few hours to two days of an alcoholic bout. In contrast to acute pancreatitis, the pain may begin gradually and persist for days or weeks. Pain is located in the epigastrium, right or left subcostal areas or around the umbilicus; characteristically it may radiate to the back between T10 and T12 and relief may be obtained by crouching forward or leaning forward over a chair. Weight loss is common and is due to malnutrition secondary to pancreatic pain, steatorrhoea and diabetes.

Diabetes develops in about a fifth of patients and steatorrhoea in a third; occasionally one of these is the presenting feature. Both these complications are more likely when the pancreas is calcified. Jaundice may arise because of obstruction to the common bile duct by fibrosis within the pancreas.

Investigation. In one-third of cases a plain radiograph of the abdomen shows calcification in the duct system or throughout the gland. A barium meal or hypotonic duodenography may show deformity of the duodenal cap as a result of oedema, and flattening and rigidity of the medial wall of the duodenum. Ultrasonography usually shows that the gland is reduced in size and demonstrates calcification and dilatation of the pancreatic ducts; when there is biliary obstruction it reveals a dilated common bile duct. These findings are also shown by computed tomography. ERCP (p. 274) also demonstrates stones and dilatation of the pancreatic ducts and is used particularly in planning surgical treatment. Pancreatic function tests may provide evidence of pancreatic insufficiency; the presence of steatorrhoea, or a diabetic glucose tolerance curve suggests that pancreatic insufficiency is severe. Estimation of serum amylase activity is of value only in an acute exacerbation.

Treatment. Pancreatic extracts are indicated when there is loss of weight, diarrhoea or abdominal discomfort; an average of 10 000 to 12 000 lipase units per meal is given. The effectiveness of this therapy is assessed by improvement in symptoms and a reduction in faecal fat. In patients who respond poorly, antacids or H_2-receptor antagonists prevent the inactivation of the pancreatic extract by gastric acid. The diet should be normal and nutritious with fat restricted to 25% of total calories. Supplements of fat-soluble vitamins are often required. For diabetes, oral hypoglycaemic agents are usually of no value; the patient is managed with diet and insulin.

The treatment of pain is often difficult . Abstinence from alcohol reduces the frequency and sometimes the severity of pain. Some authorities believe that therapy with pancreatic extract reduces the frequency and severity of pain and that these should be tried even if they are not required for reasons of malabsorption. The use of analgesics is often indicated especially before meals in order to counteract the postprandial increase in pain. Opiates may have to be used and occasionally percutaneous coeliac plexus block may be necessary.

Surgery should be contemplated for the relief of intractable pain. Drainage of the pancreatic duct into the small bowel, removal of part or most of the pancreas, or sphincterotomy are the most usual procedures. The ultimate result is so dependent on the alcoholic's ability to stop drinking that operation is not worth while in the patient who cannot do so. The indication for surgery is stronger when cysts and the possibility of cancer of the pancreas are present. The best results are obtained in those patients who are shown to have stones in the bile ducts or stenosis of the ampulla of Vater. Correction of these abnormalities may relieve pain and result in recovery of pancreatic function.

Pancreatic cysts

A pancreatic pseudocyst occurs as a complication of acute pancreatitis, chronic pancreatitis or trauma to the pancreas. A pseudocyst is a sac which contains fluid, pancreatic enzymes and blood. It usually occupies the lesser sac, displacing the stomach, and it may obstruct the duodenum. However, it can occur elsewhere in the abdomen and even in the thorax. Pseudocysts can be multiple and may resolve spontaneously. Most commonly the pseudocyst develops 1 to 2 weeks after the onset of acute pancreatitis or an acute exacerbation of chronic pancreatitis. Epigastric pain, nausea and vomiting, weight loss, fever and jaundice are likely symptoms. On examination, a smooth, tender mass is felt in the upper abdomen in about half the cases.

There is a persistent leucocytosis and raised serum amylase activity. An abdominal radiograph shows a mass in the epigastrium and a barium meal or hypotonic duodenography confirms extrinsic pressure on the stomach, duodenum and small bowel. Ultrasonography will confirm the presence of a cyst in nearly all cases.

Pseudocysts which fail to resolve spontaneously within six weeks are treated surgically by drainage into the stomach or small intestine.

Pancreatic ascites refers to ascites resulting from pancreatic duct disruption or from leaking of a pancreatic pseudocyst in patients with chronic pancreatitis. However, these events may also occur in acute pancreatitis. The pancreatic duct secretions may also track into the mediastinum and as a result, a pleural effusion may develop. The ascites presents with an increase in abdominal girth and abdominal pain. Both the ascitic fluid and the pleural fluid have a very high amylase activity. In a majority of cases, surgical treatment is necessary to resect the damaged pancreas.

Cystic fibrosis

This autosomal recessive disease is the major cause of pancreatic insufficiency and respiratory failure in childhood. Cystic fibrosis is characterised by generalised dysfunction of all exocrine glands, including those which secrete mucus. Blockage by viscid secretion causes cystic changes in the pancreas and also bronchiectasis.

Clinical features. Frequently cystic fibrosis presents in infancy with repeated attacks of respiratory infection. Defective pancreatic enzymes give rise to impaired digestion and malabsorption of fat. The stools are bulky, foamy and foul-smelling. The child is often poorly nourished. Complications include intussusception and obstruction due to faecal masses.

Increasing numbers of patients are surviving to adulthood because of better treatment of respiratory infection. The respiratory problems become progressively more important in the adolescent and adult and determine the fate of the individual; by contrast malabsorption is less troublesome. There may be bronchiectasis, recurrent spontaneous pneumothorax, recurrent haemoptysis, pulmonary fibrosis and right ventricular failure. Sometimes there is cirrhosis leading to portal hypertension. Females with cystic fibrosis may become pregnant but males are nearly always infertile.

In the child, the diagnosis is established by the finding of an increase in the concentration of sodium in the sweat (p. 816). The test is difficult to interpret after adolescence; the diagnosis is then made on the presence of chronic pulmonary disease, pancreatic insufficiency and a family history of cystic fibrosis.

Treatment. In the child, surgery may be required for a variety of complications. Replacement treatment for pancreatic insufficiency is very important to maintain adequate nutrition. The treatment of respiratory disease consists of the control of infection, postural drainage and breathing exercises. Families with cystic fibrosis require long-term support. Genetic advice should be made available to the parents (p. 15).

Carcinoma of the pancreas

The incidence of carcinoma of the pancreas is increasing in many Western countries. It is more common in males than in females and it occurs most frequently in the seventh decade. Aetiological factors are smoking, high dietary fat and occupational exposure in chemical and metal industries. Ductal adenocarcinoma is by far the commonest tumour and is located in the head of the pancreas in about 60% of cases, the body or tail in 20% and in a combination of sites in the remainder. Tumours of the ampulla of Vater obstruct the common bile duct; they should be amenable to surgery and have a better prognosis. Islet cell carcinoma (p. 301) and cystadenocarcinoma are rarer forms of cancer.

Clinical features. Apart from carcinoma of the ampulla which may bleed into the duodenum, or cause jaundice at a relatively early stage, all cancers of the pancreas are advanced by the time they cause symptoms. Epigastric pain is common, but occasionally it may be absent throughout the course of the disease. The pain is variable in type but is characteristically dull and boring and radiates through to the back. It is often intensified by food and by lying supine, especially at night. It may be relieved by crouching forward. Other symptoms include anorexia, nausea, discomfort and sometimes vomiting. These symptoms may be the only manifestations until metastases occur. Weight loss is common.

Other clinical features depend largely on the site of the growth. In the majority of cases with involvement of the head of the pancreas, jaundice is the presenting feature and may be painless and progressive. A large firm liver eventually develops. An abdominal mass is present in one-quarter of all patients and occasionally a distended gall bladder is palpable or ascites can be detected. Jaundice may not appear in cases where the lesion affects mainly the body and tail of the pancreas. The symptoms of diabetes mellitus or thrombophlebitis may occasionally be the presenting feature.

Carcinoma of the pancreas is a rapidly progressive emaciating disease especially in cases in which the head of the gland is involved, when death usually occurs within six months of the onset of obstructive jaundice.

Investigation. Pancreatic cancer may be suspected from the clinical features, a raised serum alkaline phosphatase, a diabetic glucose tolerance test and a barium meal which may show distortion or displacement of the stomach or duodenum with possible invasion by tumour. Ultrasonography is a good initial screening test for pancreatic disease but computed tomography is now the preferred method for confirming the diagnosis and deciding upon operability. In a minority of patients, it is impossible to distinguish cancer from chronic pancreatitis. In these cases, fine needle aspiration biopsy is performed percutaneously or at operation.

Duodenoscopy is important in detecting cancer of the ampulla; during this procedure, cannulation of the pancreatic duct may show stricture or obstruction of the duct and when jaundice is present, cannulation of the common bile duct may show the obstruction is within the pancreas. Occasionally malignant cells may be demonstrated in the pancreatic secretion.

Treatment. Carcinoma of the ampulla can be treated by excision of the duodenum and head of the pancreas; the prognosis in such cases is better than for cancers elsewhere in the pancreas. Radical surgery is rarely possible for pancreatic cancer. Usually the aim is to relieve obstructive jaundice by implanting the common bile duct or gall bladder into the jejunum or to forestall duodenal obstruction by gastrojejunostomy. Less than 10% of patients with cancer of the pancreas survive for one year after diagnosis and only 2% survive for two years.

Islet-cell tumours

A benign adenoma may arise rarely from the beta cells of the islets and produce hyperinsulinism with attacks of spontaneous hypoglycaemia (p. 476). Even more rare are tumours, usually malignant, from other islet cells which elaborate polypeptides, e.g. gastrin or allied substances, the secretion of which into the blood causes a variety of syndromes. The least rare is the Zollinger-Ellison syndrome (p. 291).

DISEASES OF THE SMALL INTESTINE

MALABSORPTION

A number of disorders result in malabsorption of one or more of the essential nutrients, electrolytes, minerals or vitamins. Some or all of the following features may ensue: diarrhoea, abdominal pain and distension, loss of weight, anaemia, or other evidence of specific deficiency. However, some complain only of vague ill-health, and the diagnosis may not be made for many years.

The sequence followed in this section is first to review the basic processes of absorption and the means of testing them. Then the ways in which the processes of absorption can be deranged are discussed. Finally, the clinical presentation and treatment of malabsorption in general and then of specific disorders are described.

Tests of absorption

Fat absorption takes place predominantly in the duodenum and upper jejunum. Dietary fat occurs largely in the form of insoluble long-chain triglycerides. These are emulsified mechanically in the stomach and by detergents (mainly bile acids) in the small intestine. Then pancreatic lipase hydrolyses the triglycerides to monoglyceride and fatty acids. Pancreatic bicarbonate is required to maintain the optimum pH for this hydrolysis and for the next step in fat absorption, the solubilisation of the monoglycerides and fatty acids by bile acids. This consists of their incorporation into micelles which orientate the fatty acid and monoglyceride in such a way that they can be presented to the intestinal mucosal cell for absorption (Fig. 10.2). Once in the absorptive cell, the monoglycerides and fatty acids are re-formed (re-esterified) into triglycerides which are then coated with phospholipid and protein to form chylomicrons or converted into very low density lipoproteins. Both chylomicrons and the lipoproteins pass out of the cell to be transported by the lymphatic system into the blood.

TEST OF FAT ABSORPTION. Fat excretion in the stool is measured over a 5-day period, whilst the patient is receiving a normal diet (which contains less than 100 g fat per day). The normal faecal fat excretion is less than 5 g per day–18 mmol fatty acids (p. 816).

The fat-soluble vitamins A, D and K are absorbed in the same way as dietary fat and can be used as an indirect assessment of fat absorption. For example, the plasma vitamin A level can be measured after oral administration of retinol for two or three days.

Carbohydrate absorption. Carbohydrate in the diet is in the form of starch (60%), lactose (10%) and sucrose (30%). These are digested to glucose, galactose and fructose. Glucose and galactose are absorbed into the cell by active transport mechanisms, the process requiring sodium ions and energy. The fructose molecule is too large to move across the cell membrane by simple diffusion and it is thought that it must be facilitated by a carrier.

TESTS OF CARBOHYDRATE ABSORPTION. *The glucose tolerance test* (p. 467) is sometimes used and the absence of a rise in blood glucose can indicate malabsorption, but there are so many variables that the test is difficult to interpret in the context of malabsorption.

In the *xylose absorption test*, 25 g of d-xylose are given orally after an overnight fast. Only a small proportion is metabolised and 5–8 g should be excreted in the urine over the next 5 hours.

In the *lactose tolerance test*, 50 g of lactose are given orally and blood glucose levels are measured as in the glucose tolerance test. Normally this disaccharide is broken down by intestinal lactase to glucose and galactose which are absorbed so that blood glucose levels rise. If the enzyme lactase is deficient in the intestinal mucosa, there may be no rise in blood glucose and the patient may complain of colic and diarrhoea because the unabsorbed lactose acts as an osmotic agent in the gut.

The *hydrogen breath test* is used to diagnose lactase deficiency. It has the advantage of not requiring blood samples and so is the preferred test in children. 50 g of lactose is given orally; lactose not absorbed in the small intestine passes into the colon where it is degraded by bacteria with the production of hydrogen. Hydrogen excretion in the breath is measured and this is proportional to the amount of lactose not absorbed by the small intestine.

Protein absorption. Initial hydrolysis of dietary protein molecules is performed by gastric pepsin and pancreatic enzymes. Further hydrolysis of peptides takes place at the brush border and a mixture of peptides and amino acids is absorbed into the cell. A large amount of protein, other than dietary, enters the lumen of the gastrointestinal tract each day, derived from various secretions, desquamated cells and the exudation of plasma proteins. These are absorbed by the same mechanisms as dietary protein.

TESTS OF PROTEIN ABSORPTION. Measurement of the amount of nitrogen in the stool provides a very crude estimate of the above processes. Stools are collected for 3 to 5 days and no more than 2.5 g of nitrogen per day should be excreted.

An excessive loss of nitrogen in the stool can result from the loss of albumin and other plasma proteins into the lumen of the gut. This *protein losing enteropathy* can be detected by labelling serum proteins with radioactive chromium and measuring radioactivity in the stool.

A low serum albumin level in the absence of hepatic or renal disease may indicate protein malabsorption or protein losing enteropathy. Enteric protein loss can be assessed by measuring the concentration of α_1-antitrypsin in a 3 day collection of stools and comparing the result with the serum concentration. α_1-Antitrypsin is synthesised in the liver, circulates in the plasma and is not degraded when it is lost into the lumen of the gut.

Absorption of other substances. The Schilling test (p. 505) is used in investigating the absorption of vitamin B_{12}. The serum levels of folate, iron and calcium provide an index of the absorption of these substances.

The *SeHCAT* test may be used to assess absorption of bile acids and to provide a non-invasive test of ileal function. A synthetic bile acid labelled with selenium is given by mouth and absorption is calculated from the radioactivity detected by gamma camera examination of the abdomen (or stools) or by whole body monitor.

Causes of malabsorption

1. Disorders of intraluminal digestion. Here there is an insufficiency of a digestive enzyme or detergent within the lumen of the gut. The main feature is steatorrhoea with deficiency of fat-soluble vitamins. Since the intestinal mucosal cells are normal, there is no impairment of absorption of other substances less dependent on intraluminal digestion, e.g. carbohydrate, protein, vitamin B_{12}, folate and iron.

a. DISTURBANCES OF GASTRIC FUNCTION. After gastric surgery it is possible for the correct enzymes, detergents and electrolytes to be delivered into the intestinal lumen and yet malabsorption may occur. This is because gastric emptying is no longer co-ordinated with the correct stage of digestion. For example, after gastroenterostomy or a Polya partial gastrectomy, bile and pancreatic juice may be delivered after food from the stomach has already passed down the efferent loop.

b. PANCREATIC INSUFFICIENCY. A deficiency of pancreatic lipase causes malabsorption of fat, for example, in chronic pancreatitis, cystic fibrosis and carcinoma of the pancreas.

c. DEFICIENCY OF BILE ACIDS. This may occur in two circumstances:

(i) *Interruption of the enterohepatic circulation of bile acids.* When there is disease, e.g. Crohn's, or resection of the terminal ileum, bile acids cannot be reabsorbed (p. 329) and are lost in the faeces. In the colon they prevent water and electrolyte absorption and stimulate their secretion; diarrhoea results. Synthesis by the liver cannot compensate for the loss of bile acids. There is therefore inadequate bile acid in the upper jejunum and micelles cannot be formed.

(ii) *Colonisation of the small bowel by bacteria.* The upper part of the small intestine is practically sterile under normal conditions. If a large number of bacteria are present (p. 305) bile acids are deconjugated, micelle formation becomes inefficient and steatorrhoea results. Bacteria in the small intestine can also utilise vitamin B_{12} so that it is unavailable for absorption and anaemia ensues.

2. Disorders of transport in the mucosal cells. In these disorders, the intraluminal digestive phase is normal, but the absorptive cells are not, because of:

a. *Generalised mucosal damage* from coeliac disease, tropical sprue, giardiasis, Whipple's disease or extensive Crohn's disease. In these conditions it is usual to find widespread disturbances of absorption involving xylose, folate, vitamin B_{12}, iron, calcium and amino acids in addition to steatorrhoea.

b. *Disorders with histologically normal mucosa.* Here a specific substance is malabsorbed because of the absence of a particular enzyme. Thus there may be malabsorption of lactose because of an insufficiency of lactase in the mucosa. Another example is the malabsorption of vitamin B_{12} because of a lack of intrinsic factor in pernicious anaemia.

3. Disorders of transport from the mucosal cell. These are rare and result from the blockage of the lymphatic system which is responsible for the transfer of chylomicrons from the absorptive cell to the systemic circulation. This may occur in abdominal lymphoma or tuberculosis or in the rare primary lymphangiectasia involving the mesenteric lymphatics.

Clinical features and investigation of malabsorption

Clinical features. The patient can present in various ways. In severe forms there may be general malnutrition, with loss of weight and energy and a slow deterioration in health or, in a child, a failure to grow and thrive. Abdominal distension is often a striking feature.

Steatorrhoea may be the presenting symptom. There is diarrhoea, with the passage of loose, pale, bulky and offensive stools which float on water. The patient may be anaemic due to a deficiency of iron, cyanocobalamin or of folate. Hypoalbuminaemic oedema may occur.

Haemorrhagic phenomena due to a deficiency of vitamin K may be an occasional presenting feature. Hypocalcaemia may lead to tetany and the features of rickets or osteomalacia may be present. Various other disorders due to deficiency of vitamins may be noted, such as sore tongue, angular stomatitis and dry, rough or cracked skin.

In other patients, malabsorption may be suspected because of a history of gastric surgery or intestinal resection. In mild malabsorption, there may be no diarrhoea and the condition may be recognised only after investigation for non-specific abdominal complaints or anaemia. The diagnosis may be made as a result of a barium follow-through examination in a patient with abdominal symptoms. The small intestine shows dilated loops with flocculation and segmentation of barium (Fig. 9.8).

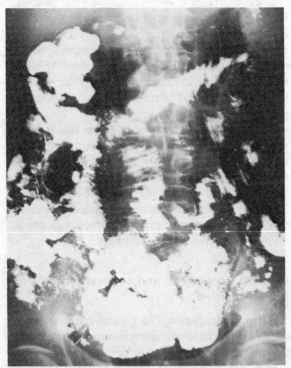

Fig. 9.8 Malabsorption. Note dilated loops, segmentation and flocculation. (Courtesy of Dr D. H. Cummack.)

Investigation. Malabsorption is confirmed by the tests of absorption which may also provide a clue as to the cause of the disorder. For example, malabsorption of several substances is likely when there is generalised disorder of the absorptive cells.

Biopsy of the jejunum may show the villous atrophy of coeliac disease. Partial villous atrophy can occur in a variety of disorders, such as tropical sprue, Crohn's disease and in mild cases of coeliac disease. If the intestinal biopsy is normal, other investigations may be necessary to provide the diagnosis, e.g. pancreatic function tests or the culture of intestinal aspirates for bacteria.

Treatment of malabsorption

A gluten-free diet must be prescribed in coeliac disease. Pancreatic insufficiency is treated by pancreatic supplements. Insufficiency of bile acids should not be treated with oral bile acids because these would pass into the colon, interfere with salt and water absorption, and so worsen the diarrhoea. The effect of the endogenous bile acids on the colon is counteracted by giving the binding agent cholestyramine in a dose of up to 12 g per day. In addition, a low fat diet is indicated because cholestyramine will usually increase the faecal excretion of fat.

Replacement therapy is necessary for those patients with anaemia, bone disease or coagulation defects. Folic acid and iron supplements are given orally and vitamin B_{12} by a monthly injection. Vitamin D and calcium supplements may be required. Glossitis and cheilosis are indications for the administration of vitamin B complex.

In severe forms of malabsorptive disease, it may be necessary to treat dehydration and electrolyte deficiency by intravenous infusions.

THE PRINCIPAL DISORDERS CAUSING MALABSORPTION

These are coeliac disease, tropical sprue, lactose intolerance, bacterial colonisation of the small intestine and Crohn's disease.

Coeliac disease

Coeliac disease is characterised by an abnormal mucosa in the small intestine, induced by a component of the gluten protein of wheat. Barley, rye and oats may also be injurious. It seems likely that local immunological responses to the gluten component are responsible.

Pathology. The mucosa of the normal small

intestine has finger-like or leaf-like villi which can be seen on histological section. In coeliac disease the mucosa at the duodeno-jejunal flexure is always abnormal and the abnormality extends distally for a variable distance. There is either (1) convolutions, like the surface of the cerebrum, which, when sectioned, appear as short wide villi, or (2) a totally flat mucosa which is termed 'subtotal villous atrophy'. In addition, the height of the epithelial cells is reduced and there is an increase in the number of plasma cells in the lamina propria. All these histological features return towards normality during treatment with a gluten-free diet.

Clinical features. Coeliac disease usually begins in the first 3 years of life. The child ceases to thrive and becomes fractious and irritable. The stools become voluminous and pale and the abdomen distended. As the disorder progresses, growth is retarded and anaemia develops.

Less commonly, the disorder may manifest itself for the first time in adult life; the presenting symptoms range from those of a mild anaemia and listlessness of long duration, to a florid malabsorptive state developing rapidly over a period of weeks. The commonest features are diarrhoea, weight loss and anaemia, usually due to combined deficiency of folate and iron. There may be peripheral neuropathy and evidence of vitamin deficiency or hypoproteinaemia. Other features are finger clubbing, dermatitis herpetiformis, amenorrhoea and infertility.

Coeliac disease predisposes to the development of lymphoma of the small intestine; colicky abdominal pain and weight loss in a previously well-controlled patient should arouse suspicion.

Treatment. A gluten-free diet must be taken indefinitely. This requires the exclusion of wheat, rye, oats and barley, and imposes severe restrictions which must be fully explained to the patient. A booklet produced by the Coeliac Society (PO Box 220, High Wycombe, Bucks.) containing diet sheet and recipes for gluten-free flour is of great value in this respect. Mineral and vitamin supplements are also given when indicated. If the patient deteriorates on a strictly supervised diet, corticosteroids may be tried; a diagnosis of lymphoma must also be considered.

Tropical sprue (p. 719)

Lactose intolerance

This disorder is being seen more often in Britain because Asian and African immigrants have insufficient lactase in the mucosa of the small intestine to digest the large amounts of lactose consumed in Britain. It may also be acquired, especially in children, as a temporary sequel to an infection of the bowel.

The patient complains of abdominal discomfort, colic and diarrhoea after the ingestion of milk or milk products. The diagnosis may be made by the lactose tolerance or hydrogen breath test. The symptoms respond to the reduction of lactose in the diet.

Bacterial colonisation of the small intestine

The effects of bacterial proliferation have been discussed on page 303. The presentation is with steatorrhoea or anaemia due to vitamin B_{12} deficiency. Radiological investigation shows a lesion causing stasis in the intestine such as jejunal diverticula, a long afferent ('blind') loop after gastrectomy or gastroenterostomy, Crohn's disease, stricture formation or a fistula between colon and small intestine.

The Schilling test is abnormal (p. 505). The glycocholic acid breath test may be used for diagnosis; bacteria in the small intestine liberate ^{14}C glycine from the labelled glycocholic acid. The ^{14}C glycine is metabolised to $^{14}CO_2$ which is measured in the breath. The diagnosis is confirmed by the correction of steatorrhoea and vitamin B_{12} malabsorption by the administration of tetracycline. Occasionally surgical correction of an abnormality may be required.

Crohn's disease

This disease is characterised by localised areas of non-specific, granulomatous inflammation of the bowel. It was formerly termed regional ileitis or enteritis. However, the eponymous designation 'Crohn's disease' is preferable since the alimentary tract can be affected anywhere from the mouth to the anus, the sites most commonly involved being, in order of frequency, terminal ileum alone, terminal ileum and right side of colon, colon alone, ileum and jejunum. The term 'inflammatory bowel disease' comprises Crohn's disease and ulcerative colitis (p. 312).

Crohn's disease may occur at any age, but most commonly between the ages of 20 and 40; it affects both sexes equally. In its chronic form, it is a debilitating disease which often interferes profoundly with a patient's life requiring repeated admission to hospital for treatment.

Aetiology. The cause is unknown. A current hypothesis is that Crohn's disease is the consequence of an abnormal immune response in the gut wall to an unidentified antigen. Crohn's disease, ankylosing spondylitis and ulcerative colitis all occur more commonly than might be expected amongst the families of patients with Crohn's disease, suggesting that all three diseases share a common but incomplete genetic basis.

Pathology. Macroscopically, the bowel is engorged and oedematous so that the lumen is markedly narrowed, sometimes enough to produce obstruction; the mucosa shows a 'cobble-stone' pattern with linear ulceration and fissuring. Characteristically, these changes are patchy; even when a relatively short segment of bowel is affected, the inflammatory process is interrupted by islands of normal mucosa, the change from the affected part being abrupt. A small lesion separated in this way from a major area of involvement is referred to as a 'skip' lesion. The affected lymph nodes are enlarged and the mesentery thickened.

Microscopically, inflammatory change involves all coats of the bowel wall. All grades of inflammation may be seen and characteristically there is oedema and hyperplasia of the lymphoid follicles. Granulomas composed of epithelioid and giant cells are seen in about 50% of cases. Another feature is deep clefts or fissures opening on to the mucosal surface and sometimes passing through the entire thickness of the bowel wall. These clefts are responsible for the fistula formation which is such a characteristic feature of the disease. Fistulae may develop between adjacent loops of bowel or between affected segments of bowel and the bladder, uterus or vagina and may appear in the perineum.

Clinical features vary and depend in part on the site and extent of the bowel affected; many other diseases may be mimicked. Crohn's disease may present acutely with features indistinguishable from acute appendicitis. At laparotomy the terminal ileum is red and oedematous and provided the abdomen is closed without resection the prognosis is relatively good.

In the chronic form of the disease, pain is the commonest symptom and may be due either to peritoneal involvement, obstruction or both. Since the terminal ileum and right side of the colon are most commonly affected, this type of pain occurs most frequently in the right lower quadrant and it may be associated with local tenderness or guarding. A mass is palpable by abdominal and frequently rectal examination. This consists of inflamed loops of bowel bound together, possibly including an abscess, and may be of any size. Colicky pain suggests obstruction, and may be associated with nausea and vomiting and excessive borborygmi. Indeed, recurrent episodes of colic due to attacks of subacute obstruction are a prominent feature in the life history of a patient with Crohn's disease; however, severe acute obstruction is uncommon.

Malabsorption and steatorrhoea can occur for a variety of reasons including loss of absorptive surface due to extensive mucosal involvement or resection, or bacterial colonisation secondary to stricture or fistula formation. Disease or resection of the terminal ileum may cause malabsorption of vitamin B_{12} as well as interrupting the enterohepatic circulation of the bile acids. The inflamed mucosa may cause a protein losing enteropathy.

Diarrhoea is frequent, but is rarely so marked as in ulcerative colitis. The stools may be formed or loose, and rarely contain frank blood, mucus or pus unless the colon is involved. In the latter case, the symptoms are indistinguishable from those of ulcerative colitis. A diagnostic feature, when present, is the occurrence of anal lesions such as oedematous skin tags or perianal abscesses and fistulae; they are more common when the colon is affected.

Weight loss is frequent and may be severe, contributing factors being reduced food intake because of anorexia, malabsorption and increased catabolism. In children growth retardation may be the principal presentation. Most patients have a moderate anaemia and low-grade fever. Other manifestations include iritis, finger clubbing, aphthous ulceration of the mouth, erythema nodosum, enteropathic arthritis (p. 569) and ankylosing spondylitis. Abnormal liver function tests are relatively common, while renal complications include hydronephrosis due to involvement of a ureter in an inflammatory mass.

Investigation. Barium meal and follow-through examination may show alteration of the mucosal pattern, deep ulceration or the pathognomonic 'string sign' due to marked narrowing of a segment of affected bowel (Fig. 9.9). In long-standing cases there may be stricture formation. The lesions tend to be discontinuous along the length of the bowel. A barium enema should be carried out since the disease may affect the small bowel and the colon simultaneously. In some patients there will be involvement of the colon segmentally or in its entirety. Crohn's disease of the colon can usually be differentiated from ulcerative colitis by the presence of shallow aphthoid or deep penetrating ulcers and discrete or eccentrically situated lesions.

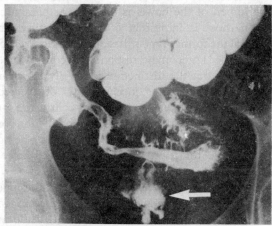

Fig. 9.9 Crohn's disease of the ileum showing marked narrowing and a fistula between the ileum and the bladder (arrow). (Courtesy of Dr G. M. Fraser.)

Culture of stool yields no specific pathogens. Microscopic examination of the faeces may reveal pus cells or red blood corpuscles and tests for faecal occult blood may be positive. Blood tests may show moderate anaemia, raised ESR, abnormal liver function tests and hypoproteinaemia. Malabsorption of vitamin B_{12} can be confirmed by a Schilling test (p. 505).

The diagnosis may be confirmed either by rectal biopsy or by excision of perianal skin tags; a rectal biopsy will sometimes show the characteristic granulomatous lesions although the mucosa appears normal to the naked eye.

Sometimes no conclusive proof of Crohn's disease is obtained, and the diagnosis can only be presumptive; such patients should be kept under observation until the natural history of the illness declares itself.

Differential diagnosis. The symptoms, signs and radiological findings are usually sufficient to suggest a lesion in the lower part of the small bowel. The other common diseases in this part of the intestinal tract are appendicitis or an appendix mass and carcinoma of the caecum. In the acute phase, it may be impossible to decide between these possibilities, so that a laparotomy may be necessary.

Ulcerative colitis is distinguished from Crohn's disease because it involves only the large bowel. The distinctive features of Crohn's disease are fistula and stricture formation, but when these are absent differentiation from ulcerative colitis may depend on demonstration of the extent and location of the disease and ultimately on biopsy. The possibility of carcinoma, either in association with or as a complication to Crohn's disease or ulcerative colitis, requires consideration.

Ileo-caecal tuberculosis may be indicated by the presence of tuberculosis elsewhere, for example, by the chest radiograph. A 'negative' tuberculin test is common in patients with Crohn's disease. Caecal amoebiasis (p. 775) actinomycosis (p. 219) and lymphoma of the ileum or colon are rarer conditions to be considered in the differential diagnosis.

Treatment. Crohn's disease is a chronic condition with remissions and relapses over many years. There is no known cure at present and treatment is largely a matter of managing particular problems as they arise and improving the general condition of the patient.

Nutrition. A low residue diet will reduce the frequency of intestinal colic and this measure alone may greatly improve the quality of life. Troublesome steatorrhoea will be improved by a low-fat diet, and when bacterial colonisation (p. 305) is suspected, intermittent courses of oral antibiotics are indicated. Supplements of iron, folic acid, calcium, zinc, vitamins and electrolytes, especially potassium, will be required when deficiencies occur. The greatest problem, however, is that of maintaining body weight and general nutrition, especially in children. Great care and encouragement is needed to ensure that the patient takes a high protein, high energy diet, if necessary by providing supplemental dietary preparations. Enteral feeding (p. 78) by naso-gastric tube can be tolerated for very long periods even in the young. In addition to improving nutrition, by 'resting' the bowel, the inflammatory process may benefit and symptoms of partial obstruction be relieved. Enteral feeding is useful also in pre-operative preparation, especially in patients with external fistulae. Occasionally total parenteral nutrition may be required in very severe cases. In addition plasma or blood infusion may be needed for the correction of severe hypo-proteinaemia.

Drugs. Corticosteroids are beneficial when there is extensive active disease which is not improving with general medical measures. However, they do not alter the long-term course of the disease. Prednisolone should be given in a dose of 40–60 mg daily in divided doses for 1 or 2 weeks depending on response, and the dose gradually reduced thereafter to 10–20 mg daily for 4 to 6 weeks and then withdrawn. Every effort should be made to stop the drug, but in the occasional case this may be difficult because of early relapse when the dose is reduced. In these circumstances, the effect of sulphasalazine (2–4 g daily) is worth a trial, much as it is used in ulcerative colitis (p. 312). Metronidazole and azathioprine have been used with variable success in patients unresponsive to other forms of therapy.

Diarrhoea may be controlled with loperamide or codeine. When the terminal ileum is extensively diseased or has been resected, cholestyramine will reduce the diarrhoea due to the cathartic effect of the unabsorbed bile acids on the colon; hydroxo-cobalamin should be given to such patients for life since dietary vitamin B_{12} will not be absorbed.

Surgical treatment. Although attacks of subacute obstruction can usually be managed conserv-atively by intestinal decompression and intraven-ous feeding, operation may be necessary if attacks occur frequently. Surgery may also be required because of abscess or fistula. With localised dis-ease, resection yields better results than bypass, but with extensive disease massive resection may result in malabsorption. Recurrence of the disease is always a danger, and therefore as much bowel as possible should be preserved. When the rectum and colon are extensively involved a total procto-colectomy as in ulcerative colitis may be the procedure of choice.

INTESTINAL OBSTRUCTION

Intestinal obstruction may be complete or incom-plete, acute or chronic, intermittent or continuous. The most important point to decide is whether the obstruction is *simple* or associated with *stran-gulation.* The latter occurs when there is interfer-ence with the blood supply to the intestine, as when the bowel is trapped or twisted. Urgent relief is required if the dangers of gangrene, perforation and peritonitis are to be avoided.

Causes. Obstruction may be mechanical, when the lumen of the bowel is blocked, or paralytic, when there is inhibition of bowel motility. In general the former type will require surgical relief, while the latter may respond to conservative measures, but the distinction is not always clear cut. Sometimes the mechanically obstructed bowel becomes exhausted and non-contractile, or it perforates at the site of the obstruction or proximally, the resultant peritonitis being responsible for paralysis of the adjacent bowel loops.

Mechanical obstruction. At all ages adhesions and hernias are common causes of obstruction. In childhood, intussusception is frequent, while in the elderly, volvulus, tumours of the large bowel and diverticular disease account for a large propor-tion of cases. Impaction of faeces in the rectum presents with spurious diarrhoea but can also cause intestinal obstruction in the aged or bedridden. In children a mass of round worms may be responsible (p. 791).

Paralytic obstruction (paralytic ileus) occurs temporarily after any abdominal operation and is a feature of shock, spinal injury and hypotension. Commonly it is due to peritonitis.

Clinical features. *Pain.* In mechanical

obstruction this is colicky and often originates at or about the site of the obstruction. Episodes of pain are accompanied by loud borborygmi. The advent of constant severe pain with tenderness is indicative of strangulation. Paralytic obstruction is associated with a dull constant pain in an abdomen which is ominously silent.

Vomiting. This is copious in high obstruction and may be late or absent in obstructions of the lower small bowel or colon. The effortless trickle of foul-smelling fluid from the corner of the mouth of the lethargic patient is seen in untreated paralytic ileus, whereas in mechanical obstruction vomiting is projectile and intermittent.

Distension. This may be absent or confined to some loops of the bowel which can be seen in the thin patient as ridges across the abdomen forming the so-called ladder pattern. Diffuse distension is late and may indicate chronic large bowel obstruction or paralytic ileus.

Bowel movements. In complete obstruction neither faeces not flatus is passed. In high obstructions, the bowels may move unaided or with enemas because of residual contents below the obstruction, while in large bowel obstruction, spurious diarrhoea may be due to a discharge of faecal-stained mucus.

Physical examination. The diagnosis of obstruction and its cause can usually be made on physical examination alone. The hernial orifices should be palpated for the presence of a tender irreducible swelling. In fat patients particular care must be taken to check the femoral regions. The presence of scars from previous abdominal operations is noted. Distension, particularly of individual loops, is significant. A distended caecum may be both seen and felt in thin patients and immediately points to a large bowel cause. Serial measurements of abdominal girth will detect progressive abdominal distension.

Tenderness anywhere in the abdomen is suggestive of peritoneal irritation and bowel strangulation. A palpable mass is associated with large bowel tumours and diverticular disease. A transient mass, felt perhaps during bouts of colic, indicates intussusception. Classically bowel sounds are increased and tinkling in mechanical obstructions, but in advanced cases they are infrequent and auscultation must be prolonged to detect the occasional tinkle. In paralytic ileus, sounds are virtually absent.

Rectal examination usually reveals an empty ballooned rectum but in low obstructions there may be blood and mucus. Obstruction due to carcinoma of the rectum is rare.

Fluid and electrolyte changes. In obstruction of the upper small bowel, fluids and electrolytes are lost because of vomiting. When the obstruction is lower down, there is stagnation in the distended bowel loops, normal absorption from the gut is interrupted, and the body is deprived of fluid even in the absence of vomiting.

Biochemically, there is haemoconcentration with loss of water and electrolytes, particularly chloride, sodium and potassium. Elderly patients may develop secondary renal failure and this will add to the electrolyte imbalance. A vicious circle develops as increasing obstruction raises the tension in the bowel and further diminishes absorption; then increasing electrolyte imbalance interferes with intestinal peristalsis rendering the obstruction more complete. Recovery is heralded by diuresis, signifying return of peristalsis and reabsorption of fluid from the lumen of the bowel.

Radiological examination. Plain radiographs, taken in the erect and supine positions, are most informative. The presence of fluid levels on the erect film, and of gas-distended loops on both films, indicate not only the diagnosis but also the site and probable cause of the obstruction (Fig. 9.10). Where the completeness of the obstruction is in doubt, serial films can be compared for any change in the gas patterns.

Treatment. If intestinal obstruction is suspected, the opinion of a surgeon should be sought, even if non-operative measures are to be used. The mainstays of treatment are decompression by gastrointestinal suction, the intravenous replacement of fluids and electrolytes, and operative relief of the obstruction. Urgent surgery is indicated for an irreducible hernia and where there is strangulation. Volvulus of the sigmoid colon is a cause of acute obstruction which can be relieved by the passage of a rectal tube.

In cases of more gradual development where there is a possibility that the obstruction can be relieved even temporarily, and in paralytic ileus, conservative measures assume greatest import-

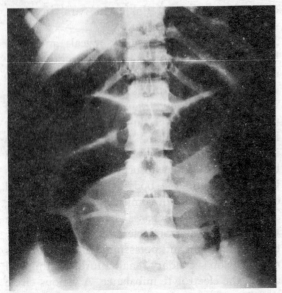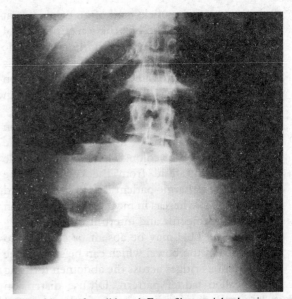

Fig. 9.10 Small bowel obstruction. Supine film on left showing dilated loops of small bowel. Erect film on right showing multiple fluid levels. (Courtesy of Dr G. M. Fraser.)

ance. Passage of a nasogastric tube in an ill and nauseated patient requires skill and patience. Once in place, continuous suction using an electric pump, and periodic checks with a syringe to confirm that the tube is patent, will achieve upper intestinal decompression.

Intravenous infusion may require to be prolonged and biochemical estimations may be frequent, so that the veins should be treated with care. Where there has been blood loss, as in carcinoma of the bowel and diverticular disease, blood transfusion is required. Throughout conservative management, accurate fluid balance charts must be kept.

PERITONITIS

Peritonitis is the reaction of the peritoneum to an irritant. Usually this is infection, although sometimes the irritation is chemical, at least initially, as when bile or duodenal contents leak into the peritoneal cavity. Appendicitis is one of the commonest causes of peritonitis and *Esch. coli* is the organism usually responsible.

Infection or chemical irritation causes the peritoneum to become congested and oedematous. There is an exudation of fluid containing large quantities of leucocytes, protein and antibodies. Dilution and destruction of the irritant is accompanied by its localisation and by the formation of adhesions. Failure of these defence mechanisms is characterised by spread of the infection and by septicaemia and toxaemia. There is still a distressingly high mortality from generalised peritonitis.

Acute peritonitis. In perforations (e.g. peptic ulcer, p. 289), the onset is sudden, with severe abdominal pain, tenderness, rigidity and shock. These initial severe features then gradually decrease; the patient appears to have improved, and the diagnosis can be missed. Then, as paralytic ileus develops and fluid collects in the peritoneal cavity, there is increasing distension, the rigidity lessens, the tenderness remains and toxicity develops.

When peritonitis is secondary to inflammation of a viscus, such as appendicitis, the initial signs are those of the underlying disease, later to be replaced by the features of peritonitis. In advanced cases, only the history of onset remains to point to the probable cause.

Established peritonitis is treated by removal of the contaminating source when it is due to such conditions as appendicitis or perforation of the bowel or gall bladder. Anaerobic infection is controlled with metronidazole. Peritoneal toilet and lavage, intravenous replacement of fluids and electrolytes, and the treatment of the concomitant ileus by nasogastric suction are also required.

While the treatment of peritonitis is that of the cause, the ideal is its prevention. Thus acute appendicitis should be diagnosed before perforation and perforated peptic ulcer should be operated upon during the stage of chemical peritonitis.

General peritonitis may resolve completely, but often it localises to form an abscess at the primary site, in the subphrenic region or in the pelvis. Persistence of fever, or continued elevation of pulse rate, white blood count and ESR, should lead to efforts to locate such residual infections, for example by ultrasonography.

Pelvic abscess usually results from localisation of a general peritonitis and forms in the lower part of the peritoneal cavity, in front of the rectum. The abscess may irritate the bladder causing frequency of micturition or involve the bowel causing diarrhoea with the passage of mucus and a feeling of incomplete emptying. It is evident on rectal or vaginal examination as a tender mass, which may discharge rectally or vaginally. Treatment with metronidazole is usually effective.

Subphrenic abscess. Localisation of pus between diaphragm and liver on the right side or between the diaphragm and the liver, spleen and stomach on the left, is a complication of peritonitis most commonly due to perforation of the stomach, duodenum or gall bladder or to operation on these organs.

There are signs of persistent infection; there may be dullness at the base of the lung and tenderness and slight oedema over the lower ribs posteriorly. Diagnosis is aided by ultrasonography or a radiograph of the diaphragmatic region which may show elevation of the diaphragm, a fluid level below it or an effusion above it. Treatment is by drainage either at laparotomy or by insertion of a drain under ultrasound control.

Tuberculous peritonitis, although now rare in Britain, is still relatively common elsewhere, notably in tropical countries. It is secondary to a tuberculous focus in the abdomen, usually in a mesenteric lymph node and it is characterised by wasting, malaise and abdominal distension. Masses caused by matted omentum and loops of bowel may be palpable. The abdomen contains fluid from which tubercle bacilli may be cultured. Diagnosis may also be made by biopsy of granulomas seen at laparotomy or laparoscopy.

In the adult, the condition may be confused with advanced malignant disease and an unnecessarily hopeless prognosis given. The response to anti-tuberculous chemotherapy (p. 230) is good and often dramatic.

ACUTE APPENDICITIS

Acute appendicitis is more common in young people. It is usually obstructive, the lumen of the appendix being narrowed by swelling of lymphoid tissue in its wall, or by stricture from previous inflammation. Obstruction is made complete by impaction of a retained faecolith leading to gangrene, perforation and a local abscess or generalised peritonitis. In other cases an oedematous inflammatory appendix mass may ensue.

Clinical features. The classical history is of the sudden onset of vague central abdominal pain followed in a few hours by shift of the pain to the right iliac fossa, where it becomes localised to McBurney's point, situated one-third of the distance along a line from the anterior superior iliac spine to the umbilicus. There is nausea and malaise. The breath is foul. There may be vomiting, but this is seldom severe and is often absent. The pulse rate is increased. In the early stages there is little elevation of temperature, so that rigors and a high fever make the diagnosis of appendicitis unlikely. Locally there is tenderness and guarding in the right iliac fossa, progressing to rigidity as peritonitis develops. Rectal examination may disclose tenderness to the right.

The 'classical' history and findings account for less than 50% of cases. Because of variations in its anatomical position the inflamed appendix may simulate other diseases of the abdomen. The patient may present with diarrhoea or with urinary or gynaecological symptoms; acute cholecystitis or perforated peptic ulcer may also be mimicked.

Non-specific mesenteric lymphadenitis may resemble appendicitis in children and adolescents. This condition is probably due to a virus. It is characterised by vague abdominal pain, slight fever and a doughy sensation on palpation. There is ill-defined tenderness in the right iliac fossa. The distinction from appendicitis may be difficult and if in doubt it is safer to operate; otherwise treatment is conservative, recovery taking place gradually over a few weeks.

In adults appendicitis may simulate other causes of a mass in the right iliac fossa (p. 307).

Treatment. The diseased appendix should be removed as early in the acute stage as possible. Attempts to temporise in the belief that mild forms of appendicitis can be distinguished from severe are dangerous, because the condition is notoriously deceptive. Even in the absence of obvious peritonitis, the acute case should have intraoperative antibiotic cover with rectal metronidazole and where there is obvious peritonitis systemic administration of ampicillin and metronidazole should be instituted.

A conservative policy is allowable only when a clearly defined appendix mass is present, without generalised abdominal signs. Once the mass has subsided, probably within 2 to 3 weeks, the appendix should be removed. Not all patients presenting with an appendix mass require antibiotics. Some need no more than rest, restriction of diet and the avoidance of purgatives. Others in whom there is more marked local tenderness, with low-grade fever and malaise, benefit from ampicillin and metronidazole.

TUMOURS OF THE SMALL INTESTINE

Tumours of the small intestine are rare, although there is some evidence that lymphoma is more likely to develop in patients who have coeliac disease. Simple tumours such as polyps and leiomyomas may cause chronic anaemia, intussusception or obstruction. They may also be found unexpectedly in the course of radiological investigation or laparotomy.

Carcinoid tumours arise from argentaffin cells. They are usually found in the appendix at appendicectomy and the prognosis is then excellent. When the primary is in the ileum, spread to the liver is common where metastases produce 5-hydroxytryptamine (serotonin) causing the carcinoid syndrome consisting of flushing, borborygmi, diarrhoea and, occasionally, fibrosis of the tricuspid or pulmonary valve. The diagnosis

is made on the clinical features and confirmed by finding an excessive amount of 5-hydroxyindoleacetic acid in the urine.

Although long-term survival is possible, even with the systemic manifestations, the primary tumour and associated lymphatic and visceral metastases should be removed whenever possible with the aim of reducing the total volume of secreting tumour. Hepatic lobectomy can be considered when spread appears localised to one lobe.

DISEASES OF THE LARGE INTESTINE

The main functions of the large bowel are the removal of water from the intestinal contents, the storage of faeces and their evacuation at controlled intervals. Continence depends on training, on the function of a sphincter mechanism in the anal canal and on rectal sensation whereby the need to defecate is appreciated.

The anal canal is sensitive to pain and touch, as is well demonstrated by the severe pain caused by fissures and inflamed piles. The rectum is insensitive to painful stimuli, so that the injection of a sclerosing agent for the treatment of haemorrhoids is painless. Rectal 'sensation' applies to an ability to appreciate distension and contraction.

In addition to clinical examination, including digital examination of the rectum, endoscopy, stool examination and radiological investigation are all important aids to diagnosis.

Ulcerative colitis

Apart from the bacillary and amoebic dysenteries and tuberculous enterocolitis, there are certain non-specific chronic inflammatory bowel diseases which are associated with ulceration of the colon. One of these is Crohn's disease which may affect both the large and the small bowel; the other, commoner disease affecting the colon, is ulcerative colitis.

Aetiology. The aetiology of ulcerative colitis is not known. The disease may be due to an abnormal immune response, possibly to bacteria or to certain foods. In a few patients withdrawal of milk from the diet may improve the diarrhoea, suggesting perhaps that the condition is due to specific allergy to milk protein. However, it seems much more likely that the improvement observed on milk withdrawal is due to a reduction in osmotic diarrhoea in patients who have developed secondary alactasia (p. 305).

A familial tendency is suggested by the increased incidence of the disease amongst relatives of patients and by the association between ulcerative colitis, ankylosing spondylitis and Crohn's disease (p. 305).

Although individual attacks of colitis often seem to be precipitated by stressful life experiences, psychological factors are not otherwise considered important in aetiology. However, the humiliation of frequent or uncontrollable bowel evacuation may induce profound psychological disturbances such as anxiety and depression and feelings of helplessness. These traits are a consequence of the disease rather than its cause, and generally decrease or disappear during remission. Indeed one of the most rewarding aspects of successful treatment, including surgery, is the remarkable improvement that may occur in the psychological well-being of the patient.

Pathology. The inflammatory process may be limited to the rectum, which is almost always involved (*proctitis*). The disease may also involve the distal colon (*distal colitis*) or the entire colon (*total colitis*). Whatever the extent of the disease, the inflammatory change is continuous throughout the affected part, in contrast to the patchy changes that occur in Crohn's disease.

In the early stages the mucosa is swollen and reddened, and punctate bleeding points may be seen. Thereafter, ulceration develops; the ulcers may be superficial or penetrate deeply, spreading longitudinally beneath the mucosa. In severe disease the mucosa may slough in parts to expose granulation tissue; the mucosa that remains becomes oedematous, hyperplastic and raised, giving the appearance of pseudopolyposis. In *acute fulminant disease* the bowel, especially the transverse colon, may be greatly dilated (*toxic dilatation*) and the bowel wall becomes thin and may rupture. In long-standing disease, the colon is shortened and generally narrowed with a lack of haustrations.

Microscopically, in contrast to Crohn's disease, inflammation is confined to the mucosa. Initially there is congestion, oedema and intra-mucosal haemorrhage. The number of goblet cells is reduced and the lamina propria is infiltrated with lymphocytes and polymorphs; the latter also accumulate in the lumen of the crypts and are termed 'crypt abscesses'. These may progress to destruction of the mucosa which is replaced by granulation tissue. Finally, on healing, the mucosa has a reduced number of crypts.

Clinical features. The disease occurs at all ages but most commonly between 20 and 40 years. The first attack is often the most severe and thereafter the disease is characterised by exacerbations and remissions although a minority of patients develop chronic symptoms. The clinical features and the management are largely determined by the extent to which the colon is involved, the severity of the inflammation and the duration of the disease.

The principal symptom is diarrhoea with loose bloody stools containing mucus and pus; defecation is often accompanied by lower abdominal discomfort, although severe pain is uncommon. Tenesmus may occur because of proctitis. Tenderness may be present on palpation of the colon, especially in the left iliac fossa; when peritoneal irritation is present, it signifies that the serosa is involved in the inflammatory process.

In severe ulcerative colitis, there is exhausting diarrhoea and dehydration. *Toxic dilatation* represents the most serious form with tachycardia, a high swinging temperature and abdominal distension. Untreated, the patient dies as a result of colonic perforation.

In chronic ulcerative colitis the bowel is permanently damaged as a result of fibrosis. The colon in such cases behaves as a rigid tube incapable of absorbing fluid properly or of acting as a faecal reservoir. There is no toxaemia, but the patient lives in chronic ill-health and with persistent diarrhoea.

When the disease is confined to the rectum, the symptoms may be trivial and consist of loose motions and perhaps blood-streaking of the stool. A severe proctitis will cause tenesmus, and frequent small loose stools, together with bleeding and mucus per rectum, but systemic disturbance is absent. Paradoxically, in distal colitis, spasm may result in constipation, with retention of faeces in the proximal colon and small hard stools.

Relapse is often associated with emotional stress, intercurrent infection or the use of anti-biotics. There is no special risk during pregnancy, when indeed it is usual for the disease to remit; in contrast there is a tendency for a severe relapse to occur early in the puerperium.

The patient is often anaemic and there may be leucocytosis and a raised ESR. In severe cases there are electrolyte disturbances and protein loss from the colon may lead to hypoalbuminaemia. Sometimes the liver function tests are abnormal. The stool should be cultured for pathogenic bacteria and a search of the mucus made for amoebae to exclude an infective cause for the colitis. Blood cultures are required if septicaemia is suspected.

Investigation. Sigmoidoscopy is essential in most cases; the mucosa appears engorged and hyperaemic and the normal vascular pattern is obliterated. In severe disease spontaneous bleeding will be seen; in less severe cases the mucosa appears intact, and bleeds only when it is gently rubbed, while in mild cases the only abnormality may be the absence of the normal vascular pattern. Rectal biopsy may be carried out to confirm the diagnosis and to exclude other causes of proctitis, such as Crohn's disease.

Radiological examination. While sigmoidoscopy confirms the diagnosis of ulcerative colitis, a double contrast barium enema will demonstrate the severity and extent of the disease. The earliest radiological change is a granular appearance of the colonic mucosa. In more severe cases ulceration and pseudopolypi will be seen (Fig. 9.11). In long-standing disease there may be shortening of the colon with narrowing of the lumen. Barium enema should not be performed in acute cases and where toxic dilatation is suspected because of the risk of perforation. In these, plain radiographs of the abdomen may allow a diagnosis to be made, since the colon will usually contain sufficient air to outline an abnormal mucosal pattern.

Complications. *Toxic dilatation* and *perforation* have already been mentioned. *Stricture* may occur at any level in the colon or rectum; on the barium enema it is usually smooth, but is sometimes difficult to distinguish from carcinoma.

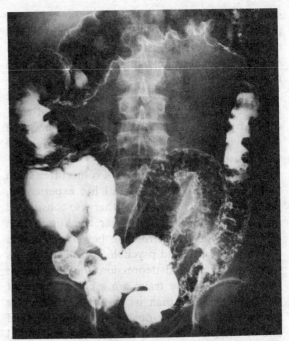

Fig. 9.11 Severe ulcerative colitis with deep ulcers and pseudopolyps affecting mainly the sigmoid colon. (Courtesy of Dr G. M. Fraser.)

Carcinoma of the colon develops more often in patients with long-standing ulcerative colitis than it does in the normal population, the risk being related to the duration, extent and age at onset of the disease. The risk increases greatly after the disease has been present for 10 years or more. It is greatest in patients with total colitis who develop the disease under the age of 20 years; in this group the risk of cancer of the colon is about 40 times greater than in a comparable normal population.

Extra-intestinal complications include entero-pathic arthritis (p. 569), aphthous stomatitis, iritis and skin lesions such as erythema nodosum and, rarely but characteristically, pyoderma gangrenosum. Septicaemia is a recurrent risk. Hepatobiliary complications include fatty liver, pericholangitis, and sclerosing cholangitis (p. 368). These complications are most common in advanced cases.

Differential diagnosis. Ulcerative colitis has to be distinguished from other causes of inflammation of the colonic mucosa namely Crohn's disease (p. 305), amoebic colitis (p. 775), bacillary dysentery (p. 753), campylobacter infections

(p. 752), and antibiotic-associated colitis (p. 44). Colitis can also occur as a result of ischaemia (p. 321) and radiation therapy. Gonorrhoea is frequently overlooked as a cause of proctitis.

Treatment. Admission to hospital is required for patients with severe bowel symptoms, especially when there are general disturbances such as weight loss, anaemia, fever or tachycardia. Such patients may require intense supportive treatment until the disease remits or as a preparation for surgery. Parenteral nutrition through a central venous line allows correction of these deficiencies in the severely wasted patient and will do much to hasten recovery after operation. The measures should include correction of dehydration and electrolyte deficiencies, especially hypokalaemia, blood and plasma infusions to correct anaemia and hypoproteinaemia, and a high protein, low residue diet.

Blood cultures should be taken initially and repeated throughout the course of the illness if fever persists. Gram-negative bacteria are the commonest organisms involved; if septicaemia is suspected parenteral administration of broad spectrum antibiotics is necessary. However, antibiotics have no special place in the primary management of ulcerative colitis; indeed a broad spectrum antibiotic may precipitate a relapse. Candidosis of the mouth and upper pharynx is common, especially in ill patients on corticosteroids and must be treated. There is no satisfactory drug for controlling diarrhoea. Codeine phosphate or loperamide may be helpful but these drugs should be avoided in severely ill patients because they may precipitate an attack of toxic dilatation of the colon.

ANTI-INFLAMMATORY DRUGS. 1. *Corticosteroids.* Although there is no specific treatment for ulcerative colitis, corticosteroids are very effective in inducing remission. Depending on the extent and severity of the disease, corticosteroids may be given as suppositories or enemas to provide topical treatment to the distal bowel, or systemically.

a. Local treatment. The preparations commonly used are prednisolone, 21-phosphatate, or betamethasone. When sigmoidoscopic examination confirms that only the rectum is involved topical treatment with corticosteroid suppositories is all that is required; the patient is instructed to insert one, two or three times daily according to severity.

Topical treatment with corticosteroid enemas may be given for distal colitis when symptoms are mild — not more than four stools per day with intermittent bleeding and little or no systemic upset. Self-administered disposable enemas are available, and the patient is taught to administer the enema twice daily, retaining the material for as long as possible. In addition sulphasalazine may be indicated. When symptoms are more severe, patients with distal colitis may require systemic corticosteroids. Either form of local treatment may be continued for 3 to 6 weeks, the duration being judged from the sigmoidoscopic appearances. Systemic absorption of corticosteroids occurs but is rarely sufficient to cause side-effects.

b. Systemic treatment. Prednisolone is given in doses of between 40–60 mg daily by mouth for 3 to 6 weeks depending on response. In severe cases corticosteroids may have to be given intravenously as hydrocortisone (100–200 mg 6 hourly). The usual contraindications to the use of these drugs must be observed (p. 455) and supplements of potassium salts should be given (p. 90). Used in this way, corticosteroids will induce remission in the majority of patients, the dose being reduced at weekly intervals as improvement takes place. Corticosteroids give rise to a sense of well-being and in addition improve appetite, so that the problem of persuading the patient to eat sufficient food is often solved; they are more effective in a first attack of ulcerative colitis, whereas corticotrophin may be more beneficial in the treatment of relapse. A long-acting form of corticotrophin (e.g. tetracosactrin zinc phosphate complex) should be used, and given in doses of the order of 1 mg daily by intramuscular or subcutaneous injection. This dosage is continued for a week after symptoms have remitted and it is then reduced at weekly intervals as in the case of corticosteroids. For convenience prednisolone may be substituted once the patient has responded adequately.

2. *Sulphasalazine* is less effective than corticosteroids but may be used in mild or moderately severe attacks in doses of 4–6 g daily. However, its principal value is that it reduces the liability

to relapse, so that once remission has been induced by corticosteroids, all patients with colitis should be maintained on a small dose of sulphasalazine (0.5 g q.i.d.) for 1 to 2 years or longer. Sulphasalazine is a combination of 5–aminosalicylic acid which is the active agent, linked to sulphapyridine acting as a 'carrier'. The compound is broken down by bacterial action in the colon, liberating 5-aminosalicylic acid which is believed to act locally. Side-effects attributed to the sulphapyridine moiety include nausea, headache, rashes, reversible sterility in the male, and very rarely haemolytic anaemia and agranulocytosis. Newer formulations using other 'carriers' for 5-aminosalicylic acid are being developed so as to avoid these side-effects.

3. *Other drugs.* Azathioprine (2.5 mg/kg) may be helpful in patients with chronic disease for whom surgery is inappropriate. Serious side-effects may occur including suppression of the bone marrow with pancytopenia, so that patients must be carefully supervised.

SURGICAL TREATMENT. If the appropriate medical measures are carried out assiduously, the majority of patients with proctitis or moderately severe colitis will pass into remission. In severe forms of ulcerative colitis, where there is toxic dilatation of the colon or perforation and in the occasional patient with severe haemorrhage, emergency surgical treatment is required. In these urgent circumstances surgery is usually restricted to colectomy with ileostomy, the rectum and distal colon being removed at a later stage when the crisis is over.

Acute ulcerative colitis which fails to respond to medical treatment, or which relapses in spite of adequate treatment, is an indication for procto-colectomy. This is also indicated in chronic forms, where the disease burns out but leaves a permanently damaged bowel, perhaps with stricture formation. Long-standing disease, particularly when the onset has been in childhood, carries a risk of carcinoma and accordingly total bowel involvement, with activity extending over more than 10 years, should lead to serious consideration of surgery.

At all stages of the disease, the timing of and preparation for surgery are important and require a joint medical and surgical approach. In emergency situations, intensive pre-operative replacement of blood, fluid and electrolytes is needed and operation is performed as soon as the patient is fit to withstand surgery. In less urgent situations, the timing of surgery depends on the degree of improvement in the patient's general condition to be expected from preoperative medical measures. Shrewd judgement is required to choose the optimum time before the patient's condition deteriorates again.

Whenever possible, in addition to a full explanation of ileostomy and its management with a demonstration of the actual appliance to be used, the patient should have the opportunity before operation of meeting someone with an established ileostomy. Modern surgical techniques and the range of ileostomy appliances available make for easy management of the stoma and allow the patient to live an almost normal life with little restriction of physical activity. To be kept in touch with advances in techniques of ileostomy care, patients should join an ileostomy association or be enrolled in a stoma therapy clinic.

When the rectum is not grossly involved it may be preserved and ileo-rectal anastomosis performed. In selected cases ileo-anal anastomosis with formation of an ileal reservoir can be used. The risk of interference with sexual function is thus reduced and the need for a stoma avoided.

Prognosis. It is extremely difficult to give a prognosis in ulcerative colitis. The extent of involvement of the colon is an important consideration, the outlook being very much better, for example, if only the rectum is involved. The immediate death rate in patients with fulminating disease, however treated, is not less than 40%, and it is high also in patients developing an attack over the age of 60. In general, the overall mortality from ulcerative colitis is of the order of 10%, but this figure can be very greatly reduced when the patient is treated by those with special experience of the disease. Thus, the mortality from total proctocolectomy done during a remission by an experienced surgeon is about 2%, whereas mortality for proctocolectomy done as an emergency procedure is 10% in the best hands, and may be 20% or 30% in those with little experience of the disease. Attention has been drawn to the risk of carcinoma in long-standing cases. Such patients should be kept under surveillance and (preferably) have periodic colonoscopic examinations to detect malignant changes.

Diverticular disease

Though diverticula occur throughout the gastro-intestinal tract, they are most common in the large bowel in middle-aged or elderly subjects. The presence of diverticula is known as *diverticulosis*; when they are inflamed the condition is known as *diverticulitis*. Such inflammation occurs almost exclusively in colonic diverticula. Because it is often difficult to separate the two conditions on clinical or radiological evidence, they are grouped together under the term '*diverticular disease*'.

Aetiology. In diverticulosis the muscular coat of the bowel is often greatly thickened, suggesting that the diverticula have formed as a result of increased intracolonic pressure. Manometric measurements support this view. It can be shown that pressure in the bowel is high and that there is an area of spasm or failure to relax at the pelvirectal junction. Dietary factors may be at least partly responsible. Diverticulosis is rare in areas of the world such as Africa and Asia where the usual diet is one of high residue; by contrast the incidence is increasing in Western countries where natural fibre is removed from the diet in the processes of food refining. Moreover there is evidence that intracolonic pressures vary with the bulk of faecal residue, a high faecal residue being associated with a low intraluminal pressure and vice versa.

Pathology. The pelvic colon is most commonly involved. Its muscle wall is thickened but the diverticula themselves are pouchings of the mucosa and have no muscle coat. It is not clear how they become inflamed. Radiological examination frequently shows the presence of a faecolith in a diverticulum, and it may be that faeces collect because of the inability of the diverticulum to contract. Faecal retention may then cause a local inflammatory reaction which may resolve spontaneously or progress to cause perforation, local abscess formation, fistula and peritonitis. When there are repeated attacks of diverticulitis, the bowel wall becomes thickened with narrowing of the lumen leading eventually to obstruction.

Clinical features. Pain or discomfort felt in the left iliac fossa is a common complaint and there may be associated local tenderness. Acute diverticulitis can give rise to severe pain, guarding and rigidity on the left side, the signs of peritonitis and obstruction being combined. Change of bowel habit, either increasing constipation or constipation alternating with diarrhoea, is frequent. This is the most important symptom of distal colonic disease and can occur with any lesion. Before middle age, bowel habits are firmly established and a definite alteration usually betokens organic disease in the colon such as carcinoma or diverticulitis and always calls for investigation. Another presenting feature may be severe rectal bleeding.

In the chronic forms, there may be symptoms of subacute obstruction with increasing abdominal distension, borborygmi and colicky pain. Spread of inflammation to the bladder may cause urinary frequency and dysuria. Occasionally a fistula to the bladder gives rise to pneumaturia and faecal contamination of the urine.

On examination, the thickened tender colon may be palpable in the left iliac fossa. A mass may be present in those patients who have developed diverticulitis, with or without abscess.

Investigation. *Sigmoidoscopy* is necessary to exclude cancer of the rectum or pelvi-rectal junction. The principal indication for *colonoscopy* is to exclude colonic carcinoma, when the radiological appearances leave room for doubt. Colonoscopic examination may be difficult because of narrowing and rigidity of the bowel, but when the suspected abnormality can be seen and a biopsy carried out, a correct diagnosis is possible. Both diverticular disease and cancer may coexist or one may mimic the other to the extent that even at operation the true diagnosis is uncertain.

Radiological examination. In diverticulosis, barium enema shows characteristic sacs along the contour of the gut (Fig. 9.12). After evacuation barium is frequently left behind in the diverticula which are clearly outlined. If diverticulitis is present, there will be narrowing, rigidity and lack of normal haustration of a segment of colon. Whether or not there are diverticula present, the main diagnostic difficulty is to distinguish the

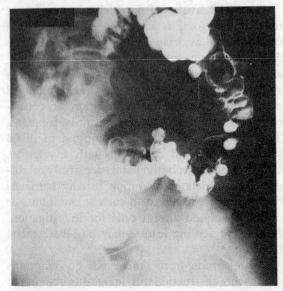

Fig. 9.12 Diverticular disease of the sigmoid colon.
(Courtesy of Dr G. M. Fraser.)

appearances from those of carcinoma and radiological differentiation may be impossible.

Treatment. Asymptomatic diverticulosis is common, is often found accidentally and requires no treatment. A high fibre diet is usually sufficient to relieve constipation. If not, a bulk laxative such as methylcellulose should be used in addition. Purgatives should be avoided.

During an attack of acute diverticulitis, bed-rest, metronidazole or ampicillin, fluids intraven-ously and orally, or even cessation of feeding and nasogastric suction may be required. Most severe attacks subside spontaneously but a few require emergency surgery which will probably be con-fined to a temporary defunctioning proximal colostomy, to be followed later by local re-section. An emergency partial colectomy may be required for acute bleeding.

Elective surgery is indicated, after recovery from an acute attack, in patients who develop obstructive features, who have complications such as fistula and in those in whom the possibility of carcinoma cannot be excluded. The treatment of choice is resection of the involved segment of pelvic colon with primary anastomosis.

Haemorrhage from the lower gastrointestinal tract

The commonest source is haemorrhoids. Bleeding per rectum may also originate in the rectum itself, in the colon or terminal ileum. With bleeding from the proximal colon or ileum, the blood may appear as melaena. The usual causes are diverticular disease, cancer of the rectum or distal half of the colon and angiodysplasia in the mucosa of the bowel wall. Less common sources of bleed-ing are polyps, ulcerative colitis and ischaemic colitis.

Rectal examination and sigmoidoscopy will detect most rectal causes of bleeding.

If bleeding is proximal to the rectum, the patient is treated conservatively, as for upper gastrointestinal haemorrhage, and in most cases bleeding will stop. Thereafter barium enema and colonoscopy will detect most lesions. If bleeding continues, angiography of the superior and inferior mesenteric arteries can be performed to detect the site of bleeding and possibly treat it by embolisation through the arterial catheter. If bleeding fails to stop, the appropriate segment of the colon can be resected.

Carcinoma of the colon and rectum

In Britain, carcinoma of the large intestine is the most common malignant tumour of the alimentary tract. In contrast it is rare in Africa and Asia. The variation in incidence of the disease between different countries has led to speculation that dietary factors and differences in bacterial flora of the bowel may be of aetiological significance. Diseases known to be clearly associated with colonic carcinoma are long-standing ulcerative colitis and familial polyposis of the colon.

Pathology. In two-thirds of patients, cancer of the large bowel occurs in the left colon or rectum. Concomitant multiple tumours are pre-sent in 2% of cases. The risk of a second cancer may reach 10% in patients with adenomatous polyps. Macroscopically the tumour may be pro-liferative and fungating, ulcerative and infiltrat-ing, polypoidal or encircling as a 'string' stricture. Perforation may occur at the site of the tumour, leading to peritonitis, localised abscess or a fistula.

Spread occurs directly in and through the bowel wall, by lymphatics and by the bloodstream through both portal and systemic circulations. Colonic carcinoma is capable of direct implant-ation on exposed surfaces, such as a suture line or area of trauma in the bowel. Metastases most commonly involve the liver.

Clinical features. Symptoms vary depending on the site of the carcinoma. In tumours of the left colon, obstruction is early. Tumours of the right colon present with anaemia, cachexia and alteration of bowel habit, but obstruction is late because of the relatively fluid nature of the bowel contents. As a consequence left-sided tumours tend to be diagnosed earlier.

Change in bowel habit, anaemia, weight loss and sometimes excessive borborygmi, abdominal distension and colicky pains indicating subacute obstruction, all point to a large bowel tumour. Some, however, are relatively symptomless until the patient presents as an emergency with obstruction.

Carcinoma of the lower rectum will almost always cause early bleeding with mucus discharge; later there is tenesmus and a feeling of incomplete emptying of the bowel. Obstruction is a feature of tumours of the pelvi-rectal junction but not the rectum proper, which is capacious and distensible.

The findings on physical examination range from no obvious abnormality to the signs of advanced malignancy. The majority of rectal tumours can be palpated on digital examination. Fresh blood in the stool should always suggest the possibility of a tumour of the rectum or pelvic colon. Occult blood is found in the stool if an ulcerating lesion is present higher in the colon.

Investigation. *Endoscopy.* More than 50% of malignant tumours of the large bowel occur in a part accessible to direct inspection with the sigmoidoscope, i.e. the rectum and the lower pelvic colon and this procedure is mandatory. The whole or part of a growth may be seen and a biopsy carried out. Colonoscopic examination is valuable when a suspicious lesion is seen more proximally on the barium enema.

Radiological examination. A barium enema will demonstrate advanced cancer as a filling defect or stricture (Fig. 9.13). For the demonstration of smaller, earlier tumours, careful preparation of the colon followed by a double contrast barium enema is necessary. A barium follow-through examination may be of value for tumours in the region of the caecum.

The *stage* of carcinoma of the rectum is defined by Dukes' classification (p. 106), and the role of

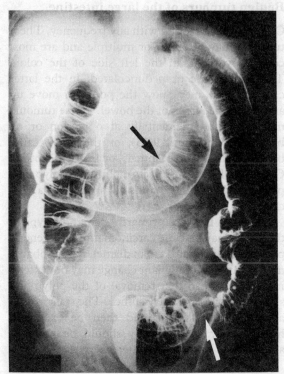

Fig. 9.13 Carcinoma of the sigmoid colon and a polyp in the transverse colon (Courtesy of Dr G.M. Fraser.)

CEA is discussed on page 103.

Treatment of choice is resection of the tumour as a one-stage procedure. If there is no colonic obstruction, or if it can be overcome by enemas, time should be spent in preparing the bowel by washouts and antibiotics. Anaemia should be corrected by pre-operative transfusion.

Carcinoma of the rectum may require total removal of the rectum with permanent colostomy and for this the patient requires pre-operative introduction to colostomy and its management. However, advances in suture techniques allow preservation of continuity in many more patients by means of a colo-rectal or colo-anal anastomosis. Success depends on early diagnosis and operation before spread has occurred and before obstruction renders the surgeon's task more complicated. The possibility of carcinoma of the colon must be considered when anyone of middle age presents with rectal bleeding, change of bowel habit or iron-deficiency anaemia.

Benign tumours of the large intestine

Only polyps are found with any frequency. These tumours may be single or multiple and are most commonly found in the left side of the colon. They are sessile or pedunculated; in the latter case the stalk may allow the polyp to move up and down the lumen of the bowel. These tumours may be found incidentally at operation or on barium enema (Fig. 9.13), or they may cause bleeding, discharge of mucus, or intussusception. Occasionally, because of its mobility, a polyp may prolapse through the anus to appear as a red, cherry-like mass.

Although they are primarily benign, polyps of the colon may become carcinomatous. In general polyps of more than 1 cm in diameter are probably malignant. The malignant change may not extend into the stalk, so that removal of the polyp and stalk at colonoscopy may suffice. The stalk as well as the polyp itself should then be examined histologically. Colonoscopy should be repeated after 2 years to exclude recurrence.

Multiple polyposis

In this condition, transmitted by autosomal dominant inheritance, there may be thousands of small polyps diffusely scattered over the mucosal surface of the colon and rectum. They appear at adolescence and become malignant in about 15 years, the patient often dying from carcinomatosis before the age of 40. The disease can be recognised by radiological or endoscopic examination from adolescence onwards of members of affected families. Prevention of carcinoma means removal of the colon and rectum with permanent ileostomy, although symptomless members of the family may find ileo-rectal anastomosis with diathermy removal of rectal polyps and periodic surveillance more acceptable.

Megacolon

Megacolon is a condition characterised by dilatation of the colon and obstinate constipation. The disease may be separated into two groups, congenital (Hirschsprung's disease) and acquired megacolon.

Hirschsprung's disease. The cause is a congenital absence of the myenteric nerve plexus in the wall of the pelvic colon and upper rectum. Occasionally the defect extends proximally. Boys are more often affected than girls and symptoms of colonic obstruction (constipation, abdominal distension and vomiting) date from birth. Symptoms may be intermittent, but even between attacks there is persistent abdominal swelling. The rectum is empty on digital examination.

Radiological examination with small amounts of barium shows a small rectum, a narrow segment above and then wide dilatation of the colon full of retained faeces. The diagnosis can be confirmed by a rectal biopsy of sufficient thickness to include muscle of the bowel wall in which the ganglion cells are situated.

Treatment is by excision of the abnormal segment of colon and rectum.

Acquired megacolon. In this group of cases, there is no defined aetiology and no particular age group. Some are examples of a milder, short segment form of Hirschsprung's disease. Others are associated with cretinism. In Chagas' disease (p. 781) autonomic ganglia in the lower colon are destroyed by a trypanosome.

Radiologically, acquired megacolon usually shows no narrowed segment, the dilatation instead extending down to the anus. The rectum is full of faeces.

Most cases can be managed conservatively, by treatment of the cause where identifiable, by high residue diets, laxatives and perhaps saline enemas. In a few patients colonic resection has been used as a last resort in the relief of obstinate constipation.

Incontinence of faeces

Incontinence is most common in elderly, debilitated or demented patients in whom the appreciation of rectal distension is diminished and the sphincteric and pelvic floor muscles are weakened. It may also be due to faecal impaction with overflow incontinence of soft faeces and require manual or instrumental disimpaction followed by the use of laxatives to prevent recurrence.

Incontinence also occurs when the sphincters and the supporting muscles are injured, for example by obstetric tear; various operative procedures are available for their repair. The sphincter mechanisms can be damaged by cancer, Crohn's disease or third degree haemorrhoids or their neurological control may be impaired by spina bifida or trauma to the lumbar spine.

There can be incontinence of faeces even when anal function is normal as in the presence of severe diarrhoea or in behavioural disturbances in children. In all instances treatment must be directed at the primary cause.

GENERAL DISEASES OF THE ALIMENTARY TRACT

Any or several components of the alimentary tract may be involved by infection, ischaemia or psychogenic disorders

Infections of the alimentary tract

Infections of the mouth due to thrush and other organisms are discussed on page 277 and gastroenteritis caused by bacterial food poisoning on page 751. Acute gastroenteritis may be caused by viruses such as rotavirus. Usually identification of the viral nature of the infection is not possible and diagnosis is presumptive on epidemiological grounds when no bacterial cause has been demonstrated.

The small intestine is involved in typhoid and paratyphoid fevers (p. 750), cholera (p. 754), staphylococcal enterocolitis (p. 742), tuberculosis (p. 226), giardiasis (p. 776), strongyloidiasis (p. 793) and ancylostomiasis (p. 792).

The principal infections involving the large intestine are bacillary dysentery (p. 753), amoebic dysentery (p. 775), antibiotic-associated colitis (p. 44) and schistosomiasis (p. 783). Some organisms, e.g. *Yersinia enterocolitica*, may infect both small and large intestines.

Abdominal infections complicating surgical or gynaecological operations and diverticulitis are commonly caused by *Bacteroides fragilis* and respond to metronidazole. Alternative therapy is provided by clindamycin or cefoxitin.

Rehydration together with oral glucose and electrolytes can be life-saving in the acute diarrhoeal illnesses which are a major cause of death in infants and children in the tropics (p. 718).

Bacterial resistance to antimicrobial agents is readily induced by their indiscriminate use in infections of the gut, many of which are not of bacterial origin. When antimicrobial therapy is indicated by the presence of systemic upset, local knowledge of sensitivity is important as resistance may have been acquired to one or more of the agents commonly used in that area.

Travellers' diarrhoea. A short attack of diarrhoea commonly affects travellers, especially in developing countries. The attack is usually acute, with watery stools and sometimes vomiting. It lasts 2 to 5 days and is self-limiting. Enterotoxigenic *Esch. coli* has been implicated in about 50% of cases and shigella in up to 20%. Other organisms, e.g. campylobacter or rotaviruses, may be involved but often the cause cannot be identified. In mild cases symptoms can be controlled by one of the synthetic narcotic analogues, loperamide or diphenoxylate. Severer cases should be treated early with co-trimoxazole or trimethoprim.

Persistence of diarrhoea after travel is a feature of giardiasis (p. 776) and amoebiasis (p. 775).

Ischaemia of the alimentary tract

The intestines are supplied by the coeliac, superior mesenteric and inferior mesenteric arteries. Of these, the superior mesenteric, which supplies the mid-gut, has poor collateral support from the other two arteries. It follows that intestinal ischaemia is usually due to sudden or slow occlusion of the superior mesenteric artery. However, it may also arise from obstruction to the venous outflow from the intestine, or from a reduction in blood flow due to shock or cardiac failure, without evidence of obstruction to the arterial or venous supply. The usual causes of blockage of the superior mesenteric artery are atheroma, thrombosis due to blood diseases, and embolism. Most cases of intestinal ischaemia occur in the elderly and in those with cardiac failure or arrhythmias.

Acute intestinal failure. This term is used to describe the consequences of acute obstruction of the superior mesenteric artery. A variable length of the small intestine undergoes necrosis of the superficial epithelium and over several hours this progresses to gangrene. The patient has abdominal pain, vomiting, watery and later bloody diarrhoea. Signs of peritonitis and hypovolaemic shock develop. There is marked leucocytosis. Early laparotomy is essential as most patients will die unless the affected bowel is resected. Occasionally, embolectomy or thrombectomy can restore the circulation and allow recovery.

Chronic intestinal ischaemia. This occurs when there is a gradual reduction of blood flow in the superior mesenteric artery with resulting impairment of the normal postprandial increase in blood flow to the small bowel. There is abdominal pain ('abdominal angina') some 30 minutes after each meal so that the patient is afraid to eat and loses weight. The condition is rare.

Ischaemia of the large intestine. Occlusion of the inferior mesenteric artery leads to ischaemia of the left colon, especially when blood flow in the superior mesenteric artery is also reduced. The disorder is termed *ischaemic colitis*. The patient presents with abdominal pain and bloody diarrhoea and the diagnosis is made by barium enema examination which shows oedema of the mucosa of the affected segment of colon. In contrast to ischaemia of the small intestine, the condition is usually transient, but in some patients it may proceed to gangrene or to stricture usually situated at the splenic flexure.

Psychogenic disorders

Disorders of the alimentary tract due to psychological disturbance are extremely common. While it can be readily shown that the blood flow as well as the secretory and motor activities of the gastrointestinal tract can be influenced by emotion, the mechanisms by which psychological distress elicits a symptomatic response from the gut are poorly understood. When psychological problems are obvious, as in anxiety or depressive states, or in the response to a stressful life experience, their relationship to symptoms can be readily confirmed. Often, however, the underlying mechanism is a long-standing emotional conflict and the connection between such problems and physical symptoms is much more difficult to establish.

Psychological disturbances can induce a great variety of individual symptoms. Anxious or stressed patients may complain of a dry mouth, or a sensation of a lump in the throat, anorexia, nausea or vomiting, aerophagy with belching, abdominal pain or discomfort, constipation or diarrhoea, or excessive flatus. Depressed patients commonly complain of a bad taste in the mouth, or of nausea, and vomiting especially on waking. Although symptoms may occur singly and are occasionally bizarre, some common patterns occur.

Nervous dyspepsia. Symptoms include pain, anorexia, nausea, retching and vomiting and belching. They may mimic peptic ulceration but in nervous dyspepsia pain tends to be continuous rather than episodic, diffuse rather than localised, worsened rather than improved by food, and not relieved by vomiting. It may be severe and is often worst on waking; it rarely occurs at night. Symptoms, though long-standing, are poorly described by the patient, and seem quite disproportionate to clinical well-being; for example, loss of appetite or vomiting is not associated with weight loss. A careful history will usually elicit features suggestive of a psychological disturbance.

Physical examination may reveal manifestations of anxiety such as labial twitching, rapid eye movements, inappropriate sweating or tachycardia. Abdominal tenderness if present is disproportionate both to clinical well-being and to the complaint. Further investigation is often necessary, but should be selected with discrimination in relation to the individual patient. This is particularly the case in patients over the age of 45, in whom a diagnosis of nervous dyspepsia should not be lightly made.

The psychological origin of the symptoms should be sought. A successful outcome depends in large part on the patient being able to accept the psychogenic origin of the symptoms, so that time spent in careful sympathetic explanation is rewarding. Many patients with nervous dyspepsia recognise their susceptibility to stress, and come to a doctor from time to time merely for reassurance. Some patients are helped by antacids or an anticholinergic such as dicyclomine (10–20 mg with meals); this may well be a placebo response.

Globus hystericus describes the sensation of a lump in the throat which is independent of swallowing and indeed may be relieved by swallowing food or drink. The symptom occurs most frequently in tense, anxious individuals, but before accepting a psychogenic basis it is necessary to exclude organic disease by a barium swallow and if necessary by endoscopy.

Psychogenic vomiting is not an uncommon manifestation of anxiety neurosis. It occurs usually on wakening, or immediately after breakfast; only rarely does it occur later in the day. It is probably a reaction to awakening and facing up to the worries of everyday life; in the young it can be due to school phobia. There may be retching alone or the vomiting of gastric secretions or food. Although psychogenic vomiting may occur regularly over long periods, there is little or no weight loss and this is of value in distinguishing it from vomiting due to organic disease of the alimentary tract. Early morning vomiting also occurs in pregnancy, alcohol abuse and depression.

It is essential in all cases to assess and, if possible, alleviate the underlying psychological disturbance. Tranquillisers and antiemetic drugs have only a secondary place.

The irritable bowel syndrome

One of the commonest disorders of the alimentary tract is that of long-standing dysfunction associated with abdominal pain for which no organic cause can be found. Bowel habit is disturbed by diarrhoea or constipation occurring alone, or alternating. Some forms of this irritable bowel syndrome are also known as *spastic colon* and *idiopathic* or *nervous diarrhoea*.

Manometric studies from the distal colon have shown various patterns. When constipation and pain are the predominant symptoms, intraluminal pressure is usually increased and there is an increased frequency of pressure waves, whereas motor activity is often reduced in patients with painless diarrhoea. These changes are not constant so that motility studies are of no value for diagnostic purposes.

Although the aetiology of the irritable bowel syndrome is uncertain, psychological disturbances, especially anxiety, are frequent; patients are often tense, conscientious individuals who worry excessively about family or financial affairs. Some relate the onset of their symptoms to an attack of infective diarrhoea; in others certain foods may precipitate symptoms.

Clinical features. The syndrome is most frequent in women between the ages of 20 and 40 years. The commonest symptom is pain referred to the left or right iliac fossa or the hypogastrium, sometimes varying in site. Pain often occurs in attacks usually relieved by defecation and sometimes provoked by food, and may be severe. Bowel habit is variable. Almost all patients notice pellet like or ribbon like stools with or without mucus at some time. Diarrhoea may be painless and characteristically occurs in the morning, and almost never at night; defecation after meals may be precipitate due to an exaggerated gastrocolic reflex. Other symptoms include abdominal distension, a sensation of incomplete emptying of the rectum, excessive flatus and audible borborygmi. Nausea, headache and tiredness may also occur.

The patient may seem anxious but is otherwise well. The descending colon may be palpable and tender. Rectal examination is normal.

Investigation. Although the diagnosis is usually suggested by the history alone, organic bowel disease has to be excluded, especially in patients developing symptoms for the first time over the age of 40 years. Sigmoidoscopy may be required to exclude an organic lesion of the distal colon. The mucosa appears normal in the irritable bowel syndrome but the colon may show marked motor activity, contracting and relaxing quite unlike the normal inert bowel. Barium enema may be indicated to exclude organic disease; there are no diagnostic radiological features in the irritable bowel syndrome. In patients whose principal complaint is painless diarrhoea, the possibility of lactose intolerance, hyperthyroidism or alcohol excess should not be overlooked.

Treatment. The patient must first be reassured on the basis of the normal findings on examination and investigation, as anxiety may precipitate or aggravate the condition and there is sometimes an underlying fear of cancer. In patients with persistent or troublesome symptoms, measures designed to modify the intestinal dysmotility are required. For constipation and pain, the patient should be encouraged to increase the roughage content of the diet and one of the hydrophilic colloids should be prescribed in a dose sufficient to ensure normal bowel movement. It is important that the patient should stop laxatives.

Pain and diarrhoea may be relieved by an anticholinergic drug such as dicyclomine or an antispasmodic such as mebeverine hydrochloride thrice daily. For patients with painless diarrhoea, improvement is commonly obtained with some dietary restriction, particularly the avoidance of fresh fruits and salads. Codeine phosphate and loperamide are useful drugs which act quickly and can be carried by the patient to use in emergency or they can be taken before any event which is known to precipitate diarrhoea.

In all patients the psychological component of the syndrome must be explained.

PROSPECTS IN ALIMENTARY DISEASE

The accurate diagnosis of most gastrointestinal diseases is now possible due to the development of sophisticated endoscopic and radiological procedures. This precision is being still further improved by developments in ultrasonography (standard and endoscopic), computed scanning and magnetic resonance imaging. All these techniques are being used increasingly to effect therapy. Thus imaging and radiographic techniques are used to control gastrointestinal bleeding and to localise, accurately, masses, abscesses and cysts which can then be biopsied or aspirated. Endoscopic procedures are being used in many different ways, for example to carry out the coagulation of bleeding points and for channelling ('stenting') strictures. There is no doubt that advances along these lines will continue. Thus lasers are being developed which can be used at endoscopy to stop bleeding from the stomach and duodenum and to reduce the mass of inoperable tumours in accessible organs, such as the oesophagus, stomach and rectum, by direct necrosis.

The ability to treat most cases of peptic ulceration with H_2-receptor antagonists and the success of highly selective vagotomy in those who require surgery, has led to more satisfactory management of the majority of such patients. It is likely that the minority of ulcers which respond poorly to H_2-receptor antagonists and patients with Zollinger-Ellison syndrome will be treated effectively with more powerful drugs such as omeprazole. There remains the significant problem of those who develop ulcers or bleeding from erosions as a result of consuming aspirin or other anti-inflammatory drugs. It is likely that an increased understanding of the components of the gastric mucosal 'barrier' and the development of drugs to strengthen it, for example the prostaglandins, will avoid these complications. The mechanisms which protect the epithelium of the entire gastrointestinal tract are also under study; this may provide new insights into diffuse conditions such as Crohn's disease, and ulcerative colitis.

Functional gastrointestinal disease remains a significant cause of illness. Our understanding of the mechanisms involved is rudimentary. The development of research into motility of the alimentary tract and the increased awareness of the large number of interacting gastrointestinal hormones and paracrine substances may eventually provide therapeutic benefits.

In some directions the surgical treatment of gastrointestinal disorders will continue to contract with the increasing efficiency and availability of medical, radiological and endoscopic alternatives. On the other hand sphincter sparing operations and other technical improvements will continue. Now that microvascular surgery and organ transplantation are established in other fields similar advances in the management of pancreatic and gut failure can be anticipated. Whilst these advances in technique offer more acceptable operations, the problem of gastrointestinal cancer remains. Chemotherapeutic agents continue to be developed. The prospect of using monoclonal antibodies as tumour 'probes' is exciting, but not yet beyond the laboratory stage. The main hope still lies in the identification of carcinogens and their elimination from the diet and environment.

G.P. Crean
D.J.C. Shearman

FURTHER READING:

Macleod J, Munro J 1986 Examination of the alimentary system. In: Clinical examination, 7th edn. Churchill Livingstone, Edinburgh. Complementary to this chapter and designed to be read in conjunction with it

Shearman D J C, Finlayson N D C 1987 Diseases of the gastrointestinal tract and liver, 2nd edn. Churchill Livingstone, Edinburgh. A new textbook primarily for clinicians

Bateson M C, Bouchier I A D 1981 Clinical investigation of gastrointestinal function. Blackwell Scientific Publications, Oxford. A guide to the more widely used tests of function for trainees and clinicians with no special expertise in gastroenterology

Sleisenger M H, Fordtran J S 1983 Gastrointestinal disease, 3rd edn. Saunders, London. The most complete reference text from the USA containing extensive bibliographies to each chapter

Clinics in gastroenterology. Saunders, London. A series of specialist volumes consisting of three numbers annually and each dealing with a specific disorder of the alimentary tract. Recommended for selective reading and as a reference library to current practice

Books and journals dealing also with hepatobiliary disease are listed on page 369

10

Diseases of the liver and biliary system

THE LIVER

ANATOMY

The liver is the largest organ in the body, weighing 1200–1500 g. Traditionally, it has been divided into right and left lobes by the falciform ligament anteriorly, the fissure of the ligamentum teres inferiorly and the fissure of the ligamentum venosum posteriorly. The right lobe is the larger and contains the quadrate and caudate lobes; the left lobe is relatively larger in infancy and contributes to the protuberant abdomen at that age.

The arterial supply is by the hepatic artery, a branch of the coeliac axis, which enters the liver in the porta hepatis and is distributed throughout the liver via the portal tracts. Its precise terminal distribution is uncertain, but most of its blood enters the sinusoids directly. In man, the hepatic artery supplies about 35% of the total liver blood flow and about 50% of its total oxygen supply. The portal vein drains the blood from the alimentary tract, spleen, pancreas and gall bladder. It also enters the liver in the porta hepatis, is distributed throughout the liver via the portal tracts and empties its blood into the sinusoids. The oxygen content of portal blood varies and is lowest during digestion. Autoregulation of blood flow by the hepatic artery compensates for variations of portal blood flow and ensures that total liver blood flow remains constant.

Histology. The liver is divided into lobules based on a central vein and peripheral portal tracts with regular radiating sinusoids separated by plates of liver cells (hepatocytes). This histological lobule has no functional correlation. The functional liver lobule or acinus comprises a group of liver cells supplied by a single hepatic arteriole and portal venule in a terminal portal tract draining through the sinusoids to several central veins on the periphery of the lobule. The central veins are tributaries of the hepatic veins which drain to the inferior vena cava.

The portal tracts contain branches of the hepatic artery, the portal vein, lymphatics and the bile ducts; the sinusoids are capillaries which are lined by endothelial and phagocytic (Kupffer) cells and which receive blood separately from the hepatic arterial and portal venous systems and convey it to the central veins; the hepatocytes (Fig. 10.1) are arranged in single-cell plates which lie between and separate the sinusoids from one another. Between the hepatocytes and the sinusoidal cells is the space of Disse which contains fluid draining to the lymphatics in the portal tracts. The space of Disse also contains unique stellate (Ito) cells responsible for the storage of vitamin A. Individual hepatocytes either line the space of Disse or abut on other liver cells; electron microscopically, the part of the membrane lining the space of Disse has irregular microvilli, while a part of the membrane adjacent to other liver cells helps to form the lining of the bile canaliculi, and here regular microvilli project into the canalicular lumen. These bile canaliculi form networks between the hepatocytes and convey bile towards the terminal bile ducts which link the intralobular bile canaliculi to the larger interlobular bile ducts in the portal tracts (Fig. 10.1).

The electron microscopic features of the liver are complex. Increasing knowledge is beginning to focus attention on the intracellular sites at which damage occurs in different forms of hepatocyte injury. Direct toxic injury (alcohol, drugs, pregnancy, Wilson's disease, Reye's syndrome) principally damages cytoplasmic organelles and causes centrilobular necrosis and fatty change; immunological damage (chronic active hepatitis, primary biliary cirrhosis, drugs) affects cell and canalicular membranes, and cholestatic injury (drugs) affects the bile secretory mechanism.

Clinical aspects. The upper border of the liver extends from the fifth rib medial to the right midclavicular line to the sixth rib in the left midclavicular line. Its lower margin crosses the epigastrium midway between the xiphisternum and the umbilicus. As the liver descends 1–3 cm in inspiration, it can normally be palpated in adults below the right costal margin during deep inspiration. Light percussion from above and from below in the right midclavicular line helps to determine liver size and is of main value in revealing a small liver. Auscultation over the liver may reveal a rub due to perihepatitis, a venous hum between the xiphisternum and umbilicus due to collateral vessels in portal hypertension, or, rarely, an arterial bruit due to hepatocellular carcinoma or acute alcoholic hepatitis.

PHYSIOLOGY

Liver cells carry out a wide variety of metabolic functions facilitated by the rich blood supply

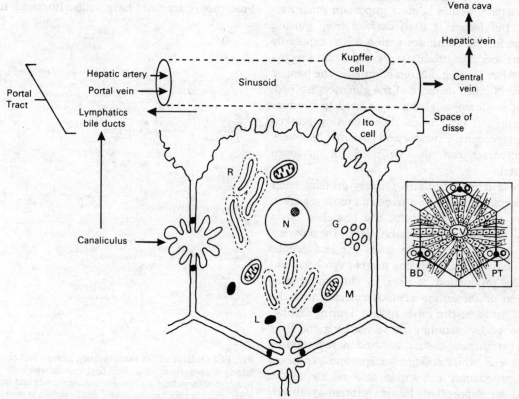

Fig. 10.1 The hepatocyte and its main related structures. The hepatocyte has a prominent nucleus and nucleolus [N] and electron microscopy shows its cytoplasm to be rich in organelles such as mitochondria [M], endoplasmic reticulum [R], lysosomes [L] and Golgi apparatus [G], responsible for complex metabolic processes. The sinusoids (capillaries) are heavily fenestrated, and are therefore highly permeable. The inset shows a lobule with plates of hepatocytes and their relationship to the central vein [CV], bile ducts [BD] and portal tracts [PR].

derived from the gut as well as the systemic circulation, and by hepatic sinusoids which are so permeable that the fluid in the space of Disse is almost the same as plasma. All hepatocytes appear capable of performing the many functions of the liver.

Carbohydrate metabolism. The liver is central to the maintenance of the blood glucose concentration which remains remarkably constant thus ensuring a steady supply of carbohydrate to extrahepatic tissues. During fasting, glucose derived from glycogen (glycogenolysis) or from newly synthesised glucose (gluconeogenesis) is added to the blood. Three-quarters is derived initially from glycogenolysis, but glycogen reserves (70–80 g) become exhausted within 24 hours of fasting and gluconeogenesis becomes steadily more important. Precursors for gluconeogenesis include lactate, pyruvate, glucogenic amino acids and glycerol. Lactate derived from extrahepatic tissues is most important quantitatively, but lactate is itself derived from glucose and as fasting continues amino acids, especially alanine, become steadily more important precursors. After feeding, insulin stimulates the hepatic uptake of a half or more of the glucose absorbed, and it is stored as glycogen or used to produce glycerol and fatty acids thus avoiding marked hyperglycaemia. Fructose and galactose in dietary carbohydrate can also be used for glycogen synthesis.

Protein metabolism. Dietary proteins enter the portal vein as amino acids and most are taken up by the liver except for the branched chain amino acids which are metabolised by the muscles. The liver utilises amino acids for endogenous hepatic protein and plasma protein synthesis and for the production of urea. A substantial proportion of the amino acids is released into the blood for the use of other tissues. During fasting, amino acids, including those reaching the liver from extrahepatic tissues, are used more for gluconeogenesis while endogenous protein synthesis, urea production and amino acid release to the blood are suppressed. Plasma protein synthesis, by contrast, varies little in relation to food intake and is a major function of the liver cells. Indeed, all the plasma albumin and most of its globulins, other than the gammaglobulins, are produced

there.

Globulins made in the liver, often exclusively, include all the coagulation factors and inhibitors of coagulation except the von Willebrand factor, many of the components of the complement system, transport proteins such as transferrin and haptoglobin and proteins with uncertain physiological function such as caeruloplasmin, α-fetoprotein, α_2-macroglobulin and α_1-antitrypsin. The result of this extensive synthetic activity is that the electrophoretic pattern of the plasma proteins is largely determined by liver function.

Lipid metabolism. Most dietary fat enters the body in chylomicrons (Fig. 10.2). Triglyceride is removed from the chylomicrons by lipoprotein lipase in the blood; the triglyceride is taken up by many tissues and the chylomicron remnants are removed by the liver. Triglyceride taken up by the liver is broken down to 2-carbon fragments which may be used in many metabolic processes. Free (non-esterified) fatty acids, liberated from

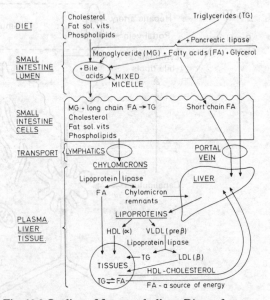

Fig. 10.2 Outline of fat metabolism. Dietary fat occurs largely in the form of long-chain triglycerides which are hydrolysed by pancreatic lipase to monoglyceride and fatty acids which are then made soluble and absorbed as micelles. In the cells of the small intestine monoglycerides and fatty acids are re-esterified into triglycerides which are coated with phospholipids to form chylomicrons to be transported by the lymphatics to the blood. Their metabolism thereafter is described on page 000.

the fat stores into the blood, are also taken up by the liver and used similarly.

Among these processes is the synthesis of new lipid molecules — triglyceride, phospholipid and cholesterol — which are combined with specific apoproteins to form lipoproteins which are released into the blood. These include very low density (pre β) lipoproteins (VLDL) and high density (α) lipoproteins (HDL). VLDL are converted by lipoprotein lipase in the blood to low density (β) lipoproteins (LDL) which transport triglyceride to muscles and other tissues as a source of energy or to the fat depots for storage. The functions of HDL are uncertain, but they may be important in cholesterol transport. The liver synthesises more cholesterol than any other organ and this can be incorporated into lipoproteins, converted into bile acids or excreted into the bile. In biliary obstruction of any severity the serum lipid concentration increases, largely due to the formation of an abnormal lipoprotein known as lipoprotein X.

Bilirubin is produced from the ferroporphyrin, haem, after removal of its iron component. Most (80%) is derived from haemoglobin breakdown by Kupffer cells in the liver and other macrophages in the spleen and bone marrow. The rest is formed by catabolism of other haem-containing proteins, particularly enzymes (e.g. cytochromes, peroxidases, and catalase) and myoglobin. This bilirubin is unconjugated, is bound to albumin in the plasma as it is not water-soluble and does not pass into the urine. It is taken up by hepatocytes, conjugated with glucuronic acid and excreted into the bile. Bilirubin diglucuronide is formed in the microsomes by the enzyme glucuronyl transferase and is water soluble. It is excreted into the bile where it constitutes 80% of the bilirubin. The remaining 20% is bilirubin monoglucuronide, and its origin is uncertain. It is excreted into bile by active transport.

Conjugated bilirubin is not absorbed in the small intestine. Bacteria in the terminal ileum and colon, however, reduce it to a group of colourless chromogens. Most of these (stercobilinogen) are excreted in the stool (100–200 mg/d). Some are absorbed from the gut and pass to the liver where most are re-excreted in the bile; a small amount

(4 mg/d) passes through the liver and is excreted in the urine where it is known as urobilinogen. Urobilinogen and its oxidation product urobilin in the urine are identical, respectively, with stercobilinogen and its oxidation product, stercobilin, in the faeces.

Bile acids. Cholic and chenodeoxycholic acids, the primary bile acids, are produced in the liver from cholesterol. They are conjugated with glycine or taurine and secreted into the bile in which they reach the duodenum. Most (95%) of the bile acids are reabsorbed into the portal blood at specific sites in the terminal ileum; they pass to the liver and are almost completely re-excreted in the bile. Small amounts reach the colon and are metabolised by the colonic bacteria. Deconjugation and changes in the structure of the primary bile acids result in the production of secondary bile acids, deoxycholic acid from cholic acid, and lithocholic acid from chenodeoxycholic acid. Most of the secondary bile acids are excreted in the faeces. However, small amounts are absorbed, reach the liver where they are conjugated with glycine or taurine, and are excreted in the bile. Bile, therefore, contains two primary bile acids — cholic and chenodeoxycholic — and two secondary bile acids — deoxycholic and lithocholic. This *enterohepatic circulation* allows large amounts of bile acid to be delivered to the intestine daily from a relatively small total bile acid pool (6 mmol; 3 g) owing to frequent recycling (10 cycles/d) through the bowel. Synthesis of new bile acid compensates only for that lost in the faeces. The hepatic capacity for bile acid synthesis is limited, and large losses from the bowel cannot be replaced. Little bile acid reaches the systemic circulation normally, but the amount increases in liver disease.

Bile acids, as they enter bile, combine to form micelles (Fig. 10.2). In the small intestine, provided the bile acid concentration remains sufficient to maintain the micellar state, this greatly increases the efficiency of fat absorption. Insufficiency of bile acids results in poor absorption of dietary fat and fat-soluble vitamins, notably vitamins D and K. Such deficiency may result from impaired synthesis in chronic liver disease, biliary obstruction, small intestinal overgrowth of bacteria capable of deconjugating and dehydroxylating bile acids, and loss of bile acids into the colon in disease of the terminal ileum or after its resection. In this last instance, the bile acids interfere with colonic water and electrolyte metabolism causing choleretic diarrhoea, while their absence from the small intestine results in steatorrhoea.

Vitamins and minerals. Several vitamins are stored in the liver; vitamin A, D and B_{12} stores are large whereas vitamin K and folate stores are small and soon disappear if the dietary intake is deficient. The liver can convert tryptophan to nicotinic acid (p. 72), and can activate vitamins as by phosphorylation of thiamin (p. 70), 25-hydroxylation of vitamin D (p. 63) and in the production of tetrahydrofolate. Vitamin K is required by hepatocytes for converting the fully synthesised procoagulants of factors II (prothrombin), VII, IX and X into active coagulation factors. This action at the end of the synthetic process explains why vitamin K does not correct coagulation deficiency due to hepatocellular disease. Normal tissue stores of iron are divided between the liver, striated muscle and the monocyte-macrophage system. Liver iron stores are found in the hepatocytes as ferritin and haemosiderin.

Hormones. The liver is an important site of hormone action and of hormone degradation. Some hormones such as insulin, glucagon, growth hormone, glucocorticoids, oestrogens, and parathormone are catabolised mainly in the liver, while others are mainly catabolised elsewhere.

Drug and alcohol metabolism. The liver is quantitatively the most important organ in drug metabolism. Two factors are particularly significant in this activity — the capacity of the liver to remove drugs from the blood and the capacity to metabolise drugs in the liver cells. The metabolism of drugs which are removed from the blood rapidly (i.e. drugs with a high clearance) depends mainly on hepatic blood flow, while the metabolism of drugs which are removed from the blood more slowly (i.e. drugs with a low clearance) depends mainly on the metabolic activity of the liver cells. Toxicity due to drugs with a high clearance is particularly likely whenever liver blood flow is reduced as in shock, cardiac failure, hepatic cirrhosis and in the elderly.

Most drugs metabolised are fat-soluble and their conversion into water-soluble substances makes them suitable for excretion in bile or urine. These conversions are carried out by enzymes of low specificity located in the microsomes. Two types of reaction occur; first, oxidation, reduction, or hydroxylation reactions, and second, conjugation reactions in which glucuronides are usually produced. Methylation, acetylation, sulphation and amino-acid conjugation may also occur.

The pharmacological results of drug metabolism vary. Barbiturates undergo oxidation with loss of activity; cyclophosphamide is metabolised from an inactive substance to an active alkylating agent; phenylbutazone is oxidised to another active agent, oxyphenbutazone; and codeine is converted in part to morphine. Conjugation, as occurs with salicylates, paracetamol and morphine, almost always causes loss of activity. Acetylation of sulphonamides makes them less soluble and therefore potentially more likely to crystallise in the urinary tract. When two drugs are being metabolised simultaneously by the same microsomal enzymes, each retards the metabolism of the other, leading to prolongation of drug action and the danger of overdosage. This is an example of one mechanism causing an undesirable drug interaction in therapy.

The action of many drugs is determined largely by their speed of metabolism in the microsomal enzyme system, the activity of which may be altered by dietary and hormonal factors. In particular, microsomal enzyme activity may be greatly increased by certain drugs they themselves metabolise, an effect referred to as *enzyme induction,* due to an increase in enzyme protein which disappears when the drug is withdrawn. Drugs producing this effect — 'inducing agents' — are many and include barbiturates, phenylbutazone and phenytoin. Enzyme induction has important therapeutic consequences, for an enzyme inducer such as a barbiturate may increase the required dose of another drug, such as warfarin. By contrast, other drugs such as cimetidine, ketoconazole and isoniazid, reduce microsomal enzyme activity and can cause toxicity from drugs given concurrently.

The liver metabolises about 90% of alcohol (ethanol) ingested, the rest being excreted by the lungs and kidneys. It is oxidised via acetaldehyde to acetate with the eventual formation of carbon dioxide. These reactions are carried out mainly by alcohol dehydrogenase, a mitochondrial enzyme, and the microsomal ethanol oxidising system. The last, like other microsomal enzymes such as γ-GT (p. 333) may be induced by drugs, including alcohol itself, and this may in part account for increased alcohol tolerance in drinkers and for their resistance to the action of micro-somally metabolised drugs. Conversely, the effects of alcohol may be enhanced when a microsomally metabolised drug such as chlormethiazole is taken concomitantly; this is a very important example of drug interaction.

Liver blood flow and the capacity to metabolise drugs can be impaired in liver disease, and care is needed to avoid overdosage, particularly with sedative drugs. The extent to which individual drugs are affected is very variable and cannot be predicted. Special care should, therefore, be taken whenever hepatic damage is present, particularly where there is evidence of severe liver damage, such as jaundice, ascites, encephalopathy, hypo-albuminaemia or a prolonged prothrombin time. Patients who have had a portal-systemic shunt are particularly sensitive to drugs, taken orally, which are normally highly cleared by the liver.

Function of the monocyte-macrophage system. Approximately 20% of the hepatic cell mass is composed of monocytes and macrophages (Kupffer cells). These cells destroy effete erythro-cytes and remove bacteria from the blood. They also have important but poorly understood im-munological functions. Antigens from the gut normally gain repeated access to the body. They are carried in the portal blood to the liver where the Kupffer cells phagocytose them and prevent their eliciting immunological responses. Kupffer cells are also very efficient at removing immune complexes from the blood. The liver, therefore, is able to prevent and suppress undesir-able immunological reactions.

Age and the liver. Hepatic structure and function alters gradually during life, and signifi-cant changes have occurred in those surviving beyond the age of about 70 years. The liver gradually gets smaller, both absolutely and in relation to the rest of the body due mainly to a reduction in the number of hepatocytes, and liver blood flow falls to about half its normal level in the elderly due in part to a fall in cardiac output. The potential for toxic reactions to drugs metab-olised by the liver is therefore probably increased. The values for liver function tests remain within normal adult ranges. The liver in the elderly is probably no more susceptible to disease than in younger people, but its reserve is less and this may be an important cause of the increased mortality of acute liver diseases in older people.

THE INVESTIGATION OF LIVER DISEASE

The reference values related to the investigations discussed in this section are given in Tables 21.3 and 21.4 (pp. 814 and 816).

Liver function tests

The term 'liver function tests' refers to a group of biochemical investigations useful in confirming that the liver is diseased, in indicating whether hepatic cells (parenchymal liver disease) or the biliary tree (obstructive or cholestatic liver dis-ease) is primarily involved, in giving an indication of the extent of liver damage and in assessing progress. The term is misleading in that many of the investigations do not measure liver functions and most liver functions are not tested in clinical practice; however, the term has become generally accepted. Liver function tests are variably abnor-mal in patients with liver disease and therefore a group of tests is usually done. It is important to realise that there are no patterns of abnormality indicative of specific diagnoses and that normality of all the commonly used tests does not prove that the liver is normal.

Bilirubin. Almost all bilirubin normally pre-sent in the blood is unconjugated. Unconjugated hyperbilirubinaemia without any abnormality of other liver function tests may result from increased bilirubin production, as in haemolysis or ineffective erythropoiesis, or from inability to transport bilirubin across the liver, as in Gilbert's syndrome. Except in the newborn, the hyperbili-rubinaemia rarely exceeds 100 μmol/l (6 mg/dl), and there is no bilirubin in the urine. Conjugated hyperbilirubinaemia without any abnormality of other liver function tests, as in the rare Dubin-Johnson syndrome, is accompanied by bilirubinuria but is uncommon.

Estimates of unconjugated and conjugated bilirubin in the blood are hardly ever necessary, and cannot be done accurately when the total serum bilirubin is less than 70 μmol/l (4 mg/dl) using generally available methods. Hyperbilirubinaemia in hepatobiliary disease is predominantly conjugated, bilirubinuria is present, and other tests of liver function are almost always abnormal. The serum bilirubin in parenchymal liver disease varies widely depending on the severity of the disease and its activity. Very high concentrations occur most frequently in biliary tract obstruction, with sustained high levels where this is due to malignant disease and more fluctuating levels where obstruction is caused by gallstones. The serum bilirubin reflects the depth of jaundice and repeated estimations may be useful in following the progress of disease.

Simple, sensitive, inexpensive dip-stick tests for bilirubin in the urine are available and useful. Unconjugated bilirubin is bound to albumin in the blood and does not pass into the urine and conjugated bilirubin is not detectable in the urine of normal persons. Consequently, bilirubinuria implies a conjugated hyperbilirubinaemia and points to hepatobiliary disease. Conversely, absence of bilirubinuria in a jaundiced patient suggests haemolysis, ineffective erythropoiesis or a congenital non-haemolytic hyperbilirubinaemia such as Gilbert's syndrome.

Urobilinogen. A dip-stick test is available to detect excessive urobilinogenuria. There is normally a diurnal variation in the urinary output of urobilinogen, maximal excretion occurring in the afternoon when tests are best performed. Since it is readily oxidised to urobilin on exposure to air at room temperature, only fresh urine samples should be used. Excess urinary urobilinogen occurs in haemolytic diseases owing to increased bilirubin excretion leading to increased urobilinogen formation; in these patients bilirubinuria is not present. Any cause of hepatic dysfunction including pyrexia and cardiac failure, or partial biliary obstruction will reduce the biliary re-excretion of urobilinogen and increase its excretion in the urine; bilirubinuria may or may not be present. No urobilinogen is found in the urine in complete biliary obstruction.

Enzymes. Liver cells contain many enzymes which may be released into the blood in various pathological processes. Measurement of the activity of these enzymes in the blood may give evidence of hepatocellular disease and of its general nature. In practice, maximal information may be obtained by measuring the activity of relatively few enzymes. It must be remembered in interpreting the results of these tests that none of the enzymes usually measured is specific to the liver and alternative sources should be considered, particularly where abnormalities have been found incidentally in patients with no clinical evidence of liver disease.

Aminotransferases. The two important enzymes in this group are aspartate aminotransferase, AST (formerly known as glutamic oxaloacetic transaminase, GOT) and alanine aminotransferase, ALT (glutamic pyruvic transaminase, GPT); both are present in the cytosol of the hepatocytes, the former also being found in the mitochondria. Normal serum contains low enzyme activity the source of which is unknown. Irrespective of the cause, whenever liver cells are damaged or killed the enzymes are liberated into the blood; this is therefore a test of the integrity of the liver cells. The highest activities are caused by any form of acute liver damage.

In viral hepatitis there is generally increased activity even in the prodromal phase and maximal levels of 10 to 100 times the normal value are usually reached in the jaundiced phase after which activity falls rapidly. Equally high activity occurs in acute hepatitis due to drugs, in acute circulatory failure and in exacerbations of chronic active hepatitis. Most patients (80%) with infectious mononucleosis or cytomegaloviral infection also have an acute hepatitis with serum aminotransferase activity raised 2 to 10 times but few develop jaundice. Hepatic damage due to paracetamol produces particularly high activities of 100 to 500 times the normal value. Serum aminotransferase activity rarely rises more than five-fold in acute alcoholic hepatitis. Patients with cirrhosis usually show only modest elevations of serum aminotransferase. In obstructive jaundice, activity may rise up to five-fold but rarely more unless cholangitis is present.

Increased serum aminotransferase activity is a very sensitive index of hepatic damage. Neither enzyme is specific to the liver, but as alanine aminotransferase is found there in much higher concentration that in other organs, increases in its activity indicate more specifically that hepatic damage is present. These enzymes are of principal value in the diagnosis of acute hepatitis and in differentiating hepatocellular from obstructive jaundice. They are of no prognostic value in either acute or chronic liver disease.

Alkaline phosphatase. This enzyme occurs in almost all tissues; in liver cells it is situated principally in the canalicular and sinusoidal membranes. Normal serum contains alkaline phosphatase activity derived mainly from bone and liver, and to a lesser extent intestine; in pregnancy additional activity of placental origin is found. When hepatocytes are damaged, relatively little alkaline phosphatase is liberated into the blood, most probably coming from cells which are killed. In hepatocellular disease, either acute or chronic, alkaline phosphatase does not usually rise more than two and a half fold. When the biliary tract is obstructed at any level, new alkaline phosphatase is synthesised in the hepatocyte membrane much of which escapes into the blood. A greatly increased blood alkaline phosphatase activity is, therefore, the main indicator of biliary obstruction though it does not give any information regarding the site of that obstruction. The alkaline phosphatase activity has no prognostic significance in liver disease.

Sometimes a raised blood alkaline phosphatase activity may be found incidentally and may be the sole abnormality. Hepatobiliary disease may be present, but it is important to ensure that the alkaline phosphatase does not have an extrahepatic origin before investigating the liver further. This may be done by electrophoretic separation of the isoenzymes of alkaline phosphase or by finding abnormal activities of enzymes more specific for the liver such as γ-glutamyl transferase or 5′ nucleotidase. Bone is the main alternative origin of a raised serum alkaline phosphatase; it results from increased osteoblastic activity, such as occurs in adolescents when it may increase up to two and a half fold, in Paget's disease, rickets, hyperparathyroidism, and in metastatic tumour in bone. Myelomatosis, though affecting bone extensively, is not associated with much bone repair, and the blood alkaline phosphatase is not usually raised. During the third trimester of pregnancy, alkaline phosphatase of placental origin may increase the serum activity up to two and a half fold.

Gamma-glutamyl transferase (γ-GT). This is a microsomal enzyme which is distributed widely in body tissues. Increased serum γ-GT activity is a sensitive index of liver abnormality. The highest activities occur in biliary obstruction, but marked increases also occur in acute parenchymal damage from any cause. In practice, γ-GT measurements give little information in patients with liver disease beyond that provided by transferase and alkaline phosphatase measurements. Serum γ-GT activity is also increased by microsomal enzyme inducing agents such as alcohol and various drugs. Increased γ-GT activity can therefore be used to detect and follow alcohol abuse in patients with little or no other abnormality of liver function provided they are not taking enzyme-inducing drugs. Increased γ-GT activity due to alcohol implies prolonged intake of more than about 60 g alcohol daily; normal γ-GT activity does not exclude prolonged intake above that level.

Plasma proteins. *Albumin* is synthesised solely in the liver. In chronic liver disease, especially cirrhosis, the serum albumin concentration is frequently low. Impaired albumin synthesis can be the cause, but this is not invariably so and other factors such as malnutrition, fever and the dilutional effect of fluid retention with ascites may be important. Low serum albumin concentrations in general detect patients with more severe liver damage, and a falling concentration is a bad prognostic sign especially when there is no ascites. Serum albumin has a long half-life (20–26 days) and consequently changes in concentration occur slowly. Thus, even in severe acute hepatitis, the serum albumin remains normal unless the illness continues for many weeks.

Globulins. It is characteristic of chronic liver disease that hyperglobulinaemia occurs in addition to hypoalbuminaemia; it may be found irrespective of changes in the serum albumin concentration in prolonged viral hepatitis or chronic active hepatitis. Once established, hyper-globulinaemia tends to persist in patients with cirrhosis. It represents a reaction of the monocyte–macrophage system in general and does not directly reflect liver cell damage.

The causes of hyperglobulinaemia are not fully understood; increases in gammaglobulins are prominent and probably reflect an increased activity of the immune system, to which many factors may contribute. In those with hypoalbumin-aemia it may represent a response to a reduced colloid osmotic pressure in the plasma. Individual immunoglobulins are variably increased, IgG mainly in chronic active hepatitis and cryptogenic cirrhosis, IgA mainly in alcoholic liver disease and IgM in primary biliary cirrhosis. Variations, however, are so frequent that Ig measurements are not of much diagnostic value.

Plasma protein electrophoresis. Various changes occur in the electrophoretic pattern of the plasma proteins in cirrhosis. The commonest are a decreased albumin and an increased gammaglobu-lin peak. There is some relation between certain electrophoretic patterns and particular forms of liver disease, but this is not precise enough to be of diagnostic value.

Coagulation factors. Severe liver damage impairs the production of several coagulation factors. This is most readily detected by the one stage prothrombin time which depends, among other things, on coagulation factors II, VII and X of liver origin. As the plasma concentration of any one of these factors has to fall to less than 30% of normal before the prothrombin time becomes abnormal, prolongation in chronic liver disease indicates severe liver dysfunction. Further-more, as the normal plasma half-life of these factors is short (5–72 hours), prothrombin time changes occur relatively quickly after liver damage and abnormalities are found in severe acute hepa-titis. Indeed, in acute hepatitis, such as viral hepatitis, the prothrombin time is a most valuable prognostic guide; an abnormal value indicates severe damage and an increasing prothrombin time indicates a progressively worse prognosis.

Bromsulphthalein (BSP) clearance. Estimation of BSP clearance from the blood is a sensitive test for hepatic dysfunction. However, the test is invalid in jaundiced patients, gives misleading results in elderly, febrile or hypo-albuminaemic patients and serious sensitivity reactions to BSP occur occasionally. These factors and the high sensitivity of enzymic tests for hepatic abnormality have led to the virtual aban-donment of the BSP test. It remains of value in the diagnosis of the Dubin-Johnson syndrome (p. 340); blood concentrations of BSP are meas-ured 45 min and 120 min after injection and a higher value at 120 min confirms the diagnosis.

Reference values. Tables 21.3 and 21.4 (pp. 814 and 816).

Other investigations of liver disease

Hepatitis A virus antigens and antibodies. Only one antigen has been found associated with the hepatitis A virus (HAV), and individuals infected with the HAV make an antibody to this antigen (anti-HAV). Anti-HAV can be found in the blood early in the clinical illness, and certainly by the time jaundice develops. It is very important in diagnosis as the HAV cannot be found readily in the blood or faeces. The mere presence of the antibody is not enough for diagnosis, as HAV infection is common in all communities and anti-body to it persists for years after infection. It is anti-HAV of IgM type, indicating a primary immune response, which is diagnostic of a recent infection; these titres fall to low levels after about 3 months. Anti-HAV (IgG) measurements can be used in studies of the prevalence of hepatitis A viral infection.

Hepatitis B virus antigens and antibodies. The hepatitis B virus (p. 344) contains several antigens to which infected persons can make immune responses. These antigens and their anti-bodies are important in identifying hepatitis B viral infection (Fig. 10.3). The hepatitis B surface antigen (HBsAg) is located in the capsular material of the virus; it can be identified by sensitive haemagglutination and radio-immunoassay meth-ods and is a reliable marker of hepatitis B viral infection. A negative test for the HBsAg makes hepatitis B virus infection very unlikely but does not exclude it (see below). It appears in the blood late in the incubation period or in the prodromal phase of acute type B hepatitis; it may be present for only a few days, disappearing even before jaundice has developed, but it usually lasts for 3–4 weeks or may persist up to 3 months. It should therefore be sought as soon as possible in acute hepatitis. Antibody to HBsAg (anti-HBs) usually appears after about 3 months and persists for many years or perhaps permanently. The presence of anti-HBs implies only that infection has occurred at some time; seroconversion alone indicates recent infection.

The hepatitis B core antigen (HBcAg) is located in the central part of the virus and is not found in the blood. However, antibody to the core antigen (anti-HBc) appears early in the illness, rapidly reaches a high titre, and then subsides gradually. Anti-HBc is initially of IgM type and IgG antibody appears later. Anti-HBc of IgM type can sometimes reveal an acute hepatitis B viral infection when the HBsAg has disappeared and before anti-HBs has developed (Figure 10.3). The central part of the virus contains another antigen, the hepatitis Be antigen (HBeAg), which appears only transiently at the outset of the illness and is followed by the production of antibody (anti-HBe). The presence of HBeAg reflects active replication of the virus in the liver.

About 5–10% of patients become chronic carriers of the hepatitis B virus after acute type B hepatitis, and they continue indefinitely with HBsAg and anti-HBc in the blood. Rarely anti-HBc alone is the sole evidence of chronic infection. In some cases the HBeAg or anti-HBe is also present (p. 344). Some healthy persons and a variable proportion of patients with chronic hepatitis (p. 351), cirrhosis (p. 353), or hepatocellular carcinoma (p. 361) are also chronic carriers of the virus. Any chronic viral carrier can transmit hepatitis, and the risk is greatest for those with chronic liver disease or with the HBeAg in the blood. The risk of transmitting infection is low for healthy carriers who have anti-HBe and close bodily contact or direct inoculation of infected blood or other body fluids is generally required.

Hepatitis B antigens and their antibodies can be used to study the epidemiology of hepatitis B virus infection.

Delta virus. This virus contains a single antigen (delta antigen) to which infected individuals make an antibody (anti-delta). Delta antigen appears in the blood only transiently, and in practice diagnosis depends on detecting anti-delta. Simultaneous infection with the hepatitis B virus and delta virus followed by full recovery is associated with the appearance of low titres of anti-delta of IgM type within a few days of the onset of the illness. This antibody generally disappears within about 2 months but persists in a few patients. Superinfection of patients with chronic hepatitis B virus infection leads to the production of high titres of anti-delta, initially IgM and later IgG. Such patients may then develop chronic infection with both viruses in which case anti-delta titres plateau at high levels.

Other viruses. Cytomegalovirus and the Epstein Barr virus (infectious mononucleosis) are occasional causes of acute hepatitis and infection can be detected by serological tests. There are no tests for non-A, non-B hepatitis viral infection.

Autoantibodies. Three autoantibodies in the blood are important in liver disease; antinuclear antibody, smooth muscle antibody and antimitochondrial antibody. Antinuclear and antimitochondrial antibodies also occur in connective tissue diseases and in autoimmune diseases, including various thyroid disorders and pernicious anaemia, while smooth muscle antibody has

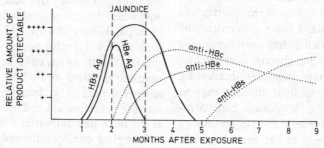

Fig. 10.3 Serological response to hepatitis B virus.

been reported in infectious mononucleosis and in a variety of malignant diseases. In liver disease, smooth muscle antibody, and to a lesser extent antinuclear antibody, may occur transiently and at low titre in acute viral hepatitis. The autoantibodies are, however, more important in chronic liver disease where they are often present for long periods and at relatively high titres. They are found particularly in chronic active hepatitis, cryptogenic cirrhosis and primary biliary cirrhosis. These autoantibodies have not previously been considered specific for liver disease, but there is increasing evidence that the antimitochondrial antibody is very strongly associated with primary biliary cirrhosis. Patients with connective tissue or autoimmune disease found to have this antibody usually prove to have asymptomatic primary biliary cirrhosis. In a patient with cholestasis, the antimitochondrial antibody is of particular value in indicating that primary biliary cirrhosis is present. Antimitochondrial antibody occurs in primary biliary cirrhosis in 95% of cases and in less than 1% of patients with obstruction of the large biliary ducts. An antimicrosomal antibody has also been described which may become important in certain forms of chronic active hepatitis. None of the autoantibodies damages liver tissue, and they are therefore unlikely to have aetiological importance.

Alpha-fetoprotein is made mainly by the fetal liver, production falling to low levels after birth. It is detected best by radioimmunoassay. The reappearance of substantial serum concentrations in adult life is almost always due to a hepatocellular carcinoma, though rarely it may be associated with other tumours, for example of the testis (p. 103). Such substantial serum concentrations can be detected in a quarter to a third of patients with hepatocellular carcinoma in Europe and North America, and in up to three-quarters of those in Africa and Asia. Lesser concentrations occur in 90% of all patients, but sometimes also in acute viral hepatitis and in chronic liver disease, particularly chronic active hepatitis. Increasing concentrations in chronic liver disease suggest hepatocellular carcinoma. Increased concentrations in the blood and amniotic fluid in pregnancy are associated with defects of the neural tube in the fetus.

Caeruloplasmin is a copper-containing globulin produced by the liver. It is important in the diagnosis of Wilson's disease in which serum concentrations are low or undetectable. Low levels may also occur in fulminant hepatic failure and in other advanced and severe chronic liver diseases, as well as in protein-losing enteropathy and malabsorption.

Copper concentrations in the liver are very high in Wilson's disease (p. 359), whereas the serum copper is low and the urine copper high. Liver copper concentrations are also high in any condition associated with prolonged biliary obstruction such as primary biliary cirrhosis.

Iron and ferritin. The serum iron concentration and the saturation of the serum iron-binding capacity are usually high when the body iron stores are increased. A high serum iron and a highly saturated iron-binding capacity in chronic liver disease suggests haemochromatosis but is not sufficient for a diagnosis as similar results occur in chronic alcoholic liver disease. The serum ferritin concentration reflects the total body iron more closely and is increased greatly in haemochromatosis. It is also the best single indication of iron overload in the asymptomatic relatives of patients. These tests can be used to follow the effects of venesection therapy. Haemochromatosis is excluded when they are all normal.

Alpha$_1$-antitrypsin deficiency, detectable by absence of the α_1 peak on serum protein electrophoresis, is a well-established cause of liver disease in infancy and childhood. Rarely, it can cause cirrhosis or emphysema (p. 346) in adults, and occasionally both diseases occur together.

Investigative procedures in liver disease.

Investigative procedures are designed to determine the site and nature of structural lesions in the liver and biliary tree and they should be used only when there is clinical or biochemical evidence of hepatobiliary disease. They range in general from the less invasive but less specific to the more specific but more invasive, and from those which examine the liver as a whole to those which look at only a part of it. Imaging is the best way of starting investigation and ultrasound has emerged as the most generally useful method.

Imaging can identify and localise disease but cannot often make specific diagnoses which require further investigations as outlined in Figure 10.4.

Ultrasonography requires a skilled operator but is particularly safe and comfortable for the patient and can be repeated as required. Its greatest single use is in examining the biliary tract in obstructive jaundice. Dilatation of the bile ducts implies a mechanical obstruction in a large duct while normal bile ducts in a patient with obvious jaundice makes a mechanical cause unlikely. Ultrasound can also be used to identify focal liver diseases such as tumours, abscesses and cysts, provided they are more than about 2 cm in diameter, and can identify more generalised liver diseases such as cirrhosis. Dilatation of the portal or hepatic veins may be seen in portal hypertension or in hepatic venous obstruction. The sensitivity of ultrasound in showing liver disease is about the same as radionuclide imaging.

Radionuclide imaging has the advantage of simplicity and is usually performed with technetium (^{99m}Tc) sulphur colloid which is taken up by the monocyte-macrophage system. It is most useful for detecting focal hepatic diseases. The uptake of colloid by the liver is much reduced when liver function is poor. The combination of an impaired patchy uptake of colloid by the liver, an increased uptake by an enlarged spleen and increased uptake by the bone marrow is very suggestive of advanced cirrhosis with portal hypertension.

Computed tomography can be used for the same purposes as ultrasound and has about the same sensitivity in detecting disease. It is unnecessarily complex for most purposes.

Magnetic resonance imaging can also be used but its value is still uncertain and it is not available widely.

Cholescintigraphy (p. 364) is a means of imaging the biliary tract using radionuclides.

Biliary radiology may be required in patients with liver disease, especially in those presenting with jaundice. Percutaneous transhepatic cholangiography (p. 364) and ERCP (p. 274) are of most value. Oral cholecystography and intravenous cholangiography (p. 364) are of no value in jaundiced patients.

Angiography. Hepatic arteriography can define the site and nature of localised liver lesions and is essential in planning hepatic surgery. Superior mesenteric arteriography can be used as a relatively safe way of examining the portal vein once contrast has passed into the venous circulation. Splenoportography and transhepatic portography can also be used to investigate the portal venous system but are now generally reserved for the investigation of portal hypertension prior to the construction of portal-systemic shunts. The portal venous pressure can be measured at splenoporto graphy or direct portography and by catheterising the hepatic veins, as the wedged hepatic venous pressure closely reflects the portal venous pressure in cirrhosis. Hepatic venography can be used to identify hepatic venous obstruction.

Paracentesis. Analysis of ascites may give useful information. In cirrhosis, the fluid is clear, the protein content usually below 30 g/l, and in the absence of infection there are less than 250 cells/mm^3. Blood-stained ascites is usually due to

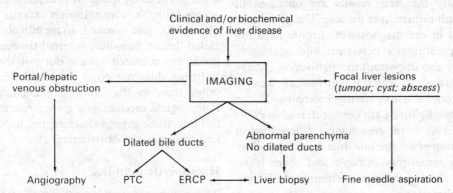

Fig. 10.4 Investigative procedures in liver disease. Suggested sequence for identifying structural lesions in the liver and biliary tract. ERCP = endoscopic retrograde cholangio-pancreatography; PTC = percutaneous transhepatic cholangiography.

malignant disease, and milky (chylous) ascites to obstruction of the cisterna chyli. Ascitic protein concentrations above 30 g/l occur in peritoneal infection, especially tuberculosis, peritoneal tumour, hepatic venous obstruction and ascites associated with pancreatic disease. Amylase activity is high in ascites caused by pancreatitis. Infections, such as spontaneous bacterial peritonitis (p. 310) or tuberculosis, can be identified by bacteriological examination and malignancy by cytology.

Liver biopsy is a relatively safe procedure in the hands of an experienced clinician. It is carried out with a special needle, usually through an intercostal space, using local analgesia. It requires a co-operative patient who will stop breathing when the biopsy is actually taken. The haemostatic mechanisms must be intact as indicated by the prothrombin time and platelet count. After the procedure, the patient remains in bed for 24 hours, regular pulse and blood pressure measurements must be recorded and blood for transfusion (2 units) should be available. The main complications are abdominal and/or shoulder pain, bleeding and, rarely, biliary peritonitis which usually occurs when there is obstruction of a large bile duct. Liver biopsy should never be done lightly as the mortality rate is about 0.05%.

Liver biopsies can be carried out in patients with defective haemostasis if this can be corrected with fresh frozen plasma and platelets or if the biopsy is obtained by the transjugular route or percutaneously under radiological control with subsequent plugging of the needle track with gelfoam.

Biopsy yields only a small sample of liver and consequently the best results are obtained in patients with diffuse liver disease. The procedure is essential in the diagnosis of chronic hepatitis and in separating its persistent and aggressive forms. It is also important in establishing a diagnosis of cirrhosis in which it may indicate a cause such as alcohol abuse or haemochromatosis.

Other investigations are now preferred in cholestasis (p. 339) as the histological differentiation of obstruction of a large bile duct from other liver diseases is sometimes difficult and there is an increased risk of biliary peritonitis following biopsy in cholestasis.

Biopsy is not usually required in acute hepatitis in which the diagnosis can normally be made on other grounds; it may be needed, however, in atypical cases. Localised disease, particularly malignancy is less accurately diagnosed unless the site of disease is first identified by one of the imaging methods, usually ultrasound. Operative liver biopsy may sometimes be valuable, as in the staging of lymphoma.

Fine needle aspiration of focal lesions in the liver can be carried out using fine-bore needles (20 to 22 gauge) guided usually by ultrasound. This can be done with minimal discomfort or risk provided the haemostatic mechanisms are satisfactory. Aspirated material is examined cytologically and histologically. The method is particularly useful for the diagnosis of tumours.

Laparoscopy can be performed under local analgesia or general anaesthesia and involves the creation of a pneumoperitoneum. The laparoscope provides an excellent view of the anterior and superior surfaces of the liver as well as some of its inferior aspect and the gall bladder. The spleen, the prominent blood vessels of portal hypertension and evidence of peritoneal disease may also be seen. Biopsies can be taken directly from diseased areas which is valuable in focal disorders, especially malignant disease. The main contraindications are haemostatic abnormalities, marked ascites and previous surgery which may have caused adhesions.

JAUNDICE

Jaundice is a clinical term referring to the yellow appearance of the skin and mucous membranes resulting from an increased bilirubin concentration in the body fluids. It is detectable when the serum bilirubin concentration exceeds 50 μmol/l (3 mg/dl); less marked hyperbilirubinaemia is called 'latent' jaundice. Internal tissues and body fluids are coloured yellow but not the brain as bilirubin does not cross the blood-brain barrier other than in the immediate neonatal period. Pathological mechanisms giving rise to jaundice fall into three groups: haemolytic, hepatocellular and cholestatic or obstructive.

Haemolytic jaundice

This results from an increased rate of destruction of red blood cells causing the production of more bilirubin. As a healthy liver can excrete a bilirubin load six times greater than normal before unconjugated bilirubin accumulates in the plasma, jaundice due to haemolysis is usually mild. Exceptions to this occur in the newborn when the hepatic bilirubin transport mechanism is immature and in patients with liver disease.

Increased bilirubin excretion leads to more stercobilinogen in the stools and to increased urobilinogen in the urine as more of this substance is absorbed from the gut. The urine rapidly becomes deep yellow on standing due to urobilin formation, and in the absence of biliary obstruction the stools are dark in colour. Pallor due to anaemia and splenomegaly due to excessive reticuloendothelial activity are usually present.

The serum bilirubin is usually less than 100 μmol/l (6 mg/dl) and the liver function tests are otherwise normal. There is no bilirubinuria because the hyperbilirubinaemia is dominantly unconjugated. Haemolysis may be due to intrinsic defects of the red blood cells or to various extracorpuscular factors (p. 511).

Hepatocellular jaundice

Hepatocellular jaundice results from inability of the liver to transport bilirubin into the bile as a result of liver cell damage. Bilirubin transport across the hepatocytes may be impaired at any point between uptake of unconjugated bilirubin into the cells and transport of conjugated bilirubin into the canaliculi. In addition, swelling of cells and oedema resulting from the disease itself may cause obstruction of the intrahepatic biliary tree. In hepatocellular jaundice the concentrations in the blood of both unconjugated and conjugated bilirubin increase, perhaps because of the variable way in which bilirubin transport is disturbed.

Acute parenchymal liver diseases, usually due to the hepatitis viruses or to drugs or alcohol (p. 341), are common causes. Immature bilirubin transport mechanisms in the newborn, especially in prematurity, and congenital defects in bilirubin transport (p. 340) are very specific metabolic defects in the liver cell causing jaundice. Chronic hepatitis and cirrhosis can also cause hepatocellular jaundice.

The clinical features vary depending on the underlying diseases. Jaundice ranges from mild to very severe.

Cholestatic jaundice

Cholestasis is a failure of bile flow, and its cause may lie anywhere between the hepatocyte and the duodenum. Jaundice becomes progressively severe in unrelieved cholestasis because conjugated bilirubin is unable to enter the bile canaliculi and also because there is a failure of clearance of unconjugated bilirubin arriving at the liver cell.

Aetiology. Causes of cholestatic jaundice are classified according to their site in the biliary tree. They can be situated in the large bile ducts, where they may be amenable to surgical treatment, or in the smaller intrahepatic bile ducts.

Large duct obstruction. The most common causes are impaction of a gallstone in the common bile duct and carcinoma of the head of the pancreas. Other causes include carcinomas of the papilla of Vater or bile duct, strictures of the bile duct (usually the result of previous surgery), metastatic tumours impinging on the bile ducts, sclerosing cholangitis and, very rarely, involvement of the common bile duct by a duodenal ulcer. Helminths occasionally migrate into the bile ducts and cause obstruction (p. 79).

Small duct obstruction. Widespread small duct obstruction is required to produce cholestatic jaundice. Drugs and alcohol are important causes which may exert their effects either on the liver cells or on the bile ducts. Other conditions causing obstruction are often primary diseases of the liver cells which also involve the small bile ducts, particularly the biliary canaliculi whose walls are formed by the hepatocytes. Such conditions include the cholestatic episodes which may occur in viral hepatitis, chronic active hepatitis, cirrhosis and the cholestasis of pregnancy. Cholestasis, sometimes with deep jaundice, may also occur for unknown reasons following surgery, in severe bacterial infections and in Hodgkin's lymphoma. Diseases involving the smaller interlobular ducts and the ductules include primary biliary cirrhosis and the pericholangitis of ulcerative colitis. Widespread secondary carcinoma in the liver sometimes produces cholestatic jaundice by impinging on bile ducts.

Clinical features. Apart from the manifestations of the causative disease, there is jaundice which, if prolonged and severe, may give the skin a greenish appearance. The stools are pale or clay-coloured due to deficiency of bilirubin and to steatorrhoea and the urine is dark due to the renal excretion of conjugated bilirubin. Some patients have generalised pruritus and accessible parts of the body may show scratch marks. Anorexia and a metallic taste in the mouth are common. Upper abdominal pain occurs particularly in large duct obstruction by a gallstone or pancreatic carcinoma.

Fever, sometimes with rigors, suggests cholangitis, which occurs most often with gallstone obstruction. A palpable gall bladder is a sign of severe biliary obstruction and is most often due to a carcinoma, usually of the pancreas. A very large and irregular liver indicates hepatic neoplasm. In prolonged obstructive jaundice, xanthomatous skin lesions, especially on the upper eyelids, occasionally appear as well as features due to secondary intestinal malabsorption; these latter include weight loss, a haemorrhagic tendency (vitamin K deficiency) and pain due to bone disease (calcium and vitamin D deficiency). In long-standing cases, clinical and biochemical evidence of biliary cirrhosis and hepatocellular failure can occur.

Congenital non-haemolytic hyperbilirubinaemia

With the exception of Gilbert's syndrome, the congenital abnormalities of bilirubin transport are very rare. In adults they all have an excellent prognosis, need no treatment and are clinically important only because they may be mistaken for more serious liver disease.

Gilbert's syndrome. This common benign condition is usually first recognised in adolescents or young adults. It probably has a varied aetiology, and in some cases is inherited as an autosomal dominant. Gilbert's syndrome generally presents as mild jaundice, occasionally following viral hepatitis from which there has been an otherwise complete recovery, or is found incidentally. Many patients have no symptoms; others suffer episodes of malaise, anorexia and upper abdominal pain, the last occasionally severe, with increases in the jaundice. These episodes may be related to infection, fatigue or fasting.

Apart from mild jaundice, examination is normal. Investigations show unconjugated hyperbilirubinaemia, generally below 100 μmol/l (6 mg/dl), with no abnormality of other liver function tests. No bilirubin is found in the urine. The peripheral blood count, reticulocyte count and the serum haptoglobin concentration are normal, giving no evidence of overt haemolysis.

The liver is normal histologically and a liver biopsy is not necessary unless there is a history suggesting liver disease.

The main cause of the unconjugated hyperbilirubinaemia is a deficiency of hepatic glucuronyl transferase; in some cases uptake of unconjugated bilirubin from the plasma may also be impaired. Glucuronyl transferase activity may be increased by phenobarbitone (60 mg b.d.) which can be used to diminish jaundice and to ameliorate other symptoms.

Crigler-Najjar syndrome. In the Crigler-Najjar syndrome (type I), there is complete absence of glucuronyl transferase from the liver. It causes severe unconjugated hyperbilirubinaemia and kernicterus in the newborn leading to early death, though a few patients have survived to adulthood. This autosomal-recessive condition is very rare. A milder form (type II), due to partial deficiency of the enzyme, also occurs. Jaundice is less severe, kernicterus is rare and most survive to adult life. This condition is autosomal-dominant and is also very rare.

Dubin-Johnson syndrome. This very rare autosomal recessive condition is caused by a reduced ability to transport organic anions, such as bilirubin glucuronide, into the biliary canaliculi. It causes malaise and variable mild jaundice. The hyperbilirubinaemia is of the conjugated type and bilirubin is found in the urine.

Other organic anions which are poorly transported include BSP (p. 334), which can be used to diagnose the condition, and the contrast agents for biliary radiology so that the gall bladder, though normal, is frequently visualised poorly or not at all on cholecystography. Liver biopsy shows a characteristic dark pigment in the centrilobular hepatocytes. The prognosis is excellent.

Rotor syndrome. This very rare condition causes mild jaundice, due to conjugated hyperbilirubinaemia, and bilirubinuria. The liver is normal histologically and BSP clearance is unimpaired. It is probably caused by poor uptake and storage of bilirubin by the liver cells. The prognosis is excellent.

Effect of drugs on bilirubin metabolism

Numerous drugs and chemicals affect bilirubin metabolism. In normal adults, drugs interfering with bilirubin disposal produce only mild hyperbilirubinaemia, sometimes without jaundice, but more marked jaundice may occur where the ability to metabolise bilirubin is impaired. This occurs in the newborn, where hyperbilirubinaemia may become sufficient to cause kernicterus (p. 652), in those with congenital non-haemolytic hyperbilirubinaemia and in patients with chronic liver disease such as cirrhosis. Hyperbilirubinaemia disappears readily when the drug is stopped.

The main sites at which drugs may interfere with bilirubin metabolism are shown in Table 10.1. Sulphonamides and salicylates displace unconjugated bilirubin from the binding sites on serum albumin; given to a newborn child with haemolytic disease or to the mother in late pregnancy, they may precipitate the development of kernicterus without increasing the serum bilirubin. Drugs which raise the serum bilirubin may increase either its unconjugated or conjugated

forms depending on whether they act prior to or at the stage of conjugation or thereafter. Unconjugated hyperbilirubinaemia occurs when drugs produce haemolysis, impair transport from the plasma to the conjugating site or reduce conjugation itself. Conjugated hyperbilirubinaemia occurs when transport of conjugated bilirubin into the biliary canaliculus is impaired; drugs which do this also reduce BSP transport and increase BSP retention in the blood. Inducing agents, such as phenobarbitone, can increase the capacity of the liver to conjugate bilirubin so that patients on long-term treatment with such agents, e.g. epileptics, tend to have low serum bilirubin concentrations.

Oral contraceptives usually contain an oestrogen capable of causing cholestasis and a progestogen. Most preparations currently available contain very small amounts of oestrogen and jaundice is rare. Those who develop jaundice due to oral contraceptives frequently also develop cholestasis of pregnancy and both conditions may reflect an unusual hepatic reaction to a steroid agent. This may have a genetic basis as both conditions show a similar geographic distribution.

ACUTE PARENCHYMAL DISEASE OF THE LIVER

Aetiology. In acute parenchymal liver disease (acute hepatitis) there is a sudden episode of widespread damage in which variable numbers of hepatocytes undergo necrosis. These episodes are

Table 10.1 Effects of drugs on bilirubin metabolism. Sites of action of some drugs *reducing* the plasma protein binding of bilirubin or its uptake, transport, conjugation or excretion by hepatocytes.

Site of action			
Plasma	Hepatocyte		
Protein binding	*Uptake and transport*	*Conjugation**	*Excretion into canaliculus*
Sulphonamides	Rifampicin	Novobiocin	Sulphadiazine
Salicylates	Filix mas		Oral contraceptives
	Cholecystographic media		Methyltestosterone
			Anabolic steroids (C-17α alkyl substituted testosterones)
Unconjugated bilirubin		Conjugated bilirubin	

*Phenobarbitone *increases* conjugation of bilirubin.

due largely to infective or toxic agents.

INFECTIONS. The most important infective causes are the hepatitis A and B viruses, the delta virus and the non-A, non-B viruses. Cytomegalovirus, Epstein Barr virus and yellow fever virus occasionally cause clinically apparent acute hepatitis. Other viruses, however, have been implicated only rarely. Less frequently non-viral agents such as *Leptospira icterohaemorrhagiae* (Weil's disease), *Toxoplasma gondii* (toxoplasmosis) and *Coxiella burneti* (Q fever) may cause acute hepatitis. Bacteria usually produce a liver abscess (p. 362) rather than an acute hepatitis.

TOXIC SUBSTANCES. Most substances causing acute hepatitis are drugs. Usually, liver damage caused by drugs is due to idiosyncratic reactions (i.e. not related to the dose of the drug and occurring in only a few individuals). Among the drugs more commonly responsible are: chlorpromazine and other phenothiazines, phenelzine and other monoamine oxidase inhibitors, imipramine, amitriptyline, erythromycin, isoniazid, rifampicin (and occasionally other antituberculous drugs), halothane, methyldopa, phenylbutazone, indomethacin, chlorpropamide and thiouracil. Liver damage due to drugs is reported increasingly, and any drug should be suspected.

A few drugs cause liver damage in all people in a dose-related manner. These include tetracycline, especially in pregnancy or in those with renal dysfunction, and paracetamol which is often used in self-poisoning.

Potent liver poisons include carbon tetrachloride and yellow phosphorus. Where there are strict rules regarding their use, damage due to these agents is rare. Occasionally severe liver damage occurs from eating poisonous fungi (*Amanita phalloides*). Alcohol is by far the most important liver toxin; in addition to chronic liver damage it may produce acute alcoholic hepatitis.

METABOLIC ABNORMALITY. Acute hepatitis can occur in Wilson's disease (p. 359) and in pregnancy usually during the third trimester.

CIRCULATORY DISTURBANCES. Acute hepatic damage, sometimes sufficient to cause jaundice, may be caused by any form of shock or by right ventricular failure particularly when it is severe or develops rapidly.

Pathology. Lesions found in hepatitis due to viruses and most drugs are similar. Cell damage throughout the liver is the dominant abnormality, particularly in centrilobular areas, though individual lobules are variably affected. Damaged hepatocytes have a swollen granular appearance, while dead ones become shrunken and deeply stained, sometimes losing their nuclei to form eosinophilic Councilman bodies; these bodies, originally described in yellow fever, suggest acute hepatitis. The lobules may be infiltrated with mononuclear cells. Polymorphonuclear leucocytes and fatty change are not seen. The portal tracts are enlarged with a predominantly mononuclear cell infiltrate.

More severe damage is accompanied by collapse of the reticulin framework, particularly between the central veins and portal tracts which become linked to one another; this is known as bridging or subacute hepatic necrosis. Very severe damage results in destruction of whole lobules (massive necrosis) and is the lesion underlying fulminant hepatic failure. Cholestasis is occasionally very prominent.

Sometimes, the main histological abnormality is fatty change. This occurs in damage due to carbon tetrachloride, tetracycline and a number of other direct toxins. Rarely, severe fatty degeneration of the liver is encountered in pregnancy or as a metabolic disturbance in Reye's syndrome in children (p. 347).

VIRAL HEPATITIS

Viral hepatitis is almost always caused by one or other of the hepatitis viruses, namely the A, B, non-A, non-B and delta viruses. Hepatitis due to cytomegalovirus or Epstein Barr virus accounts for only about 1% of cases. Viruses give rise to illnesses which are similar in their clinical and pathological features and which are frequently anicteric or asymptomatic.

Acute type A hepatitis

Aetiology and epidemiology. Type A hepatitis is due to a virus which can now be cultured though currently this is done only for research purposes. It may belong to the picornavirus group of enteroviruses (p. 726). It is highly infectious and is usually spread by human faeces entering the body via the oral route directly or indirectly. Infected persons excrete viruses in the faeces for about 2 weeks before the onset of illness and for 5 to 7 days thereafter. Children are most commonly affected and conditions of overcrowding and poor sanitation facilitate spread. In occasional outbreaks, water, milk and shellfish have been the vehicles of transmission. Though faeces is the usual source, infection can also be spread by blood and by homosexual activity, especially in men. The sources in the community appear to be persons incubating or suffering from the disease; a carrier state, analogous to that for hepatitis B virus, has not been identified. The incubation period of type A hepatitis is about one month.

Clinical features. In the case of average severity, prodromal symptoms precede the development of jaundice by a few days to 2 weeks. They are the usual manifestations of an acute infectious disease, and include chills, headache and malaise. Gastrointestinal symptoms may be prominent; anorexia and distaste for cigarettes are common and early complaints, and nausea, vomiting and diarrhoea may follow. A steady upper abdominal pain occurs as a result of stretching of the peritoneum over the liver as the organ enlarges; the pain is severe in some patients. Initially physical signs are scanty; the liver is usually tender, though not readily palpable, enlarged cervical lymph nodes may be found and splenomegaly may occur, particularly in children.

Dark urine and a yellow tint to the sclerae herald the onset of jaundice. As obstruction to the biliary canaliculi develops, the jaundice deepens, the stools become paler, the urine darker and the liver more easily palpable. At this time the appetite often improves and gastrointestinal symptoms diminish in intensity. Thereafter the jaundice usually recedes, the stools and urine regain their normal colour, the liver enlargement regresses and, in the course of 3 to 6 weeks, the great majority of cases gradually recover.

Milder cases occur or the disease may run an anicteric course which is recognised by known contact with a definite case or by the association of vague gastrointestinal complaints or malaise with bilirubinuria and biochemical evidence of hepatic dysfunction.

Investigation. A serum aminotransferase activity exceeding 400 units/l, even before jaundice develops, is the most striking abnormality. The serum bilirubin reflects the degree of jaundice, the alkaline phosphatase activity rarely exceeds 250 units/l (30 KA units/dl) unless marked cholestasis develops, and the albumin concentration is normal. The prothrombin time is increased in severe cases and in these circumstances is a good guide to prognosis. Bilirubinuria is an early finding, occurring in the prodromal phase and usually continuing into the convalescent period. Urobilinogenuria appears just before jaundice, disappears at the height of the jaundice owing to intrahepatic cholestasis and reappears early in convalescence as a sign of recovery. Mild proteinuria may be present. The while cell count is normal or low in uncomplicated cases, sometimes with a relative lymphocytosis; this is of some value in differentiation from Weil's disease (p. 761). Serological tests allow a specific diagnosis to be made (p. 334).

Differential diagnosis is discussed on page 348.

Course and prognosis. Almost all patients make a full recovery. During convalescence 5–15% relapse with a return of symptoms and signs; these cases of *relapsing hepatitis* almost always subside spontaneously. More frequently, the serum aminotransferase activity increases without any return of clinical illness; these asymptomatic 'biochemical' relapses also subside spontaneously. Either from the onset or during the course of the illness, more severe jaundice of a clinically and biochemically obstructive type may develop and it may follow a prolonged course. Liver biopsy shows the features of hepatitis with prominent cholestasis and no evidence of chronic liver damage. This clinical syndrome is known as *cholestatic viral hepatitis* and, though it may continue for many months, the prognosis is good.

Following clinical and biochemical recovery, debility for 2 to 3 months is common. Sometimes, particularly in anxious patients, there may be prolonged malaise, anorexia, nausea and right hypochondrial discomfort without clinical, biochemical or histological evidence of liver disease. This syndrome, which may be exacerbated by too frequent clinical and biochemical assessment, is known as the *posthepatitis syndrome*; it is not due to liver disease and should be treated by reassurance.

Death from acute type A hepatitis is uncommon. In young adults, the mortality is around 0.2%. With increasing age, however, the frequency of severe episodes and death increases so that over the age of 60 years mortality reaches about 3%. Evidence regarding mortality during pregnancy is conflicting; most reports suggesting an increased mortality are derived from countries in which the standard of living is low. In Europe and North America the mortality in pregnant women is probably not increased. Those who die of the acute illness do so after developing *fulminant hepatic failure* (p. 347). Rarely, *aplastic anaemia* may occur several months after recovery from viral hepatitis. Prolonged carriage of the virus and the development of chronic liver disease are not features of hepatitis A infection.

Treatment and prevention. There is no specific therapy; general measures applicable to all forms of acute hepatitis are discussed on page 349. Although for many years patients have been treated in general medical wards without cross-infection occurring, indicating that isolation is not essential, precautions for preventing the spread of enteric infections are advisable.

The most effective prophylactic measures are to improve social conditions, particularly over-crowded and unhygienic situations. Individuals can be protected from infection for about 3 months by immune serum globulin provided this is given very soon after exposure to the virus. Its use can be considered for those at particular risk such as close contacts, the elderly, those with other major disease and perhaps pregnant women. Prevention can be effective in an outbreak of hepatitis, for example in a school or nursery, as injection of those at risk prevents secondary spread, for example to families. Persons travelling to endemic areas may be protected by immune serum globulin for about 3 months. The protective effect of immune serum globulin is attributed to its anti-HAV content. A vaccine against type A hepatitis virus is not available.

Acute type B hepatitis

Aetiology and epidemiology. Type B hepatitis is due to a virus which cannot yet be grown but which can be transmitted to certain primates, such as the chimpanzee, in which it can replicate. It comprises a capsule and a core containing DNA and a DNA polymerase enzyme. The virus and an excess of its capsular material circulate in the blood where it can be identified (p. 334).

Blood and certain blood products are the main sources of infection. Coagulation factor concentrates which are manufactured from a plasma pool and cannot be sterilised are a particular hazard and account for the high incidence of hepatitis in haemophilia. Only blood products subjected to pasteurisation (albumin solutions, γ-globulin fraction) can be regarded as largely free of risk. Spread may follow transfusion of infected blood or blood products or injections with contaminated needles, a mode of spread most common among parenteral drug abusers who share needles. Tattooing or acupuncture can also spread this disease if inadequately sterilised needles are used.

The ability to identify the hepatitis B virus has shown that it may cause sporadic infections which cannot be attributed to parenteral modes of spread. Infected serum can transmit disease orally and the discovery of the HBsAg or viral DNA in body fluids, such as saliva, urine, semen and vaginal secretions, suggests many alternative modes of spread. Close personal contact seems necessary for transmission of infection and sexual intercourse, especially in male homosexuals, is an important route. Finally, the virus may be spread from mother to child; transmission at or soon after birth seems more likely than transplacental spread. In addition to those incubating or suffering from the disease, some asymptomatic individuals carry the virus in the blood over long periods, perhaps for life.

Individuals with hepatitis B viral disease are not all equally infectious. Patients with acute hepatitis are highly infectious for at least as long as the HBsAg is in the blood. Patients with chronic hepatitis are much more infectious when the HBeAg, viral DNA or DNA polymerase are in the blood and least infectious when the anti-HBe is present.

The incubation period of acute type B hepatitis is about 3 months.

The main pathology is in the liver (p. 342).

Clinical features. The clinical features are

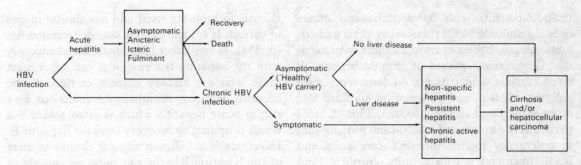

Fig. 10.5 HBV infection. Range of possible clinical outcomes.

similar to, but usually more severe than those of type A hepatitis. Transient rashes, including urticaria, may occur and arthralgia is common in the prodromal period. Though these can occur in type A hepatitis, they are much more suggestive of type B hepatitis. The mortality depends on the virulence of the virus, the age of the patient and any underlying disease. In about 5–10% of cases chronic hepatitis B carriage follows the acute episode.

Some patients may develop diseases of other organs including polyarteritis nodosa, glomerulo-nephritis and, in childhood, papular acroderma-titis. Otherwise complications are as in type A hepatitis. The range of possible sequelae, in contrast, is very different (Fig. 10.5).

Chronic asymptomatic carriers. Some individuals usually with no history of acute hepa-titis and lacking clinical evidence of liver disease are chronic carriers of the hepatitis B virus. They all have the HBsAg and anti-HBc in the blood, some also have the HBeAg and others anti HBe. The frequency of chronic carriers in Western Europe, North America and Australia and New Zealand is about 0.1%, but higher frequencies are found in South America (1–2%), in Mediter-ranean countries and India (3–5%) and in sub-Saharan Africa and the Far East (5–15%). Vertical transmission of the virus from mother to baby at or soon after birth is considered the commonest means of transmission in high incidence areas. Most asymptomatic chronic carriers have normal liver function tests and need not undergo liver biopsy as significant histological abnormalities are uncommon. Persistent biochemical abnormalities

and active liver disease on liver biopsy are more common in those with the HBeAg or DNA polymerase in the blood, and liver biopsy should be considered.

The prognosis for chronic asymptomatic car-riers is uncertain, but the virus can be carried for many years without severe chronic liver disease occurring. Some develop chronic hepatitis and cirrhosis. All are at increased risk of hepatocellular carcinoma, and at least in the Far East the risk for chronic carriers of the virus is some 250 times that of the uninfected population.

Patients with impaired immune responses are very liable to become chronic carriers; this occurs particularly in Hodgkin's disease and other lym-phomas, in those on immunosuppressive drugs, in patients on long-term dialysis, and in institu-tionalised patients with Down's syndrome.

Treatment. No specific treatment is available for acute HBV infection. Chronic infection can be treated in specialist centres with drugs such as interferon when there is HBeAg in the blood and particularly when active liver disease is present. Supportive therapy is described on page 349.

Prevention. Hepatitis B vaccines capable of producing active immunisation in all but about 5% of normal individuals are available. These vaccines are made by purifying HBsAg from the plasma of chronic hepatitis B virus carriers in such a way as to exclude the hepatitis B virus itself. They give a high degree of protection and have proved safe so far, but they are expensive. Vaccination can be considered in those at special risk of infection who are not already immune as evidenced by anti-HBs in the blood. Such persons include patients with haemophilia and others needing multiple blood transfusion, drug addicts, homosexuals, babies born to mothers with hepatitis B infection, spouses of chronic hepatitis B virus carriers, and patients on long-term renal dialysis. Medical and paramedical staff are also often at increased risk of infection. This includes particularly dentists and medical and nursing staff in emergency rooms, intensive care areas and renal, liver and oncology units. Surgeons and obstetricians are obviously also at risk. Laboratory staff are protected best by stringent technical precautions in handling blood products. The vaccine is ineffective in those already infected by the hepatitis B virus.

Type B hepatitis can be prevented or minimised by the intramuscular injection of hyperimmune serum globulin prepared from blood containing anti-HBs. Where available, it should be given within 24 hours, or at the most a week, of exposure to infected blood in circumstances likely to cause infection; these include accidental needle puncture, gross personal contamination with infected blood, oral ingestion or contamination of mucous membranes, or exposure to infected blood in the presence of cuts and grazes. Vaccine can be given together with hyperimmune globulin (active-passive immunisation).

Post-transfusion type B hepatitis can be largely prevented by scrupulous blood transfusion technique, by using volunteer donors and excluding those with a history of jaundice and by screening all blood for the HBsAg. Non-A, non-B hepatitis viruses are now the cause of 90% of post-transfusion hepatitis, though type B virus hepatitis still occurs occasionally. Sterile needles and syringes should always be used and, if disposable equipment is not available, should be autoclaved for 20 minutes at 120°C. Thorough washing followed by boiling in water for 20 minutes is an acceptable emergency procedure. Strict precautions should be observed by all persons involved in handling human blood.

Delta hepatitis

The delta virus is an RNA virus which has no independent existence, depends on the hepatitis

B virus to replicate itself and has similar modes of spread. It is identified by anti-delta antibodies (p. 335). It can infect individuals simultaneously with the hepatitis B virus, or it can superinfect those who are already chronic carriers of the hepatitis B virus. Simultaneous infections give rise to acute hepatitis which is often severe but which is limited by recovery from the hepatitis B. Infections of individuals who are chronic carriers of the hepatitis B virus can cause an episode of acute hepatitis or the development of progressive chronic hepatitis. Those individuals become chronic carriers of the hepatitis B and delta viruses.

Delta virus has a world-wide distribution but is endemic in the Mediterranean basin where it is transmitted mainly by close personal contact and occasionally by vertical transmission from mothers who also carry the hepatitis B virus. Parenteral drug abuse is the main association outside endemic areas.

Non-A, non-B hepatitis

The existence of non-A, non-B hepatitis was recognised once infection with the hepatitis A and B viruses could be excluded by specific serological methods. The responsible agent or agents cannot yet be identified, but they can transmit infection in humans and confer specific immunity. Non-A, non-B hepatitis is diagnosed by excluding hepatitis A and B, cytomegaloviral, and Epstein Barr viral infections. It may cause up to a quarter of sporadic cases of acute viral hepatitis and it is known to cause 90% or more of post-transfusion hepatitis in North America, Europe and Australia and New Zealand. Post-transfusion hepatitis caused by plasma can be virtually eliminated by limiting plasma pool sizes to 10 donors, but this is more difficult to achieve in the production of coagulation factor concentrates which carry a relatively high risk of hepatitis.

Long and short incubation forms of the disease occur, the clinical features are similar to those of type A and type B hepatitis and a chronic carrier state can follow infection. Immune serum globulin, useful in type A hepatitis, may also prevent or ameliorate non-A, non-B hepatitis the contribution of which to the production of chronic liver disease is not yet known.

Fulminant hepatic failure

Fulminant hepatic failure is a rare syndrome in which hepatic encephalopathy, characterised by mental changes progressing from confusion to stupor and coma, results from sudden severe impairment of hepatic function. The syndrome is defined further as occurring within 8 weeks of onset of the precipitating illness, in the absence of evidence of pre-existing liver disease, to distinguish it from those instances in which hepatic encephalopathy represents a deterioration in chronic liver disease.

Aetiology and pathology. Acute viral hepatitis is the commonest cause, drugs (p. 342) being the next most frequent. Rarely, it occurs in pregnancy, in Wilson's disease, following shock or from poisons such as carbon tetrachloride. Reye's syndrome (p. 347) causes fulminant hepatic failure in children and adolescents.

Extensive parenchymal necrosis is the most common lesion (p. 342). In fatal cases, less than 30% of the liver cells appear viable histologically and often few such cells are seen. Severe fatty degeneration is characteristic of fulminant hepatic failure caused by tetracycline, pregnancy and Reye's syndrome.

Clinical features. Cerebral disturbance (encephalopathy) is the cardinal manifestation of fulminant hepatic failure. Its cause is unknown, but it is thought to be due to toxic substances, including ammonia, nitrogenous compounds which may act as false neurotransmitters and fatty acids. The earliest features are reduced alertness and poor concentration progressing through behavioural abnormalities such as restlessness, aggressive outbursts and mania, to drowsiness and coma. Confusion, disorientation, inversion of sleep rhythm, slurred speech, yawning, hiccoughing and, in the late stages, convulsions may occur. More general symptoms include weakness, nausea, and vomiting. Right hypochondrial pain is only an occasional feature.

Examination shows jaundice which develops rapidly and is usually deep in fatal cases. Jaundice is not seen in Reye's syndrome, and sometimes death occurs before it develops in this and other causes of fulminant hepatic failure. Fetor hepaticus, a sweet musty odour to the breath, may be present and is said to be due to methyl mercaptan. A flapping 'hepatic' tremor of the extended hands is characteristic. The liver may be enlarged initially, but later becomes impalpable. Hepatic dullness on percussion may disappear indicating much shrinkage and a bad prognosis. Splenomegaly is uncommon and never prominent. Ascites and oedema occur in a few patients surviving a week or more. Severe haemostatic disturbance predisposes to purpura and bleeding. Upper gastrointestinal erosions are frequent making gastrointestinal bleeding common and sometimes fatal. Neurological examination may show pupillary abnormalities, chorea, muscle spasticity and extensor plantar responses. Other features include fever, sweating, hypotension, tachycardia, hyperventilation and renal failure.

Reye's syndrome is a rare acute encephalopathy in children with fatty degeneration of the liver developing after an infectious illness such as influenza or chickenpox which has often been treated with aspirin. Vomiting is common but jaundice exceptional.

Investigation. The serum bilirubin reflects the degree of jaundice. Initially, serum aminotransferase activity is high, as in acute viral hepatitis, but with progression of damage activity falls; this investigation has diagnostic but not prognostic significance. The prothrombin time rapidly becomes prolonged as coagulation factor synthesis fails; this is the laboratory test of greatest prognostic value, a progressive and marked prolongation being a very bad sign. Alkaline phosphatase activity is variable. Serum albumin concentration remains normal unless the course is prolonged. Increased serum and urine amino acids are characteristic but are not generally measured. White blood cell counts vary, leucocytosis occurring even in the absence of infection. The urine contains protein, bilirubin and urobilinogen.

Liver biopsy is contraindicated because of the severe haemostatic deficiency and because it rarely gives information required for management. Viral causes are sought serologically. Wilson's disease (p. 359) should always be considered in patients under 35 years old.

Course and progress. The progress of fulminant hepatic failure is closely related to the encephalopathy. When only minor signs are present and drowsiness is not prominent some two-thirds of patients survive. Once the patient is comatose only 10 to 20% survive. The prognosis is worse with increasing age and, perhaps, when due to certain agents such as halothane. In fatal cases, death usually occurs within a week. Life-threatening complications, some amenable to conservative therapy, may arise in the course of the illness. These include profound hypoglycaemia, cerebral oedema, respiratory failure, hypothermia, bacterial infections, bleeding due to coagulation disorders, pancreatitis and renal failure with severe oliguria. Electrolyte disturbances, particularly hyponatraemia, hypokalaemia and alkalosis, may also occur. The great majority of those who recover from fulminant hepatic failure regain normal hepatic structure and function.

Treatment. There is no specific therapy. Supportive measures are described on page 349.

Differential diagnosis of acute parenchymal disease of the liver

Most patients with acute parenchymal liver disease are suffering from viral hepatitis. This diagnosis depends on the clinical features described above, a history of contact with a jaundiced person or of transfusion, or damage to the skin when handling blood within an appropriate incubation period, the results of liver function tests, and serological tests particularly for the A and B hepatitis viruses. The possibility of drug-induced hepatitis should always be considered, the diagnosis depending on exposure to the drug within 2 weeks of the onset of symptoms with no other detectable cause for the illness.

In the pre-icteric phase there may be confusion with other acute generalised infections, acute abdominal emergencies when pain is present, or gastroenteritis. Especially in young persons, there may be confusion with infectious mononucleosis (p. 522) and cytomegaloviral infection (p. 730).

Weil's disease (p. 761) may cause severe jaundice. In contrast to viral hepatitis, there is a polymorphonuclear leucocytosis and protein, blood and casts are found in the urine. The diagnosis is made by demonstrating a rise in specific antibodies, and leptospires may be isolated from the blood or urine.

Large-duct biliary obstruction, usually due to a stone or a neoplasm, causes jaundice which is sometimes difficult to differentiate from that due to viral hepatitis. This is particularly so when an episode of viral hepatitis becomes prolonged and obstructive features develop. Clinically, a patient over 40 years old, previous attacks of abdominal pain, the gradual onset of fluctuating or progressive jaundice, marked pruritus, weight loss and right upper quadrant abdominal pain or a palpable gall bladder indicate a large duct obstruction. Leucocytosis or a positive test for blood in the stool also suggest large-duct obstruction. Liver function tests are of greatest value at an early stage; in viral hepatitis serum alkaline phosphatase does not usually exceed 250 units/l (30 KA units/dl) and serum aminotransferase activity almost always exceeds 400 units/l, while in biliary obstruction the reverse usually obtains. This laboratory differentiation becomes less clear as the disease progresses, however, and in biliary obstruction cholangitis may increase serum aminotransferase activity.

Ultrasonography is the most important investigation as it can show whether or not the bile ducts are dilated. Liver biopsy is indicated when the bile ducts are not dilated and percutaneous transhepatic or retrograde cholangiography when they are (Fig. 10.4). The HBsAg and the antimitochondrial antibody must always be sought. Where viral hepatitis is a possibility, laparotomy should be avoided as such patients withstand anaesthesia and surgery poorly.

Treatment of acute parenchymal disease of the liver

Aetiological factors. It is important to detect drug-induced acute hepatitis so that the drug may be stopped and the patient warned to avoid its use in future. Penicillin, given early, is effective in Weil's disease (p. 761). In most cases, however, nothing can be done to eliminate the cause of the disease.

Bed-rest. When symptoms are marked, bed-rest should be advised, the patient rising to the toilet if desired. Thereafter, the younger patient may be up and about taking care only to avoid exhaustion. For those in whom the risks of hepatitis may be greater, bed-rest should be prolonged until symptoms and signs have disappeared and liver function tests have returned substantially towards normal. These patients include those over 50 years, the pregnant, and those with other major disease.

Diet. A good general diet containing some 3000 kcal daily is desirable. Initially, owing to anorexia and nausea, this is usually not tolerated, in which case a light diet supplemented by fruit drinks and glucose is usually acceptable. The content of the diet should be dictated largely by the patient's wishes; however, a good protein intake should be encouraged. If vomiting is severe, intravenous fluid and glucose may be required for a few days.

Drugs. Those metabolised in the liver should be avoided where possible, a principle applying especially to sedative and hypnotic agents. Alcohol must be avoided during the illness and should not be taken in the ensuing 6 months. Oral contraceptives may be resumed after clinical and biochemical recovery.

In patients with marked malaise, anorexia or vomiting prednisolone may cause rapid regression of symptoms with return of appetite. In this small group of patients, it may be given provided the HBsAg test is negative as there is some evidence that corticosteroids may lead to chronic HBV infection. The dose is reduced rapidly from 20 mg daily as symptoms remit.

Fulminant hepatic failure. There is no specific treatment but certain measures should be instituted as soon as possible once encephalopathy occurs. The patient's life is sustained in the hope that hepatic regeneration will take place spontaneously. There should be close observation so that steps may be taken quickly to correct complication as they occur.

Encephalopathy is treated by withdrawing all nitrogen intake, by reducing the nitrogen-producing colonic flora with neomycin (1 g orally 4–6 hourly), and by increasing faecal output with lactulose (p. 357). If tests for stool blood are positive the colon should be washed out. Electro-encephalography may be used to follow the course of the encephalopathy. Sedative drugs must be used with very great care, restlessness and excitement being best controlled, if necessary, with diazepam.

Cerebral oedema is a frequent cause of death and is difficult to diagnose as it often develops rapidly and rarely causes papilloedema. It can present as a sudden respiratory arrest. Unequal or abnormally reacting pupils, local or general myoclonus or focal fits, increasing hyperventilation, decerebrate posturing, and fixed dilated pupils all point to cerebral oedema and the appearance of any one indicates the need for treatment. Mannitol 20% (1 g/kg body weight) should be infused intravenously over half an hour, and the dose repeated if the clinical signs are not reversed. Most patients need two doses (range 1–4) for any one episode of cerebral oedema.

Nutrition. Calories are provided as glucose (300 g/d) either orally, or by nasogastric tube, or into a large central vein as a 10–20% solution (0.6–1.2 mol/l). Fluid and electrolyte therapy depends on maintenance of accurate fluid balance records and on daily measurements of serum urea, sodium, potassium and bicarbonate. Saline must be used cautiously to avoid sodium overload, and potassium deficiency, which occurs readily, should be corrected. The blood glucose should be measured 4 hourly in the severe phase as potentially fatal hypoglycaemia often occurs; its treatment may require large amounts of glucose. Estimations can be made simply by using dip-stick tests, but some checks by a laboratory method should also be made. Capillary blood is used for dip-stick tests and precautions to avoid infection, particularly wearing gloves, should be taken in obtaining samples.

Haemorrhage. As these patients have poor vasomotor control, early detection of bleeding and rapid correction of blood volume by transfusion are required. This is facilitated by regular recordings of pulse, blood pressure, hourly urine output and if possible central venous pressure. Impaired haemostasis leads to bleeding, particularly from the gastrointestinal tract. Intramuscular injections are best avoided. The development of a bleeding tendency is detected by regular haemoglobin, platelet count, prothrombin time and faecal occult blood measurements. Treatment is discussed on page 357. Cimetidine (50 mg i.v. hourly) or ranitidine (50 mg i.v. 8 hourly) should be given to prevent gastrointestinal bleeding.

Infection is common and serious. As fever and leucocytosis may result solely from the liver disease itself, they are no guide and regular blood, urine, and throat cultures and chest radiographs should be carried out. Prophylactic antibiotics should not be used. If infection is strongly suspected gentamicin and cefuroxime may be given once specimens have been taken for culture.

Other measures. A close watch on the respiration is needed as initial hyperpnoea may rapidly become apnoea, requiring tracheostomy and assisted ventilation. Renal failure, revealed by a rising blood urea or creatinine, may eventually require dialysis. The temperature must be measured 4 hourly as hypothermia can follow central loss of temperature control.

Fulminant hepatic failure requires intensive patient care, access to varied specialised help, and a hospital with great technical resources. Many special treatments have been tried. None is of proven value and some involve the risk of infecting staff; they include corticosteroids, exchange transfusion, plasmapheresis and haemodialysis. Liver transplantation has occasionally been successful.

CHRONIC PARENCHYMAL DISEASE OF THE LIVER

There are two main forms of chronic parenchymal liver disease: 1. chronic hepatitis, which comprises chronic persistent hepatitis and 2. chronic active hepatitis, and cirrhosis.

Aetiology. There are many causes of chronic hepatitis and cirrhosis. In Britain, cirrhosis is usually associated with alcohol abuse, chronic active hepatitis or primary biliary cirrhosis. No cause can be found in 30% of cases (cryptogenic cirrhosis). Haemochromatosis accounts for about 5% of patients and all other causes are rare.

Alcohol. The mechanism whereby alcohol damages the liver is unknown; it is now, however, accepted as a direct liver toxin in man and in other primates. The production of cirrhosis requires a prolonged intake of alcohol of about 80 g or more daily for 5 to 15 years. Women may be at greater risk of liver damage than men, and a daily alcohol intake may be more likely to cause cirrhosis than episodic drinking.

Infection. Rarely, patients can develop cirrhosis over a few months or years after viral hepatitis. In some patients with chronic hepatitis or cirrhosis, the proportion showing marked geographic variation (0–30%), the HBsAg is found persistently in the blood and in such cases the hepatitis B virus is the causative agent. Superinfection with delta virus increases the chances of progressive chronic hepatitis in these patients. The non-A, non-B viruses can cause chronic infection and are likely causes of chronic liver disease. The hepatitis A virus does not cause chronic liver disease.

Immunological factors. Some patients with chronic liver disease of unknown cause have abnormal serum antibodies (p. 334). Though the autoantibodies themselves are not cytotoxic, their presence has suggested that liver damage may be produced by abnormal immune mechanisms. Currently, the possibility that sensitised lymphocytes may do this is being investigated. Immune reactions are also likely to be important in chronic liver disease caused by the hepatitis B virus.

Metabolic disorders. These include excess hepatic deposition of iron in haemochromatosis and of copper in Wilson's disease. Alpha$_1$-antitrypsin deficiency may cause chronic liver disease in children or in adults, but most other metabolic conditions involving the liver manifest themselves first in childhood, e.g. glycogen storage and fibrocystic disease.

Drugs. Chronic hepatitis and cirrhosis have been reported in patients on long-term treatment with methotrexate or methyldopa. Other drugs (e.g. phenylbutazone, sulphonamide) have been cited occasionally.

Cholestasis. Prolonged obstruction anywhere in the biliary system may cause cirrhosis. In primary biliary cirrhosis, obstruction results from damage to interlobular bile ducts. Cirrhosis from large-duct obstruction may occur with biliary strictures or in sclerosing cholangitis. Neoplastic lesions do not cause cirrhosis as survival is short.

Congestion. Prolonged hepatic congestion can

eventually cause cirrhosis. This is rare, as death usually occurs before cirrhosis develops. Congestion may be due to hepatic venous outflow obstruction (p. 361) or chronic heart failure.

Malnutrition. This often occurs secondarily in patients with cirrhosis, but it is unlikely that it is primarily responsible for cirrhosis. Permanent liver damage does not follow marasmus or kwashiorkor.

Pathology. CHRONIC HEPATITIS. Two types of chronic hepatitis are recognised histologically. Their names — persistent hepatitis and aggressive hepatitis — are easily confused with the clinical syndromes they underlie — chronic persistent hepatitis and chronic active hepatitis; this should be avoided.

In *persistent hepatitis* the essential feature is an infiltration of chronic inflammatory cells confined to the portal tracts which may be expanded or show short fibrous septa extending into the parenchyma. Changes in the hepatocytes are absent or slight; there may be small foci of liver cell necrosis with inflammatory cell infiltration (spotty necrosis) and sometimes the residual changes of viral hepatitis. Lobular architecture is normal and cirrhosis only rarely develops.

In *aggressive hepatitis,* the histological process underlying the clinical condition chronic active hepatitis, both the portal tracts and the parenchyma are involved, lobular architecture is distorted and cirrhosis often develops. The portal tract infiltration of mononuclear cells extends irregularly into the surrounding parenchyma so that swollen liver cells become isolated in the inflammatory cell infiltrate. This process of hepatocyte destruction is called 'piecemeal necrosis' and it leads to septum formation linking portal tracts and central veins. The ensuing disruption of lobular architecture is accompanied by the development of regenerative nodules and then by cirrhosis. Changes in the rest of the parenchyma are variable and resemble those of persistent hepatitis. These changes do not occur diffusely and may be more advanced in some areas than others, a point to be considered in interpreting biopsies.

CIRRHOSIS. Here, widespread death of liver cells resulting from many causes is accompanied and followed by progressive fibrosis, regenerative (nodular) hyperplasia of surviving hepatocytes, and distortion of liver architecture resulting in portal-systemic vascular shunts. The whole liver is involved, though not necessarily every lobule. Cirrhotic livers have an infinitely variable appearance limiting the usefulness of anatomical classifications. Currently, a simple classification into micronodular, macronodular and mixed cirrhosis is used.

Micronodular cirrhosis is characterised by regular connective tissue septa, regenerative nodules approximating in size to the original lobules (1 mm in diameter) and involvement of every lobule. This form, also previously called portal, septal, nutritional, monolobular, or Laënnec's cirrhosis, is characteristic but not pathognomonic of the parenchymal damage induced by alcohol.

In *macronodular cirrhosis* the connective tissue septa vary in thickness and the nodules show marked differences in size, the larger ones containing histologically normal lobules. This form was previously called posthepatitic or postnecrotic cirrhosis.

Mixed cirrhosis shows features of both micronodular and macronodular cirrhosis. None of these types of cirrhosis is static; micronodular cirrhosis may, for example, develop into a macronodular stage.

CHRONIC HEPATITIS

It is important not to confuse gradually resolving acute hepatitis with chronic hepatitis. As there is no certain way to avoid this by clinical assessment or investigation, including biopsy, a diagnosis of chronic hepatitis should only be made firmly once liver disease has been present on clinical or other grounds for at least 6 months.

Chronic persistent hepatitis

Aetiology and pathology (persistent hepatitis) are discussed on page 351. Symptoms are mild and comprise fatigue, poor appetite, fatty food intolerance and upper abdominal discomfort, especially over the liver. The condition may be asymptomatic and revealed by biochemical tests done for other reasons. There may or may not be a history of acute hepatitis. Examination may show slight hepatomegaly, but is often normal. There are no features of chronic liver disease.

Serum bilirubin is normal or slightly raised, serum aminotransferase is raised up to fivefold and alkaline phosphatase is generally normal. Serum albumin and globulin are normal. The HBsAg may be present but autoantibodies are not found. Liver biopsy shows persistent hepatitis.

Differentiation should be made from the post-hepatitis syndrome (p. 344) and Gilbert's syndrome (p. 340), as well as from the pericholangitis associated with Crohn's disease and ulcerative colitis (p. 312). The prognosis is usually excellent, the patient should be reassured and no treatment is required. Rarely, progression to chronic active hepatitis or cirrhosis may occur.

Chronic active hepatitis

Chronic active hepatitis (CAH) is in general more severe than chronic persistent hepatitis. Its aetiology and pathology (aggressive hepatitis) are discussed on page 351.

Clinical features. The most florid forms of the disease occur predominantly in females in the second and third decades. The onset is usually insidious with fatigue, anorexia and jaundice. In about a quarter of cases, the onset is acute, resembling viral hepatitis which, however, does not resolve normally. Other features include fever, arthralgia and epistaxis. Amenorrhoea is the rule.

On examination, the general health appears good; jaundice is mild to moderate or occasionally absent but signs of chronic liver disease, especially spider telangiectasia and hepatosplenomegaly, are almost always present. Sometimes a 'Cushingoid' face with acne, hirsutism and pink cutaneous striae, especially on the thighs and abdomen, are present. Bruises may be seen. Though liver disease usually dominates the clinical syndrome, many associated conditions occur in florid CAH emphasising its essentially systemic nature. These include migrating polyarthritis of large joints, a variety of rashes, most non-specific but including inflammatory papules and urticaria, lymphadenopathy, thyroid disorders such as Hashimoto's thyroiditis, thyrotoxicosis and myxoedema,

Coombs'-positive haemolytic anaemia, pleurisy, transient pulmonary infiltration, ulcerative colitis and glomerulonephritis. Some patients have Sjögren's syndrome (p. 557).

Less severe CAH has become recognised increasingly, and now most patients with CAH have these milder syndromes. Indeed, CAH is recognised incidentally in some. Fewer signs of chronic liver disease are found and sometimes the physical examination is normal. CAH due to hepatitis B viral infection is usually associated with this less florid form of disease. It occurs most often in males over 30 years of age and comes to attention when an episode of acute viral hepatitis fails to resolve, with the features of cirrhosis, or even incidentally in an asymptomatic individual. Examination often reveals little of note; hepatomegaly is the most common abnormality, jaundice is slight or absent and fewer than a third of patients have spider telangiectasia or splenomegaly. Systemic features other than arthralgia are uncommon.

Investigation. Liver function tests vary; the activity of the disease is indicated by the serum aminotransferase activity, and the severity of liver damage is reflected in the serum albumin concentration and the prothrombin time. Aminotransferase activity in relapses of florid disease is usually more than 10 times increased and hypoalbuminaemia and marked hyperglobulinaemia are common. The serum bilirubin reflects the degree of jaundice but usually does not exceed 100 μmol/l (6 mg/dl). The serum alkaline phosphatase activity reflects the degree of intrahepatic cholestasis. Autoantibodies are found especially in patients with florid disease; antinuclear antibodies are found in half the patients, smooth muscle antibodies in two-thirds and antimitochondrial antibodies in a quarter. The HBsAg and the serum ceruloplasmin and alpha$_1$-antitrypsin concentrations should be measured.

Diagnosis and prognosis. Differentiation from acute viral hepatitis can be impossible when CAH presents with an acute exacerbation. An acute hepatitis showing unremitting activity (aminotransferase increased at least tenfold, or increased at least fivefold with serum gammaglobulin increased at least twice) for 10 weeks is likely to be due to CAH, but in all cases the diagnosis should not be considered certain until a biopsy done at least 6 months after the onset is examined. Drugs should always be sought as a cause and Wilson's disease (p. 359) and α_1-antitrypsin deficiency must be excluded.

Most patients eventually progress to cirrhosis with the development of portal hypertension (p. 353), ascites (p. 354) and encephalopathy (p. 354). The course of CAH associated with autoantibodies is marked by exacerbations and remissions, and about half the patients die of liver failure within 5 years if no treatment is given. CAH due to hepatitis B viral infection progresses more slowly and usually without exacerbations.

Treatment. Corticosteroids are life-saving in CAH of unknown cause, particularly during exacerbations of active symptomatic disease associated with autoantibodies. Initially, prednisolone 30 mg/d is given orally and the dose reduced gradually as the patient and liver function tests improve. Maintenance therapy is required for at least a year after liver function tests have become normal, and even then relapse often occurs if the drug is withdrawn. Side-effects from prednisolone are uncommon at a maintenance dose of 10 mg/d or less. Azathioprine 50–100 mg/d orally may be added to the therapy to allow the dose of prednisolone to be reduced to this level. Ascites, encephalopathy and portal hypertension are treated (p. 356). Corticosteroids are less important in asymptomatic CAH with mild activity and are contraindicated in CAH due to hepatitis B virus infection.

CIRRHOSIS OF THE LIVER

Aetiology and pathology are discussed on pages 350 and 351.

Clinical features. These vary greatly and may include any combination of manifestations described below. None is specifically related to particular causes of cirrhosis, though florid spider telangiectasia, gynaecomastia and parotid enlargement are more common in alcohol-associated cirrhosis. Autopsy experience shows that cirrhosis may be entirely asymptomatic, and in life it may be found incidentally at surgery or with minimal features such as isolated hepatomegaly. Enlarge-

ment of the liver tends to be more common in the early stages of the disease, disappearing as hepatocyte destruction and fibrosis reduce liver size. The patient may complain of weakness, fatigue or weight loss. Non-specific digestive symptoms such as anorexia, nausea, vomiting and upper abdominal discomfort may occur as does gaseous abdominal distension. Otherwise, clinical features are due mainly to portal hypertension and/or hepatic insufficiency.

Portal hypertension results from destruction and distortion of the hepatic vasculature leading to obstruction of blood flow. Its cardinal features are splenomegaly, hypersplenism and a portal-systemic collateral circulation. Cirrhosis is the commonest cause of portal hypertension in Europe, North America and Australia and New Zealand, but there are many other causes (p. 360).

Splenomegaly is seldom marked in adults, the tip rarely reaching more than 5 cm below the costal margin. In childhood and adolescence it may be much more marked. When the spleen is not enlarged clinically or radiographically, portal hypertension is unlikely.

Haematological changes. Moderate leucopenia and thrombocytopenia frequently occur with splenomegaly and are attributed to hypersplenism (p. 541). Anaemia may occur and when hypochromic is usually due to blood loss from the gut. Macrocytes and target cells are common; though the marrow is usually normoblastic, megaloblastic anaemia sometimes occurs. Megaloblastic changes are usually due to nutritional folate deficiency; vitamin B_{12} deficiency is rare.

Collateral circulation occurs where there are portal-systemic communications. These are in the distal oesophagus and proximal stomach, in the anus and distal rectum, in the falciform ligament and between the colonic, omental, splenic and retroperitoneal veins. Collateral vessels may be seen on the anterior abdominal wall and rarely they radiate prominently from the umbilicus ('caput medusae'). A venous hum can occasionally be heard over a large umbilical collateral vessel. The most important collateral vessels are in the oesophagus and stomach (oesophagogastric varices) as they can cause bleeding which is usually severe and acute, but occasionally occult and chronic. Bleeding may occur from varices elsewhere in the gut but this is very rare. The presence of oesophagogastric varices establishes a diagnosis of portal hypertension. Special radiological procedures can demonstrate the patency of the splenic and portal veins, assess the extent of collateral circulation and allow the portal pressure to be measured (p. 337).

Ascites in cirrhosis is due to a combination of liver failure and portal hypertension. Liver failure leads to salt and water retention by decreasing renal blood flow. This produces both a reduced glomerular filtration rate with excessive tubular resorption of water and sodium, and an increased renal release of renin leading to secondary hyperaldosteronism. Failure of the liver to metabolise aldosterone intensifies the secondary aldosteronism and failure to metabolise vasopressin reduces renal water clearance. Hypoalbuminaemia lowers the colloid oncotic pressure of the plasma, encourages the formation of oedema and may contribute to a poor renal blood flow. Portal hypertension and lymphatic obstruction in the liver predispose to the localisation of fluid in the abdomen.

Jaundice is mainly due to failure of bilirubin metabolism. Intrahepatic cholestasis may also be a contributing factor. In cirrhosis jaundice is generally mild or absent. Increasing jaundice implies progressing liver failure.

Circulatory changes usually consist of increased peripheral and reduced visceral blood flow especially to the kidneys. The cause for this is unknown. Increased peripheral blood flow is indicated by palmar erythema. Arteriolar changes result in cutaneous *spider telangiectases*; these lesions comprise a central arteriole, which may raise the skin surface, from which small vessels radiate. They are usually confined to the area above the nipples and occur especially on the face, necklace area, forearms and dorsum of the hands. At an early stage they may appear as white spots on cooling the skin.

Reduced arterial oxygen saturation is frequent and central cyanosis may occur; this is probably due to the development of pulmonary venoarterial shunts and similar shunts may predispose to the development of clubbing of the fingers.

Endocrine abnormalities. Gynaecomastia, sometimes unilateral, may occur. It can result from the liver disease or may be induced by spironolactone

therapy. Loss of libido occurs in both sexes; there is impotence and testicular atrophy in men and breast atrophy and irregular menses or amenorrhoea in premenopausal women.

Haemorrhagic tendencies are found in advanced liver failure and are due largely to underproduction of coagulation factors (p. 542). Thrombocytopenia may also occur particularly when splenomegaly is present. It is seldom sufficient to cause spontaneous bleeding but may aggravate bleeding from other causes such as varices. Serum fibrinogen concentration is not reduced until the terminal stages, though occasionally fibrinolysis may be significant. Bruising, purpura, epistaxis, menorrhagia or gastrointestinal bleeding can all occur.

Skin pigmentation. Generalised hyperpigmentation due to increased melanin deposition can occur in any form of cirrhosis, but especially in haemochromatosis and after prolonged cholestasis.

Dupuytren's contracture may be more frequent in patients with cirrhosis but the statistical evidence for this is poor.

Fever. About a third of cirrhotic patients have a low-grade fever not due to infection.

Hepatic (portal-systemic) encephalopathy. The mental and neurological features described in fulminant hepatic failure (p. 347) occur in cirrhosis in a more chronic and intermittent fashion. This complication sometimes overshadows the liver disease and leads to a diagnosis of primary mental disorder. Rarely, irreversible central nervous system changes occur with paraplegia, parkinsonism, epileptic fits and dementia.

In addition to liver failure, another factor is that the collateral venous circulation in cirrhosis bypasses the liver and allows nitrogenous substances from the gut to reach the systemic circulation thereby increasing the tendency to encephalopathy. Where anastomoses are extensive, encephalopathy may even occur despite relatively good liver function; this is rare in cirrhosis alone, but may be seen following a surgical portal-systemic shunt.

Encephalopathy in the cirrhotic patient may be precipitated by various factors including sedatives, too aggressive diuretic therapy, a high protein diet, infection, trauma (e.g. surgery), gastrointestinal bleeding, hypokalaemia and constipation.

Renal failure consequent on liver failure can occur in cirrhosis. The kidneys themselves are intrinsically normal, and renal failure is thought to result from a diminished renal flood flow. The condition is called functional renal failure of cirrhosis or the *hepatorenal syndrome*. It occurs in advanced cirrhosis, almost always with ascites, and uraemia is characterised by the absence of proteinuria or abnormal urinary sediment, a urine sodium less than 10 mmol/d and a urine/plasma osmolality ratio greater than 1.5. The prognosis is very poor.

Investigation. The serum bilirubin may be normal; increases are very variable. Bilirubinuria may or may not be present, but excessive urobilinogenuria is usual. Serum aminotransferase activity is usually slightly increased by up to threefold and serum alkaline phosphatase is raised similarly. All these tests may be normal and they are of no prognostic value. The serum albumin is reduced and the prothrombin time remains prolonged in spite of parenteral vitamin K in those with poor liver function; these tests, especially sequential results, are of considerable value as deteriorating levels indicate a poor outlook. The serum globulin is raised. BSP retention is almost always increased, though falsely normal values may occur in hypoalbuminaemia.

It is particularly important to detect causes of cirrhosis requiring specific treatment, e.g. haemochromatosis and Wilson's disease.

Differential diagnosis. Alternative diagnoses to be considered depend on how the patient presents, for example with haematemesis (p. 288) or ascites (p. 354). In those with hepatomegaly, secondary carcinoma should be especially considered where enlargement is gross, irregular and hard and where the spleen is not palpable. The site of the primary tumour may be found. A primary liver tumour is also possible (p. 361). Cardiac failure, tricuspid valve disease and constrictive pericarditis should be sought especially where the liver is large, smooth and tender. Rarer causes of hepatomegaly include lymphoma, leukaemia, amyloidosis, sarcoidosis, abscess and hydatid cyst. In the tropics, kala azar, malaria or schistosomiasis may be present.

Prognosis. Although cirrhosis is a progressive disease, the rate of deterioration varies and the outlook is related to many factors. The prognosis is better where the cause of cirrhosis can be corrected, as in alcohol abuse, haemochromatosis and Wilson's disease. Worsening liver function evidenced by jaundice or ascites indicates a poor prognosis unless a treatable cause such as bleeding or infection is present. Encephalopathy not associated with an extensive collateral circulation is a poor prognostic sign and, as with ascites, a poor response to therapy is ominous. Acute bleeding from oesophageal varices is fatal in about 50% of cases. Marked hypoalbuminaemia (below 25 g/l), hyponatraemia (below 120 mmol/l) not due to diuretic therapy and a prolonged prothrombin time are bad prognostic signs. The course of cirrhosis is uncertain as unforeseen complications such as severe infection or hepatocellular carcinoma may lead to death.

Treatment is discussed on page 356.

BILIARY CIRRHOSIS

Biliary cirrhosis results from prolonged obstruction anywhere between the small interlobular bile ducts and the papilla of Vater.

Primary biliary cirrhosis. This disease affects predominantly women, usually in middle age. It was previously considered rare, but is now recognised as relatively common, affecting about 1 in 40 000 in Britain. A chronic granulomatous inflammation of unknown cause destroys the interlobular bile ducts in the liver with the eventual development of cirrhosis. Immune complexes are found in the blood but their importance in producing liver damage is unknown.

Pruritus is the commonest initial complaint and may precede jaundice by months or even years. When the patient is jaundiced, pruritus is almost always present. Although there may be abdominal discomfort, the abdominal pain, fever and rigors of large bile-duct obstruction do not occur. Diarrhoea resulting from malabsorption of fat, and pain and tingling in the hands and feet due to lipid infiltration of peripheral nerves occasionally occur. Bone pain or fractures due to osteomalacia from malabsorption or osteoporosis (hepatic osteodystrophy) are often prominent later.

Initially patients are well-nourished, but considerable weight loss can occur as the disease progresses. Scratch marks may be found. Jaundice is only prominent late in the disease when the patient may become a bottle-green colour. Xanthomatous deposits occur in a minority especially around the eyes, in the hand creases and over the elbows, knees and buttocks. Hepatomegaly is virtually constant. Splenomegaly occurs later as portal hypertension develops. The disease generally lasts 5 to 10 years in symptomatic patients terminating in liver failure or alimentary bleeding from oesophageal varices.

The diagnosis is based on the clinical picture, on liver function tests showing cholestasis, especially a very high serum alkaline phosphatase activity greater than 250 units/l (30 KA units/dl), and on a positive antimitochondrial antibody test. It is confirmed by liver biopsy and by the absence of dilated bile ducts on ultrasonography.

The widespread availability of liver function and immunological tests has led to increasing recognition of asymptomatic primary biliary cirrhosis, especially in patients with related disorders such as thyroid and connective tissue diseases. These patients generally have a good prognosis, especially if they do not have oesophageal varices.

No specific therapy is available. Corticosteroids, azathioprine and penicillamine have all been tried but none is effective and all may have serious adverse effects. Palliative measures, e.g. for pruritus, are described on page 358.

Secondary biliary cirrhosis. This develops after prolonged large duct biliary obstruction due to gallstones, bile duct strictures and, occasionally, sclerosing cholangitis (p. 368). There is chronic cholestasis with episodes of ascending cholangitis or even liver abscess (p. 362). Finger clubbing is common and xanthomas and bone pain may develop. Cirrhosis, ascites and portal hypertension are late features.

Treatment of hepatic cirrhosis

Although no treatment can reverse cirrhosis or even ensure that no further progression occurs, medical therapy can promote improved general health and alleviate symptoms. The main problems are to detect treatable causes, to correct malnutrition, to control fluid retention, encephalopathy and alimentary bleeding and to manage chronic cholestasis. There is no satisfactory treatment for the hepatorenal syndrome.

Aetiological factors. Treatable conditions such as alcohol abuse, drug ingestion, haemochromatosis and Wilson's disease should always be sought. Relief of biliary obstruction will prevent biliary cirrhosis.

Nutrition. In the absence of encephalopathy or ascites, a high energy (3000 kcal/d), protein-rich (80–100 g/d) diet should be advised. Where cholestasis is not a feature, fat intake need not be restricted. Alcohol must be forbidden. When a good diet is taken, vitamins and other supplements are not required.

Ascites. Treatment of ascites and oedema may relieve symptoms but does not improve the prognosis and, if over vigorous, may lead to encephalopathy or renal failure which can be fatal. Sources of excessive sodium intake should be sought and corrected first. These may be very salty foods, sodium-containing drugs such as certain antacids (sodium bicarbonate, magnesium trisilicate mixture, and magnesium carbonate mixture) alginates, salicylates, and effervescent calcium, or sodium-retaining drugs such as carbenoxolone, non-steroidal anti-inflammatory agents and steroid hormones. Thereafter, in milder cases salt restriction alone may be sufficient. By using salt in cooking while avoiding salt at table, especially salty foods such as soups, ham and bacon, daily salt intake may be reduced to about 2 g of sodium chloride daily (40 mmol of sodium).

More severe ascites requires diuretics. Initially, a potassium sparing drug such as spironolactone (100 mg/d) should be used. Triamterene (100 mg/d) is an alternative. Additional diuresis may be obtained from a medium potency diuretic such as bendrofluazide. Potassium supplements may not be necessary with this drug combination but hypokalaemia should be avoided as it may precipitate or worsen encephalopathy.

Patients with marked ascites should be admitted to hospital. They generally have more severe liver dysfunction and require more vigorous therapy to which they are apt to react adversely. Bed-rest, restriction of water intake to 1 l/d, restriction of salt to 20 mmol of sodium daily (1 g salt) and potassium supplements may induce diuresis. If this does not occur within 4 days spironolactone or triamterene should be added and potassium intake reduced or stopped. Only when large doses of spironolactone (400 mg/d) have failed should high potency diuretics such as frusemide (40–160 mg/d) be used. Treatment should aim to produce a weight loss of 0.5–1 kg/d, and regular checks should be made of the blood urea and electrolyte concentrations.

Occasionally patients do not respond to treatment; many are continuing to take salt and this should be checked. The temptation to remove fluid by paracentesis alone must be resisted as patients tolerate this poorly; up to 5 litres may be removed without risk to relieve abdominal discomfort and respiratory distress caused by gross ascites. Paracentesis with reinfusion of salt-poor albumin or of an ultrafiltrate of the ascitic fluid is sometimes used. Intravenous infusion of salt-poor albumin (25 g) alone over 3 hours with frusemide (40–80 mg i.v.) may also initiate diuresis in resistant cases. Ascites unrelieved by medical therapy can often be helped by a LeVeen shunt which carries ascites directly to the central veins.

Hepatic encephalopathy. Episodes of encephalopathy develop in many patients with cirrhosis and are usually readily reversed until the terminal stages occur. The principles of treatment are as in fulminant hepatic failure (p. 347). In severe cases all dietary protein is stopped or reduced below 20 g/d, and glucose (300 g/d) is given orally or parenterally. As encephalopathy improves, dietary protein is increased by 10–20 g/d on alternate days to an intake of 40–60 g/d which is usually the limit in these cirrhotic patients.

Lactulose (15–30 ml t.i.d.) is given to produce two stools daily. Lactulose is a disaccharide which reaches the colon intact and is then split by colonic bacteria. It produces an osmotic laxative effect, reduces the pH of the colonic content thereby limiting colonic ammonia absorption and promotes the incorporation of nitrogen into bacteria. If the effect of lactulose is disappointing then neomycin (1 g/4–6 hourly) may be added. Neomycin, which acts by reducing bowel flora, is also used as an alternative to lactulose if diarrhoea becomes troublesome. Although neomycin is poorly absorbed a careful watch should be kept for ototoxic effects from long-term use especially if there is any uraemia.

Variceal bleeding. Acute bleeding from oesophagogastric varices is frequently severe. Blood transfusion is required, and every effort should be made to avoid hypotension which reduces liver blood flow and can produce significant liver damage. When initial bleeding has been controlled, its source should be determined by endoscopy as about a quarter of patients with varices are bleeding from some other lesion, especially acute gastric erosions. Measures to stop the bleeding include the reduction of portal venous pressure and local procedures such as the application of pressure to the varices, sclerotherapy, embolisation of vessels feeding the varices and transection of the varices. The risk of rebleeding can be reduced by shunt surgery or by sclerotherapy.

REDUCTION OF PORTAL VENOUS PRESSURE. *Vasopressin* helps to arrest bleeding by constricting the splanchnic arterioles and thereby reducing portal pressure and blood flow. It can be given intravenously in a dose of 20 units in 100 ml of 5% glucose over 15 minutes, and this may need to be repeated 3–4 times at hourly intervals as the drug is destroyed rapidly. Abdominal colic, evacuation of the bowels and facial pallor from general arteriolar constriction indicate that vasopressin is active, and absence of these suggests an inert preparation. Vasoconstriction can cause angina, arrhythmia and even myocardial infarction and vasopressin should not therefore be used in patients with ischaemic heart disease. Vasopressin can also be given by intravenous infusion 0.4 unit/minute until bleeding stops or for 24 hours and then 0.2 unit/minute for a further 24 hours. Cessation of bleeding is judged from nasogastric aspiration and from the pulse and blood pressure.

Terlipressin is a more costly alternative to vasopressin with certain advantages. Terlipressin itself is not active, but vasopressin is released from it over several hours in amounts sufficient to reduce the portal pressure without producing systemic, including cardiac, effects. It is given in a dose of 2 mg intravenously every 6 hours until bleeding stops and then 1 mg every 6 hours for a further 24 hours.

Somatostatin reduces splanchnic blood flow, probably by inducing vasoconstriction, and in a dose of 250 μg i.v. followed by 250 μg hourly can stop bleeding from oesophageal varices. It seems to have fewer side-effects than vasopressin but it is much more expensive.

Propranolol has been advocated as a medical means for reducing portal venous pressure and preventing variceal bleeding but its efficacy remains to be proved.

LOCAL MEASURES to control acute variceal bleeding include balloon tamponade, sclerotherapy, variceal embolisation and oesophageal transection.

Balloon tamponade is achieved with a *Sengstaken tube* possessing two inflatable balloons which exert pressure on the lower oesophagus and gastric fundus. It is passed by mouth and inflation, initially of the gastric balloon alone, may control bleeding. The *Minnesota tube* allows secretions to be aspirated from the upper oesophagus when the balloons are inflated.

Sclerotherapy can be used to stop acute bleeding but its main role is the prevention of recurrent bleeding.

Transhepatic embolisation entails passing a catheter through the liver into the portal vein and obliterating the collateral vessels by injecting sclerosing material. This method requires specialised facilities not widely available.

Oesophageal transection of the varices can be done relatively easily with a stapling gun, though it carries some risk of subsequent oesophageal stenosis. Emergency portal-systemic shunt surgery has a mortality of 50% or more and is rarely practicable.

PREVENTION. Recurrent variceal bleeding is the rule rather than the exception in patients who have had bleeding from oesophageal varices, and treatment to prevent this is needed.

Portal-systemic shunt surgery was previously the treatment of choice as it effectively prevents bleeding provided the shunt remains patent. There has, however, been increasing dissatisfaction with treatment as the operations do not prolong life and often cause troublesome hepatic encephalopathy perhaps because the total shunts used previously divert all the portal blood away from the liver. More recently, *selective shunts*, particularly the distal splenorenal (Warren) shunt, which decompresses the varices while preserving much of the portal blood flow to the liver have been developed. The distal spleno-renal shunt prevents rebleeding, induces much less encephalopathy and is currently the favoured operation.

Shunts should be considered only for those under 60 years of age with good liver function evidenced by good general health, no ascites or evidence of encephalopathy, serum bilirubin less than 35 μmol/l (2.0 mg/dl), and serum albumin over 35 g/l. There is no place for the prophylactic use of shunt operations in patients with varices who have not bled.

Sclerotherapy. The relative ease of endoscopy with fibreoptic instruments has led to a resurgence of interest in injection sclerotherapy. Varices are injected with a sclerosing agent as soon as practicable after bleeding is controlled, and injections are repeated every 1–2 weeks thereafter until the varices are obliterated. Regular follow-up is then necessary to allow treatment of any recurrence of varices. The treatment is not free of risk as injections can cause ulceration and stricture formation, but, in general, morbidity is low; even those with poor liver function can be treated and recurrent bleeding is largely prevented. There is also some evidence that this treatment can prolong life.

Chronic cholestasis. Where this is associated with irremediable large duct biliary obstruction, treatment is required for pruritus, steatorrhoea and cholangitis.

Pruritus, believed to be due to bile acids, is the main symptom demanding relief. This is best achieved with the anion-binding resin cholestyramine, which reduces the bile acids in the body by binding them in the intestine and increasing their excretion in the stool. A dose of 4–16 g/d orally is used. The powder is mixed in orange juice and the main dose (8 g) is taken with breakfast when maximal duodenal bile acid concentrations occur. Cholestyramine may bind other drugs in the gut (e.g. anticoagulants); the latter should therefore be taken one hour before the binding agent.

Cholestyramine is sometimes ineffective,

especially in complete biliary obstruction. Terfenadine, an antihistamine (60 mg b.d.), or ultraviolet therapy may help in such cases. Methyltestosterone (25 mg/d sublingually) or, for women, norethandrolone (10 mg t.i.d.) may also be effective though both reversibly increase cholestasis at the canalicular membrane and jaundice worsens.

Steatorrhoea. Prolonged cholestasis is associated with steatorrhoea and malabsorption of fat-soluble vitamins and calcium. Steatorrhoea can be reduced by limiting fat intake to 40 g/d. Medium chain triglyceride supplements can be used to augment calorie intake. Monthly injections of vitamin K_1 (10 mg), vitamin D (calciferol 2.5 mg; alfacalcidol 1 μg/d orally) and calcium supplements should also be given, the last as effervescent calcium gluconate (2–4 g/d). This preparation, however, contains much sodium and, where there is fluid retention, calcium gluconate alone should be used.

Cholangitis requires treatment with antibiotics which can be given continuously if attacks occur frequently.

MISCELLANEOUS DISEASES OF THE LIVER

Primary haemochromatosis. This is an uncommon disease in which excessive iron absorption over years leads to a gross increase in total body iron from the normal level of 4 g to 20–60 g. It is caused by a genetic defect associated with certain of the histocompatibility antigens. Iron is deposited widely: the important organs involved are the liver, pancreas, endocrine glands and heart. In the liver, iron deposition occurs first in the peripheral hepatocytes extending later to all hepatocytes. The gradual development of fibrous septa leads to the formation of irregular nodules and finally regeneration results in macronodular cirrhosis.

Clinical features generally occur in men aged over 45 years, menstruation and pregnancy providing protective mechanisms in women in whom the disease is ten times less common. There may be manifestations of hepatic cirrhosis, diabetes mellitus or heart failure. Leaden-grey skin pigmentation due to excess melanin and iron occurs especially in exposed parts, axillae, groins and genitalia, hence the term 'bronzed diabetes'. Impotence, loss of libido and testicular atrophy are also common.

The serum iron concentration is increased and the serum iron binding capacity is usually over 70% saturated. The serum ferritin is also high (p. 336). The diagnosis is confirmed by liver biopsy, and the iron content of the liver can be measured (p. 816).

Haemochromatosis must be distinguished from other forms of cirrhosis, especially that due to alcohol in which there may be excess liver iron. Differentiation must also be made from other causes of excess body iron discussed below.

Treatment is by weekly venesection of 500 ml (250 mg iron) until the serum iron is normal; this may take 2 years or more. Thereafter, venesection is done to keep the serum iron normal. Other therapy includes that for cirrhosis and diabetes mellitus. Other family members should be investigated and any with asymptomatic disease treated.

Secondary haemochromatosis. Many conditions are associated with widespread secondary siderosis. Though they may cause features similar to haemochromatosis, these are rare and the history suggests the true diagnosis. Primary conditions include chronic haemolytic disorders, sideroblastic anaemia (p. 503), multiple blood transfusion (generally over 150 litres) and dietary iron overload (p. 59). Marked hepatic siderosis may also occur in alcoholic cirrhosis.

Wilson's disease (hepato-lenticular degeneration) is a rare but important autosomal recessive condition caused by an abnormality of copper metabolism. Normally, dietary copper is absorbed from the stomach and proximal small intestine, and is rapidly taken up into the liver where it is stored and incorporated into caeruloplasmin which is secreted into the blood. The functions of caeruloplasmin are unknown. The accumulation of excessive copper in the body is prevented by its excretion, and the most important route is via the bile. The precise nature of the metabolic defect in Wilson's disease is unknown, but it results in a failure of copper excretion in the bile leading to its accumulation in the body. There is almost always a failure of synthesis of caeruloplasmin also, though occasional patients with Wilson's disease have a normal plasma caeruloplasmin concentration. The amount of copper in the body at birth in Wilson's disease is normal but thereafter it increases steadily; the organs most affected by this are the liver, the basal ganglia of the brain and the eyes.

Clinical features usually arise between the ages of 5 and 30 years. Hepatic disease occurs predominantly in childhood and early adolescence while neurological damage causes basal ganglion syndromes (p. 652) in later adolescence. These manifestations can occur alone or simultaneously. Most patients presenting with Wilson's disease have Kayser-Fleischer rings, though these may be detectable only by slit-lamp examination; they are the most important single clinical pointer to the diagnosis. Kayser-Fleischer rings are characterised by greenish-brown discolouration of the corneal margin appearing first at the upper periphery. They eventually disappear when treatment is given. Other manifestations include haemolysis, renal tubular damage and osteoporosis, but these are virtually never presenting features.

The clinical features of liver damage are not specific. Episodes of acute hepatitis can occur, especially in children, and may progress to fulminant hepatic failure. Chronic persistent hepatitis and chronic active hepatitis can also develop, and eventually cirrhosis with liver failure and portal hypertension.

Investigation. Any patient under 35 years of age with recurrent hepatitis, chronic hepatitis or cirrhosis of unknown cause should be investigated for Wilson's disease. A family history of hepatic or neurological disease and Kayser-Fleischer rings are the most important clinical clues to the diagnosis, and a low serum caeruloplasmin concentration is the best single laboratory test. However, any cause of liver failure can lead to a low serum caeruloplasmin and occasionally the serum caeruloplasmin is normal in Wilson's disease. Other features of a disordered copper metabolism should therefore be sought; these include a low serum copper concentration, a high urine copper excretion (p. 818) and a very high hepatic copper content (p. 816). Rarely, it may be necessary to demonstrate failure of the liver to incorporate radioactive copper into caeruloplasmin.

Treatment. The copper-binding agent penicill-

amine is the drug of choice in Wilson's disease. The dose given must be sufficient to produce cupriuresis and most patients require 1.5 g/d (range 1–4 g). The dose can be reduced once the disease is in remission, but treatment must continue for life and care taken to see that reaccumulation of copper does not occur. Young women should continue to take the drug during pregnancy as it is not teratogenic. Serious toxic effects of penicillamine (p. 562) are fortunately rare in Wilson's disease. If they do occur triethylene tetramine dihydrochloride is the next drug of choice.

The *prognosis* of Wilson's disease is excellent provided treatment is started before irreversible damage is done, and the long-term complication of hepatocellular carcinoma does not occur as it does in haemochromatosis. Siblings of patients with Wilson's disease should also be investigated and treatment should be given to any who have the disease even if it is asymptomatic.

Non-cirrhotic portal hypertension. Portal hypertension is virtually always due to obstruction to the portal blood flow somewhere in the portal venous system. Splenomegaly with hypersplenism (p. 541) and a collateral circulation are the main consequences irrespective of the cause. The obstruction may be outside the liver (extrahepatic presinusoidal) in the portal or splenic vein where the result is the development of collateral vessels bypassing the obstruction as well as portal hypertension. Umbilical infection in the neonatal period is believed to be an important cause but other conditions leading to thrombosis include polycythaemia vera, malignant invasion from adjacent organs, pancreatitis and abdominal trauma.

Obstruction in the portal tract (intrahepatic presinusoidal) may also be responsible and causes include schistosomiasis, congenital hepatic fibrosis, myeloproliferative disease, exposure to arsenic or vinyl chloride and primary biliary cirrhosis. Mixed intrahepatic obstruction is usually caused by cirrhosis but other causes include the Budd-Chiari syndrome and polycystic disease of the liver.

Cirrhosis is the commonest cause of portal hypertension in Europe and North America, but schistosomiasis is the commonest cause worldwide. Portal hypertension due to increased portal blood flow, as with a splenic arteriovenous fistula, is exceptionally rare.

Congenital hepatic fibrosis is a rare condition in which broad fibrous bands are found in the liver. Most patients have associated cystic renal disease. Many die in early childhood of renal failure. Those who survive maintain good liver function but often develop gastrointestinal bleeding due to portal hypertension, usually presenting between 5 and 30 years of age.

Hepatic venous outflow obstruction is an uncommon condition. It can occur in the larger hepatic veins (*Budd-Chiari syndrome*) and obstruction may be due to thrombosis, especially in polycythaemia vera and in women taking oral contraceptives, to invasion by tumours of the liver, kidney, or adrenal, or to congenital venous webs. In up to three-quarters of patients no cause can be found for the obstruction. The same syndrome may develop in constrictive pericarditis or right ventricular failure. Obstruction may also follow damage to the central hepatic veins in *veno-occlusive disease*. This can be due to ingestion of toxic alkaloids in 'bush tea' infused from plants and has been attributed increasingly to cytotoxic drugs.

The condition generally develops fairly rapidly with abdominal pain, tender hepatomegaly and ascites. Liver biopsy shows severe centrilobular congestion. Hepatic venous obstruction can be demonstrated ultrasonically and angiographically. Mild cases can recover completely but severer cases often die rapidly or go on to develop cirrhosis.

The liver in protozoal and helminthic infections. Protozoal infections associated with liver changes include malaria, trypanosomiasis, visceral leishmaniasis, toxoplasmosis and amoebiasis; the last is the most important as it causes liver abscesses which respond promptly to treatment (p. 362). In some cases of persistent malarial infection gross splenomegaly and portal hypertension develop (p. 773).

Schistosomiasis is the most significant helminthic infection as it causes portal hypertension (p. 783). Echinococcosis, giving rise to hydatid liver cysts (p. 789), is the next most important. Rarely the roundworm, *Ascaris lumbricoides* (p. 791), may obstruct the common bile duct, and

liver flukes (p. 786) may cause inflammation and adenocarcinoma of the bile ducts.

FOCAL DISEASES OF THE LIVER.

Tumours of the liver

Primary malignant tumours. *Hepatocellular carcinoma (hepatoma)* is the principal primary liver tumour. Its incidence shows great geographic variation, being common in Africa and S.E. Asia but rare in temperate climates. Chronic hepatitis B viral infection has emerged as the most important cause world-wide, and chronic carriers of the virus have a much increased risk of the disease (p. 345). Ingestion of aflatoxin-contaminated foods may also be important in tropical countries (p. 720). Hepatocellular carcinoma occurs predominantly in males, and in 80% of cases cirrhosis is present. Cirrhosis may be of any type, but hepatocellular carcinoma appears most commonly in haemochromatosis and alcoholic cirrhosis, dominantly male diseases, and rarely in primary biliary cirrhosis, which mainly affects women. Other aetiological factors include exposure to toxins such as thorotrast and arsenic which usually produce angiosarcomas but which may also cause hepatocellular carcinomas. Oestrogens and androgens may cause adenomas or rarely hepatocellular carcinomas.

Macroscopically, the tumour may be a single mass or there may be multiple tumour nodules. Microscopically, the tumour is made up of trabeculae of well-differentiated cells resembling hepatocytes. Bile secretion by tumour cells may be seen and is diagnostic.

Deterioration in a patient with cirrhosis should always lead to suspicion of hepatocellular carcinoma, the clinical features of which include weakness, anorexia, weight loss, fever, abdominal pain, abdominal mass and ascites. Hepatocellular carcinomas are vascular so that a bruit may be heard over the liver or intra-abdominal bleeding may occur. Metabolic abnormalities are recognised increasingly and include polycythaemia, hypercalcaemia, hypoglycaemia and porphyria cutanea tarda.

The detection of high concentrations of α-

fetoprotein (p. 561) in the blood is virtually diagnostic. Imaging almost always reveals a filling defect(s) and the diagnosis may be confirmed by liver aspiration or biopsy. Surgical removal requires a tumour confined to one lobe in the absence of cirrhosis and is rarely feasible; the possibility should always, however, be considered. Doxorubicin (p. 109) can provide useful palliative therapy.

Other primary tumours are rare; they include haemangioendothelial sarcomas and cholangio-carcinoma (p. 368).

Secondary malignant tumours are common and usually originate from carcinomas in the bronchus, breast, abdomen or pelvis. They may be single or multiple. Peritoneal dissemination frequently results in ascites.

Symptoms of the primary neoplasm are absent in about half the cases. Hepatomegaly may suggest cirrhosis, but splenomegaly is rare. There is usually rapid liver enlargement with fever, weight loss and jaundice. A raised alkaline phosphatase activity is the commonest abnormality but the liver function tests may be normal. Ascitic fluid has a high protein content, may be blood-stained and cytology may reveal malignant cells.

Imaging (p. 536) usually reveals filling defects and the diagnosis is confirmed by liver aspiration or biopsy. The tumour in the liver determines the prognosis and investigations to identify an asymptomatic primary lesion are pointless except in the rare instance of a solitary liver deposit amenable to resection.

Benign tumours. Hepatic adenomas are rare vascular tumours which may present as an abdominal mass or with abdominal pain or intra-peritoneal bleeding. They are more common in women and may be caused by oral contraceptives.

Abscesses of the liver

These are either pyogenic or amoebic (p. 775); both have similar clinical features. Pyogenic abscesses may result from:
1. Ascending infection in biliary obstruction (cholangitis)
2. Haematogenous spread via
   a. The portal vein from intra-abdominal foci of infection such as appendicitis, diverticulitis, pelvic abscesses, inflammatory bowel disease and umbilical infection
   b. The hepatic artery from other sites in the body
3. Direct extension from contiguous disease such as cholecystitis, pancreatitis and perforating peptic ulcer
4. Trauma such as a penetrating wound
5. Infection of a pre-existing lesion such as a liver tumour or cyst.

Liver abscesses due to suppurative appendicitis in young people are now infrequent whereas abscesses in older people due to biliary obstruction are relatively common, especially in compromised patients. Abscesses vary greatly in size. Single lesions are more common in the right lobe and multiple abscesses are most often due to biliary obstruction. A wide variety of bacteria can be involved and infection with several organisms occurs in about a third of cases. *Esch. coli* and streptococci are the most frequent and anaerobes are also often present.

Clinical features. Fever and sometimes rigors, and weight loss occur. Mild jaundice may be present but obvious jaundice develops only with large abscesses causing biliary obstruction. Pain is the commonest symptom, usually on the right side but sometimes it radiates to the right shoulder or is pleural. Hepatomegaly is found in more than half the patients and tenderness can usually be elicited by gentle percussion over the organ. Abnormalities are present at the base of the right lung in about a quarter of patients. Atypical presentations are common and explain the frequency with which the diagnosis is made only at autopsy.

Liver imaging is the most revealing investigation and shows 90% or more of symptomatic abscesses. A leucocytosis is frequent, alkaline phosphatase activity is usually increased and the serum albumin is often low. The chest radiograph may show a raised right diaphragm and collapse or effusion at the base of the right lung.

Treatment includes antibiotics and drainage of the abscess. Pending the findings from the culture of pus aspirated from the abscess, treatment should commence with a combination such as ampicillin, gentamicin and metronidazole.

Aspiration or drainage with a catheter placed in the abscess under the guidance of ultrasound is increasingly preferred to surgical drainage, but the latter may be required for those who fail to respond. Untreated liver abscesses are invariably fatal.

Cysts of the liver

Solitary cysts are rare, probably congenital, vary greatly in size and occur more frequently in the right lobe.

Polycystic disease is characterised by many cysts of variable size; half the patients have associated polycystic disease of the kidneys (p. 410). Cysts may be found elsewhere as in the pancreas and lungs. Some patients have cerebrovascular aneurysms.

Hepatic cysts are usually found incidentally, often during imaging done for some other purpose. Occasionally a large cyst may cause upper abdominal pain, nausea, vomiting and a palpable mass. Complications are rare and include obstructive jaundice, infection, torsion, bleeding and rupture. Portal hypertension may occur in the polycystic form. Liver function tests are usually normal.

THE GALL BLADDER AND BILE DUCTS

ANATOMY AND PHYSIOLOGY

The junction of interlobular bile ducts forms the right and left hepatic ducts which exit from the liver in the porta hepatis. These join immediately to form the common hepatic duct which, with the common hepatic artery and portal vein, lies in the free edge of the lesser omentum. The common hepatic and cystic ducts join to form the common bile duct which varies in length (2–9 cm) depending on where the junction occurs. The common bile duct, passing towards the duodenum, may be sub-divided into supraduodenal, retroduodenal, intrapancreatic and intraduodenal portions; it is, however, more useful to separate it into a thin-walled, wide-lumened proximal part up to 8 mm in diameter on ultrasonography, and a thick-walled, narrow-lumened distal part 1–3 cm in length which may taper to a thread radiologically. The thick-walled segment starts just outside the duodenal wall; it may be seen radiologically as a notch and is formed by the muscular choledochal sphincter (sphincter of Oddi) which is separate from the pancreatic duct sphincter. The common bile and pancreatic ducts usually fuse in the duodenal submucosa to enter the second part of the duodenum at the apex of the papilla of Vater.

The gall bladder is a pear-shaped sac of about 50 ml capacity situated under the right hepatic lobe. Its fundus lies close to the tip of the right ninth costal cartilage, its body and neck passing posterosuperiorly into the cystic duct which runs in a series of S-bends to join the common hepatic duct. Congenital abnormalities of the biliary system are rare but biliary atresia or a choledochal cyst may occur. Most anomalies are variations of normal anatomy.

The liver secretes bile continuously, producing 1–2 litres daily at a pressure of 15–25 cm of water. As the resting pressure in the common bile duct is somewhat higher than that in the gall bladder, bile enters the latter where it is concentrated about 10-fold by water and electrolyte absorption. The intraluminal pressure in the common bile duct is probably maintained by the choledochal sphincter. Bile duct pressures above 30 cm of water inhibit bile secretion. Reflux of bile into the pancreatic duct often occurs normally.

The gall bladder receives an autonomic nerve supply, mainly from the vagus; acetylcholine causes contraction of gall-bladder muscle and it is likely that vagal innervation controls gall-bladder tone while the sympathetic nerve supply has little or no effect. Gall-bladder contraction is due mainly to cholecystokinin secreted by the duodenal mucosa in response to food (p. 271). The choledochal sphincter normally opens and closes rhythmically; cholecystokinin and glyceryl trinitrate cause it to relax, while secretin and the analgesic drugs morphine, pethidine and pentazocine cause contraction. Of the analgesic drugs, pentazocine causes least sphincteric contraction.

INVESTIGATION

Radiological investigation. *A plain radiograph* may show stones in the gall bladder or bile ducts, the soft tissue mass of an inflamed gall bladder, gas in the biliary tree (due to a fistula into the intestine following the recent passage of a stone) or pancreatic calcification. Between 10–30% of gallstones are radio-opaque.

Cholecystography. An iodine-containing compound is used which is absorbed from the gut, excreted into the bile and concentrated in the gall bladder so that it becomes radio-opaque; it is given the night before the investigation. The normal gall bladder shows as a homogeneous ovoid opacity. Non-opaque gallstones may show as 'filling defects' within the opaque area; much less commonly a tumour may do the same. Failure of the gall bladder to opacify is a frequent finding in gall-bladder disease (non-functioning gall bladder). However, failure to take, or vomiting of, the tablets, gastric outflow obstruction, diarrhoea, occasionally intestinal malabsorption, poor liver function or a serum bilirubin above 35 μmol/l (2 mg/100 ml) can produce the same result. In addition, for unknown reasons, a normal gall bladder may fail to opacify in up to 20% of patients; for this reason the test should then be repeated if the gall bladder is non-functioning, doses of the contrast medium being given on each of the 2 days prior to the test. If the gall bladder still fails to opacify, it is virtually certain to be diseased.

Intravenous cholangiography. This is no longer regarded as a reliable investigation because the extent of opacification of the biliary tree is much less than that achieved by direct forms of cholangiography so that gallstones cannot be excluded by this method. Furthermore allergic reactions are fairly frequent.

Percutaneous transhepatic cholangiography is of value in patients with obstructive jaundice and it may be done if the prothrombin time and platelet count are satisfactory. Under local analgesia, a narrow bore needle is passed into the liver and contrast material is injected under radiological control until a bile duct is entered. Where there is large-duct obstruction, the dilated biliary tree is usually entered readily allowing a demonstration of the site and often the nature of the obstruction. Less frequently the biliary tree is shown to be normal. Failure to enter the biliary tree cannot be taken to exclude fully a large duct obstruction.

While narrow-bore needles have reduced the risk of biliary leakage and peritonitis, facilities for surgery should be available.

Operative cholangiography. The biliary tree should always be defined by injecting contrast material during operations on the biliary tract, either via the cystic duct or directly into the common bile duct.

Endoscopic retrograde cholangiopancreatography. (ERCP, p. 274).

Ultrasonography is a sensitive method for detecting gallstones and tumours in the gallbladder, and it can reveal cholecystitis by showing thickness of the gall bladder wall. Ultrasonography is a particularly useful investigation in pregnancy. It is also the best initial investigation of jaundice because it accurately demonstrates dilatation of the biliary tree due to mechanical obstruction

Cholescintigraphy is a safe means of demonstrating biliary excretion and can be used to detect bile duct obstruction and cholecystitis. ^{99m}Tc-labelled radionuclides, which are rapidly concentrated in the biliary system, are injected intravenously. Non-visualisation of the gall bladder in association with the clinical picture of acute cholecystitis indicates a blocked cystic duct and supports the diagnosis of acute cholecystitis.

Choledochoscopy allows the direct inspection of the common bile duct at surgery and is a useful adjunct to operative cholangiography in avoiding the retention of stones in the common duct. It can also be used to remove retained stones via a T-tube track.

GALLSTONES

Gallstone formation is the commonest disorder of the biliary tract and it is unusual for the gall bladder to be diseased in the absence of stones.

Epidemiology and pathology. The prevalence of gallstones is not known because in most instances they are asymptomatic but about 15–20% of the adult population in Britain are affected, the frequency being greater than 40% in those over 60 years. In those less than 40 years there is a 3:1 female preponderance whereas in the elderly the sex ratio is about equal. Gallstones are common in North America, Europe and Australia, but less frequent in India and the Far East, and rare in African blacks. In prosperous countries the incidence of symptomatic gallstones seems to be increasing and occurring at an earlier age.

In the past, gallstones have been classified by their macroscopic appearance into metabolic, inflammatory and mixed types. Biochemical analysis, however, has shown this to be misleading. In countries where gallstones are common, cholesterol is the most usual and frequently the major component irrespective of appearance. In Western countries cholesterol gallstones account for up to 75% of stones and contain between 50–98% of cholesterol. The remaining 25% of stones are calcium bilirubinate (pigment stones) which are either black or brown in colour. While in some cases the cause for pigment stones is haemolysis or infection in the biliary tree, the cause is unknown in the majority of patients in Western communities.

Aetiology of cholesterol gallstones. Formation of these is due mainly to physico-chemical changes in bile predisposing to cholesterol precipitation. Cholesterol, which is insoluble in water, is held in solution in bile by its association with bile acids and phospholipid in the form of mixed micelles (p. 301). In gallstone disease, the liver produces bile containing reduced amounts of bile acid relative to cholesterol. The bile therefore becomes saturated or even supersaturated with cholesterol. Such bile is termed lithogenic. These changes precede gallstone formation and may be due to either a reduction in the size of the bile acid pool associated with reduced bile acid secretion into the bile or an absolute increase in cholesterol secretion as in obese patients. Although the liver produces the abnormal bile, the gall bladder is important in gallstone formation because it provides a site for cholesterol precipitation and a reservoir for gallstone growth. Factors promoting or inhibiting crystal formation are important. Infection and inflammation in the gall bladder may enhance the tendency to form stones.

Certain conditions predispose to gallstone formation, e.g. obesity and high parity in younger women. Disease or loss of the terminal ileum and long-term cholestyramine therapy leads to loss of bile acids in the faeces; cirrhosis is associated with the formation of pigment stones. Diets to lower serum cholesterol and the long-term use of oral contraceptives also increase the frequency of gallstones.

Clinical features. The great majority of gallstones give rise to no symptoms and remain silent during the patient's lifetime. Symptomatic gallstones manifest either as biliary pain ('colic') or cholecystitis. In the former there is pain in the right upper quadrant, pain radiating to the right chest posteriorly or right shoulder-tip pain. In acute cholecystitis there are additionally fever, nausea and vomiting with marked tenderness and guarding in the right upper quadrant. The pain may last for hours or days and be induced by food.

Fatty food intolerance, 'dyspepsia' and flatulence are not reliable symptoms of gallstones. Thus 'gallstone dyspepsia' is a misnomer and not an indication for cholecystectomy.

Occlusion of the cystic duct may result in a mucocele of the gall bladder which may be palpated in the right upper quadrant. If the material becomes infected an empyema of the gall bladder ensues with marked tenderness, rigors, fever and leucocytosis.

A gallstone passes into the common bile duct in 10–15% of patients and may cause obstructive jaundice. Upper abdominal pain is present in three-quarters of these patients and there is frequently a history of biliary pain. Biliary infection causes fever in one-third of cases; ascending cholangitis may then be severe, giving rise to liver abscesses or to septicaemia with shock. Obstruction is usually incomplete so that the faeces remain pigmented and both bilirubin and excess urobilinogen are present in the urine. Occasionally, a gallstone may obstruct the common bile duct in the absence of abdominal pain or fever and mimic a pancreatic or biliary neoplasm. In other instances, it may be associated with an attack of acute pancreatitis (p. 296).

Rarely, a larger gallstone which has reached the intestinal tract, usually via a cholecystenteric fistula, may cause intestinal obstruction usually at the terminal ileum. The clinical features are those of small intestinal obstruction with or without a history of biliary pain. Abdominal radiographs show small intestinal obstruction, perhaps the gallstone and sometimes gas in the biliary tree indicating a biliary-enteric fistula.

Investigation. In the presence of bile-duct obstruction there will be bilirubinuria and elevation of serum bilirubin, marked increase of alkaline phosphatase and gamma-glutamyl transferase activity (p. 333) and only moderate increases of transaminase. Abdominal radiographs occasionally show gallstones. Cholecystography will reveal either gallstones or a non-functioning gall bladder. Ultrasonography should be used when cholecystography fails to show gallstones in a patient with suggestive symptoms. It usually demonstrates dilated bile ducts where stones are causing jaundice, and transhepatic or retrograde cholangiography or ERCP may then be needed.

Treatment. The most satisfactory treatment is cholecystectomy with the removal of any stones elsewhere in the biliary tract. Stones lodged in the common bile duct can be removed via a sphincterotomy carried out at endoscopy; this is a very important consideration in the management of elderly and infirm patients.

The medical dissolution of gallstones is effective only with small radiolucent cholesterol stones in a gall bladder which functions on cholecystography. The success rate in properly selected patients approaches 70%; but less than 30% of patients are suitable for therapy. It takes 6 months to 2 years to dissolve stones, and long-term prophylaxis thereafter is probably required. This form of treatment may, however, have a role when surgery is inadvisable or refused. Two drugs may be used; both are naturally-occurring bile acids, chenodeoxycholic acid (12–15 mg/kg/d) and ursodeoxycholic acid (8–10 mg/kg/d). The latter may come to be preferred because it causes less diarrhoea and less disturbance of liver function tests. Patients need to be followed with 6-monthly cholecystography.

The management of the truly silent, asymptomatic gallstone is unclear. Whether or not cholecystectomy should be carried out remains controversial, but it should be considered only in those with no contraindication to surgery.

ACUTE CHOLECYSTITIS

Aetiology and pathology. Acute cholecystitis is almost always associated with obstruction of the gall bladder neck or cystic duct by a gallstone. Occasionally, obstruction may be by mucus, a worm, or rarely by a neoplasm. Initially, the inflammation is sterile being perhaps due to chemical irritation from an increasing concentration of the bile in the gall bladder. Later, enteric organisms, especially *Esch. coli* and *Strep. faecalis*, reach the gall bladder by unknown routes and secondary infection occurs. Culture of gall bladder contents within 24 hours of the onset of symptoms yields organisms in 30% of patients, whereas after 72 hours organisms are obtained in about 80%. Acute cholecystitis in the absence of stones is rare; it may develop in typhoid and paratyphoid fever during bacteraemia, or after major trauma, burns or surgery.

All degrees of inflammation occur from mild congestion to gross swelling and tenseness of the gall bladder with ulceration of its wall. Occasionally, perforation takes place or the gall bladder may become distended with pus (empyema). Prolonged obstruction of the cystic duct may also lead to distension of the gall bladder by mucus (mucocele); the patient may experience right upper abdominal discomfort and the gall bladder may be palpable. Rarely, gas forms in the wall (emphysematous cholecystitis), a condition more frequent in males and in diabetes mellitus.

Clinical features. The disease occurs at any age and is seen increasingly in persons aged under 40 years. The cardinal feature is upper abdominal pain mainly in the epigastrium and right hypochondrium. It is commonly severe, causing restlessness, pallor, sweating and vomiting. Its onset is sudden and it increases quickly to its maximum intensity. The pain is not truly colicky in nature and usually remains intense for up to an hour, though it may persist for many hours unless relief is obtained from powerful analgesics. There may be a history of previous similar pain.

Examination shows right hypochondrial tenderness and rigidity, worse on inspiration (Murphy's sign). Occasionally the gall bladder is palpable. Fever is present and rigors may occur. Jaundice is seen in a minority of patients and is usually slight.

Medical therapy is followed by recovery in 80–90% of patients though recurrences are common. Sometimes there is deterioration due to the development of empyema, perforation and peritonitis or ascending cholangitis. In such an event increasing abdominal pain and rigidity, high fever, tachycardia and hypotension occur.

Investigation. A plain radiograph of the abdomen may show gallstones. Cholecystography should not be performed as it fails to reveal the gall bladder and ultrasonography usually shows gallstones. Radionuclide biliary scintigraphy is the method of choice as failure of the gall bladder to fill indicates obstruction of the cystic duct. The serum amylase may be slightly raised and a moderate leucocytosis is common. Bilirubinuria may or may not be present.

Differential diagnosis has to be made from other causes of severe upper abdominal pain. These are mainly perforated peptic ulcer, acute pancreatitis and appendicitis especially if retrocaecal. Myocardial infarction and right basal pneumonia should always be considered. Investigations useful in this differentiation are the raised serum amylase in acute pancreatitis, chest and abdominal radiographs, and an electrocardiogram. Occasionally there may be confusion with renal colic, herpes zoster, epidemic myalgia, pleurisy and acute intermittent porphyria.

Treatment. This consists of bed-rest, relief of pain, antibiotics and maintenance of fluid balance. Severe pain is relieved best by morphine 10–20 mg intramuscularly. Increased tone of the choledochal sphincter due to this drug may be minimised by atropine 0.6 mg intramuscularly. Less severe pain can be relieved by pethidine 100 mg or pentazocine 30 mg intramuscularly. Effective relief of pain may require repeated doses of analgesic every 2–3 hours. Provided persistent vomiting is not present, oral fluids can be given. Nasogastric aspiration is required only when there is persistent vomiting, in which case fluid must be given by the intravenous route. Co-trimoxazole or an antibiotic is prescribed in the elderly and when there is marked fever or leucocytosis. The development of complications may require emergency surgery but only in less than 10% of cases.

Early operation is advocated as the definitive treatment for acute cholecystitis. Therapy is begun as above, and cholecystectomy done once the acute illness has been controlled and during that same hospital admission. The results of such therapy are similar to those of conservative treatment in which the inflammation is allowed to resolve spontaneously and surgery is undertaken 3 months after the acute episode. It does, however, require only the one hospital admission, and it obviates the possibility of recurrent attacks.

Postcholecystectomy syndrome. Where cholecystectomy is carried out for acute cholecystitis in the presence of gallstones, at least 70% of patients get complete relief of symptoms. When symptoms persist or biliary pain recurs, radiological examination of the biliary tree for gallstones or unrecognised neoplasia should be performed. Endoscopic retrograde cholangiopancreatography is specially valuable. In some patients, neither this nor investigation for other diseases such as peptic ulcer or pancreatitis shows any abnormality. The patients are then often considered to suffer from a functional abnormality of the biliary tree — 'biliary dyskinesia'. In some, sphincterotomy may be helpful if there is radiological or manometric evidence of spasm of the lower choledochal spinchter. In others, antacids, simple analgesics, sedatives, avoidance of foods clearly followed by symptoms and reassurance should be tried. In many patients with the postcholecystectomy syndrome the indications for cholecystectomy were incorrect, namely fat intolerance or flatulence.

MISCELLANEOUS DISEASES OF THE GALL BLADDER AND BILIARY TRACT

Cholesterolosis of the gall bladder. In this condition lipid deposits in the submucosa and epithelium appear as multiple yellow spots on the pink mucosa. The changes are restricted to the gall bladder, symptoms are due to associated gallstones and the condition is recognised only at operation.

Adenomyomatosis of the gall bladder. Here there is hyperplasia of all elements in the gall bladder wall usually localised to the fundus where it shows as a filling defect on cholecystography. Localised adenomyomatosis is responsible for folding of the gall-bladder fundus, the 'phrygian cap'. Adenomyomatosis may also be generalised in which case cholecystography shows a distorted gall bladder. Frequently there are associated gallstones. Although in most cases there are no symptoms, recurrent biliary pain sometimes occurs. Polyps may be demonstrated by cholecystography or ultrasound. In symptomatic patients, treatment is by cholecystectomy though where there are no gallstones operation should not be performed before excluding other diseases, especially peptic ulcer and pancreatitis.

Sclerosing cholangitis. In this condition there is fibrotic obliteration of the extra- or intrahepatic duct system. It may be primary, associated with ulcerative colitis or retroperitoneal fibrosis, or secondary to cholelithiasis or biliary surgery. There is gradually progressive cholestasis and abdominal pain punctuated by episodes of cholangitis. Secondary biliary cirrhosis may occur. The diagnosis can be made at ERCP when material for cytology can be obtained or by biopsy of the bile ducts at laparotomy.

Choledochal cyst. This cystic dilatation occurs in the common bile duct. It almost always presents by the age of 30 years with episodes of jaundice or abdominal pain. A mass is sometimes palpable in the right hypochondrium. Treatment is surgical, usually by drainage of the cyst or, rarely, excision.

Tumours of the gall bladder and bile ducts

Benign tumours are uncommon and usually found incidentally at operation or autopsy. Cholesterol polyps, sometimes associated with cholesterolosis of the gall bladder, papillomas and adenomas are the main types.

Carcinoma of the gall bladder is a rare tumour occurring more often in women and above the age of 65 years. It usually is in the fundus or neck of the gall bladder and some 90% are adenocarcinomas. The remainder are anaplastic or, rarely, squamous tumours. Gallstones are usually also present and these are held to be important in the aetiology of the tumour.

There may be a history of repeated attacks of biliary pain followed by general deterioration in health, and weight loss or the patient may present with jaundice. The gall bladder or a mass is palpable in the right hypochondrium in half the patients.

Liver function tests most frequently show cholestasis. Gall-bladder calcification, detectable on an abdominal radiograph, is strongly associated with cancer. Endoscopic retrograde or percutaneous transhepatic cholangiography may be helpful but frequently the diagnosis is made only at laparotomy.

In the majority of patients, the tumour is inoperable and survival is short.

Cholangiocarcinoma is an uncommon tumour arising anywhere in the biliary tree from the small intrahepatic bile ducts to the papilla of Vater. It is not associated with cirrhosis. Virtually all the tumours are adenocarcinomas of varying degrees of differentiation and often with a marked connective tissue stroma.

Clinically, obstructive jaundice is the usual presenting feature unless the tumour involves only the right or left hepatic duct or an intrahepatic radical. Half the patients have upper abdominal pain and weight loss. Intrahepatic tumours are diagnosed as described for hepatocellular carcinoma (p. 361) with the exception that alpha-fetoprotein is hardly every found. Transhepatic or retrograde cholangiography are the best methods for diagnosing large duct tumours preoperatively. Tumours above the junction of the hepatic ducts are often missed at operation despite operative cholangiography which may not show the intrahepatic ducts.

It is rarely possible to remove the tumour surgically, but a bypass procedure to relieve itching is worthwhile as these tumours often grow only slowly. Biliary obstruction, particularly when pruritus is present, can be relieved by passing a drainage tube (stent) through the tumour by a transhepatic or perendoscopic retrograde route. This is applicable particularly to elderly patients and to those who are unfit for surgery.

Carcinoma at the papilla of Vater needs to be differentiated from cholangiocarcinoma and carcinoma of the pancreas (p. 300) as resection is often possible and consequently prognosis is much better. Papillary carcinomas present with obstructive jaundice and occult blood is often found in the faeces. They can be identified and biopsied at duodenoscopy, and their resectability assessed by ERCP and, if necessary, by CT imaging.

PROSPECTS IN HEPATOBILIARY DISEASE

The last 15 years have seen the development of serological means for identifying the hepatitis A and B viruses, and for identifying the recently discovered delta virus. Methods are now needed for identifying the non-A, non-B viruses, especially as they can cause chronic infection and may therefore cause chronic liver disease. Several serological possibilities have been investigated but no progress has been made in producing a reliable test for these viruses.

The production of effective vaccines against hepatitis B viral infection has been an important advance. This vaccine could have a major impact on reducing chronic viral infection, chronic liver disease and hepatocellular carcinoma especially in countries where chronic hepatitis B viral infection is common, as in Asia. Production of vaccine is limited as the starting material is plasma from chronic carriers of the hepatitis B virus and current research aims to produce viral components synthetically which should eventually allow the production of large amounts of a much less costly vaccine.

Considerable efforts are being made currently to find measures to eradicate chronic hepatitis B viral infection. Treatment so far has been aimed at ending active viral replication which is associated with progressive damage in the liver and with high infectivity. Successful treatment results in loss of viral DNA and DNA polymerase from the blood and seroconversion of HBeAg to anti-HBe. Promising results have been obtained with adenine arabinoside and interferon. No treatment eliminates the virus totally perhaps because it becomes incorporated in the genome of the host cell.

In chronic liver disease, prevention must be the long-term objective. Much will depend on how society faces the problem of alcohol abuse. Where disturbance of immunity seems to be an aetiological factor, recent observations indicate that the T lymphocyte has a significant role and advances in this area may lead to more rational therapy.

The development of a liver support system for the management of patients with liver failure has, as yet, met with only limited success. Difficulties include perfecting such materials as polymer-coated charcoal capable of adsorbing substances toxic to the liver. Progress in this field is urgently required if we are to reduce the very high mortality in acute liver necrosis and also to facilitate liver transplantation. The latter has reached the stage where about 50% of suitable patients survive more than a year with an excellent quality of life. Drugs such as cyclosporin may improve the results in the future.

Much effort continues to be expended upon the aetiology of gallstone disease with the emphasis mainly on factors promoting and inhibiting nucleation and stone growth. The widespread introduction of ultrasonography and its use as an epidemiological tool will undoubtedly provide a better understanding of risk factors and the natural history of cholelithiasis. Technological developments in the endoscopy of the biliary tree continue to advance rapidly and the place of conventional surgery in biliary tract disease will increasingly come under review. But the main goal of clinicians — a convenient, safe, and non-invasive method for permanently removing gallstones — remains as elusive as ever.

JOHN RICHMOND
N.D.C. FINLAYSON
I.A.D. BOUCHIER

FURTHER READING:

Sherlock S 1985 Diseases of the liver and biliary system, 7th edn. Blackwell Scientific Publications, Oxford. A classic, single-author account of clinical and investigative hepatology

Shearman D J C, Finlayson N D C 1988 Diseases of the gastrointestinal tract and liver, 2nd edn. Churchill Livingstone, Edinburgh. A textbook primarily for clinicians

Bouchier I A D, Allan R N, Hodgson H J F, Keighley M R B 1984 Textbook of gastroenterology. Baillière Tindall, London. For further information about the gall bladder, gut and pancreas

Wright R, Millward–Sadler G H, Alberti K G M M, Karran S (eds) 1985 Liver and biliary disease, 2nd edn. Baillière Tindall, London. A very comprehensive reference book

Schiff L (ed) 1982 Diseases of the liver, 5th edn. Lippincott, Philadelphia. A very comprehensive reference book

Popper H, Schaffner F (eds) 1986 Progress in liver diseases, vol VIII. Grune and Stratton, New York

Gut and Gastroenterology. These journals provide original articles and reviews about hepatobiliary disease as well as gastroenterology

11

Diseases of the kidneys and genito-urinary system

ANATOMY AND PHYSIOLOGY

The kidneys are each composed of approximately one million nephrons, the basic structure of one of which is illustrated in Figure 11.1.

The blood supply of the kidneys is relatively large and amounts to about one-quarter of the cardiac output at rest, i.e. 1300 ml per minute. The afferent arterioles which give rise to the glomerular capillaries arise from branches of the renal artery. Emerging from the glomeruli the capillaries unite to form the efferent arterioles which then supply blood to the proximal and distal convoluted tubules surrounding the glom eruli. The medulla is supplied by arterioles which arise from those glomeruli situated in the deeper regions of the cortex.

For a short distance the afferent arterioles and distal convoluted tubules are in contact. At this point the tubular cells become tall and columnar, forming the macula densa and the wall of the arteriole is thickened by cells which contain large secretory granules. These structures together constitute the *juxtaglomerular apparatus* which is intimately concerned in the regulation of the volume of the extracellular fluids and blood pressure.

The effective filtration pressure of about 12 mmHg within the glomerular capillaries results in the filtration of fluid from the plasma into Bowman's capsule. This fluid is identical in its composition with plasma except that it normally contains no fat and very little protein. The filtrate thus formed then flows through the various parts of the tubule and is modified according to the needs of the body by tubular secretion and by the selective reabsorption of its constitutents.

Functions of the kidneys

In health the volume and composition of the body fluids vary within narrow limits and the kidneys are largely responsible for maintaining this state. The various renal functions are conveniently considered under the following headings and some are shown diagrammatically in Figure 11.1.

Regulation of the water content of the body. About two-thirds of the water filtered by the glomerulus is reabsorbed iso-osmotically in the proximal tubules. The remainder passes through the distal nephron where its reabsorption is regulated by vasopressin (p. 426) In the presence of vasopressin the distal convoluted tubules and collecting ducts become permeable to water which is then passively reabsorbed in response to the high concentration of sodium, chloride and urea which exists in the medullary interstitium. The urine thus becomes concentrated. In the absence of vasopressin the distal nephron is impermeable to water. In these circumstances tubular reabsorption of sodium chloride without water in the ascending limb of Henle's loop and the distal convoluted tubule results in the formation of a dilute urine. Disorders of the water-regulating mechanism which result in oliguria or polyuria are described on pages 374 and 432.

Regulation of the electrolyte content of the body. The electrolyte content is kept remarkably constant as a result of selective reabsorption and secretion of ions by the renal tubules. In the proximal convoluted tubule and pars recta about 65% of the filtered sodium is reabsorbed by a complex combination of active and passive transport mechanisms and a large part of the filtered chloride is reabsorbed by a passive mechanism linked to the primary active transport of sodium. The cells of the proximal tubule cannot sustain an osmotic gradient and consequently 2/3 of the filtered water is reabsorbed passively in association with the electrolytes. Most of the remaining sodium and chloride is reabsorbed,

without water, in the thick ascending limb of Henle's loop—a process essential for creation of the medullary gradient upon which concentration of the urine depends. Unabsorbed sodium passes into the distal convoluted tubules and collecting ducts where its reabsorption along with chloride or 'in exchange' for potassium or hydrogen ions is enhanced by the hormones of the adrenal cortex, particularly aldosterone. The cells lining this part of the nephron can sustain a large concentration gradient for sodium between the tubular and peritubular fluids. Thus in a sodium depleted individual the concentration of sodium in the

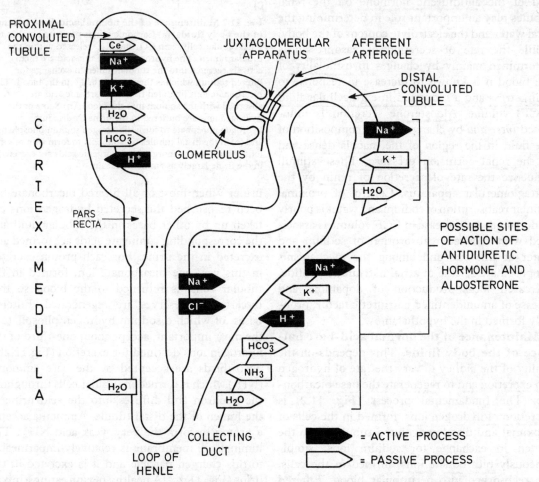

Fig. 11.1 Some of the events concerned in urine formation. In the proximal convoluted tubule about two-third ? the filtered sodium, chloride, potassium and water are reabsorbed. The greater part of the filtered bicarbonate is also reabsorbed here by a process which involves the secretion of hydrogen ions. Sodium and chloride are reabsorbed without water in the ascending limb of the loop of Henle; the loops function as counter-current multipliers and are largely responsible for the hyperosmolality of the medullary interstitium. In the distal convoluted tubule and collecting duct, potassium is transported into the cells and diffuses into the lumen in response to an electrochemical gradient. Hydrogen ions and ammonia are also secreted there and water is passively reabsorbed in the presence of antidiuretic hormone.

urine can be reduced almost to zero.

More than 90% of filtered potassium is reabsorbed in the proximal tubule and the ascending limb but the precise mechanisms are not known. Urinary potassium is largely derived from diffusion from the distal tubular cells. An electrochemical gradient is created by active transport of potassium from the peritubular fluid into the cells, a process stimulated by aldosterone, while an intraluminal potential negative with respect to the peritubular fluid favours diffusion of potassium into the lumen.

The dual actions of the adrenocortical hormones and of the antidiuretic hormone on the renal tubules play an important role in determining the total water and the electrolyte content of the body. While the rate of secretion of vasopressin is determined mainly by changes in osmolality of the blood it is known to increase in response to pain, stress and a reduction in extracellular fluid (ECF) volume. Aldosterone secretion is influenced *inter alia* by changes in the composition of the fluid in the region of the macula densa and in the renal perfusion pressure. These stimuli influence the rate of secretion of renin by the juxtaglomerular apparatus. Control of proximal tubular reabsorption of sodium and water is poorly understood. An increase in ECF volume is associated with reduced reabsorption of sodium and water at this site and among the mechanisms proposed are release of atrial natriuretic peptide, increased local production of dopamine and release of an unidentified natriuretic factor, probably formed in the hypothalamus.

Maintenance of the normal acid-base balance of the body fluids. This depends on the ability of the kidney to vary the rate of hydrogen ion excretion and to regenerate the base bicarbonate. The fundamental process (Fig. 11.2) is secretion of hydrogen ions, formed in the cells of proximal and distal convoluted tubules, into the lumen in exchange for sodium ions; simultaneously bicarbonate ions, formed in the cells, are reabsorbed into peritubular blood. Filtered bicarbonate ions are reabsorbed by this mechanism (Fig. 11.2a) up to a threshold of a plasma concentration of 25 mmol/l. When the plasma concentration rises above this level, reabsorption is incomplete and the excess is eliminated in the

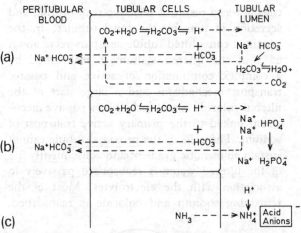

Fig. 11.2 **Maintenance of the normal acid-base balance of the body fluids.** (a) Carbonic acid is generated within the renal tubular cells from CO_2 and H_2O released within the tubular lumen. The hydrogen ions of this acid are then actively secreted into the tubular lumen in exchange for filtered sodium which is then reabsorbed into the blood. The bicarbonate ions liberated from the carbonic acid are absorbed with the sodium into the blood. (b) Some of the hydrogen ions are buffered in the urine by disodium hydrogen phosphate to form dihydrogen sodium phosphate and (c) in the distal tubules by ammonia to form ammonium ions. Anions of the inorganic and organic acids are excreted in the urine largely as ammonium salts.

urine. When most or all filtered bicarbonate has been reabsorbed the secreted hydrogen ions are taken up by other bases in the tubular fluid and the corresponding conjugate acids are formed and excreted in the urine. For each proton excreted in this way one bicarbonate ion, formed in the tubular cells, is returned to the blood so that bircarbonate reserves are regenerated. Filtered bases, of which disodium hydrogen phosphate is the most important, accept about one-third of the hydrogen ions destined for excretion (Fig.11.2b). Two-thirds are accepted by the base ammonia (NH_3) which is formed in tubular cells throughout the nephron and diffuses into the acid urine in the lumen of the distal tubule. Ammonia accepts a proton to form the very weak acid NH_4^+. The luminal cell membrane is relatively impermeable to this charged particle and it is excreted in the urine (Fig. 11.2c). A healthy person eating a mixed diet excretes 40–80mmol of hydrogen ions in the urine daily. When the rate of production of protons is increased (e.g. in diabetic ketoacidosis) the healthy kidney produces larger quantities of ammonia and up to 500 mmol/l of hydrogen ions may be excreted in the urine, mainly as NH_4^+. By contrast when a diet consisting mainly of fruit and vegetables is taken, disodium hydrogen phosphate and bicarbonate are excreted in the urine and tubular secretion of hydrogen and ammonium ions is suppressed.

Retention of other substances vital to body economy, e.g. glucose, amino acids, phosphate, bicarbonate, proteins. Glucose is normally reabsorbed so completely by the proximal tubules that none can be detected in the urine by clinical tests. Renal glycosuria (p. 468) is a benign defect of tubular reabsorption in which glucose appears in the urine in the presence of normal blood glucose levels. More rarely other congenital or acquired abnormalities of tubular transport result in abnormal loss in the urine of amino acids, phosphate, sodium, potassium, calcium and water. These defects may occur singly or in combination. Examples are cystinuria, familial hypophosphataemia, nephrogenic diabetes insipidus and the Fanconi syndrome, a disease which usually does not present until the third decade of life.

In health only a small amount of protein (0.2g/l) reaches the fluid in Bowman's capsule. The volume of glomerular filtrate, however, is so great that if this small amount were not reabsorbed, more than 36 g of protein rather than the normal 50 mg would be excreted in the urine in 24 hours.

Excretion of waste metabolic products, toxic substances and drugs. The end-products of metabolism, especially those of protein, include urea, uric acid, creatinine, phosphates and sulphates, and are excreted in the urine.

Hormonal and metabolic functions. The juxtaglomerular apparatus secretes renin, which converts angiotensin to angiotensin I. Angiotensin II, formed from the latter by a converting enzyme, probably plays an important part in regulation of the intrarenal circulation. Angiotensin II also increases the rate of aldosterone secretion by the adrenal cortex and also causes systemic vasoconstriction. This may be one mechanism by which renal ischaemia produces hypertension.

The kidney is the main source of erythropoietin necessary for normal erythropoiesis (p. 494) and it is also responsible for the formation of 1,25 dihydroxycholecalciferol (p. 63). Two prostaglandins (PGE_2 and PGI_2) are also produced within the kidney. Both are powerful vasodilators; PGI_2 is probably a mediator in renin release. Both may be concerned in the control of the renal circulation.

INVESTIGATION OF RENAL DISEASE

In many patients suffering from renal disease, symptoms and signs are not referred to the anatomical site of the kidneys. This is due to the fact that clinical features of renal disease most frequently arise from abnormalities in the chemical composition of the body or from hypertension, anaemia or metabolic bone disease. Their true origin therefore may be suspected only after the detection of urinary abnormalities and the importance of a routine examination of the urine cannot be overemphasised.

The tests which may be of value include the determination of the volume of urine passed in 24 hours, the detection of the presence of abnormal urinary constituents and bacteriological examination. Under certain standardised conditions the determination of the specific gravity or osmolality and pH of urine is of value. Chemical examination of the blood is mandatory and in addition it may be necessary to obtain further information by tests of glomerular and tubular function.

The urethra and bladder can be inspected by urethroscopy and cystoscopy and catheterisation of the ureters can provide samples of urine from each kidney.

Radiological examination includes a plain radiograph of the abdomen, excretion urography (intravenous pyelography), retrograde pyelography and renal angiography. Further information can be obtained by ultrasonic, radio-isotope and computed scanning, and by renal biopsy.

Examination of the urine

Urinary volume. In health and in temperate climates the volume of urine excreted usually lies within the range of 800–2500 ml per 24 hours. There is a limit to the power of the kidneys to concentrate urine and on a normal diet a minimum volume of 500 ml is required to excrete the solid urinary constituents which consist mainly of urea and electrolytes.

Oliguria is the production of insufficient urine

to enable solute to be excreted in adequate amounts and the *milieu intérieur* of the body to be preserved. If the concentrating power of the kidneys is seriously reduced or if the solute to be excreted is increased above the normal, as occurs, for example, in severe infections or after traumatic injury, a daily output of as much as 2–3 litres of urine may be insufficient. Oliguria develops in conditions associated with a reduction in renal blood flow and rate of glomerular filtration, e.g. sodium and water depletion, hypotension, cardiac failure, acute glomerulonephritis, acute tubular necrosis and other organic diseases of the kidneys. In these circumstances urine flow sometimes ceases completely and *anuria* develops. Anuria from this cause should be distinguished from urinary retention. In the latter case distension of the bladder will be found on examination of the abdomen and confirmed if necessary by catheterisation.

Polyuria denotes a persistent increase in urinary output. It must be distinguished from frequency of micturition, which is the frequent passage of small quantities of urine without an increase in the total volume.

There are two basic mechanisms which give rise to polyuria and which occur alone or in combination. It may be due (1) to the excretion of an abnormally large amount of solute which interferes with reabsorption of water in the nephron, or (2) to a reduction in the ability of the kidney to concentrate urine so that an increased volume of water is needed to eliminate a given amount of solute. The second defect may arise because of lack of circulating vasopressin or insensitivity of the concentrating mechanism within the kidney to its action. Polyuria occurs in the following clinical circumstances:

1. Diabetes mellitus in which an osmotic diuresis occurs because of glycosuria due to hyperglycaemia.

2. Chronic renal disease with uraemia where, in the remaining functioning nephrons, the GFR is increased. This, and the high blood levels of substances such as urea, creatinine, phosphate and sulphate results in an increased filtered load per nephron of poorly reabsorbable substances which act as osmotic diuretics.

3. Conditions in which there is decreased responsiveness of the distal nephron to vasopressin, e.g. in some cases of chronic renal disease (amyloidosis, myelomatosis, some patients with chronic obstructive nephropathy or chronic pyelonephritis), during the recovery phase of acute renal failure, in hypercalcaemia, in potassium depletion and in inherited nephrogenic diabetes insipidus.

4. Drugs which may induce unresponsiveness to vasopressin; these include lithium carbonate and amphotericin.

5. Diabetes insipidus of neurohypophyseal origin in which there is diminished secretion of vasopressin.

6. Inhibition of vasopressin secretion due to excessive drinking of fluid either from choice because of psychological disturbance or, rarely, as a result of a lesion of the hypothalamus.

7. The elimination of oedema, e.g. in recovery from heart failure or the nephrotic syndrome.

Concentration of the urine. The concentrating mechanism can be tested by measuring the osmolality or specific gravity of a specimen of urine obtained after water deprivation or administration of vasopressin. *Urine osmolality* is determined by the number of particles of solute in a kilogram of water and is essentially independent of the type of solute present. *Urine specific gravity* is an approximate measure of osmolality but depends not only on the number of particles but also on their molecular weights. In health when urea and sodium chloride are the main urinary solutes specific gravity is an approximate measure of osmolality. In uncontrolled diabetes mellitus the specific gravity is raised out of proportion to the osmolality because of the presence of large amounts of urinary glucose (MW 180).

The ability to concentrate urine is best determined by measuring the osmolality of a specimen obtained after 22 hours of food and water deprivation and it should not be less than 900 mOsm/kg (SG 1.026). This procedure is unpleasant, potentially dangerous in patients with impaired renal function and rarely necessary for clinical purposes. Instead several pre-breakfast samples are obtained daily for a few days and if the osmolality in any one reaches 700 mOsm/kg (SG approx. 1.021) no further investigation is necessary.

Those who fail this test undergo water deprivation from 16.00 hours and the first two urine samples passed next morning after rising are tested. The osmolality in at least one should be not less than 700 mOsm/kg in the young or 600 mOsm/kg in the elderly. Alternatively 20 μg of desmopressin can be instilled into each nostril at 17.00 hours and the urine passed immediately before retiring and after rising next morning should achieve the same minimal osmolality. This drug should not be used in patients with cardio-vascular disease.

Dilution of the urine. A number of conditions (p. 91) interfere with the ability to produce a dilute urine and to excrete water normally. Occasionally it is desirable to test these functions by giving the patient 1000 ml of water to drink within 20 minutes. Urine is then collected at 20 minute intervals for 4 hours. A healthy individual excretes at least 750 ml of urine in this time and the osmolality of one sample should be less than 150 mOsm/kg (SG less than 1.003). This test may be dangerous in patients with adrenal insufficiency and the result is readily invalidated by pain or emotional disturbance which lead to the release of vasopressin.

Reaction of the urine and acid excretion. In health urinary pH ranges from about 4.3 to 8.0. A very high pH (over 8.0) nearly always indicates urinary tract infection with an organism which forms ammonia from urea. In certain cir-cumstances the ability of the renal tubules to excrete hydrogen ions is depressed. This may be due to failure to form a very acid urine or inability to secrete a sufficient quantity of the buffer base ammonia. Failure to reduce the pH of the urine to less than 5.3 following oral administration of ammonium chloride is characteristic of both proximal and distal renal tubular acidosis either of which can occur as an inherited or acquired defect. Distinction between the two forms of the disorder requires more elaborate investigation. In chronic renal failure the ability to form urine of pH less than 5.3 is commonly retained but excretion of the ammonium ion is reduced and this defect can be demonstrated after administration of ammon-ium chloride.

Abnormal constituents of urine detectable by routine examination. PROTEIN in the urine, detectable by dipstix or salicylsulphonic acid

almost invariably indicates the presence of disease of the kidneys. Its magnitude bears little relation to the overall level of renal function. Significant proteinuria does not occur in disease of the lower urinary tract, though a small amount can be detected in severe urinary tract infection or in obvious haematuria. Small amounts of protein are usually found in the urine in chronic renal disease, in the course of febrile illness and in heart failure. Larger amounts of protein (3 g/d or more) are found in the nephrotic syndrome and invariably indicate glomerular disease.

The great bulk of the urinary protein is albumin and larger molecular weight plasma proteins are present in only small amounts. The pattern of proteinuria can be determined and an index of selectivity assessed. *A highly selective proteinuria* is one in which the larger molecular weight proteins are virtually absent, while a *non-selective proteinuria* is one which the larger proteins are found in significant amounts. The degree of selec-tivity is an indication of the amount of glomerular damage and is of help in predicting the response to be expected to the administration of cortico-steroids.

Postural (Orthostatic) Proteinuria. In a number of apparently healthy children and adolescents, and less commonly in adults, protein is excreted in the urine in variable but usually small amounts without associated disease of the kidneys. The urine formed while these individuals are recum-bent at night is free from protein so that examin-ation of the first specimen voided immediately on rising in the morning is normal. However urine formed while the individual follows the usual daytime activities or following vigorous exercise is found to contain protein. Tests of renal function show no abnormality and further investigations are not justified. It should be remembered that postural proteinuria sometimes occurs in the pre-sence of organic renal disease.

Bence Jones protein. Many patients suffering from one of the monoclonal gammopathies (p. 540) excrete light chains (Bence Jones protein) in their urine. These proteins are not detected by dipstix and can be best identified by immunoelec-trophoresis of urine.

BLOOD is found in the urine in a wide variety of clinical conditions; haematuria commonly indicates serious disease of the urinary tract and the cause must always be sought without delay. The appearance of the urine varies with the amount of blood and is normal to the naked eye when only traces are present. When larger amounts of blood are present the urine may be smoky in appearance, bright red or reddish-brown. The brown discolouration is due to the formation of acid haematin from haemoglobin.

Microscopic examination of the urine for red cells should be performed on the sediment obtained after centrifugation of a freshly voided specimen. They are found in varying number in acute glomerulonephritis, infective endocarditis, malignant hypertension, polyarteritis nodosa or systemic lupus erythematosus affecting the kidney, renal tuberculosis, congenital cystic disease, haemorrhagic disease, renal infarction and trauma to the kidneys. Red cells occur in the urine also in inflammation and tumours of the kidney and of the urinary tract, in benign hyperplasia and carcinoma of the prostate, and in the presence of urinary calculi. Red cells are absent, or very scanty, in minimal lesion and membranous glomerulonephritis and in most cases of the nephrotic syndrome due to other causes.

Many of these conditions can be diagnosed by the presence of characteristic symptoms and signs in addition to haematuria. When haematuria is the sole or presenting symptom the cause is most likely to be renal carcinoma, papilloma of the bladder, benign prostatic hypertrophy or, in some localities, schistosomiasis (p. 783).

When blood appears only at the beginning of micturition, the rest of the urine voided being clear, the source of bleeding is distal to the bladder. When blood is uniformly mixed with the urine, it may have come from any part of the urinary tract other than the urethra. Renal colic accompanying haematuria indicates that the bleeding is renal or ureteric in origin.

Haematuria may be mimicked by other rarer causes of discolouration of the urine:

1. *Haemoglobinuria,* which accompanies various intravascular haemolytic disorders (p. 510) and occurs occasionally in normal people after strenuous exercise. The urine gives the chemical tests for haemoglobin, but no red cells are present on microscopic examination of the centrifuged deposit of a fresh sample of urine.

2. *Myoglobinuria* occurs when lesions of skeletal muscle result in rhabdomyolysis with release of myoglobin into the circulation. No red cells are seen in the sediment, chemical tests for haemoglobin are positive but myoglobin can be distinguished from haemoglobin by spectrometry.

3. *Acute intermittent porphyria* results in large amounts of porphobilinogen being excreted in the urine. Fresh urine from such cases may appear normal, but on standing for some hours a dark red colour may develop. The presence of porphobilinogen may be suspected from the red colour produced by the addition of Ehrlich's aldehyde reagent. In contrast to that produced by urobilinogen, this colour is not extracted by chloroform.

4. *Beetroot, senna, dyes* used to colour sweets and *phenolphthalein* used in proprietary purgatives are rarer mimics of haematuria.

PUS CELLS AND BACTERIA. Pus cells may be found in the urine in inflammation of any part of the urinary tract. The urine should always be examined under the microscope and cultured when urinary tract infection is suspected. In obtaining the specimen for culture it is best to avoid catheterisation. A midstream specimen (MSU) should be obtained from both male and female patients, and a culture should be made of this within 2 hours (p.392). Suprapubic aspiration of the bladder is easily performed, without local anaesthetic, when the bladder is full. This is a useful technique for obtaining an uncontaminated sample of urine, particularly from small children. Quantitative culture of the urine should be performed; bacterial counts of more than 100 000/ml indicate significant infection in a properly obtained MSU. The presence of any bacteria in suprapubic aspirate must be considered significant.

CASTS are cylindrical structures of microscopic size which are found in the urinary sediment. They are formed in the renal tubules by the coagulation of protein. Red blood corpuscles or epithelial cells may be impressed upon this matrix, producing blood and epithelial casts respectively; such casts are found in the early stages of acute glomerulonephritis and other diseases in which there is glomerular inflammation. Granular casts are formed by degeneration of the impressed cells. Epithelial and granular casts are indicative of inflammation and degeneration of the renal tubules. Hyaline casts are formed by coagulated protein without the addition of cellular elements and are found in chronic glomerulonephritis and occasion-

ally in small numbers in normal urine, especially after vigorous exercise.

OTHER ABNORMALITIES. Glycosuria (p. 467); biliuria and urobilinogenuria (p. 332).

REFERENCE VALUES. Table 21.6 (p. 818).

Chemical analysis of the blood

With progressive impairment of renal function the composition of the body fluids becomes abnormal. These abnormalities may be detected by blood analyses. The products of metabolism which in health are excreted in the urine are retained in the blood, and the concentration of urea, creatinine and the anions such as phosphate and sulphate increases. Determination of the concentration of blood urea gives a useful indication of the degree of renal failure, but it should be remembered that it does not rise above the accepted normal maximum until renal function is reduced by at least 50%.

The diminishing capacity of the kidneys to excrete hydrogen ions results in their accumulation in the blood, and the severity of the consequent metabolic acidosis may be estimated by measurement of arterial [H^+] and the concentration of plasma bicarbonate. Estimation of plasma sodium, potassium, calcium and protein concentrations is of value in certain circumstances.

REFERENCE VALUES. Table 21.3 (p. 814).

Renal Clearance. The ability of the glomeruli to perform their function is best studied by the measurement of renal clearance where clearance $C = UV \div P$, U and P being the urinary and plasma concentration of any given substance and V the minute volume of urine. If a substance in the plasma passes freely through the glomerular filter and is neither absorbed nor excreted by the tubules, the quantity excreted in the urine (UV) is identical with the amount filtered by the glomeruli; the clearance of such a substance therefore equals the rate of glomerular filtration (GFR). The polysaccharide, inulin, appears to be excreted in this way and its clearance is used to estimate GFR, which for the average adult is about

120ml/min. A similar value is obtained using the clearance of 51CrEDTA. In clinical practice, however, the clearance of creatinine, which approximates to that of inulin, is usually carried out by collecting all the urine passed in a 24 hour period and withdrawing one sample of blood during the day of collection.

Radiological and imaging investigation

A *plain radiograph* of the abdomen should always be taken before proceeding to excretion urography. Provided the kidneys are adequately outlined by perirenal fat it can give an indication of renal size, shape and position. It can also demonstrate radio-opaque calculi or other areas of calcification such as nephrocalcinosis. It will not, however, provide any indication of renal function.

Excretion urography is carried out by the intravenous injection of an organic iodine-containing compound, about one third of which is excreted largely by glomerular filtration within the first hour. It is particularly useful to demonstrate the size, shape and position of the kidneys but two risks must be borne in mind. The patient may develop an allergic reaction to the iodinated dye. The examination should be undertaken with non-ionic contrast agents in patients with known atopy, diabetes mellitus or renal insufficiency and in those who have a history of adverse reactions to contrast agents. In addition, it is common practice to dehydrate the patient before this examination in order to increase the concentration of dye within the kidney and collecting systems and obtain a better picture. The need for this has been largely superseded by the development of agents which allow the use of greater volumes of contrast medium so that good pictures can be obtained without water deprivation. In some patients, dehydration results in significant reduction in renal function and it is therefore strictly contraindicated in children and in patients with diabetes mellitus, renal failure and multiple myeloma.

Following the injection, films are taken at timed intervals. There is first an increase in the radiographic density of renal substance (nephrogram) as the contrast medium is concentrated in the renal tubules. In the adult, healthy kidneys usually measure 11–14 cm in length and a useful guide is that the bipolar diameter is similar in length to that of three lumbar vertebrae. The renal cortical thickness can be assessed and any focal or generalised cortical defect seen, such as the scars of chronic pyelonephritis. In significant unilateral renal artery stenosis, early films will show a delay on the stenotic side, in the nephrogram which will subsequently become more dense and persist longer compared with the normal side. Thus in hypertensive patients who are being investigated for unilateral renal disease it is important to obtain early films to detect this difference. Within a few minutes the contrast begins to be excreted into the calyceal system, pelvis and ureters, which are best demonstrated within the first 20 minutes. Abnormalities in the renal papillae such as renal papillary necrosis may be seen and the appearance of the pelvi-calyceal system, ureters and bladder will indicate the presence of partial or complete obstruction or of any structural abnormalities. Clubbed calyces and slow excretion are commonly found in chronic urinary obstruction. When obstruction is severe, there is often distension of the pelvis and thinning of the renal cortex and there may be extravasation of contrast medium into extrarenal tissue. In renal tuberculosis, calcification and cavitation are common. Pools or streaks of contrast medium within the pyramids without calyceal deformity suggest medullary sponge kidney. Polycystic disease causes bilateral renal enlargement and the calyceal structure is stretched and spidery.

Pyelography. *Retrograde pyelography* is used mainly to investigate lesions of the ureter and to define the cause of obstruction. Contrast medium is injected under screening control into ureteric catheters inserted during cystoscopy. This allows direct inspection of the bladder and ureteric orifices and may be of particular value when developmental abnormalities are present. Because of the risk of introducing infection to the upper renal tract this examination should not be undertaken in the presence of acute urinary infection.

Antegrade pyelography requires percutaneous insertion of a fine catheter into the pelvi-calyceal system. This allows detailed examination of the pelvi-calyceal system and ureters and localisation of any obstruction. The procedure can be extended to allow percutaneous drainage of an obstructed system and prevent further loss of renal function. It is particularly valuable when ultrasound examination suggests distension of outflow system.

A micturating cystogram is of importance in the investigation of urinary infection in childhood. It will demonstrate vesico-ureteric reflux and give information about its severity as well as delineating lesions of the bladder neck and urethra.

Renal angiography is used to demonstrate the anatomy of the renal arterial system and is particularly useful in assessing renal artery stenosis, fibromuscular hyperplasia and arteriovenous malformations. In patients with a renal mass, it is of the value in determining whether the blood supply to the mass suggests a malignant lesion. Angiography is carried out following percutaneous catheterisation of the femoral artery with the catheter tip advanced to above the origin of the renal arteries or to within one or other renal artery. The technique of digital subtraction angiography allows for visualisation of the arterial system after an intravenous injection of contrast but as yet this technique cannot show fine details of the arterial tree. It can, however, be used in those patients in whom arterial puncture is likely to be hazardous. Angiography can be extended to carry out balloon angioplasty to dilate the artery in patients with arterial stricture. In addition, arterial embolisation can be undertaken in patients with malignant renal tumours.

Renal ultrasound is useful in assessing renal size and cortical thickness and for demonstrating focal scarring of the cortices. It also distinguishes solid renal tumours from cystic lesions and hydronephrosis. Polycystic kidney disease is readily diagnosed by ultrasound which is an excellent screening test for this condition. Dilatation of the pelvi-calyceal system and ureters, renal calculi and nephrocalcinosis are readily identified. In the assessment of patients suspected of having malignant renal tumours ultrasound can give additional information by demonstrating extension of tumour to the inferior vena cava, the regional lymph nodes or the liver. Ultrasound has many advantages being quick, inexpensive and harmless. Since there is no exposure to ionising radiation or intravenous contrast agents it is particularly useful for repeated follow-up studies.

Portable equipment is of special value in investigating patients unfit to travel.

Computed tomography is less widely available than ultrasound but it is particularly helpful in the diagnosis of masses in the Kidney and retroperitoneal tissues. The information obtained can be increased by the use of contrast agents. In patients with renal malignancy, extension of the tumour to the perirenal tissue, retroperitoneal space, renal vein or inferior vena cava can be readily identified. It is of value in assessing the extent of renal trauma, particularly when vascular damage is suspected.

Radionuclide studies require injection of radiopharmaceuticals which are taken up and excreted by the kidney thereby giving some assessment of function. The use of ionising radiation, however, restricts the frequency of follow-up studies. Static and dynamic techniques are available, the former using a radioactive compound which is taken up and retained by the renal parenchyma. Static imaging is employed to demonstrate the extent of functioning renal tissue and is particularly useful in the presence of mass lesions or areas of infarction.

Dynamic scanning employs radioactive substances which are taken up by the kidney and then excreted through the collecting systems, ureters and bladder. Computer analysis of uptake and excretion allows assessment of the renal vascular supply, the degree and rate of excretion and the presence of any obstruction. It is helpful in assessment of renovascular hypertension and when assessing obstructive uropathy. A major use is in the assessment of primary non-function in a renal transplant where it is important to differentiate between inadequate renal perfusion and acute tubular necrosis.

Renal biopsy

The technique of renal biopsy has greatly increased understanding of renal disease and in particular, knowledge of glomerulonephritis. Tissue obtained can be examined by light and electron microscopy; immunoglobulins, complement and fibrin can be identified by the use of immuno-fluorescence microscopy. Biopsy is especially useful in diagnosis in patients with proteinuria of unknown origin, in unexplained renal failure when the kidneys are of normal size, in suspected systemic disease associated with abnormal urinary constituents and in haematuria in which lesions of the lower urinary tract have been excluded. In experienced hands it is a safe procedure, but should be carried out only in patients possessing two kidneys and after the exclusion of any bleeding disorder by an appropriate coagulation screen. Hypertension, if present, should be under control.

GLOMERULAR DISEASES

Introduction

The term glomerulonephritis is used to identify a group of diseases in which the disease affects the glomerulus and is often inflammatory in nature. Glomerulonephritis can be considered as 'primary' when the major problem appears to start in the glomerulus or 'secondary' when involvement is part of a systemic disease. This distinction, while convenient, is somewhat artificial as primary glomerulonephritis may well have systemic effects while it is not uncommon in certain systemic diseases for the glomerular involvement to be the initial feature. Systemic lupus erythematosus, polyarteritis, Henoch-Schönlein disease, diabetes mellitus and amyloidosis frequently involve the kidney.

The classification of glomerulonephritis was in the past confused because glomerular diseases were identified by clinical presentation. The introduction of percutaneous renal biopsy provided a detailed histological classification which has been further expanded following development of immunohistological techniques and electron microscopy. It is now recognised that there is poor correlation between the clinical presentation and the histological appearances. For instance, a patient with a proliferative glomerulonephritis may present with the acute glomerulonephritis syndrome, the nephrotic syndrome, renal failure or hypertension while a patient with the nephrotic syndrome may have an underlying proliferative, membranous, mesangiocapillary or minimal change glomerulonephritis or systemic diseases. Renal biopsy carefully examined by light microscopy, immunohistological techniques and electron microscropy, provides the most accurate diagnostic information.

Patients with glomerular disease may present with any one of a number of clinical syndromes. The clinical hallmarks are proteinuria, haematuria, hypertension and impairement of renal function. In different types of glomerular diseases, these cardinal features are present to a variable extent, and not all will be present in all patients.

Pathogenesis of glomerulonephritis

In the majority of cases of glomerulonephritis there is clear histological evidence of inflammation; in others, such as minimal lesion glomerulonephritis, there is no evidence of an inflammatory process. In some circumstances the causative factors are known and the pathogenesis understood, in others we are ignorant of both.

Experimental models of glomerular disease have been very useful in furthering the understanding of the pathogenesis of glomerulonephritis. Two main processes are involved:

1. Immune complexes are deposited in the glomerular capillary wall or mesangium either because of 'trapping' of circulating complexes or by the formation of complexes in situ by the reaction of circulating antibody with 'fixed' or 'planted' antigens (usually endogenous).

2. There is binding in the glomerular capillary basement membrane of antibodies directed against specific antigens in the glomerular basement membrane.

When an antigen excites antibody formation there is, normally, an excess of antibody in the complexes formed and these are large and insoluble and are removed rapidly by macrophages. When complexes are relatively small and soluble they may circulate for long periods and eventually become deposited in the glomerular capillary walls. This situation usually occurs where there is a modified immune response and when there is relative antigen excess or antigen-antibody equivalence. It is possible therefore that patients who develop immune complex glomerulonephritis suffer from some minor defect of their immune system which results in the formation of abnormal complexes. The site of deposition within the glomerulus depends on the size, solubility and electrical charge of the particles, and upon the electrical charge of the capillary basement membrane. Following the interaction of antigen and antibody the complement system is activated and an inflammatory response develops. This involves attraction of polymorphs with liberation of inflammatory substances and proteases leading to the formation of further leucotactic proteins and peptides (p. 26). The glomerular response to the deposited material depends upon the site of deposition and other factors, but in most cases there is an increase in number and functional activity of cells in the mesangium. This appears to be due both to proliferation of intrinsic mesangial cells and to infiltration of monocytes. Platelets are also involved and they may produce mitogenic substances which further stimulate proliferation; they also produce platelet factor 4 which is chemotactic. The extent of this inflammatory response will depend upon the site of complex formation, the duration of complex formation and the ability of the glomerulus to remove the products of inflammation.

In a small number of cases of glomerulonephritis, a circulating antibody directed against antigens of glomerular capillary basement membrane can be detected. The pathogenesis of this is unknown but in some patients appears to follow viral infection of the respiratory tract. Deposition of the antibody severely disrupts the integrity of the capillary wall, consequently fibrinogen and other materials pass through to the urinary space and stimulate the formation of epithelial crescents. The result is a crescentic glomerulonephritis of a type known clinically as Goodpasture's syndrome.

In a number of instances of glomerulonephritis the casual antigen is known but it has become apparent that no single agent produces a uniform glomerular response. Furthermore, even in well-defined forms of glomerulonephritis, the rate of progression of the disease varies greatly from patient to patient. It is possible that the glomerular response to a specific insult is genetically determined and this theory is supported by the fact that a number of forms of glomerulonephritis are associated with particular HLA types. Furthermore in some instances the HLA may give some indication as to prognosis, e.g. HLA-B8 and

DRw3 are associated with a poor prognosis in patients with membranous glomerulonephritis. It is most likely that most glomerulonephritis is the result of some environmental factor, such as viral or bacterial antigens, acting in a susceptible patient who is relatively immuno-incompetent due to inherited or acquired factors.

CLINICAL PRESENTATION

Acute glomerulonephritis syndrome ('acute nephritis')

This syndrome is characterised by the sudden onset of haematuria, proteinuria, oliguria and hypertension which in some cases develops 7–20 days after a streptococcal infection. The infection itself may be slight or may even pass unnoticed and there is no relationship between its severity and the probability of development of acute nephritis. Acute nephritis also occurs in infective endocarditis and after viral infections. Renal biopsy shows it may be the mode of presentation of mesangiocapillary glomerulonephritis, IgA nephropathy and a number of systemic diseases, particularly vasculitis.

In children the onset is usually abrupt, a striking feature being swelling of the face, which is part of a generalised oedema caused by sodium and water retention. It is most marked around the eyes because the skin is more loosely attached to the subcutaneous tissues here and because the patient can usually lie flat. Ankle oedema is also present. There may be breathlessness due to pulmonary oedema and, in severe cases, pleural effusions. Occasionally there is discomfort in the renal angles or upper abdomen and there may be fever, anorexia, vomiting and headache. There is usually a moderate rise in blood pressure and, in a few cases, hypertensive encephalopathy.

In adults the onset is less dramatic and a history of infection is less common. The majority present with haematuria; in others the initial complaint may be progressive tiredness and slowly developing oedema of the legs.

The output of urine is usually reduced, due to a fall in glomerular filtration rate and increased tubular reabsorption of sodium and water. Anuria

may occur in severe cases. Characteristically the urine is slightly discoloured with a 'smoky' appearance but occasionally it is red. Proteinuria is usually non-selective (p.375) and seldom exceeds 3 g daily. Microscopic examination of the urinary deposit reveals red cells, leucocytes and blood, epithelial and granular casts. Erythrocyte casts are characteristic and are formed in the tubules by binding of red blood cells with Tamm Horsfall mucoprotein. In the early stages the urine is concentrated. The GFR is usually transiently reduced and the concentration of the urea in the blood raised.

In favourable cases complete recovery occurs and this is likely in the majority of children. The acute manifestations lessen in the course of 3 or 4 days, the temperature, pulse and blood pressure fall to normal. Diuresis occurs, and the oedema, haematuria and number of casts in the urine diminish. Small amounts of blood and protein may persist in the urine for several weeks or months.

Differential diagnosis. The acute glomerulonephritis syndrome must be distinguished from:

1. *Angio-oedema*, in which sudden swelling of the eyelids is a frequent feature. This condition is usually associated with swelling of the lips or tongue; urinary abnormalities are absent. The patient may be known to have an allergic history.

2. *Acute pyelonephritis*, in which oedema is absent and pain and tenderness in the lumbar region are associated with frequency of micturition. The urine contains micro-organisms, more pus cells than erythrocytes and red cell casts are absent.

3. *Haematuria* due to tuberculosis or tumours of the kidney or urinary tract in which oedema does not occur and there are no red cell casts in the urine.

Treatment. Patients suffering from this syndrome should remain in bed until haematuria, hypertension and oedema have diminished or disappeared. When the blood urea is raised the intake of protein should be reduced to 40 g daily. When oedema is present fluid should be restricted to 500 ml daily plus the volume of the previous day's urine. Daily intake of sodium should be restricted to 100 mmol ('no added salt' diet). If oedema is severe diuretics may be necessary. Any focus of infection is treated and after the acute stage is over eradicated under antibiotic cover. Hypertension does not require treatment in most cases but hypertensive encephalopathy should be treated.

Nephrotic syndrome

The nephrotic syndrome is characterised by heavy proteinuria, hypoproteinaemia and generalised oedema. The usual explanation for its development is given below. Normally only a small amount of protein crosses the glomerular capillary wall and this is reabsorbed in the proximal tubules. When the permeability of the glomerular capillary wall is increased the amount of protein presented to the tubules exceeds their reabsorptive capacity and protein spills over into the urine. Protein reabsorbed by the tubules is catabolised and therefore the net loss of protein to the patient is always greater than can be accounted for by the measured urinary loss. If the loss of protein exceeds the rate of hepatic synthesis hypoproteinaemia will ensue. This reduces plasma colloid osmotic pressure and as a result there will be an accumulation of fluid in the extravascular space. Hypovolaemia then leads to stimulation of the renin-angiotensinaldosterone system causing increased tubular reabsorption of sodium and to a rise in ADH secretion causing increased water reabsorption. Consequently there is intense conservation of sodium and water by the kidney, which in the presence of a low plasma colloid osmotic pressure, results in further accumulation of fluid in the interstitial spaces.

Lipoproteins and other proteins such as fibrinogen and other coagulation factors are increased. This may help to account for the increased incidence of atherosclerosis and thrombosis in patients with the nephrotic syndrome.

Patients present with gradually increasing oedema. The oedema is generalised, first involving the subcutaneous tissue and later serous sacs. The face is characteristically pale and puffy. General health may remain good but eventually is progressively impaired with increased liability to infection of the oedematous tissues or serous cavities. Protein malnutrition may occur.

The urine usually contains protein in moderate amounts but occasional patients excrete as much as 30 g/d. Granular and hyaline casts are seen on microscopic examination, red cells being scanty or absent. In the early stages renal function is usually normal. Plasma cholesterol is slightly raised and the plasma may look milky due to an increase in fat and lipoproteins. Both the plasma albumin and the total plasma proteins are greatly reduced.

The course and prognosis depends on the underlying renal lesion which can be determined by renal biopsy.

Treatment is directed at relief of oedema. Patients should be advised to take a diet to which no salt is added (100 mmol sodium intake). In patients with normal renal function a liberal intake (90–100 g/d) of protein is indicated in an attempt to make good the urinary loss. In patients whose renal function is already impaired there is evidence that an increased intake of protein is associated with hyperfiltration in the remaining functioning glomeruli which may result in glomerular sclerosis and renal failure.

Diuretics are of great value in controlling oedema. The most commonly used drugs act in: (1) the thick ascending limb of the loop of Henle (loop diuretics — frusemide, bumetanide, ethacrynic acid); (2) the first part of the distal convoluted tubule (thiazides, chlorthalidone, metolazone); (3) the late distal tubule (potassium-sparing diuretics — spironolactone, amiloride, triamterene). When oedema is mild a satisfactory diuresis can usually be obtained by using drugs acting on the early distal tubule. They have the advantage of inducing a fairly gentle diuresis so that they are particularly useful for patients who are working. In more severe oedema it is frequently necessary to start treatment with a loop diuretic but these have the disadvantage that they induce a large diuresis rapidly. Some patients find that this renders them housebound for up to 4 hours after taking the drug.

In a number of patients with severe oedema a combination of agents is required to achieve effective diuresis. This is necessary because, when there is a strong stimulus to retain sodium, it is essential to block sodium reabsorption at more than one site in the nephron. For example, frusemide will inhibit reabsorption of sodium in the ascending limb thereby delivering more sodium to the distal nephron; when there is marked secondary aldosteronism much of the sodium will be reabsorbed in this portion of the tubule and only when an aldosterone antagonist has been added will effective diuresis occur. In a few patients combined diuretic therapy with three drugs is required and in such a situation it is essential to employ drugs which act at different sites. In patients who are profoundly oedematous it may be necessary to give intravenous albumin to increase the plasma colloid osmotic pressure temporarily in order to obtain a diuresis. When an oedema-free state has been achieved patients can frequently maintain it on a much smaller dose of diuretic.

Asymptomatic proteinuria

This can be defined as the chance detection of proteinuria during routine urine testing, usually in young people who are undergoing medical examination for employment or insurance purposes. The proteinuria may be orthostatic (p. 375), or induced by exercise when it is usually of no sinister significance. In other circumstances proteinuria may indicate underlying glomerular disease. In such patients renal biopsy is indicated if the proteinuria exceeds 2 g daily, if there is associated hypertension, haematuria or impaired renal function, if the plasma complement is reduced or when the underlying renal disease has to be clearly defined for employment, insurance or any other purpose.

Recurrent haematuria

Painless recurrent haematuria is most commonly confused with the acute glomerulonephritis syndrome. In recurrent haematuria, however, there is no latent period between the associated infection and appearance of macroscopic haematuria. In most patients, there are repeated episodes of macroscopic haematuria usually appearing within 1 or 2 days of the development of a mucosal inflammatory illness. The macroscopic haematuria usually lasts for 2–3 days and between episodes microscopic haematuria can often be detected. Proteinuria rarely exceeds 2 g/d and hypertension and oliguria are uncommon. It occurs most commonly in young adults and is most frequently associated with IgA nephropathy (p. 385).

In some patients, recurrent haematuria is associated with unilateral or bilateral loin pain (the 'loin pain haematuria syndrome'). This most commonly occurs in young women. On light microscopy, renal biopsy reveals no significant glomerular abnormality, except for slight mesangial cell increase in some cases. There is often deposition of complement (C3) in arterioles. The aetiology and pathogenesis is unknown, but some patients exhibit an exaggerated immune complex reaction.

Other clinical presentations

Hypertension. A number of patients presenting with the typical acute glomerulonephritis syndrome will have hyptension. In others the finding of hypertension is the first indication of glomerular disease. In the absence of a typical acute glomerulonephritis, this usually indicates a long-standing glomerulonephritis and, not uncommonly, there is associated impairment of renal function.

Acute renal failure (p. 401). This can be caused by a number of glomerular diseases, most commonly by crescentic glomerulonephritis, vasculitis and disseminated intravascular coagulation.

Chronic renal failure. At the time of presentation a number of patients have severe renal impairment (p. 397) which has clearly developed over many months or years. These patients usually have bilateral small smooth kidneys and a presumptive diagnosis of progressive glomerulonephritis is made on the basis of significant proteinuria, haematuria and hypertension in the absence of any other obvious cause of impaired renal function. Renal biopsy is usually inadvisable in view of the high risk of bleeding. Furthermore, it may be difficult to determine the precise histological category. In any event, it is unlikely that treatment in such circumstances will result in significant improvement in function.

Table 11.1 Glomerular diseases. GN = glomerulonephritis.

Histopathology	Common presenting feature	Prognosis
Proliferative GN		
1. Diffuse proliferative GN	Acute GN syndrome	Resolution in majority of children; prognosis less good in adults
2. IgA Nephropathy	Recurrent haematuria	Usually a benign course; a minority develop renal failure
3. Mesangiocapillary GN	Nephrotic syndrome	Slow development of renal failure
4. Focal or segmental GN	Haematuria; acute GN syndrome	Good. Small minority develop renal failure
5. Crescentic GN	Acute GN syndrome	Rapid development of renal failure
Minimal lesion GN	Nephrotic syndrome; asymptomatic proteinuria	Reversible with corticosteroids or cyclophosphamide
Membrane GN	Asymptomatic proteinuria; nephrotic syndrome	25% spontaneous resolution 50% slow development renal failure
Focal and segmental glomerulosclerosis	Nephrotic syndrome	Frequent progression to renal failure

HISTOLOGICAL PRESENTATION

'Primary' glomerulonephritis

There are a number of clinical syndromes in which it would appear that the glomerulus is primarily involved in the disease process. Accurate diagnosis can only be achieved following renal biopsy. Three main histological types are recognised: *proliferative, membranous* and *minimal lesion glomerulonephritis*. The majority of cases of glomerulonephritis belong to the proliferative group (>70%) and this group can be further subdivided according to certain histological appearances (Table 11.1). It includes several variants, namely IgA nephropathy, mesangiocapillary glomerulonephritis, focal and segmental glomerulonephritis and crescentic glomerulonephritis, one form of which is Goodpasture's syndrome. This classification is a useful working structure but it must be remembered that many of these histological patterns may also be found in other conditions, e.g. in systemic lupus erythematosus there may be either a proliferative or membranous glomerular lesion.

Proliferative glomerulonephritis

In proliferative glomerulonephritis there is a varying degree of proliferation of mesangial, epithelial and sometimes endothelial cells, which is associated, in some cases, with infiltration with polymorphonuclear leucocytes and monocytes. It may occur following an infection, e.g. post-streptococcal or postviral glomerulonephritis. However, in the majority of cases it is not possible to identify the antigen which has stimulated the development of the appropriate antibody and subsequently of immune complex formation. Numerous infections are associated with glomerulonephritis and although the streptococcus has been widely implicated, its incidence in Europe has declined significantly. It is still, however, common in developing countries where the site of infection is usually the skin. Proliferative glomerulonephritis may occur at any age and in either sex. It can present in many different ways but most commonly does so as acute glomerulonephritis or the nephrotic syndrome. The clinical features appear to depend mainly on the severity of the underlying disease. In the majority of patients unselective proteinuria is present, and may be sufficient to cause the nephrotic syndrome. Haematuria is universal and the presence of red cell casts on urine microscopy is diagnostic. In the majority of patients renal function is normal, but some will develop significant impairment of function and a small proportion proceed to chronic renal failure.

Histologically two main groups can be identified although these may represent a continuous spectrum rather than distinct entities:

1. Severe proliferative changes (sometimes called diffuse endocapillary proliferative glomerulonephritis) in which there is a marked increase of mesangial cells associated with variable infiltration with polymorphonuclear leucocytes and macrophages. On immunofluorescence microscopy, immunoglobulins, complement and fibrin can usually be identified in the capillary walls and/or mesangium indicating the inflammatory nature of the condition. On electron microscopy subepithelial immune complex deposits ('humps') may be observed on the basement membrane (Fig. 11.3). Frequently electron-dense deposits can be observed within the mesangium. In some patients capsular adhesions and small crescents may be seen in a few glomeruli.

2. Mild to moderate cellular proliferation (sometimes called mesangial proliferative glomerulonephritis) in which there is a less marked mesangial cell increase associated with a variable increase in mesangial matrix. On immunofluorescence microscopy, immunoglobulins may be detected within the mesangium in association with complement. There is variable inflammatory cell infiltrate and the appearances are of a relatively benign condition.

The natural history of proliferative glomerulonephritis is variable and depends upon the severity of the glomerular lesion, the degree of renal impairment at the onset and the presence of hypertension. No specific therapy has yet been developed for this condition and treatment is therefore entirely symptomatic. A search should be made for any underlying infection and appropriate treatment instituted. Therapy should aim at good control of blood pressure with hypotensive drugs and relief of oedema with diuretics.

The prognosis is variable. In patients presenting with the acute glomerulonephritis syndrome resolution occurs in most children but the prognosis is less good in adults. Patients who present with asymptomatic proteinuria usually have a good prognosis but the greater the degree of proteinuria and the longer it persists the poorer the prognosis. Patients who, at the time of diagnosis, have hypertension or impaired renal function are more likely to progress to renal failure.

IgA nephropathy

IgA nephropathy can be considered as a variant of proliferative glomerulonephritis in which the predominant immunoglobulin deposited in the glomerulus is IgA and its site of deposition is usually in the mesangium with occasionally some in the glomerular capillary wall. It was first described about 20 years ago by Berger and co-workers from Paris and has been subsequently reported in many countries although the incidence varies considerably. It is prevalent in Japan where it accounts for 30–40% of primary glomerulonephritis and also in Southern Europe where it accounts for 20–35%. In Britain and North America it is detected in approximately 10% of renal biopsies. The geographical differences may be accounted for by different biopsy practice but in view of the known association with HLA-Bw35 and DR4 it is possible that population genetics play an important part.

It most commonly presents as recurrent haematuria in young adult males. In the majority of patients the episodes of macroscopic haematuria are closely associated with mucosal infections, usually of the upper respiratory tract. Between episodes of macroscopic haematuria, microscopic haematuria is common. In a small proportion of patients the haematuria is associated with loin pain. Minor proteinuria is common but approximately 20% of patients may develop a nephrotic syndrome. Older patients most commonly present with hypertension or chronic renal failure. The pathogenesis is unknown but in view of the close association between the episodes of macroscopic haematuria and mucosal infections, it is possible that mucosal IgA plays some part. It is likely that there is mesangial deposition of IgA immune complexes or aggregates of IgA secreted by lymphocytes in mucosal tissues in response to stimulation by bacterial or viral antigens.

On light microscopy the most common appearance is that of a diffuse and mild mesangial proliferative glomerulonephritis. In others these changes are restricted to some lobules of some glomeruli producing a focal and segmental mesangial proliferation. Commonly mesangial IgA deposition (Fig. 11.4) is associated with complement (C3) and IgG and IgM. The diffuse increase in mesangial matrix may progress to focal

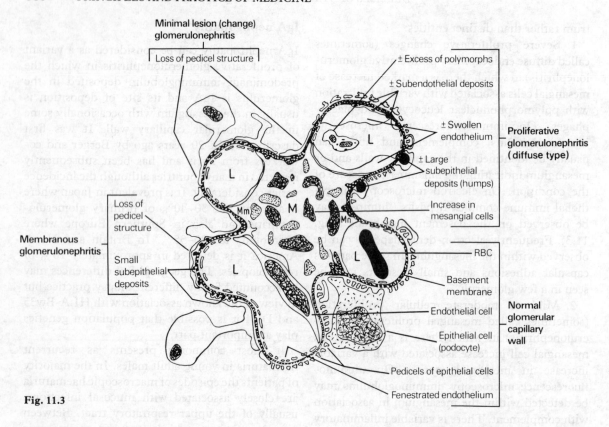

Minimal lesion (change) glomerulonephritis
Loss of pedicel structure

± Excess of polymorphs
± Subendothelial deposits
± Swollen endothelium

Proliferative glomerulonephritis (diffuse type)

± Large subepithelial deposits (humps)
Increase in mesangial cells

Membranous glomerulonephritis
Loss of pedicel structure
Small subepithelial deposits

RBC
Basement membrane

Normal glomerular capillary wall

Endothelial cell
Epithelial cell (podocyte)
Pedicels of epithelial cells
Fenestrated endothelium

Fig. 11.3

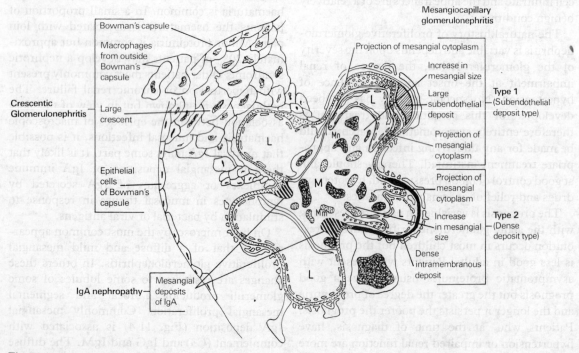

Bowman's capsule
Macrophages from outside Bowman's capsule

Mesangiocapillary glomerulonephritis

Projection of mesangial cytoplasm
Increase in mesangial size
Large subendothelial deposit

Type 1 (Subendothelial deposit type)

Crescentic Glomerulonephritis
Large crescent

Projection of mesangial cytoplasm

Epithelial cells of Bowman's capsule

Projection of mesangial cytoplasm
Increase in mesangial size

Type 2 (Dense deposit type)

Dense intramembranous deposit

IgA nephropathy
Mesangial deposits of IgA

Fig. 11.4

glomerulonephritis (below). No specific therapy has been shown to affect the natural history of this condition. It usually follows a benign course and after an interval of 5–10 years many patients become asymptomatic. As the episodes of macroscopic haematuria are associated with upper respiratory tract infections, long-term antibiotic therapy and/or tonsillectomy have been advocated, but have not been shown to be of value.

Although IgA nephropathy has been considered to be a relatively benign condition long-term follow-up studies indicate that approximately 25% of patients may develop some renal functional impairment and, in Britain, about 10% progress to end-stage renal disease and require chronic dialysis. The features which indicate a poor prognosis are the presence of proteinuria in excess of 3.5 g daily, hypertension, older age onset and the appearance of focal glomerulosclerosis on biopsy. IgA nephropathy has been known to recur in transplanted kidneys.

Mesangiocapillary glomerulonephritis

In mesangiocapillary glomerulonephritis (MCGN) the glomeruli which are diffusely involved show a marked enlargement of mesangial tissue due to both cellular proliferation and to a disproportionately large increase in matrix. This gives the glumeruli a lobular appearance. The capillary lumen is often diminished and may be displaced to the periphery of the lobule. Electron microscopy reveals two main subgroups. In type 1 large subendothelial deposits are present and the mesangial cytoplasm extends from the mesangium to the capillary wall (Fig. 11.4). There is the formation of a new layer of basement membrane on the luminal side giving the capillary walls the appearance of having a double contour. In type 2 the capillary wall is thickened due to the deposition of electron-dense linear deposits in the lamina densa of the basement membrane (Fig.

11.4). Similar deposits can be found in Bowman's capsule and tubular basement membrane.

The two types have many clinical similarities. They most commonly present between the ages of 15 and 25 years and there is slight female preponderance. The clinical presentation is usually with acute glomerulonephritis and although some may present with recurrent haematuria only, a few patients present with nephrotic syndrome. Hypertension and impaired renal function are frequently present at diagnosis. Many have hypocomplementaemia. In type 1 this is due to classical pathway activation whereas in type 2 the alternate pathway is involved due to the presence of a nephritic factor (p. 22).

The pathogenesis is unclear. In some instances it would appear that type 1 MCGN follows streptococcal infections or is associated with bacterial endocarditis or an infected ventriculoatrial shunt. The activation of complement would suggest that it is immune complex mediated and some accounts have reported the presence of circulating complexes. In type 2 MCGN the nephritic factor is an IgG autoantibody and it is likely that the consequent low C3 predisposes to glomerular disease.

There is no specific treatment for either type 1 or type 2 MCGN. A number of regimens have been suggested including steriods, immunosuppresive drugs, anticoagulants and antiplatelet drugs but none has been shown to be of particular value.

In both types the prognosis is poor, approximately 75% of patients progressing to end-stage renal failure over a variable period. However, a number of patients retain stable renal function. Development of hypertension or increasing proteinuria are poor prognostic signs. Type 2 MCGN frequently recurs in transplanted kidneys.

Focal and segmental glomerulonephritis

This condition is characterised by proliferative and sometimes necrotic changes which occur in

Fig. 11.3 Glomerulonephritis (GN). A composite diagram in which the normal capillary wall is contrasted with the pathological changes found in proliferative, minimal lesion and membranous GN [L = capillary lumen; M = mesangium; Mn = mesangial nucleus; Mm = mesangial matrix column]. (Courtesy of Department of Pathology, University of Edinburgh.)

Fig. 11.4 Glomerulonephritis (GN). A composite diagram showing a section of Bowman's capsule, the walls of 4 capillaries and the related mesangium to illustrate the pathological changes found in IgA nephropathy, crescentic and mesangiocapillary GN [L = capillary lumen; M = mesangium; Mn = mesangial nucleus; Mm = mesangial matrix column]. (Courtesy of Department of Pathology, Unversity of Edinburgh.)

segments of some but not all glomeruli. 'Focal' is used to indicate that only some glomeruli are affected and 'segmental' indicates that only a segment of the glomerulus is involved.

The most common presenting feature is haematuria or acute glomerulonephritis. Focal and segmental glomerulonephritis occurs most commonly in young adults and proteinuria is frequently associated with systemic disease such as Henoch-Schönlein purpura, microscopic polyarteritis, Wegener's granulomatosis and bacterial endocarditis.

Histologically the appearances are of mesangial cell proliferation confined to a percentage of glomeruli and usually to only part of the tuft. In some instances the lesions may be necrotising and occasionally small crescents are present. The pathogenesis in cases unassociated with other systemic diseases is unknown.

There is no specific treatment. A search should be made for underlying systemic disease which might be amenable to therapy. The prognosis is generally good and only a small minority progress to renal impairment. In patients in whom there is an underlying systemic disease, the prognosis is that of the systemic disease.

Crescentic glomerulonephritis

In this form of proliferative glomerulonephritis the most striking feature is the presence of large cellular epithelial crescents occuring in 70% or more of glomeruli (Fig. 11.4). These large crescents are associated with glomerular ischaemia and the remaining glomerular tuft usually shows no proliferation and is frequently distorted.

Clinically crescentic glomerulonephritis occurs most commonly in adults presenting as acute glomerulonephritis or acute renal failure. There is no association with any specific agent although many patients appear to have had a preceding viral illness. Renal failure is common and hypertension is usually mild and proteinuria minor. There is usually a fairly rapid clinical course with development of severe functional impairment.

The pathogenesis is unknown but it is most likely that the initiating event is immunologically mediated and that there is a rupture of the capillary basement membrane with subsequent leakage of fibrinogen into Bowman's space. This acts as a stimulus to the parietal epithelial cells to divide and thereby form crescents. Monocytes and polymorphs accumulate in Bowman's space.

There is no universally successful treatment for this condition although high dose prednisolone, pulse methylprednisolone, cyclophosphamide and plasma exchange have all been advocated. The most beneficial would appear to be pulse intravenous methylprednisolone, 1 g daily for 3 days, followed by conventional high-dose corticosteroid therapy. The majority of patients deteriorate very rapidly and haemodialysis is often required early in the illness. Although a number of patients have been shown to respond to steriod therapy, the majority will develop renal failure.

Goodpasture's syndrome

This is a variety of proliferative glomerulonephritis in which there is immune-mediated glomerular damage due to the presence of a circulating antiglomerular basement membrane antibody which in most instances results in a crescentic glomerulonephritis.

Clinically it usually presents as acute renal failure and occurs most commonly in young adult males and during springtime. There is cross-reactivity between the glomerular basement membrane and pulmonary basement membrane; some patients have associated intrapulmonary haemorrhage and may present with haemoptysis. In such patients the chest X-ray reveals pulmonary infiltration and there may be significant impairment of lung function. In the majority of patients irreversible renal failure develops rapidly. On biopsy the appearances are usually those of crescentic glomerulonephritis and immunofluorescence microscopy reveals a linear deposition of IgG along glomerular capillary walls.

The diagnosis should be established as early as possible since plasma exchange combined with immunosuppression is highly effective in patients who still retain renal function. After oliguria develops, plasma exchange is ineffective and should be undertaken only for life-threatening intrapulmonary haemorrhage.

The prognosis is poor; when oliguria develops

there is likely to be any recovery of renal function even with the most intensive therapy. Intrapulmonary haemorrhage carries a poor prognosis and may occur in these patients in association with any intercurrent febrile illness.

Membranous glomerulonephritis

In membranous glomerulonephritis the glomerular capillary basement membrane is uniformly thickened and there is no significant proliferation of cells or at most a minor mesangial cell increase.

Most patients present with the nephrotic syndrome although some cases are detected because of asymptomatic proteinuria. Membranous glomerulonephritis is most common in middle age and in males. Proteinuria usually exceeds 3.5 g daily and is non-selective. Hypertension occurs in approximately one-third of patients and renal failure develops in approximately 50%. Membranous glomerulonephritis is found in association with a number of conditions (Table 11.2). It is important to search for any underlying condition, particularly a malignant neoplasm.

Table 11.2 Conditions associated with membranous glomerulonephritis.

Infections:	Malignancy:
Malaria	Carcinoma (lung, breast,
Syphilis	gastrointestinal)
Hepatitis B	Lymphoma
Drugs:	Systemic disease:
Gold	Diabestes mellitus
Mercury	SLE
Penicillamine	
Captopril	

On light microscopy there is a diffuse regular thickening of the capillary basement membrane of all glomeruli which on electron microscopy reveals numerous small subepithelial electron-dense deposits (Fig. 11.3). On immunofluorescence microscopy these deposits contain immunoglobulins and complement and in some cases, where there is an underlying predisposing cause, relevant antigens may be detected, e.g. tumour antigens. The pathogenesis is most likely the *in situ* formation of immune complexes due to the presence of circulating antigen and low avidity antibody.

A number of regimes have been reported to be beneficial in treatment including high-dose alternate day steriod therapy, immunosuppressive drugs, chlorambucil, antiplatelet agents and anticoagulants. As in any condition where a wide variety of different regimes is advocated it is likely that none is very successful. In view of the fact that only 50% of patients will progress to renal failure, it is best to reserve any therapy for those in whom deterioration is documented and to consider any such therapy experimental. Treatment for the control of blood pressure and oedema should be undertaken.

The prognosis is variable, approximately 50% of patients progressing to impaired renal function while 25% have complete remission. Patients who present with a severe nephrotic syndrome, impaired renal function or hypertension and male patients and older patients, appear to have an increased risk of developing renal failure. The presence of HLA-B8 or DRw3 is associated with a poor prognosis.

Minimal lesion glomerulonephritis

In minimal lesion glomerulonephritis the morphological changes are minor and in many the renal biopsy appears normal on light microscopy. In some, however, there is a very slight proliferation of mesangial cells. On electron microscopy there is usually a moderate to marked loss of epithelial pedicel structure (Fig. 11.3) with consequently a smearing of the epithelial cytoplasm along the glomerular capillary basement membrane. This appears to be a non-specific change and may be a reflection of the severe proteinuria.

Clinically the lesion occurs most commonly in children between 3 and 15 years. It may, however, occur in adults. It usually presents as a nephrotic syndrome associated with selective proteinuria (p. 375). Hypoproteinaemia is common and there is frequently a compensatory increase in beta-2 globulins and cholesterol. Haematuria and hypertension are rare. Renal function is usually normal although in some children where there is significant hypovolaemia there may be prerenal acute renal failure. A number of patients are atopic.

The pathogenesis is unknown but it is thought to be immunologically related because of the universal satisfactory response to steriod therapy and because relapses are frequently associated with intercurrent infections. It is likely that the condition results from many different stimuli producing increased suppressor T cell activity. There is an association with HLA-B12 and DRw7.

In children the diagnosis can be made without renal biopsy by finding selective proteinuria in the absence of haematuria, impaired renal function or hypertension. In adults diagnostic biopsy is required. Symptomatic treatment consists of diuretic therapy to control oedema. This sometimes requires to be combined with infusions of albumin. Specific treatment is with corticosteroids which are most commonly given as prednisolone 60 mg/m^2 orally, daily for 4 weeks or until proteinuria disappears. When the urine has been free from protein for 2 weeks, prednisolone should be gradually reduced to zero over 4 weeks. Some 30% of patients will have a relapse within 3 years and for those who have frequent relapses and require repeated courses of steriod the use of alternate day prednisolone therapy may reduce the incidence of steriod toxicity. For patients who have frequent relapses or develop unacceptable steriod side-effects, cyclophosphamide 75 mg/m^2 daily for 8 weeks may be of value.

Minimal lesion glomerulonephritis characteristically has a remitting and relapsing course. In time a number of patients will undergo spontaneous remission but steroid therapy is indicated because of the complications of chronic hypovolaemia and the risk of infections in patients who are grossly oedematous. Relapses occurring many years later are recognised but even in the long term there does not seem to be any deterioration of renal function.

Focal and segmental glomerulosclerosis

The term 'glomerulosclerosis' refers to partial or total replacement of a glomerulus by hyaline material, which in most cases is excess mesangial matrix. In some circumstances this appears to develop in glomeruli which are chronically ischaemic whereas in other cases it seems to result from a previous focal proliferative glomerulonephritis. There is, however, a separate entity, focal glomerulosclerosis, in which there is no underlying condition to account for the sclerosis which is typically focal and segmental.

In focal glomerulosclerosis the patient presents with the nephrotic syndrome and in the early stage the condition may be clinically indistinguishable for minimal lesion glomerulonephritis but later haematuria, hypertension and renal failure are common. It can occur at any age, but is most common in children and young adults. Unlike other forms of glomerulonephritis, focal glomerulosclerosis appears initially to affect the juxtamedullary glomeruli. In these glomeruli there is an increase in mesangial matrix which gradually expands to destroy the surrounding lobule and then further until global sclerosis occurs. In time similar lesions appear in glomeruli throughout the cortex. The pathogenesis of this condition is unknown.

There is no specific treatment but hypertension and oedema require attention. Regular follow-up of patients is mandatory in view of the frequent progression to renal failure. Unfortunately recurrence in transplanted kidneys is well recognised.

RENAL INVOLVEMENT IN SYSTEMIC DISEASES

Certain systemic diseases, e.g. SLE, vasculitis, amyloidosis and diabetes mellitus (p. 481), are frequently accompanied by significant renal involvement. In most instances the disease involves small blood vessels or capillaries and the vascular structure of the kidney makes it particularly vulnerable. In many patients, the systemic manifestations will be apparent before any renal abnormality is found while in a small number, the presenting features will arise from renal involvement, the more widespread systemic manifestations becoming apparent only later. In either event, it would be wise to consider that once renal involvement is manifest, the prognosis worsens significantly.

Systemic lupus erythematosus. Clinical renal disease is present in approximately 40% of patients at presentation and this incidence increases with time. However, even at initial presentation there is evidence of renal involvement in almost all patients subjected to renal biopsy.

The renal lesion is most frequently due to deposition of immune complexes containing DNA and anti-DNA. Most commonly there is an associated diffuse proliferative glomerulonephritis which may vary in severity from a mild proliferation to necrosis and crescent formation. Some 20% of patients show a focal glomerulonephritis whilst in 15% the appearances are those of membranous glomerulonephritis. Wire loop lesions in the capillary walls are highly suggestive of SLE and haematoxylin bodies (disordered nuclei of cells damaged by autoantibodies) are specific to SLE.

SLE is a multisystem disease of remission and exacerbation and thus may present in differing ways with clinical features which are liable to change. Clinically proteinuria is the most common sign of renal involvement (p. 574). It may be asymptomatic or sufficient to produce a nephrotic syndrome. Haematuria is also common but usually microscopic. Hypertension occurs in approximately 20% of patients and renal failure may present as an acute or chronic illness. Steroid and other therapy (p. 575) is indicated. The prognosis of SLE is variable and to some extent dependent upon the type and severity of renal involvement. In patients whose renal biopsy reveals normal histology or only minor changes, the prognosis is good. Focal glomerulonephritis usually has a relatively benign course with a 5-year survival of approximately 65%. Patients with a membranous lesion also have a good prognosis. Those patients who exhibit a diffuse proliferative appearance, particularly when associated with crescents or necrosis, have a poor prognosis.

Vasculitis is inflammation of blood vessels, frequently associated with necrosis. It may affect arteries, capillaries or veins alone or in combination. The inflammation usually leads to a reduction in lumen with consequent ischaemia. There is no satisfactory classification because the clinical and pathological manifestations frequently overlap and therefore the various syndromes represent a spectrum rather than distinct entities. Vasculitis may exist as a primary condition or may complicate an underlying disease due to immune stimulation or as a consequence of drug therapy. Renal involvement is common in polyarteritis nodosa and Wegener's granulomatosis, it is variable in microscopic polyarteritis and Henoch-Schönlein purpura and uncommon in all other forms of vasculitis.

In *polyarteritis nodosa* (p. 193) haematuria is a feature and in some patients loin pain develops due to areas of renal infarction. *Microscopic polyarteritis* is a multisystem inflammation of capillaries. Renal involvement is variable consisting of either focal or segmental proliferative glomerulonephritis with or without fibrinoid necrosis or a crescentic glomerulonephritis. Hypertension is less common than in the nodosa form and the clinical presentation is usually as an acute glomerulonephritis or acute renal failure. Treatment is with corticosteroids but in both forms the prognosis is poor, renal failure being the commonest cause of death.

Wegener's granulomatosis is a variant of polyarteritis characterised by granulomatous lesions in the upper respiratory tract and lungs associated with fibrinoid necrosis of blood vessels and a focal proliferative glomerulonecrosis. Frequently the clinical presentation is with nasal symptoms and renal manifestations tend to occur late. The condition responds to cyclophosphamide which may have to be on a long-term basis.

Henoch-Schönlein purpura (p. 570) may involve the kidneys within 4 weeks of its onset and cause either asymptomatic proteinuria, haematuria, acute glomerulonephritis, nephrotic syndrome or acute renal failure. Children are more commonly affected than adults and in them the prognosis is good whereas approximately 50% of adults progress to renal failure.

Amyloidosis. This multisystem disease may be generalised or localised and may be primary or secondary to conditions such as rheumatoid arthritis, chronic suppuration, lepromatous leprosy or myelomatosis. When the kidney is involved the extracellular deposits of fibrils and protein damage glomerular capillaries and cause proteinuria which, in 30% of patients, will be sufficient to cause a nephrotic syndrome. Renal amyloidosis may also produce a renal tubular acidosis of either a proximal or distal type or nephrogenic diabetes insipidus. Renal failure is common and approximately 50% of patients will progress to terminal renal failure within 6 months of renal involvement becoming manifest. There is no satisfactory treatment.

INFECTIONS OF THE KIDNEY AND URINARY TRACT

The urinary tract, like the respiratory and digestive tracts, ends on the body surface and therefore can never be sterile throughout its length. However, when the tract is anatomically and physiologically normal and local and systemic defence mechanisms are intact, organisms are confined to the lower end of the urethra. Stasis of urine in any part of the tract is thus an important cause of urinary tract infection. The latter is defined by the presence of more than a hundred thousand organisms per ml in the midstream sample of urine and may be asymptomatic and found on routine examination. More commonly urinary tract infections induce symptoms which cause the patient to seek medical advice. Indeed such patients account for 1.2% of all consultations in general practice. In the individual patient the extent to which the urinary tract has been invaded cannot be determined with certainty on clinical grounds. However, only a minority of patients with recurrent infections of the lower urinary tract develop deterioration of renal function later in life and it is thus likely that in many cases infection is confined to the lower urinary tract. Even when there is unequivocal involvement of the kidneys, subsequent chronic renal failure is very rare in adults with anatomical and functionally normal urinary tracts.

INFECTIONS OF THE LOWER URINARY TRACT

Aetiology. Community surveys suggest that the prevalence of urinary tract infection in women is about 3% at the age of 20 and that it increases by about 1% in each subsequent decade. About 50% of women suffer from symptoms of lower urinary tract infection sometime during their adult lives. In males such infections are rare except in the older age group where urinary tract obstruction due to prostatic hypertrophy is relatively common. In women colonisation of the urethra and bladder with organisms derived from the faecal flora is facilitated by the short urethra. In 80–90% of cases the infection is due to *Esch. coli* and the remainder to proteus, pseudomonas species, streptococci or staphylococci. Certain strains of *Esch. coli* are particularly well adapted to invade the urinary tract because they possess surface pila which allows them to adhere to the urothelium. Sexual intercourse, which causes minor trauma to the urethra and facilitates retrograde spread of organisms from the introitus into the bladder, and inadequate perineal hygiene, are predisposing factors. Instrumentation of the bladder readily introduces organisms and should be avoided if possible; when essential it should be carried out with strict aseptic technique. Urine is an excellent culture medium and multiplication of organisms introduced into the bladder is limited by regular and complete bladder emptying and probably by secretion of IgA by the bladder mucosa. Residual urine left after micturition interfers with the bactericidal action of mucosal IgA; thus the patient who is unable to void completely because of obstruction below the bladder, gynaecological abnormalities or pelvic floor weakness is susceptible to infection. Patients with ureteric reflux also have residual urine because urine expelled into the ureters during voiding returns to the bladder when the organ relaxes.

Clinical features. There is often an abrupt onset of frequency of micturition and dysuria. Scalding pain is felt in the urethra during micturition and cystitis often gives rise to suprapubic pain during and for a few moments after voiding. After the bladder has been emptied there may be an intense desire to pass more urine due to spasm of its inflamed wall. Suprapubic tenderness is often present and the urine may have an unpleasant odour and appear cloudy. Gross haematuria may occur but systemic symptoms are usually slight. The diagnosis is made on the basis of the characteristic clinical features and the demonstration that a midstream urine contains pus cells and more than 100 000 organisms/ml.

Treatment. Ideally the results of urine culture should be available before specific therapy is given but if the patient is in acute discomfort a midstream specimen of urine should be sent for culture and treatment started while awaiting the result. Since infection is usually due to *Esch. coli* initial use of trimethoprim or ampicillin is rational and the antibiotic can be changed if a resistant organism is found on culture or if the response is unsatisfactory. Symptomatic relief usually occurs within 48 hours and it is not necessary to continue the drug for more 4 or 5 days. A high fluid intake is desirable and administration of sodium bicarbonate (2 g four times a day) to alkalinise the urine may help to relieve dysuria. A midstream urine should be sent for culture about 3 weeks after the end of the antibiotic course to determine whether the infection has been eradicated because relapse or recurrence of infection is relatively common.

In patients in whom the urinary tract is normal, particularly women with recurrent infection induced by sexual intercourse, freedom from attacks can usually be achieved by taking a single nightly dose of a suitable antibiotic after voiding and before going to bed. This regime should be started after completion of a curative course of treatment and continued for several months. Ampicillin, trimethoprim, nalidixic acid or cyclo-serine are examples of suitable drugs. Some women with recurrent infection remain free from attacks if they practice pre- and post-coital mictu-rition and maintain good perineal hygiene. Appli-cation of an antiseptic cream such as 0.5% cetri-mide to the peri-urethral area before intercourse may provide protection. If these simple measures fail the patient should take long-term prophylactic antibiotics as indicated above.

Possible causes of failure to respond to treat-ment or relapse include:

1. Inability to void urine completely as a result of obstruction below the base of the bladder, paraplegia or some other neurological lesion cystocele or urethrocele.

2. Continued re-infection from above (e.g. pyelonephritis associated with calculi) or from the genital tract (e.g. cervicitis or prostatitis).

3. Involvement of the bladder by (a) malignant tumour arising from the bladder or adjacent organs, (b) vesical calculus, (c) inflammation from adjacent structures (e.g. diverticulitis).

4. Post-menopausal atrophy of the urethra due to lack of oestrogen.

5. Infection with organisms resistant to the antimicrobal agent used (e.g. trichomonas, *Myco. tuberculosis*).

Asymptomatic or covert bacteriuria is defined as the presence of more than 1000 000 organisms/ml in the midstream urine of appar-ently healthy asymptomatic patients. Surveys indicate that approximately 1% of children under the age of 1, 5% of schoolgirls, 0.03% of school-boys and men and about 3% of non-pregnant adult women have covert bacteriuria. There is no evidence that asymptomatic bacteriuria is a cause of chronic interstitial nephritis (chronic pyelonephritis) in non-pregnant adults in whom the urinary tract is normal. When it occurs in infants, pregnant women or in anyone with an abnormal urinary tract, antibiotic treatment is required.

Urethral syndrome is the term applied to patients, usually female, who have symptoms suggestive of urethritis and cystitis and in whom no bacteria are cultured from the urine. Possible explanations include infection with organisms not readily cultured by ordinary methods (e.g. chlamydia, certain anaerobes), allergy to vaginal deodorants and disinfectants, and congestion of the urethra related to sexual intercourse.

Acute prostatitis gives rise to frequency and dysuria often accompanied by considerable sys-temic disturbance and perineal pain. On digital examination, per rectum, the prostate gland is usually very tender. The diagnosis is confirmed by obtaining a positive culture from urine or from urethral discharge obtained after prostatic massage. The treatment of choice is trimethoprim, erythromycin or tetracycline, all of which pene-trate prostatic secretions.

INFECTIONS OF THE UPPER URINARY TRACT

Aetiology. Bacterial infection of the renal parenchyma is usually due to ascent of organisms from the lower urinary tract via the ureter although in a few cases, notably in the newborn, it is blood borne. About 75% of infections are due to *Esch. coli*, the remainder being due to klebsiella, streptococci, staphylococci or the pro-teus group of organisms. Upper urinary tract infection is commonly associated with obstruction of the urinary tract but in adult women and in infants it can occur without evidence of such a lesion. The presence in the kidney of cysts or of scars due to previous inflammation facilitates establishment of bacteria, perhaps because such lesions cause obstruction of nephrons. Once organisms are established in the renal medulla their eradication is difficult because the high tissue osmolality interferes with the bactericidal activity of plasma, with the mobilisation of leucocytes and with phagocytic capacity.

Acute pyelonephritis

Pathology. The renal pelvis is acutely inflamed and there is often co-incident cystitis. On section small cortical abcesses and linear streaks of pus in the medulla are often evident. Histological examination shows focal infiltration of the renal tissue by polymorphonuclear leucocytes and many polymorphs in tubular lumina.

Clinical features. Commonly there is a sudden onset of pain in one or both loins, radiating to the iliac fossa and suprapublic area. In some cases, particularly in children, pain is confined to the epigastrium or iliac fossae. There may be dysuria and strangury with frequent passage of small amounts of scalding cloudy urine due to associated cystitis. In most cases the temperature rises rapidly to 38–40°C with general manifestations of fever. A rigor may occur and there may be vomiting. Tenderness and muscular guarding are usually present in the renal angle and lumbar region. Characteristically there is a leucocytosis. Microscopic examination of the urine reveals numerous pus cells and organisms, some red cells and epithelial cells.

Acute pyelonephritis in infants and children, like infections of the throat and middle ear, often presents as fever without localising symptoms. The initial feature may be a convulsion but apathy, abdominal distension and diarrhoea sometimes occur. In the febrile child the urine should always be examined for pus cells and organisms.

Acute necrotising papillitis may very rarely follow a severe attack of acute pyelonephritis. Fragments of renal papillae may then be excreted in the urine and can be identified histologically. This complication, which may lead to acute renal failure, is particularly liable to occur in diabetic patients, in paraplegics and in those addicted to analgesics.

Differential diagnosis. Acute pyelonephritis should be distinguished from acute appendicitis, salpingitis, cholecystitis and diverticulitis in which pus and organisms are not present in the urine. Less commonly nowadays it may be mimicked by *perinephric abscess* due to infection by *Staphylococcus aureus*. In this condition there are marked pain and tenderness in the renal region and there may be bulging of the loin on the affected side. Fever and polymorphonuclear leucocytosis occur and the patient is often extremely ill. Urinary symptoms are absent and there are no pus cells or organisms in the urine. An untreated perinephric abscessa may eventually point and discharge in the loin or groin.

Treatment depends upon the infecting organism and its sensitivity. Ideally this information should be available before specific therapy is begun but when the patient's condition demands treatment, administration of trimethoprim, cotrimoxazole or ampicillin, all of which are active against *Esch. coli*, can be started and the drug altered later if indicated by the results of the culture or by a poor clinical response. In the very severe case and if *Esch. coli* septicaemia occurs, an aminoglycoside should be used. Four weeks after completion of the treatment a midstream urine should be examined to ensure that the infection has been eradicated. If this has not been accomplished further treatment with an appropriate antibiotic is required.

In every case of the possibility of underlying abnormality of the renal tract must be kept in mind. Excretion urography should be performed in all men and children who present with a first attack of acute pyelonephritis and in women who have recurrent attacks. If an abnormality is found further investigation and treatment are required.

Chronic pyelonephritis

Chronic (infective) pyelonephritis is a form of chronic interstitial nephritis resulting from recurrent urinary tract infections. The morphological changes in the kidney are not entirely diagnostic, but the most important feature is the presence of coarse scars, each of which is associated with retraction of the related papilla and dilatation of the corresponding calyx. These features can be identified by excretion urography or radionuclide scanning or on examination of the kidney at operation or autopsy. Histological features are not significantly different from those of chronic ischaemia or of non-infective chronic tubulointerstitial nephritis (p. 406). The incidence of chronic pyelonephritis is not known. About 20% of patients in Europe requiring dialysis or transplant for the treatment of end-stage renal disease are said to have chronic pyelonephritis but the precise criteria used to make the diagnosis are not known so there is doubt about the accuracy of the figures.

Aetiology. In the absence of anatomical abnormalities of the urinary tract acute pyelonephritis in patients over the age of 5 does not lead to serious chronic renal disease. Possibly the most important predisposing factor is the presence of severe *vesico-ureteric reflux* (VUR) in children. Reflux of urine from the bladder into the ureter during voiding is normally prevented because the ureter passes through the vesical wall obliquely and is therefore occluded during contraction of the bladder muscle. Abnormalities of the intramural section of the ureter allow reflux to occur and this is an important means whereby organisms from the bladder may reach the kidney. VUR may be unilateral or bilateral, and its severity varies. In mild cases small amounts of urine pass a short distance up the ureter during voiding and return to the bladder after the cessation of micturition to form residual urine. In more severe cases reflux occurs up the entire length of the ureter; this results in a rise in intrapelvic pressure and then the orifices of the compound renal papillae are forced open and urine refluxes into the renal parenchyma as far as the cortex. It is thought that the scars of chronic infective pyelonephritis arise as a result of this intraparenchymal reflux, particularly if the urine is infected. VUR is commonly congenital, but can arise as a result of obstructive lesions at the bladder neck. It is thought to occur in utero, and it is likely that the scars of chronic infective pyelonephritis are formed during the first year of life. In young children with recurrent urinary tract infections the scars are found in 8–13%, and VUR is usually demonstrable on the side of the scarred kidney. Reflux diminishes as the child grows and may disappear; it is rarely demonstrable in an adult with a scarred kidney due to infection in childhood. Intrarenal reflux in young children reduces the rate at which the kidney grows.

When urinary tract infection occurs in the presence of *obstruction* due to any cause, permanent damage may result in any age group. In *pregnant women* permanent renal damage may possibly result from urinary tract infection. The hormonal changes of pregnancy cause reduced ureteric motility and ureteric dilatation and may also facilitate establishment of infection in the renal parenchyma. About 5% of pregnant women have asymptomatic bacteriuria and if no antibiotics are given acute pyelonephritis occurs in 40% of such cases; hence the importance of treating asymptomatic bacteriuria in pregnancy.

When scarring has occured, destruction of renal tissue usually continues even in the absence of recurrent infections. Why this happens is not known. Possible explanations include damage to remaining functioning glomeruli by progressive ischaemia resulting from lesions of blood vessels sustained during acute infection, survival of bacterial variants in the hypertonic medullary tissue or the development of progressive chronic tubulo-interstitial nephritis (p. 406).

Pathology. The changes may be unilateral or bilateral, and of any grade of severity. The fully developed case usually shows gross scarring of the kidneys, which may be much reduced in size with narrowing of the cortex and medulla. Renal scars are juxtaposed to dilated calyces. Histologically there is patchy fibrosis with chronic inflammatory cell infiltration, tubular atrophy, periglomerular fibrosis and eventual disappearance of nephrons. The arteries and arterioles may show sclerosis and narrowing. These changes are not diagnostic.

Clinical features. In many cases no symptoms arise directly from the renal lesions, and the patient may consult the doctor because of lassitude, tiredness and vague ill-health or for symptoms of uraemia or arterial hypertension. The discovery of hypertension or proteinuria on routine examination may be the first indication of the presence of the disease. Symptoms arising from the urinary tract, however, may also be present and include frequency of micturition, dysuria and aching lumbar pain. Occasionally weakness and fainting may occur if the renal disorder is accompanied by excessive salt loss in the urine. The urine may contain pus cells, a small amount of protein and many epithelial cells, though in some cases it may be normal.

Investigation. The intravenous urogram shows the diagnostic features. The kidneys are reduced in size and there is localised contraction of the renal substance associated with clubbing of adjacent calyces. Culture of the urine should be carried out in all cases. When infection is present *Esch. coli* is the commonest organism. Other agents include proteus, *Pseudomonas aeruginosa* and staphylococci. Investigations such as rectal and vaginal examination, cystoscopy and urography must be carried out to determine whether there is underlying abnormality causing obstruction to the flow of urine. A micturating cystogram will disclose any vesico-ureteric reflux. Renal function should be assessed by investigation of the blood urea, plasma electrolytes and creatinine clearance. In some cases it may be necessary to assess the capacity to acidify the urine or to conserve sodium.

Course and prognosis. The course is usually a long one and is sometimes punctuated by acute exacerbations. The infection is difficult to eradicate, even when underlying mechnical obstructions are found and relieved.

Pyonephrosis may occur, especially in the presence of renal calculi. It is characterised by persistent lumbar pain, intermittent pyrexia, often with rigors, emaciation, pyuria, and, if both kidneys are involved, uraemia; one or both kidneys may become palpable.

Some cases progress to chronic uraemia, which may be alleviated for a year or two by treatment. In elderly, diabetic or paraplegic patients a fulminating infection may be the immediate cause of death.

Treatment is similar to that described for the acute disease. The chronic infection is usually more difficult to eradicate. Attempts should be made to remove obstructive lesions or renal calculi by appropriate surgical procedures. An antibiotic to which the organism is sensitive should be given for 7 days (p. 394). If the infection is not eradicated suppressive treatment may be required for many months, the antibiotic used being given in smaller doses and as indicated by the changing pattern and sensitivity of the organisms in the urine.

Ampicillin, trimethoprim and nalidixic acid are valuable for this purpose. Double micturition should be practised by patients with vesico-ureteric reflux. Control of hypertension is essential.

When the renal infection is unilateral or if pyonephrosis has developed, nephrectomy may be indicated; rarely, high blood pressure may be cured by the removal of the diseased kidney. The role of surgery in the correction of vesico-uretic reflux is undecided, particularly because the reflux tends to disappear as the child grows older.

A moderate degree of uraemia may be present which progresses little for months or years. This is especially so when hypertension is absent or minimal. Cases with more severe renal impairment should be treated as indicated on page 399. Patients who lose excessive amounts of sodium in the urine become depleted of sodium and water and this increases the uraemia. Clinical improvement can be achieved in such cases by giving 5–10 g of salt daily by mouth. The limit to the additional salt is set by the occurrence of systemic or pulmonary oedema, or by an aggravation of hypertension. Sodium bicarbonate may be substituted in part for sodium chloride when acidosis is severe.

Renal tuberculosis

Tuberculosis of the kidney is invariably secondary to tuberculosis elsewhere and occurs as a result of blood-borne infection. The initial lesion develops in the renal cortex and if untreated may ulcerate into the pelvis with consequent involvement of the bladder, epididymes, seminal vesicles and prostate. The disease tends to occur in young people and may manifest itself with recurrent haematuria and dysuria due to secondary involvement of the bladder. In addition the general features of tuberculosis, i.e. malaise, fever, lassitude and weight loss, may be present. Chronic renal failure may result from destruction of kidney tissue or be due to obstruction of the urinary tract when lesions heal by fibrosis.

Culture of the urine by ordinary methods may be sterile in spite of pyuria and indeed sterile pyuria is an indication to perform special cultures for tubercle bacilli. The extent of the infection should be ascertained by cystoscopic examination, by urography and by culture of the urine from both ureters. Chemotherapy should be given as for tuberculosis elsewhere (p. 230). Partial or total nephrectomy or epididymectomy may be necessary in those in whom the disease has advanced to the stage of producing serious destruction of tissue.

CHRONIC RENAL FAILURE

Chronic renal failure is the irreversible deterioration in renal function which results from a diminished mass of effective functioning renal tissue. The ensuing impairment of the excretory, metabolic and endocrine functions of the kidney leads to the development of the clinical syndrome of *uraemia*. The kidney plays a centrol role in maintaining the *milieu interieur* and the consequences of chronic renal failure are therefore widespread. As the condition develops, the composition of the body fluids becomes abnormal, particularly with regard to its water and salt content, its acid-base equilibrium, and the concentration of nitrogenous compounds normally excreted by the kidney. Anaemia, metabolic bone disease, neuropathy and gastrointestinal abnormalities develop. Associated hypertension is common and most patients have increased susceptibility to infection and evidence of general deterioration of metabolic functions.

The social consequences of chronic renal failure are considerable. In Britain approximately 55 new patients per million of the adult population progress to terminal renal failure each year. The introduction of long-term dialysis and transplantation has transformed the outlook for such patients and these techniques must be regarded as among the most significant medical advances of this century.

Aetiology. Chronic renal failure may be caused by any condition which destroys the normal structure and function of the kidney. In many patients the condition progresses insidiously over a number of years and frequently it is impossible to determine the underlying renal disease. Conditions which can lead to chronic renal failure are:

1. *Congenital and inherited diseases*. These include polycystic disease, and rare inherited forms of glomerulonephritis such as *Alport's syndrome* in which a progressive glomerulonephritis is associated with perceptive nerve deafness and sometimes with abnormalities of the eye such as cataracts.

2. *Glomerulonephritis*. Proliferative glomerulonephritis (including mesangiocapillary glomerulonephritis) and membranous glomerulonephritis, focal glomerulosclerosis and systemic conditions such as polyarteritis, systemic lupus erythematosus, amyloidosis and diabetes mellitus frequently progress to uraemia.

3. *Hypertension*. Essential hypertension may occasionally lead to nephrosclerosis and uraemia and should certainly be considered if there is a family history of high blood pressure. Many uraemic patients are hypertensive and it is frequently difficult to determine whether this is primary or secondary. In the accelerated phase of hypertension, whatever its cause, evidence of renal disease is invariably present and renal function deteriorates rapidly.

4. *Infections of the urinary tract*. When recurrent infections occur in pre-school children, in pregnant women or in patients with abnormalities of the urinary tract they may result in a form of chronic interstitial nephritis with cortical scarring, and renal failure may ensue later. Tuberculosis, particularly if diagnosed late, may cause renal failure because of caseation in the kidney or development of obstructive uropathy due to fibrosis at the vesico-ureteric junction.

5. *Other forms of chronic interstitial nephritis*. Excessive intake of analgesics causes a form of chronic interstitial nephritis which, in severe cases, can lead to papillary necrosis and loss of renal substance. A number of patients with end-stage renal failure have chronic interstitial nephritis of unknown origin.

6. *Urinary tract obstruction* may occur from lesions from within the lumen such as calculi, lesions in the wall of the urinary tract such as neuromuscular defects or tumours and also from external compression due to conditions such as retroperitoneal fibrosis and retroperitoneal or pelvic tumours.

7. *Schistosomiasis* (p. 783) is a common cause of chronic renal failure in endemic areas in Africa and the Middle East.

Pathogenesis of uraemia. Disturbances in water, electrolytes and acid-base balance undoubtedly contribute to the clinical picture in patients with chronic renal failure but the exact pathogenesis of the clinical syndrome of uraemia is unknown. Almost any substance present in abnormal concentration in the plasma of patients with chronic renal failure has been suspected of being a 'uraemic toxin'. It is most likely that the syndrome is caused by accummulation in body fluids of a number of substances among which must be included phosphate, parathyroid hormone, urea, creatinine, guanadine, phenols and indols. There is no satisfactory way of assessing the biological toxicity of the different substances retained by uraemic patients but it must be assumed that the uraemic toxins are substances excreted by the normal kidney, particularly since symptoms improve following regular dialysis.

Clinical features. In the early stages of the disease, the patient may be asymptomatic and the existence of renal insufficiency may be revealed by discovery of proteinuria, anaemia, hypertension or a raised blood urea during the course of routine examination. When renal function deteriorates slowly it is not uncommon for patients to remain asymptomatic until the glomerular filtration rate (GFR) has fallen to less than 15 ml per minute. Later, because of the widespread effects of progressive renal failure, symptoms and signs are referable to almost every system and patients present with complaints which at first sight may not suggest their renal origin. The most frequent symptoms are loss of energy and weakness (often due to anaemia), breathlessness on exertion (due to anaemia or hypertension) and polyuria. Anorexia, nausea, vomiting and diarrhoea due to disordered intestinal motility are common and associated hypertension may cause headaches and visual disturbances. Pruritus results from metastatic calcification of the skin, pallor from anaemia and pigmentation from retention of urochromes which are normally excreted in the urine. Loss of libido results from endocrine disturbances such as hyperprolactinaemia. Lastly, most patients complain of a vague feeling of ill-health which they find difficult to describe. None of these symptoms alone is indicative of underlying renal disease but the occurrence of more than one should suggest the possibility of renal failure.

The rate of progression to end-stage renal failure is very variable but inevitably as the disease advances, renal function deteriorates and uraemia increases, the patient looks more ill and the anaemia becomes more severe. With the exception of those who develop cardiac failure and those in whom the chronic stage of the disease has followed rapidly upon the initial oedematous stage, the patients are not only free from oedema but may exhibit signs of water and sodium depletion. The skin and tongue are dry and the blood pressure may fall from its previous high value. Acidosis contributes to the dyspnoea and respirations are deep (Kussmaul's respiration). Later, hiccoughs, pruritus, muscular twitchings, fits, drowsiness and coma may ensue.

ANAEMIA is a common feature and to some extent reflects the severity of the biochemical disturbance. Several factors contribute, including (1) a reduced dietary intake of iron and other haematinics due to anorexia and dietary restrictions, (2) impaired intestinal absorption of iron, (3) diminished erythropoiesis due to the toxic effects of uraemia on the marrow precursor cells, (4) reduced red cell survival and (5) increased blood loss due to capillary fragility and poor platelet function. Plasma erythropoietin is usually within the normal range but this is inappropriately low for the degree of anaemia. When chronic renal failure occurs in patients with polycystic kidneys, anaemia is less severe — possibly because the large kidneys produce more erythropoietin. Treatment is limited to correction of any existing iron deficiency.

RENAL OSTEODYSTROPHY. Some patients complain of ill-defined bone pain and in a few marked skeletal deformities occur. These features are due to the metabolic bone disease which accompanies uraemia and consists of a mixture of osteomalacia, hyperparathyroid bone disease (osteitis fibrosa) osteoporosis and osteosclerosis. Osteomalacia results from failure of the kidney to convert cholecalciferol to its active metabolite 1,25 dihydroxycholecalciferol. A deficiency of the latter leads to diminished intestinal absorption of calcium, hypocalcaemia and reduction in the calcification of osteoid. Osteitis fibrosa results from secondary hyperparathyroidism, the parathyroid glands being stimulated by the low plasma calcium and possibly also by hyperphosphataemia. In some patients the stimulus to the parathyroid glands is sufficiently marked to induce tertiary or autonomous hyperparathyroidism and severe bone fibrosis and cyst formation may occur. Osteoporosis occurs in many patients possibly related to the mild malnutrition which is frequently associated with uraemia. Osteosclerosis occurs mainly in the sacral area, at the base of the skull and in the vertebrae; the cause of this unusual reaction is not known.

MYOPATHY. There is frequently a generalised muscle weakness in uraemia, most likely caused by a combination of poor nutrition, hyperparathyroidism, vitamin D deficiency and disorders of electrolyte metabolism.

NEUROPATHY. The functions of peripheral nerves and of the autonomic nervous system are impaired in uraemia. There is a demyelination of medullated fibres, the longer fibres being involved earlier. Sensory neuropathy may cause paraesthesiae and motor neuropathy may present as foot drop. Development of uraemic autonomic neuropathy may in part explain the frequency of disorders of gastrointestinal motility and the occasional occurrence of postural hypotension in the absence of sodium and water depletion. Clinical manifestations of neuropathy appear very later in the course of chronic renal failure. They improve and may, indeed, resolve when dialysis is started.

ENDOCRINE FUNCTIONS. These are generally depressed. In the female, amenorrhoea is common and in both sexes there is loss of libido presumably due to the associated hyperprolactinaemia.

CARDIOVASCULAR DISORDERS. *Hypertension* develops in approximately 80% of patients with chronic renal failure because of increased activity of the renin-angiotensin system, sodium retention and secondary aldosteronism. It is important to control such hypertension, since the elevated blood pressure causes further vascular damage in the kidney thus increasing renal impairment. *Atherosclerosis* is common and a number of factors, including abnormalities of lipid and carbohydrate metabolism, contribute to its development. In association with the atherosclerosis, and particularly if there is tertiary hyperparathyroidism, vascular calcification may devlop and may be sufficiently severe to cause loss of adequate per-

fusion to the limbs. *Pericarditis* is a very common finding in untreated end-stage renal failure.

ACIDOSIS. Declining renal function is associated with a diminished ability to excrete hydrogen ions and a resultant metabolic acidosis which is commonly asymptomatic. Nevertheless, wherever possible, the plasma bicarbonate should be maintained at or above 18 mmol/l by giving sodium bicarbonate supplements. Sustained acidosis results in protons being buffered in bone thereby aggravating the uraemic osteodystrophy.

INFECTIONS. Both cellular and humeral immunity are impaired, and thus increased susceptibility to infection is the rule. Urinary tract infections are very common and must be treated promptly as they may lead to further destruction of functioning renal tissue. Opportunistic infections may occur but are relatively uncommon until late in the course of renal failure.

Investigation and treatment. The management of chronic renal failure falls into three distinct parts:

1. Investigations to determine the nature of the underlying renal disease and to detect any reversible factors which are exacerbating the uraemic state.

2. Measures designed to limit adverse effects of loss of renal function and when possible to prevent further renal damage.

3. In patients with progressive destruction of renal tissue, there comes a point when some supportive measure in the form of either dialysis or transplantation is required.

When the patient first presents a detailed history and physical examination are required with particular attention being paid to the cardiovascular and genito-urinary systems. It is important to consider all possible underlying causes and both the family history and the drug history are important. Wherever possible, the nature of the underlying disease should be determined by undertaking appropriate biochemical, radiological and biopsy investigations. Occasionally treatment of the underlying renal disease arrests the progress of renal failure, e.g. treatment of renal tuberculosis. The degree of functional impairment should be assessed and the extent of any systemic complications documented.

In every case a search must be made for reversible factors which exacerbate the biochemical disturbance and these should be corrected. Renal perfusion is diminished in the presence of sodium and water depletion, following haemorrhage and when there is untreated cardiac failure or uncontrolled hypertension. The GFR is also reduced in urinary tract obstruction. Renal function can be depressed, reversibly, by nephrotoxic drugs (p. 412). Infection at any site increases protein metabolism and raises the blood urea, while infection in the urinary tract may cause reversible reduction in renal function.

In patients with established irreversible renal failure, a number of measures can be undertaken which will reduce symptoms and may slow the progression to terminal renal failure.

HYPERTENSION AND CARDIAC FAILURE. Hypertension must be controlled but over-zealous treatment must be avoided and the blood pressure reduced gradually. In the majority of patients, the best results will be obtained by maintaining the diastolic pressure in the region of 90 mmHg. Cardiac failure should be treated along the usual lines, great care being taken to modify the dose of any drugs used (p. 000).

DIET. When the serum creatinine consistently exceeds 300 μmol/l or the blood urea 25 mmol/l, dietary protein restriction should be instituted. In the adult the intake should be restricted to approximately 40 g daily and an adequate intake of carbohydrate (250 g) and fat (60 g) provided giving an energy value of at least 1700 kcal. It is not advisable to reduce the dietary protein intake further except in those patients who are unsuitable for long-term dialysis who should receive 20 g/d.

FLUID. The daily fluid intake will depend on the nature of the underlying disease. In view of the impaired concentrating power, a large volume of urine, about 2.5 l/d, is needed to excrete end-products of metabolism and a fluid intake of 3 l/d is desirable. Fluid restriction is necessary only when the GFR is less than 5 ml/min or cardiac failure is present. Patients with cystic disease, obstructive uropathy or rare tubular lesions who have marked polyuria will require additional fluid.

ELECTROLYTES. In the absence of oedema, cardiac failure or hypertension, sodium restriction is contraindicated. Excessive loss of sodium in the urine (salt-losing nephropathy) occurs in some forms of renal failure but not in chronic glomerular disease. Patients with salt-losing nephropathy readily become depleted of sodium and water, particularly if there is an episode of vomiting. When this occurs fluid and electrolytes must be given intravenously. The volume and nature of the fluid required depends on the severity of the sodium and water depletion (p. 85) and the degree of acidosis (p. 96).

Generally in patients with glomerular diseases, and/or hypertension, a diet containing about 100 mmol of sodium per day ('no added salt' diet) should be prescribed. When the creatinine clearance has fallen below 10 ml/min, potassium restriction is often required and is achieved by advising the patient to avoid high potassium foods.

OSTEODYSTROPHY. The plasma calcium and phosphate concentrations should be kept as near to normal as possible. Hypocalcaemia can be corrected by giving 0.25–1 μg/d of alfacalcidol, a synthetic analogue of vitamin D. The plasma calcium must be monitored regularly and the dose adjusted to prevent hypercalcaemia. Hyperphosphataemia, due to impaired phosphate excretion, is common in uraemia and the plasma phosphate can be reduced by the use of agents, such as aluminium hydroxide, which bind phosphate ions in the intestine. To prevent aluminium toxicity, the dose of aluminium hydroxide should be kept to a minimum and should only be administered at meal times. Hyperparathyroid bone disease responds well to such measures but in severe osteitis fibrosa parathyroidectomy is usually indicated. Osteomalacia is frequently reistant, presumably because of some other inhibitory factors acting on the bone calcification site. The osteoporotic and osteosclerotic components of renal osteodystrophy have no satisfactory treatment.

Dialysis and transplantation. The introduction of regular intermittent haemodialysis has prolonged the lives of many patients with chronic renal failure. Haemodialysis should be started when, despite adequate medical treatment, the symptoms of uraemia have become troublesome, preferably before the patient has developed serious consequences of uraemia such as severe osteodystrophy, pericarditis, neuropathy or cachexia from prolonged anorexia. Repeated access to blood vessels is achieved by establishing an arteriovenous fistula, usually in the forearm. Haemodialysis is usually carried out for 4 to 6 hours three times weekly and many patients can be trained to carry out their treatment at home. Patients on haemodialysis usually notice a gradual reduction of their uraemic symptoms during the first 6 weeks of treatment. Blood, chemistry, however, does not return to normal, anaemia, although improved, persists, and osteodystrophy may progress. Nevertheless, many patients lead relatively normal and active lives and prolonged survival in excess of 20 years is now regularly reported.

CONTINUOUS AMBULATORY PERITONEAL DIALYSIS (CAPD) is a form of long-term dialysis involving the introduction of a permanent intraperitoneal catheter to the abdominal cavity. Normally 2 litres of sterile isotonic dialysis fluid are introduced into the peritoneal cavity and left for a period of approximately 6 hours. The fluid is then drained and fresh dialysis fluid introduced. This cycle is repeated four times daily during which time the patient is fully mobile and able to undertake normal daily tasks. Initially this technique was introduced as a less expensive form of dialysis but the costs are actually very similar to those of home dialysis. However, it is particularly useful in young children, in elderly patients with cardiovascular instability and in patients with diabetes mellitus. Its long-term use may be limited by episodes of peritonitis but many patients have now been treated very satisfactorily for up to 5 years without serious complications.

RENAL TRANSPLANTATION. Offers the possibility of restoring normal kidney function and thereby correcting the many metabolic abnormalities of uraemia. The graft is usually taken from a cadaver donor or from related siblings or parents. ABO compatibility is essential and it is customary to select donor kidneys on the basis of HLA compatibility. Results of transplantation have improved significantly in the past few years. The 3-year graft survival is now in the region of 70 to 80% while 3-year patient survival is approximately 90%. Long-term immunosuppressive therapy, however, is required and this is associated with an increased incidence of infections, particularly opportunistic infections, and a greatly increased incidence of malignant neoplasm, especially of the skin. Nonetheless, trans-

plantation does offer the best hope of complete rehabilitation and is the most cost effective of all the options.

Prognosis. Unless some form of supportive therapy such as dialysis or transplanatation is available chronic renal failure is eventually fatal. When the serum creatinine persistently exceeds $300 \mu mol/l$ there is usually a progressive deterioration in renal function, irrespective of aetiology. The rate of deterioration is very variable from patient to patient, in part related to the aetiology and the development of hypertension, but it is relatively constant for any particular patient. A plot of the reciprocal of the serum creatinine concentration against time allows the physician to determine when the serum creatinine will reach a value in the region of $1000 \mu mol/l$, and dialysis will be required. Such a plot will also detect any unexpected worsening of the renal failure.

Information about the long-term prognosis for patients on dialysis or following transplantation is lacking because these techniques have been available only for the past 30 years and technology is changing rapidly. Continuous ambulatory peritoneal dialysis (CAPD) has been available for less than 10 years and so no long-term information is available. However, in spite of these limitations dialysis and transplantation can be considered as highly effective forms of treatment with a 5-year survival of approximately 80% for home haemodialysis, 65% for a transplanted kidney, 55% for hospital haemodialysis and 45% for CAPD. It should be remembered that these figures are not directly comparable because of patient selection and the fact that many older patients and those with systemic disease (e.g. diabetes mellitus) are treated by CAPD. However, they can be used as a guide and clearly indicate how the management of end-stage renal disease is very much better than that of many other potentially fatal diseases such as carcinoma.

ACUTE RENAL FAILURE

Acute renal failure (ARF) is characterised by an acute and usually reversible deterioration of renal function which develops over a period of days, or, rarely, weeks and results in uraemia. A marked reduction in urine volume is usual but not invariable. The clinical features are determined by the underlying condition and by the rapidly developing uraemia and many patients present complex problems of diagnosis and management. Many of the disorders giving rise to acute renal failure carry a high mortality but, if the patient survives, renal function usually returns to normal or near normal.

Classification. Normal renal function depends upon adequate glomerular perfusion, formation of a filtrate which is modified by tubular cell activity and excretion of the urine. ARF may be due to disruption of any of these processes and it is convenient to consider it as being *prerenal, renal* or *postrenal*. In prerenal ARF the kidneys are inadequently perfused and the GFR is greatly diminished. This may be due to a poor cardiac output, vascular disease limiting renal blood flow, or hypovolaemia resulting from haemorrhage or severe fluid depletion. Renal causes of ARF include diseases of the renal arterioles, the rapidly progressing types of glomerulonephritis, injury to tubular cells (acute tubular necrosis) by toxins or ischaemia, intraluminal obstruction of nephrons from precipitation of crystals or protein and acute interstitial nephritis due to infections or drug reactions. Postrenal ARF is caused by obstruction of the urinary tract at any point in its course. Prompt identification of the cause of prerenal or postrenal ARF and introduction of appropriate treatment will often lead to restoration of renal function. The longer the period of inadequate perfusion or obstruction the more likely it is that actual damage to kidney tissue will occur.

ACUTE RENAL FAILURE DUE TO PRE-RENAL DISORDER

Pathogenesis. The kidney receives approximately 25% of the cardiac output at rest and if cardiac output falls, regional vasoconstriction will occur limiting the blood flow to organs other than the heart and brain. Initially skin blood flow is diminished and this is followed by reduction in perfusion to the gastrointestinal tract and muscles. When the renal blood supply is restricted glomerular filtration will be reduced by selective cortical vasoconstriction and oliguria results.

Aetiology. The most important causes of pre-renal ARF are:

1. Reduced circulating blood volume due to

a. Haemorrhage from any cause including complications of pregnancy, trauma and gastrointestinal bleeding.

b. Loss of plasma as in burns and crushing injuries.

c. Sodium and water depletion (p. 85):

(i) From the gastrointestinal tract in severe vomiting, diarrhoea, acute intestinal obstruction, paralytic ileus, pancreatitis, fistulae, etc.

(ii) In urine due tok excessive treatment with diuretics, diabetic ketoacidosis, etc.

(iii) From the skin due to sweating, severe dermatitis.

2. Reduction of cardiac output (cardiogenic shock) or increase in the size of the vascular bed (septic shock).

3. Intravascular haemolysis or rhabdomyolysis (breakdown of skeletal muscle) in which substances are released which are capable of reducing the renal circulation.

4. Diseases involving the major renal vessels, such as thrombosis of the renal arteries, occlusive embolus of the aorta or renal arties or aortic aneurysm, which result in renal underperfusion.

Clinical features. Patients often present with marked reduction of blood pressure and signs of inadequate peripheral perfusion. However, ischaemia and prerenal ARF may occur in the absence of systemic hypotension. The cause of the circulatory disturbance is usually obvious but it must be remembered that significant concealed blood loss can occur into the gastrointestinal tract, following trauma (particularly where there are fractures of the pelvis or femur) and into the uterus in concealed accidental haemorrhage. It is also difficult to assess the magnitude of the loss of intravascular fluid into tissue after crushing injuries or in severe inflammatory dermatoses. The diagnosis is made on the basis of the history and clinical findings. In patients with previously normal kidneys who have not been given diuretics in the recent past the urine is highly concentrated, the osmolality exceeding 600 mOsm/kg, and the urinary concentration of sodium is less than 20 mmol/l. In such patients the urine/plasma urea ratio exceeds 10:1. These findings depend on the kidneys' ability to respond to inadequate perfusion by intense conservation of sodium and water. They will therefore not be found in patients in whom renal impairment existed before the acute episode. There is a progressive increase in blood urea and plasma creatinine.

Treatment of prerenal acute renal failure requires that the cause of the disorder be established and rectified. When hypovolaemia is present the circulation must be restored, as rapidly as possible, by replacing blood, plasma or sodium and water as indicated. It may be necessary to monitor central venous or pulmonary wedge pressure to determine the rate of administration of fluid. Provided treatment is intituted early, restitution of the renal blood fow will usually be accompanied by a return of renal function. If oliguria persists in spite of the return of the circulation to normal then the reversible structural changes of acute tubular necrosis (below) are likely to have developed. In a few cases, particularly those complicated by disseminated intravascular coagulation (p. 551), irreversible cortical necrosis may occur.

ACUTE RENAL FAILURE DUE TO INTRINSIC RENAL DISEASE

The most common cause of this condition is acute tubular necrosis due to acute ischaemia or to the effects of toxic agents such as drugs or bacterial endotoxins. In addition, ARF sometimes develops in conditions which affect the intrarenal arteries and arterioles such as hypersensitivity vasculitis, accelerated hypertension and disseminated intravascular coagulation. A number of glomerular diseases, particularly those which run a rapid course such as crescentic nephritis or focal necrotising proliferative glomerlonephritis also produce acute deterioration in renal function and there is now good evidence that acute tubulo-interstitial nephiritis (p. 406) often due to drugs, causes ARF.

Acute tubular necrosis

There are two varieties of acute tubular necrosis, the more common ischaemic type and a type caused by poisons such as heavy metals which injure cells. Although the aetiology of acute ischaemic tubular necrosis varies, the common factor in all cases is a diminution in the supply of oxygen and essential nutrients to the tubular cells which are metabolically active. This results in reduction of cell function and eventually in necrosis of small numbers of tubular cells. Fortunately these have the capacity to regenerate and to reform the basement membrane. Thus, providing the patient can be kept alive during the regeneration phase, kidney function usually returns to near normal values.

Pathogenesis. The initial insult causes disruption of the cell membrane leading to intracellular anoxia and consequently to a rapid influx of calcium ions. This disturbs mitochondrial respiration, leading to anaerobic glycolysis and intracellular acidosis. If this process continues it causes denaturation of intracellular protein, lysozomal disruption and cell death. This leads to small focal breaks in the tubular basement membrane, and consequent escape of tubular contents into the interstitial tissue.

During shock, renal blood flow is greatly reduced. Measurements of renal blood flow made during the established phase of acute renal failure (oliguric phase) indicate that when the circulation is restored in shocked patients, renal blood flow rises to about 20% of normal and remains at that level until the onset of renal recovery. During the oliguric phase there is a significant selective reduction in cortical blood flow due in part to interstitial oedema and in part to swelling of the endothelial cells of glomeruli and peritubular capillaries. These factors result in an increase in vascular resistance. Cortical blood flow may be further reduced by the action of local and systemic vasoconstrictors such as thromboxane, vasopressin, noradrenaline and angiotensin II.

It follows that a number of factors contribute to the persistent oliguria in acute renal failure. Reduced glomerular perfusion limits the rate of filtrate formation. In addition the tubular lumina may be obstructed due to formation of casts composed of necrotic tubular cells and Tamm Horsfall protein, and to external compression resulting from the raised intrarenal pressure resulting from interstitial oedema. Disruption of the tubular basement membrane allows back diffusion of tubular fluid into the interstitial space. It is likely that in the pathogenesis of the oliguric phase all these mechanisms have some part to play although their relative importance may vary depending on the nature of the primary insult.

After a period of about 10–20 days, renal function returns. There is often a transient diuretic phase in which the urine output increases rapidly and remains excessive for several days before returning to normal. This may be due to the fact that the normal medullary concentration gradient has been dissipated during the period of oliguria. Maintenance of the medullary gradient depends not only on tubular transport but also on the continued delivery of filtrate to the ascending limb of the loop. Both these factors are disturbed during the acute phase of ARF; the medullary concentration gradient is gradually 'washed out' and is not re-established until glomerular filtration and tubular function are at least partly restored. Not all patients exhibit the diuretic phase which is to some extent dependent on the severity of the renal damage and the rate of recovery.

Pathology. The pathological appearances are dependent upon the stage of the illness. In established cases, the kidneys may be enlarged and the cortex is often paler than normal, compared to the relatively dark medulla. Histologically the glomeruli appear relatively normal, although on electron microscopy there may be endothelial cell swelling and some fibrin deposition. The most obvious abnormality is the presence of scattered breaks in tubular basement membranes, sometimes associated with visible necrosis of associated tubular cells. Actual tubular cell necrosis is surprisingly insignificant but many tubules are lined by swollen vacuolated cells. Late in the syndrome the tubular epithelial cells will appear flattened, and during the regenerative phase there may be evidence of mitotic activity. There is frequently interstitial oedema and infiltration with macrophages, plasma cells and fewer polymorphs. In cases where the condition has been caused by drugs, the interstitial inflammatory appearances are more marked, and constitute an acute tubulo-interstitial nephritis (p. 206).

Clinical features are those of the causal condition together with those of rapidly developing uraemia. In many patients, there is an obvious underlying cause such as trauma or an episode of septicaemia. In the majority of patients the urine volume is greatly reduced to between 50 and 500 ml daily during the oliguric phase. Anuria (urine volume less than 50 ml daily) is rare in acute tubular necrosis and usually indicates acute urinary tract obstruction. In about 20% of cases the urine volume is normal or increased but the urine contains little nitrogen. This results from a combination of a GFR of only a few ml per minute and a gross reduction of tubular function. Thus despite an apparently good urine output the daily load of metabolic waste products cannot be excreted, the blood urea and plasma creatinine rise and the clinical picture of uraemia develops. During an episode of ARF the rate at which the blood urea and creatinine rise is determined by the rate of tissue breakdown.

In patients who are suffering from severe infections or who have undergone major surgery or trauma the daily increment of blood urea exceeds 5 mmol/l. Disturbances of water, and electrolyte and acid-base balance arise as a consequence of loss of kidney function. Hyperkalaemia is common particularly when there is massive tissue breakdown, haemolysis or metabolic acidosis and since it predisposes to ventricular arrhythmias it must be promptly controlled. Patients may have dilutional hyponatraemia at the time of presentation. Some have received inappropriate amounts of intravenous fluid but in many cases hyponatraemia is due to continued drinking in the presence of oliguria. Hypocalcaemia is also common and is thought to be due to reduced production of 1,25 dihydroxycholecalciferol by the kidneys. Metabolic acidosis develops except in patients in whom there has been excessive vomiting or aspiration of gastric contents.

At first the patient may feel well but after some days, if treatment is inadequate, the features of uraemia appear. Initially these are anorexia, nausea and vomiting. Apathy is followed by mental confusion and later muscular twitching, fits, drowsiness, coma and bleeding episodes occur. The respiratory rate is frequently elevated due to acidosis, pulmonary oedema or respiratory infection. Pulmonary oedema may be due to administration of excessive amounts of intravenous fluids. However, there is evidence that the permeability of pulmonary capillaries is increased in uraemic patients. Moreover damage to pulmonary capillaries which occurs during shock also predisposes to the development of pulmonary oedema (adult respiratory distress syndrome, p. 213). Anaemia, which is common, may be due to excessive blood loss, haemolysis or decreased erythropoiesis. Many patients have an increased bleeding tendency due to disordered platelet function and disturbances of the coagulation cascade. Gastrointestinal haemorrhage may occur, often late in the illness, from mucosal erosions throughout the length of the gastrointestinal tract. Severe infections often complicate the course of ARF because humeral and cellular immune mechanisms are depressed by uraemia.

Treatment. The principles are:

1. Institution of initial emergency measures to prevent death from hyperkalaemia, shock or pulmonary oedema.

2. Determination of the underlying cause of the condition and institution of appropriate treatment.

3. Maintenance of a satisfactory clinical and metabolic state during the oliguric phase.

4. Careful control of fluid and electrolyte balance during the diuretic recovery phase.

EMERGENCY RESUSCITATIVE MEASURES. In a significant number of cases hyperkalaemia is present when the patient is first seen and this must be corrected to prevent life-threatening cardiac arrhythmia. When there is evidence of a reduced circulating blood volume, prompt transfusion with appropriate fluids is essential and this often requires monitoring of central venous or pulmonary wedge pressure. Patients who present with severe pulmonary oedema usually require haemodialysis or peritoneal dialysis to remove sodium and water.

DETERMINATION OF THE CAUSE OF ARF. In many cases the underlying cause is obvious. When this is not the case a wide range of investigations, including renal biopsy, may be needed to establish the diagnosis.

TREATMENT OF THE OLIGURIC PHASE. In established acute renal failure, the main aims are to control fluid and electrolyte balance, maintain nutrition, prevent gross distortion of the body chemistry and protect the patient from infection. Patients with severe acute renal failure are seriously ill and require skilled nursing, preferably in single rooms designed to prevent cross-infection. Particular attention must be paid to the care of the skin and the mouth, and to prevention of infection of in-dwelling intravenous lines. Plasma urea, creatinine and electrolytes should be estimated and cultures of blood, urine and wounds carried out daily. Great care must be exercised in the use of drugs (p. 412). In all but the mildest cases some form of dialysis will be required.

WATER AND ELECTROLYTE BALANCE. Following initial resuscitation, the patient should be maintained on a daily fluid intake equal to the volume of the urine output plus 500 ml to replace insensible loss. In febrile patients an increased allowance is required to replace the fluid lost through sweating. As no electrolytes are lost the intake of these substances should be minimal but should abnormal losses of fluid occur, as in diarrhoea, additional fluid and electrolytes will be required. If possible the patient should be weighed daily. Large changes in body weight, or the development of oedema, or, alternatively, of signs of water and electrolyte depletion, indicate the need for a reappraisal of water and electrolyte intake.

PROTEIN AND ENERGY. In patients in whom it is hoped to avoid dialysis, dietary protein is restricted to about 40 g/d and attempts are made to suppress endogenous protein catabolism to a minimum by giving as much energy as possible in the form of fat and carbohydrate. For this purpose a diet restricted in its protein and electrolyte content may be supplemented by preparations containing glucose polymers. In the event of severe anorexia or vomiting, oral treatment should be stopped and parenteral nutrition given (p. 78).

In patients who are hypercatabolic, it is often necessary to resort to parenteral nutrition in order to maintain a suitable intake of energy and nitrogen. This usually involves giving a greater volume of fluid than would be required to maintain water balance and as a consequence more frequent dialysis or haemofiltration may be necessary.

DIALYSIS. It is fairly generally agreed that the blood urea should be kept below 30 mmol/l during an episode of ARF. It this cannot be achieved by dietary measures some form of dialysis is essential. In patients in whom the blood urea is rising rapidly haemodialysis is required. Peritoneal dialysis also is an effective means of correcting fluid balance and the metabolic disturbances in all but the most severe cases. It is particularly useful in small children and patients with cardiovascular disturbances.

Haemodialysis is effective in correcting the metabolic abnormalities but requires vascular access, cardiovascular stability and adequate blood pressure. The frequency with which haemodialysis is undertaken is dependent upon the rate of rise of blood urea. Haemofiltration is a technique similar to haemodialysis but which is better tolerated particularly in patients with cardiovascular instability. A newer technique of continuous spontaneous arteriovenous haemofiltration has been introduced where a highly permeable membrane filter is employed to remove an ultrafiltrate of plasma which is replaced by reinfusing an appropriate volume of a modified ringer lactate solution. This technique is employed on a 24-hour basis and is of particular value in those patients who require long-term parenteral nutrition.

RECOVERY PHASE. After approximately 10–20 days, there is a return of renal function. In a number of patients there is the rapid onset of a diuretic phase when the urine output is frequently 3–5 litres daily. This diuretic phase persists for 3–4 days and probably results from the washout of the normal medullary concentration gradient. During this time the concentration of blood urea tends to remain constant whereas the creatinine may slowly fall. Sufficient fluid must be given to replace the increased loss of water in the urine and frequently it is necessary to give it by vein as patients are rarely able to drink enough. Supplements of sodium chloride and sodium bicarbonate are usually needed during the diuretic phase to compensate for increased urinary loss. In some patients, potassium salts may also be required. After a few days, the urine volume falls as the concentrating mechanism is restored. This is associated with a gradual return of the ability to conserve sodium and potassium and to regenerate bicarbonate. The blood urea and serum creatinine fall to normal and as the renal function improves, the patient can start on a normal diet.

Prognosis. The high mortality from acute renal failure of ischaemic origin has been greatly reduced by the measures described above. Prognosis depends on the speed and efficiency with which the therapy is put into operation, the prompt recognition and effective treatment of complicating infection and the nature and severity of the condition precipitating the syndrome. In cases of uncomplicated acute renal failure such as those due to simple haemorrhage, the mortality should now be negligible even when haemodialysis is required. In severe renal failure, complicated by serious infection of multiple injuries, it is still about 70%, the outcome being determined by the severity of the underlying disorder and the complications rather than by the renal failure itself. Development of infection or of gastrointestinal haemorrhage increases the mortality significantly.

Other causes of ARF

When acute renal failure arises as a result of renal disease other than acute tubular necrosis the clinical picture is that of the underlying condition complicated by the features of acute uraemia. Frequently the diagnosis is not immediately obvious and renal biopsy must be performed to define the nature of the kidney pathology. Management is along the lines already discussed, but in addition specific treatment of the underlying renal disease may be required. Thus steroids, immunosuppressive drugs and rarely plasma exchange may be of value in acute renal failure due to hypersensitivity vasculitis and crescentic glomerulonephritis. Control of the blood pressure is critical when acute renal failure is due to accelerated hypertension.

Acute tubulo-interstitial nephritis is a well-recognised cause of acute renal failure. It results most commonly from hypersensitivity to drugs such as penicillin, ampicillin, sulphonamides or rifampicin and other manifestations of hypersensitivity such as fever, arthralgia, rashes, marrow depression, eosinophilia and disturbance of liver function may be present. Renal biopsy usually shows an acute tubulo-interstitial nephritis associated with marked interstitial oedema and infiltration with inflammatory cells, including eosinophils.

Any drugs suspected of causing the condition must be stopped. There is some evidence that resolution is speeded up in drug-induced cases by administration of steroids. Following an episode of acute tubulo-interstitial nephritis there may be a degree of permanent renal damage.

POSTRENAL ACUTE RENAL FAILURE

Acute renal failure may result from obstruction (p. 407) at any point in the urinary tract. In the presence of two functioning kidneys, ureteric obstruction causes uraemia only when it is bilateral. The diagnosis may be suggested by a history of previous urinary symptoms such as loin pain, haematuria, renal colic, nocturia or difficulty in micturition. However, in many instances, the onset is clinically silent and the cause of obstruction discovered only after appropriate investigation. In contrast to the oliguria of acute renal failure associated with tubular necrosis, anuria is common and is always suggestive of an obstructive cause.

In patients with anuria, ultrasound examination of both kidneys and ureters should be done as soon as possible. When ureteric dilatation or hydronephrosis is found, percutaneous nephrostomy can be undertaken to decompress the urinary system. This frequently results in a considerable diuresis and a satisfactory improvement in the disordered blood chemistry. Indeed relief of obstruction is sometimes accompanied by a massive diuresis which necessitates a high fluid and electrolyte intake. Antegrade pyelography can be undertaken through the nephrostomy and may reveal the cause of obstruction. Alternatively cystoscopy and retrograde pyelography can be done. In a number of instances the obstruction is caused by a malignant pelvic neoplasm such as carcinoma of the cervix or the recto-sigmoid junction. Such lesions may be palpable on rectal or vaginal examination. Unfortunately the disease is often so advanced that active intervention is seldom advisable.

When the obstruction has been relieved and the blood chemistry has returned to near normal the underlying cause must be defined and treated.

OBSTRUCTION OF THE URINARY TRACT

Obstruction to the flow of urine from the kidney through the pelvis, ureter, bladder and urethra is a common disorder; it causes stasis and a rise in pressure within the urinary tract which predisposes to infection, stone formation and renal failure. Obstruction may occur at any level but is most often found at the pelvi-ureteric junction, in the ureter, at the neck of the bladder or in the urethra. Obstruction at the pelviureteric junction causes hydronephrosis; obstruction of the ureter results in hydroureter and later hydronephrosis; obstruction of the bladder neck or urethra distends the bladder, causes hypertrophy of its muscle seen on cystoscopic examination as trabeculation, and hydroureter and hydronephrosis. If obstruction is unrelieved, slow progressive destruction of renal tissue occurs. Superimposed infection may cause cystitis or pyelonephritis in which renal damage may become more rapid.

Aetiology. Obstruction may be due to an organic lesion in the lumen or in or around the wall of the urinary tract or it may arise because of a congenital neuromuscular defect at the pelvi-ureteric junction, ureter or bladder neck preventing the contraction wave and therefore the flow of urine. Vesico-ureteric reflux is an important complication in infancy. Organic causes include stone, blood clot, tumour, or fibrosis following infection. An aberrant renal artery, retroperitoneal fibrosis, inadvertent ligation of the ureter at operation, carcinoma of the cervix, prostatic enlargement or phimosis may compress the lumen from outside.

Clinical features vary with the cause and site of the lesion and in particular whether it is above or below the bladder. When the obstruction is supravesical, renal colic may occur, especially if the onset is sudden. More commonly the obstruction is gradual and an aching pain in the loins, sometimes aggravated by drinking, develops. Superimposed infection causes systemic manifestations with fever and dysuria. Haematuria is common. Transmission of the increased hydrostatic pressure to the kidney in partial obstruction interferes with the counter-current concentrating mechanism and may result paradoxically in polyuria. Occasionally a hydronephrotic kidney is palpable. Sometimes the patient presents only with anuria and acute renal failure, and the diagnosis is made only after excretion urography or ultrasound examination reveals dilated kidneys or ureters.

When the obstruction is below the bladder, there is difficulty in micturition and the urinary stream is thin in calibre and poor in force. Complete urinary retention may occur with consequent distension of the bladder, which may be visible as a swelling of the lower abdomen and palpable; anuria or overflow incontinence may ensue. In the latter event catheterisation reveals the presence of residual urine in the bladder after the patient has voided.

Treatment. In all cases the ultimate objective is to remove the source of obstruction. This is often possible, as in the case of a stone, prostatic hypertrophy or urethral stricture. In the first instance it is necessary to relieve the obstruction in order to alleviate symptoms and preserve renal function. The action required varies with the nature of the underlying disease, but sometimes it may be dealt with temporarily by draining the kidney, i.e. nephrostomy, the ureter, i.e. ureterostomy, or the bladder, i.e. suprapubic or urethral catheterisation. Temporary drainage of the obstructed kidneys can often be achieved by inserting fine catheters into the renal pelvis under ultrasound control. Antibiotics should be given if infection is severe but it is preferable to wait until the obstruction has been removed or relieved.

When the hydronephrosis or pyonephrosis affects one kidney and this is severely damaged, nephrectomy is indicated. When obstruction affects both kidneys and is irremediable appropriate treatment for renal failure should be given.

RENAL AND VESICAL CALCULI AND NEPHROCALCINOSIS

Aetiology. Renal calculi consist of aggregates of crystals and small amounts of proteins and glycoprotein but their genesis is poorly understood. In Britain, stones in which the crystalline component consists of calcium oxalate are the most common and accounted for 39.4% of 1000 calculi analysed in a London series. In this series 13.8% of stones contained both calcium oxalate and calcium phosphate, 13.2% calcium phosphate and 15.4% magnesium ammonium phosphate. Small numbers of cystine stones and uric acid stones were found. Different types of stone occur in different parts of the world and dietary factors probably play a part in determining the varying patterns. In developing countries bladder stones are common, particularly in children. By contrast, in industrialised developed countries the incidence of childhood bladder stone is low and renal stones in adults are more common. A recent survey in Scotland found that 4% of the population had stones in the urinary tract but prevalence varies in different areas. It is surprising that renal and vesical calculi and nephrocalcinosis do not occur more frequently since some of their constituents are present in urine in a concentration in excess of their maximum solubility in water. However, urine contains glycoaminoglycosans, pyrophosphate and citrate and these substances, by forming complexes, may keep otherwise insoluble salts in solution in the urine.

Certain conditions are frequently associated with stone formation:

1. A climate or an occupation which necessitates living or working under conditions where excessive loss of water from sweating occurs. The high concentration of the constituents of stones in the diminished volume of urine results in their precipitation.

2. Obstruction of the urinary tract or urinary infection predisposes to the formation of phosphate stones.

3. Hypercalciuria increases the liability to form stones containing calcium oxalate and calcium phosphate. Hypercalcaemia occurs when there is an excessive intake of dietary calcium, prolonged immobilisation, hyperparathyroidism, Cushing's syndrome, renal tubular acidosis, sarcoidosis, multiple myeloma or vitamin D intoxication. The condition known as idiopathic hypercalciuria is due to one of two abnormalities, excessive absorption of calcium from the gut or reduced reabsorption of filtered calcium in the renal tubules.

4. Calcium oxalate is the commonest constituent of renal calculi and a high intake of oxalate, which is contained in fruits and vegetables, or increased intestinal absorption of oxalate, such as occurs in ileal disease, predispose to stone formation.

5. Certain rare inherited disorders lead to production of stones, e.g. cystine stones in cystinuria and oxalate stones in hyperoxaluria.

6. Conditions such as gout and myeloproliferative disorders, which cause increased excretion of uric acid, predispose to the formation of uric acid stones.

The pH of the urine influences the extent to which some of these conditions induce stone formation; thus an alkaline urine tends to increase precipitation of calcium phosphate and may be responsible for the occurrence of calcium phosphate stones in patients with renal tubular acidosis. In contrast the solubility of uric acid and cystine is reduced when the urine is acid. Today, however, in prosperous countries the majority of calculi occur in healthy young men in whom investigations reveal no single cause for stone formation. It is likely that multiple aetiological factors are present in such cases and that an alteration in the relative proportions of crystalloids and glycoaminoglycosans in the urine is of particular importance.

Pathology. Urinary concretions vary greatly in size. There may be particles like sand anywhere in the urinary tract or large round stones in the bladder. Staghorn calculi fill the whole renal pelvis and branch into the calyces; they are usually associated with hydronephrosis and chronic pyelonephritis. Most renal stones contain calcium but the nature of the salt varies with their origin. Deposits of calcium may also be present throughout the renal parenchyma, giving rise to nephrocalcinosis. This is especially liable to occur in cases of chronic pyelonephritis, renal tubular acidosis, hyperparathyroidism, vitamin D intoxication, and in healed renal tuberculosis.

Clinical features vary according to the size, shape and position of the stone, and the presence and nature of the underlying condition. Renal calculi or nephrocalcinosis may be present for many years and yet themselves give rise to no symptoms. While nephrocalcinosis never gives rise to pain, the most common complaint arising from renal calculi is an intermittent dull pain in the loin or back, increased by movement or a sudden jolt. Some abnormal constituents of the urine, e.g. red cells, protein or pus cells, can be found at one time or another.

Renal colic. When a stone is small enough to enter the ureter and large enough to obstruct it, an attack of renal colic develops. The patient is suddenly aware of a pain in the loin, which soon radiates round the flank to the groin and often into the testis or labia in the sensory distribution of the first lumbar nerve. The pain steadily increases in intensity to reach a maximum in a few minutes. The patient is restless, and generally tries, unsuccessfully, to obtain relief by assuming various positions, both lying and sitting, and by pacing about the room. There is pallor, sweating, and often vomiting, and the patient may groan in agony. Frequency and haematuria may occur.

Without treatment the intense pain usually subsides within 2 hours but may continue unabated for several hours or some days. In many cases the pain is constant during the attack, though slight fluctuations in severity may occur. Contrary to what is often believed, it is rare for attacks to consist of intermittent severe pains, coming and going every few minutes for some hours.

Investigation. The diagnosis of renal colic is usually easily made from the history and by the finding of red cells in the urine. All patients suspected of having renal calculus, including those with renal colic, should have a radiological examination of the urinary tract, including a retrograde urogram in some instances. If there is doubt about the cause of the abdominal pain, an intravenous urogram during the attack may be helpful. When the pain is due to a stone in the ureter, the radiograph shows a dense renal shadow with delay in the appearance of the dye in the renal pelvis. Appropriate investigations should be undertaken to discover the presence of any underlying condition which might be responsible for the development of renal calcification or lithiasis.

Treatment and prevention. The immediate treatment of renal pain or renal colic is rest in bed, the application of warmth to the site of pain, and the administration of analgesic drugs, e.g. pethidine (100 mg) or morphine (15–30 mg), and antispasmodic drugs, e.g. atropine sulphate (0.8 or 1.2 mg). These should be given intramuscularly and may be repeated once within 2 hours.

Attempts to dissolve calculi in the kidneys have not been successful but an extremely expensive piece of apparatus called a lithotripter is available in a few centres and using this machine many calculi can be broken up, in vivo, by application of shock waves to the body surface. The small piece of stone are then passed in the urine. The technique cannot be used unless there is free drainage of the urinary tract below the stone. Stones in the renal pelvis can be removed by open operation or via a percutaneous nephrostomy. Stones in the ureter usually pass naturally and operative removal may result in stricture and its complications. When, however, pain persists or becomes intolerable the stone can often be removed by endoscopy via the bladder or via a percutaneous nephrostomy depending on its site. Urgent intervention is required in the event of anuria or if infection or hydronephrosis develops.

Suitable medical or surgical measures should be instituted for the correction of any primary cause of renal lithiasis that may have been discovered. Preparations containing vitamin D must be avoided. In idiopathic hypercalciuria due to excessive absorption of calcium a diet low in calcium, by reducing the intake of milk and cheese, is advisable. In idiopathic hypercalciuria of renal origin, bendrofluazide in a dose of 5 mg/d reduces urinary calcium excretion by about 30%. In recurrent oxalate stones the elimination from the diet of articles which have a very high content of oxalate, such as rhubarb and spinach, may be worthy of trial. Persons who have passed several uric acid or urate stones, as may occur in gout or in patients with leukaemia, benefit from allopurinol (p. 528) which also has a place in treating calcium oxalate stone disease to which urates may contribute.

Since the distribution of phosphorus occurs so widely in foodstuffs, dietary restriction for the treatment of phosphate calculi is unlikely to be of any value. Phosphatic calculi are found only in alkaline urine, hence acidifying the urine by administering ammonium chloride daily may be effective. In contrast, cystine and urate stones may be prevented or sometimes dissolved by making the urine persistently alkaline, especially if combined with a high output of urine.

Lastly, the most important therapeutic and prophylactic measure for all forms of stones is the provision of an adequate fluid intake which assists in preventing deposition of crystalloids in the renal tissue. A daily output of urine of at least 3 litres is advisable hence the intake of fluid should be approximately 4 litres daily. If the climate or the patient's occupation causes much sweating the fluid intake requires to be greatly increased.

CONGENITAL ABNORMALITIES OF THE KIDNEYS

Congenital anomalies of the urinary tract affect more than 10% of infants and, unless they are immediately lethal, some are prone to lead to complications in later life. About 1 in 500 infants is born with only one kidney and, although usually compatible with a normal life, it is often associated with abnormalities in other organs.

Polycystic disease

This genetically determined abnormality of renal structure may be associated with other congenital abnormalities, e.g. cystic liver (p. 363). There are two modes of inheritance. The infantile form is very rare and is inherited as an autosomal recessive; it is usually fatal within the first year of life. The commoner or adult type is inherited as an autosomal dominant trait. It may be found during infancy, but symptoms often do not develop until adult life. Both kidneys are affected, are several times the normal size and consist of masses of cysts, predominantly cortical, with a variable amount of renal parenchyma which often shows extensive fibrosis and arteriolosclerosis.

The clinical features include pain in the renal angles, haematuria, uraemia and usually a slowly developing arterial hypertension. Often one or both kidneys can be palpated and the surface may be nodular. In addition to polycystic disease, other diseases in which the kidneys may be palpable are hydro- or pyonephrosis, solitary cyst, renal carcinoma and other tumours. It should be remembered, however, that in some normal people all of the right kidney, and occasionally the lower pole of the left kidney may be felt on clinical examination. This is particularly true in slim women. On the other hand, pathologically enlarged kidneys are not always palpable. When a kidney can be felt, as in polycystic disease, it may be possible to appreciate departures from the normal size, smooth surface and firm consistency. Diagnosis can be confirmed by ultrasound or retrograde pyelography.

In course, prognosis and treatment, polycystic disease resembles chronic glomerulonephritis and death frequently occurs in middle age from uraemia, cerebrovascular accident or cardiac failure.

Medullary cystic disease

Medullary cysts are found in two widely different conditions. In *medullary sponge kidney* the cysts are confined to the collecting ducts in the renal papillae. Affected patients are usually middle aged and present with pain, haematuria or urinary tract infection. The diagnosis is made on radiographic examination in which, following excretion urography, contrast media is seen to fill dilated or cystic tubules, which are sometimes calcified. The prognosis is generally good.

In *uraemic medullary cystic disease* small cortical cysts are also present and these lead to progressive destruction of the nephrons; this condition occurs in younger patients and there is often a family history. Sometimes affected kidneys are salt-losing; this aggravates the degree of renal failure but, even when treated appropriately, serious renal failure is usual.

Renal tubular acidosis

Renal tubular acidosis (RTA) results from a failure of either reabsorption of bicarbonate in the proximal tubule or of acidification of the urine in the distal tubule. There may be little or no overall reduction in renal function. Although renal tubular acidosis may be a congenital condition it may also be secondary to a variety of conditions (Table 11.3).

Distal renal tubular acidosis (classical or type 1). In the distal form the ability to form a very acid urine is lost and the urine pH cannot be reduced below 5.4 even in the presence of severe systemic acidosis. This is due to failure of the distal tubules either to generate or to secrete hydrogen ions. Two forms have been described. In the first, known as complete RTA there is a persistent hyperchloraemic acidosis and in the second, incomplete form, the plasma bicarbonate

Table 11.3 Causes of renal tubular acidosis.

Distal RTA (type 1)	*Proximal RTA (type 2)*
Primary	
Familial autosomal dominant	Sporadic Familial
Secondary	
Renal diseases	Renal diseases
Pyelonephritis	Nephrotic syndrome
Medullary sponge kidney	Transplanted kidney
Hydronephrosis	
Sickle cell disease	
Transplanted kidney	
Drugs	Drugs
Lithium	Tetracycline
Amphotericin	Carbonic anhydrase
	inhibitors
Dysproteinaemias	Dysproteinaemias
Amyloidosis	Amyloidosis
Hyperglobulineamia	
Cryoglobulinaemia	
Disordered calcium	Disordered amino acid
metabolism	metabolism
Vitamin D intoxication	Cystinosis
Hyperparathyroidism	Tyrosinosis
Immunologically mediated	Heavy metals
Chronic active hepatitis	Cadmium
Primary biliary cirrhosis	Lead
Sjögren's syndrome	Copper
SLE	Mercury

is normal but the ability to excrete an acid load is impaired. Distal RTA may be asymptomatic or patients may present with anorexia, fatigue, muscle weakness, osteomalacia, nephrocalcinosis and nephrolithiasis. Renal sodium wasting due to diminished hydrogen/sodium exchange in the distal tubule is relatively common and potassium depletion may result from stimulation of the renin-angiotensin-aldosterone system consequent on volume depletion from sodium wasting. Frequently there is hypercalciuria, increased excretion of phosphate and recurrent stone formation. Young children pesent with failure to thrive, polyuria, dehydration and constipation.

Treatment consists of determining and dealing with the underlying cause where possible (Table 11.3). Bicarbonate supplements should be given in a dose sufficient to keep the plasma bicarbonate in excess of 18 mmol/l. It is often convenient to give a mixture of sodium and potassium bicarbonate. Calcium supplements and alfacalcidol are used to treat any associated osteomalacia.

Proximal renal tubular acidosis (type 2). This may occur as an isolated defect (primary or isolated proximal RTA). More commonly it is part of a syndrome in which there are multiple defects in proximal tubular function and patients have, in addition, glycosuria, aminoaciduria, phosphaturia and uricosuria. There is an impairment of the proximal tubular sodium/hydrogen exchange leading to decreased bicarbonate reabsorption and consequently a marked reduction in plasma bicarbonate. Once the plasma bicarbonate concentration has fallen to very low levels (about 10–12 mmol/l) the reduced filtered load of this ion can be reabsorbed by the proximal tubular cells, and the amount of bicarbonate leaving the distal tubule is negligible. In these circumstances it is possible to demonstrate that the distal tubular cells are capable of secreting hydrogen ions against a gradient so that a very acid urine can be formed. There is frequently associated hyperchloraemia, potassium depletion and hypocalcaemia.

Treatment of any underlying cause should be instituted (Table 11.3). As in type 1 RTA, the plasma bicarbonate should be maintained about 18 mmol/l with appropriate supplements of sodium and potassium bicarbonate. Where necessary, calcium supplements and alfacalcidol should be given.

DRUGS AND THE KIDNEY

Drug-induced renal disease

The susceptibility of the kidney to damage by drugs stems from the fact that it is the route of excretion for many water soluble compounds including drugs and their metabolites. These are delivered in large amounts to the kidney which receives 25% of the cardiac output, and drugs such as the cephalosporins may reach high concentrations in the renal cortex as a result of proximal tubular transport mechanisms while others, like aspirin, are concentrated in the medulla because of the operation of the counter-current system.

Damage to the kidney may arise in the course of treatment with a large variety of drugs and a number of different lesions may result. An accur-ate drug history is therefore essential in all patients, particularly those in whom there is unexplained impairment of renal function.

Potential causes of renal failure. Acute renal failure may arise as a result of drug-induced *proximal tubular necrosis* occurring during treatment with the aminoglycosides, some cephalosporins, tetracyclines or iodinated contrast media. In these cases the recommended dose has often been exceeded. There is, however, reason to believe that elderly patients, patients with extracellular fluid depletion and those receiving loop diuretics may be particularly susceptible to this type of injury. Opiates and antihypertensives cause a fall in blood pressure with consequent reduction in renal blood flow and occasionally precipitate *acute ischaemic renal failure* (p. 403). Another cause of acute renal insufficiency is an *acute tubulo-interstitial nephritis* (p. 406) induced by drugs such as penicillins, sulphonamides, allopurinol and phenylbutazone. Patients with tubulo-interstitial nephritis often have other manifestations of hypersensitivity such as fever, rash, arthralgia and eosinophilia, and in such cases microscopic haematuria is common. Less severe degrees of this condition produce mild renal impairment and proteinuria. The relatively soluble sulphonamides in use today rarely cause urinary tract obstruction by precipitating in the renal tubules, but occasionally hypersensitivity to these drugs induces *polyarteritis*. Renal failure due to *intravascular coagulation* occurs rarely from the use of oral contraceptives, and is not always reversible.

Analgesic nephropathy. The occurrence of chronic renal insufficiency due to long-continued ingestion of analgesics is an important cause of chronic renal failure. Phenacetin was the major culprit but other analgesics such as aspirin or non-steroidal anti-inflammatory drugs may be responsible particularly when given in combination or when given to dehydrated individuals. The pathological changes affect the cortico-medullary junction predominantly, with diffuse interstitial fibrosis and tubular atrophy. A variable interstitial infiltration of lymphoid cells, plasma cells, macrophages and sometimes eosinophils is present. Ultimately there is a loss of tubules in the cortex and medulla. Acute papillary necrosis is a common feature. The changes probably result from ischaemia due to interference with blood flow through the postglomerular vessels of juxta-medullary glomeruli. This may be related to reduced intrarenal levels of vasodilator prosta-glandins. A recognised complication is the development of carcinoma of the renal pelvis.

Most of the patients are women who suffer from anxiety or have personal problems. They are commonly apprehensive and smoke or drink alcohol to excess. Other patients have taken analgesics for many years for headache, rheumatoid arthritis or osteoarthrosis. Symptoms include polyuria and thirst and the features of recurrent urinary tract infection. Renal colic or ureteric obstruction and acute renal failure may be caused by the passage of fragments of necrotic renal papillae which can be recognised by microscopic examination of the urine. Many patients present for the first time with features of chronic renal failure.

Apart from the history of drug ingestion, the diagnosis can sometimes be made by the characteristic radiological appearance of the papillae on retrograde pyelography. The contrast medium is seen as a small tract within the papillary substance; later the papillae may separate, giving a ring shadow. There is often microscopic or macroscopic haematuria and sterile pyuria may be present. Proteinuria is usually less than 1 g in 24 hours. Provided the analgesic is withdrawn sufficiently early there is a reasonable prospect of some recovery of renal function; otherwise irreversible renal failure develops. Treatment therefore consists of withdrawing the offending drug and, if necessary, substituting another analgesic. When renal function is severely impaired the general management of patients with chronic renal failure should be instituted.

Miscellaneous lesions. Drug-induced *glomerulonephritis*, often presenting as the nephrotic syndrome, occasionally complicates treatment with penicillamine, gold or captopril. A variety of drugs is capable of producing relatively discrete *disturbances of tubular function*. Thus, distal renal tubular acidosis and loss of potassium may result from administration of amphotericin, and lithium may reduce renal concentrating power and cause polyuria. *Obstruction* of the urinary tract due to retroperitoneal fibrosis has been reported following practolol and methysergide, while intrarenal obstruction can result from deposition of uric acid in tubules following treatment of myeloproliferative disease.

Use of drugs in patients with impaired renal function

Adverse reactions to drugs are significantly more common in patients with impaired renal function. In these circumstances urinary excretion of many drugs and their metabolites is reduced. In addition uraemia is associated with alterations in the distribution of drugs in body fluids, reduced binding of drugs by plasma albumin and changes in metabolism of drugs by the liver.

Drugs should never be given to patients with impaired renal function unless specific indications for their use exist. The least toxic alternative should be chosen and the British National Formulary or other reference (p. 820) consulted to find the recommended dose for use when renal function is impaired and also the likely adverse effects of the drug. Commonly used drugs the dose of which needs to be reduced in renal failure include cephalosporins, cimetidine, hydralazine, digoxin, co-trimoxazole, aminoglycosides, narcotic analgesics, aspirin and phenylbutazone. During therapy a careful watch must be kept for any adverse effects and the drug stopped or the dose reduced should they develop. Measurements of the concentration of the drug in plasma are sometimes helpful in monitoring drug dosage (p. 818).

TUMOURS OF THE KIDNEY AND GENITO-URINARY TRACT

Renal carcinoma is the most common tumour of the kidney and is most frequently found in adult men. It was formerly called a hypernephroma on the mistaken view that it arose from adrenal rest tissue within the kidney. Haematuria is the most frequent presenting feature and blood clots may give rise to renal colic. Sometimes the tumour causes vague pain in the abdomen or flank and it may also be responsible for long continued fever. Occasionally patients present first with symptoms arising from metastases in the lungs, liver or bones. On rare occasions polycythaemia occurs, and this is believed to be due to excessive production of erythropoietin. The tumour may be palpable and is defined by radiological investigation and ultrasonography. Early surgical treatment affords the only prospect of cure.

Nephroblastoma (Wilm's tumour) is the second most common malignant tumour of the kidney and presents in the first decade, and often the first year of life. It most commonly presents as an abdominal mass sometimes discovered accidently by the patient. Haematuria tends to occur late in the disease. The tumour is radiosensitive and responsive to chemotherapy (p. 111). The best hope of cure is early diagnosis.

Tumours of the renal pelvis, ureter and bladder are histologically similar and are almost always transitional cell carcinomas. They tend to spread locally by direct invasion but also by implantation to other parts of the urinary tract. While some are benign, e.g. papillomas, all urinary tract tumours are liable to recur even after apparently adequate treatment. The bladder is by far the most common site and epidemiological studies have shown that it is particularly likely to develop in patients who work in industries such as dyeing and printing where there may be exposure to aniline and in areas endemic for urinary schistosomiasis (p. 783). Haematuria is almost always the sole presenting symptom of these tumours. Features due to obstruction to the urinary tract also occur and symptoms of urinary tract infection may be superimposed.

Diagnosis is made by cystoscopy, biopsy and radiography. Bladder tumours are treated by diathermy or radiotherapy or chemotherapy (p. 109). The last may be used systemically or intravesically. Cystectomy with transplantation of the ureters to the colon or skin may be necessary.

Prostatic carcinoma usually presents with symptoms of urethral obstruction similar to those of benign prostatic hypertrophy. On digital examination of the rectum the prostate is felt to be very hard and the median furrow may be obliterated. Spread through the capsule and metastases in bone occur and are often associated with a rise in the plasma acid phosphatase.

Treatment varies with the stage of the disease and consists of prostatectomy or deprivation of the testicular androgens on which the growth depends by measures such as orchidectomy or oestrogen therapy. Painful gynaecomastia may be a troublesome side-effect of the latter.

Benign enlargement of the prostate gland is of unknown cause but it may be associated with a fall in androgen secretion. It is most commonly found in men over 60 years. Histologically the inner zone of the gland undergoes hyperplasia and hypertrophy and there is an increase in the fibromuscular stroma. The enlarged prostate obstructs the outflow of urine from the bladder by compressing, displacing, distorting and elongating the prostatic urethra with the effects on bladder and renal function referred to on page 407.

The clinical features are those of progressive obstruction to urinary flow. Acute urinary retention may arise if the gland suddenly increases in size because of superimposed infection or congestion, or when cardiac failure develops in the elderly. Then the patient has a sudden desire to micturate but is unable to do so, the bladder becomes tense and is tender. More chronic retention may pass unnoticed for some time but there is a gradual increase in the volume of the urine which remains in the bladder after micturition. Haematuria and bleeding from the urethra may also occur and may be the presenting symptom. On rectal examination the prostate may feel large, elastic and is uniform in consistency; however, when the median lobe alone is affected, the prostate feels normal and the condition can be recognised only by cystoscopy. Transurethral resection of prostatic tissue is the treatment of choice to relieve outflow obstruction.

Testicular tumours now constitute the commonest form of malignant disease in men aged 25–34 years. A seminoma presents as a painless and often uniform, rapid enlargement of the testis. A teratoma causes more nodular changes and may secrete gonadotrophic hormones producing gynaecomastia. A testicular tumour may be overlooked if it is obscured by a hydrocele or if the examination is inadequate. Spread to the abdomen and lungs can occur and cause death but with early diagnosis testicular cancer is curable. Seminomas can be treated successfully by orchidectomy and radiotherapy. Chemotherapy is usually required for teratomas in which the prognosis is potentially poorer. However, with appropriate therapy, cure is now possible for the majority of patients. Tumor markers may be helpful in assessing response to treatment and for monitoring remissions (p. 101).

Sexual disorders of endocrine origin

These are discussed on pages 458 to 461.

SEXUALLY TRANSMITTED DISEASES

The Venereal Diseases Regulations of 1916 defined the venereal diseases as syphilis, gonorrhoea and chancroid. These are still the legally defined venereal diseases in Britain. The incidence of syphilis fell after World War II and remains at a low level. Gonorrhoea also decreased after this war, but started to increase again in the late 1950s. At the same time the incidence of other conditions started to rise. These included viral infections (e.g. herpes simplex and warts), chlamydial infections (e.g. non-gonococcal urethritis), parasitic conditions (e.g. scabies and pediculosis pubis), protozoal conditions such as trichomoniasis and fungal infections such as candidosis. Recently other diseases have been recognised to be sexually transmitted, including hepatitis and AIDS. The incidence of gonorrhoea is now declining, but these other conditions have continued to increase.

Spread and control

The fundamental factor in spread is the acquisition of infection from one sexual partner and its transmission to another. This in turn depends on the availability of partners. The most important influence in the number of partners is population movement including the migration of people from rural to urban areas and worldwide travel. Other social factors which promote spread of disease include affluence, alcohol consumption, increased leisure, personal freedom, prostitution, and ignorance. The last leads to failure to recognise infection and the continuing change of partners despite infection. Other important factors in transmission include asymptomatic disease in women and homosexual men, antimicrobial treatment and modern contraception. Unfortunately antimicrobial resistance leads to treatment failure and the spread of resistant infection. Oral contraceptives and the intrauterine device, provide no barrier to infection.

High risk groups for sexually transmitted disease include men aged 18 to 34 years and women aged 16 to 24 years, frequent travellers, prostitutes, homosexuals, members of the armed forces, merchant navy and air crew, and entertainers of all sorts. These diseases affect all socioeconomic groups; no-one is immune.

Control of sexually transmitted disease in Britain is founded primarily on good clinical medicine and most patients attend specialist clinics. The basis of clinical practice is accurate diagnosis, effective treatment and careful follow-up to confirm cure. Secondly, control depends on the identification of potentially infected contacts and ensuring they attend for examination and treatment. Education is also important in control. Serological screening of blood donors and antenatal women is undertaken, but screening is less important in Britain than in countries with less well developed clinical services.

SYPHILIS

Syphilis is a chronic infection due to *Treponema pallidum*. It is systemic from the beginning, runs a chronic course characterised by florid features at some times but by long periods of latency at other times. Syphilis is infectious during the first 2 years when it may be transferable to the fetus; it responds well to penicillin and certain other antimicrobials.

The classification is shown in Table 11.4

The subdivision between early and late syphilis

Table 11.4 Classification of syphilis.

Acquired	Early	Primary
		Secondary
		Early latent
	Late	Tertiary
		(benign gummatous)
		Quarternary
		(Cardiovascular p. 192
		and neurosyphilis p. 640)
Congenital	Early	
	Late	
	Stigmata	
	(or scars)	

is 2 years. The course is variable and may be latent throughout. At any time syphilis may develop clinical features so all cases must be treated.

Clinical features. ACQUIRED SYPHILIS. *Early stage; primary.* After an incubation period (with extremes of 9 to 90 days but commonly 14 to 28 days) the primary lesion or chancre develops at the site of infection, usually on the genitalia or, in homosexuals, at the anus. A small pink macule appears which soon becomes papular and ulcerates. The regional lymph nodes are moderately enlarged, discrete, rubbery, painless, and not tender.

Early stage; secondary. The primary chancre tends to heal and 6 to 8 weeks later symptoms of generalised infection appear with malaise, headache and low fever. Four cardinal signs appear — a rash, condylomata lata, lymphadenopathy and mucous patches — though any of them may be absent:

1. A rash is present in 75% of patients. This starts as a faint macular eruption on the trunk and proximal limbs; it develops into a generalised papular rash which is characteristically dull red, polymorphic and symmetrical, does not itch and may become scaly.

2. Condylomata lata are large flat papules that develop in warm moist areas such as around the anus.

3. Lymphadenopathy is found in 50% of patients and may be generalised. The nodes resemble those found in primary syphilis.

4. Mucous patches are found in 30% of patients; they are superficial ulcers on the mucous membranes of the genitalia, mouth and throat. They may have a characteristic white base and narrow red margin and may coalesce to form 'snail track' ulcers. Alternatively they may be so superficial as to be scarcely visible.

In over 30% of cases changes occur in the cerebrospinal fluid indicating involvement of the nervous system; clinical features of low grade meningitis may rarely be present, sometimes with cranial nerve palsies. Rarely the eyes, bones, joints (p. 572) or abdominal viscera may be affected. After several months the secondary changes gradually disappear to be followed by a latent period.

Late stages. Latency may persist for many years.

The *tertiary stage* takes 10 or more years to develop and mainly affects skin and subcutaneous tissues, mucous membranes and submucosa, and bones, (e.g. skull). Lesions run a long benign course. The characteristic pathological finding is called a gumma.

Quartenary stage. Cardiovascular syphilis (p. 192) and neurosyphilis (p. 640) usually take longer to develop characteristic features and may lead to the patient's death.

CONGENITAL SYPHILIS. The fetus may contract syphilis from an infected mother. There is no primary stage. The disease may be so severe that the child is born dead, or vesicles and bullae may present on the skin at birth. The child may appear normal at birth but fails to thrive, and within a few months develop a rash and signs of syphilitic disease of bone, joints (p. 572), liver, kidneys and other organs. In a third group of cases the disease remains latent for years until lesions of bones, joints and teeth, iritis, keratitis, nerve deafness, juvenile tabes or general paralysis appear.

Congenital syphilis is now rare in Western countries, where screening in antenatal clinics and treatment of a syphilitic woman during pregnancy usually ensure the birth of a normal baby.

Investigation. In the primary and secondary stages *T. pallidum* may be found in the chancre, papules or mucous patches by squeezing a drop of serum from one of these lesions and examining it under a microscope fitted with a dark ground condenser.

The serological tests for syphilis give positive results from about the fourth week and are always strongly positive in the secondary stage. Nonspecific antigen is used in screening tests such as the cardiolipin Wasserman reaction (CWR) or preferably the Venereal Disease Research Laboratory (VDRL) test. Hence the specificity and sensitivity of such tests is variable. False positive results may be found in infectious mononucleosis, systemic lupus erythematosus and other generalised diseases, while negative results may be observed in older patients with late syphilis. For diagnosis additional tests are required which use specific treponemal antigen e.g. *T. pallidum* haemagglutination assay (TPHA) and the fluorescent treponemal antibody-absorbed (FTA-ABS) test. Any patient in whom latent syphilis is suspected should have all these tests repeated on two separate samples of blood, the CSF should be examined to exclude neurological disease, and chest radiographs taken to exclude calcification of the ascending aorta which indicates cardiovascular disease.

Course and Prognosis. Syphilis can run a very variable course. The primary stage may not be present or may not be noticed. The secondary stage may also be transient or absent. Many cases are found in the latent stage following serological testing and in 60% of these the disease does not progress unless the immunological balance is disturbed by some systemic disease. Modern anti-microbial therapy gives cure rates of 95 to 99%.

Differential diagnosis. Primary syphilis must be considered in the differential diagnosis of all genital ulcers, common causes of which include herpes simplex, erosive balanitis and trauma. Less common causes of genital ulcers include scabies and secondary syphilis.

The macular rash of secondary syphilis may resemble a drug eruption, rubella and skin conditions such as pityriasis rosea and lichen planus. The papular rash may resemble drug rashes, scabies, acne vulgaris and, when scaly, psoriasis. Condylomata lata must be distinguished from condylomata acuminata or viral warts (p. 421). Ulcers in the mouth or throat may be confused with herpes simplex, aphthous ulcers, ulcerative stomatitis or the ulceration in agranulocytosis, while ulcers on the genital mucosa may be confused with herpes simplex and erosive balanitis (p. 421). Lymphadenopathy may suggest infectious mononucleosis or a lymphoma.

Syphilis has to be distinguished on clinical grounds from yaws, endemic (non-venereal) syphilis and pinta. These granulomatous diseases, caused by spirochaetes morphologically indistinguishable from *T. pallidum*, are described on pages 762 to 764.

Treatment. *T. pallidum*, though remaining very sensitive to penicillin, needs prolonged treatment. Hence longer acting forms such as procaine penicillin are used. A patient with primary syphilis requires 600mg of procaine penicillin daily for 10–12 consective days. For secondary, tertiary or latent syphilis the course should be continued for 14 or 15 days and for cardiovascular and neuro-syphilis (p. 640) it should be prolonged for 21 days. In large patients the dose should be increased to 900 mg or 1.2 g of procaine penicillin especially in neurosyphilis. Tetracycline should be given to patients allergic to penicillin; for early syphilis, latent syphilis and tertiary syphilis 500 mg of oxytetracycline four times daily for 15 days is recommended while for cardiovascular and neuro-syphilis the course should be continued for 21 to 28 days. All patients must be followed up to ensure cure. Contact tracing is an important part of management.

GONORRHOEA

Gonorrhoea is due to the Gram-negative diplococcus *Neisseria gonorrhoeae* which infects the columnar epithelium of the genital tract, rectum, pharynx and eyes. The incubation period is usually 2 to 10 days.

Clinical features. In the male the anterior urethra is the most common site for infection. Anterior urethritis usually causes dysuria and a purulent discharge; occasionally symptoms are mild or absent.

In females the lower cervical canal is the site most commonly infected but the urethra and rectum are also involved in about half the cases. There may be vaginal discharge and dysuria, but 50% of the women have no symptoms.

The homosexual male may have rectal infection which is often asymptomatic. He may also have asymptomatic pharyngeal infection; heterosexual men and women occasionally have pharyngeal gonorrhoea.

Investigation. Gonorrhoea may be suspected clinically but diagnosis depends on laboratory investigations. Gram-negative intracellular diplococci may be seen in stained pus from infected tracts and this allows rapid diagnosis in the outpatient clinic. Confirmation by culture of exudate on selective media in the laboratory is important.

Course and prognosis. Symptoms gradually resolve without treatment but it is not known how long patients remain infectious. The longer the delay in treatment the more likely is the development of complications. Most patients in Western countries seek treatment early so complications are rare. Infection may spread to the posterior urethra and occasionally along one vas deferens to the epididymis causing acute epididymitis and rarely epididymo-orchitis. Infection in the cervical canal may spread to the fallopian tubes (salpingitis) and to other pelvic structures and may lead to sterility. Pelvic infection may be associated with perihepatitis characterised by right hypochondrial pain and tenderness.

Bacteraemia is rare causing fever, joint pains and a rash—sparse peripheral haemorrhagic pustules surrounded by erythema, though other skin lesions may occur. Acute gonococcal arthritis (p.571) and septicaemia are now extremely rare in the Western world. Infection of the conjunctiva of infants born to infected mothers causes purulent conjunctivitis and damage to sight (ophthalmia neonatorum). This too is rare in the Western world but remains an important cause of blindness in many tropical areas.

Differential diagnosis. Gonococcal urethritis must be differentiated from non-gonococcal urethritis (below) by a Gram stained smear and culture of the discharge. The same investigations taken from the cervix, urethra and rectum allow the differentiation of gonorrhoea in the female from other causes of dysuria such as urinary infection (p. 392) and other causes of vaginal discharge such as trichomoniasis or candidosis (p. 767). Rectal infection rarely causes clinical proctitis and therefore a Gram stained smear and culture are essential for diagnosis. Interpretation of pharyngeal smears is complicated by saprophytic neisseria so only cultures are taken from the throat.

Treatment. A single intramuscular injection of 2.4 g of procaine penicillin plus 1 g of probenecid by mouth, or 2 g of ampicillin plus 1g of probenecid together by mouth is usually sufficient to cure most uncomplicated infections in Britain. Co-trimoxazole, preferably 8 (480 mg) tablets in a single oral dose or 3 doses of 5 tablets at 12-hourly intervals, may be given to patients who are allergic to penicillin. If one of these treatments fails it is important to establish if the patient is infected with a gonococcus which is relatively resistant to penicillin or with one of the strains,

rare in Britain, totally resistant to penicillin. Relatively resistant strains usually respond to 4.8 g of intramuscular procaine penicillin or to 3.5 g of ampicillin orally, each given with 1g of probenecid. Totally resistant strains respond to cefuroxime, cefoxitin or cefotaxime (p. 42). Patients allergic to penicillin may be given spectinomycin (p. 44). Cases with complications need multiple dose therapy such as 2 g of ampicillin plus 1 g of probenecid followed by 500 mg of ampicillin plus 500 mg of probenecid 6 hourly for 14 days.

It is essential to establish cure of gonorrhoea, and any accompanying infection, by repeating culture of secretions from infected sites. Tracing contacts is also important in the management of gonorrhoea.

NON-GONOCOCCAL INFECTION

Non-gonococcal urethritis

In Britain, urethritis in males is more commonly non-gonococcal than gonococcal in origin. About half the non-gonococcal cases may be due to *Chlamydia trachomatis*, a member of the genus *Chlamydia* which also cause lymphogranuloma venereum (p. 419), and other diseases (p. 737); a small proportion is due to *Ureaplasma urealyticum*. A few cases are caused by trauma or herpes simplex virus; the remainder are of undetermined origin. Non-gonococcal urethritis also occurs in Reiter's disease (p. 567). The incubation period of non-gonococcal urethritis varies from a few days to a few weeks.

Clinical features resemble those of gonorrhoea but are milder. As indicated by the name the usual investigations are to exclude gonorrhoea by Gram stain and culture of infected secretions. Where available, urethral exudate may be cultured for chlamydiae.

Untreated non-gonococcal urethritis runs a prolonged low grade course. Local complications are rare and resemble those due to gonorrhoea.

Treatment is with 250 mg of oxytetracycline 6-hourly for 14 days. Cure rates are lower than in syphilis or gonorrhoea; refractory cases may be given 250 g of erythromycin stearate 6-hourly for 14 days.

Non-gonococcal genital infection in women

Chlamydiae may infect the cervical canal. It is therefore important to examine and treat partners of infected men. Uncomplicated genital chlamydial infection in women causes no symptoms or signs. Treatment is with 250 mg of oxytetracycline or erythromycin 6 hourly for 14 days.

Chlamydiae may spread upwards and cause pelvic infection; this is a more common cause of pelvic infection than gonorrhoea. Treatment is with 500 mg of oxytetracycline or erythromycin 6-hourly for at least 14 days. A woman with cervical chlamydial infection may infect her baby at birth usually causing eye infection and occasionally pharyngeal infection and pneumonia.

LYMPHOGRANULOMA VENEREUM

Lymphogranuloma venereum is caused by *Chlamydia trachomatis*; it is sexually transmitted and is widely distributed in the tropics. The different types of *C. trachomatis* can be identified by serotyping and since this method became available cases have been recognised in temperate climates.

Clinical features. A small transient genital ulcer appears 1 to 5 weeks after infection. The regional lymph nodes enlarge and become matted together, tender and adherent to the deep tissues and to the overlying skin which may develop a characteristic dusky pink colour. There may be fever, weight loss, and rarely a macular rash and hepatosplenomegaly.

Infection may spread to the pelvic nodes. If the condition is untreated, abscesses and sinuses may develop. Proctitis and rectal ulceration, multiple sinuses and fistulae may occur. Healing is with scarring and lymphoedema may follow.

Investigation. The diagnosis may be confirmed by isolating *C. trachomatis* and by demonstrating a rise in serum antibodies preferably by means of the microimmunofluorescent test, or by the complement fixation test. Syphilis must be excluded by dark ground examination for *T. pallidum* and by serological tests.

Treatment. Once syphilis has been excluded most cases respond well to 500 mg of oxytetracycline 6-hourly for 14 days. Severe cases may require a larger dose initially and chronic cases need more prolonged treatment. Inguinal abscesses require aspiration but incision should be avoided. When sinuses have formed excision is necessary.

CHANCROID

Chancroid is due to a small Gram negative bacillus, *Haemophilus ducreyi*, 1–2 microns in length and characteristically seen on stained smears in chains arranged like fish in shoals. The disease is sexually transmitted. It is said to be common in the tropics but most cases are diagnosed clinically and over-reporting may occur.

Clinical features. The incubation period is usually 1 to 8 days. Genital lesions start as small painful tender papules which soon form shallow irregular tender ulcers. The inguinal lymph nodes enlarge, soften and suppurate; they may become adherent. Malaise and fever occasionally accompany the local signs.

If the condition is neglected, inguinal abscesses form and occasionally genital ulcers progress to cause tissue destruction.

The multiple, tender irregular genital ulcers with suppurating lymph nodes may suggest the diagnosis but chancroid must be differentiated from primary and secondary syphilis, lymphogranuloma venereum, granuloma inguinale and genital herpes.

Investigation. *H. ducreyi* may be recognised in Gram stained smears of exudate from the genital ulcers. The organism may also be cultured but special media are required. Syphilis must be excluded because primary and secondary stages tend to be common where chancroid is found.

Treatment. This may be: 500 mg erythromycin stearate b.d. for 14 days; 2 g of sulphadimidine initially followed by 1 g 6-hourly for 7 to 14 days, 2 tablets of co-trimoxazole b.d. for 7 to 10 days, 1 g of streptomycin i.m. daily for 7 to 14 days; or 500 mg of oxytetracycline 6-hourly for 10 to 20 days. Bathing with saline will suffice for the genital lesions. Serological tests should be repeated after 3 months to ensure coincidental syphilis has not been missed. Inguinal abcesses may need aspiration.

GRANULOMA INGUINALE

Granuloma inguinale is due to *Donovania granulomatis* and is characterised by bipolar Donovan's bodies 1 to 2 microns long demonstrable in mononuclear cells in scrapings from the genital lesion. The disease is sexually transmitted and occurs almost exclusively in coloured people in tropical and subtropical areas.

Clinical features. The incubation period varies from a few days to 3 months. The genital lesion starts as a small papule which enlarges to form a granulomatous ulcer which spreads to surrounding areas such as thighs, perineum and natal cleft. Lesions have a velvety appearance, varying in colour from pale pink to deep red. Granulomas develop in the inguinal region resembling enlarged lymph nodes. If the genital lesions become secondarily infected this may lead to actual lymph node enlargement. Occasional extragenital lesions occur.

Untreated lesions may continue for years to spread at the periphery and leave an unhealthy scar which tends to break down. Fibrosis may lead to stenosis of the urethra, anus or vagina.

Well developed granuloma inguinale may be characteristic. It is important to differentiate it from primary and secondary syphilis, and from lymphogranuloma venereum, chancroid and genital herpes simplex.

Investigation. The diagnosis may be confirmed by taking a scraping from the margin of the genital lesion, staining by Giemsa's method and then identifying Donovan's bodies microscopically. A biopsy may also be taken. Syphilis must be excluded by dark ground examinations for *T. pallidum* and by serological tests.

Treatment. This may be with 1g of streptomycin intramuscularly twice daily for 10 to 20 days or 500 mg of oxytetracycline for 14 to 21 days. Oxytetracycline should be avoided until syphilis has been excluded and serological tests for syphilis should be repeated 3 months after treatment.

SEXUALLY TRANSMITTED VIRAL DISEASES

Anogenital Herpes simplex

This condition is due to *Herpes simplex* virus and resembles labial herpes or cold sores. The virus is spread by contact usually during sexual intercourse.

Clinical features. There is often a relatively severe initial or primary attack with local discomfort followed by a crop of vesicles on the external genitals. The vesicles soon rupture and are often followed by further crops. The lesions may be widespread on the genitals with regional lymph node enlargement, fever and malaise. There may be root pains in the second and third sacral dermatomes and occasionally retention of urine. In homosexual men, and rarely in heterosexuals and females, the anus may be affected.

The initial illness lasts 2 to 4 weeks and in about half the patients there are recurrent attacks. These follow the same sequence of local discomfort and then a cluster of vesicles covering an area of about one square centimetre breaking down to form erosions and then healing. The frequency of recurrences lasting 2 to 7 days thereafter gradually decreases.

A woman with active disease may infect her baby during delivery. There may also be a link between genital herpes and subsequent carcinoma of the cervix.

The virus may be cultured from vesicular fluid or from scrapings from fresh erosions. Syphilis must be excluded.

Treatment. Lesions always heal and local bathing with saline and treatment of secondary infection with 2 tablets of co-trimoxazole twice daily for 7 days will usually suffice. Antiviral drugs have not yet an established place in the treatment of this condition but acyclovir (p. 46) may shorten the severe initial attack.

Other sexually transmitted viral diseases

AIDS. This is discussed on page 726.

Hepatitis. HB antigen is commonly sexually transmitted between homosexual men. Hepatitis is usually transient and subclinical with only minor biochemical abnormalities. A few men develop chronic active hepatitis or cirrhosis. A vaccine has been introduced which gives a high degree of protection against the spread of hepatitis B among homosexuals (p. 344).

Hepatitis A and non-A non-B hepatitis may also spread among homosexuals.

Cytomegalovirus disease of a subclinical type is widespread among homosexuals who occasionally develop mild clinical disease. Cytomegalovirus disease may also spread heterosexually.

Warts are common on the genitals and anus and spread by sexual contact. There is a link between genital warts and subsequent carcinoma, especially if the cervix is involved. *Molluscum contagiosum* is also found on and near the genitals and is sexually transmitted.

MISCELLANEOUS CONDITIONS

Under this heading some conditions are included which are not sexually transmitted but have to be considered in the differential diagnosis of those that are.

Balanitis. This strictly means inflammation of the glans penis; the undersurface of the prepuce is often also involved, when the correct term is balanoposthitis. It is more common in men with a long or tight prepuce who have difficulty with hygiene. *Candidia albicans, Trichomonas vaginalis, streptococci* and some anaerobic bacteria cause balanitis. The affected areas are either generally or patchily erythematous with erosions in severe cases. There may be a white or purulent exudate. Diagnosis is from the clinical appearance. If one of the causes can be recognised, appropriate therapy should be given plus local saline bathing; if no cause can be identified then saline bathing alone will suffice. Diabetes mellitus, broad spectrum antimicrobials, corticosteroids and antimitotic drugs may predispose to candidosis.

A characteristic form called circinate balanitis occurs in Reiter's disease (p. 567) with well defined, round erosions which may coalesce. Balanitis xerotica obliterans is a local form of the skin condition lichen sclerosus et atrophicus; initially there is patchy erythema but later there is atrophy leading to meatal stenosis and phimosis.

Genital ulceration. Acute genital ulceration occurs in the Stevens Johnson syndrome (p. 45), while recurrent genital ulceration occurs in Behçet's syndrome (p. 569). In the latter condition healing takes place leaving characteristic irregular scars often called 'splash' scars from their appearance.

Vaginal Discharge. This is a common complaint and may be due to a variety of causes including chemicals such as antiseptics in the bath water, physical trauma, or infective agents such as *Candida albicans, Trichomonas vaginalis* or bacteria. *C. albicans* produces a thick white adherent discharge and itch. *T. vaginalis* produces a thin yellow discharge and irritation. Anaerobic bacteria and *Gardnerella vaginalis* produce a malodorous off-white discharge. The different micro-organisms can be identified by microscopy and culture; local antifungals are given for candidosis and metronidazole for trichomoniasis and anaerobic and Gardnerella infections.

Infestations and other skin conditions. *Scabies* (p. 801) is commonly sexually transmitted between young adults and it is important to remember contact tracing in its management. The lesions are modified on the genitals where the burrows are coiled to produce a dull red papule.

The crab louse, *phthirus pubis* is not confined to the pubic area but may be found in other body hair such as the eyelashes. Characteristic crab-like adult lice and nits (eggs attached to hairs) are seen, better with a magnifying glass than by the naked eye. The adult causes an itch or the patient may notice the parasite. Diagnosis is made by recognising lice or nits and treatment is by local application of benzyl benzoate or gammabenzene hexachloride lotion.

Skin conditions which may affect the genitals include lichen planus, psoriasis, seborrhoeic dermatitis and tinea cruris. They can usually be recognised from their appearance, and from that of the rash elsewhere. A number of premalignant skin conditions have been recognised histologically; clinically they appear as persistent red patches. Any such lesion, with no identifiable cause, not responding to therapy, should be biopsied if it persists for more than 3 months. Squamous cell and basal cell carcinomas appear on the genitals either as persistent warty growths or ulcers.

Special problems in homosexuals. Homosexuals form a special high risk group. They change partners frequently and have a high prevalence of AIDS (p. 726), early syphilis, gonorrhoea, hepatitis B and other forms of hepatitis, and infectious mononucleosis. They may also be infested with *Entamoeba histolytica* and other intestinal organisms.

PROSPECTS IN NEPHROLOGY

The last 25 years have seen major advances in understanding the nature of renal disease and in its therapeutic control. Since 1950, renal transplantation and haemodialysis for acute and chronic renal failure have passed through a tentative and experimental phase and become established clinical procedures. Studies of renal biopsies by light, electron and immunofluoroescence microscopy have transformed concepts of glomerular disease; knowledge of immunological mechanisms are beginning to clarify the origin of glomerular damage, and awareness that the kidney acts as an endocrine organ has increased understanding of some forms of hypertension, of vitamin D resistance and renal osteodystrophy and of renal anaemia. Progress in the foreseeable future is likely to consist of a steady consolidation of these foundations. Knowledge of renal structure will be further advanced by the use of scanning electron microscopy and the application of immunofluorescent techniques to electron microscopic preparations.

A fuller understanding of the factors which control renal blood flow, glomerular filtration rate and sodium and water excretion is slowly being achieved. This will influence the management of many renal disorders notably acute and chronic renal failure and the nephrotic syndrome.

In recent years there have been a number of technical advances. Development of the lithotripter has made it possible to disintegrate stones in the urinary tract in vivo. This has led to a widening of the accepted indications for intervention in patients with stone disease and has to some extent simplified the problem of dealing with patients with recurrent calculi. In expert hands the technique of balloon angioplasty provides an alternative to surgery in patients with renal artery stenosis. Steady miniaturisation of artificial kidneys using improved sythetic membranes and adsorbents with the ultimate aim of producing a portable, round-the-clock working artifical kidney is likely to continue.

ANNE T. LAMBIE
A.M. DAVISON
(*Diseases of the kidneys and genito-urinary system*)
R.N. THIN
(*Sexually transmitted diseases*)

FURTHER READING:

Diseases of kidney and genito-urinary system:
Macleod J, Munro J 1986 Clinical examination, 7th edn. Churchill Livingstone, Edinburgh. For further information about examination of the kidneys and the urine.
Forrester J M 1986 Companion to medical studies, 4th edn, vol 1. Blackwell Scientific Publications, Oxford. For information about anatomy and physiology of the kidney.
Brenner B M, Rector F L 1981 The kidney, vols 1 & 2. Saunders, Philadelphia. A reference book with a physiological background.
Brenner B M, Lazarus J M 1983 Acute renal failure. Saunders, Philadelphia. A compehensive reference book.
Avery G S 1980 Drug treatment. Adis Press. For information about drugs and renal disease (ch 21 Wright N, Robson J S).
Kidney International. The journal of the International Society of Nephrology covers a wide range of clinical and experimental opics and contains good reviews.
Nephrology, Dialysis, Transplantation. The journal of the European Society of Nephrology also covers a wide range of topics but is more clinically oriiientated than Kidney International.

Sexually transmitted diseases:
King A Nicol C, Rodin P 1982 Venereal diseases, 4th edn. Baillière Tindall, London.

12

Endocrine and metabolic diseases

Rapid progress in our understanding of the physiology of the endocrine system has had a major impact on the investigation and treatment of many endocrine disorders. Part of this progress has stemmed from improvements in the methods used for the assay of hormones. The introduction of highly specific and sensitive radio-immunoassays has enabled the clinician to diagnose endocrine dysfunction accurately. The relative simplicity of most of these assays has meant that large numbers of samples can be processed. This has resulted in a service which has allowed physicians distant from specialist centres to practise a high standard of endocrinology. Indeed, as endocrinology permeates nearly all clinical disciplines it is becoming increasingly important for all doctors to be aware of the advances in this field. Such knowledge should lead to the earlier detection of endocrine disease and hence to a reduction of the morbidity associated with it.

Unicellular organisms such as coliform bacilli can produce hormones (e.g. insulin) and it would seem likely that evolution has led to a change in the role of these 'hormones'. Initially they were probably part of an autocrine system within the unicellular organism. This led to an isocrine system where secretory products of adjacent cells had a local action on each other. With the development of specialised hormone secreting cells the paracrine system emerged. In this the specialist cell secretes a hormone which acts locally on other cells. A classic example is the pancreatic islet which contains cells secreting insulin, glucagon, pancreatic polypeptide or somatostatin. These are arranged in such a way that the secretion of one cell, such as that secreting somatostatin, can directly modulate an adjacent insulin-secreting cell. Increasing complexity and size of multicellular organisms resulted in the evolution of the endocrine system where groups of specialist cells formed glands which secreted hormones directly into the bloodstream. These chemical messengers then had a specific effect at a distance from the site of secretion on certain responsive tissues or target organs.

The practice of clinical endocrinology is changing rapidly as a result of the isolation and synthesis of hormones which has stemmed from advances in the techniques of protein chemistry and recombinant DNA technology. The last few years has seen the purification and synthesis of two new hypothalamic releasing hormones, one for ACTH and the other for growth hormone; the isolation of the insulin gene has allowed the bacterial synthesis of human insulin. Human growth hormone has also been produced by this technique and has now replaced growth hormone purified from human pituitary tissue. This is because the latter preparation may have been contaminated with a slow virus responsible for the development of Creutzfeldt-Jakob disease (p. 462). The somatostatin gene has been chemically synthesised and can be inserted into a plasmid vector (p. 17). Transformed *Escherichia coli* can thus be used to synthesise somatostatin. Clearly this technique will rapidly lead to the in vitro synthesis of all the important polypeptide hormones.

Understanding of the mechanisms of hormone

action will lead to still further advances in endo-crinology. For example, the pulsatile release of the gonadotrophin releasing hormone is critical in determining its effect. Long-acting analogues of it not only do not stimulate but actually inhibit gonadotrophin release. Conversely, giving the naturally occurring releasing hormone sub-cutaneously in a pulsatile manner by a minipump can be used to induce puberty or to treat certain types of infertility.

For the student, clinical endocrinology is a most exciting subject in which disease processes can be readily understood by knowledge of basic physiology and anatomy. For the doctor and the patient there is the satisfaction that most endocrine diseases can be accurately diagnosed and respond to the appropriate therapy.

THE HYPOTHALAMUS AND THE PITUITARY GLAND

ANATOMY AND PHYSIOLOGY

The pituitary gland is enclosed in the sella turcica, bridged over by the diaphragma sellae, with the sphenoidal air sinuses below, and the optic chiasma in the subarachnoid space above. The gland is composed of two lobes, anterior and posterior, and is connected to the hypothalamus by the infundibular stalk carrying the portal vessels from the median eminence of the hypo-thalamus to the anterior lobe of the pituitary gland and nerve fibres to the posterior lobe.

The anterior lobe

The anterior lobe consists of three main histolog-ical types of cell as identified by conventional staining: chromphobe, acidophil and basophil. However, the correlation between these types of staining and hormone secretion is not close. Through the action of its seven hormones, four of which act on target endocrine glands while the remainder act primarily on target tissues, the anterior pituitary affects growth, thyroid activity, sexual function, lactation, the metabolism of water, carbohydrate, protein and fat, as well as skin pigmentation.

Hormones of the anterior lobe. Secretion of each of these hormones is influenced by a stimulus provided by the hypothalamus, either in the form of a releasing hormone or factor, or by an inhibitor which suppresses secretion or by both (Fig.12.1).

The secretion of the hypothalamic factors in turn is dependent upon a wide variety of stimuli of nervous, metabolic, physical or hormonal origin, in particular from the appropriate target organs of the pituitary hormones, the thyroid gland, the adrenal cortex and the gonads.

TSH. The thyrotrophin releasing hormone (TRH) is a tripeptide formed in the hypothalamus, like the other hypothalamic releasing or inhibiting factors and passes through the portal system of vessels connecting the hypothalamus to the pituitary gland, where it promotes the secretion of the thyroid stimulating hormone (TSH).

In its turn TSH stimulates the thyroid gland to produce the thyroid hormones thyroxine (T_4) and triiodothyronine (T_3). These hormones then exert a negative feedback control over TRH and TSH secreton. Even though T_4 is a prohormone which is then converted to the biologically active T_3, the pituitary secretion of TSH is more affected by circulating T_4. This is because of rapid conver-sion of T_4 to T_3 by the pituitary.

LH AND FSH. The gonadotrophin releasing hormone GnRH is a decapeptide and acts on the pituitary to release both luteinising hormone (LH) and follicle stimulating hormone (FSH). Despite the fact that there is only one releasing hormone, LH and FSH can be secreted independently. This depends on the feedback of gonadal steroids on the pituitary which modulates the response to the releasing hormone.

The effect of sex steroids on feedback control differs in males and females. In men testosterone and probably dihydrotestosterone can inhibit LH secretion. In women the rising level of oestradiol during the phase of follicular development triggers the mid-cycle surge of LH—a phenomenon known as positive feedback. Endogenous opiates also appear to play a role in determining LH pulse frequency. Thus the opiate antagonist naloxone increases the frequency in patients with hypo-thalamic amenorrhoea such as that associated with excessive exercise.

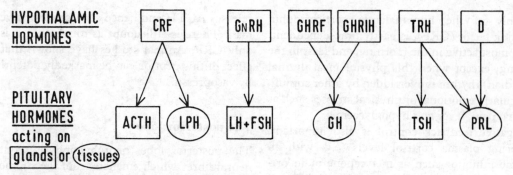

HYPOTHALAMIC
HORMONES

PITUITARY
HORMONES
acting on
glands or tissues

Fig. 12.1 The principal direct relationships between the hypothalamus and the anterior pituitary. Hypothalamic releasing [R] and inhibiting [I] activities are described as hormones [H] when they have been chemically identified and synthesised, and as factors [F] while their recognition still depends upon biological activity determined by bioassays.

Hypothalamic hormones
CRF: Corticotrophin releasing factor
GnRH: Gonadotrophin releasing hormone
GHRF: Growth hormone releasing factor
GHRIH: Growth hormone release inhibiting hormone
          (somatostatin)
TRH: Thyrotrophin releasing hormone
D: Dopamine (Prolactin release inhibiting factor)

Anterior pituitary hormones
ACTH: Adrenocorticotrophic hormone (corticotrophin)
LPH: β-lipotrophin
LH: Luteinising hormone
FSH: Follicle stimulating hormone
GH: Growth hormone
TSH: Thyroid stimulating hormone (thyrotrophin)
PRL: Prolactin

In contrast to LH the control of FSH secretion is mainly by inhibin, a polypeptide which is secreted by the testis and the ovary. Ovine inhibin has been purified and characterised.

GnRH appears to be secreted in an intermittent manner leading to pulses of gonadotrophin secretion. This pattern of secretion is critical. Continuous administration of GnRH downregulates receptors on the pituitary gonadotrophs and therefore paradoxically inhibits gonadotrophin secretion. Thus long-acting analogues of GnRH are being used for the treatment of hormone dependent prostate and breast cancer and may have a role as contraceptives. Conversely pulsatile administration of GnRH is proving to be an important way of treating certain types of hypogonadotrophic infertility.

GH (growth hormone) is controlled by a dual system, namely growth hormone releasing factor (GHRF) and an inhibitory hormone (GHRIH). Growth hormone releasing factor has been isolated from pancreatic tumours found in patients with acromegaly, and has been shown to be similar to that present in the hypothalamus. Infusion of the pancreatic factor releases growth hormone without affecting other anterior pituitary hormones.

The major effects of growth hormone are mediated by an insulin-like growth factor (IGF 1), whose original name was somatomedin C. This polypeptide circulates in the blood bound to a specific carrier protein. The liver is a major source of IGF 1 production.

GHRIH is a tetradecapeptide known also as somatostatin and has many other actions, apart from its effect on growth hormone, including inhibition of endocrine secretions (gastrin, TSH and glucagon) and of exocrine secretions (gastric acid and pancreatic enzymes). It is also produced in sites other than the hypothalamus such as the gastrointestinal tract and the delta cells of the pancreatic islets.

PRL (prolactin) secretion differs from that of other anterior pituitary hormones in that it is under predominantly inhibitory control. The inhibitory factor is dopamine which is secreted by the hypothalamus into the portal system. Thus cutting the pituitary stalk leads to an elevation of prolactin secretion but inhibits the secretion of all the other anterior pituitary hormones. Administration of TRH stimulates prolactin as well as TSH release but there is little evidence that TRH normally controls prolactin release.

ACTH (corticotrophin). The secretion of the adrenocorticotrophic hormone (ACTH) and presumably of the hypothalamic corticotrophin releasing factor (CRF), is partly time-dependent, being most active in the morning, and least in the evening, except when this physiological diurnal (circadian) rhythm is overridden by other stimuli, particularly emotional or physical stresses such as trauma, pain, fever and hypoglycaemia.

Negative feedback control is also important. Lowering plasma cortisol levels (e.g. with an enzyme inhibitor such as metyrapone or in primary adrenal failure) stimulates the release of CRF and hence ACTH. This effect of cortisol seems to be exerted both at the level of the hypothalamus and the pituitary.

LPH. β-melanocyte stimulating hormone (β-MSH) is now known to be an artefact created by extracting the pituitary under harsh conditions. The β-MSH amino acid sequence is contained within β-lipotrophin (LPH) which is the C-terminal part of the ACTH precursor molecule, pro-opiocortin. This core sequence is also present within ACTH (α-MSH) and in the N-terminal part of pro-opiocortin (γ-MSH) (Fig.12.2). Thus there are several molecules derived from pro-opiocortin which may function as melanocyte stimulating hormones and cause pigmentation of the skin and mucous membranes by increasing melanin synthesis in the melanocytes.

The C-terminal part of β-LPH (61–91) is β-endorphin, one of the endogenous substances with morphine-like actions. The first five amino acids of β-endorphin are the same as those of the pentapeptide opioid, metenkephalin. Current evidence suggests, however, that metenkephalin is not derived from β-endorphin but from another precursor molecule.

The secretion of ACTH and β-LPH is under the control of CRF. A 41 amino acid peptide has been isolated, sequenced and synthesised which

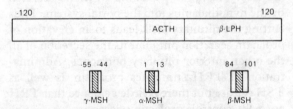

Fig. 12.2 ACTH/LPH precursor. The hatched areas represent the common core sequence within different molecules, each of which can stimulate melanocytes.

releases ACTH and hence cortisol when given to man. There is still doubt as to whether it is the only CRF. Animal studies have shown that the effect of this peptide can be markedly potentiated by vasopressin.

The posterior lobe

The posterior lobe (neurohypophysis) contains neural fibres which emanate from the supraoptic and paraventricular nuclei of the hypothalamus.

Hormones of the posterior lobe. The neurohypophysis secretes two hormones, arginine vasopressin (AVP) — here referred to as vasopressin — and oxytocin together with their specific bonding proteins (neurophysins). The principal action of vasopressin is to increase the reabsorption of water by the renal tubules, and because of this action it is also known as the antidiuretic hormone (ADH). The secretion of vasopressin is controlled by three main mechanisms. A rise in plasma osmolality stimulates vasopressin release which in turn results in water retention to preserve homeostasis. A fall of about 15% in plasma volume without any change in osmolality can also stimulate vasopressin secretion by activating volume receptors in the thorax. In addition the central nervous system also can play a role. Pain, for example, produces an antidiuresis.

The role of oxytocin in the male is unknown. In the female it has traditionally been thought to be important in parturition and the expression of milk from the breast but its role in parturition has been questioned.

INVESTIGATION OF PITUITARY FUNCTION

All the protein and peptide hormones of the pituitary gland can be measured in body fluids by radio-immunoassay and access to a laboratory with a full range of these assays is critical for the proper evaluation of pituitary function. Approximate adult reference values for hormone concentrations in the plasma are given on p. 817. In addition the hypothalamic hormones, TRH, CRF and GHRF have been synthesised and can be used clinically to stimulate the release of the appropriate pituitary hormones. Furthermore, assays for the hormones produced by the target glands of the pituitary are available. Thus it is possible to assess very fully and specifically the functional activity and the secretory capacity of the pituitary gland and its target organs. Several pituitary hormones, namely TSH, ACTH, GH, and gonadotrophins are available in suitable forms for the investigation and treatment of endocrine disorders, and are useful in distinguishing between primary insufficiency of the adrenal cortex, the thyroid gland and the gonads, and secondary failure due to reduced or absent secretion of one or more pituitary trophic hormones.

One of the fundamental principles of the investigation of endocrine disorders is that if high levels of a hormone are suspected then an appropriate suppression test should be used. Conversely if there is hormone deficiency a stimulation test is normally required. Thus in assessing the increased production of growth hormone in acromegaly a *glucose tolerance test* is performed with measurement of growth hormone at half-hourly intervals for 2 hours along with measurement of blood glucose. Under physiological conditions growth hormone secretion is promptly suppressed by a rise in the blood glucose while there is either absent suppression or a paradoxical rise in patients with pituitary tumours secreting growth hormone.

BASAL FUNCTION OF ANTERIOR PITUITARY. Assessment should include measurement of serum thyroxine, an 09:00 plasma cortisol, plasma prolactin, and plasma testosterone in the male and oestradiol in the female.

GH. When assessing the ability to secrete growth hormone in suspected hypopituitarism, insulin-induced hypoglycaemia (*insulin tolerance test*) is usually employed. The test has the additional advantage that it stimulates the secretion of ACTH and hence cortisol. Prolactin is also released. Insulin-induced hypoglycaemia is also used in the assessment of growth hormone secretion in children of short stature. In immediately prepubertal children the growth hormone response may be impaired and the test may need to be repeated after priming with a sex steroid, testosterone for boys and ethinyloestradiol for girls.

The insulin tolerance test is safe provided it is not used when hypoglycaemia could be dangerous,

e.g. in patients with ischaemic heart disease or epilepsy or with severe hypopituitarism where the basal 09:00 plasma cortisol level is less than $180 \, nmol/l \, (7 \, \mu g/100 \, ml)$. The usual dose of insulin is 0.15 units/kg. It is important to achieve adequate hypoglycaemia (blood glucose $< 2.2 \, mmol/l$ $(40 \, mg/100 \, ml)$). Blood samples are taken at 0, 30, 45, 60, 90 and 120 minutes for the measurement of blood glucose, plasma cortisol and growth hormone.

GH response to GHRF is of value in distinguishing patients who lack the releasing hormone (the usual cause of isolated growth hormone deficiency) from those who have primary pituitary disease.

ACTH. Release of ACTH and hence of cortisol can be tested by giving CRF. This, however, unlike the insulin test, does not test the integrity of the hypothalamus. It may be useful in distinguishing pituitary-dependent Cushing's disease (exaggerated ACTH response) from the ectopic ACTH syndrome (no reponse).

TSH, PRL, LH and FSH. The ability of the pituitary to secrete TSH and PRL can be tested by TRH given intravenously and by measuring the serum TSH and PRL concentration before the drug and after 20 and 60 minutes. GnRH can be given intravenously at the same time and the plasma LH and FSH measured also. This test demonstrates that the gonadotrophins can be secreted in response to the releasing hormone. To test the ability of the hypothalamus to produce the releasing hormone, the anti-oestrogen clomiphene is given and the gonadotrophin response measured.

The need to measure prolactin during dynamic function tests is debatable. In prolactin deficiency it may be of value. In prolactin excess the response may indicate the cause. Thus in patients with prolactin-secreting pituitary tumours the prolactin response to TRH is usually blunted.

INVESTIGATION OF POSTERIOR PITUITARY FUNCTION. This is considered in the section on diabetes insipidus.

TUMOURS OF THE PITUITARY GLAND

Pathology. Pituitary tumours may be macro-adenomas (associated with enlargement of the pituitary fossa or involvement of the adjacent structures) or microadenomas less than 10 mm in diameter. Adenomas may be _functional_ or _non-functional_. They may also produce hypofunction of the rest of the pituitary through _pressure atrophy;_ such failure of function may be progressive and sequential with the secretion of growth hormone and luteinising hormone declining first, followed by FSH, TSH and ACTH.

Excess production of a pituitary hormone may not necessarily be due to a tumour but to _hyperplasia_ of the secreting cells on account of a disorder in hypothalamic control (excess production of a releasing hormone or insufficient production of an inhibiting hormone) or following ectopic production of the releasing hormone.

In the case of _GH_, excess production is usually due to an _acidophil_ (or mixed acidophil and chromophobe) _macroadenoma_ of the pituitary. On the other hand, excess secretion of _ACTH_ (and of β-lipotrophin) is usually associated with a _microadenoma_ or _hyperplasia of basophil_ (or mixed basophil and chromophobe) cells with little or no evidence of enlargement of the pituitary fossa, except in cases of long standing or in Nelson's syndrome (p. 429).

Prolactin-secreting tumours are the _most common_ of the pituitary adenomas. They may be acidophil (densely granulated) or more commonly chromophobe (sparsely granulated). It is important to understand that the conventional classification of pituitary tumours based on the staining characteristics of the cells may be misleading. Thus many tumours with hormone secretion have little stored hormone and hence are chromophobe. For this reason the increased sensitivity of immunohistochemistry is useful in characterising these tumours. Specific antibodies against the pituitary hormones can then be used to localise hormones.

Craniopharyngiomas are tumours, usually cystic, developing in _cell rests of Rathke's pouch_, and may be located within the sella turcica, or commonly in the suprasellar space, where they frequently _calcify_. In either situation their clinical presentation is likely to be due to _pressure_ on adjacent structures, e.g. the visual pathways.

Primary carcinoma of the pituitary gland is rare, but a _metastatic tumour_ from a primary in the _breast, lung, kidney_ or elsewhere may occur in the hypothalamus and reduce pituitary function.

Other tumours, for example pinealoma, ependymoma or meningioma, may occasionally be associated with some disturbance of pituitary function. Granulomatous lesions of the pituitary or hypothalamus such as sarcoidosis or syphilis may mimic pituitary tumours.

Clinical features. These vary, depending on the type of lesion in the pituitary gland and the effect of that lesion on surrounding structures. Enlarging tumours of the gland may present with signs attributable to increased output of hormones or to failure of secretion. Some tumours secreting hormones compress the remaining pituitary tissue, so that there may be failure of some functions of the gland in the presence of an excess of others. Headache is the most constant but least specific symptom.

Involvement of an _optic nerve_, the optic chiasma, or an optic tract leads to impaired visual fields. _Bitemporal hemianopia_ is the most characteristic finding associated with _pressure_ upon the _chiasma_ (Fig. 15.4, p. 602). Optic atrophy may be apparent on ophthalmoscopy. Diplopia and strabismus may follow pressure on the third, fourth or sixth cranial nerves.

Some tumours expand sufficiently to interfere with ADH secretion and so cause diabetes insipidus. Damage to the posterior pituitary _per se_ will not normally produce diabetes insipidus as vasopressin secretion by the hypothalamus continues. Thus if there is _diabetes insipidus_ it usually indicates that the tumour has a _suprasellar extension_. Tumours which expand upwards to impinge on the _hypothalamus_ may cause _obesity_ and _disturbance of sleep_, _thirst_, temperature control and _appetite_.

Investigation. Enlargement of the sella turcica and erosion of the clinoid processes may be detected on _radiological examination_, or suprasellar calcification may be seen in a craniopharyngioma. A 'double floor' of the sella may be present if the tumour is expanding downwards with one side of the pituitary fossa being larger than the other. _Computed tomography_ may be helpful. Cisternography is another useful investigation to determine the suprasellar anatomy. In this a water-soluble contrast medium is injected by cisternal puncture and used to outline the superior aspect of a pituitary tumour or to define a hypothalamic lesion.

Treatment. If there is evidence of pressure on the visual pathways then urgent treatment is required. Many tumours can be decompressed by a trans-sphenoidal approach. In addition bromocriptine (p. 430) can shrink prolactinomas and more rarely growth hormone secreting tumours and surgery thereby avoided.

When there is hyperfunction of the pituitary sufficiently severe to affect the patient's welfare and prognosis, then treatment aimed at either destroying the tumour, or affecting its capacity to grow or secrete should be considered. In Cushing's disease (pituitary dependent Cushing's syndrome), prolactinomas and acromegaly it may be possible by trans-sphenoidal surgery selectively to remove an adenoma and leave sufficient pituitary tissue to maintain normal function. Alternatively, suppression of growth and, to a less predictable extent, of secretory capacity may be achieved by external radiotherapy usually with a linear accelerator. The implantation of yttrium in the pituitary fossa is an alternative form of radiotherapy used only in certain specialist centres. The same is true for proton beam therapy.

SYNDROMES DUE TO ANTERIOR PITUITARY HYPERSECRETION

Gigantism and acromegaly. Hypersecretion of growth hormone by acidophil cells may very rarely develop before the epiphyses have united and produce gigantism. Much more frequently it occurs in adult life, after union of the epiphyses, to cause acromegaly (large extremities). If hypersecretion begins in adolescence and persists into adult life, gigantism and acromegaly may be associated.

Acromegaly is characterised by an increase in the size of the bones which is clinically evident in the hands, feet, supraorbital ridges, sinuses and the lower jaw. The skin becomes thick and coarse; the subcutaneous tissues increase in depth, while enlargement of the tongue, lips, nose and ears may be conspicuous. The viscera, for example the heart, thyroid and liver, enlarge. Excessive sweating is common. Carbohydrate tolerance is reduced in about 30% of cases to the extent that

diabetes mellitus develops.

As the disease progresses, the patient often develops arthritis (p. 571), kyphosis and muscular weakness. Arterial hypertension is a common complication. The disease tends to progress slowly over several years, but patients are frequently seen in whom the progress of the condition has apparently been arrested, or a phase of hyperpituitarism may pass into hypopituitarism. Alternatively growth hormone excess may continue but deficiencies of other pituitary hormones may result from the effect of the tumour on the normal pituitary.

Because of the difficulty in assessing the activity of the disease clinically, growth hormone levels should be measured, usually during a glucose tolerance test.

Bromocriptine, a long-acting dopamine agonist, is used to reduce GH levels as an adjunct to pituitary surgery or irradiation. The response is a paradoxical one in that dopamine elevates rather than reduces GH in normal subjects.

Cushing's disease. Hypersecretion by basophil cells, or sometimes by chromophobe cells, leads to Cushing's disease (p. 450). This condition used to be treated by bilateral adrenalectomy. In the years thereafter some patients develop hyperpigmentation and an aggressive pituitary tumour which is usually locally invasive (Nelson's syndrome). For this reason most patients are now treated by trans-sphenoidal surgery. In about 75% of cases an adenoma is found and can be selectively removed. The remaining patients may have hyperplasia of ACTH secreting cells of unknown aetiology and may required total hypophysectomy. It is important to make sure that the patient does not have a tumour secreting ACTH ectopically (e.g. bronchial carcinoid) as these can be mistaken for pituitary-dependent Cushing's syndrome.

Hyperprolactinaemia syndrome. This may result from a number of different causes apart from prolactinomas. Many drugs either antagonise the action of dopamine (phenothiazines, butyro-phenones, metoclopramide) or deplete the hypothalamus of dopamine (methyldopa), and elevate prolactin levels. Oestrogens also raise prolactin levels and account for the progressive hyperprolactinaemia in pregnancy. TRH stimulates prolactin secretion but it is not clear whether this is why some patients with primary hypothyroidism have hyperprolactinaemia. In renal failure prolactin levels are commonly elevated. The reason for this is obscure. Very high levels of prolactin are nearly always indicative of a pituitary tumour.

Clinical features. Hyperprolactinaemia may be associated with galactorrhoea and therefore the breasts in both sexes must be examined. Hippocrates was one of the first to observe that milk secretion was associated with decreased gonadal function. Thus in women amenorrhoea, oligomenorrhoea, deficient luteal phase progesterone production or menorrhagia may all be associated with hyperprolactinaemia. It is important to measure prolactin in cases of unexplained infertility.

In men hyperprolactinaemia usually presents with loss of libido or impotence. Unfortunately at this stage many have a macroadenoma often with associated visual field defects.

Treatment with bromocriptine or newer drugs such as pergolide will lower prolactin levels and usually restore gonadal function to normal. In some patients with pituitary tumours this will not happen because of gonadotrophin insufficiency. In others there may be high levels of gonadotrophins with a premature menopause.

Treatment with a dopamine agonist may also rapidly reduce the size of large prolactin-secreting pituitary tumours. Patients with visual field defects may thus avoid the need for urgent pituitary surgery. However, once the tumour has been reduced in size definitive treatment, usually with radiotherapy, but sometimes surgery, is required.

For microprolactinomas the choice is between medical treatment with drugs such as bromocriptine or trans-sphenoidal surgery. The results of surgery in major centres are good (initial cure rates of about 80%) but there is some evidence of recurrence. Prolactinomas may rapidly enlarge during pregnancy and such patients must be carefully supervised.

Precocious puberty. True precocious puberty results from the premature activation of the hypothalamic-pituitary-gonadal axis and needs to be distinguished from precocious pseudopuberty associated with gonadal or adrenal tumours or congenital adrenal hyperplasia (p. 454). True precocious puberty is usually idiopathic in girls and there is frequently a positive family history. In boys it is more commonly indicative of central nervous system disease. Long-acting analogues of gonadotrophin releasing hormone are now being used to treat precocious puberty and thus improve the adult height prognosis and avoid the physical and psychological problems.

SYNDROMES DUE TO ANTERIOR PITUITARY HYPOSECRETION

Hypopituitarism

Aetiology. At one time destruction of the anterior lobe of the hypophysis was commonly due to infarction and this was often a sequel to post-partum haemorrhage (*Sheehan's syndrome*). Improvements in obstetrical care have greatly reduced the incidence of this accident and hypopituitarism is now most commonly due to a chomophobe adenoma. Other causes include tumours, trauma, granulomas (syphilis, tuberculosis, sarcoidosis) and craniopharyngioma. Some cases may be due to an autoimmune hypophysitis. Surgical treatment or radiotherapy of tumours of the pituitary gland is often followed by partial or complete hypopituitarism calling for replacement therapy, and hypophysectomy is sometimes performed in the treatment of malignant disease elsewhere, for example carcinoma of the breast.

Clinical features. In all causes of hypopituitarism, LH secretion tends to be lost early in the course of the disease. In the male impotence and loss of libido are early symptoms. Later in the established disease there may be gynaecomastia, decreased frequency of shaving and absent or scanty axillary and pubic hair.

Symptoms of adrenal insufficiency may be noted, but the changes in serum electrolytes found in severe adrenal insufficiency do not occur in hypopituitarism and the blood pressure is usually not so low. This is because aldosterone continues to be secreted by the glomerulosa layer of the adrenal cortex, since this function is largely independent of corticotrophin. Cortisol production, however, falls to a minimum because the essential corticotrophic stimulus from the pituitary gland is inadequate. In contrast to the pigmentation of the skin in Addison's disease, a striking degree of pallor is usually present due to capillary vasoconstriction and the absence of melanin.

Coma is liable to develop if patients with hypopituitarism are inadequately treated. It usually follows some mild infection or injury, in the same way that an Addisonian crisis may follow some relatively trivial stress. The coma may be due to one or more of the effects of hypopituitarism. These include lack of growth hormone resulting in increased sensitivity to insulin and hence hypoglycaemia. Water intoxication is another factor, due to a disturbance of water control in patients with adrenal insufficiency. Hypothyroidism is also a component in the causation of coma; hypothermia with a rectal temperature as low as 32°C or less may develop.

Investigation is discussed on page 426.

Treatment. The aim should be to provide adequate substitution therapy, according to the deficiencies demonstrated, so that the patient can lead a normal life. Cortisol should be given by mouth in doses of 20 mg in the morning and 10 mg in the evening or according to the cortisol blood profile. Thyroid hormone, if required, should be given orally as thyroxine 0.15 mg daily. It is dangerous to give thyroid hormone to patients with adrenal insufficiency until they have been protected by cortisol against the possibility of an Addisonian type of crisis. Excessive doses of corticosteroids may result in the development of Cushing's syndrome. Because aldosterone secretion is maintained, mineralocorticoid replacement therapy is not required.

Sex hormone replacement therapy is indicated to restore normal sexual function and to prevent the development of osteoporosis. In men depot preparations of testosterone are effective either by subcutaneous implant every few months or by monthly intramuscular injections. Testosterone undecanoate can be given by mouth but produces variable blood levels and is expensive. In women cyclical oestrogen therapy is indicated in premenopausal patients with gonadotrophin deficiency. Ethinyloestradiol (20 μg daily) is given for 3 out of 4 weeks and a progestogen such as medroxyprogesterone acetate (5 mg daily) for the 4th week.

In patients requiring fertility, gonadotrophin therapy may be given. This can result in hyperstimulation of the ovary with multiple ovulation. Careful monitoring of the oestrogen response to the gonadotrophin will usually avoid this. Very promising results have been reported with pulsatile GnRH therapy in many patients with hypopituitarism. This suggests that a complete absence of pituitary gonadotrophs is rare.

Growth hormone deficiency

In children hyposecretion of GH causes short stature. The term 'dwarfism' has been discarded by many clinicians because of its unpleasant connotations. Pituitary tumours are an uncommon cause of GH deficiency in children compared with a genetic inability to secrete GH which is usually due to a lack of growth hormone releasing factor. Other causes of GH deficiency include craniopharyngioma.

In children with short stature it is essential that accurate records of height and weight are kept and entered on a percentile chart. If the child is below the 3rd percentile for height or is crossing the percentiles then further investigation is indicated. Radiographs of the non-dominant hand and wrist are compared with a standard atlas. With GH deficiency a delayed bone development will be found. GH secretion can be investigated by insulin-induced hypoglycaemia (p. 427).

Children in whom GH secretion has been shown to be absent may be treated by biosynthetic human growth hormone. The response to this therapy is judged by serial readings recorded on standard height and weight charts.

Differential diagnosis of short stature. Growth may be delayed or impaired for many reasons. Tallness and shortness of stature have genetic components and it is therefore necessary to enquire about parental heights. A chromosomal abnormality is responsible for Turner's syndrome (p. 9). Persistent stunting of growth is a recognised association with chronic intrauterine growth retardation, premature birth, anoxic forms of congenital heart disease, chronic liver, pulmonary or renal disease, many chronic infections, and persistent undernutrition (p. 57). Emotional deprivation may also be a cause of growth failure.

Short stature of hypothalamic or pituitary origin must also be distinguished from:

1. *Corticosteroid excess.* Cushing's syndrome in childhood is associated with short stature. This must be kept in mind when a child is given long-term corticosteroid therapy.

2. *Cretinism and juvenile hypothyroidism.* If these conditions are not recognised and treated promptly, stunting of growth will occur (p. 442).

3. *Short stature due to malabsorption.* In many such patients there is no clinical evidence of malabsorption. Investigations which may be required are indicated by the causes given on p. 303.

4. *Achondroplasia or dyschondroplasia.* These hereditary disorders of endochondral ossification are characterised by failure of the long bones of the arms and legs to grow properly, while the trunk and head develop normally. Patients with these conditions are sexually and intellectually normal.

Other anterior pituitary deficiencies

Gonadotrophin hyposecretion may result from an isolated deficiency of GnRH or from damage to the hypothalamus or pituitary and may cause delayed puberty. This has to be distinguished from delayed puberty of constitutional origin in which case there is often a family history to support the diagnosis.

Isolated deficiencies of *thyrotrophin releasing hormone* or *corticotrophin releasing factor* are very rare being much more commonly the result of conditions causing hypopituitarism.

DIABETES INSIPIDUS

This uncommon disease is characterised by the persistent excretion of excessive quantities of urine of low specific gravity, and by constant thirst. Diabetes insipidus (DI) can be subdivided into two main types, cranial DI in which there is deficient production of the antidiuretic hormone, arginine vasopressin (AVP), and nephrogenic DI in which the renal tubules are unresponsive to vasopressin.

Aetiology. Cranial DI may rarely result from a genetic defect in vasopressin production with a dominant mode of inheritance. There is also a recessive condition in which DI may be associated with diabetes mellitus. More commonly cranial DI develops after damage to the hypothalamus or with high stalk lesions. This may occur with large tumours of the pituitary, with hypothalamic damage due to conditions such as histiocytosis-X or a craniopharyngioma, and as a sequel to basal meningitis or trauma. In panhypopituitarism, the symptoms of diabetes insipidus may not be apparent until corticosteroid therapy has been provided because an adequate level of corticosteroids is required for DI to be expressed. In some patients no cause can be found.

Nephrogenic DI may be inherited as a sex-linked recessive condition or may be acquired. Hypokalaemia, hypercalcaemia, heavy metal poisoning and lithium therapy may all block the renal response to vasopressin.

Clinical features. The most marked symptoms are polyuria and polydipsia. The patient may pass 5–20 or more litres of urine in 24 hours. The urine is clear and of low specific gravity and osmolality, i.e. usually less than the plasma osmolality.

The diagnosis of cranial DI depends on demonstrating that a rise of plasma osmolality induced by withholding fluids is not accompanied by a normal rise in the osmolality or specific gravity of the urine, but that when vasopressin is given, such a rise does occur. The latter test is necessary in order to show that the kidney is capable of concentrating the urine which it cannot do in nephrogenic DI.

Water deprivation test. This may be required to differentiate the polyuria of diabetes insipidus from that found in psychogenic polydipsia. The test should be carried out during the day and should not normally last more than 8 hours. No coffee, tea or smoking is allowed beforehand. The patient should be weighed at the start of the test and at intervals during it. If the weight falls by more than 3% the test should be stopped. An increase in weight suggests the possibility of surreptitious drinking. During the procedure plasma and urine samples are taken for measurement of osmolality. At the end of test, if there has not been an antidiuresis, vasopressin is given and the urine osmolality followed over the next four hours.

In cranial DI the pre-testing plasma osmolality is usually high and with fluid deprivation often exceeds 300 mOsm/kg. The urine osmolality of the DI patients is usually less than that of the plasma at the end of the test but rises when vasopressin is given whereas in normal subjects urine osmolality after 8 hours fluid deprivation is about 800 mOsm/kg and does not increase when vasopressin is given.

In psychogenic polydipsia the initial plasma osmolality is usually below normal and the urine osmolality fails to rise normally with water deprivation. The renal response to exogenous vasopressin is also impaired because of the effect of long-term over-hydration on the kidney.

Treatment. This is usually with the long-acting analogue of vasopressin, desmopressin (DDAVP). The amount of vasopressin required to keep the patient in water balance must be determined by measuring the fluid output. Desmopressin is given intranasally; $10–20\,\mu g$ once or twice daily elicits a response as effectively as vasopressin given by injection.

A variety of other drugs have been used. Chlorpropamide, the oral hypoglycaemic agent, enhances the renal responsiveness to vasopressin and can be used either in mild DI or in severe DI when large doses of DDAVP are required. As might be anticipated hypoglycaemia can be a problem. An alternative drug with a similar action is carbamazepine. Thiazide diuretics remain the only effective drug therapy for nephrogenic DI and reduce urine volume in this condition by about 50%.

Inappropriate secretion of ADH

This is discussed on page 91 with other causes of water excess and their treatment.

THE THYROID GLAND

Anatomy and physiology. The thyroid gland consists of an isthmus and two lateral lobes, and lies in front of and on either side of the upper part of the trachea and the laminae of the thyroid cartilage. Posteriorly it is closely related to the recurrent laryngeal nerves which lie between the trachea and the oesophagus; the gland is separated from these nerves by its fibrous sheath. The thyroid gland is provided with a rich blood supply through the superior and inferior thyroid arteries. The parathyroid glands are usually to be found lying on the posterior aspect of the thyroid, in its substance or in the sheath of the gland and in relation to the upper cornu of the thymus.

T_3 and T_4. The thyroid hormones, triiodothyronine (T_3) and thyroxine (T_4), are dipeptides containing respectively 3 and 4 atoms of iodine in each molecule. Both are normally stored in the colloid vesicles as thyroglobulin (Fig.12.3). T_3 is metabolically more active than T_4 in that it is effective in smaller doses and acts more rapidly. Only a small proportion of circulating T_3 is secreted directly by the thyroid, approximately 85% arising from extra-thyroidal monodeiodination of T_4. Alternatively T_4 may be monodeiodinated to reverse-T_3 (rT_3) which appears to have no metabolic activity but is a potent inhibitor of T_4 conversion to T_3. More than 90% of both T_3 and T_4 in the serum is bound to serum proteins, mainly to the specific transport protein, thyroxine binding globulin (TBG), but also to albumin and,

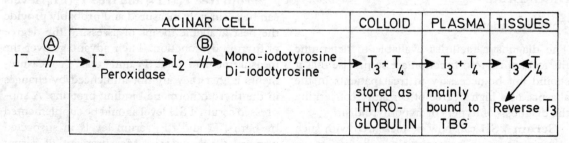

Fig. 12.3 Synthesis of thyroxine (T_4) and of triiodothyronine (T_3). The main sites of block induced by (A) potassium perchlorate and (B) by carbimazole, methimazole and the thiouracil group of drugs are also shown.

in the case of T_4 alone, to thyroxine binding prealbumin. The conversion of T_4 to T_3, possibly at the site of action, may be necessary before metabolic activity can be expressed. The action of the thyroid hormones is to increase the rate of metabolism of most tissues. They also supplement the metabolic effects of catecholamines. It is only free T_4 and free T_3 that can diffuse out of the vascular spaces and be metabolically effective.

TSH and TRH. Thyroid function is controlled by thyrotrophin, the thyroid stimulating hormone (TSH) secreted by the anterior pituitary gland which in turn is controlled by thyrotrophin releasing hormone (TRH) secreted by the hypothalamus. TRH has been synthesised and is available for clinical use. There is also a negative feed-back mechanism whereby the levels of free T_3 and free T_4 influence the secretion of TSH by the anterior pituitary. The synthesis and release of thyroid hormones from the colloid into the circulation are stimulated by TSH.

Calcitonin is a polypeptide hormone secreted by the parafollicular C (calcitonin) cells of the thyroid gland. When administered by injection, it lowers the serum calcium concentration. Its main effect on bone is to inhibit resorption, so that in these two important respects it could be regarded as a physiological antagonist of parathyroid hormone. It is secreted in very large quantities by medullary carcinomas of the thyroid gland, without however producing significant hypocalcaemia, and after complete removal of the source of the hormone, namely the thyroid gland, hypercalcaemia is not a feature.

THE INVESTIGATION OF THYROID DISORDERS

Thyroid function

The diagnostic facilities available to determine the level of thyroid function are so precise that it should not be necessary to treat patients in the absence of a high degree of certainty concerning the diagnosis of hyper- or hypothyroidism.

Serum TSH can now be measured with such sensitivity, using monoclonal antibodies in an immunoradiometric assay (TSHirma), that the suppressed levels which occur in primary thyrotoxicosis can be detected. In the presence of a normally functioning hypothalamo-pituitary axis, changes in the serum TSHirma level are the most sensitive index of changes in thyroid function. Thus a suppressed TSHirma would indicate the earliest phase of thyrotoxicosis while an elevation in the serum TSHirma would be the earliest change in the development of primary hypothyroidism. Having detected an alteration in the serum TSHirma level it is therefore necessary to establish the significance of that alteration by measurement of the levels of thyroid hormones in the serum.

The serum level of TSHirma in patients with untreated hypopituitarism have not yet been adequately reported. In ill euthyroid subjects serum TSH levels may be suppressed and this should not be mistaken for subclinical thyrotoxicosis. The reliability of using TSHirma levels as a sole routine screening test for thyroid function within the context of a large routine service laboratory has yet to be established.

TRH test. Here the plasma TSH level is measured before and 20 minutes after the intravenous injection of $200\,\mu g$ TRH. In primary thyrotoxocosis the secretion of TSH by the anterior pituitary is suppressed. While this could not be discerned by techniques that were available until recently, these earlier techniques could detect the failure of the plasma TSH levels to rise more than $1\,mU/l$ in response to TRH. With the development of the TSHirma assay the need for TRH tests has largely been supplanted. The TRH test should however be retained as an arbiter when there may be doubt about the validity of the detection of a suppressed TSHirma level and in the investigation of suspected pituitary disorders.

Serum free T_3 (fT_3) and free T_4 (fT_4) levels can be accurately measured and probably provide the best available means of assessing the degree of thyroid dysfunction. Their advantage over the measurement of total T_3 and total T_4 measurements is that they are not influenced by changes in the thyroid hormone binding proteins. A suppressed serum TSH level should be supplemented by both fT_3 and fT_4 serum levels in suspected primary thyrotoxicosis. Measurement of serum fT_4 on its own is not sufficient as a normal result may be obtained in the presence of a raised fT_3 level (T_3 thyrotoxicosis), and a raised fT_4 level may be found in the presence of a normal fT_3 level when the patient has impaired conversion of fT_4 to fT_3. In patients taking thyroxine replacement therapy the fT_4 level is frequently raised in the presence of a normal fT_3 level in a euthyroid subject. In some patients the development of primary thyrotoxicosis can be traced through the presence of a suppressed TSHirma with normal fT_3 and fT_4 levels, to T_3 thyrotoxicosis and finally to a situation when both fT_3 and fT_4 are raised. fT_3 levels may be reduced in an ill patient due to the increased production of rT_3. Free thyroid hormone levels may also be disturbed by the presence of antibodies to thyroid hormones to give misleading results. Confidence in the interpretation of thyroid function biochemistry is greatly enhanced by a group of results conforming to a recognised pattern. By using tests as a group the chances of missing hypopituitarism or making a wrong diagnosis on the basis of the single spurious result are greatly reduced.

Total serum thyroxine (tT_4) measured by competitive protein binding or radio-immuno-assay is not influenced by exogenous iodine, but is altered by factors which affect the concentration of thyroid hormone-binding proteins (TBG). Thus, concentrations may be raised in people with normal thyroid function when levels of TBG are increased in pregnancy, oestrogen administration or as a congenital anomaly. Decreased levels of TBG may be due to the nephrotic syndrome, androgen therapy, liver failure or be inherited. TBG may appear to be low if binding sites are saturated with drugs such as salicylates, sulphonyl-ureas and phenytoin. Alternatively these drugs may increase the catabolism of T_4, thus lowering the total T_4 levels. Serum tT_4 levels are still extensively used in routine laboratories as many of the large service laboratories have their own inexpensive inhouse assays, not dependent on the purchase of expensive commercial kits as presently usually required for measurement of free thyroid hormone levels and TSHirma.

Total serum tri-iodothyronine (tT_3) is subject to the same limitations as serum tT_4 in relation to the level of TBG and albumin, although to a lesser extent. As with fT_3, it may be depressed in illness so that a low result may be recorded in an ill euthyroid subject.

T_3 resin uptake, free thyroxine index and effective thyroxine ratio. The need for these tests to overcome problems relating to changes in thyroid hormone binding has largely disappeared with the development of serum TSHirma, fT_3 and fT_4 assays.

The uptake of radioactive iodine or technetium. The overactive gland synthesising excess T_4 has an increased uptake of iodine which can be shown by measuring the proportion of an oral tracer dose of ^{131}I (half-life of 8 days) taken up by the thyroid gland in a given time (e.g. 4 hours) by using an appropriate 'counter' over the neck. Alternatively, an isotope of technetium (^{99m}Tc) may be used intravenously with the thyroid uptake measured at 20 minutes, giving an even smaller dose of radiation which can be regarded as insignificant. When ^{123}I is available, its use has emerged as the isotope of choice for thyroid imaging and uptake studies. It provides a detail of iodine scanning with only slightly more radiation exposure than technetium and only about 3% that of ^{131}I. However it is more difficult and costly to obtain.

The major fallacies in such studies are caused by iodine deficiency or enzyme deficiency beyond the stage of iodide uptake (which can give an increased uptake measurement without the presence of thyrotoxicosis) and iodine excess (which can give a low uptake measurement in spite of the presence of thyrotoxicosis). The source of excess iodine may be X-ray contrast media, iodinisation programmes, or iodine containing drugs such as amiodarone. Another cause of low iodine uptake thyrotoxicosis may be an acute autoimmune thyroiditis with release of stored thyroid hormones into the serum, but suppressed thyroid cell function. It is necessary to know how avid is the uptake of iodine by the thyroid before treating a thyrotoxic patient with radioactive iodine.

A radionuclide scan of the thyroid using ^{131}I, ^{99m}Tc or ^{123}I will indicate the distribution of functioning thyroid tissue. Such scans are useful in determining the nature of a solitary thyroid nodule — whether it is functional ('hot') or non-functional ('cold'). They may also be useful in deciding whether a goitre is multinodular or diffuse and whether there is a retrosternal extension of functioning tissue. The nature of a suspected maldevelopment, e.g. sublingual thyroid, can also be determined. In vivo isotope tests should not be done in women who may be pregnant and in children only when essential, using ^{123}I or ^{99m}Tc.

Choice of test or combination of tests is made in the light of the foregoing and in relation to the individual problem and the local resources. The optimal group of tests to assess the thyroid function would be serum TSHirma, fT$_3$ and fT$_4$, supplemented by TRH test in suspected secondary hypothyroidism and TSH receptor antibody tests in establishing whether a suppressed TSHirma in the presence of normal thyroid hormone levels reflects subclinical Graves' disease.

The nature of a goitre

The following tests may be helpful in elucidating the nature of a euthyroid goitre (enlargement of the thyroid gland):

Radiographs of the neck and thoracic inlet will indicate the presence of a significant goitre, whether it is compressing or displacing the trachea, and if there is a retrosternal extension. It will also show if an adenoma or the wall of a cyst is calcified. A lateral view will show if there is a retrotracheal extension of the goitre that may sometimes occur in Hashimoto thyroiditis.

Ultrasonography of the thyroid may determine whether a solitary 'cold' area on radionuclide scanning is purely cystic (and therefore almost certainly benign) or partially cystic (and therefore suspicious of being malignant).

Examination of the vocal cords will confirm if a change in the voice is due to damage to a recurrent laryngeal nerve by a large or malignant goitre.

Serum autoantibodies to thyroid cytoplasm or to thyroglobulin in high titre are indicative of Hashimoto thyroiditis in the appropriate clinical context.

Needle biopsy of the thyroid may be indicated if the nature of a goitre is still in doubt. Multiple biopsies may be taken under local anaesthetic, but the limitations of small biopsy specimens, with the possibility of a false negative report, must be remembered.

HYPERTHYROIDISM

The clinical condition consequent upon overproduction of T$_3$ or of both T$_3$ and T$_4$ is referred to as hyperthyroidism or thyrotoxicosis. In a significant minority of patients the excess production of thyroid hormone is confined to T$_3$ (T$_3$ thyrotoxicosis) but it is likely that a greater number of cases have an initial phase of excess T$_3$ production followed by an overproduction of both T$_3$ and T$_4$, and it is usually at the latter stage that the diagnosis is made.

Aetiology and pathology. The serum TSHirma levels in patients with primary thyrotoxicosis are either reduced or undetectable. Cases of secondary thyrotoxicosis due to excess TSH production by pituitary tumours are exceptionally rare.

In many patients with hyperthyroidism the IgG autoantibody, human specific TSH receptor antibody, can be detected in the serum and it is possible that antibodies that can stimulate the TSH receptor (thyroid stimulating immunoglobulin, TSI) may be the cause of hyperthyroidism in most instances of Graves' disease (type I thyrotoxicosis), as defined below. Other evidence of autoimmune activity directed against the thyroid gland in hyperthyroidism is the presence of lymphocytic infiltration in the gland which may be negligible, focal or extensive. There is an increased prevalence of HLA-DR3 in Graves' disease which thus appears to be an autoimmune hyperthyroidism occurring in a genetically preselected population.

In the majority of patients with hyperthyroidism the thyroid gland is either diffusely hyperactive (*Graves' disease*) or the gland consists of multiple active nodules interspersed with inactive areas (type II thyrotoxicosis). This latter state is probably the outcome of alternate stimulation and degeneration or results from the development of thyrotoxicosis upon a multinodular goitre. Toxic nodular goitres tend to occur in older patients and diffuse goitres in younger subjects. In a small percentage of patients, thyrotoxicosis is due to the presence of a hyperactive solitary nodule (type III thyrotoxicosis) with suppression of the remainder of the gland through the normally functioning feed-back mechanism.

Histologically, in Graves' disease, the thyroid vesicles are reduced in size and relatively empty of colloid; the epithelium is tall and columnar in contrast to the flat cuboidal epithelium of the normal gland. The vascularity is markedly increased.

Clinical features. Thyrotoxicosis is found much more frequently in women than in men (8:1), usually in the third to sixth decades, but it may occur at any age. There may or may not be a clinically detectable goitre. The increased blood supply to the thyroid often causes a bruit, and sometimes a thrill.

Most of the clinical features of thyrotoxicosis may be explained in terms of excess production of T_3 or of $T_3 + T_4$, although it is possible that T_4 is nothing more than a prohormone. The increased metabolism accounts for the loss in weight in spite of the increased appetite that is so often a striking feature in the clinical history. Occasionally, however, the patient overcompensates in terms of food intake and may gain weight.

Thyroid hormones potentiate the action of catecholamines. The increased cardiac output required to meet the metabolic demands, together with the effect of T_3 and T_4 on the sympathetic nervous system, tends to produce a tachycardia, or, particularly in elderly patients, arrhythmias such as atrial fibrillation or ectopic beats. The patient may complain of palpitations with or without the symptoms of cardiac failure. Sinus tachycardia, persisting during sleep, is one of the earliest and most constant signs. The pulse pressure is increased and a collapsing pulse and capillary pulsation may be detectable. In the older patient cardiovascular manifestations may be the only clinical evidence of hyperthyroidism.

There are other consequences of the effect of excess thyroid hormones on the beta-adrenergic receptors. Patients commonly complain of increased frequency of bowel motions, usually with formed stools. Retraction of the upper eyelids and a fine tremor of the fingers may occur, while the hands are often hot and sweaty because of the increased metabolic rate and the need to lose excess heat. Intolerance of warm environments is characteristic. Thyrotoxic patients, although they are hyperdynamic, have a low efficiency in terms of what they achieve. They suffer from an inability to relax both mentally and physically; anxiety is frequent.

Less common clinical features that cannot be so readily explained in terms of disturbed physiology include exophthalmos (p. 441), pretibial myxoedema and finger clubbing, reduced fertility and menstrual irregularities. In addition there may be thyrotoxic myopathy (p. 666), which recovers when normal thyroid function is restored.

In some cases thyrotoxicosis undergoes spontaneous remission within a period of months or years, while in other cases it follows a prolonged or intermittent course.

Thyrotoxic crises are now uncommon, as cases of hyperthyroidism are recognised and treated earlier and more effectively. They may be seen shortly after thyroidectomy in patients who have not been adequately prepared for operation or in patients who have been operated on for some other disability without hyperthyroidism having been recognised. Alternatively a crisis may be precipitated by a severe infection. The patient in crisis suffers from severe mental and physical exhaustion with delirium, delusions or mania, dehydration, ketosis, tachycardia, cardiac failure and fever.

Hyperthyroidism in the newborn and in children. Thyrotoxicosis may occur rarely in the newborn when it is thought to be due to the transplacental transmission of thyroid stimulating antibody. This form of hyperthyroidism is self-limiting. If thyrotoxicosis occurs before epiphyseal fusion there is an increase in the growth rate so that affected children are unusually tall for their age.

Investigation. The serum fT_3, fT_4 and TSHirma levels should be measured in all cases of suspected thyrotoxicosis if the facilities are available, as it is important to be certain of the diagnosis before embarking on a prolonged course of drugs or using a destructive form of therapy. Reliance should not be placed on a single test which is necessarily liable to laboratory error nor should the tests be done individually in series according to the results obtained at each step, if this leads to unacceptable delays in treating the patient. While a normal TSHirma, that is technically accurate, excludes primary thyrotoxicosis, a suppressed level by itself does not establish the diagnosis.

Treatment. Three effective methods of treating thyrotoxicosis are available: (1) antithyroid drugs, such as carbimazole, initially supplemented as necessary by beta-adrenergic blocking agents, for example propranolol; (2) surgery, after a euthyroid state has been achieved with antithyroid drugs or under propranolol and potassium iodide cover; (3) radioactive iodine, with or without the use of propranolol or antithyroid drugs.

ANTITHYROID DRUGS. The site of action of the different antithyroid drugs is indicated in Figure 12.3. Most commonly used are those that block the organic binding of iodine to tyrosine, carbimazole in Europe and its active metabolite, methimazole, in North America. Other drugs which act in this way are propyl and methyl thiouracil, which may occasionally be useful in the event of hypersensitivity to the drug of first choice.

Carbimazole is given initially in full suppressive doses of 15–20 mg at 8-hourly intervals for 3 to 4 weeks, according to the severity of the condition and the size of the goitre. Thereafter the dose can gradually be reduced, and, as the patient's clinical state responds, the aim should be to maintain a euthyroid state with as little of the antithyroid drug as possible; this ranges between 5–30 mg given once daily. Overtreatment with antithyroid drugs will result in TSH production by the anterior pituitary with a risk of increase in size of the thyroid. In patients in whom the natural history of the underlying process is one of exacerbation and remission, stable control may be achieved with drugs only when an excessive dose of carbimazole (but not greater than 45–60 mg/d) is combined with continuous thyroxine administration in a dose of 0.15 mg/d. The patient's response should be monitored by measuring serum levels of fT_3, fT_4 and TSHirma. Ideally all three tests are required to assess whether too much or too little antithyroid drug has been taken, in view of the fact that the serum TSH may remain suppressed for weeks or months following prolonged thyrotoxicosis even although a euthyroid state had been achieved. On the other hand, an elevation in the serum TSH level in the presence of a normal fT_4 would be an indication of excessive dosage of the antithyroid drug.

If antithyroid drugs are being used as definitive therapy they should be continued for at least 1 year and restricted to patients who do not have a large goitre. By selecting cases in this way about 50% of thyrotoxic patients will go into lasting remission and will not require further therapy. The probability of remission or relapse after 6–12 months' treatment with antithyroid drugs can be assessed by determining whether TSH receptor antibodies are still present in the serum.

Carbimazole, methimazole and the thiouracil group of drugs as well as potassium perchlorate, may produce toxic effects, of which the commonest is a rash and the most serious are the blood dyscrasias, agranulocytosis being most frequent. Patients taking these drugs must be told to report a sore throat and to stop the drug immediately until it is clear whether agranulocytosis has occurred.

Potassium perchlorate induces blood dyscrasias more commonly than other antithyroid drugs, including red cell aplasia which is usually lethal. For this reason, potassium perchlorate should be used only as a temporary expedient if hypersensitivity to other drugs has occurred and if radioactive iodine therapy or surgery under propranolol cover are not acceptable alternatives. It should never be used in a dose greater than 1g/d.

Potassium iodide has no place as an antithyroid drug except in preparation for subtotal thyroidectomy (in combination with propranolol or when the patient has already been made euthyroid with carbimazole or methimazole), or in the management of thyrotoxic crisis.

BETA-ADRENOCEPTOR ANTAGONIST DRUGS are very useful as they can produce much symptomatic improvement by countering the effect of T_3 and T_4 on catecholamine action. Thus anxiety, palpitations, increased bowel activity, lid retraction and finger tremor may be alleviated with propranolol, 40–80 mg 6 hourly. It can therefore be useful during the interval of several weeks which is required for antithyroid drugs or radioactive iodine to be fully effective provided there are no contraindications to its use such as cardiac failure, asthma, or insulin dependent diabetes. In severe thyrotoxicosis much higher doses (up to 1 g/d or more) may be required but must be used with care.

SURGICAL TREATMENT. Provided the necessary expertise is available, partial thyroidectomy is the treatment of choice if the patient is considered too young for radioactive iodine therapy (i.e. during the reproductive years) and antithyroid drugs have failed, or if there have been sensitivity reactions to antithyroid drugs. A thyrotoxic patient younger than 40 years with a large goitre should be treated by surgery rather than by antithyroid drugs.

Men relapse more frequently after prolonged antithyroid drug therapy than women and some authorities advocate surgery as the treatment of choice in men under the age of 40, irrespective of the size of the goitre. The patient may state a preference once the possibilities have been explained. For a woman a thin thyroidectomy scar may be more acceptable cosmetically than a goitre.

Preparation for thyroidectomy is either by propranolol in increasing dosage until beta-blockade has been achieved, or by carbimazole until euthyroid. In either event potassium iodide is given for 10–14 days before surgery in a dose of 60 mg twice daily. It makes the gland firmer and less vascular and the operation easier. The effects of potassium iodide are transitory so that it is important to reserve the drug for use in the circumstances described. Potassium iodide by itself should not be used to try and achieve a euthyroid state except in thyrotoxicosis crisis.

If propranolol is used substantially as preoperative preparation it is essential that tachycardia is controlled (by increasing the dose above 80 mg 4 times per day if necessary), that the dose on the morning of operation is not omitted and that propranolol is continued for 7 days after operation. Before surgery, evidence for adequate beta-blockade should be demonstrated on exercise tolerance. Some thyrotoxic patients are very resistant to beta-blockade by propranolol; the high doses of the drug in these subjects should be reduced immediately after surgery when the serum levels of fT_4 and fT_3 will drop rapidly. The advantages of propranolol preparation are greater flexibility in the timing of surgery, less blood loss and quicker permanent control of the thyrotoxicosis.

Postoperative complications: 1. Hypothyroidism and hyperthyroidism. Some 80% of thyrotoxic patients treated by subtotal thyroidectomy should have no complications. In some 15% there will be either recurrence of the thyrotoxicosis or postoperative hypothyroidism requiring continuous thyroxine replacement therapy. The relative proportion of each depends on the amount of thyroid tissue left at operation. Thyrotoxic patients with high titres of thyroid complement fixing antibody in the serum before operation tend to have an appreciable degree of lymphocytic infiltration in the gland and tend to develop hypothyroidism postoperatively. While the majority of patients who become hypothyroid after surgery do so within the first 6 months or a year, there is a low but steady further incidence with each year after surgery making annual review of the patient desirable. Transient hypothyroidism may occur in the first few months following surgery, presumably due to the suppression of the hypothalamo-pituitary axis following a prolonged period of elevated serum T_4 and T_3 levels.

2. *Damage to a recurrent laryngeal nerve* occurs in a small percentage of patients and will produce temporary hoarseness with subsequent appreciable recovery as the other vocal cord compensates. The normal function of both vocal cords should be confirmed before surgery and checked after surgery.

3. *Hypoparathyroidism.* The parathyroid glands may be rendered temporarily ischaemic by interruption of their blood supply or they may be inadvertently removed, producing transient or permanent hypoparathyroidism respectively. The late onset of hypoparathyroidism is a complication of partial thyroidectomy which should be looked for in the follow-up of surgical patients, as cataract and mental disturbance may develop insidiously in the presence of persistent mild hypocalcaemia. On account of the high incidence of recurrent laryngeal nerve damage and of hypoparathyroidism following second operations, thyrotoxic patients who relapse after surgery should be treated with radioactive iodine.

RADIOACTIVE IODINE is widely used in the treatment of thyrotoxic patients over the age of 40 years and also for younger patients who for some other reason appear to have a short life expectancy or who have been sterilised. It has no established complications other than hypothyroidism in the years following therapy. The incidence of thyroid cancer or leukaemia following ^{131}I therapy has not increased. Although an effect on the spontaneous mutation of the gametes in the ovary or testis has not been proved it is difficult to disprove and therefore the administration of radioactive iodine to persons of reproductive age who have not been sterilised should be discouraged unless there is no suitable alternative. Patients with atrial fibrillation who have only a suppressed serum TSHirma and normal serum fT_3 and serum fT_4 levels should not be given destructive thyroid therapy until the significance of this biochemical situation is more clearly understood.

Dosage. The assessment of the appropriate therapeutic dose of [131]I (half-life 8 days) presents some difficulties for the following reasons. The amount of functional thyroid tissue is not easy to assess with accuracy, the amount of radiation to the gland following a given dose can be assessed only by time-consuming dynamic studies, and even if a predicted amount of radiation per gram of thyroid tissue could be given, there remains the variation in radiosensitivity among thyroid glands of different patients. For these reasons the empirical assessment of dosage using clinical criteria gives results as good as those dependent on sophisticated physical methods, provided that an avid uptake of the isotope by the gland has been established.

Using a dose as small as 185 MBq (5 mCi) [131]I with a diffuse uptake of the isotope as shown on a scan in a small thyroid or as high as 555–1100 MBq (15–30 mCi) for a large multinodular gland, the patient's thyrotoxicosis will be controlled in some 70% of cases following a single oral administration. It may take 2 months or longer for the dose to be effective. If the thyrotoxicosis is severe, more rapid relief may be obtained by the addition of propranolol. Carbimazole should preferably not be given prior to the administration of ^{131}I as there is some evidence that it reduces the effective radiation dose by virtue of the enzyme block which it induces. When given after ^{131}I, carbimazole masks the effectiveness of the ^{131}I and makes the assessment of the need for a further dose of ^{131}I more difficult. The use of carbimazole in conjunction with ^{131}I should therefore be reserved for patients with cardiac failure or asthma, in whom propranolol is contraindicated.

After 2 months a further dose of ^{131}I should be given in the 30% who have not responded adequately to the first dose, using a 50 to 100% higher dose in order to avoid the undesirable occurrence in a few patients of the need for repeated doses of the isotope. Large doses of ^{131}I should be given to thyrotoxic patients with cardiac failure or atrial fibrillation to ensure prompt control of thyroid function with a single dose, even though this will produce a high incidence of hypothyroidism. The patient's thyroid state can then be stabilised by replacement doses of thyroxine.

Thyrotoxicosis associated with a solitary 'hot' nodule should be treated with a large dose of [131]I (if the patient is over 40 years) or by excision of the nodule.

Hypothyroidism following radioactive iodine therapy. The continuing incidence of new cases for many years makes regular review essential. The overall incidence of hypothyroidism may be of the order of 50% at 7 years depending on the dosage of ^{131}I given. Transient hypothyroidism with low serum TSH levels may occur in the first 6 months after ^{131}I therapy due to the suppression of TRH and TSH secretion consequent upon sustained elevated fT_4 and/or fT_3 levels before therapy. Subsequent to that a rise in the serum TSH level is an early warning that hypothyroidism may develop with low serum T_4 levels.

THYROTOXIC CRISIS. Treatment consists of: intravenous fluid and glucose; parenteral hydrocortisone on account of possible adrenocortical exhaustion; sedation and suppression of hyperpyrexia; digoxin for cardiac failure; propranolol if cardiac failure is not pronounced; intravenous potassium iodide 60 mg twice daily as the most rapidly acting antithyroid drug; and reduction of body temperature by tepid sponging. Antithyroid drugs such as carbimazole are administered as soon as the patient is capable of taking medicines orally. Precipitating causes must be dealt with, e.g. acute infection. Prevention and early recognition are essential if deaths are to be avoided.

HYPERTHYROIDISM IN CHILDREN AND IN PREGNANCY. As the results of thyroidectomy in children and young teenagers may be less satisfactory than in adults and as radioactive iodine therapy is contraindicated in this age group, treatment should be with carbimazole or methimazole for as many years as is necessary.

In pregnancy, hyperthyroidism may be treated with antithyroid drugs or by surgery provided the operation can be carried out in the middle trimester after appropriate preparation with antithyroid drugs and preoperative potassium iodide. If antithyroid drugs are used throughout it is important to give the smallest dose that will control the thyrotoxicosis and to use an index of thyroid function that is not altered by pregnancy (e.g. serum TSHirma, fT_3 and fT_4). Towards term, the dose of antithyroid drugs should be further reduced in the hope of withdrawing them for the last 3 weeks of pregnancy. In this way the uncommon complication of the fetus being born with a goitre may be avoided.

The mother's serum should be tested for TSH-receptor antibodies. The baby should be checked for neonatal thyrotoxicosis. If antithyroid drugs are to be continued after pregnancy the baby must not be breast fed. Thyrotoxicosis may relapse in the postnatal months after being quiescent during pregnancy.

Exophthalmos

Autoimmune mechanisms involving the extra-ocular muscles, the retro-orbital fat and connective tissue are thought to be important in the pathogenesis of endocrine exophthalmos (*Graves' ophthalmopathy*). Defined as the protrusion of one or both eyeballs, exophthalmos may be detected clinically in the majority of cases by observing the white sclera both above and below the iris. In other cases periorbital oedema, which is frequently also present, may obscure this sign. The degree of protrusion and especially any progression or regression of exophthalmos should be recorded by use of an exophthalmometer.

Exposure of the cornea as a consequence of the eyelids failing to close properly will result in keratitis producing a feeling of grit in the eye and excessive watering. The conjunctiva may become injected and oedematous. Weakness of the extra-ocular muscles may give rise to an ophthalmoplegia with double vision, which is often first detected when the patient is asked to look upwards and outwards.

In some patients exophthalmos may precede the development of frank thyrotoxicosis and present a problem in differential diagnosis, especially if the exophthalmos is unilateral when orbital or retro-orbital tumours and infections may require consideration. CT scanning is particularly helpful in this context. Support for an endocrine aetiology may be obtained by eliciting a family history of thyroid disease or by demonstrating a suppressed serum TSHirma level or thyroid or gastric antibodies in the serum. Autoantibodies to eye muscle antigen, although described, are not diagnostically useful at the present time.

Treatment. In a small minority of cases the exophthalmos takes a relentlessly progressive course so that the increased intra-orbital pressure causes a severe aching in the eyes and reduction in visual acuity with papilloedema. Pressure within the orbit must be relieved urgently if permanent deterioration in vision is to be avoided. Decompression of the orbital cavity by surgical means may be required, but large doses of oral prednisolone together with cyclophosphamide and plasma exchange may obviate the need for surgery. Fortunately, in most cases exophthalmos is less severe; its progression ceases and there is a prolonged phase of gradual improvement although the eyes seldom return to the normal state.

In mild cases, chloramphenicol eye drops and the wearing of slightly tinted spectacles with protective side pieces to the frames will prevent the irritation of glare, dust and wind. In more severe cases lateral tarsorrhaphy, stitching together the outer margins of the eyelids, may be required, thereby improving their appearance and preventing exposure keratitis.

In relation to the treatment of thyrotoxicosis it is particularly important that hypothyroidism is avoided as this does seem to aggravate any associated exophthalmos.

HYPOTHYROIDISM

Hypothyroidism may be primary due to causes within the thyroid gland itself or, less commonly secondary, due to failure of TSH production following pituitary or hypothalamic disease. Hypothyroidism, especially when it is due to primary thyroid failure, is often, but not necessarily, associated with myxoedema, a thickening of the skin or other tissues by deposition of mucopolysaccharide giving the patient a characteristic appearance. When hypothyroidism is secondary to pituitary insufficiency, myxoedema is unusual.

Aetiology. Spontaneous primary hypothyroidism is much less common than thyrotoxicosis and principally affects middle-aged females, although it can occur in either sex at any age. It may be associated with a goitre or with thyroid atrophy. The commonest cause of spontaneous goitrous hypothyroidism in an adult female is Hashimoto's thyroiditis. It is believed that Graves' disease, Hashimoto's thyroiditis and primary atrophic hypothyroidism belong to a continuous spectrum of disease. This is characterised by a common familial trait towards organ specific autoimmune disease and by the frequent occurrence in the serum of thyroid and gastric parietal cell antibodies. The natural history of Graves' disease in the absence of destructive forms of therapy is the incipient development of hypothyroidism over a period of one or several decades, a further indication that both belong to the same spectrum of autoimmune thyroid disease. Less commonly hypothyroidism may be associated with other types of goitre, for example in dyshormonogenesis (p. 444). Hypothyroidism commonly occurs as a sequel to ^{131}I therapy for thyrotoxicosis. It may also be induced by certain drugs (p. 444).

Clinical features. ADULTS. In contrast to thyrotoxicosis the symptoms are the result of decreased metabolism, with slowing of mental and physical activity. The onset is gradual and often mistaken for ageing. On questioning, the patient may admit to sensitivity to cold, constipation, gain in weight, tiredness, vague generalised pains, deafness, forgetfulness or disordered menstrual function. The patient may also complain of tingling in the fingers from compression of the median nerve in the carpal tunnel.

In an advanced case the face appears swollen with puffy eyelids, thick lips and an enlarged tongue. There is often a malar flush but elsewhere the skin is pale as a consequence of thickening with myxoedema or of anaemia. Sweating is conspicuously absent and the skin is dry and readily

flakes on rubbing. The hair tends to be more sparse than normal and lustreless. Speech is slow, monotonous and husky or, in advanced instances, deep and croaky.

Characteristically the pulse rate is slow, but if the condition has progressed to cardiac failure, tachycardia may be found. Commonly there is evidence of coronary artery disease with angina pectoris or ECG changes of myocardial ischaemia. On radiological examination the heart is frequently seen to be enlarged; in some cases there may be a pericardial effusion which is usually reversible with treatment.

Marked slowing of the recovery phase of the ankle jerk due to delayed relaxation of the calf muscles is a useful clinical sign. Patients with severe hypothyroidism may show frank psychosis with hallucinations and delusions ('myxoedema madness') or pass into a state of coma. In a severe case, failure to control body temperature is one of the most lethal complications; mortality rises markedly as the body temperature falls below 32°C.

CHILDREN. While it is easy to detect the disease in its advanced state a high index of suspicion is required to avoid missing the early case and to prevent many years of unnecessary ill health. Hypothyroidism presents as a deterioration in performance at school, lack of interest in games and an arrest or slowing of growth. These features will precede the development of clinically obvious myxoedema. As in adults there may or may not be a goitre.

INFANTS. Failure of thyroid development is responsible for the condition of *cretinism*. The defects leading to this state may be inherited as autosomal recessives: in the heterozygous state the child may be goitrous only, but in the homozygous state both goitrous and a cretin. Cretinism also occurs in areas of endemic goitre (p. 60).

It is important to diagnose the state and initiate thyroxine replacement therapy as early as possible. The development of the brain is dependent on the thyroid hormones so that delay in starting treatment will inevitably lead to permanent mental impairment which will be the more severe the longer the delay. The diagnostic features are failure to achieve the normal milestones of development, constipation, poor feeding and a characteristic cry. Only in advanced cases will the child develop the obvious features of cretinism, which include a coarse facies with a broad flat nose, thick lips and a large tongue protruding from the mouth, and a pot belly with umbilical hernia.

Investigation. The measurement of serum fT_4 should be combined with a serum TSH measurement. The measurement of serum fT_3 is not helpful in suspected hypothyroidism.

All patients with untreated primary hypothyroidism have an elevated serum TSH level but not all patients with an elevated serum TSH necessarily have a significant degree of hypothyroidism. Many apparently normal subjects, especially the elderly, have a raised serum TSH but normal thyroid hormone levels associated with thyroid autoantibodies in the serum. Such patients may be regarded as having subclinical hypothyroidism due to autoimmune thyroiditis. As the rate of progression to overt hypothyroidism with low serum fT_4 levels may be very slow, such individuals probably do not require any treatment but should be kept under observation.

While a normal or low serum TSHirma level may be associated with secondary hypothyroidism due to pituitary or hypothalamic disease, a normal serum TSHirma level would exclude primary hypothyroidism. A TRH test in the presence of a normal or low serum TSHirma may be helpful in deciding whether secondary hypothyroidism is due to pituitary or hypothalamic disease. Screening of neonates for elevated serum TSH levels facilitates the early detection of cretinism. In many countries this is done using blood from a heel-prick. The filter paper sample is then assayed for TSH.

Radiographs of the epiphyses in children, or of ossification centres in the wrist or heel in infants, will indicate whether the bone age is delayed relative to the chronological age. Hypothyroidism in young people is invariably associated with impaired bone development; fragmentation of the epiphysis at the head of the femur is a striking radiological sign.

Treatment. In uncomplicated adult cases treatment with thyroxine should start with 0.05 mg/d increasing to 0.1 mg/d after 3 weeks provided cardiac failure or angina have not arisen. After a further 3–6 weeks the dose may be increased to 0.15–0.2 mg/d. This is the normal full replacement dose, but a few patients may require up to 0.3 mg thyroxine/d. Patients must understand that their well-being depends on continued treatment and must not stop thyroxine when they feel better. There is no advantage in divided doses or taking tablets that consist of a mixture of T_3 and T_4.

In a patient known to have ischaemic heart disease it will usually be desirable to keep the dose of thyroxine between 0.05 and 0.1 mg/d and to use a beta-adrenergic blocking agent such as propranolol. In patients with secondary hypothyroidism it is essential to treat any adrenocortical insufficiency before starting thyroxine.

Myxoedema coma with hypothermia. Small doses (10–20 μg) of triiodothyronine may be given intravenously 8 hourly together with hydrocortisone and glucose. The body temperature should be restored very slowly to a level of 32°C; above this level active warming should be abandoned in favour of heat conservation using a space blanket or foil.

GOITRE

This term is applied to any enlargement of the thyroid gland and on clinical examination its size, shape, consistency, symmetry, irregularity of surface, mobility and the presence of a bruit should be established. The level of thyroid activity should be determined by the tests already described.

Goitre associated with thyrotoxicosis will not be discussed further. The diagnosis of the common condition of simple goitre is arrived at by the exclusion of other causes, such as Hashimoto's thyroiditis, subacute thyroiditis, dyshormonogenesis, or carcinoma of the thyroid gland.

Hashimoto's thyroiditis is characteristically a firm diffuse enlargement of the thyroid gland with or without hypothyroidism. It may give rise to an aching discomfort in the neck and to mild dysphagia. It occurs most commonly in middle-aged women. In almost all cases the serum contains antibodies to thyroglobulin or to the microsomal fraction of thyroid cytoplasm, frequently in high titre. The ESR is often elevated. Histologically the gland consists of rather small thyroid vesicles with columnar epithelium showing a varying degree of eosinophilic granularity, infiltration by lymphocytes and plasma cells, sometimes with germinal centre formation and an increase in the fibrous tissue stroma.

In most instances there will be a satisfactory regression in the size of the goitre in response to thyroxine 0.2 mg/d, which can be hastened by giving 20 mg prednisolone 8-hourly for 10 days only. Adults with Hashimoto's thyroiditis should remain on life-long thyroxine therapy irrespective of whether or not they were initially hypothyroid. In adolescence, Hashimoto's thyroiditis may be transitory.

Subacute (de Quervain's) thyroiditis is a painful condition generally associated with some thyroid enlargement. It is thought to be due to a viral infection (e.g. Coxsackie B). Thyroid function is suppressed and histologically the characteristic feature is the presence of giant cells. The ESR may be markedly elevated and thyroid antibody tests are generally negative. The condition tends to regress spontaneously but may be persistent. Thyroxine 0.2–0.3 mg/d should then be given to suppress TSH secretion and, in some cases, it may be necessary to give a course of oral corticosteroids.

Dyshormonogenesis. The patient who has a partial enzyme defect related to one of the steps in the synthesis of thyroid hormones (Fig.12.3) is likely to develop a goitre in response to continued TSH secretion induced by the low serum thyroxine. While all these defects are rare, the commonest and the easiest to detect is a genetically determined defect in the binding of iodine to tyrosine which, when associated with nerve deafness, is known as *Pendred's syndrome.*

Drug-induced goitre may be due to lithium or para-aminosalicylic acid and is often associated with hypothyroidism. It may be due to iodine or iodine containing drugs such as amiodarone when the goitre may be associated with either hypothyroidism or hyperthyroidism.

Tumours of the thyroid gland. CARCINOMA is uncommon, forming about 1% of all cases of cancer in Britain. The tumours may be well-differentiated papillary or follicular carcinomas (or a mixture of the two) or be anaplastic. Advanced cancers are obvious by their hardness, irregularity, adhesion to surrounding tissues and associated lymphadenopathy. Early carcinoma of the thyroid gland presents as a single nodule which almost invariably has poorer function than the surrounding normal thyroid tissue. If the nodule is sufficiently large it will be detectable as a 'cold' area on radioisotope scanning. It is not possible to distinguish clinically between a single nodule that is malignant and one that is benign; all single (solitary) nodules should therefore be removed for histological examination. As thyroid histology in terms of establishing the presence or absence of malignant disease can be difficult, there would appear to be little point in carrying out fine needle biopsy and compounding the problems by the provision of small specimens.

Well-differentiated thyroid tumours should be treated by total thyroidectomy followed by life-long oral thyroxine 0.2–0.3 mg/d according to the patient's age. Metastases from a well differentiated tumour may take up sufficient radioactive iodine, after all normally functioning thyroid tissue has been ablated by surgery and ^{131}I, to allow effective therapy with a further large dose of ^{131}I. Non-functioning secondaries can be treated by local radiotherapy. Anaplastic tumours may show a good initial response to radiotherapy, but invariably recur.

Medullary carcinoma of the thyroid arises from the parafollicular C-cells; although rare, it is of particular interest as it is associated with high levels of plasma calcitonin, prostaglandins or 5-hydroxytryptamine, causing symptoms such as flushing, borborygmi and diarrhoea. Patients with this form of thyroid cancer may have neuromas on the tongue, lips or eyelids, Marfanoid skeletal proportions (p. 192), and, occasionally, phaeochromocytomas.

Total thyroidectomy and removal of affected lymph nodes are required. The tumour is not very radiosensitive. It does not take up ^{131}I. Relapse can be detected by calcitonin assay.

BENIGN TUMOURS. Solitary 'cold' lesions in the thyroid may consist of adenomas or cysts; they can usually be differentiated by isotope scanning and ultrasonography. Calcification in cysts is common. Cysts without an admixture of solid constituents may be aspirated and the fluid sent for cytology. Haemorrhage occasionally occurs into adenomas and for this reason, in addition to the risk of malignancy, their removal is justified.

Simple goitre may occur sporadically, but in certain parts of the world it is found more frequently and is then referred to as endemic goitre (p. 60). The aetiology is believed to be closely related to iodine deficiency, mainly in the diet. An intermittent shortage in supply of iodine to the gland over prolonged periods is thought to result in the multinodular character of long-standing goitres. Less commonly factors in the diet or water such as excess calcium may interfere with iodine absorption; goitrogens in the diet may prevent concentration of iodine by the thyroid. When the secretion or release of thyroid hormones is suppressed, the goitre results from continuing increased secretion of TSH.

A small, soft diffuse, simple goitre may occur at puberty or during pregnancy and may regress spontaneously thereafter, but in other cases it persists. If already present, it may enlarge further at these times. A simple goitre of long standing may achieve considerable size, become grossly nodular and give rise to obstructive symptoms, particularly if there is a retrosternal extension. Deviation of the trachea may be noted clinically or radiologically and obstruction at the thoracic inlet may lead to venous engorgement of the head and neck. Bruits and thrills do not occur in simple goitres. Cretinism is associated with endemic goitre in areas where iodine deficiency is severe.

The treatment of sporadic simple diffuse goitre at puberty should be with thyroxine for 1 to 2 years and not potassium iodide. An adequate dietary intake of iodine should be ensured (p. 60). Multinodular simple goitres are unlikely to respond to thyroxine and may require partial thyroidectomy for cosmetic reasons, or if obstructive symptoms are present or likely to occur. Postoperative life-long treatment with thyroxine may prevent a recurrence, although hypothyroidism after partial thyroidectomy for simple goitre is uncommon.

An adequate intake of iodine, particularly in the early years of life, is the only really satisfactory way of preventing sporadic simple goitre. The incidence of endemic goitre can be greatly reduced by correcting iodine deficiency, for example, by legislation that ensures that table salt contains traces of iodine (p. 60).

THE PARATHYROID GLANDS

Anatomy and physiology. These glands, usually four in number, each measure about 5 mm in diameter. Their relation to the thyroid gland is described on page 433. The parathyroid glands control the concentration of calcium and inorganic phosphorus in the blood, both by enhancing the removal of mineral from the skeleton, and by promoting the excretion of phosphorus by the kidney.

Calcium occurs in plasma in two forms, 'diffusible' and 'non-diffusible'. The former consists of ionised calcium, and a small amount of non-ionised calcium salts of organic acids. From the point of view of neuromuscular function and the occurrence of tetany, as well as the secretion of parathyroid hormone, it is the ionised plasma calcium concentration which is important. The non-diffusible fraction is that portion which is bound to the plasma albumin.

Assays of parathyroid hormone (PTH) are becoming more widely available but many still have considerable overlap between the normal range and hyperparathyroidism. In such cases a 'normal' PTH value is often said to be abnormal or inappropriate for the high plasma calcium. Calcitonin and vitamin D metabolites also affect the metabolism of calcium and phosphorus, and must be considered in disorders of these elements. Controversy continues regarding the reliability and relevance of calcitonin assays, except in the diagnosis of medullary carcinoma of the thyroid gland.

HYPERPARATHYROIDISM

Primary hyperparathyroidism is usually due to a single parathyroid adenoma. Very occasionally it may be caused by simple hyperplasia or multiple adenomas: a functioning parathyroid carcinoma can also occur.

Secondary hyperparathyroidism is due to hypertrophy of the glands and is found in chronic renal failure which causes hypocalcaemia followed by an increase in parathyroid activity. Secondary hyperparathyroidism also occurs as a sequel to osteomalacia, malabsorption or rickets.

Tertiary hyperparathyroidism is used to describe the cases of the secondary variety of long standing in which a continuing stimulus is responsible for parathyroid hyperplasia being replaced by autonomous function in one or more parathyroid adenomas.

Osteitis fibrosa or *von Recklinghausen's disease of bone* occurs in the rare event of hyperparathyroidism involving the bones to such an extent that cyst formation occurs. Such patients usually have vitamin D deficiency and the bone lesions can be healed by vitamin D therapy.

Clinical features. Mild, asymptomatic hyperparathyroidism is not uncommon, particularly after middle age. Patients with more severe hypercalcaemia frequently complain of weakness, loss of appetite, nausea, vomiting, constipation, drowsiness or confusion. Some of these patients also have a peptic ulcer, the symptoms from which may obscure those of hyperparathyroidism. Acute pancreatitis is sometimes a presenting feature. When bone involvement is marked, backache is a common complaint. Pseudo-gout (p. 581) may occur as can hypertension.

Renal calculi frequently form in association with the increased excretion of calcium in the urine. While many patients with hyperparathyroidism develop symptoms due to renal calculi, relatively few presenting with renal calculi are due to increased parathyroid activity. In other cases of hyperparathyroidism deposits of calcium form in and around the renal tubular epithelium (nephrocalcinosis). Tubular reabsorption of water may be impaired as a consequence or from the direct effects of hypercalcaemia producing nephrogenic diabetes insipidus with polyuria and polydipsia. In cases of long standing, and in those with associated pyelonephritis, the renal disease may progress to uraemia in spite of the relief of the hyperparathyroidism.

Physical examination is usually unhelpful. Occasionally a parathyroid tumour is sufficiently large and suitably placed to be palpable or even visible as a swelling in the region of the thyroid gland. Calcification may be present at the corneoscleral junction or in the conjunctiva, seen more readily with a slit-lamp.

MULTIPLE ENDOCRINE NEOPLASIA. A parathyroid adenoma may coexist with secreting adenomas or hyperplasia elsewhere. In multiple endocrine neoplasia type I the patients have hyperparathyroidism, pancreatic islet cell tumours (gastrinoma or insulinoma) and pituitary adenomas (usually prolactinomas). In multiple endocrine neoplasia type II the features are medullary carcinoma of thyroid, phaeochromocytoma and hyperparathyroidism. In type III in addition to the medullary carcinoma and phaeochromocytoma there are mucosal and submucosal neuromas usually involving the lips and tongue. Hyperparathyroidism is rare in type III.

Investigation. *Hypercalcaemia and related findings.* Hypercalcaemia is the most significant chemical finding. The fasting plasma calcium may be considerably increased above the upper limit of normal (p. 814). It may be necessary to carry out estimations at intervals in doubtful cases, since hypercalcaemia may be episodic. A tourniquet should not be used in obtaining samples since this may be responsible for raising the plasma calcium. If the plasma albumin is low the value for the plasma calcium should be adjusted upwards.

Causes of hypercalcaemia other than hyperparathyroidism include metastatic malignant disease of bone and cancer, without bone secondaries, producing a PTH-like polypeptide. A number of factors have been identified as activating osteoclasts and thus producing hypercalcaemia. They are at least 100 times more potent than PTH in increasing bone resorption and have been found in some patients with malignancy and hypercalcaemia. Other factors produced by tumour in bone may have a local or paracrine effect. In about 10% of patients with hypercalcaemia, prostaglandins may be involved, and drugs that inhibit prostaglandin production, such as indomethacin, can lower serum calcium.

Patients with sarcoidosis and hypercalcaemia have elevated levels of the active vitamin D metabolite, 1,25-dihydroxycholecalciferol. Less common causes of hypercalcaemia include overdosage with vitamin D, hyperthyroidism, and immobilisation especially in patients with increased bone turnover as in Paget's disease.

The plasma inorganic phosphate is usually lowered in hyperparathyroidism and the plasma chloride elevated. The plasma alkaline phosphatase, an index of osteoblastic activity, may be raised (p. 814) depending on the degree of involvement of bone.

Radiological examination. In the early stages there may be demineralisation and subperiosteal erosions may be noted in the phalanges. These are most marked on the radial side of the middle phalanx. There may also be resorption of the terminal phalanges. A 'pepper-pot' appearance may be seen in lateral radiographs of the skull. Cystic changes are rare. In nephrocalcinosis scattered opacities may be visible within the renal outline. There may be soft tissue calcification elsewhere.

Localisation of parathyroid tumour. Ultrasonography and occasionally arteriography can be helpful in locating the site of an adenoma. Computed tomography may show a mediastinal adenoma but is of little value in the neck. The uptake of radioactive thallium by the parathyroid tumour may be useful. As thallium is also taken up by the thyroid a separate thyroid scan has to be performed with technetium and the image subtracted from the thallium scan to reveal the parathyroid uptake. These localising procedures are not usually performed before the first neck exploration but can be of particular value if re-exploration is required.

Parathyroid hormone radio-immunoassay. As discussed, an inappropriately high plasma PTH, even within the normal range, in the presence of hypercalcaemia, is indicative of hyperparathyroidism. Such assays may also be helpful in localising small tumours by identifying high concentrations of parathyroid hormone in blood obtained from specific veins in the root of the neck or mediastinum.

Treatment. Removal of a solitary adenoma is usually sufficient to produce clinical cure, provided advanced renal disease is not already present. Patients with multiple adenomas or generalised hyperplasia of all the parathyroids may be difficult to manage, especially when the glands lie in unusual situations such as the superior mediastinum, but surgical treatment offers the only prospect of cure.

The current management of hyperplasia is to remove all four glands and to transplant some of this tissue to the forearm. If hypercalcaemia returns then part of the transplant can be excised under local anaesthetic. Patients with bone involvement may, following removal of the tumour, show the 'hungry bones' syndrome characterised by tetany with hypocalcaemia and sometimes hypomagnesaemia. It is not certain whether people, especially the elderly, with mild symptomless hypercalcaemia come to any harm from the continued presence of a parathyroid tumour.

Some patients with severe primary hyperparathyroidism may present as a medical emergency with hypercalcaemia. Adequate rehydration is an essential first step in management. Such patients often have a fluid deficit of several litres and when this has been replaced plasma calcium will usually fall to a level where surgery can be considered. Saline administration produces a calcium diuresis but care must be taken not to overload the circulation. Intravenous phosphate used to be given to lower calcium but has the danger of producing ectopic calcification. Oral phosphate is safer.

HYPOPARATHYROIDISM

This unusual condition may arise from a variety of causes, but with each the clinical feature in common is tetany. Biochemically, a depressed concentration of calcium and a raised concentration of phosphate in plasma are characteristic.

Postoperative hypoparathyroidism. A transitory form of the disorder is common after a partial thyroidectomy, presumably due to interference with the blood supply of the parathyroid glands. After a complete thyroidectomy permanent hypoparathyroidism may occur. Hypoparathyroidism may be transient following removal of a hyperfunctioning parathyroid adenoma, the other three parathyroid glands having been suppressed by the high calcium levels.

Infantile hypoparathyroidism may be transient and associated with maternal hyperparathyroidism or calcium deficiency. It persists in thymic aplasia (Di George syndrome, p. 32).

Idiopathic hypoparathyroidism may develop at any age, and is sometimes associated with autoimmune disease of the adrenal, thyroid or ovary especially in young people. In addition to tetany other features include psychoses, cataracts, aberrant calcification and moniliasis, particularly of the finger nails.

Pseudohypoparathyroidism is the term applied to a congenital variety in which there is tissue resistance to the effects of parathyroid hormone. The PTH receptor is normal but there is a defective post-receptor mechanism. Pseudohypoparathyroidism presents with the biochemical features of hypoparathyroidism, and in addition aberrant calcification, cataracts, mental retardation and skeletal abnormalities, for example small, stocky stature and short 4th and 5th metacarpals. These patients have elevated levels of plasma parathyroid hormone and high concentrations of calcitonin have been found in their circulation and in their thyroid glands.

Treatment. Commercial preparations of parathyroid hormone available for the treatment of parathyroid insufficiency are unsatisfactory because they have to be given by frequent injections, and soon become ineffective because of antibody formation. In the acute phase, calcium is given intravenously as for tetany; substitution therapy for persistent hypoparathyroidism and for pseudohypoparathyroidism is provided by calciferol. In some patients it is difficult to control the serum calcium. These can usually be successfully treated with $1,25\text{-}(OH)_2D_3$ in doses ranging from $0.25\text{--}1\,\mu g/d$ or with $1\text{--}2\,\mu g/d$ of $1\alpha\ OH\text{-}D_3$ (p. 64).

Tetany

Aetiology. There is an increased excitability of peripheral nerves due either to a low plasma calcium concentration or to alkalosis in which the proportion of the plasma calcium in the ionised form is decreased, although the total calcium concentration remains unaltered. Magnesium depletion should also be considered as a possible contributing factor, particularly in the malabsorption syndrome.

CAUSES OF DEPLETION OF PLASMA CALCIUM. (1) *Inadequate intake or absorption of calcium.* This occurs in rickets, osteomalacia and the malabsorption syndrome. (2) *Hypoparathyroidism.* (3) *Chronic renal failure* where, although the plasma calcium is often low, coincident acidosis usually prevents tetany. (4) *Pancreatitis* may also be associated with hypocalcaemia.

CAUSES OF ALKALOSIS. (1) *Repeated vomiting* of acid gastric juice, as in gastric outlet obstruction from peptic ulceration. (2) *Excessive quantities of absorbable alkalis* given by mouth especially when associated with repeated vomiting. (3) *Hyperventilation*, commonly due to hysteria, lowers the arterial P_{CO_2}. (4) *Primary hyperaldosteronism* (p. 452).

Clinical features. In *children* a characteristic triad of carpopedal spasm, stridor and convulsions occurs, though one or more of these may be found independently of the others. The hands in carpal spasm adopt a characteristic position. The metacarpophalangeal joints are flexed, the interphalangeal joints of the fingers and thumb are extended and there is opposition of the thumb (*main d'accoucheur*). Pedal spasm is much less frequent. Stridor is caused by spasm of the glottis.

Adults complain of tingling in the hands, feet and around the mouth. Less often there is painful carpopedal spasm while stridor and fits are rare.

Latent tetany may be present when signs of overt tetany are lacking. It is best recognised by eliciting *Trousseau's sign*. Inflation of the sphygmomanometer cuff on the upper arm to more than the systolic blood pressure is followed by characteristic spasm in the forearm muscles within 4 minutes. A less specific sign of hypocalcaemia is that described by *Chvostek* in which tapping over the branches of the facial nerve as they emerge from the parotid gland produces twitching of the facial muscles.

Treatment. *Control of tetany.* Injection of 20ml of a 10% solution of calcium gluconate slowly into a vein will raise the plasma calcium concentration immediately. An intramuscular injection of 10 ml may also be given to obtain a more prolonged effect. In severe cases of alkalotic tetany, intravenous calcium gluconate often relieves the spasm, while more radical treatment of the alkalosis, which will vary with the cause, is being applied. If tetany is not relieved by giving calcium the administration of magnesium may be required.

Correction of alkalosis. 1. In persistent vomiting, intravenous isotonic saline is the most effective treatment.

2. When alkalis have been given to excess their withdrawal may suffice to stop the tetany, but if not, ammonium chloride 2 g should be given 4-hourly by mouth until relief has been obtained.

3. The inhalation of 5% carbon dioxide in oxygen may be prescribed for the correction of the alkalosis of hyperventilation, or more simply, the patient should be made to rebreathe expired air from a suitable bag. The hysterical patient should also have appropriate psychotherapy (p. 689).

Treatment of the underlying condition. When tetany follows removal of a parathyroid adenoma and if there is any residual parathyroid tissue, this usually undergoes compensatory hypertrophy. In the interval parenteral or oral calcium with or without vitamin D may be required. If all the parathyroid tissue has been removed, prolonged replacement therapy with calciferol is commonly used to maintain a normal plasma calcium concentration. One tablet (1.25 mg) daily is usually adequate, but less, or more, may be required. The maintenance dose is determined by monitoring of the plasma calcium at intervals, as persistent hypercalcaemia which might follow prolonged high doses of vitamin D can lead to widespread metastatic calcification and eventually renal failure.

In chronic renal failure with hypocalcaemia the logical treatment is with either $1,25\text{-}(OH)_2D_3$ or $1\alpha\text{-}OH\text{-}D_3$ (p. 448). Treatment may also be required for rickets (p. 65), osteomalacia (p. 68) or malabsorption (p. 304).

THE ADRENAL GLANDS

Anatomy and physiology. The adrenal glands lie in relation to the upper poles of the kidneys. Each consists of an inner medulla which secretes adrenaline and noradrenaline and an outer cortex of three layers. These, from without inwards, are the zona glomerulosa, zona fasciculata and zona reticularis (Fig. 12.4). Although over 40 steroid compounds have been extracted from the adrenal cortex, the principal hormones are cortisol (glucocorticoid), aldosterone (mineralocorticoid) and androstenedione, androsterone and dehydroepiandrosterone (androgens).

Adrenocorticotrophic hormone (ACTH, p. 425) alters the rate of biosynthesis and secretion of the glucocorticoid cortisol from the zona fasciculata and reticularis. ACTH also increases the secretion of the adrenal androgens. Aldosterone secretion by the zona glomerulosa is primarily controlled by the renin-angiotensin mechanisms. Acute elevation of ACTH levels will stimulate aldosterone but chronic ACTH excess, as in pituitary-dependant Chushing's syndrome, does not.

The *glucocorticoids* have effects which are antagonistic to insulin, tending to raise the blood sugar by converting amino acids derived from protein breakdown into glucose (gluconeogenesis). Glucocorticoids such as cortisol have other important actions including the suppression of inflammatory reactions which may occur in response to injury, infection or immunological mechanisms. Glucocorticoids are also lipogenic and have some mineralocorticoid effects especially when used in pharmacological doses.

Aldosterone produces retention of sodium and increased excretion of potassium and if given in pharmacological doses over a prolonged period also causes hypertension. Weight for weight, aldosterone has far greater mineralocorticoid activity than the glucocorticoids.

In addition to *androgens*, the adrenal cortex also synthesises *oestrogen* and *progesterone* in small quantities in both sexes. The nitrogen-retaining (anabolic) activity of the androgenic hormones is antagonistic to the catabolic effect of the glucocorticoids.

HYPERFUNCTION OF THE ADRENAL GLAND

Cushing's syndrome. This can be defined as the symptoms and signs associated with prolonged exposure to inappropriately elevated plasma corticosteroid levels. The patients may be divided into two main groups depending on whether or not the condition derives from exposure to excessive ACTH.

1. ACTH dependent causes of Cushing's syndrome:

a. Iatrogenic—administration of excessive quantities of ACTH or its synthetic analogues.

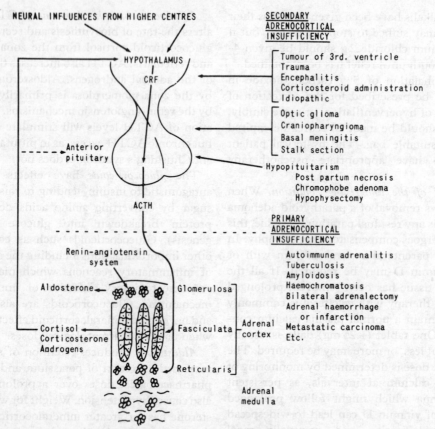

Fig. 12.4 Causes of primary and secondary adrenocortical insufficiency.

b. Pituitary-dependent bilateral adrenocortical hyperplasia, conventionally called *Cushing's disease*.

c. The ectopic ACTH syndrome — secretion of ACTH by malignant or benign tumours of non-endocrine origin, e.g. bronchial carcinoma.

2. Non-ACTH dependent causes of Cushing's syndrome:

a. Iatrogenic — administration of supraphysiological doses of corticosteroids.

b. Adenomas or carcinomas of the adrenal cortex.

Cushing's syndrome associated with pituitary-dependent adrenocortical hyperplasia and adrenal tumours is four times more common in women than in men with a peak age incidence between 35 and 50 years. This contrasts with the male predominance and later age incidence found in Cushing's syndrome secondary to the ectopic production of ACTH.

Clinical features. These can be interpreted largely in terms of the action of the glucocorticoids. Thus the gluconeogenic effect is seen as an elevation of the blood glucose level and glycosuria; a proportion of patients develop diabetes. The effect on the blood sugar is however not invariable because of other mechanisms that counteract any disturbance in carbohydrate metabolism, such as insulin secretion. The breakdown of protein to form glucose is reflected in the reduction of muscle, bone and connective tissue, leading to weakness, proximal myopathy, osteoporosis, easy bruising and purple striae of the skin over the abdomen, buttocks and thighs. Osteoporosis may be sufficiently severe to produce backache; radiological changes in the vertebral bodies may progress to collapse, kyphosis and shortening of stature.

The most striking features of Cushing's disease are the rounded plethoric appearance (moon face), central obesity and 'buffalo hump' (accumulation of fat at the lower part of the back of the neck) due to redistribution of body fat. There is also arterial hypertension caused by sodium retention. The loss of potassium may contribute to muscular weakness. The overproduction of adrenal androgens may lead to the development of hirsutism and acne in some patients with perhaps temporal recession of hair in females. Amenorrhoea or other disorders of menstrual function are common. Mental symptoms, in particular depression, may be prominent.

The pituitary gland in Cushing's disease is seldom grossly enlarged either in the presence of hyperplasia or of an adenoma of the basophil or chomophobe cells and usually no enlargement may be detectable on a radiograph of the pituitary fossa.

In an adrenocortical tumour affecting the zona fasciculata/reticularis, the clinical features will depend on the type of steroid that the tumour is synthesising. If it is glucocorticoids almost exclusively the clinical features will be indistinguishable from the other causes of Cushing's syndrome, whereas if the tumour is making androgens predominantly the female patient will be virilised, with pronounced hirsutism, deepening of the voice, recession of the hair on the forehead, acne and clitoral enlargement, possibly with increased libido. In males an adrenal tumour may induce feminisation, e.g. gynaecomastia, if the tumour is mainly making oestrogens. Although many adrenocortical adenomas are benign, functional carcinomas also occur with metastases to other organs.

When ectopic ACTH is the cause of Cushing's syndrome the striking features are the rapid development of brown pigmentation due to the very high plasma levels of ACTH and LPH (p. 426). Frequently such patients show a marked alkalosis and potassium depletion. Characteristically they do not appear cushingoid (moon face and central obesity) presumably because of the short survival time of the underlying malignant process. With benign tumours secreting ACTH, such as a bronchial carcinoid, the clinical presentation may be indistinguishable from pituitary-dependant Cushing's syndrome.

Investigation. Disordered function of the zona fasciculata/reticularis is almost invariably reflected in an alteration of the normal circadian rhythm of cortisol secretion with high levels of serum cortisol in the evening. However, the demonstration of such an abnormality does not establish the diagnosis since stress, obesity or depression may produce similar findings.

In subjects with normal adrenocortical function the secretion of cortisol should be readily suppressible with biologically active analogues of cortisol such as dexamethasone. These substances do not contribute to the measurement of endogenous serum cortisol by radio-immunoassay. Normal subjects and patients suffering from simple obesity will show suppression of cortisol secretion following 0.5 mg oral dexamethasone 6-hourly for 48 hours. The majority of patients with Cushing's disease will show significant suppression following 2.0 mg dexamethasone 6-hourly for 48 hours, while most patients with adrenal tumours and the ectopic ACTH syndrome will fail to do so at this dosage. A useful screening test can be done as an outpatient by taking 2.0 mg dexamethasone orally at 23:00 and reporting to the clinic at 09:00 on the following morning when the serum cortisol is measured. In normal individuals and in simple obesity the morning rise in serum cortisol is suppressed, i.e. serum cortisol less than 170 nmol/l.

The estimation of urinary free cortisol either in a 24-hour urine sample or the measurement of the free cortisol:creatinine ratio in a single early-morning sample of urine may be useful in distinguishing between Cushing's syndrome and simple obesity.

The response in the serum cortisol levels following insulin hypoglycaemia is helpful in distinguishing between patients with true Cushing's syndrome (no response) and those who are stressed or severely depressed and who might show loss of circadian rhythm and resistance to dexamethasone suppression (normal response).

When abnormal production of adrenal androgens is suspected, specific steroid measurements by radioimmunoassay are to be preferred to the measurement of urinary 17-oxosteroids. Examples are the measurement of dehydroepiandrosterone in suspected adrenocortical carcinoma, or measurement of cortisol, ACTH and 17α-hydroxyprogesterone in congenital adrenal hyperplasia due to C21-hydroxylase deficiency (p. 454).

Cause of excess activity of the zona fasciculata/ reticularis. Some indication of this may be obtained by radioimmunoassay of the plasma ACTH concentration. Moderately elevated levels are seen in Cushing's disease, low or undetectable levels occur in adrenal adenoma and strikingly high levels are usually found in the ectopic ACTH syndrome. Computed tomography of the abdomen and chest is the technique of choice to show the adrenal anatomy and to locate a suspected ectopic ACTH secreting tumour in patients with proven Cushing's syndrome, especially a small (<1.5 cm) lung tumour. Benign adrenal tumours may also be localised by scintigraphic scanning using labelled cholesterol. Only occasionally is adrenal vein sampling for estimation of the serum cortisol required. Both glands should be studied as 10% of adenomas are bilateral.

Treatment. This clearly depends on establishing the cause of overactivity of the zona fasciculata/reticularis. The treatment of Cushing's disease by removal of a pituitary adenoma is discussed on page 429. The adrenal which is the site of an adenoma or carcinoma should be excised. In the case of the ectopic ACTH syndrome the primary tumour should be removed if feasible. Transitory improvement may be achieved by using metyrapone (which inhibits the enzyme 11-beta-hydroxylase that is involved in the final step in the synthesis of cortisol), or aminoglutethimide to block cortisol synthesis together with appropriate electrolyte replacement with particular reference to potassium.

Hyperaldosteronism

Overactivity of the zona glomerulosa may be primary in origin or secondary to some other pathological process. In *primary hyperaldosteronism*, usually associated with an adenoma and known as *Conn's syndrome*, the most consistent symptom is weakness, often episodic, and attributable to potassium deficiency. Polyuria and polydipsia, also due to the effects of potassium depletion and impaired renal tubular reabsorption of water, commonly occur. Tetany may be an occasional presenting symptom precipitated by the metabolic alkalosis associated with potassium depletion. The blood pressure is usually raised and the condition may be mistaken for essential hypertension, or for myasthenia gravis because of the weakness. Oedema is most unusual although its presence might be anticipated from the sodium retaining effect of aldosterone. Primary aldosteronism should be treated by removal of the affected gland or if this is not possible, spironolactone should be given.

Secondary hyperaldosteronism occurs in salt depletion, in cirrhosis of the liver with ascites, in the nephrotic syndrome, in severe cardiac failure especially with diuretic therapy and in malignant hypertension. The use of spironolactone in management is discussed on page 92. Secondary aldosteronism may also occur in unilateral renal ischaemia due to renal artery stenosis, and can be improved or cured by surgery or transluminal angioplasty.

In primary hyperaldosteronism plasma renin activity is suppressed with elevated aldosterone levels, whereas in secondary hyperaldosteronism both renin and aldosterone are high. In primary hyperaldosteronism computed tomography of the adrenals, isotope scanning and adrenal vein catheterisation may all be helpful in distinguishing an adenoma from hyperplasia of the zona glomerulosa.

INSUFFICIENCY OF THE ADRENAL CORTEX

Inadequate secretion of the adrenocortical hormones may be primary from acquired disease of the adrenals (Addison's disease) or from congenital deficiency of the enzymes required for the synthesis of adrenocortical hormones (congenital adrenal hyperplasia). It may be secondary to failure of ACTH secretion due to pituitary or hypothalamic disorders (Fig.12.4).

Addison's disease

Autoimmune adrenal failure and, much less commonly, tuberculous destruction of the adrenals are the main causes of Addison's disease in the developed countries, while other causes listed in Figure 12.4 are rare.

Autoimmune adrenal failure (previously referred to as 'idiopathic' or 'simple' atrophy) affects females twice as frequently as males and may occur at any age. It is characterised by adreno-cortical antibodies in the serum, by cell mediated hypersensitivity to adrenocortical antigens, the presence of HLA-B8 and HLA-DR3 and by a high incidence of other organ-specific autoimmune diseases such as thyrotoxicosis, Hashimoto's thyroiditis, primary atrophic hypothyroidism, pernicious anaemia, premature ovarian failure, idiopathic hypoparathyroidism and also insulin dependent (Type I) diabetes. Histologically both adrenals show atrophy of the cortical cells in all three zones with lymphocytic infiltration and increase in fibrous tissue. The medulla is not significantly affected. The adrenals are usually smaller than normal and appear atrophic.

In tuberculous destruction of the adrenal there is caseation with giant cells, and calcification which may be detected radiologically in long-standing cases.

Clinical features. The onset of adrenal insufficiency may be acute or chronic, or more commonly acute following upon chronic. The main clinical features of chronic primary adrenal insufficiency are weakness, weight loss, hyper-pigmentation with or without vitiligo, hypotension and gastrointestinal disorders. The invariable symptoms of tiredness and malaise, both physical and mental, gradually increase. Loss of weight does not occur until the adrenal failure is well advanced and then it is invariable. Anorexia, nausea and constipation alternating with diarrhoea occur with increased frequency as the disease progresses. Eventually in adrenal crisis the gastro-intestinal complaints may be the outstanding feature and an erroneous diagnosis of severe gastro-enteritis may be made; pain may simulate an acute abdomen. A wrong diagnosis may cost the patient her or his life.

Pigmentation of the skin is often the clinical sign that first raises the suspicion of primary hypoadrenalism. A history of its recent onset is more significant than pigmentation of long standing. This feature is due to increased melanin and is most obvious in regions normally pigmented and exposed to light or pressure, e.g. face, neck, back of hands, knuckles, elbows and knees, or in areas of the body subject to friction and in skin creases, particularly in the palms. The mucous membranes of the mouth, the conjunctivae and the vagina may also become pigmented. Scars that have been present before the onset of primary adrenal failure remain unpigmented in contrast to those that are acquired after the onset of adrenal failure. Pigmentation may precede the other features of hypoadrenalism by many years. It often manifests itself initially by the patient acquiring a much better suntan than usual and the tan taking longer to disappear. The progressive pigmentation is due to increased secretion of LPH (p. 426) by the pituitary which occurs simultaneously with augmented ACTH release and to ACTH itself (Fig. 12.2). Vitiligo, patchy areas of depigmentation of the skin surrounded by increased pigmentation, occurs in 10 to 20% of patients with Addison's disease, particularly in dark-skinned races.

The patient may give a history of very slow recovery from an illness or operation, having escaped an acute crisis at such a time. Likewise, there may be a history of extreme sensitivity to drugs such as morphine or pethidine.

Hypotension is almost invariable whether the patient is erect or supine. It is uncommon for a patient with primary adrenocortical failure to have a systolic blood pressure greater than 110 mmHg before replacement therapy is started. Normal reflex maintenance of the blood pressure is impaired and dizziness and syncope may result from postural hypotension.

Reactive hypoglycaemia after a carbohydrate meal may occur, cortisol being one of the physiological antagonists of insulin. Hypoglycaemia is usually manifest by tiredness and lethargy, the patient having more than usual difficulty in getting up in the morning.

Loss of body hair, especially in the female, is occasionally found but is generally not so marked as in hypopituitarism. Menstrual disorders, usually amenorrhoea, are common during the onset of the disease. A significant proportion of patients with autoimmune Addison's disease suffer from premature failure of ovarian function on account of an immunological reaction against antigens that are shared between the adrenal cortex and the steroid producing cells of the ovary.

Secondary adrenal insufficiency

The secretion of ACTH and TSH is more resistant to pituitary damage than is the secretion of the gonadotrophins or growth hormone, so that patients with adrenal insufficiency secondary to organic pituitary disease generally show clinical features of impaired gonadotrophin secretion or of growth hormone secretion if the patient is of appropriate age for such manifestations. There is usually marked loss of axillary and pubic hair and the skin is fine provided hypothyroidism is not pronounced. A patient with secondary adrenal insufficiency will differ from one with Addison's disease by showing pallor instead of increased pigmentation of the skin. Because the secretion of aldosterone is largely independent of the pituitary, the blood pressure is better maintained than in primary adrenal insufficiency and the threat to life is less marked. Otherwise the symptoms are similar to those of primary adrenal insufficiency. In the absence of ACTH secretion the zona fasciculata/reticularis undergoes disuse atrophy.

Adrenal insufficiency induced by the prolonged use of therapeutic doses of corticosteroids is discussed on page 457.

Congenital adrenal hyperplasia

The synthesis of cortisol and aldosterone involves a series of enzymatic steps involving hydroxylases (Fig. 12.5). Congenital adrenal hyperplasia with insufficiency may present at birth, in infancy, or in childhood, depending on the type and severity of the hydroxylase deficiency. The fall in the secretion of cortisol will activate the anterior

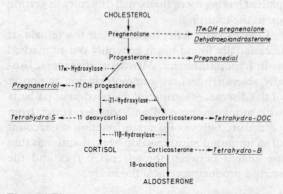

Fig. 12.5 The enzymatic steps involved in the synthesis of cortisol and aldosterone in the adrenal cortex and the urinary metabolites (underlined in italics) that are likely to be increased should there be an enzyme block at the next enzymatic step.

pituitary to secrete ACTH with increased stimulation of the enzymatic steps preceding the block. This usually means the production of large quantities of androgenic steroids.

The commonest enzyme deficiency is that of the 21-hydroxylase. In about one third of cases there is mineralocorticoid deficiency which if untreated may result in severe salt depletion and death in the first few weeks of life.

At birth, female infants may show signs of virilisation with clitoral hypertrophy and variable degrees of fusion of the labia. Male infants particularly may die from adrenocortical insufficiency, because the genital stigmata to be seen in female infants are not present to provide a warning of adrenal disease. If the enzyme defect is less severe the patient may survive infancy and present in childhood with evidence of precocious puberty. Growth may be abnormally advanced at first but is restricted later by early fusion of the epiphyses. Thus patients with mild examples of the enzyme defects usually come under supervision when ambiguous external genitalia, excessive tallness, premature appearance of secondary sexual characteristics or libidinous tendencies arouse parental anxieties.

Investigation of adrenal insufficiency

The symptoms and signs of adrenal insufficiency are so non-specific that confirmation of the diagnosis must be sought whenever suspicion arises. Tests of adrenocortical function are based on: (1) the metabolic effects of corticosteroids; (2) the measurement of serum cortisol levels in the resting state and following stimulation; (3) measurement of ACTH levels in the plasma.

1. **Metabolic effects.** Patients with Addison's disease, in contrast to those with secondary adrenal insufficiency, may show alteration in their serum electrolytes with depressed sodium and elevated potassium and urea levels; this is by no means invariable even in advanced cases and must not be depended upon for diagnosis. Some degree of hypoglycaemia may occur but this also is of little diagnostic value.

2. **Cortisol levels.** Provided the patient is not in crisis or approaching crisis, time may be taken to determine the presence or absence of a circadian

rhythm in plasma cortisol levels by taking blood at 09:00 and 23:00 for 2 or 3 consecutive days for determination of serum cortisol levels before treatment is started. Low levels and the absence of a diurnal rhythm could be due to a lesion at any point in the hypothalamic-pituitary-adrenal axis. Normal levels and a normal rhythm would suggest that the whole axis is normal, but the possibility exists that, while overall function is maintained, there has been a significant reduction in reserve function which could be of paramount importance in times of stress. For this reason, if either primary or secondary adrenal insufficiency is suspected clinically, the circadian rhythm studies should be supplemented by stimulation tests.

ACTH test. The stimulation tests should be done in a logical sequence, starting with the administration of ACTH or a potent analogue. The preparation of choice is tetracosactrin which consists of the biologically active first 24 amino acids of human ACTH and has an action of about 30 minutes when given in a dosage of $250\,\mu g$ intramuscularly. Glucocorticoids taken within the previous 12 hours may invalidate the test. In normal subjects the serum cortisol level at 30 minutes reaches at least 550 nmol/l with an increment above basal which exceeds 200 nmol/l. A normal response excludes primary adrenocortical insufficiency, but an impaired or absent response requires further investigation using tetracosactrin depot. Special care should be taken in patients with a history of allergic disease in view of occasional hypersensitivity reactions to tetracosactrin depot.

In primary adrenal insufficiency (Addison's disease) there is little or no response to depot tetracosactrin. For practical purposes the criteria for primary adrenal insufficiency would be failure of the serum cortisol levels to rise above 700 nmol/l by 5–12 hours after the third intramuscular injection of 1.0 mg tetracosactrin depot given on three consecutive mornings. In secondary adrenal insufficiency there is a characteristic stepwise increase in serum cortisol levels on each day of tetracosactrin depot administration.

Since highly biologically active analogues of cortisol, such as betamethasone or prednisolone, do not cross react in the radio-immunoassay for cortisol, tetracosactrin stimulation tests can be effectively carried out even though the patient may have recently started replacement therapy using these analogues.

Insulin-induced hypoglycaemia (p. 427) should be the next procedure in a patient in whom secondary adrenocortical insufficiency is suspected. Unless radio-immunoassay of ACTH is readily available, a normal adrenal response to ACTH stimulation should have been demonstrated before giving insulin because a cortisol rise in response to hypoglycaemia depends upon ACTH secretion and the patient is thus being used for bioassay. Normal peak values of cortisol induced by insulin show a mean of 785 nmol/l with a range of 560–1060 nmol/l, the increment being a mean of 420 with a range of 200–670 nmol/l.

3. **Measurement of serum ACTH levels.** In the presence of low levels of serum cortisol, if the plasma ACTH level is high, one would have strong evidence of primary adrenocortical insufficiency.

Treatment of adrenocortical insufficiency

All patients with adrenocortical insufficiency will require replacement therapy with a glucocorticoid, while the majority of patients with Addison's disease will also need a mineralocorticoid. In congenital adrenal hyperplasia, full replacement doses of glucocorticoid will suppress ACTH secretion and prevent excessive formation of metabolites with consequent regression of the clinical features. If the enzymic block demands it, a mineralocorticoid should be added.

Cortisol (hydrocortisone) is the drug of choice for routine glucocorticoid replacement therapy. Cortisone acetate, although widely used, has the disadvantage that it has to be metabolised by the liver to cortisol before having any physiological action. Abnormal liver function results in reduced conversion of cortisone acetate to cortisol and the possibility of impaired liver function is particularly relevant in cases of secondary adrenal insufficiency taking oral androgens for concomitant hypogonadism.

Other synthetic glucocorticoids, e.g. prednisone, prednisolone, dexamethasone and betamethasone, are useful in keeping a patient in good health while adrenal function tests are being done, but have the disadvantage in long-term therapy that they do not react in the radio-immunoassay for cortisol so that their blood levels cannot be monitored by this method. Cortisol, cortisone acetate and the synthetic glucocorticoids have a biological action of some 6 to 8 hours.

Maintenance treatment. It is best to give the glucocorticoid medication in a regime which mimics the normal circadian variation of cortisol output. For most patients this would be 20 mg cortisol at breakfast time and 10 mg at about 18:00. The equivalent doses of cortisone acetate would be 25 mg and 12.5 mg respectively. While it is not possible to be dogmatic about how much glucocorticoid any individual may require as absorption and metabolism may vary, the regime described will meet the needs of most patients. To assess the requirements of those whose response appears to be unsatisfactory a *cortisol profile* should be carried out. Serum cortisol levels should be estimated before and half an hour, 1 hour and then at 2-hourly intervals after an oral dose of 20 mg of cortisol, or whatever dose seems to be clinically indicated. The plasma level usually reaches a peak after 30–60 minutes and the amount of cortisol should be adjusted to give a peak of 700–830 nmol/l and a level of about 165 nmol/l before the evening dose.

Fludrocortisone is the most useful mineralocorticoid for maintenance therapy, and the dose should be adjusted according to the serum electrolytes, the state of hydration of the patient and the blood pressure. Most patients require 0.05–0.15 mg in a single oral morning dose. The signs of overdosage of mineralocorticoid are those of sodium retention (p. 92) and potassium depletion (p. 89). The occasional patient who is unable to tolerate fludrocortisone may be given a long-acting preparation intramuscularly, e.g. deoxycortone pivalate 50–100 mg every 2 to 4 weeks.

Secondary adrenocortical insufficiency. The regime to be followed is the same as in Addison's disease except that a mineralocorticoid is not required as aldosterone production is little affected. Any associated condition due to lack of other trophic hormones will require therapy along the usual lines.

During periods of stress, e.g. trauma, infection or operations, it is necessary for the dose of glucocorticoid to be increased to mimic what would happen in an individual with normal function of the hypothalamic-pituitary-adrenal axis. Thus if a patient develops severe coryza or influenza the dose of oral steroids should be increased to twice their normal maintenance level for 2 to 3 days. Should gastroenteritis with or without vomiting occur the oral glucocorticoid should be changed to intramuscular hydrocortisone at an increased dose level. Consequently patients with impaired adrenal function, either primary or secondary, should have available ampoules of hydrocortisone hemisuccinate for injection which are not outdated and which they know how to use.

Precautions. Every patient on oral steroids of whatever form should have a card or preferably a bracelet giving details of the diagnosis, steroid dosage and the medical attendant's address. Should the patient be involved in an accident and be taken unconscious to a casualty department a disastrous outcome may be avoided if information that the patient is taking steroids is available. Even the most minor operation is a potential hazard to a patient with adrenocortical insufficiency. On no account should such a patient be given morphine or pethidine. For dental extraction the patient should be admitted to hospital for the day and given twice the normal dose of glucocorticoid on the day of the extraction and possibly the following morning. Normal replacement dosage may then be resumed provided there are no complications. Larger doses of steroids and more careful monitoring of cortisol levels are required before and after more major surgery.

ADRENAL CRISIS. This is a medical emergency. If promptly treated with intravenous hydrocortisone (as sodium succinate or sodium phosphate) and intravenous fluids there is in most cases a dramatic improvement over 12 to 24 hours in a previously moribund patient. Occasional cases will need more protracted treatment depending upon how quickly the precipitating cause, e.g. infection, is brought under control.

The intravenous fluids should consist of 5% glucose in isotonic saline to correct hypoglycaemia and sodium loss. Hydrocortisone is best given parenterally over the first 24–48 hours until gastrointestinal symptoms subside and oral medication will be retained. The initial dose should be

100 mg intravenously 6 hourly for the first 24 hours and then 50 mg 6 hourly for the next 24 hours. If progress is satisfactory, oral cortisol can be given thereafter in a dose of 20 mg 8 hourly which can then be further reduced in a stepwise fashion by 10 mg daily until normal maintenance levels are reached. Below 40 mg of oral cortisol per day a mineralocorticoid is best added to the therapeutic regime, initially in a single morning dose of 0.1 mg fludrocortisone.

Prognosis. With modern therapy the life expectancy of patients with adrenal insufficiency should be normal, within the limits imposed by any associated disease such as pituitary tumour, or other disorders such as insulin dependent diabetes mellitus which may coexist with auto-immune adrenal insufficiency. Otherwise the main risk to life is the avoidable occurrence of adrenal crisis and delay in its prompt management.

CORTICOSTEROIDS AND ACTH IN THE TREATMENT OF DISEASE

Corticosteroids. Extensive use is made of the anti-inflammatory actions of corticosteroids and their synthetic analogues. The doses of steroid analogues therapeutically equivalent to 20 mg cortisol for an anti-inflammatory effect are cortisone (25 mg), prednisolone (5 mg), betamethasone (0.75 mg) and dexamethasone (0.75 mg). Of these prednisolone is the most commonly used for purposes other than replacement therapy. It is widely prescribed in the treatment of connective tissue diseases, of autoimmune disorders and conditions involving other forms of immune reaction as discussed under the heading of the various diseases.

DANGERS OF CORTICOSTEROID THERAPY. The use of corticosteroids in doses exceeding those required for replacement therapy carries risks which must be balanced against the therapeutic advantages. These risks can be subdivided into: (1) the undesirable metabolic consequences that cannot be separated from the anti-inflammatory effect of the steroid and (2) the suppression of the hypothalamic-pituitary-adrenal (HPA) axis that may follow the use of pharmacological doses.

1. *The metabolic consequences* are those that are encountered in Cushing's syndrome and are more pronounced the higher the dose and the longer the treatment. Thus, although certain corticosteroid analogues may have slightly less mineralocorticoid activity than cortisol, fluid retention, moon face, hypertension, central obesity and striae may all be induced. The glucocorticoid action not infrequently precipitates diabetes mellitus. Osteoporosis is an insidious but frequent complication of long-term therapy as a result of a decrease in bone formation and an increase in bone resorption especially in the spine and ribs. As in Cushing's syndrome, mental symptoms may be troublesome, ranging from euphoria to severe depression.

Corticosteroids may modify the normal response to a major illness so that pain, tenderness, fever or a raised ESR may be abolished, while the response to inflammation and therefore the defences against infection may be poor and healing impaired. In this way treatment with these drugs may be responsible for masking the more typical and sometimes dangerous consequences of a variety of illnesses. For example, oral corticosteroids may induce peptic ulceration with perforation without pain, and the physical signs indicative of inflammation in the peritoneal cavity may not be present. Another example is the reactivation of latent tuberculosis.

2. *The suppression of the HPA axis* following prolonged corticosteroid therapy in doses greater than 7.5 mg prednisolone per day or its equivalent may be persistent, especially with regard to the hypothalamic-pituitary portion of the axis. This may make it difficult to withdraw steroid, the patient being as vulnerable as someone with secondary adrenocortical insufficiency due to organic pituitary disease. Stimulation of the adrenal cortex in such cases is usually possible with adequate ACTH dosage, but there is no known way of producing a comparably strong and prolonged stimulus to the hypothalamic-pituitary axis.

WITHDRAWAL OF CORTICOSTEROIDS. It should first be ensured that the adrenal cortex is functional by giving tetracosactrin depot (p. 455). Then, after gradually reducing the dosage of oral steroid, a maintenance dose of 20 mg cortisol should be given at 08:00–09:00 and no cortisol in the evenings; the hypothalamo-pituitary axis will then have no exogenous steroid to suppress the secretion of CRF or ACTH in the early hours of the morning. In this way a normal diurnal rhythm may be restored and the HPA axis should thereafter respond normally to stress. This may take many months to achieve, while in other cases, normal function may be restored shortly after steroid therapy has been withdrawn.

ACTH. Because it can be such a difficult task to withdraw corticosteroid therapy, attempts have been made to use synthetic ACTH preparations such as tetracosactrin depot in place of oral corticosteroids. When used in appropriate doses, there is evidence that therapeutically useful elevation in the plasma cortisol level may be achieved in some patients without suppression of the HPA axis. However, this may be only a reflection of the amount of corticosteroid secreted in response to this stimulus. In children ACTH therapy has the distinct advantage over treatment with oral steroids in that it causes less inhibition of growth.

The incidence of mooning of the face and obesity is similar with oral corticosteroids and ACTH. Peptic ulceration and bruising are commoner with corticosteroids, and hypertension, pigmentation and acne with ACTH. In view of the serious risks involved very careful consideration must be given before either is employed and the practitioner must be convinced that the therapeutic benefits outweigh the disadvantages.

PHAEOCHROMOCYTOMA
Phaeochromocytomas are tumours of chromaffin tissue which secrete catecholamines; noradrenaline nearly always predominates over adrenaline. The tumours, most of which are benign, may occur at any site along the sympathetic chain, but 90% are found in the adrenal glands. Rarely the lesions may be multiple. Phaeochromocytoma is an uncommon tumour but of considerable interest because of its pharmacological effects. The clinical presentation depends upon the relative amounts of noradrenaline and adrenaline secreted. The most common sign is hypertension which may be sustained or, characteristically, paroxysmal with associated episodes of extreme skin pallor, sweating, palpitations, headache, epigastric pain and chest discomfort. Apprehension is common during a paroxysm.

Diagnosis depends on the demonstration of increased levels of catecholamines or their metabolites in the urine or plasma, e.g. metanephrine and normetanephrine. The location of the tumour can be shown by scanning or angiography.

Treatment is by excision of the tumour if it can be identified or, failing this, alpha and beta receptor blockade may be used. In order to avoid hypertension and arrhythmias during induction of anaesthesia and handling of the tumour at operation, the pre-operative preparation of the patient with alpha and beta adrenergic blocking agents (phenoxybenzamine and propranolol) is essential. Emergencies associated with hypertensive crises should be dealt with by the intravenous administration of phentolamine in doses of 5 mg or by infusion of sodium nitroprusside. Careful preparation before and during operation should prevent any severe fall in blood pressure resulting from hypovolaemia. If hypotension persists noradrenaline should be given intravenously in saline.

SEXUAL DISORDERS IN THE MALE
These may present in many forms. Some are due to faults arising in the mechanism of sex determination as early as conception, others to errors later in sexual differentiation of the embryo and fetus, and after birth, in sexual development. Abnormalities of the sex chromosomes may be associated with failure of sexual development so that the individual may show some of the characteristics of both sexes (intersex). The term hermaphroditism is reserved for patients in whom male and female gonadal tissue is found to coexist; it occurs much less commonly than the intersexes.

The anatomical characteristics of the male are influenced by essential hormonal factors, particularly androgen secretion. The personality and behaviour of the male are further attributes which must be considered in assessing the individual patient's needs. A few only of the more common sexual disorders occurring in the male will be discussed here. Sexually transmitted diseases are described on pages 415 to 421, and psychosexual disorders on pages 675 and 697.

Hypogonadism
This term is used to include failure of one or both of the main functions of the testis, namely the

production of spermatozoa and the secretion of androgens. The defect may involve only impaired spermatogenesis in the seminiferous tubules. If the interstitial (Leydig) cells are affected the secretion of testosterone is reduced or abolished. Tubular dysfunction is then inevitable as testosterone is required for spermatogenesis.

Aetiology. Hypogonadism may arise from hypothalamic or pituitary disease (hypogonadotrophic hypogonadism) or from primary testicular disease (hypergonadotrophic hypogonadism). Hypogonadotrophic hypogonadism with an apparently normal pituitary gland appears to be due to failure of the hypothalamus to secrete gonadotrophin releasing hormone. This isolated deficiency of GnRH is often associated with an absent sense of smell (Kallmann's syndrome). Any type of pituitary disease may be associated with gonadotrophin deficiency and hence hypogonadism. Impotence is a common presentation of hyperprolactinaemia. Lowering prolactin levels with bromocriptine may restore potency.

Primary testicular failure may be due to trauma, tuberculosis, gonococcal infections, syphilis, malignant disease or orchitis as in mumps. Maldescent or failure of descent will also lead to failure of the tubular epithelium to develop. Haemochromatosis, cirrhosis of the liver and oestrogen administration may all be associated with testicular insufficiency. The disorder may also be due to abnormalities of the sex chromosomes (p. 8). Many cases remain, however, for which an aetiological diagnosis is still not possible, and these form the majority of patients who present with infertility as their only complaint (idiopathic oligospermia).

Clinical features. The results of failure of function of the interstitial cells depend upon the age of the patient at the time of the onset of the disease. When this occurs *before puberty* the external genitalia and the secondary sex characteristics fail to develop. In these circumstances the epiphyses of the long bones do not close at the usual age and in consequence the patient may grow to an excessive height. The typical prepubertal eunuch develops into a tall man with a hairless face, a high-pitched voice, small genitalia and an immature personality. Some pubic hair is present and is the result of adrenal androgen production — the adrenarche.

When the onset of the disease is *postpubertal* the changes are less striking. Growth is not affected and there is regression rather than disappearance of the secondary sex characteristics. The external genitalia undergo partial atrophy. Fatigue, loss of initiative and libido and impotence are the usual complaints. In some patients, particularly when the deprivation is sudden as after surgical castration, there may be 'menopausal symptoms' such as hot flushes and profuse sweating, unless replacement therapy is provided.

Treatment. Hypogonadism due to deficiency of androgens may be corrected by replacement therapy with testosterone. A satisfactory and most economical form of therapy is the implantation of 200–600 mg of testosterone, in pellets, into the anterior abdominal wall. Renewal may be required after 6–8 months. Alternatively depot intramuscular injections of testosterone can be given. An oral preparation, testosterone undecanoate, is available but is expensive. In cases of deficiency of the germinal epithelium, due to lack of FSH associated with pituitary disease, increased spermatogenesis may be achieved by treatment with human chorionic gonadotrophin and purified LH and FSH which have been obtained from menopausal urine. When the FSH deficiency results from hypothalamic failure, pulsatile GnRH therapy via a portable infusion pump can be given. Several months of treatment is necessary to achieve adequate spermatogenesis.

Cryptorchidism

Cryptorchidism (undescended testis) usually occurs in otherwise normal boys but may be the presenting feature of hypogonadotrophic hypogonadism. Highly retractile testes, particularly in an obese boy, may be mistaken for cryptorchidism. If the glands remain in the inguinal canal they are more liable to trauma than if situated in the scrotum. The seminiferous tubules will fail to develop in an undescended gland, and if the condition is bilateral, sterility will follow. Even in testes which remain undescended into adult life the interstitial cells function normally, so that the secondary sex characteristics develop in the usual way. A course of chorionic gonadotrophin should be given at about 6 years of age. Alternatively GnRH can be given intranasally for 1-4 weeks. With inguinal testes the success rate for descent is about 40% which is similar to that with gonadotrophin. If medical treatment is unsuccessful the testis or testes should be placed in the scrotum surgically.

In maldescent the testis takes an abnormal route and is liable to develop malignancy. Such testes should either be brought down into the scrotum or, if discovered in the adult, removed.

Impotence

Erectile dysfunction or failure (impotence) is thought to be due to psychological causes in the majority of cases. The incidence of this condition increases with age; vascular disease involving the internal pudendal artery or its branches is common in these patients. This alone may be the cause of the impotence or a trigger for psychological dysfunction. Impotence may also be an early symptom in diabetes mellitus, multiple sclerosis and tabes dorsalis. Endocrine causes of impotence are uncommon and there is usually an associated loss of libido.

Full investigation is necessary to determine whether there is primary or secondary testicular dysfunction. If there is secondary hypogonadism then hypothalamic-pituitary function apart from that relating to the gonads must be assessed. Androgen therapy will usually restore potency and libido. In some patients hyperprolactinaemia without gonadotrophin deficiency will be present; this condition responds to bromocriptine therapy. If infertility is a problem in secondary hypogonadism then gonadotrophin or, in some patients, gonadotrophin releasing hormone will usually be required.

Infertility in the male

The husband is responsible for the infertility of approximately one half of all childless marriages. There is usually defective development of the germinal epithelium in the seminiferous tubules, with oligospermia or azoospermia. Infertility may follow hypogonadism due to any of the causes already described. Chemotherapy with agents such as cyclophosphamide may produce azoospermia which also occurs with oestrogen or anti-androgen therapy. Less obvious is the effect of drugs such as sulphasalazine which may also produce oligospermia. Antibodies to sperm (p. 28) may explain a small number of cases of male infertility but in the majority the primary cause is unknown.

In azoospermic patients due to primary testicular dysfunction FSH levels will be high. A normal level suggests obstruction as the cause of azoospermia. Testicular biopsy and analysis of the seminal fluid may be helpful. A reduced fructose concentration in semen suggests that there is obstruction to fluid coming from the seminal vesicles. This and other types of obstruction may be amenable to surgery.

Results of treatment with gonadotrophins, clomiphene or androgens have been disappointing. Artificial insemination using sperm from the oligospermic husband is nearly always unsuccessful and patients may opt for artificial insemination by a donor. In severe oligospermia in vitro fertilisation has resulted in normal pregnancies.

SEXUAL DISORDERS IN THE FEMALE

Many conditions regarded as primarily gynaecological may have much wider implications. *Primary amenorrhoea*, for example, may provide an important indication of systemic disorder; it may be due to a chromosomal anomaly such as Turner's syndrome or it may be due to an auto-immune reaction against antigens shared between the steroid producing cells in the ovary and in the adrenal cortex. Hermaphroditism may present with amenorrhoea. Congenital adrenal hyperplasia, if unrecognised and untreated in childhood, pituitary tumours and developmental disorders in the genital tract may all require full gynaecological and endocrine assessment for precise diagnosis.

Secondary amenorrhoea also requires further investigation, but it is so common a feature of a wide range of conditions that by itself it has little diagnostic value. Hyperprolactinaemia must be considered as should anorexia nervosa when amenorrhoea is associated with weight loss.

Risks of oral contraception. A low level of mortality is associated with all major reversible methods of fertility control, including oral contraception (OC), compared with the risk of death from pregnancy and delivery in women using no such methods. The use of OC may be associated with coronary artery disease, hypertension, cerebrovascular accident, deep vein thrombosis, pulmonary embolism and neoplasia of the cervix of the uterus. These risks vary with the individual and with the duration of use and the composition of the OC.

Immediate undesirable effects which may influence the woman's acceptance of OC include weight gain, jaundice (p. 341), bleeding occurring during courses of treatment (breakthrough bleeding) and failure to bleed between courses. These complaints may subside after the first few months. Other troublesome effects include depression and decreased libido. The incidence of all these problems has diminished as the dose of oestrogen in the commonly used oral contraceptives has been reduced.

Sexually transmitted diseases are described on page 415 and *psychosexual disorders* on page 697.

Disorders of the menopause

The cessation of the menstrual cycle occurs in most women in the Western world between the ages of 45 and 50; it is the result of the gradual failure of the ovaries to produce oestrogens and progesterone. As a consequence the pituitary gland becomes more active and produces FSH and LH in greater quantity. Assays for these hormones are of value in distinguishing amenorrhoea due primarily to failure of the ovaries from amenorrhoea due to failure of the pituitary to secrete gonadotrophins.

Clinical features. The ease with which a woman adapts herself to the change of circumstances associated with the menopause varies widely. In some the reduction of oestrogen secretion is associated with psychological symptoms; in others adjustment is readily achieved and may be unattended by any emotional reaction. In the group of patients who are troubled by symptoms, anxiety, emotional instability, irritability, insomnia, and particularly hot flushes and sweating are common complaints. Depression is frequent and occasionally may be severe with suicidal tendencies.

Obesity may first appear, or, if previously present, may increase. Hirsutism, especially the appearance of hair on the upper lip and chin, is not uncommon. Osteoporosis may present for the first time in the early years after the menopause usually with back pain. This condition occurs more commonly in women who have had a premature menopause and have not been given oestrogen. Pruritus vulvae is a complication which is frequently associated with changes in the mucous membranes of the genital tract. Leukoplakia vulvae may develop, and if untreated may progress to carcinoma. Senile vaginitis may cause considerable distress from dyspareunia, dysuria and vaginal discharge, especially if complicated by secondary infection.

Treatment. The essential treatment is explanation of the nature of the condition, coupled with specific treatment for the complications. Features attributable to oestrogen deficiency call for replacement therapy with a synthetic oestrogen such as ethinyloestradiol. The daily dose required to suppress menopausal symptoms in different individuals varies from 10 to 50 μg daily, but 20 μg is often adequate; this should be given in courses lasting for 21 days, repeated if necessary after an interval of 7 days. The need to add a progestogen to the oestrogen is a matter of controversy. The patient must be warned that this treatment may be followed by vaginal bleeding as in a normal menstrual period. Other appropriate measures, such as treatment of obesity or depression may also be required.

DIABETES MELLITUS

Diabetes mellitus is a clinical syndrome characterised by hyperglycaemia, due to deficiency or diminished effectiveness of insulin. This can arise in many different ways and the diagnostic label 'diabetes mellitus' includes numerous different disorders. Lack of insulin, whether absolute or relative, affects the metabolism of carbohydrate, protein, fat, water and electrolytes, sometimes with grave consequences. The long-standing metabolic derangement is frequently associated with permanent and irreversible functional and structural changes in the cells of the body, those of the vascular system being particularly susceptible. The changes lead in turn to the development of well-defined clinical entities, the complications of diabetes, which most characteristically affect the eye, the kidney and the nervous system.

Diabetes mellitus is the most common of the endocrine disorders. The prevalence in Britain is over 1%, although about half of those affected remain undetected.

Aetiology. On the basis of aetiology two main categories of diabetes are recognised, namely primary and secondary diabetes.

PRIMARY DIABETES. The great majority of cases seen belong to this group, which consists of two main clinical types: *insulin-dependent diabetes mellitus*—IDDM (Type I) most frequent in those less than 50 years old and rapidly fatal without treatment with insulin and *non insulin dependent diabetes mellitus*—NIDDM (Type II) occurring mainly in the middle-aged and elderly and compatible with long survival without treatment. Although the precise aetiology is still uncertain, in both types it is the susceptibility to diabetes, rather than diabetes *per se*, which is inherited and heredity and environment interact to determine which of those with a genetic predisposition actually develop the clinical syndrome and the timing of its onset. However, both the pattern of inheritance and environmental factors differ in IDDM and NIDDM as is discussed in detail below.

SECONDARY DIABETES. A minority of cases of diabetes occur as a result of a recognisable pathological process or secondary to the treatment of some other condition.

1. *Pancreatic diabetes*. Diseases such as pancreatitis, haemochromatosis and carcinoma cause destruction of the pancreas and lead to impaired secretion and release of insulin. Diabetes will also follow pancreatectomy.

2. *Insulin antagonists*. Diabetes may occur in conditions where there is an abnormal concentration of hormones antagonistic to the action of insulin in the circulation.

a. *Growth hormone* can produce permanent diabetes in experimental animals and about 30% of patients with acromegaly are diabetic.

b. *Adrenocortical hormones*, such as cortisol, raise the concentration of glucose in the blood by increasing gluconeogenesis and by inhibiting utilisation of glucose by the peripheral tissues. Thus, many patients with Cushing's syndrome show impaired carbohydrate tolerance and diabetes may be precipitated by ACTH or corticosteroid therapy. Conversely increased sensitivity to insulin is an important feature of Addison's disease and of hypopituitarism.

c. *Adrenaline* raises the blood glucose concentration by increasing the breakdown of liver glycogen and by suppressing the secretion of insulin. Patients with phaeochromocytoma frequently show a diabetic blood glucose curve on glucose tolerance testing and the incidence of these uncommon tumours is relatively high among diabetic patients.

d. *Thyroid hormone* in excess will aggravate the diabetic state and some patients with hyperthyroidism show impaired glucose tolerance.

e. *Gestational diabetes* refers to the hyperglycaemia which can occur temporarily during pregnancy in individuals who have an inherited liability to develop the disorder. During normal pregnancy there is an increased production of hormonal antagonists to insulin such as human placental lactogen, which in turn demands an increased rate of secretion and release of insulin. A failing pancreas may be unable to meet this demand.

3. *Iatrogenic diabetes*, in those genetically susceptible, may be precipitated by various forms of therapy, notably with corticosteroids, and thiazide diuretics.

4. *Liver disease*, particularly cirrhosis and hepatitis, may be associated with impaired glucose tolerance.

Aetiology of IDDM. The increased risk of developing IDDM is HLA linked and is primarily associated with the D locus (p. 29). Associations with alleles at other loci occur because of linkage disequilibrium (p. 30). Two established axes of increased and one of reduced susceptibility have been identified. The relative risk of developing IDDM associated with Dw3-DR3 is 7.39, with Dw4-DR4 9.23, with DR3-DR4 14.26, and with Dw2-DR2 0.12. The HLA-DR determinants are probably in linkage disequilibrium with immune response (Ir) genes which are thought to exist on chromosome 6 within the HLA region. Since there is at present no way of defining Ir genes in man, the HLA antigens serve as 'markers' for genes which confer increased and reduced susceptibility to IDDM. Affected siblings of diabetics usually have one, and in many cases both haplotypes in common, irrespective of the HLA determinants that make up the haplotype.

It is postulated that the Ir genes control the immune response to environmental factors capable of damaging the β cells of the pancreatic islet. Susceptible individuals react abnormally to assault by viruses or other cytotoxic agents which leads to β cell destruction either directly or by initiating an immune reaction. Islet cell antibodies (ICA) are present in the plasma of over 80% of patients with newly diagnosed IDDM, but it is uncertain whether these are responsible for, or result from β cell damage. Prospective family studies suggest that immune-mediated destruction of the pancreatic β cells involving both humoral and cell-mediated immunological processes occurs over a prolonged period, sometimes extending over several years. Hyperglycaemia occurs only when 90% of the β cell mass has been destroyed.

The possibility of heterogeneity within IDDM was suggested by the demonstration of two separate HLA-DR linked axes of susceptibility. Two subtypes of IDDM have been identified. *Type 1a* is more common and occurs predominantly in those less than 30 years of age. The primary association is particularly with HLA-DR4 and slightly more males are affected. Viruses are probably responsible for initiating β cell destruction and autoimmune phenomena such as ICA are transient and may result from, rather than cause, pancreatic damage. Treatment with conventional insulin preparations is associated with a high plasma titre of insulin-binding antibodies (IBA) in this type of diabetes.

Type 1b is less common, occurs mainly in women over the age of 30 years, and is primarily associated with HLA-DR3. ICA tend to persist, other autoimmune diseases coexist with this type of diabetes more often than can be accounted for by chance and in cases where these disorders are not present thyroid, gastric, intrinsic factor, and adrenal antibodies are frequently found. There is often a strong family history of autoimmune disease.

Aetiology of NIDDM. NIDDM is not HLA linked and there is no evidence that autoimmunity or viruses have anything to do with its development. Studies with twins and sibships have shown that genetic factors are more important in the development of this type of diabetes than in IDDM, but there is little information about what is inherited. Progress in this field has been hampered by heterogeneity within NIDDM, lack of genetic markers and the association and interaction of environmental factors such as obesity, diet, inactivity, and pregnancy, which probably play a critical role in the clinical expression of NIDDM.

The insulin gene, situated on the short arm of chromosome 11, has been investigated as a possible genetic marker for NIDDM. However, although one allele seems to affect blood glucose homeostasis its relationship to the development of NIDDM is uncertain.

Simple deficiency of insulin cannot entirely account for the diabetic syndrome in NIDDM. Increased hepatic production of glucose and resistance to the action of insulin are characteristic of this type of diabetes. Insulin resistance is also seen in obesity and the majority of middle-aged diabetic patients are obese. Most of the evidence supports the view that obesity is diabetogenic in those genetically predisposed to the disorder and that the rising incidence of diabetes in older people is largely related to the increasing prevalence of obesity in the population as a whole. However, obesity cannot account for all the insulin resistance in obese patients with NIDDM, and many non-obese, non-insulin dependent patients are also insulin resistant.

Insulin resistance may be due to any one of three general causes: an abnormal insulin molecule, an excessive amount of circulating antagonists and target tissue defects. The last is the common cause of insulin resistance in NIDDM. The specific mechanisms underlying this insulin resistant state are heterogeneous. In patients with relatively mild impairment of glucose tolerance the defect in insulin action is associated with a decreased number of cellular insulin receptors. Patients with more severe hyperglycaemia usually combine a reduced number of receptors with a post-receptor defect in the action of insulin and the latter seems to be the predominant abnormality. Increased amounts of circulating hormonal antagonists are not thought to be primarily involved in the aetiology of either IDDM or NIDDM. However, uncontrolled diabetes is associated with increased plasma concentration of antistorage hormones such as growth hormone, and glucagon, and the normal suppressive effect of oral carbohydrate on the secretion of these hormones is diminished. Treatment of the diabetes abolishes these abnormalities which are thought to be secondary to absolute or relative deficiency of insulin. Other types of insulin resistance are extremely rare. They include a syndrome in which antibodies are directed against the insulin receptor.

It should be noted that increased hepatic production of glucose and/or decreased peripheral utilisation of glucose cannot lead to sustained hyperglycaemia unless the pancreatic islets fail to adapt to the situation. Although the maximum, absolute, plasma concentration of immunoreactive insulin may be relatively normal in patients with mild NIDDM it is low in relation to the plasma glucose and a delay in the insulin response to glucose is commonly seen during a glucose tolerance test. This defect in insulin secretion appears to be selective for glucose since the response to other stimuli such as amino acids and sulphonylurea drugs is normal. It is not known whether the β cell abnormality is due to intrinsic structural or metabolic change within the islet or whether it is caused by some imbalance in neuro-endocrine input or by a change in the sensitivity of the β cell to glucose.

Chemical pathology. Whatever the aetiology, in all cases of diabetes hyperglycaemia results from deficiency of insulin. This is absolute in IDDM and relative in NIDDM. Increased gluconeogenesis and lipolysis follow as compensatory reactions under the influence of such hormones as growth hormone, glucagon and adrenocortical hormones, in what is basically a situation of glucose lack. Thus the hyperglycaemia characteristic of diabetes arises from two main sources, namely a reduced rate of removal of glucose from the blood by the peripheral tissues and an increased rate of release of glucose from the liver into the circulation.

CONSEQUENCES OF HYPERGLYCAEMIA AND GLYCOSURIA. When the glucose concentration in the blood exceeds the capacity of the renal tubules to reabsorb it from the glomerular filtrate, glycosuria occurs. In most people the level of blood glucose at which this happens is approximately 10 mmol/l (180 mg/100 ml). Glucose increases the osmolality of the glomerular filtrate and thus prevents the reabsorption of water as the filtrate passes down the renal tubular system. In this way the volume of urine is markedly increased in diabetes and *polyuria* and *nocturia* occur. This in turn leads to loss of water and minerals which results in *thirst* and *polydipsia*. Severe depletion of water and electrolytes may ensue.

CONSEQUENCES OF POOR GLUCOSE UTILISATION. Impaired utilisation of carbohydrate results in a sense of *fatigue*, and causes two main compensatory mechanisms to operate in an attempt to provide alternative metabolic substrate. Both of these lead to loss of body tissue, that is *wasting*, which may occur in spite of normal or even an increased intake of food, and which is additional to any loss of weight resulting from loss of body fluid. The compensatory mechanisms are:

1. *Increased glycogenolysis and gluconeogenesis.* As glycogen and protein are catabolised, glucose, nitrogen, water and electrolytes, particularly potassium, are released from cells into the extracellular space. An increased urinary excretion of potassium, magnesium and phosphorus therefore occurs.

2. *Increased lipolysis.* This is seen as a raised fasting plasma concentration of non-esterified fatty acid (NEFA), and a diminished fall in plasma NEFA in response to a carbohydrate load. The extent to which increased lipolysis occurs is proportional to the degree of insulin deficiency. If the latter is marked, the normal response to feeding, namely suppression of lipolysis, may be lost and the plasma concentration of NEFA may remain constantly elevated.

Fatty acids are taken up by the liver and degraded through eight steps within the mitochondria of the liver cells. Each stage yields one molecule of acetyl coenzyme A. Normally most of these molecules enter the citric acid cycle by condensing with oxaloacetic acid, but in severe diabetes more is formed than can enter the citric acid cycle. Instead acetyl coenzyme A is converted to acetoacetic acid. Most of this is then reduced to beta-hydroxybutyric acid, while some is decarboxylated to acetone. These ketone bodies, when formed in small amounts, are usually oxidised and utilised as metabolic fuel. However, the rate of utilisation of ketone bodies is limited. When the rate of production by the liver exceeds that of removal by the peripheral tissues, then the blood level rises.

Ketone bodies increase the osmolality of the plasma and so also lead to the withdrawal of water from the cell. They are acids which dissociate almost completely at physiological pH releasing hydrogen ions into the body fluids. The fall in pH is countered by the buffers of the blood, the most important being bicarbonate. The dissociation of carbonic acid is reduced, and the ratio of bicarbonate ions to carbonic acid falls, and measurement of plasma bicarbonate will show a lower value than normal. This state is called *ketoacidosis*. The rise in hydrogen ion concentration and increase in PCO_2 in the arterial blood stimulate pulmonary ventilation so that clinically hyperpnoea or 'air hunger' is observed.

The extent to which the clinical features of dehydration and ketoacidosis are seen in the individual will depend on such factors as the speed at which the condition develops and the extent to which the patient increases the intake of fluid, as well as on the degree of insulin deficiency present. Insulin exerts its anticatabolic effects at a lower concentration than that required for its anabolic actions. This means that when insulin deficiency is partial, as in patients with NIDDM, the anticatabolic effect of insulin may be relatively well preserved while its anabolic action is more seriously defective. In these circumstances lipolysis is not markedly accelerated and the concentration of ketone bodies in the blood remains relatively normal despite significant hyperglycaemia.

Pathology. In IDDM there is degeneration of pancreatic islet tissue, from which the beta cells have largely disappeared, leaving behind a variable number of alpha cells and a majority of small undifferentiated cells. The few remaining beta cells show evidence of excessive activity; the nuclei

are commonly enlarged with degranulation of the cytoplasm. These appearances of the pancreas are consistent with the extremely low plasma insulin levels found in these patients.

In NIDDM the moderate reduction in the total mass of islet tissue which is commonly seen does not appear to be sufficient in itself to account for the degree of impaired carbohydrate tolerance present. On the other hand, the observation that in many cases the beta cells, despite prolonged hyperglycaemia and their reduced number, fail to develop cytological signs of hyperactivity, suggests that in these diabetics the beta cells may be relatively insensitive to the stimulus of an elevated blood glucose.

Long-standing diabetes is commonly associated with an abnormal thickening of the basement membrane of the capillaries throughout the body. This *per se* is not pathognomonic of diabetes. It occurs for example as part of the normal ageing process; however the increased permeability of the thickened basement membrane in diabetes is a unique pathological feature. The main clinical and pathological impact of this microangiopathy is to be found in the retina, kidney and nervous system (pp. 480–484).

Clinical features. Two main types of diabetes have long been recognised, and it is now clear that the level of plasma insulin correlates well with the clinical picture and the type of treatment subsequently required.

1. IDDM usually develops during the first 40 years of life in patients of normal or less than normal weight. The majority develop severe symptoms of diabetes acutely, over a period of several weeks or months and if treatment with insulin is withheld they rapidly develop fatal ketoacidosis.

2. NIDDM usually appears in middle-aged or elderly patients who are often obese and in whom hyperglycaemia can usually be controlled by dietary means alone or, if not, by an oral hypoglycaemic compound. Insulin is detectable in the plasma of nearly all patients in this category, and they are therefore less prone to develop ketosis. In this sense the disease is less severe than IDDM; however, the complications associated with long-term diabetes occur in both types. Many patients with NIDDM have a long history of mild symp-

toms which may come and go, and which may frequently be ignored or misdiagnosed for years before the true diagnosis is made.

Apart from patients with established clinical diabetes, two other categories are recognised.

1. *Potential diabetics* are persons with a normal glucose tolerance test who nevertheless have an increased liability to develop diabetes for genetic reasons, e.g. the children of two diabetic parents; a sibling who has one or both haplotypes in common with an insulin-dependent diabetic sib; the non-diabetic member of a pair of identical twins where the other is diabetic.

2. *Latent diabetics* are persons in whom the glucose tolerance test is normal, but who are known to have given an abnormal result under conditions imposing a burden on the pancreatic beta cells, e.g. during pregnancy, infection or other severe stress, mental or physical, during treatment with cortisone or other diabetogenic drugs, or when overweight.

PRESENTATION. Diabetes may be discovered in one of several ways:

1. Many patients are first noted to have glycosuria in the course of some routine examination. They may have had few or no symptoms, and no abnormal physical signs may be found.

2. Some patients present complaining of some or all of the classical symptoms of diabetes, including thirst, polydipsia, polyuria, nocturia, tiredness, loss of weight, white marks on clothing, pruritus vulvae or balanitis, impotence, a change in refraction usually in the direction of myopia and parasthesiae or pain in the limbs.

The severity of many of the classical symptoms of clinical diabetes are directly related to the severity of glycosuria. If relatively mild hyperglycaemia has developed slowly over many years the renal threshold for glucose will rise, glycosuria may be slight, and the symptoms of diabetes correspondingly trivial.

3. Diabetes may first present as a fulminating ketoacidosis associated with an acute infection or even without evidence of a precipitating cause, and in such cases epigastric pain and vomiting may be the presenting complaints. This is more likely to occur in IDDM and such cases are acute medical emergencies.

4. Patients may present with symptoms due to the complications of diabetes.

PHYSICAL SIGNS depend very much on the mode of presentation. Cases without complications will usually show no abnormal physical signs attributable to diabetes. In some cases vulvitis or balanitis may be found, since the external genitalia are especially prone to infection by fungi (Candida) which flourish on the skin and mucous membranes contaminated by glucose.

In the fulminating case the most striking features are those of dehydration. The intraocular pressure may be obviously reduced. A rapid pulse and a low blood pressure may then be anticipated. Breathing may be deep and sighing in the acidotic patient; the breath is usually fetid and the sickly sweet smell of acetone may be noticeable. Apathy and confusion may be present or there may be stupor or even coma.

Evidence of complications of diabetes may be noted. Ophthalmoscopy may show the typical appearance of diabetic retinopathy (p. 481). The most constant early signs of diabetic neuropathy are loss of the ankle jerks, and impaired vibration sense in the legs (p. 483). The presence of diabetic nephropathy (p. 481) may be indicated by proteinuria in addition to glycosuria.

Potential and latent diabetic patients usually complain of no symptoms and show no abnormality on examination. However, certain features are recognised as being characteristic of potential diabetes without necessarily implying that such individuals will progress to clinical diabetes. For example genetically constituted potential diabetics are predisposed to coronary and peripheral arterial disease. They may show abnormal lipid patterns in response to oral contraceptives. They have a high incidence of still-born or abnormally large and heavy babies and babies with congenital defects. Potential and latent diabetics may be much overweight at a time when there is no detectable abnormality in terms of carbohydrate intolerance.

Diagnosis. By definition hyperglycaemia remains the *sine qua non* of the diagnosis of diabetes mellitus. In the individual case when the classical symptoms are present, the diagnosis is often beyond reasonable doubt by the time the history taking and physical examination are complete, and it may then be confirmed by the finding of marked glycosuria, with or without ketonuria, and a random blood sugar greater than 14.0 mmol/l (250 mg/100 ml). However, in many cases, particularly those with NIDDM who have few if any symptoms, and where glycosuria is frequently discovered by chance, the diagnosis is less obvious and a glucose tolerance test will be required.

URINE TESTING. *Glycosuria.* For individual screening purposes sensitive and glucose-specific dip-stick methods are available. Clinistix consists of a paper stick impregnated with an enzyme preparation which turns purple when dipped in urine containing glucose. No other urinary constituent gives this reaction: it therefore provides a rapid and specific qualitative test for glucose. A positive response indicates that the urinary glucose concentration exceeds 0.55–1.11 mmol/l (10–20 mg/100 ml), but does not measure the amount accurately. Semiquantitative measurement of urinary reducing activity can be obtained using copper reduction methods, most conveniently with the Clinitest tablet.

If a sample collected during the 2 hours following a meal is examined, then more of the milder cases of diabetes will be recognised than if an overnight specimen is tested. The most serious disadvantage in the use of the urine test diagnostically arises from individual variations in renal threshold, so that on the one hand some undoubtedly diabetic people have a negative urine test for glucose due to a raised renal threshold, and on the other those with a low renal threshold give a false positive test. In order to distinguish cases of this type from patients with mild diabetes, suitable tests of carbohydrate tolerance are required.

Detection of ketone bodies in urine. Clinically important amounts of ketone bodies can be recognised by the nitroprusside reaction which is conveniently carried out using Acetest tablets or Ketostix test papers. Ketonuria may be found in normal people who have been fasting for long periods, who have been vomiting repeatedly or who have been eating a diet very high in fats and low in carbohydrate. Ketonuria is therefore not pathognomic of diabetes, but if both ketonuria and glycosuria are found, the diagnosis of diabetes is practically certain.

RANDOM BLOOD SUGAR. In many cases the diagnosis of diabetes can be made with the help of a single blood sugar estimation, which may be used as the final confirmatory test when the symptoms strongly suggest the diagnosis. In these circumstances a random blood sugar exceeding 14.0 mmol/l (250 mg/100 ml) is almost certain to indicate diabetes. However, a random blood sugar below this level does not exclude diabetes, and in this case some degree of standardisation of the conditions under which the blood sugar is measured is necessary. In practice, the oral glucose tolerance test is the cornerstone of the diagnosis of diabetes unless a grossly elevated single blood sugar measurement, with or without clinical symptomatology, has already made this clear.

THE ORAL GLUCOSE TOLERANCE TEST (Fig. 12.6). The patient, who should have been on an unrestricted carbohydrate intake of at least 150 g for 3 days or more, fasts overnight. Out-patients should rest for at least half an hour before starting the test, and should remain seated and refrain from smoking during the test. A sample of blood is taken to measure the fasting blood glucose level and 50–100 g glucose dissolved in 250–350 ml of water is then given by mouth. Thereafter samples of blood are collected at half-hourly intervals for at least 2 hours, and their glucose content is estimated.

The WHO Expert Committee on Diabetes (1985) recommended that a 75 g glucose load should be used and that the following concentrations of glucose in venous whole blood (estimated by a specific enzymatic assay) should be

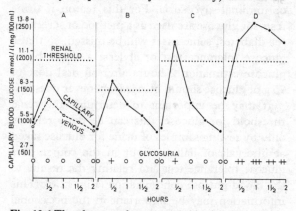

Fig. 12.6 The glucose tolerance test: blood glucose curves after 75 g glucose by mouth, showing (A) normal curve, (B) renal glycosuria, (C) alimentary (lag storage) glycosuria and (D) diabetes mellitus of moderate severity.

accepted as normal or diabetic respectively. Values for plasma glucose are about 15% higher than those for whole blood.

Glucose concentration mmol/l (mg/100 ml)

	Normal	Diabetic
Fasting	<5.5 (100)	>6.7 (120)
2 hours after glucose	<6.7 (120)	>10.0 (180)

Intermediate readings indicate the need for further evaluation of the patient, including the history obtained. It may be necessary to keep the patient under observation and to repeat the test at a later date. In pregnancy those with intermediate readings should be treated as diabetic since even minimal hyperglycaemia is associated with an increased fetal loss rate.

Differential diagnosis of glycosuria. *Renal glycosuria.* Apart from diabetes, the commonest cause of glycosuria is a low renal threshold for glucose, or renal glycosuria. Renal glycosuria also commonly occurs temporarily in pregnancy, due probably in this case to an increase in the glomerular filtration rate. Renal glycosuria is a benign condition unrelated to diabetes, and is not accompanied by the symptoms associated with glycosuria in diabetes, i.e. thirst and polyuria.

Renal glycosuria is a much more frequent cause of glycosuria than diabetes in young persons, particularly in the age group 20 to 30 years, when they are commonly examined prior to entering the armed services, professions and industry. In the older age groups the reverse holds, and significant hyperglycaemia can occur without any or minimal glycosuria. For this reason if urine tests for glucose are used as a method of screening for diabetes, some cases will be missed, so that a glucose tolerance test or at least a single blood glucose estimation 2 hours after an oral dose of 75 g of glucose should be used whenever possible.

It may be important to determine the renal threshold for glucose; this can be done reliably only by testing samples of urine for glucose taken at intervals of half an hour in the course of a glucose tolerance test and relating the results to the blood glucose concentration (Fig. 12.6). This information may be important in the occasional diabetic with a low renal glucose threshold who, if attempts are made to control the diabetes on urine tests alone, may be kept in a persistent state of hypoglycaemia.

Alimentary (lag storage) glycosuria. In some individuals an unusually rapid but transitory rise of blood glucose follows a meal and the concentration exceeds the normal renal threshold; during this time glucose will be present in the urine. This response to a meal or to a dose of glucose is traditionally known as 'lag storage', although alimentary glycosuria is a better term; it is not uncommon as a cause of symptomless glycosuria. It may occur in otherwise normal people or after a partial gastrectomy, when it is due to rapid absorption, or in patients with hyperthyroidism or hepatic disease. This type of blood glucose curve is usually regarded as benign and unrelated to diabetes; although the peak blood glucose is abnormally elevated, the value 2 hours after oral glucose is normal (Fig.12.6).

Carbohydrate deprivation can lead to the development of a diabetic type of blood glucose curve with associated glycosuria in normal people. It would seem, however, that the daily carbohydrate intake has to be less than about 50 g before it has a notable effect. This effect of a low carbohydrate intake may be of importance clinically in relation to the diagnosis of diabetes in a person on a weight reducing diet or if acutely ill with a low daily intake of food.

The management of diabetes mellitus

Aims of treatment. The ideal treatment for diabetes would allow the patient to lead a completely normal life, to remain not only symptom-free but in good health, to achieve a normal metabolic state, and to escape the complications associated with long-term diabetes. Nowadays diabetic patients rarely die in ketoacidosis, but the major problem which has emerged is the chronic invalidism, due to disease of both large and small blood vessels (p. 480), of many of those whose duration of life has been extended.

Although the relationship between the degree of control and the development of serious diabetic complications is not a simple one, it would appear that the vascular abnormalities are secondary to the metabolic abnormalities occurring in diabetes, since they are found in both primary and secondary diabetes and can be produced experimentally in animals rendered diabetic by various methods. Moreover data from clinical studies strongly suggest that although genetic factors may affect the susceptibility to develop complications, the incidence of serious retinopathy is related to the degree of diabetic control achieved. It is therefore incumbent on all those who are involved in looking after diabetic patients to strive in every way to achieve as good control as is practicable in terms of blood glucose concentration. The immediate aims of treatment are therefore, first, the abolition of symptoms of diabetes, second, the correction of hyperglycaemia while avoiding hypoglycaemia and, third, the attainment and maintenance of an appropriate body weight.

Patients should realise as early as possible that it is upon themselves that success or failure will depend. The doctor can only advise. As adherence to a diabetic regimen demands from the patient self-discipline and a sense of purpose, every effort should be made to ensure that the object of each aspect of management is understood. Accordingly, time must be spent on the education of the patient, and the doctor must be responsible for ensuring that all diabetic patients are educated to the limit of their abilities and that as far as possible they have adjusted adequately to their condition and have sufficient knowledge to undertake the day-to-day management of their diabetes competently.

As soon as the diagnosis is certain the patient should be told and instruction and treatment begun forthwith. The average patient suffers initially from an acute anxiety reaction for which explanation is the best remedy. Moreover understanding is likely to lead to better cooperation in treatment.

Type of treatment. There are three methods of treatment, namely diet alone, diet and oral hypoglycaemic drugs and diet and insulin. Each obliges the patient to adhere to a lifelong dietary regimen. Approximately 60% of new cases of diabetes can be controlled adequately by diet alone, about 20% will need an oral hypoglycaemic drug and another 20%, mainly younger patients, will require insulin. The principles governing the choice of therapeutic regimen when a diabetic patient is seen for the first time are discussed on page 474. A patient may pass from one group to another temporarily or permanently.

Diet. GENERAL PRINCIPLES. The treatment of all diabetic patients, especially those who require insulin, involves some dietary adjustment if control is to be satisfactory. By regulating the amount and the time of food intake, particularly of carbohydrate, and by dove-tailing the dose of insulin, or of oral hypoglycaemic agent, an attempt is made to keep the blood glucose concentration within the normal range throughout the day and night. It is obvious that if the intake of food varies from day to day it is impossible to work out a steady insulin or other regimen to cover it. Patients should understand that this is the main reason for dietary restriction and not the exclusion of certain 'bad' (sugary) foods.

If one is to achieve a fixed daily intake and avoid the monotony of a static diet sheet, some kind of exchange system is necessary; this is the basis for the construction of nearly all diets in use today. Many doctors are intimidated by the number and variety of diet sheets published and feel that, since they are not trained dietitians, they cannot treat diabetes. A dietitian is certainly most helpful but is not indispensable; the basic principles of an exchange system of dietary treatment are simple, although the education of a patient in their use is time-consuming.

The first step in preparing any dietary regimen is to map out a time-table of the patient's day including a description of the usual meals. This is an essential step and one which is too often omitted. The total daily requirement of calories must next be decided. The diet must be nutritionally adequate for the patient's needs, and it must, therefore, be estimated for each individual patient after considering such factors as age, sex, actual weight in relation to desirable weight (Table 21.2, p. 813), activity, occupation and financial resources. An approximate range for the various groups might be (1) an obese, middle-aged or elderly patient with mild diabetes 1000–1600 kcal daily, (2) an elderly diabetic but not overweight, 1400–1800 kcal daily, (3) a young, active diabetic, 1800–3000 kcal daily. The body weight must be maintained at or slightly below the ideal for the patient's height. Thus the calorie range of group 2 may have to be extended if it is not sufficient to maintain weight, and young patients in group 3 who are overweight may have to reduce their daily intake to below 1800 kcal.

Next the proportion of calories derived from carbohydrate, protein and fat must be allocated. The approximate ratio in the British national diet is, protein 12%, fat 42% and carbohydrate 46%. Although sucrose should be eliminated from the diet the percentage of calories derived from carbohydrate should usually be increased slightly, those from protein increased if this is practicable, and those from fat reduced. In most diabetic diets, therefore, the percentage of calories derived from carbohydrate should be about 50%, from protein 15% and about 35% from fat.

The daily intake of *carbohydrate* to be prescribed ranges from the minimum sufficient to prevent ketonuria, that is, 100 g daily, to a maximum of 240–300 g. The upper limit is imposed by the fact that under normal circumstances it is difficult to achieve satisfactory blood glucose levels throughout 24 hours with a daily carbohydrate intake greater than this. If the daily intake of carbohydrate is 240 g, approximately 50 g carbohydrate will usually be provided by each of the three main meals and 30 g by each of three snacks. A simple method of calculating the carbohydrate content of the diet is to allocate a figure equivalent to one-tenth of the total calories plus approximately 30–50 g to carbohydrate. Thus, if a diet of 1800 kcal is prescribed it should contain about 210–230 g of carbohydrate (p. 810). All the carbohydrate eaten should be in the form of starch. Readily absorbed carbohydrates, such as glucose and sucrose, should generally be avoided because they produce a sudden rise in the blood glucose. A high intake of fibre will increase satiety and reduce constipation and may help to lower serum lipid and blood glucose.

The consumption of *protein* is largely determined by social and economic considerations and will frequently be lower than would be considered desirable. If this is the case, every effort should be made to increase the protein intake and to try to ensure that some protein is eaten at each main meal. An adequate consumption of protein is necessary in children and adolescents to ensure satisfactory growth, and since amino acids stimulate the beta cells of the pancreas to secrete insulin, in both normal subjects and those with NIDDM, a smaller rise in blood glucose occurs when carbohydrate is consumed along with protein. In both categories of diabetic patients consumption of protein will also promote satiety and so help them to keep more strictly to their carbohydrate allowance. A minimum amount of protein should therefore be specified in all diabetic diets, but in the case of those who are not obese it should be emphasised that more may be taken if desired. The daily consumption of protein will usually lie in the range of 60–110 g.

The *fat* intake should be adjusted to bring the total calories to the level desired, and will usually amount to 50–150 g daily. Because diabetic patients have an increased risk of death from ischaemic heart disease which may be related to the amount of saturated fat in the diet, the total amount of fat should be restricted even in those who are not obese. Plasma lipids, particularly cholesterol, should be checked regularly and if significantly elevated the diabetic diet may be appropriately modified (p. 489).

When the patient's requirements have been assessed the figures must be translated into practical and comprehensible instructions for the patient with the help of a diet sheet (p.810). Each patient should be given a list of exchanges with instructions regarding the meals at which they may be taken. The diet sheet and exchanges must be discussed with the patient repeatedly and with a relative if necessary until the system is fully understood.

TYPES OF DIET. Basically there are two types of diet: (1) measured, in which the amount of food to be eaten at each time of the day is specified, and (2) unmeasured, in which the patient is supplied with a list of foods grouped in three categories: foods with a high sucrose content which are to be avoided altogether; foods containing carbohydrate in the form of starch which are to be eaten in moderation only; and non-carbohydrate foods which may be eaten as desired.

Measured diets. In these diets the portions of food may be measured either by weighing with scales or more simply by using household measures. Measured diets are required for two groups of patients, (a) those who require insulin or an oral hypoglycaemic agent, and (b) those who are overweight and require a strict reducing regimen. Patients should if at all possible weigh out the portions of food initially. They should be provided with simple dietetic scales for this purpose. After a few weeks most patients are capable of assessing the weight of portions with sufficient accuracy by eye, and regular weighing becomes less necessary. However, it is often valuable to check visual assessments by weighing from time to time.

Group (a). A method of constructing a diet of 1800 kcal suitable for such patients is described on page 810. It is important to realise that the exchanges or portions employed as units are arbitrary and are decided mainly in the light of the food habits of the population as a whole. The British Diabetic and Dietetic Associations have recommended that the carbohydrate unit should contain 10 g carbohydrate. In Britain the staple carbohydrate food is bread, and the basic carbohydrate exchange for the purposes of calculation is therefore taken to be 20 g ($\frac{2}{3}$oz) bread which contains 10 g carbohydrate, along with 2 g protein and $\frac{2}{3}$g fat. This is the reason why a carbohydrate exchange contains some protein and fat in addition to carbohydrate. Note also that a protein exchange contains some fat.

Group (b). Diabetics who are obese should be urged to accept a reducing regime (p. 80). The method of achieving reduction in weight is the same for obese diabetic patients as for those with simple obesity. The diet on page 809 will meet the needs of many. The portions in this diet can be weighed with scales but more usually are dispensed using household measures as described in this diet. It should be explained that such a strict diet is to be followed only temporarily until the standard weight is reached; thereafter the diet may be increased, and if the patient is sufficiently intelligent, advice can then be given on how to avoid monotony by using a list of exchanges for diabetic diets (p. 811).

Unmeasured diets. If insulin or oral hypoglycaemic agents are not required and marked obesity is not present it may not be necessary for the patient to follow such an accurate diet. Sometimes it may be impracticable to do so because of the patient's mental, visual or other physical incapacity or unwillingness to cooperate. Many patients develop the disease when they are already middle-aged or elderly and have a mild type of diabetes often associated with moderate obesity. For such patients an unmeasured diet of the type described on page 811 may be adequate.

Alcohol. There is no medical objection to taking alcoholic drinks in moderation provided the patient realises that account must be taken of their caloric value and carbohydrate content. Beer may contain 10–30 g of carbohydrate per half litre (1 pint approx.) and with the alcohol this will provide 150–400 kcal, depending on the strength of the beer. Sweet wines and cider all have a high carbohydrate content, and spirits such as whisky and gin, while free of carbohydrates, contain about 70 kcal per 30 ml.

Sweetening agents. Advice may also be asked about sweetening agents and so-called diabetic foods and drinks. Saccharin has been employed as a sweetening agent for many years. It has no caloric value. Sorbitol, a glucose derivative, aspartame (formed from aspartic acid and phenylalanine) and fructose are also added to 'diabetic' foods and drinks for sweetening purposes. In moderate quantities none will interfere with the action or requirements of insulin. If a patient is having difficulty in reducing weight or in maintaining a normal weight, then the use of substitutes for sugar should be discouraged, since they may perpetuate the patient's desire to eat sweet foods and thus make it more difficult to tolerate dietary restrictions. Diabetic chocolate has a high fat content and this must be taken into account.

Oral hypoglycaemic drugs. A number of compounds are effective in reducing hyperglycaemia in patients who would otherwise require insulin. The sulphonylureas, tolbutamide and chlorpropamide, and to a lesser extent the biguanide, metformin, have a place in the management of about 20% of diabetic patients. Although their mechanism of action is different, the action of both groups depends upon a supply of endogenous insulin, and it is therefore futile and dangerous to attempt to control IDDM with these compounds.

SULPHONYLUREAS. These drugs are valuable in the treatment of patients with NIDDM who fail to respond to simple dietary restriction and who are not overweight. Although their initial hypoglycaemic action is associated with an increased amount of immunoreactive insulin in peripheral plasma, their long-term hypoglycaemic effect seems to be mainly due to extrapancreatic actions. These include reduced hepatic release of glucose and improved sensitivity to insulin, possibly due to an increase in the number of peripheral insulin receptors.

Tolbutamide is the mildest, and probably also the safest, of the sulphonylureas. Since its effective action does not exceed 6 to 8 hours it should be administered two to three times a day. The dose varies between 1 and 2 g daily. It is very well tolerated and toxic reactions such as rashes occur only rarely. Tolbutamide is a useful drug in the elderly where the risk and the consequences of inducing hypoglycaemia are increased. Unfortunately, the relapse rate is relatively high.

Chlorpropamide has a biological half-life of about 36 hours, and an effective concentration can be maintained in the blood by a single dose at breakfast. The usual maintenance dose is between 100 and 375 mg daily; larger doses should not be used on a long-term basis, since above this level there is an increased risk of toxic effects, such as jaundice, rashes, and blood dyscrasia.

If alcohol is taken following chlorpropamide an unpleasant flushing of the face occurs in some patients. This is a dominantly-inherited trait associated with NIDDM. The demonstration that this reaction can be blocked with naloxone suggests that these patients may have inherited an unusual sensitivity to endorphins.

Chlorpropamide may lead to severe hypoglycaemia, which can be very refractory to treatment. Great care must be taken to avoid this, particularly in elderly patients, and once glycosuria has been abolished and symptoms relieved, the daily dose of chlorpropamide must be reduced to the minimum required to maintain control. In fact many patients who require 375–500 mg daily initially can be maintained on a long-term basis on 100 mg or less per day.

Other sulphonylureas such as acetohexamide, tolazamide, glibenclamide, glipizide and glymidine are more expensive and usually offer little advantage over chlorpropamide but may be useful in individual patients.

BIGUANIDES. The biguanides, metformin and phenformin, are less widely used in Britain than the sulphonylureas, because of the higher incidence of side-effects, particularly gastrointestinal symptoms and because there have been a significant number of deaths from lactic acidosis in patients taking these drugs, particularly phenformin. However, metformin is useful in two clinical situations. Firstly, since its administration is not associated with an increase in weight it may be preferred when it is essential to treat a patient with NIDDM who is overweight but in whom hyperglycaemia persists despite efforts to adhere to a diet and reduce weight. Secondly, as the hypoglycaemic effect of the biguanides appears to be synergistic with that of the sulphonylureas, there is a place for combining the two when the sulphonylureas alone have proved inadequate and when, as happens with 5 to 10% of patients, initial success is followed after several months, or even years, by loss of control.

Metformin is given with food in two or three daily doses of 0.5–1.0 g each. Its use is contraindicated in patients with impaired renal or hepatic function and in those who take alcohol in excess, as the risk of lactic acidosis occurring is significantly increased in such patients. Its administration should be discontinued, at least temporarily, if any other serious medical condition develops, and treatment with insulin substituted.

CLINICAL USE OF SULPHONYLUREAS AND BIGUANIDES. Patients may be started on an oral hypoglycaemic drug as soon as it is clear that dietary measures alone are inadequate. Evidence of some response is usually apparent within a week, though a full response may not occur for considerably longer. Diabetics treated successfully in this way for prolonged periods may ultimately need an alteration of dose or a change of regime temporarily or permanently; in particular they may require insulin to meet the need created by a severe infection, an operation or other stress.

There is some evidence that those taking an oral hypoglycaemic drug are at increased risk of dying from ischaemic heart disease. This may be due to a high incidence of ventricular fibrillation in diabetic patients on oral therapy who sustain a myocardial infarct. Efforts should therefore be made to control as many patients as possible by diet alone for this and other reasons (p. 474). Furthermore those taking oral hypoglycaemic drugs who develop a myocardial infarct should have these replaced by insulin during the acute illness and have a longer period of close supervision, preferably in a coronary care unit.

Insulin. With one or more of the preparations of insulin available it is usually possible to keep the blood glucose within reasonable, although not physiological, limits throughout the day and night without undue risk of hypoglycaemia.

Two main therapeutic forms of insulin are available, (1) unmodified, rapid-onset, short-acting and (2) modified or depot, delayed-onset, long-acting preparations. There are various varieties of each type some of which are shown in Table 12.1. The older insulins contain varying amounts of glucagon, pro-insulin, altered insulin and other peptides, which are largely responsible for the insulin-binding antibodies found in the plasma of all patients treated with these insulins. Highly purified, 'monocomponent' or 'single peak' insulins prepared from pig and cattle pancreases and human insulin, synthesised by recombinant DNA technology, are now available which are much less antigenic and are superseding the older preparations. Care must be taken to avoid hypoglycaemia when transferring patients from the older to the newer preparations, and the higher the dose of conventional insulin, the stricter the supervision required.

UNMODIFIED INSULINS. These are clear solutions in contrast to the depot insulins which are cloudy. When injected subcutaneously, unmodified insulin is effective in 20-30 minutes and its action continues for approximately 6 hours (Table 12.1). Unmodified insulin is essential in (1) new cases with severe dehydration or ketoacidosis, (2) emergencies associated with ketosis, such as acute infection, gastroenteritis and some surgical operations, (3) the treatment of nearly all young patients and (4) in any situation where intravenous insulin is required.

MODIFIED (DEPOT) INSULINS. These preparations are cloudy solutions. Their delayed and prolonged action can be achieved in two main ways. In isophane preparations insulin is adsorbed on to a large protein molecule, protamine, in the presence of zinc. When injected subcutaneously the protamine-zinc-insulin complex breaks up slowly in the tissues gradually releasing the bound insulin over a period of 12–24 hours. Insulin zinc suspensions do not contain foreign protein. The duration of their action depends on the size and form of the insulin crystals as well as on the rate at which these crystals are dissolved and absorbed. The former is achieved by carefully controlling the conditions of precipitation; the latter is delayed by buffering with acetate and by adding small

Table 12.1 Insulins: types, preparations and duration of action.

Type	Proprietary preparations		Species	Approximate hours of action
Unmodified. Rapid onset				
Soluble or regular insulin (acid)	Soluble insulin	(Wellcome)	Cattle	
Neutral insulins	Neusulin	(Wellcome)	Cattle	
	Velosulin	(Nordisk)	Pig	'Short'
	Humulin S	(Eli Lilly)	Human (biosynthetic)	6
	Actrapid MC	(Novo)	Pig	
	Actrapid HM	(Novo)	Human (semisynthetic)	
Modified (Depot). Delayed onset				
Isophane type insulins	Neuphane	(Wellcome)	Cattle	
	Insulatard	(Nordisk)	Pig	'Intermediate'
	Humulin I	(Eli Lilly)	Human (biosynthetic)	12
Insulin zinc suspensions	Monotard MC	(Novo)	Pig	
	Protophane HM	(Novo)	Human (semisynthetic)	
Isophane type insulin	Humulin Zn	(Eli Lilly)	Human (biosynthetic)	'Long'
Insulin zinc suspensions	Ultratard MC	(Novo)	Pig	16 +
	Ultratard HM	(Novo)	Human (semisynthetic)	24 +

All these insulins are available in highly purified form and in three strengths: 40, 80 and 100 international units/ml. Soluble insulin is also supplied as a solution containing 20 i.u./ml. In Britain and the USA only 100 i.u./ml strength is available for routine clinical use. In many parts of the world neutral unmodified insulins have superseded soluble insulin which is strongly acid and more antigenic.

amounts of zinc.

Examples of preparations of insulin are listed in Table 12.1. Most patients with IDDM do best by taking unmodified insulin along with one of the intermediate depot insulins before breakfast and repeating this combination before the evening meal. The unmodified and depot insulins prepared by each individual manufacturer may be mixed in one syringe for injection but preparations of different manufacturers should not be mixed.

In practice one must be prepared to try combinations of the various insulin preparations, and to vary the time at which they are administered in the light of the results of blood glucose estimations at different times of the day until smooth control is achieved over 24 hours. It is impossible to forecast the response of a patient to insulin, and the daily dose required to establish control varies widely from patient to patient.

Choice of therapeutic regimen. Although the regimen eventually adopted in each case of diabetes is chosen by a process of trial, the age and weight of the patient at diagnosis indicate with a high degree of probability the type of treatment likely to be required. The chief indications for the main types of therapeutic regimen are:

1. Practically all young patients who develop diabetes before the age of 40 require treatment with insulin. The majority will be best controlled by taking unmodified insulin along with one of the depot insulins in the morning, and a second dose of unmodified insulin, or of unmodified and depot insulin before the evening meal. Examples of suitable combinations of commercial preparations are Velosulin and Insulatard or Actrapid MC and Monotard MC or Humulin S (soluble) and Humulin I (isophane) taken twice daily.

2. The majority of patients developing the disease over the age of 40 can and should be controlled by diet alone. This applies particularly to obese patients, but others who are not overweight may also do well on dietary therapy alone.

3. Those over the age of 40 who fail to achieve satisfactory control by dietary measures alone will usually respond well to a sulphonylurea if they are not obese, or to a biguanide if they are obese. If adequate control is not achieved by one drug, a combination of sulphonylurea and biguanide may be tried. If this fails insulin will be required.

It must be stressed again that obese patients should be treated by dietary restriction and weight reduction rather than by the administration of insulin or an oral hypoglycaemic agent. The advent of the 'insulin era' has obscured the remarkable improvement in glucose tolerance which usually results from reduction in weight. Insulin and the sulphonylureas increase the appetite, and thus may increase weight and intensify the total disability.

Initiation of treatment. It is desirable that the patient learns to manage all aspects of the disorder as quickly as possible, and this can best be done on an outpatient basis while leading a relatively normal existence at home and at work. However, patients being stabilised on insulin have to be seen daily at first and if this is not practicable, admission to hospital will be necessary. Hospital admission will also be necessary for patients with severe ketoacidosis. The therapeutic plan must include measures directed at any of the complications to which the diabetic is prone and which may already be present at diagnosis, namely coronary artery disease and hypertension, obliterative arterial disease, nephropathy, retinopathy, cataract, neuropathy, pulmonary tuberculosis and other infections, particularly of the skin and urinary tract (p. 483).

A practical point worth mentioning, since it may give rise to distress if not anticipated, is that blurring of vision, which may occur in a severe diabetic before treatment, may become noticeably worse after starting treatment with insulin or tablets. It is due to transitory osmotic abnormalities in the eye, especially the lens, and may persist for as long as several weeks after initiating treatment.

PATIENT'S EDUCATION. Every patient who is capable of learning must be taught how to perform urinary or, preferably, capillary blood glucose estimations and tests of urinary ketones, to keep a record of the results and to understand their significance.

All patients requiring insulin must learn to measure their dose of insulin accurately with an insulin syringe, to give their own injections and to adjust the dose themselves on the basis of urine and/or blood tests and other factors such as illness, unusual exercise and insulin reactions. They should be made to experience an insulin reaction (p. 476).

All patients must have a working knowledge of diabetes, i.e. they must be able to recognise the symptoms associated with marked glycosuria and to understand their significance. They must be told that many drugs have undesirable effects on the diabetic state, as may also such other factors as illness of any kind or emotional upset. They should be advised to consult their doctor or clinic at once as soon as they are aware of any deterioration in health or tests which does not respond rapidly to the simple measures that they take themselves.

All patients must know how to take care of their feet, and learn to treat any infected lesion with respect. Regular chiropody is important especially for elderly patients.

Education of the patient is time-consuming and repeated practical demonstrations may also be required. It may be supplemented by reading appropriate booklets. It is only in this way that diabetic patients can safely undertake all normal activities while maintaining good control of their disease. If the patient is a child, or is blind, mentally defective or otherwise incapable, instructions must be given to a parent or other attendant.

It is a wise precaution for diabetic patients who are taking insulin or oral hypoglycaemic drugs to carry a card with them at all times stating their name and address, the fact that they are diabetic, the nature and dose of any insulin or other drugs they may be taking, and, in addition, giving the name, address and telephone number of their family doctor and any special diabetic clinic they may be attending. Suitable cards are provided by the British Diabetic Association for the use of members.

SUPERVISION OF PATIENT. Diabetics should be seen at regular intervals for the remainder of their lives. The object is to check the degree of control and if necessary to make appropriate alterations in treatment and to watch for any complications. Records should be kept so that the doctor is immediately on the alert if changes in health occur. The frequency of visits is determined by the severity of the disability and the reliability of the patient. For the general practitioner with diabetic patients scattered over a wide area, this supervision may be difficult. For this reason and because of the need to develop and apply new and better techniques for the control of diabetes, many hospitals arrange diabetic clinics.

ASSESSMENT OF CONTROL. At the patient's regular visit to the diabetic clinic or general practitioner, the degree of control should be assessed by considering the patient's weight in relation to standard weight, the results of urine and/or blood glucose tests, the concentration of glycosylated haemoglobin (HbA_1) and the presence or absence of symptoms of either hyper- or hypoglycaemia.

Proper assessment of control is impossible unless in the course of normal activity the patient tests samples of urine or preferably blood regularly. By selecting suitable times for the tests and tabulating the results, it is easy for the doctor or the experienced patient to decide whether the dose of insulin or hypoglycaemic drug should be changed, or whether the carbohydrate content of the diet or the time when it is taken should be altered.

Urine testing. Semiquantitive preprandial urine testing is the time-honoured method of assessing control. This is usually done using Clinitest tablets or Diastix strips. The former method is more inconvenient but is more accurate particularly when ketonuria is present since this inhibits colour development in the Diastix strip. The Diabur 5000 test strip avoids these problems. Diabetics taking insulin should test samples of urine obtained before breakfast, before the midday and evening meals, and at bedtime (prior to a bedtime snack if this is taken). The patient must empty the bladder and discard the urine about 30 minutes before passing a specimen for testing. Patients treated by diet alone or with oral hypoglycaemic agents should test the first morning specimen and a sample passed about 2 hours after the main meals of the day. The majority of all the above specimens should be either free of glucose or contain $\frac{1}{4}\%$ or less.

While the patient is being stabilised, tests will have to be carried out three or four times daily; when control is established the frequency can be greatly reduced. One daily preprandial test taken serially at different times of the day is much more informative about the state of control than a single test carried out at the same time daily. Alternatively, three or four tests can be performed on a single day once or twice weekly.

Blood glucose estimations. Since there is often a poor correlation between simultaneous urinary and blood glucose estimations it is preferable to measure the blood glucose concentration at different times of the day when assessing control. Many patients can be taught to take capillary blood samples and measure the blood glucose concentration in these by means of enzyme impregnated sticks (e.g. Dextrostix or BM Glycemie 20–800), if possible with a simple colorimetric meter, to improve accuracy. In assessing the result it is important to consider the interval between taking the sample and the last meal and also previous physical activity. The aim should be to keep the fasting blood glucose level less than 7.0 mmol/l (126 mg/100 ml) and the post-prandial peak under 10.0 mmol/l (180 mg/100 ml).

Glycosylated haemoglobin (HbA$_1$). When haemoglobin from a normal adult is passed through a chromatographic column it separates into the major component HbA (92–94% of the total) and several minor, faster-moving components collectively known as HbA$_1$ (6–8% of the total). These are structurally identical to HbA except for the addition of a glucose group to the terminal amino acid of the β chain. This is a post-synthetic, non-enzymatic reaction and the rate of synthesis of HbA$_1$ is a function of the blood glucose concentration. Since the glucose linkage is relatively stable, HbA$_1$ accumulates throughout the life span of the erythrocyte and its concentration reflects the mean blood glucose concentration over the previous few months. Measurement of HbA$_1$ can therefore be used as a supplement to urine tests and blood glucose estimations to monitor the degree of diabetic control achieved.

Insulin reactions and hypoglycaemia. If unmodified insulin is administered to a normal person the blood glucose falls, producing symptoms that may begin to appear when the concentration is about 2.7 mmol/l (50 mg/100 ml) and are fully developed at about 2.2 mmol/l. In diabetics who are constantly hyperglycaemic, the same symptoms may develop at higher levels, e.g.

6.6 mmol/l or more. The symptoms may include any one or more of the following: a feeling of being weak and empty, hunger, sweating, palpitation, tremor, faintness, dizziness, headache, diplopia and mental confusion. Abnormal behaviour, leading occasionally to arrest on a charge of being drunk and disorderly, may also occur. Alternatively, and particularly in children, there may be lassitude and somnolence or muscular twitchings. Eventually coma, sometimes with convulsions, may follow.

Hypoglycaemia induces secretion of adrenaline, and this in turn causes tachycardia and tremor. Adrenaline, by mobilising liver glycogen, combats the hypoglycaemia. This homeostatic reaction partly explains why patients rarely die of hypoglycaemic coma from too much unmodified insulin. By contrast, coma is dangerous when it arises from a large dose of depot insulin or from an overdose of a sulphonylurea, particularly chlorpropamide. The latter condition, although relatively uncommon, is resistant to treatment, since the drug reduces the hepatic release of glucose, and because the half-life of the drug is so long. The brain is dependent on the blood glucose for the energy necessary for its activity. Permanent brain damage may result from prolonged hypoglycaemia which should be prevented from recurring by prompt reduction of the dose of insulin or of sulphonylurea.

Hypoglycaemia due to overdosage with unmodified insulin comes on rapidly, at the time when the insulin is having its maximum effect that is, through the morning or in the early evening, and usually elicits classical symptoms and responds rapidly to treatment. Reactions from excessive depot insulin given before breakfast usually occur in the later afternoon, at night or early next morning. These reactions may begin gradually with little adrenaline response, become persistent and profound and respond more slowly to treatment. The predominant warning symptoms are very variable and include headache, malaise, night sweats, nausea leading sometimes to troublesome vomiting, mental confusion and drowsiness, especially in the morning.

TREATMENT OF HYPOGLYCAEMIC REACTIONS. Since hypoglycaemia can easily be corrected if recognised early, diabetic patients should experience the condition under supervision. In this way they learn to recognise the early symptoms. They must be made to realise that the most frequent causes of the condition are unpunctual meals and unaccustomed exercise, and seek to avoid both or to make adjustments to meet these circumstances. They should always carry some tablets of glucose or a few lumps of sugar for use in an emergency. Unless an attack of hypoglycaemia is adequately accounted for, the patient should reduce the next and subsequent doses of insulin by 20% and seek medical advice.

If the patient is so stuporous that swallowing is impossible an intravenous injection of 25 g of glucose (50 ml of a 50% solution) should be given. This may have to be repeated. Alternatively, the insulin-dependent patient may be given a subcutaneous or intramuscular injection of 1 mg of glucagon, repeated if necessary after 10 minutes. This raises the blood glucose by mobilising liver glycogen, and has the advantage of convenience in that it can be given by anybody capable of using a syringe, but it may not be effective in severe and prolonged hypoglycaemia due to depot insulins. In addition to increasing hepatic glycogenolysis, glucagon stimulates the secretion of insulin and therefore should not be used to treat hypoglycaemia induced by an oral hypoglycaemic agent.

As soon as the patient is able to swallow, glucose should be given orally. Full recovery may not occur immediately. Further, when hypoglycaemia has occurred in a diabetic using a depot preparation of insulin or a sulphonylurea, particularly chlorpropamide, the possibility of relapse within a day or more should be anticipated.

Repeated episodes of hypoglycaemia may lead to permanent intellectual deterioration; accordingly, adjustments to prevent recurrences are essential.

THE COMPLICATIONS OF DIABETES MELLITUS

Diabetic ketoacidosis

Prior to the discovery of insulin more than 50% of diabetic patients ultimately died of ketoacidosis. Today this complication is preventable and accounts for less than 2% of diabetic deaths. However, both the incidence and the mortality rate are still regrettably high. Failure of the patient to understand the disease, and failure to appreciate the significance of symptoms of poor control are the most common causes. Thus its prevention is largely a problem of education of patients and at times of their physicians. A clear understanding of the biochemical disorder involved (p. 464) is essential for its efficient treatment which should aim at having the patient out of danger within 24 hours.

Water and mineral depletion. The deficit of total body water in a severe case may be about 6 litres. About half of this is derived from the intracellular compartment and occurs comparatively early in the development of acidosis with relatively few clinical features; the remainder represents loss of extracellular fluid sustained largely in the later stages. It is at this time that marked contraction of the size of the extracellular space occurs, with haemoconcentration, a decrease in the plasma volume, and finally a fall in blood pressure with associated renal ischaemia and oliguria.

The concentration of sodium and potassium in the serum gives very little indication of total body losses, and may even be raised due to disproportionate losses of water. Sodium loss, mainly from the extracellular space, may amount to as much as 500 mmol. Potassium loss from the cells may be 400 mmol or more. The concentration of potassium in the plasma in these circumstances is dependent on the balance between catabolism of protein and glycogen and haemoconcentration on the one hand, and urinary excretion on the other. Since the former generally exceeds the latter plasma potassium is likely to be high initially, in spite of a total body deficit. However, within a few hours of beginning treatment with insulin, there is likely to be a precipitous fall in the plasma potassium. At least three mechanisms are responsible for this; dilution of extracellular potassium by the administration of potassium-free fluids, the movement of potassium into the cells as the result of insulin therapy, and the continuing renal loss of potassium.

Ketoacidosis. The mechanism of the development of this state has been described (p. 464).

Apart from the clinical findings, its severity can be rapidly assessed by measuring the plasma bicarbonate, less than 12 mmol/l indicating severe acidosis. The hydrogen ion concentration in the blood is an even more valuable guide but it may not be as readily available. There are no simple and accurate quantitative methods for the determination of plasma ketones.

Clinical features. Any form of stress, particularly an acute infection, can precipitate severe ketoacidosis in even the mildest diabetic. The most common cause is neglect of treatment due to carelessness, misunderstanding or illness, and failure to adjust the therapeutic regimen in the event of an acute infection.

The symptoms of diabetic ketoacidosis invariably include intense thirst and polyuria. Constipation, cramps and altered vision are common. Sometimes, especially in children, there is abdominal pain, with or without vomiting. Hence diabetic ketoacidosis is important in the differential diagnosis of the acute abdomen. Weakness and drowsiness are commonly present, but it should be remembered that the state of consciousness is very variable and a patient with dangerous ketosis requiring urgent treatment may walk into hospital. For this reason the term diabetic ketoacidosis is to be preferred to 'diabetic coma', which suggests that there is no urgency until unconsciousness occurs. In fact it is imperative that energetic treatment is started at the earliest possible stage.

The signs include a dry tongue and soft eyeballs due to dehydration; 'air hunger' indicated by long, deep, sighing respirations; a rapid, weak pulse, and low blood pressure; sometimes abdominal rigidity and tenderness; the smell of acetone in the breath; ultimately coma supervenes.

INVESTIGATION. This shows (1) ketonuria and severe glycosuria; (2) blood glucose usually between 22.2 and 44.4 mmol/l (400 and 800 mg/100 ml), but it may be much higher and in some cases lower; (3) low, plasma bicarbonate and blood pH; (4) low normal or raised serum sodium and potassium; (5) leucocytosis.

Hyperglycaemia and ketoacidosis do not always necessarily correlate well. Even at a level of blood glucose as low as 19.4 mmol/l (350 mg/100 ml), life-threatening acidosis may be present. In con-

trast diabetic coma can occur, usually in elderly patients, with extreme hyperglycaemia and dehydration but no ketoacidosis (p. 480). This is known as *hyperosmolar diabetic coma*.

Treatment. Ketoacidosis should be treated with urgency in hospital. Intravenous therapy is required since even when the patient is able to swallow, fluids given by mouth may be poorly absorbed. Establishing an intravenous infusion can be technically difficult because of collapsed veins, but cutting down and tying in a cannula should be avoided if at all possible, because the veins may be needed again.

Treatment must be checked against the blood concentration of glucose, potassium and bicarbonate estimated at intervals at first of not longer than 2 hours. Only in this way can the metabolic disorder be corrected accurately and rapidly. The aim should be to overcome with all speed: (1) ketosis, by means of insulin to permit glucose utilisation; (2) shock, acidosis, and water and electrolyte depletion, by means of appropriate intravenous fluids; (3) infection, if present, by means of antibiotics.

Only unmodified insulins should be used. Ketosis and dehydration render the comatose patient relatively resistant to insulin. The conventional treatment of diabetic ketoacidosis has, therefore, involved the use of large doses of unmodified insulin. It is now known that such large doses of insulin are unnecessary and that low-dose regimens are just as effective, are less complicated and may be safer.

An infusion of saline is started and 20 units of unmodified insulin given by intramuscular injection immediately and 4–6 units hourly thereafter, either by intramuscular injection or intravenous infusion, preferably using a constant-rate pump (Fig. 12.7). The blood glucose concentration should fall by 3–6 mmol/l/h. If there is no fall in the blood glucose concentration by two hours after starting treatment, then the dose of insulin should be doubled until a satisfactory response is obtained. When the blood glucose concentration has fallen to 10.0 mmol/l (180 mg/100 ml) 5% glucose should replace or be added to the saline infusion and the dose of insulin reduced to 1–4 units i.v. hourly, or 8–16 units 4 hourly by subcutaneous injection.

Time (hours)	Insulin Units (U) (unmodified preparation)		IV Fluid	IV Potassium rate of infusion: mmol/hour
	Intramuscular	Intravenous (rate of infusion: units/hour)		
0	20 U		*Isotonic (0.9%) saline 1.0 litre in 30 minutes	Check urinary output Obtain results for plasma electrolytes
	6 U	6 U/hour	0.5 litre in 30 minutes	If plasma concentration (mmol/l) is:
				>6 6–4.5 4.5–3 <3
	*If plasma Na⁺ > 155 mmol/l give 0.45% saline.		Give mmol K⁺/h	↓ ↓ ↓ ↓
				0 13 26 39
1	6 U	6 U/hour	0.5 litre in 30 minutes 0.5 litre/hour	
				Monitor plasma concentration every 1–2 hours and change infusion rate accordingly
2	6 U If fall in blood glucose <3 mmol/l/h switch to IV	6 U/hour If fall in blood glucose <3 mmol/l/h double rate	0.5 litre/hour	
3	CONTINUE 6 U every hour UNTIL blood glucose concentration 1–4 U hourly	6 U/hour <10 mmol/l, then give 1–4 U/hour	0.25 litre/hour 5% glucose: 0.25 litre/hour	

NB: Average fluid deficit = 6 litres — 3.0 litres from Extra-cellular compartment replaced by NaCl
— 3.0 litres from Intra-cellular " " by glucose

Procedures: Intravenous line; catheterise after 3 hours if no urine passed; nasogastric tube to keep stomach empty. Central venous pressure line if cardiovascular system compromised so that volume of IV fluid can be adjusted

Monitor: Blood glucose and electrolytes hourly for 3 hours and then 2–4 hourly; temperature, pulse, respiration, BP hourly; urinary output; urinary ketones; ECGs, blood osmolality, arterial pH, in some cases

Fig. 12.7 Management of diabetic ketoacidosis. These guidelines for a typical, 'average' case should be modified appropriately in the individual patient after considering the blood biochemistry and clinical features.

The deficit of extracellular fluid, which is usually about 3 litres, should be made good by infusion of saline isotonic with plasma (0.9% NaCl). A suitable regimen is 1 litre in half an hour, 1 litre in 1 hour, and then 1 litre in 2 hours until there is clinical improvement (Fig. 12.7). Elderly patients or those with cardiovascular disease will require modification of this regimen and monitoring of central venous pressure may be necessary. If during the treatment the serum sodium rises above 150 mmol/l, 0.45% saline should be given.

In cases which are also severely acidotic (pH < 7.0), 500 ml of the isotonic saline may be replaced by isotonic sodium bicarbonate (1.4%) and this may be repeated if the pH remains <7.1 mmol/l. Under no circumstances, however, should correction of the total deficit be attempted since there is some evidence that rapid correction of acidosis in diabetic ketoacidosis may aggravate tissue hypoxia and also reduce the level of consciousness by causing a paradoxical acidosis of the cerebrospinal fluid. The combined administration of bicarbonate and insulin will also increase the risk of hypokalaemia and potassium should be given along with bicarbonate.

The intracellular deficit of water, usually about 2–3 litres, must be replaced by using 5% glucose and not by more saline. It is best given when the blood glucose is approaching normal. It is important to continue the intravenous glucose together with appropriate doses of insulin until the ketonuria has disappeared and the water deficit has been made good.

Acute circulatory failure should be treated as described on page 143.

Every patient in diabetic ketoacidosis is potassium depleted and nearly all will require intravenous potassium (p. 89) to prevent the development of dangerous hypokalaemia during the course of treatment. As the serum potassium is often high at presentation, potassium therapy should be started cautiously and carefully monitored by frequent estimations of plasma potassium (Fig. 12.7). ECGs are sometimes helpful, a decrease in the height of the T wave indicating a falling plasma potassium. Approximately 80 mmol of potassium may safely be given by vein in the first 16 hours, but much more than this may be required and sufficient must be given to maintain a normal plasma concentration. It is customary to add 1.5 g potassium chloride (20 mmol potassium) to each 500 ml of fluid given intravenously. Once oral feeding has started potassium chloride (p. 89) should be given 4-hourly for 2 to 3 days to restore the total body deficit.

In a stuporous or comatose patient, gastric aspiration should be undertaken to avoid the risk of inhaling vomitus. The stomach will often contain a large amount of brown fluid containing altered blood.

Infections must be carefully sought and vigorously treated since it may not be possible to abolish ketosis until they are controlled.

Once ketosis has been overcome and the salt and water deficit made good (usually in about 24 hours), feeding by mouth can be started with frequent small fluid feeds each containing 25 g carbohydrate. Two examples of such feeds are:

1. 100 ml ($3\frac{1}{2}$ oz) fruit juice plus 15 g ($\frac{1}{2}$ oz) of cane sugar or glucose.

2. 200 ml (7 oz) milk plus 10 g ($\frac{1}{4}$ oz) cereal plus 7 g ($\frac{1}{4}$ oz) sugar.

Sufficient insulin should be given to prevent further ketonuria or glycosuria. Control of blood glucose can be lost very quickly and frequent blood glucose estimations are needed. Unmodified insulin should be given before each oral feed, even if the urine is free of sugar and only very small doses are required.

HYPEROSMOLAR, NON-KETOTIC DIABETIC COMA. Treatment differs from that of ketoacidotic coma in two main respects. These patients seem to be relatively sensitive to insulin and it is probably best to give approximately half the dose of insulin usually employed in diabetic ketoacidosis. Once it is known that plasma osmolality is high (calculated by the formula 2 × sodium mmol/l + glucose mmol/l = 285 mOsm/l normally) 0.45% saline should be given until the osmolality approaches normal, when 0.9% should be substituted.

COMA DUE TO LACTIC ACIDOSIS. Clinically the patient is likely to be a diabetic taking a biguanide, who is very ill and overbreathing, but not so profoundly dehydrated as is usual in coma due to ketoacidosis, and whose breath does not smell of acetone. Ketonuria is no more than mild, yet plasma bicarbonate and pH are markedly reduced. Diagnosis is confirmed by a high (usually > 5.0 mmol/l) concentration of lactic acid in the blood.

Treatment is with large amounts of intravenous bicarbonate; as much as 2500 mmol may be needed. Insulin is given by continuous intravenous infusion and glucose added when the blood level falls to about 10.0 mmol/l. Dialysis may be required in very severe cases (pH < 7) if sodium overload results from the administration of large quantities of sodium bicarbonate. Despite such measures the mortality in this condition is greater than 50%.

Differential diagnosis of coma in a diabetic. Confusion between coma due to hypoglycaemia and that associated with ketosis should seldom arise; the distinction is clear (Table 12.2). Diabetic coma may occasionally pass undetected into hypoglycaemic coma through too enthusiastic treatment; likewise, vomiting induced by hypoglycaemia from a depot insulin may continue until diabetic coma develops.

Hyperosmolar, non-ketotic diabetic coma and coma due to lactic acidosis are distinguished by the features given above.

Vascular disorders
Vascular disease, arterial, arteriolar and capillary, is the largest and most intractable problem in clinical diabetes. Arterial disease is easily the commonest cause of death in diabetics over the age of 50, while nephropathy accounts for more than half the deaths under 50. Strict control probably offers the best chance of delaying the

Table 12.2 Differences in coma due to hypoglycaemia and ketoacidosis in IDDM.

	Hypoglycaemic coma	*Coma with ketosis*
History:	no food; too much insulin; unaccustomed exercise	too little or no insulin; an infection; digestive disturbance
Onset:	in good previous health; related to last insulin injection	ill-health for several days
Symptoms:	of hypoglycaemia; occasional vomiting from depot insulins	of glycosuria and dehydration; abdominal pain and vomiting
Signs:	moist skin and tongue full pulse normal or raised BP shallow or normal breathing brisk reflexes	dry skin and tongue weak pulse low blood pressure air hunger diminished reflexes
Urine:	no ketonuria no glycosuria, if bladder recently emptied	ketonuria glycosuria
Blood:	hypoglycaemia normal plasma bicarbonate	hyperglycaemia reduced plasma bicarbonate

onset and progress of the vascular complications of diabetes.

Atherosclerosis occurs commonly and extensively in diabetes. The pathological changes in diabetics are not specific in a qualitative sense but they occur earlier and are more widespread than in non-diabetics. Thus diabetics are more prone at an earlier age than other people to myocardial infarction and hypertension. The peripheral pulses in the legs are often diminished or impalpable, and particularly in elderly patients, intermittent claudication and ischaemic changes in the feet are frequently present. Defective circulation in the legs resulting in poorly nourished tissues predisposes to gangrene. If a painless peripheral neuropathy is present, the patient will tend to ignore or neglect injuries and other damage to the tissues. Diabetic gangrene usually starts in one foot, following a trivial injury. A great deal can be done to prevent these complications by instructing diabetics with a poor circulation to wear properly fitting shoes, to use bed-socks rather than hot water bottles, never to cut their own corns and 'to keep the feet as clean as the face'. The services of a skilled chiropodist are invaluable.

Diabetic nephropathy

A specific type of renal lesion may occur as a result of the changes in the basement membrane of the glomerular capillaries—*diabetic glomerulosclerosis*. There are two types, diffuse and nodu-

lar. The former is the more common and consists of a generalised thickening of the basement membrane. The nodular type is a development of this, in which rounded masses of hyaline material (Kimmelstiel-Wilson bodies) are superimposed upon the diffuse lesion. Diabetic glomerulosclerosis can be seen by light microscopy in about 70% of diabetic patients at autopsy. Even with well-established diabetic glomerulosclerosis the patient may exhibit only slight to moderate proteinuria. In some cases, however, marked proteinuria and the nephrotic syndrome develop with increasing renal failure.

There is no definite way of preventing or modifying the progression of nephropathy once this is clinically apparent as proteinuria. However any associated hypertension must be controlled. In the later stages the management is the same as in other forms of chronic renal failure (p. 399).

Diabetic retinopathy

Retinopathy is the commonest long-term complication of diabetes. In most cases it produces no symptoms but it can cause blindness and in Britain diabetic retinopathy is now the most common cause of blindness in the middle-aged.

Clinical features. Microaneurysms, venous abnormalities, haemorrhages, exudates and new vessel formation occur in varying combinations in different patients (Plate II). Abnormalities of the capillary bed, which are not clinically visible,

PLATE I

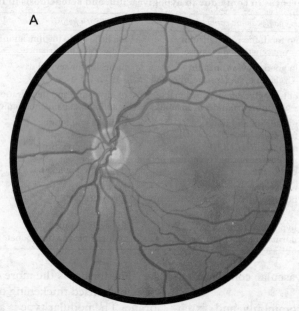

A. Normal retina. Painting of left eye showing arteries and veins, the white optic cup in the centre of a clean cut disc surrounded by a scleral ring (a normal variant). The darker red avascular area beyond the temporal side of the disc is typical of a normal macula. (Courtesy of Professor C. I. Phillips.)

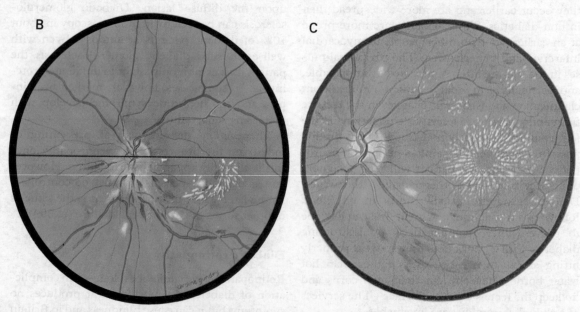

B. Hypertensive retinopathy. The upper half of this painting shows the retinal blood vessels in hypertension of moderate severity. The arteriolar blood column is narrower than normal and some sheathing of the upper temporal and nasal branches is shown. Variations in breadth of the arteriolar blood column indicates an irregular lumen. Veins at arterial-venous crossings are narrowed ('nipping'), partly because of pressure by arterioles and also because opacity of the arterial wall obscures the venous blood column. The lower half of the painting shows severe hypertensive retinopathy. Haemorrhages and soft exudates are added to the abnormalities seen in the upper half and these are more marked. (Courtesy of Professor C. I. Phillips.)

C. Severe hypertensive retinopathy. Retinal painting showing haemorrhages, two soft exudates, numerous hard exudates including a macular star, and irregularity of the calibre of the arterioles.

PLATE II

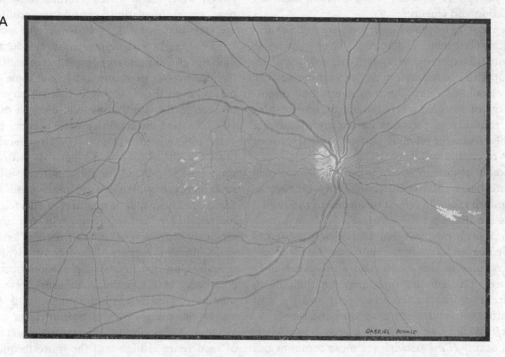

GABRIEL DONALD

A. Diabetic retinopathy. Retinal painting showing microaneurysms, haemorrhages, hard exudates and dilated veins.

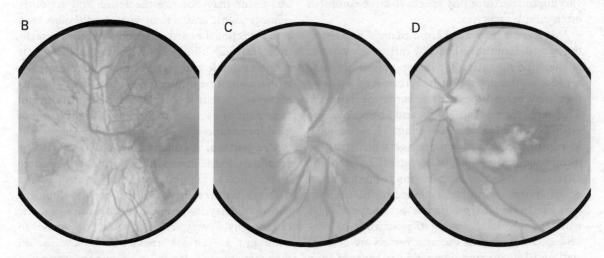

B. Advanced proliferative diabetic retinopathy. Retinal photograph showing heavily vascularised sheets of fibrous tissue forming in the vitreous and mainly derived from the optic disc.

C. Papilloedema. Retinal photograph showing swelling of the disc and haemorrhages on or very near the disc.

D. Thrombosis of retinal vein. Photograph showing haemorrhages and exudates in the territory of the lower temporal branch of the central retinal vein. There is also pathological cupping of the disc due to raised intra-ocular pressure which predisposes to retinal thrombosis. (Courtesy of Professor C. I. Phillips.)

are the earliest lesions. They include capillary dilatation and closure.

In most cases *microaneurysms* are the earliest clinical abnormality detected. They appear as minute, discrete, circular, dark-red spots near to, but apparently separate from, the retinal vessels. They look like tiny haemorrhages but photography of injected preparations of retina show that they are in fact minute aneurysms arising mainly from the venous end of capillaries near areas of capillary closure.

Venous abnormalities are among the commonest manifestations of diabetic retinopathy. Dilatation, irregularity and increased tortuosity of the retinal veins are all seen.

Haemorrhages, most characteristically occurring in the deeper layers of the retina and hence round and regular in shape, are also a relatively early feature. The smaller ones may be difficult to differentiate from microaneurysms and the two are often grouped together as 'dots and blots'.

Soft exudates, similar to those seen in hypertension, occur. *Hard exudates* are more common and are specific to diabetic retinopathy. They are yellow, with irregular, sharply defined edges, varying in size from tiny specks to large confluent often circular patches.

New vessels may arise from mature vessels on the optic disc or the retina. The earliest appearance is that of fine tufts of delicate vessels forming arcades on the surface of the retina. As they grow they may extend forwards towards the vitreous. They are fragile, readily leak and at first have no visible connective tissue covering. They are liable to rupture, causing haemorrhage which may be intraretinal, preretinal (subhyaloid) or into the vitreous. Serous products leaking from these new vessel systems stimulate a connective tissue reaction. This *retinitis proliferans* first appears as a white cloudy haze among the network of new vessels. As it extends the new vessels are obliterated and the surrounding retina is covered by a dense white sheet. At this stage bleeding is less common but retinal detachment can occur due to contraction of adhesions between the vitreous and the retina.

CLASSIFICATION. Patients with only microaneurysms, retinal haemorrhages and exudates are classified as having *simple* or *background retino-pathy*, while those with preretinal haemorrhage, new vessel formation, or fibrous proliferation are classified as having *proliferative* or *malignant retinopathy*. As with nephropathy, the duration of diabetes is the most important factor influencing the occurrence of retinopathy and some abnormality, even if only a single microaneurysm, can be seen in the fundi of at least 60% of diabetics who have had the condition for 30 years.

INTERFERENCE WITH VISION. In general, prognosis for vision is good for patients with simple retinopathy and bad for those with proliferative retinopathy, of whom half are blind within 5 years. Microaneurysms, abnormalities of the veins, blot haemorrhages and exudates will not interfere seriously with vision unless they are associated with macular oedema or directly involve the macula. Unfortunately all these lesions occur most commonly in the perimacular area. New vessels may be completely symptomless until sudden visual loss occurs from a haemorrhage into the vitreous. Although these frequently clear, the risk of recurrence is high and the more frequent the haemorrhage the slower and less complete the recovery. New vessel formation is treatable. Fibrous tissue may obscure the retina and seriously damage sight, and retinal-vitreal adhesions may pull the retina forward and produce retinal detachment causing blindness. Retinitis proliferans is the irreversible end-stage of diabetic retinopathy which cannot be influenced by any form of treatment at present available. Early detection and treatment of new vessel formation is therefore of vital importance.

Prevention. As microangiopathy seems to be secondary to the metabolic abnormality and there is evidence to suggest that good control of the diabetes reduces the chance of its development and may delay its progression to severe diabetic retinopathy, every effort should be made to maintain a normal metabolic state in all diabeticpatients. It is a common error to suppose that diabetes which is 'mild', i.e. treated by diet alone, carries little risk of complications. Whatever the type of diabetes, duration of the disorder and sustained hyperglycaemia are the main factors associated with the development of microangiopathy.

Treatment. There is no specific treatment

of simple retinopathy. The diabetes and any hypertension must be well controlled. Clofibrate will clear hard exudates from the retina but will not affect any underlying neuronal degeneration. It may be of value in preventing further exudation but the possible benefits must be weighed against the risks (p. 490).

In simple retinopathy visual loss results from macular exudates, haemorrhage or oedema. Photocoagulation can be used to destroy abnormally leaking vessels in the perimacular area and thus reduce oedema. Coagulation of the centre of rings of hard exudates may hasten absorption of the exudates.

The primary aim in treating proliferative retinopathy is to destroy new vessels by photocoagulation before vitreous haemorrhage, macular damage or retinal detachment occur. Light coagulation of new vessels on the retina can be done under local anaesthesia, and in skilled, experienced hands is a simple procedure which carries little risk and can be very effective. All diabetic patients must therefore have their eyes examined regularly, every 6 to 12 months, by a competent observer. Once there is evidence of progression of simple retinopathy, and particularly whenever new vessels are seen, the patient must be referred to an ophthalmologist for further supervision and treatment.

Cataract. Very rarely a specific type of opacity of the lens (cataract) occurs in young diabetics whose disease has not been adequately controlled. Senile cataract also occurs in elderly diabetics, but is said to be no more common than in other people in this age group.

Infections

Poor control of diabetes is associated with a lowered resistance to infection. Alternatively latent diabetes may be unmasked by a severe infection such as a carbuncle or pneumonia. Glucose tolerance may return to normal, at least temporarily, when the infection is controlled by appropriate antimicrobial therapy. Cleanliness is a special virtue in the prevention of skin infection which is common in diabetes.

Pulmonary tuberculosis. If a diabetic under treatment shows unexplained loss of weight, increase in insulin requirements or symptoms of pulmonary disease, clinical and radiological examination of the lungs should be undertaken. Early diagnosis of tuberculosis and its specific treatment facilitates control of the diabetes.

Urinary tract infections. The presence of glucose in the urine provides a favourable medium for the growth of bacteria. Persistent infections of the urinary tract frequently occur. Specific therapy is required both for the urinary tract infection and the glycosuria.

Candidosis (p. 767) is a common cause of pruritus vulvae in the diabetic woman. In the majority, abolition of glycosuria brings rapid relief. In a few cases local nystatin cream and pessaries may be required.

Diabetic neuropathy

This is a common complication in diabetic patients. It is symptomless in the majority but causes severe disability in a few. Like retinopathy, neuropathy is related to the duration of diabetes and the degree of metabolic control. It can be divided into somatic and visceral or autonomic types. None of the classifications is entirely satisfactory since sensory, motor and autonomic nerves can be involved in varying combinations so that mixed syndromes frequently occur.

Clinical features. SYMMETRICAL, MAINLY SENSORY, POLYNEUROPATHY may be chronic or acute and is frequently asymptomatic. In a minority of patients, symptoms include paraesthesiae in the feet and sometimes in the hands, aching or lancinating pain in the lower limbs worse at night, burning sensations in the soles and difficulty in walking. Physical signs commonly include loss of tendon reflexes in the lower limbs, diminished vibration sense distally and 'glove and stocking' impairment of other modalities of sensation. There may be chronic and perforating ulcers in the feet and painless arthropathy (Charcot's joints). There may also be some motor involvement causing muscle weakness and wasting. On investigation both sensory and motor conduction velocity are reduced.

ASYMMETRICAL, MAINLY MOTOR, POLYNEUROPATHY (DIABETIC AMYOTROPHY) presents as severe, progressive, asymmetrical weakness and wasting of the proximal muscles of the lower (and occasionally also the upper) limbs. It is commonly accompanied by severe pain and sometimes there may be marked loss of weight (neuropathic cachexia).

MONONEUROPATHY. Either motor or sensory function may be affected within a single peripheral or cranial nerve. Those most commonly involved are the third and sixth cranial nerves resulting in diplopia, the ulnar and median nerves with entrapment in the carpal tunnel and the sciatic and lateral popliteal nerves leading to foot drop.

AUTONOMIC NEUROPATHY is not necessarily associated with somatic neuropathy. Either parasympathetic or sympathetic fibres or both may be affected in one or more systems in an individual patient. In the *cardiovascular system*, postural hypotension may occur as a result of damage to the sympathetic vasoconstrictor supply to the arteries in the lower limbs and splanchnic bed. There may also be resting tachycardia and loss of heart rate variation on deep breathing and standing up from the horizontal position. In the *gastrointestinal* tract there may be oesophageal atony, gastroparesis, and nocturnal diarrhoea with faecal incontinence. *Genito-urinary* autonomic neuropathy commonly causes impotence and may also result in an atonic bladder with recurrent urinary tract infection and overflow incontinence. *Sudomotor* phenomenon include profuse perspiration of the head and neck following ingestion of cheese or curry, drenching noctural sweats, and anhidrosis leading to fissures in the feet. *Vasomotor* phenomena include loss of peripheral vasomotor responses (patients complain of constantly cold feet) and dependent oedema due to loss of vasomotor tone and increased vascular permeability. *Pupillary* abnormalities include decreased pupil size, resistance to mydriatics and delayed or absent response to light. *Loss of awareness of hypoglycaemia* due to sympathetic neuropathy is common in long-standing diabetes and causes practical problems in the management of patients with IDDM.

Treatment. Symptomatic relief and a degree of functional improvement can sometimes be achieved in symmetrical sensory polyneuropathy by normalising the blood glucose concentration (e.g. by continuous subcutaneous infusion of insulin). The administration of aldose reductase inhibitors to control the accumulation of sorbitol in nerves has been shown to improve nerve conduction velocity and symptoms in a few patients. On the whole, however, treatment for the minority of patients who develop troublesome symptoms is disappointing. Severe pain and paraesthesiae may lead to depression resistant to analgesics and antidepressants.

In diabetic amyotrophy the prognosis is good with intensive treatment and most patients recover over a period of months or years.

The development of autonomic neuropathy is less clearly related to poor metabolic control than somatic neuropathy and improved control rarely results in amelioration of symptoms. The 5-year mortality is 50%.

SPECIAL PROBLEMS IN THE MANAGEMENT OF DIABETES MELLITUS

Diabetes in children. Fortunately diabetes is not common in childhood, but when it occurs it always requires treatment with insulin. The therapeutic problem of matching the dose of insulin to the food intake raises practical difficulties but the principles of treating children with diabetes are the same as for adults who have IDDM. It is important to achieve as good control of the diabetes as possible and children and their parents need to be educated in the management of the disorder to the limit of their ability.

Diet. The nutritional needs of diabetic children are essentially no different from those of other children. Because of growth caloric requirements of children are large in proportion to their size, by comparison with adult standards. It may be difficult to provide enough calories because children's preferences for foods are often unpredictable. On the other hand the child must not become too fat; hypoglycaemia due to too much insulin can lead to excessive appetite and hence to obesity. Diabetic children should not usually have sugar or sweets, but otherwise the diet need differ little from that of their friends. It is important that everything possible should be done to avoid distinguishing them from their contemporaries. A dietitian can do much to help the child and the parents.

Once trained, they may take part in the same range of activities as their peers, provided that appropriate supervision is arranged. The British Diabetic Association runs special camps for diabetic children.

Insulin. Day-to-day requirements for insulin are often very variable. Children's emotions and activities fluctuate unexpectedly — sometimes wildly active and sometimes sulking. This may have an important effect on their daily needs for insulin; excessive activity may result in hypoglycaemia, whilst lethargy may lead to hyperglycaemia. The latter may also be caused by any one of the numerous infectious diseases to which all children are prone. A combination of unmodified insulin and one of the depot insulins before breakfast, repeated before the main evening meal is a suitable arrangement for most diabetic children, providing the necessary flexibility. Children and parents need to have sufficient knowledge to make daily alterations in the dose of insulin on the basis of the results of preprandial urine or blood tests and factors such as exercise and illness.

Diabetes in pregnancy. If a diabetic woman wishes to have a child there is no reason, apart from genetic aspects (p. 488) why she should avoid pregnancy, provided that she suffers from none of the more serious complications of diabetes and provided she remains constantly under expert medical care. Nevertheless pregnancy in a diabetic woman carries certain definite risks. In the later stages of pregnancy she may develop an excessive accumulation of amniotic fluid; in addition the fetus is sometimes unusually large leading to difficulty in labour. Moreover the chances that a diabetic mother may lose her baby, either from a stillbirth or in the early neonatal period, are greater than those of a non-diabetic mother, even with the most careful supervision. Congenital malformation is more common in insulin-dependent diabetic pregnancy and now accounts for the majority of deaths.

The proper treatment of a pregnant diabetic patient requires the close and co-ordinated supervision of a team consisting of physician, obstetrician, anaesthetist, nurse and dietitian. The sooner the pregnancy is diagnosed the better. Some non-pregnant diabetic women often miss one or more menstrual periods, especially if their disease is poorly controlled. For this reason a laboratory test for pregnancy is often helpful. There are grounds for suggesting that oral hypoglycaemic agents might be teratogenic, and any diabetic patient who is taking these drugs and wishes to become pregnant should change to insulin.

Good control of the diabetes is the key to a successful pregnancy. A normal blood glucose concentration (HbA_1 8% or less) before and at the time of conception and throughout the pregnancy should be the aim. Further education of the patient may be needed in the proper management of her diet and insulin while at home. The diet, at first at least, need differ in no important respect from the diabetic diet to which she has been accustomed, but may need adjustment later, particularly with additional milk. Practical problems may be created for the physician and dietitian by bouts of vomiting that may occur in the early stages of pregnancy, and by the peculiar food fads which some pregnant women develop. The administration of highly purified unmodified and depot insulin before breakfast, unmodified insulin before the main evening meal, and an intermediate depot insulin at bedtime is the best regimen for most pregnant diabetic patients.

After the diagnosis of pregnancy the patient should be seen at first at fortnightly and later at weekly intervals. Continued control of the diabetes may be complicated by other factors. First, the renal threshold for glucose often falls as pregnancy advances. This is a normal phenomenon, but in the diabetic it means that the tests for glycosuria are even more unreliable than usual. Further, in the later stages of pregnancy, lactosuria may occasionally occur and may lead to confusion. For these reasons and because good diabetic control is mandatory, most patients will benefit from being taught to estimate their own blood glucose concentration. If excessive amounts of glucose are lost in the urine because of the lowered renal threshold, it may be necessary to give additional carbohydrate feeds between meals and sometimes at night, covered by suitable amounts of unmodified insulin to avoid ketosis. Then, too, the requirements for insulin usually increase as pregnancy advances. Frequent estimations of blood glucose are needed to ensure that an increase in insulin dosage, based on misleading urine tests, is not producing hypoglycaemia; or alternatively, that hyperglycaemia is not insidiously building up through failure to give enough insulin to meet an increase in insulin requirements.

Because of the risk in late pregnancy of sudden intrauterine death, pregnancy in a diabetic woman has hitherto seldom been allowed to proceed to term. Today with better metabolic control later delivery is possible and most are now delivered between the 38th and 39th week after induction of labour or if necessary by Caesarean section. Estimation of the lecithin/sphingomyelin ratio in the amniotic fluid is helpful in choosing a date for delivery. If the ratio is above 2.0 the risk of respiratory distress in the infant is low.

On the morning of delivery the usual breakfast and insulin should be replaced by an intravenous infusion of 10% glucose with 10 units of unmodified insulin added to each 500 ml. This should be given at a rate of 100 ml hourly. The blood glucose should be monitored at intervals of 1–2 hours and the rate of infusion and the dose of insulin adjusted to keep the blood glucose concentration at about 6.0 mmol/l. An alternative method is to give the insulin separately from the glucose infusion, by means of a constant-rate infusion pump at a rate of 1–2 units hourly. Whatever method is used administration of insulin should be stopped immediately on delivery and subcutaneous insulin resumed according to need as determined by urine and blood tests. Little or no insulin may be required for 12 hours after delivery. Thereafter, the pre-pregnancy dose can be gradually resumed.

A final word of warning is necessary. It has already been indicated that sugar in the urine is not unusual during normal pregnancy, either because of a fall in the renal threshold for glucose or through lactose appearing in the urine. The finding, however, of reducing substances in the urine of a pregnant woman should never be lightly dismissed as a normal phenomenon. Full clinical investigation to exclude diabetes is essential; otherwise a preventable catastrophe may follow. Since even minimal hyperglycaemia in pregnancy is associated with an increased fetal loss, the diagnostic criteria for diabetes in pregnancy are more stringent than those recommended for non-pregnant subjects (p. 468).

Diabetes and surgery. Any surgical operation, however minor, and the accompanying anaesthetic cause metabolic stress which the diabetic is less well able to meet than the normal person. Operations under local anaesthesia do not usually require special treatment of the diabetes. For operations under general anaesthesia two points must be kept in mind: the need to provide an adequate supply of energy for the tissues, and the need to be constantly on the alert for acidosis.

In practice there are two separate problems related to elective and emergency surgery:

1. ELECTIVE SURGERY IN A STABILISED DIABETIC. All diabetics should be admitted to hospital about 3 days before even a minor operation. During this period the control of the diabetes can be checked thoroughly. Provided a diabetic goes to the theatre in good condition, there is unlikely to be any significant change in the blood glucose, plasma bicarbonate or ketone levels during the operation.

A diabetic who is not on insulin can usually be managed without special care other than careful postoperative observation of the clinical state, glycosuria, ketonuria and blood glucose concentration. However, care must be taken to avoid hypoglycaemia in those taking a sulphonylurea and conversely insulin may be required if significant loss of control occurs.

In the case of insulin treated patients it is desirable that the operation should take place as early as possible in the morning. The patient should receive no breakfast and nothing by mouth before operation and the normal dose of insulin should be omitted. Before being transferred to the theatre the fasting blood glucose level should be determined. If this lies between 7.0 and 10.0 mmol/l (120 to 180 mg/100 ml) and surgery is minor, then no glucose or insulin need be given. If the level is below 5.0 mmol/l, then about 25 g of glucose should be given intravenously, preferably in hypertonic solution, in order to prevent possible hypoglycaemia (from the action of the previous day's depot insulin) during the operation. If the fasting blood sugar is over 10.0 mmol/l then some insulin will be required. About one third of the usual total daily dose is indicated, in the form of unmodified insulin, but its administration can usually be postponed until after operation. If a major surgical procedure is to be performed, intravenous 5% glucose or glucose saline should be given at a rate of 500 ml over 4 hours, along with unmodified insulin i.v. Either 12 units can be added to each 500 ml glucose or 1–3 units hourly can be given separately from the glucose infusion by a constant-rate infusion pump. The blood glucose concentration should be estimated frequently and the dose of insulin adjusted appropriately.

Recovery from the anaesthetic must be carefully supervised. The sooner the patient returns to the usual diet the better. This interval may be a few hours or several days, depending on the nature and severity of the operation. Within a few hours of recovery from the anaesthetic many patients are able to take fluid or semi-fluid feeds containing 25 g carbohydrate (p. 480) at 3- to 4-hourly intervals covered by suitable doses of unmodified insulin. After a major operation some insulin-dependent diabetics may need to have most of their energy requirements supplied as glucose, either intravenously or by mouth. If all has gone well, a single determination of the fasting blood glucose each morning will suffice. If recovery is stormy, measurements may be necessary at 4-hourly intervals or even more frequently. The determination of the plasma bicarbonate and electrolytes in the blood will also be helpful. The insulin dosage will depend on these findings, and until stability has been regained only unmodified insulin should be used.

Each specimen of urine must be tested for sugar and ketone bodies. If ketosis develops it is essential to take immediate steps to increase the metabolism of glucose by adjusting the dose of insulin.

2. DIABETES AND SURGICAL EMERGENCIES. Circumstances vary so much that it is impossible to consider them except in the most general way. The essentials are to maintain the oxidation of glucose by the tissues at a sufficient rate and to combat acidosis and electrolyte disturbances when they occur. This can be done effectively only if the state of the diabetic control is assessed continuously and accurately. A laboratory service that can provide rapid results is thus essential. As long as the surgical condition remains untreated

and the 'metabolic stress' continues, the diabetic condition is likely to get worse. Once the patient's surgical condition is under control a prompt response may be expected to appropriate therapy for the diabetes.

Prevention of diabetes mellitus

NIDDM is a disease of the prosperous, and in wealthy countries it is one of the major health problems. The hardships of the Second World War were associated with a marked decline in the incidence of NIDDM in European countries; rationing of both food and petrol was probably responsible. The importance to health of sufficient exercise and of avoiding dietary excess has been stated repeatedly. Diabetes, like obesity and atherosclerosis, is likely to arise in genetically predisposed persons who eat too much and exercise too little. Excess of dietary carbohydrate may strain the limited capacity of the pancreas to produce insulin, especially if it is in the form of sugar or other refined carbohydrate; excess of dietary fat may accelerate the complications of diabetes; atherosclerosis is a common cause of death in diabetics. In any event the public should be warned primarily against an overall excess of calories.

Investigation of the HLA system has shown that certain individuals have an increased risk of developing IDDM and that genetic factors may also play a part in susceptibility to develop complications. These genetic characteristics of susceptibility and the relevant environmental factors need to be defined more precisely before appropriate preventive measures can be taken.

SCREENING. It is much easier to control the disease and to maintain the health of the patient in a state which allows a normal life to be led, if the diagnosis is made early. In many patients the biochemical changes can be detected before the symptoms are sufficiently severe to make them seek medical advice. Any screening technique is expensive and should be used only if it is likely that a significant number of new diabetics will be recognised. High-risk groups, for example the first degree relatives of known diabetics, the obese and the mothers of babies weighing more than 4.5 kg at birth, will give a particularly high yield.

The prevalence of diabetes in different communities varies from 0.5 to 5%. These figures vary widely according to the social and economic state of the people and the educational and medical services available.

Urine testing has been widely used as a screening procedure. As up to 3% of people may have renal glycosuria and so will have to be recalled for blood tests, and as a number of undoubted diabetics will be missed owing to their raised renal threshold for glucose, this is an unsatisfactory procedure. Whenever practicable, estimation of the blood glucose 2 hours after 75 g glucose orally is recommended as the screening procedure.

Quite apart from screening high-risk groups it is not difficult to make out a case for a routine test of the urine for glucose in every full clinical examination; and all those with glycosuria (albeit of minor degree) should be considered diabetic until proved otherwise.

GENETIC COUNSELLING. Diabetic patients will often consult their doctor about the advisability of having children. They can be told that the risks of pregnancy and delivery are little greater for a diabetic mother than for a normal woman, provided she submits to the strict discipline required. The chances that she will produce a healthy baby are also good, but not quite so good as for a normal mother. The chances that her child will subsequently develop diabetes are higher than normal (p. 16) but most diabetics have healthy children, and how strongly a doctor should word these necessary warnings is a matter for judgement in each case. The family history, the severity of the disease in the parents and their educational and economic background, must all be considered.

Conclusion. The management of a patient with diabetes mellitus offers a special opportunity for good medical practice, there being few other chronic diseases in which efficient management makes so much difference to the patient's life. The problems presented by the aetiology of diabetes and its long-term complications continue to offer some of the most demanding and fascinating challenges in medical research today.

OTHER METABOLIC DISEASES

Metabolism is as fundamental as life itself; in medicine the term is usually restricted to disorders which can best be described in biochemical terms.

Many metabolic disorders are acquired. Others are congenital. The genetic aetiology of numerous inborn errors of metabolism has been identified with abnormalities of the structure or function of DNA and the pattern of their inheritance mapped by the study of a particular biochemical disorder. The vast majority of inborn errors of metabolism are rare and it would be inappropriate to describe them here. The reader will find much further information in specialised textbooks (p. 492).

Metabolic disorders may be classified in various ways, for example by the mode of inheritance or by the chemical factors involved. The specific enzyme deficiency responsible for the disorder, or the body system principally affected may be named. Disorders of carbohydrate, protein or amino acid, lipid or mineral metabolism may be predominant features, and a few examples of these are given below.

Carbohydrate. Diabetes mellitus is by far the most frequent and important disorder of carbohydrate metabolism. Rare genetic errors lead to abnormalities in the metabolism of galactose (galactosaemia), fructose (fructosuria), and glycogen (glycogen storage diseases, such as von Gierke's disease, p. 580).

Amino acids. Inborn errors account for many relatively rare diseases such as cystinuria (p. 373) and the Fanconi syndrome (p. 373). Phenylketonuria is also rare but leads to mental retardation if not detected in the neonatal period and treated with a special diet.

Purines. Gout is a classical example of a metabolic disorder and is described on page 579, along with other causes of arthritis.

Lipids are complex substances among which cholesterol and triglyceride are the most useful indices for the detection and monitoring of hyperlipidaemia. Lipids circulate as lipoproteins (chylomicrons, low and high density lipoproteins), while free fatty acids are bound to albumin (p. 328). Analysis of fasting serum lipids and particularly of lipoproteins provides a useful classification of the hyperlipidaemias as devised by WHO, and based particularly on the work of Fredrickson (Table 12.3). In this classification there are five major types (I–V) of hyperlipidaemia due either to genetic defects in lipid metabolism or to

Table 12.3 Classification of hyperlipidaemia. LDL = low density lipoproteins, VLDL = very low density lipoproteins, N = normal. β refers to electrophoretic mobility.

Fredrickson type	Lipoproteins elevated	Lipids		Treatment group
		Cholesterol	Triglycerides	
I	Chylomicrons	N or +	+	3
IIa	LDL	+	N	1
IIb	LDL, VLDL	+	+	2
III	abnormal VLDL (broad β pattern)	+	+	2
IV	VLDL	N or +	+	2
V	Chylomicrons VLDL	+	+	2

environmental factors such as diet, alcohol and drugs, including oestrogens and cortico-steroids. Measurement of lipoproteins is usually not necessary for management which can generally be determined by clinical observation along with measurement of fasting serum cholesterol and triglyceride.

Hyperlipidaemias

Primary hyperlipidaemia. Such patients can for most clinical purposes be placed in one of three groups. Two of these are metabolically heterogeneous but treatment can usually be allocated on a group basis.

Group 1 consists of those with hypercholesterol-aemia and normal triglycerides (Fredrickson's Type IIa). The serum is clear, and low density (β) lipoproteins increased. Most patients have mild to moderate hypercholesterolaemia (7–10 mmol/l) and physical signs are usually absent although early arcus senilis or xanthelasma may be present. The disorder is relatively common in Britain and is a risk factor for ischaemic heart disease. It is usually weakly inherited and environ-mental factors, such as the dietary intake of saturated fat and cholesterol, are probably important in its aetiology.

About 5% of patients with hypercholesterol-aemia have a more sharply defined disorder trans-mitted as an autosomal dominant and present from birth. Serum cholesterol levels range from 8–16 mmol/l in heterozygotes and from 16–32 mmol/l in the rare homozygotes. In this dis-order clinical stigmata of hyperlipidaemia are

frequent. Tendon xanthomas and arthritis (p. 573) are common. Arcus senilis and xanthelasma on the eyelids are often prominent and 50% have ischaemic heart disease by the time they are 50 years old.

Group 2 comprises those with predominant hypertriglyceridaemia (Fedrickson's Types IIb, III, IV and V). The serum is cloudy, triglyceride and very low density (pre-β) lipoproteins increased, and cholesterol may be normal or, if increased, the rise is usually less pronounced than that of triglyceride. Specific physical signs are uncommon although xanthomas can occur. Obes-ity, impaired carbohydrate tolerance and hyper-uricaemia often coexist. There is a strong associa-tion with ischaemic heart disease and this group is also relatively common in Britain.

Group 3 is represented by Fredrickson's Type I. This is a rare disorder consisting of chylo-micronaemia resulting from deficiency of extra-hepatic lipoprotein lipase.

Secondary hyperlipidaemia occurs in association with diabetes mellitus, and in hypo-thyroidism, the nephrotic syndrome, biliary obstruction and pancreatitis.

Treatment. Control of *primary hyperlipid-aemia* always requires dietary measures. Obesity must be corrected in every case. The low calorie diet on page 809 can be appropriately modified in relation to the fat content.

Groups 1 and 2 should have a fat-modified diet in which the intake of cholesterol is restricted and the total fat intake is reduced to provide about 36% of the total calories. The intake of saturated fat is reduced, while the intake of polyunsaturated fat is increased to provide a polyunsaturated: saturated fat ratio of more than 1:1. A list of foods to be avoided is given on page 811. An abnormal sensitivity to carbohydrate and/or alcohol is responsible for inducing hyperlipidaemia in some of those in Group 2 who will require to restrict their consumption of sucrose and alcohol, even if they are not obese.

Group 3 patients improve dramatically with restriction of fat intake to about 25 g daily.

If dietary measures alone are insufficient to control the hyperlipidaemia, Group 1 patients should first be given cholestyramine. An incomplete response in these patients may be improved by the addition of nicotinic acid. Patients in Group 2 usually respond to nicotinic acid. Indications for the use of clofibrate came under scrutiny when two extensive clinical trials of this drug for the primary prevention of ischaemic heart disease revealed an increased mortality from ischaemic heart disease, cerebrovascular disorders and neoplasms, particularly of the respiratory and gastrointestinal tracts, among treated individuals. This excess mortality is unexplained but the use of clofibrate should be strictly confined to the few cases of severe hyperlipidaemia which have failed to respond to the measures outlined above and where the clinical benefit seems likely to be greater than the risk associated with medication. Those in this category are likely to include patients with the relatively uncommon Fredrickson's Type III hyperlipoproteinaemia (broad-β-band disease) which is associated with early-onset peripheral vascular disease and cardiac ischaemia and those with severe endogenous hypertriglyceridaemia (Fredrickson's Type IV or V hyperlipoproteinaemia) where there is a risk of acute relapsing pancreatitis when the plasma triglyceride concentration exceeds 6–7 mmol/l.

Secondary hyperlipidaemia usually responds to treatment of the underlying condition when this is possible.

PROSPECTS IN DIABETES MELLITUS

The scale of the clinical problem presented by diabetic patients with disease of both large and small blood vessels, the mounting evidence that

although genetic factors may increase individual susceptibility the excess mortality and morbidity incurred by these patients is secondary to the metabolic disturbance, the introduction of better methods of assessing diabetic control, the realisation that at present normal or near normal metabolism is achieved in only a minority of treated diabetic patients, and an increased understanding of the deficiencies and limitations of conventional treatment have led to a search for better methods of treatment and for possible ways of preventing diabetes.

Obese patients with NIDDM represent about half the total diabetic population. Although they frequently have marked hyperglycaemia it is possible to restore normal metabolism in most of these patients by effective dietary treatment leading to significant reduction in weight and this form of treatment has no disadvantage whatsoever. However, published reports and daily clinical experience suggest that in practice the results of treatment are particularly poor in this large group of patients. This is due partly to lack of skilled advice in relation to diet at diagnosis and partly to the difficulty of maintaining motivation on a long-term basis. Essential components of effective therapeutic programmes have included a permanent dietitian attached to the diabetic clinic as an integral part of the team, individually prescribed diets, close supervision, and education of patients in both the nature of the relationship between obesity and diabetes and the potential hazards of non-compliance. The development of better methods of delivering effective treatment and of educating and motivating this group of patients to change their way of life is the top priority here.

Conventional treatment of patients with IDDM using subcutaneous injections of insulin is far from ideal since it is not only inconvenient and inflexible, but also achieves normal or near normal metabolism in only a minority of patients. Such treatment makes unrealistic demand on some patients, for example adolescents, a proportion of whom have low self-esteem and become depressed and negative in their outlook.

The need to raise morale and motivation is increasingly recognised, for example by avoiding hospital admission wherever possible, by providing a 'hotline' advice service and special informal clinics for young people, and by encouraging the creation of self-help groups.

Improved control can be achieved with battery-powered portable pumps, providing continuous subcutaneous, intramuscular or intravenous infusion of insulin. In these systems insulin is delivered at fixed rates (a low basal rate and one or more higher rates before main meals) with no reference to the blood glucose concentration. Like conventional treatment their successful use requires a high degree of patient motivation and has the particular disadvantage that if the pump fails the onset of ketosis tends to be more rapid than with conventional treatment because there is no subcutaneous depot of insulin. These systems are unsuitable for general therapeutic use at present since they are still relatively large and unreliable, do not invariably incorporate an automatic failure alarm, and lack a glucose sensor device.

'Artificial pancreas' systems consist of three basic components: a mechanism for estimating the blood glucose concentration, an insulin delivery pump, and a computer controller which regulates the administration of insulin on the basis of the blood glucose level. Ideally such a device should be small enough for implantation and measure blood glucose without consuming blood. Existing systems use blood and are large, extracorporeal, relatively unreliable and very expensive. They have few clinical applications, but have some use as an investigative tool.

Use of pancreatic transplantation as a treatment for IDDM is associated with many problems. These relate particularly to the exocrine pancreas, the supply of human organs, and the autoimmune destruction of implanted insulin secreting cells. Several approaches have been tried to overcome the digestion of tissue by the secretions of the exocrine pancreas. These include ligation of the pancreatic duct or injection of inert material into the ductal system, but none has been entirely successful. Immunosuppression is required, probably on a permanent basis to avoid both graft rejection and autoimmune destruction of the transplanted endocrine pancreatic tissue, whether whole organ or isolated islets. Use of the latter avoids the problems associated with the exocrine pancreas, but there are difficulties such as the supply, purification and storage of islets. Attempts have been made to enclose islets in semipermeable membrane capsules to protect against both rejection and autoimmune destruction.

From a public health standpoint the only cost-effective way of dealing with IDDM is to prevent it. Immunosuppression using a variety of methods has been tried in newly diagnosed patients with IDDM. Cyclosporin gives the best results but considerable variation is reported in different studies and in individual patients within studies and it seems clear that, as in transplanted patients, immunosuppression is required on a long-term basis. Elucidation of the precise sequence of events leading to autoimmune destruction of the endocrine pancreas and the identification of accurate predictive markers for the development of clinical disease as distinct from genetic susceptibility, offer the hope that a rational therapeutic approach based on more specific immuno-modulation in the pre-diabetic period will emerge.

JOYCE D. BAIRD
Diabetes mellitus and other metabolic diseases

W.J. IRVINE
Diseases of the thyroid and adrenal glands

C.R.W. EDWARDS
Diseases of the hypothalamus, pituitary, and parathyroid glands and sexual disorders

FURTHER READING:

Endocrinology:
Edwards C R W 1986 Integrated clinical science: endocrinology. Heinemann, London. This book provides the undergraduate with both the basic science and clinical aspects of endocrinology including diabetes mellitus.
Hall R, Anderson J, Smart G A, Besser M 1980 Fundamentals of clinical endocrinology, 3rd edn. Pitman Medical, London. A very good general textbook
Williams D H 1981 Textbook of endocrinology. Saunders, Philadelphia. A large comprehensive source of reference of particular value to the postgraduate student
Belchetz P E 1984 Management of pituitary disease. Chapman and Hall, London. A useful book covering all aspects of the physiology and pathophysiology of the pituitary

Diabetes mellitus:
Alberti K G M M, Krall L P 1985 The diabetic annual, 1. Elsevier, Amsterdam
Keen H, Jarrett R J 1982 Complications of diabetes, 3rd edn. Arnold, London

Nattrass M 1986 Recent advances in diabetes. Churchill Livingstone, Edinburgh

Metabolic disorders:

Beaumont J L, Carlson L A, Cooper G R, Fejfar Z, Fredrickson D S, Stasser T 1970 Classification of hyperlipidaemias and hyperlipoproteinaemias. Bulletin of the World Health Organization 43: 891. This is a definitive classification agreed by a WHO specialist committee.

Lewis B 1976 The hyperlipidaemias. Clinical and laboratory practice. Blackwell Scientific Publications, Oxford

Bondy P K, Rosenberg L E 1980 Metabolic control and disease, 8th edn. Saunders, London

Stanbury J B, Wyngaarden J B, Fredrickson D S 1980 The metabolic basis of inherited disease, 5th edn. McGraw-Hill, New York

Periodicals:

Most textbooks have a problem in keeping up to date in areas of rapid progress and endocrinology is one of these. Students thus need to consult journals for recent advances. In addition to the general medical periodicals which frequently publish endocrine articles the most valuable clinical journals are the Journal of Clinical Endocrinology and Metabolism, and Clinical Endocrinology.

13

Diseases of the blood

BLOOD FORMATION

Blood cells are formed both in the liver and the spleen up to the fifth month of fetal life. Thereafter normal formation of the red cells, the granular series of white cells and the platelets takes place increasingly in the medullary cavity of bones and from birth onwards is restricted to these sites. Lymphocytes originate in the bone marrow. Some migrate to the thymus where they are processed to become T lymphocytes and are found in the interfollicular areas of lymph nodes, spleen and circulating in blood. Others, which become B lymphocytes, migrate to the follicular areas of lymph nodes and spleen.

During childhood there is a progressive diminution in the amount of red haemopoietic marrow so that in the young adult it is confined to the heads of the femur and humerus, to flat bones such as the sternum, ribs and ilia and to the vertebrae, the rest of the marrow cavity being occupied by fat. The red marrow may extend into the shafts of the long bones, replacing the fat, when there is an increased demand for blood formation. Blood cells have a finite life span and require to be continuously replaced. Newly formed cells are provided by actively proliferating cell systems in the marrow, spleen and lymph nodes.

There is evidence which suggests that all blood cells are derived from a totipotent haemopoietic stem cell (THSC). Cells which will mature into lymphocytes appear to arise from this cell at a very early stage of differentiation and cells destined to become the 'myeloid' elements at a slightly later stage (Fig. 13.1). In the latter, pluripotent myeloid stem cells (PMSC) are formed which, in turn, give rise to cells committed to one or another maturation pathway such as the erythroid, granulocyte/monocyte and megakaryocyte cell systems. On the lymphoid side, pre-B and pre-T stem cells are formed which mature to become B and T lymphocytes respectively. Normally, the THSC and the PMSC are in an inactive (G_0) phase, but can be stimulated to cell production and self-replication when depletion of more differentiated elements occurs. The stem cells are not clearly recognisable in the marrow until they are fully committed to a maturation pathway. Given a suitable environment, individual primitive blood cells will become colony-forming units (Fig. 13.1) which mature along certain lines. Such cells, like the more primitive stem cells, are probably capable of self-sustaining replication as well as providing cells for maturation. They appear to be susceptible to humoral influences and cell-cell interaction which stimulate and control proliferation. Certain disease states which involve the totipotent stem cell affect all the haemopoietic cell lines while other disorders may affect only one or other of the lines. The latter are, in some instances, easier to treat since there is the possibility of regenerating normal marrow from the totipotent stem cells.

Of the three types of cell found in the blood, erythrocytes and platelets are true blood cells. They differ from most other cells in the body in that they have no nuclei. Leucocytes are cells which use the blood to migrate from the marrow

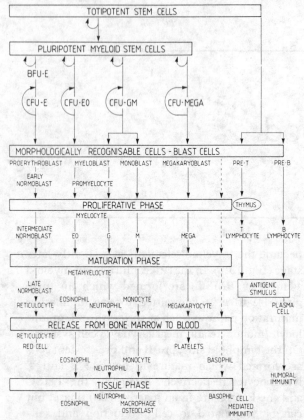

Fig. 13.1 Origin and development of blood cells.
Curved arrows represent self-replication. BFU-E = burst
forming units — erythroid; CFU = colony forming unit;
CFU-E = CFU erythroid; CFU-EO = CFU eosinophil;
CFU-GM = CFU granulocyte–monocyte; CFU-MEGA =
CFU-megakaryocyte; EO = eosinophil; G = granulocyte;
M = monocyte; MEGA = megakaryocyte.

or other production sites to the tissues where they
function. Thus leucocytes in the circulation form
only a very small fraction of the total white cell
mass.

The red blood cells (erythrocytes)

The earliest identifiable red cell precursor in the
marrow is the pro-erythroblast, a large cell with
a nucleolated nucleus and deeply basophilic cytoplasm. This cell undergoes a series of divisions
rapidly so that the daughter cells do not have
time to regrow between divisions and become
progressively smaller. At the same time, maturation proceeds with the formation of haemoglobin in the cytoplasm. Early, intermediate and late

normoblasts can be identified (Fig. 13.1).

Proliferation ceases at the intermediate normo-
blast stage and maturation is then completed
with condensation of the nuclear chromatin and
eventual ejection of the nuclear remnant. At this
stage the cell still has the capacity to synthesise
haemoglobin, due to the presence of ribosomes in
the cytoplasm. This ribosomal material gives the
cell a faintly bluish colour with Romanowsky
stains. Supravital staining with new methylene
blue causes condensation of the ribosomes to form
reticular material which makes these cells easy to
identify, and they can be counted as *reticulocytes*.
The reticulocyte matures into an adult red cell in
about 3 days and is released to the circulation
about half way through this period. Under stress,
marrow reticulocytes can be released sooner, raising the reticulocyte count without an increase in
erythropoiesis. These 'marrow' reticulocytes can
be recognised as they have a much more dense
central aggregate of reticulum with supravital
stains. Usually an absolute increase in the number
of reticulocytes reflects increased erythropoiesis.
After the first few days of life there are, in health,
no nucleated red cells in the peripheral blood.
The presence of normoblasts indicates excessive
or abnormal blood formation or irritation of the
bone marrow by invasion with foreign elements.

The mature erythrocyte is a circular biconcave
disc with a mean diameter of 7.2 μm. There is an
excess of membrane which is partly responsible
for the biconcave shape but the maintenance of
this shape requires energy supplied by glycolysis.
This unusual morphology gives the red cell considerable plasticity enabling it to pass through
capillaries and other structures of small diameter.
In some disorders red cells may lose membrane
becoming progressively more spherical and rigid.
As a result it is more susceptible to destruction
particularly in the spleen, which is uniquely
adapted to filtering out such cells. The spleen also
removes inclusion bodies from red cells without
destroying the cells.

The red cell membrane is a complex dynamic
structure, one function of which is to maintain
high levels of potassium and low levels of sodium
in the cell by means of the ionic pumps. The
surface of the membrane also carries antigenic
determinants for the various blood groups.

Iron is essential for haemoglobin synthesis. Other factors which influence erythropoiesis include vitamin B$_{12}$ (p. 504), folate (p. 504), thyroxine, vitamin C, androgens and possibly trace elements such as copper and manganese.

Erythropoiesis is controlled by a hormone, erythropoietin, produced mainly in the kidneys. There cells, which are probably located in the tubules, monitor the provision of oxygen to the tissues and respond to hypoxia by the production of erythropoietin. It acts mainly on the stem cells stimulating increased activity.

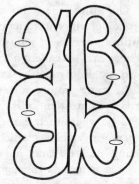

Fig. 13.2 Haemoglobin A (schematic). Each alpha and beta globin chain carries a haem moiety in its folds.

Haemoglobin

Haemoglobin in the erythrocyte provides the oxygen transport mechanism of the blood. Red cells also convey carbon dioxide from the tissues to the lungs buffering the carbonic acid formed in the red cell (p. 95). Haemoglobin is a complex molecule, a conjugate of a red pigment (haem) with protein (globin). Haem is formed under the control of the enzyme ALA synthetase by the condensation of glycine and succinyl coenzyme A to form amino levulinic acid. There follows a series of synthetic steps which build the porphyrin ring, at the end of which the enzyme haem-synthetase (ferrochelatase) inserts iron into the ring and haem is formed. Each step in this synthetic pathway requires its own enzyme, deficiency of which gives rise to various forms of porphyria.

The globin fraction of normal adult haemoglobin (haemoglobin A) consists of four paired polypeptide chains, two alpha chains of 141 amino acids and two beta chains of 146 amino acids (Fig. 13.2). Haemoglobin F, the fetal haemoglobin, differs by having two gamma chains instead of beta chains. Haemoglobin A2, which is found in small amounts of between 2–3% of the total haemoglobin in adults, has two delta chains instead of beta chains. Each globin chain carries one haem moiety in a specially constructed 'pocket' formed by the folds of the chain.

One molecule of oxygen is carried by each haem fraction in the haemoglobin molecule which is therefore capable of carrying four molecules of oxygen. Beta, gamma and delta chains are incapable of accepting oxygen to their haem pockets until the alpha chains have taken up oxygen. When this occurs a configurational change in the haemoglobin molecule prises open the haem pockets of the other chains, allowing them to accept oxygen. Thus the more oxygen the haemoglobin molecule has, the more easily it acquires further oxygen until saturated. In the tissues the reverse occurs, easy loss becoming more difficult as haemoglobin becomes desaturated. This function can be influenced further by a byproduct of glucose metabolism, 2–3-diphosphoglycerate (2–3-DPG). The concentration of 2–3-DPG in the red cell affects the avidity of the haemoglobin molecule for oxygen by reversible combination with deoxygenated haemoglobin. Increased levels of 2–3-DPG decrease haemoglobin's oxygen affinity and improve release to the tissues. Under hypoxic conditions, 2–3-DPG levels in the red cells increase as a compensatory mechanism. This is the first step in acclimatisation at high altitude; it occurs within 24–48 hours, long before there is any increase in red cell numbers stimulated by increased erythropoietin production.

The white blood cells (leucocytes)

White blood cells are found in the blood as they migrate from bone marrow to the tissues. In any one individual the number is remarkably constant showing only minor diurnal variation. There are five morphologically distinct types of white cell. Three of these, known as granulocytes or polymorphonuclear leucocytes, are characterised by specific granules in their cytoplasm. A fourth type of cell, the monocyte, is closely related to the granulocytes. The fifth is the lymphocyte, a distinct cell, morphologically and functionally.

The granular series (*polymorphonuclear leucocytes*). These are so called because of the granules shown by Romanowsky stains in the cytoplasm of the more mature forms. Granulocytes are derived from stem cells in the bone marrow (Fig. 13.1), where their earliest recognisable precursors are myeloblasts which have large nuclei containing nucleoli and no cytoplasmic granules. Myeloblasts mature through promyelocyte, myelocyte and metamyelocyte stages with coarsening of nuclear chromatin and development of cytoplasmic granules. In later stages of maturation the nucleus becomes kidney shaped and finally segments into lobes connected by thin chromatin strands. The cells are classified as neutrophil, eosinophil or basophil according to the staining reactions of their granules.

The production of granulocytes is probably regulated by humoral influences, such as colony stimulating factor, at least some of which are produced locally in the marrow microenvironment by mononuclear phagocytic cells and fat cells. There appears to be a close and inverse relationship between the numbers of monocytes and neutrophils.

Immature granulocytes, such as myelocytes, are found when the production of leucocytes is being stimulated by severe pyogenic infection and an increase in the cytoplasmic granulation may also be seen (toxic granulation). In adults the appearance of more primitive forms in the blood, such as myeloblasts and promyelocytes, indicates a serious disturbance of marrow function such as invasion by metastases or neoplastic change as in leukaemia.

Neutrophil granulocytes are phagocytic cells which ingest bacteria and fungi. Once mature, neutrophils may be held in the marrow for varying periods as part of a reserve pool of cells. Sooner or later the cells migrate out of the marrow and circulate in the blood for, on average, about 7 hours. They leave the circulation by adhering to the capillary endothelium (marginating) and migrating through the vessel wall into the tissues. It is thought that this is promoted by chemotaxis. A considerable proportion of neutrophils in the blood may be marginated. Certain stress factors

such as exercise and emotion may return these cells to the circulating blood causing a rise in white cell count. Their granules contain lysozyme and other substances which are discharged into the vacuole created by the ingestion of bacteria and which assist in the killing and digestion of the bacteria. The products of autodigestion from cells killed by organisms (pus cells) are potent stimulants of fresh neutrophil formation by the marrow. Pyrogens are also released. Neutrophils ingest uric acid crystals and may disintegrate in the process, liberating tissue damaging substances and causing local inflammation.

Apart from responding to infection, neutrophils also produce a vitamin B_{12} binding protein, transcobalamin III, which explains the high levels of vitamin B_{12} in the serum in conditions in which there is a greatly increased number of neutrophils, e.g. chronic myeloid leukaemia.

The degree of segmentation of neutrophils varies from unsegmented to five segments. The number of segments appears to have no functional importance. A failure to segment, with the formation of 'band' cells, occurs in toxic conditions and under such circumstances the degree of segmentation tends to diminish. This is called a 'shift to the left'. A 'shift to the right', in which there is increased segmentation, occurs in disorders such as vitamin B_{12} and folate deficiency and also in iron deficiency.

Mature neutrophil granulocytes account for more than 50% of the total leucocytes in the peripheral blood in a healthy adult; a huge reserve is held in the marrow and they are also present in large numbers in various organs and tissues.

Eosinophil granulocytes are also produced in the marrow. Factors influencing this are poorly understood but T lymphocytes appear to exert some control. Eosinophils are also phagocytic but less actively so than neutrophils. They are associated with allergic reactions, ingest antigen-antibody complexes and are concerned in processes involving foreign proteins, such as hypersensitivity reactions and in association with parasitic infections.

Basophil granulocytes are poorly phagocytic. The Fc portion of the IgE molecule is attached to specific binding sites on their surface. Activation of this by antigens results in degranulation of the cell with the release of histamine. Thus basophils participate in immediate hypersensitivity reactions in the same way as mast cells (tissue basophils) as described on page 24. Basophils also contain heparin which may be released to participate in lipid metabolism.

Monocytes derive from the same precursor elements that produce the granulocyte. They partially mature into cells with an irregularly shaped nucleus in a cloudy blue cytoplasm containing numerous minute red granules. Monocytes are motile and phagocytic and migrate into the tissues where they develop further into various types of macrophages such as tissue macrophages, Kupffer cells, osteoclasts and possibly fat cells. There they constitute the *monocyte–macrophage system*, previously known as the reticuloendothelial system, which removes debris as well as micro-organisms and collects and presents antigenic material to lymphocytes (p. 23).

Lymphocytes originate from committed stem cells in the bone marrow. Some migrate to the thymus where they are processed to become T lymphocytes. Others become B lymphocytes and a few become cytotoxic killer cells. About 75% of circulating lymphocytes are T cells. The rest are B cells and a few are 'null' cells showing neither T nor B characteristics. Both B cells and T cells respond to antigenic stimuli by transformation, in the case of B lymphocytes to plasma cells producing immunoglobulin. Their functions are described on page 23.

The platelets (thrombocytes)

Platelets are derived from megakaryocytes in the bone marrow. Megakaryocytes are very large cells containing multilobulated nuclei and granular cytoplasm from which the platelets are formed by budding. With Romanowsky staining, platelets are seen as small (2–4 μm), hyaline, non-nucleated bodies with blue or purple granules. Platelet life span is estimated to be about 10 days and destruction is mostly in the spleen if the platelet is not used in haemostasis. Production appears to be regulated by thrombopoietins. The main role of platelets is in haemostasis by adhering to areas of vascular injury and promoting aggregation of more platelets. Aggregation goes through primary

(reversible) and secondary (irreversible) stages with shape change and release of thromboxane A2 and other factors required in blood coagulation (p. 542).

Normal haemotological values

These are given in Table 21.8 (p. 819).

Blood destruction

Destruction of all formed elements of the blood occurs in the monocyte-macrophage system. The survival time of the mature erythrocytes in the peripheral blood is approximately 110 to 120 days. This is the period estimated by cross-transfusion experiments and represents the mean life span. A more practical technique for investigational use is one in which red cells labelled with ^{51}Cr are transfused and the time taken for half of the radioactivity to disappear is measured. By this method the half-life of the radioactivity in the red cells is 25 to 35 days and is shorter than the true half-life because of the elution of chromium from the cells. As red cells age their enzyme activity declines, the cells become defective and are removed from the blood and broken down in the monocyte-macrophage system. The degradation of haemoglobin yields iron from haem which is mostly utilised by the marrow for synthesis of fresh haemoglobin. The iron-free residual pigment, biliverdin, is converted to bilirubin and carried by the plasma to the liver for excretion. The globin is recycled.

The life span of granulocytes is probably about 3 to 4 days, of which less than 24 hours is spent in the circulation. The life span of monocytes and lymphocytes is less certain. It appears that there are short lived lymphocytes (3 days) and long lived lymphocytes (e.g. memory cells, p. 23) which may re-enter the circulation at intervals for many years.

Terms relating to blood disorders

Microcytosis means that the average size of the red cells is reduced. It is commonly found in iron deficiency anaemia and other disorders of haemoglobin synthesis.

Macrocytosis means that the average size of the

red cells is greater than normal. It is seen, for instance, in megaloblastic anaemias but its occurrence does not necessarily mean megaloblastic change in the marrow.

Hypochromia exists when the red cells contain less than the normal amount of haemoglobin. They stain less deeply and show greater than normal central pallor. The mean corpuscular haemoglobin concentration (MCHC) is below normal. Hypochromia is commonly associated with microcytosis and is a characteristic feature of iron deficiency anaemia.

Anisocytosis means inequality in the size of the red cells. It is found in many forms of anaemia but is most prominent in megaloblastic anaemia.

Poikilocytosis means marked irregularity in the shape of the red cells. It is never present without anisocytosis and usually reflects dyserythropoiesis.

Elliptocytosis means elliptical red cells; *ovalocytosis* refers to a less marked abnormality. Such cells are found in small numbers in a variety of disorders such as megaloblastic and hypochromic anaemias. When the majority of cells are oval or elliptical it indicates a hereditary disorder of dominant type which is usually clinically benign; in less than 10% of cases, a haemolytic state exists and may cause anaemia.

Target cells are abnormally flat red cells with a central mass of haemoglobin surrounded by a ring of pallor and an outer ring of haemoglobin. They are commonly associated with liver disease, impaired splenic function (hyposplenism) and haemoglobinopathies.

Polychromasia and reticulocytosis. Young red cells when stained by the Romanowsky method have a faint bluish colour (*basophilia*) due to residual ribosomal material. A blood film in which such cells are present in increased numbers along with those of normal pink colour is said to show polychromasia. This, like reticulocytosis (p. 494), indicates increased production of new red cells by the bone marrow.

Punctate basophilia. Pathologically damaged young red cells may show several deep blue dots in the cytoplasm with Romanowsky staining. Such punctate basophilia may be found in any severe anaemia, but the presence of many of these cells is most commonly seen in β-thalassaemia and

chronic lead poisoning where it may occur when the anaemia is slight.

Nucleated red cells are usually normoblasts and are found in the blood when erythropoiesis is very vigorous or when there is irritation of the bone marrow, as in leukaemia, or infiltration by secondary tumour.

Leucocytosis means an increase in the total number of white blood cells (over $11.0 \times 10^9/l$ in adults). This may take the form of a polymorphonuclear leucocytosis in which the increase is due to the outpouring of many young neutrophil granulocytes, as occurs in the presence of pyogenic infections. Alternatively it may take the form of a lymphocytosis, as is frequently found in whooping cough. Infants commonly respond to infections by producing a lymphocytosis.

Leucopenia means a decrease in the total number of white cells below $4.0 \times 10^9/l$ and usually involves a reduction only of the granulocytes (*neutropenia*). Leucopenia is found in tuberculosis, enteric fever, many acute viral infections, brucellosis and in hypoplastic and aplastic anaemia. Occasionally leucopenia is found in overwhelming infections and is a bad prognostic sign. In a small number of patients it may be constitutional and represent no threat to health. In others it may be early evidence of developing acute leukaemia.

Eosinophilia is the term used when the number of eosinophil granulocytes exceeds $0.4 \times 10^9/l$. Eosinophilia is found most commonly in infections with worms, in allergic diseases, Hodgkin's lymphoma and polyarteritis nodosa. Rarely it may be familial or idiopathic.

Monocytosis refers to a monocyte count exceeding $0.8 \times 10^9/l$ and is found in advanced tuberculosis, malaria and in some neutropenic states.

Thrombocytopenia means a diminution in the number of blood platelets and is clinically significant only below a figure of $100 \times 10^9/l$. Capillary bleeding tends to occur when the platelet count falls below $40 \times 10^9/l$ but there is a poor correlation between the platelet count and a bleeding tendency.

Leucoerythroblastic is used to describe a blood picture in which primitive granulocytes and erythroblasts are simultaneously present in the peripheral blood. It is usually but not necessarily associated with anaemia and reflects bone marrow irritation, as in malignant infiltration of the marrow, or disordered haemopoiesis, as in myelofibrosis.

Extramedullary haemopoiesis means that production of blood cells takes place outside the normal sites. It occurs not uncommonly in the first year of life when the available bone marrow space is insufficient to allow for an increased demand for blood formation.

DISEASES OF THE RED BLOOD CELLS

THE ANAEMIAS

Anaemia may be defined as a state in which the level of haemoglobin in the blood is below that which is expected, taking into account both age and sex. At birth the haemoglobin is high (20 g/dl) because fetal haemoglobin has a higher oxygen affinity. After birth lower affinity haemoglobin A replaces haemoglobin F and the haemoglobin level rapidly drops, partly by removal of effete red cells and partly by reduced production, reaching about half the birth level when the baby is 3 months of age. Thereafter the average level rises gradually until the child reaches puberty when a further rise occurs which is more marked in males than females. Adult males have haemoglobin levels on average 2 g/dl higher than adult females. This reflects the stimulus of androgens on erythropoiesis. It is possible for a haemoglobin level of 12 g/dl to be regarded as anaemic in an adult male, but normal in an adult female. In practice, most adults who are otherwise in reasonably good health function satisfactorily if the haemoglobin is above 10 g/dl, provided this lower level has not appeared quickly. The presence of symptoms related to anaemia depends partly on its severity but also on how rapidly the anaemia developed. Thus a patient who has a reduction of haemoglobin from 13 g/dl to 8 g/dl in 1 week may have severe symptoms, while another patient whose anaemia has developed slowly to a similar level over months may be asymptomatic.

Aetiology. Anaemia may be caused by:

1. Loss of blood, which may be either acute or chronic (haemorrhage).

2. Inadequate production of normal red cells by the bone marrow (hypoplasia; aplasia).

3. Excessive destruction of red blood cells (haemolysis).

Most anaemias are multifactorial in their aetiology and many causes are relatively rare. The vast majority of anaemias are due to failure of haemoglobin synthesis as a result of iron deficiency, the commonest reason for which is blood loss. This simple approach to the anaemias helps to guide the clinician in planning investigation as it reflects what is happening. Alternatively, anaemias can be classified on the basis of the morphology of the red cell as (1) normocytic (2) microcytic and (3) macrocytic.

Clinical features of anaemia reflect the diminished oxygen carrying capacity of the blood. Their severity depends on the degree of anaemia and the rapidity of its development, but are independent of its type.

The symptoms of anaemia are fatigue, lassitude, breathlessness on exertion, palpitations, anorexia, taste disturbances, tinnitus, dizziness, dimness of vision, headache, insomnia and paraesthesiae in the fingers and toes. Myocardial hypoxia causes angina pectoris, especially in older patients with coronary artery disease. Signs include pallor of the skin and, much more significantly, of mucous membranes, tachycardia, cardiac dilatation, systolic murmurs and, in severe cases, oedema in dependent parts.

ANAEMIAS DUE TO BLOOD LOSS

Classification:

1. Acute (large volume over short period).
2. Chronic (small volumes over long period).

ACUTE BLOOD LOSS. A healthy adult can lose about half a litre of blood without ill effect. This is the basis of the blood transfusion service. When more than half a litre of blood is lost, compensatory mechanisms come into play which reduce blood flow to peripheral structures such as skin and muscle, and conserve the supply for central organs. The pulse rate rises and blood pressure is maintained. The patient is pale, cold and sweating and usually has to lie flat in order to maintain the cerebral circulation; hypovolaemic shock may ensue. At this stage the haemoglobin level of the blood is unchanged and in some cases may be higher than before the acute blood loss. If no further bleeding occurs, plasma production replenishes the volume, diluting the remaining red cells, and anaemia appears in about 24–36 hours. If blood loss is very severe, compensatory mechanisms fail and irreversible hypovolaemic shock supervenes, progressing to death. Anaemia may not have had time to appear.

The primary problem in acute blood loss is lack of blood volume which must be replaced by transfusion of whole blood, red cell concentrate, plasma or plasma substitutes. The anaemia which appears later, if red cells are not given or if plasma or plasma substitutes are used, will be corrected in the ensuing few weeks by increased red cell production unless the body iron stores are depleted. When acute blood loss is associated with other diseases, which themselves impair erythropoiesis, recovery of haemoglobin may be slow and the anaemia may become chronic. Immediately after acute blood loss there may be a transient leucoerythroblastic blood picture. A few days later a reticulocytosis of 5–10% develops, subsiding gradually as the haemoglobin level recovers. A transient rise in platelet count may also be observed.

CHRONIC BLOOD LOSS in contrast to the acute process, does not give rise to reduction in blood volume or to anaemia since the body has time to compensate by increased plasma and red cell production. Eventually, however, the continued loss of red cells causes depletion of iron stores, red cell production is impaired, and anaemia appears.

ANAEMIAS DUE TO INADEQUATE PRODUCTION OF RED CELLS

Classification: Inadequate production of red blood cells may be caused by:

1. Deficiency of essential factors: iron, vitamin B_{12}, folate or erythropoietin.

2. Toxic factors: inflammatory disease, hepatic and renal failure, drugs.

3. Endocrine deficiencies: hypothyroidism, hypoadrenalism, hypopituitarism, hypogonadism.

4. Invasion of bone marrow: leukaemia, secondary carcinoma, fibrosis.

5. Disorders of developing red cells: sideroblastic anaemia, other idiopathic refractory anaemias, hereditary disorders of haemoglobin synthesis (thalassaemia).

6. Failure of stem cells: aplastic anaemia, frequently drug induced.

Iron deficiency anaemia

Iron deficiency is by far the commonest cause of anaemia in most parts of the world.

Iron metabolism. Iron is essential for the synthesis of the haem fraction of haemoglobin. It is also present in myoglobin and enzymes such as the cytochromes. Iron in food (p. 59) is absorbed from the upper small intestine, mainly in the ferrous form, but it can also be absorbed as haem from red meat. Iron readily takes the ferric form in which it cannot be absorbed but the low pH of the stomach contents helps to preserve it in the ferrous form.

All cells obtain iron from the iron transport system (*transferrin*) in the blood by transfer across their membrane. The intestinal mucosal cell is no exception but it also receives iron by absorption from the gut lumen. When body stores of iron are adequate the intestinal mucosal cell is well supplied with iron from the blood, and absorption from the gut is discouraged. When demands for iron increase, or the body stores are low, the mucosal cell becomes iron depleted and avid for iron and therefore absorption from the gut increases.

Iron absorbed by the intestinal mucosal cell goes into a labile pool within the cell from which it may be complexed with apoferritin to form a ferritin store (p. 501). It may also go to mitochondria in the cell or pass to the blood transport system with which the labile pool in the cell is in dynamic equilibrium. Iron for erythropoiesis comes mainly from the iron transport system and almost all iron absorbed from the gut goes preferentially to the bone marrow and is used by the developing red cells. Increased erythropoiesis associated with a variety of disorders may promote iron absorption even when iron stores are increased. Thus some forms of prolonged anaemia, not due to blood loss or iron deficiency, can be associated with excessive iron stores.

Haem absorbed by the mucosal cell is split in the cell and iron liberated. The iron is then treated in the same way as that absorbed by other means. Iron obtained from the catabolism of haemoglobin from destroyed red cells is recycled either to the bone marrow, or if there is excess, to the iron stores. Iron is stored in cells in two forms, (1) *ferritin* from which iron is fairly readily available, and (2) *haemosiderin* which is a more stable form and constitutes the bulk of the iron stores. Haemosiderin is probably formed by the degradation of ferritin and can be stained by the Prussian blue reaction. This is used to provide a crude measurement of iron stores in the body.

Iron is lost from the body as the intestinal mucosal cells are sloughed off into the gut. A small amount is also excreted in sweat and urine. The total daily loss amounts to about 1 mg.

Aetiology. Iron deficiency usually results from either loss of iron due to bleeding, and inadequate diet (p. 59) or malabsorption (p. 303). Occasionally it may be excreted in the urine in the form of haemosiderin. Of these causes, losses due to bleeding in greater amounts than can be balanced by absorption is by far the commonest.

There are periods in life when iron deficiency may be regarded as almost physiological. At birth the normal infant has a store in the form of a very high haemoglobin level and in addition some iron is available in the liver. This is adequate for erythropoietic requirements in the first few months of life. Thereafter a mild degree of deficiency appears since milk is a very poor source of iron. If weaning is delayed for 1 or 2 years, as is the custom in certain parts of the world, deficiency may become marked. If the child is weaned to a good diet, the deficiency is fairly quickly corrected. When prematurity and haemorrhage from the cord at birth deprive the infant of the normal store of iron, deficiency may appear sooner and be more severe.

In adolescents, in whom a marked growth spurt occurs, iron requirements may outstrip absorption. Food fads are not uncommon at this age and may contribute.

Menstruation causes an average loss of 30 mg of iron each month requiring approximately 1mg a day increased absorption above normal needs.

Although this loss disappears during pregnancy, the mother requires additional iron for the fetus, the placenta, her own increased red cell mass and blood loss at parturition. The daily requirements will be about 2.5 mg plus her own basic requirement of 1 mg a day giving a total of 3.5 mg. This increased demand for iron rises as pregnancy progresses and is therefore greatest in the second half of pregnancy. Because of these factors iron deficiency is much more common in females than males during the reproductive years.

In post-menopausal women and adult men the commonest cause of iron deficiency is gastrointestinal bleeding, e.g. from erosions associated with non-steroidal anti-inflammatory drugs, and ulcers. Hookworm infection is very common and is the main cause of iron deficiency in many parts of the world.

At all ages, a diet containing insufficient food rich in iron (p. 59) can cause or contribute to iron deficiency anaemia. Elderly people living alone, particularly men, are prone to allow their dietary habits to deteriorate and, for example, eat little or no meat.

Clinical features. In many cases there are no symptoms and the deficiency may be discovered incidentally. In others vague symptoms of tiredness are insufficient to make the patient seek medical help. The symptomatology of severe iron deficiency is mainly that of anaemia (p. 499). However, there are some characteristic features. Angular stomatitis, glossitis and brittle finger nails are relatively common. Flattening or concavity of the nails (koilonychia), is sometimes seen in addition to the evidence of nail cracking. Dysphagia is rare but when present should raise the possibility of a post-cricoid web (Plummer-Vinson syndrome). Pica, the eating of strange things, such as coal, earth, or foods in great excess such as tomatoes or greens, is more common than generally realised and may be uncovered only if the patient is specifically asked. Splenomegaly is uncommon unless the anaemia is severe but may reflect other disease such as portal hypertension, of which the iron deficiency is also symptomatic.

Investigation. BLOOD COUNTS AND INDICES. The first abnormality to appear is microcytosis. Later, hypochromia occurs due to a reduced amount of haemoglobin in the red cells. Evidence of red cell dysplasia is seen by the finding first of oval and elliptical cells and later of poikilocytes. Some target cells may be found but often indicate other problems (p. 498). The haematological findings are a reduced haemoglobin with normal or slightly reduced red cell count, a low mean cell volume (MCV) of less than 76 fl, a low mean cell haemoglobin (MCH) of less than 27 pg, a normal or reduced mean corpuscular haemoglobin concentration (MCHC) and blood film evidence of microcytes, hypochromia and elliptocytosis. The white cell and differential counts are usually normal, although hypersegmentation of the neutrophils commonly occurs. The ESR is usually lower than would be expected for the degree of anaemia or associated disease. A raised platelet count suggests that bleeding may be the cause of the deficiency.

Haematological indices vary according to whether they are produced by electronic counters such as the Coultercounter model S or by manual means. In the latter case, the MCV will not be satisfactory in many instances, as it depends on accurate red cell counting and the MCHC is then the index to use. Since the MCH, which is also dependent on an accurate red cell count, reflects both cell size and haemoglobin saturation, it is a less useful index.

The iron binding capacity of the blood reflects the level of the iron transport protein, transferrin, which is normally about one-third saturated with iron. Saturation below 15% indicates iron deficiency and above 50%, iron overload, or failure to utilise available iron as in pernicious anaemia. Serum ferritin is present in minute quantities and is measurable only by radio-immunometric means. The range is wide in both sexes, mean values being higher in males. The levels, which correlate well with body iron stores, are very low in iron deficiency and raised in iron overload.

Bone marrow iron stores are found to be empty when stained by the Prussian blue technique.

DIAGNOSIS OF THE CAUSE OF IRON DEFICIENCY. Once iron deficiency has been established, a cause should be sought. The direction of the investigations will obviously be influenced by the age and sex of the patient, the history and the findings on examination. Excessive menstrual loss and repeated pregnancy are common causes. In the absence of any clear lead, evidence of gastrointestinal blood loss should first be sought with faecal occult blood tests, barium meal and enema and endoscopy. Negative barium studies should not be accepted as evidence of the absence of lesions. ^{51}Cr-labelled red cells may be used to demonstrate blood loss into the gut. The patient's blood is labelled and reinfused. The radioactivity in the stool provides an accurate measurement of the amount of blood lost.

In tropical countries hookworm infection and schistosomiasis must be considered as likely causes but additional factors will require to be sought. In patients in whom there is a known cause of intravascular red cell destruction, such as a prosthetic heart valve, the urine should be tested for haemosiderin. Where malabsorption is suspected, investigation should follow appropriate lines (p. 301).

Treatment. It is self evident that the patient who is iron deficient requires iron. Almost all patients can be treated by the oral route and the cheapest preparation is dried ferrous sulphate given as a tablet containing 200 mg of the salt (60 mg elemental iron) three times a day. A small proportion of patients develop 'indigestion', constipation or diarrhoea and then more expensive proprietary preparations may be tried. There are many of these and there is probably little to choose between them except that preparations employing a delayed release effect are to be avoided. They may give rise to less side-effects probably because of reduced release at the best absorption site. For the patient who cannot swallow tablets, proprietary liquid preparations may be used and are generally palatable.

Evidence of a response to oral medication usually appears in under 2 weeks. If no response is seen, it may be that the patient is not taking the tablets for a variety of reasons. A check may be made by examining the stool which will be grey or black if the patient is taking the iron.

The rise in reticulocyte count associated with response to iron therapy is usually modest and seldom above 10%. After the haemoglobin level has returned to normal, iron should be continued for at least 6 months and in some cases a year in order to replenish iron stores. In cases of malabsorption, almost continuous therapy may be required or the parenteral route utilised.

PARENTERAL IRON THERAPY. This should be used only after iron deficiency has been clearly demonstrated. Preparations of iron for injection should not be used except when one or other of the oral preparations cannot be tolerated or is found to be ineffective. The parenteral route of administration is suitable for the few patients who are genuinely unable to take iron by mouth because of pain, vomiting or diarrhoea, or who are unable to absorb iron because of some disorder of the gastrointestinal tract. It may also be used for patients who are shown or suspected to be unreliable in taking oral preparations. Iron given by injection has also been used for the treatment of the anaemia of rheumatoid arthritis, for the correction of severe anaemia in the late stages of pregnancy and following major operations.

The recommended single dose of iron-sorbitol is 1.5 mg of iron per kg of body weight given daily. It is assumed that about 250 mg of iron are required to increase the haemoglobin level by 1 g/dl of blood but the total dosage of iron should not exceed 2.5 g. Iron-sorbitol should be given by intramuscular injection and never intravenously.

Iron-dextran is seldom given intramuscularly because of local irritation and of reports of sarcomatous change in animals. It can be given intravenously by what is known as the 'total dose infusion method' in a suitable diluent. Alarming systemic anaphylactic reactions can occur.

Hypochromic anaemia of chronic disease

A blood film similar to that of iron deficiency anaemia may be due to chronic inflammatory or neoplastic diseases and is associated with abundant stores of iron in the marrow. There is inhibition of mobilisation of iron for haemoglobin formation. The microcytic, hypochromic blood picture is associated with a low serum iron but also a normal or low iron binding capacity; the saturation of the iron binding capacity is usually less reduced than is found in iron deficiency anaemia with a similar level of serum iron. Saturation of the iron binding capacity below 15% almost always means iron deficiency. Although iron can be observed in the storage cells in the marrow virtually no sideroblasts are seen. Serum

ferritin levels are normal reflecting the true state of the body iron stores.

Sideroblastic anaemias

These are rare conditions in which red cell production is impaired by disordered iron metabolism. The term sideroblast refers to a developing erythroblast which can be shown to have one or two iron granules in the cytoplasm. A siderocyte is a red cell containing iron granules. The iron granules are free in the cytoplasm and not associated with organelles. Both are normal findings. In certain pathological states iron accumulates in the mitochondria and appears as a ring of granules round the nucleus and is the characteristic cell of the sideroblastic anaemias.

Aetiology. Sideroblastic anaemias occur in two forms:

1. A hereditary condition which usually shows a sex-linked mode of inheritance, produces a microcytic, hypochromic blood picture very similar to that of iron deficiency, is unresponsive to iron therapy and is a benign disorder.

2. An acquired group of anaemias of which many are idiopathic, occurs mainly in the elderly. Others are associated with a variety of disorders, including inflammatory disease (e.g. rheumatoid arthritis), malignant disease, pernicious anaemia, myxoedema, drugs such as isoniazid, and rarely pyridoxine deficiency.

Clinical features are those of anaemia. Often an unsuccessful attempt has been made to treat the patient with iron, particularly in the hereditary form which mimics iron deficiency. The diagnostic feature of all these conditions is the finding of ring sideroblasts within the bone marrow. With satisfactory management patients with the idiopathic acquired type can survive for a number of years but some develop acute myeloblastic leukaemia indicating that the sideroblastic anaemia was a pre-leukaemia condition.

Treatment includes the withdrawal of iron therapy. In some patients venesection may result in an improvement if iron overload is present. Rarely the disorder is caused by pyridoxine deficiency and then response will be observed to doses as small as 1 mg daily. Other cases respond to massive doses of pyridoxine up to 600 mg daily;

improvement may be slow and treatment should not be abandoned in less than 3 months. When these measures are unsuccessful, transfusions with red cell concentrate may be required for the rest of the patient's life. In cases where the disorder is secondary to remediable disease, specific treatment usually corrects the sideroblastic disorder.

THE MEGALOBLASTIC ANAEMIAS

Haemopoietic tissue is one of a number of rapidly proliferating tissues in which DNA synthesis is intense. Both vitamin B_{12} and folate are essential for DNA synthesis and deficiency of one or both causes disordered cell proliferation. Haemopoiesis is particularly susceptible and division of cells is delayed and eventually halted. Morphological changes appear in the marrow cells. In the red cell series these changes are described as megaloblastic because the cells appear abnormally large. Changes also occur in the granulocyte precursors and megakaryocytes and disordered morphology can be seen in other rapidly dividing cells such as those of the gastrointestinal tract.

Normally in red cell production, cell division occurs rapidly. Between divisions the cells do not have time to regrow to their full size and a progressive decrease occurs. When DNA synthesis is reduced, the time between divisions is increased, more cell growth occurs and the cells become larger. In red cell precursors, haemoglobin production appears to be one of the factors limiting proliferation. Once a certain haemoglobin level has been reached, division stops. Thus in megaloblastic disorders not only do the red cell precursors have time to grow to a larger size, but they also undergo less divisions because there is no inhibition of haemoglobin formation. The end products are abnormally large and misshapen red cells which are well haemoglobinised.

As megaloblastic change becomes worse, increasing numbers of erythroblasts fail to mature and are destroyed in the marrow (ineffective erythropoiesis). Even in normal marrow a small proportion of developing cells suffer this fate but in advanced megaloblastic change the majority of the cells never mature to red cells. This massive destruction of cells in the marrow liberates large amounts of enzymes among which lactate dehydrogenase rises to very high levels in the blood. Eventually, in the absence of treatment, cell production fails. Excessive doses of antimetabolites which interfere with DNA synthesis and which are used in the treatment of cancer (p. 109) have similar effects and may induce severe dysplasia.

Vitamin B_{12} is a cobalt-containing porphyrin known as a cobalamin. In man the absorption of vitamin B_{12} from the lower ileum is facilitated by gastric intrinsic factor, a glycoprotein synthesised by gastric parietal cells, which complexes with vitamin B_{12}. Intrinsic factor is not absorbed. Vitamin B_{12} after absorption is bound to a carrier protein, transcobalamin, which transports it to the tissues where it is taken up by cells and the vitamin B_{12} released by degradation of the complex.

Folates and interaction with vitamin B_{12}. Folic acid (pteroylglutamic acid) and related compounds are known as folates. Folic acid as such is available as a medicinal compound but the body obtains folates by the breakdown of polyglutamates in food to monoglutamates in the small intestine or mucosal cell. In the plasma folate appears as methyl tetrahydrofolate which is changed to tetrahydrofolate (THF) by a pathway for which vitamin B_{12} is essential. Without this, active folate coenzymes are poorly formed. 5,10 methylene THF is the form essential for the synthesis of DNA. Dihydrofolate from this step is reconverted to THF by dihydrofolate reductase, an enzyme inhibited by the folate antagonist, methotrexate. Formyl THF (folinic acid) will bypass both the metabolic blocks created by vitamin B_{12} deficiency or methotrexate and act as an antidote to this drug. Folinic acid or folic acid must not be used in treating vitamin B_{12} deficiency as they will accelerate neurological damage although they may correct the anaemia.

Deficiency of vitamin B_{12}. This vitamin is obtained mainly from animal foodstuffs. Vegetables alone are an inadequate source. Requirements of vitamin B_{12} in the normal person amount to 1–2 μg daily. Deficiency takes at least 3 years to appear as there are large stores in the liver. It occurs because:

1. The diet may be inadequate (true vegans).

2. There may be intrinsic factor deficiency due to gastric atrophy as in pernicious anaemia, gastrectomy or, rarely, to congenital deficiency without gastric atrophy.

3. There may be disease of the terminal ileum reducing or eliminating the absorption site, e.g. Crohn's disease.

4. Vitamin B$_{12}$ may be removed from the gut either by bacterial proliferation in blind loops or by parasites such as the fish tapeworm (p. 789).

Addisonian pernicious anaemia

The term Addisonian pernicious anaemia should be limited to megaloblastic anaemia due to a failure of secretion of intrinsic factor by the stomach other than from surgery. This disease is rare before the age of 30, occurs mainly between 45–65 years and affects females more than males.

Pathology. The marrow morphology reflects the failure of DNA synthesis with extensive maturation arrest of the red cell precursors and disparity in the maturation of nucleus and cytoplasm. Granulocyte precursors are often diminished in number and giant metamyelocytes are seen. Megakaryocytes may also be reduced in number and show dysplastic changes. There is evidence of increased blood destruction — including unconjugated hyperbilirubinaemia and increased deposition of iron (haemosiderin) in the liver, spleen, kidneys and bone marrow. The gastric mucosa is thin and atrophic. In untreated or inadequately treated cases degenerative changes in the posterior and lateral tracts of the spinal cord may be found (subacute combined degeneration).

Clinical features. The onset is insidious and the degree of anaemia is often great before the patient consults the doctor. In addition to the symptoms of anaemia there may be intermittent soreness of the tongue and periodic diarrhoea.

The patient generally appears well nourished despite the fact that weight loss is a common feature. The skin and mucous membranes are pale and in severely anaemic cases the skin and conjunctivae may show a lemon yellow tint. The surface of the tongue is usually smooth and atrophic, but sometimes it is red and inflamed. The spleen may be palpable. In many cases

paraesthesiae occur in the fingers and toes and occasionally there are signs of subacute combined degeneration (p. 657), which can appear before the anaemia. Dementia may also occur. In females there may be infertility. The urine contains excess of urobilinogen.

Investigation. Examination of the stained blood film shows a macrocytic blood picture. There is marked anisocytosis and poikilocytosis and in more advanced cases, fragmented red cells. Nucleated red cells sometimes show the features of megaloblastic change and can be found in the blood film, particularly if a 'buffy coat' preparation is made. This latter technique is useful if it is not possible to examine the bone marrow.

The reticulocyte count is usually low in absolute terms. Results expressed as a percentage must be assessed in relation to the reduced number of red cells. The absolute count is usually less than $100 \times 10^9/l$. Leucopenia is frequently present and is due to neutropenia. Hypersegmentation of the neutrophils is common. The platelet count is often within normal limits but may be reduced and occasionally severe thrombocytopenia is seen.

With modern counting equipment and the widespread availability of blood counts, this disorder is often diagnosed before anaemia appears as the result of finding a raised MCV. Consequently more florid, advanced cases are now seen less often.

Diagnosis is achieved in the first place by demonstrating that the patient has a megaloblastic anaemia, based on the finding of a macrocytic blood picture with the features mentioned above, a megaloblastic marrow and a low serum vitamin B$_{12}$ level. Serum folate levels may be raised. A *Schilling test* will demonstrate that there is a failure of vitamin B$_{12}$ absorption due to a lack of gastric intrinsic factor. The fasting patient is given 1 μCi of cobalt labelled vitamin B$_{12}$ orally and at the same time 1000 μg of vitamin B$_{12}$ is administered intramuscularly. The injected material saturates the binding proteins in the patient's blood so that vitamin B$_{12}$ absorbed from the gut is lost in the urine. Urine is collected for 24 hours (48 hours if the patient has renal disease) and the radioactivity in the urine measured and related to the dose given orally. Normal subjects excrete more than 15% of the administered radioactivity in the 24 hour urine specimen. Patients with pernicious anaemia usually excrete less than 8% and very often less than 1% of the administered dose. The test is then repeated adding intrinsic factor to the oral dose of labelled vitamin B_{12}. If the defect in absorption is corrected, it is reasonable to assume that the patient has a failure of intrinsic factor production. Uncommonly the correction is poor due to high levels of anti-intrinsic factor antibodies in the stomach contents and higher doses of intrinsic factor may be required. Alternatively poor correction may indicate disease in the ileum. The Schilling test can be used for diagnostic purposes, even after the patient has been treated and is in remission.

Other tests which contribute to making a diagnosis of pernicious anaemia are the finding of intrinsic factor antibodies in the plasma in 50% of cases and the demonstration of pentagastrin fast achlorhydria, although often this unpleasant test is omitted if the results of the Schilling test are clear. Parietal cell antibodies are found in 80% of patients with pernicious anaemia but are diagnostically unhelpful as they are also found in many who do not have the disease.

Treatment. GENERAL. The decision to give a blood transfusion is based on general principles concerning the clinical state of the patient. When the haemoglobin level is so low as to endanger life, e.g. under 4 g/dl, it should be seriously considered. In all types of chronic anaemia of sufficient severity to require transfusion the blood should be given very slowly, preferably as red cell concentrate, because of the danger of producing cardiac failure. A diuretic should be given simultaneously with the red cell concentrate.

SPECIFIC. Hydroxocobalamin should be given in a dosage of 1000 μg twice during the first week, then 1000 μg weekly until the blood count is normal. Within 48 hours of the first injection the bone marrow shows a striking change from a megaloblastic to a normoblastic state. Within 2 to 3 days the reticulocyte count begins to rise, reaching a maximum between the fifth and tenth days. If there is coexisting inflammatory disease the response may be delayed. There is a brief peak of red cell output due to the maturation of the large number of cells held in maturation arrest by the vitamin B_{12} deficiency. Depending on the initial erythrocyte count the proportion of reticulocytes may rise above 50% but soon falls to below 10% as more normal production is resumed.

In some cases the rapid regeneration of the blood depletes the iron reserves of the body and recovery is halted. To prevent this occurring, ferrous sulphate (200 mg t.i.d.) should be given soon after the commencement of treatment. A combined deficiency of vitamin B_{12} and iron is recognised by the presence of macrocytosis and hypochromia — a dimorphic blood picture.

If a patient diagnosed as have pernicious anaemia fails to respond to the parenteral administration of adequate doses of hydroxocobalamin, it suggests that the diagnosis is wrong. The patient may be suffering from one of the other types of megaloblastic anaemia which may be partially or completely refractory to hydroxocobalamin. Such cases may respond to folic acid.

MAINTENANCE TREATMENT. The patient suffering from pernicious anaemia must be given regular doses of hydroxocobalamin indefinitely (1000 μg i.m. every 3 months). Theoretically the interval between doses may be longer but there is no merit in seeking the minimum effective dose. Blood counts should be done once a year and the assessment should never be made solely on clinical impression or on the haemoglobin level alone. With the maintenance of a normal blood count by adequate specific treatment the patient has a normal expectancy of life. There is, however, a statistically significant increase in deaths from gastric carcinoma in patients with pernicious anaemia. Patients with subacute combined degeneration of the cord should be given monthly hydroxocobalamin (p. 657).

Other causes of megaloblastic anaemia due to vitamin B_{12} deficiency

Dietary insufficiency is rare except in countries where meat and other animal foodstuffs are not eaten for religious or other reasons. The deficiency is readily corrected by parenteral administration of vitamin B_{12}. Thereafter the vitamin may be given by mouth.

Gastrectomy. Total resection of the stomach results in a complete loss of intrinsic factor production and therefore failure to absorb vitamin B_{12}. The patient will require life-long vitamin B_{12} injections. Partial gastrectomy reduces vitamin B_{12} absorption, in some cases to the point that deficiency occurs. Gastritis may, in part, be responsible. The Schilling test often demonstrates reduced absorption. One annual injection of 1000 μg of hydroxocobalamin is adequate prophylaxis for a patient who has had a partial gastrectomy.

Disease of the terminal ileum should be suspected if the Schilling test is not corrected by the addition of adequate amounts of intrinsic factor.

Bacterial colonisation of the small intestine (p. 305) results in an abnormal Schilling test, both without and with intrinsic factor; this is corrected by the administration of tetracycline.

Megaloblastic anaemias due to folate deficiency

Folate occurs mainly in the form of polyglutamates in both vegetable and animal foodstuffs. Much is destroyed by cooking and body stores are relatively small, lasting only a few weeks. It is absorbed mainly in the jejunum. Its metabolism thereafter has been described on page 504. Folate deficiency arises from:

1. Inadequate intake. Diets which totally lack fresh vegetables and meat or which consist of overcooked food, may not provide enough folate.

2. Disease of the upper small bowel. This may occur in coeliac disease or tropical sprue; very rarely extensive resection of the small bowel has a similar effect.

3. The body's demands exceeding intake.

a. When there is very active cell proliferation, e.g. haemolytic anaemia, leukaemias and other neoplastic disease, during periods of acute or chronic infection and in extensive psoriasis.

b. Pregnancy, when the demands of the fetus and placental growth require large amounts of folate. In this situation folate is taken by the fetus in amounts adequate for its needs, even when the mother is folate deficient. There is no evidence that the fetus is ever affected by folate deficiency in the mother.

4. Interference with the dihydrofolate reductase system (p. 504). This enzyme system may be blocked by certain drugs, particularly methotrexate. In theory trimethoprim may also do this but a real danger appears to exist only in patients deficient in folate from another cause.

5. An unexplained mechanism. Alcohol and the antiepileptic drugs phenytoin and primidone may cause folate depletion by an unknown mechanism not related to (4).

Prevalence. Approximately 60% of all cases of megaloblastic anaemia in Britain are due to folate deficiency. The majority of those suffering from vitamin B_{12} deficiency have pernicious anaemia. In tropical countries most megaloblastic disease is due to folate deficiency associated with malnutrition and pregnancy. Addisonian pernicious anaemia appears to be relatively uncommon in the tropics and in some areas is quite rare.

Clinical features are those of anaemia and of the underlying cause. Glossitis is less common than in vitamin B_{12} deficiency. Neurological problems are very rare.

Investigation. The blood and bone marrow findings in megaloblastic anaemia due to folate deficiency are indistinguishable from those in vitamin B_{12} deficiency as described for pernicious anaemia but serum and red cell folate levels are low. However, when the onset of folate deficiency has been recent and acute, the red cell folate, which reflects the patient's folate status over the previous 3 months, may still be within normal limits. Likewise, patients who have received folate therapy for a day or two will have a high serum folate level but may still show evidence of their past deficiency in the red cell folate. Serum folate should always be measured on a fasting specimen. The vitamin B_{12} level in the serum may also be marginally reduced for reasons that are not clear. The Schilling test, however, is normal and the vitamin B_{12} level returns to normal with folate therapy provided there is not a true vitamin B_{12} deficiency from another cause. Once folate deficiency has been established an explanation should be found among the causes already mentioned.

Treatment. A daily dose of 5 mg of folic acid by mouth is sufficient; for maintenance therapy 5 mg once a week is almost always adequate. Folic acid must never be given, other than with vitamin B_{12}, in Addisonian pernicious anaemia or other vitamin B_{12} deficiency anaemias, because of the risk of aggravating or precipitating neurological features of vitamin B_{12} depletion. In pregnancy, megaloblastic change due to vitamin B_{12} deficiency is very rare indeed. It is therefore reasonable to give folate supplements $(350 \, \mu g/d)$ to pregnant women. When a drug such as methotrexate inhibits dihydrofolate reductase, it is possible to employ folinic acid to overcome the metabolic block.

PRIMARY IDIOPATHIC APLASTIC ANAEMIA

This is a rare but grave disease of the stem cells which fail to a varying degree, producing serious hypoplasia of the marrow elements. An immunological mechanism may be responsible.

Clinical features. The disorder may occur at any age, the peak incidence being around 30 years. The onset is insidious and the clinical problems are due to the reduction or virtual absence of production of red cells, granulocytes and platelets. Infections and haemorrhage are the most troublesome complications and may prove lethal. Bleeding occurs in the skin and mucous membranes. Haematuria and epistaxis are common. Intracranial bleeding is always a risk. Necrotic mouth and throat ulcers and monilial infections reflect the neutropenia.

Investigation. Known causes of hypoplastic and aplastic anaemia must first be excluded. A careful inquiry into exposure to drugs, chemicals and radiation should be made. A history of viral illness, particularly hepatitis, may be important. A full blood count demonstrates a pancytopenia. Neutropenia is the most marked aspect of the leucopenia, although leucopenia may not be the first development. The anaemia is normocytic, normochromic and often marked. Platelet production is often the most severely affected and the last to recover. The bone marrow should be examined by aspiration and trephine. The latter provides a better assessment of cellularity; aspirate may be difficult to obtain (dry tap). Studies with ^{59}Fe show poor clearance of the isotope from the blood, poor uptake and utilisation by the marrow and no extramedullary haemopoiesis.

Treatment. In children and adults up to 50 years the possibility of bone marrow transplantation (p. 509) should be considered urgently. No blood products from relatives should be given until compatibility testing has been completed in order to avoid the risk of immunisation against potential donor antigens. Bone marrow transplantation now carries a better prognosis than when the disease is treated in a more conservative manner.

For patients for whom bone marrow transplantation is not possible, there are two aspects to management. The first is supporting the patient by replacement therapy. This consists of maintaining a reasonable haemoglobin level and is the least of the problems because transfusion of red cell concentrate can be given regularly. Vigorous antimicrobial therapy for infection and platelet transfusions for bleeding are required as outlined in the management of acute myeloblastic leukaemia (p. 525). Corticosteroids may be used to reduce bleeding but carry the risk of promoting infection.

The second aspect is an attempt to stimulate haemopoiesis and promote recovery. Androgenic steroids with low virilising activity are employed; these include oxymetholone by mouth or nandrolone decanoate intramuscularly. High doses of methyl prednisolone may also be used. Red cell production and to a lesser extent granulocyte production benefit most from these drugs which unfortunately have undesirable and troublesome side effects when used over long periods. This is particularly so in children in whom secondary sexual characteristics may be stimulated and premature fusion of epiphyses may occur if the treatment is not suitably curtailed. Androgens may also cause cholestasis; fluid retention and prostatic enlargement may occur. Intravenous antilymphocyte or antithymocyte globulin may be given where an autoimmune process is thought to be an aetiological factor. Risks include anaphylaxis and serum sickness.

Prognosis. The course tends to be prolonged. Spontaneous improvement and recovery may occur and is one reason why treatment should be vigorous and prolonged. Androgens may be ineffective in the early phase of the disease but become effective later and should not be abandoned because of initial failure. The prognosis is undoubtedly poor and more than 50% of patients die usually within the first year after diagnosis. Patients who survive longer than 1 year have a better chance of remission. In a few patients leukaemia supervenes and it is probable that these have been cases of leukaemia presenting in an aplastic or hypoplastic phase.

Secondary pancytopenia

This condition may be due to:

1. Idiosyncrasy to certain drugs such as chloramphenicol, indomethacin, sulphamethoxypyridazine and tolbutamide or to certain industrial chemicals and insecticides chiefly benzene and its derivatives such as trinitrophenol, trinitrotoluene and gamma-benzene hexachloride.

2. The majority of drugs used in the chemotherapy of malignant disease.

3. X-rays and radioactivity.

4. Replacement of the bone marrow by abnormal cells such as tumour or by fibrous tissue.

5. Viral infections, particularly hepatitis.

6. Deficiency states such as severe lack of vitamin B_{12} or folate.

The clinical features and methods of diagnosis are the same as for primary idiopathic aplastic anaemia. The noxious agent if identified should be removed but otherwise treatment is as for the idiopathic form. Bone marrow transplantation may be required in young patients who have HLA matched sibling donors.

BONE MARROW TRANSPLANTATION

This is the only therapeutic measure which holds out the hope of 'cure' for persons with a variety of haematological disorders, particularly those with neoplastic disorders affecting the totipotent or pluripotent stem cell compartment and those with a failure of haemopoiesis (aplastic anaemia) or a major inherited defect in blood cell production (e.g. thalassaemia). Healthy marrow from a donor is injected intravenously into a recipient who has been suitably 'conditioned' with chemotherapy and radiotherapy. Conditioning ablates the recipient's haemopoietic tissue. The injected cells will 'home' to the marrow and will produce enough erythrocytes, granulocytes and platelets for the patient's needs in about 3–4 weeks. It takes longer, months, or even years, to regain good lymphocyte function and immunological stability. During this period the patient is at great risk from opportunistic infections.

The best donors are histocompatible siblings and the best results are obtained in patients under 20. Older patients can be transplanted, but results become progressively worse with age. The patient must be sufficiently stable psychologically to contend with a period of aggressive therapy during the transplantation process. The patient should be free of other disorders which might seriously limit life span.

Bone marrow transplantation is not a particularly difficult or complicated procedure but it requires highly specialised supervision and supportive facilities and a fully trained staff. It is best done in units established for the care of acute leukaemias under the primary care of haematologists, with the cooperation of immunologists, microbiologists, radiotherapists and a full laboratory service.

Indications. Transplantation may be syngeneic (identical twin donor) or allogeneic (nonidentical donor). Disorders for which allogeneic transplantation is currently offered include: severe aplastic anaemia, severe immunodeficiency syndromes, acute myeloblastic leukaemia in first remission, acute myelofibrosis, T and B cell lymphoblastic leukaemia in first remission and chronic myeloid leukaemia in chronic phase. Transplantation is also a possibility for acute lymphoblastic leukaemia (common type) in second remission, resistant acute leukaemia and selected patients with lymphoma.

Autografting in which the patient's own marrow is harvested to be given back again after intensive therapy may be used for disorders which do not primarily involve the haemopoietic tissues or in patients in whom very good remissions have been achieved. For chronic myeloid leukaemia, autografting with the patients own chronic phase cells harvested and stored at the time of presentation has been used to treat the disease when it enters the acute phase.

GVH disease. If the graft is successful, problems of graft-versus-host (GVH) disease and interstitial pneumonitis may cause serious morbidity and death. Even low-grade GVH disease, which is probably advantageous in terms of survival, can reduce the quality of life.

GVH disease is due to the cytotoxic activity of donor T lymphocytes becoming sensitised to their new host which they regard as foreign. This may produce either an acute or chronic form of GVH disease. The acute form usually appears 14 to 21 days after the graft, although it may appear earlier or up to 70 days later. It is associated with diarrhoea, hepatitis, cholestasis and exfoliative dermatitis. All these features may vary from being mild to lethally severe. The occurrence appears to be associated with infection, although the relationship is not fully understood. Methotrexate, cyclosporin, antithymocyte globulin and high dose corticosteroids have all been used to treat the disorder. The more severe forms prove very difficult to control.

Chronic GVH disease may follow acute GVH disease or arise independently; it occurs later than acute GVH disease. It often resembles a connective tissue disorder, although in mild cases a rash may be the only manifestation. Chronic GVH disease is usually treated with azathioprine and corticosteroids.

ANAEMIAS DUE TO EXCESSIVE RED CELL DESTRUCTION

Haemolytic anaemias

Red cell turnover is a normal physiological process, red cells having an average survival of 120 days. Various abnormalities either in the red cell or its environment may shorten its life-span and more rapid replacement is then required. Anaemia develops when marrow output no longer compensates. The increased output of new red cells is reflected in a raised reticulocyte count which gives an indication of the severity of the process. Under more extreme stress, nucleated red cells may be released.

The catabolic pathways for haemoglobin degradation are unimpaired but overloaded. There is an increase in unconjugated bilirubin in the blood and increased reabsorption of urobilinogen from the gut, which is excreted in the urine in increased amounts. Bile does not appear in the urine. The level of bilirubinaemia is not greatly increased and jaundice is mild (p. 338).

Intravascular haemolysis liberates haemoglobin into the plasma where it is bound mainly by the α-2 globulin, haptoglobin, to form a complex too large to be lost in the urine. It is taken up by the liver and degraded there. Some haemoglobin is partially degraded and bound to albumin to form methaemalbumin. This is the basis for the *Schumm's test* for haemoglobin in the plasma.

If all the haptoglobin has been consumed, free haemoglobin may be lost in the urine. In small amounts this is reabsorbed by the renal tubules where the haemoglobin is degraded and the iron stored as haemosiderin. Sloughing of the renal tubular cells gives rise to haemosiderinuria which always indicates intravascular haemolysis. When greater amounts of haemoglobin are lost through the kidneys haemoglobinuria occurs, giving the urine a black appearance.

Extravascular haemolysis occurs in the phagocytic cells of the spleen, liver, bone marrow and other organs. It may not result in much depletion of haptoglobin. Furthermore inflammatory disease increases haptoglobin levels as does steroid therapy. Ahaptoglobinaemia may occur as an inherited disorder. For these reasons estimation of the haptoglobin level in the blood is not always easily interpreted. Nevertheless absence of haptoglobin is a strong indicator of haemolytic disease.

Blood and marrow findings. The peripheral blood shows a moderate macrocytosis and polychromasia due to the reticulocytosis. Specific red cell abnormalities may give a clue to the type of haemolytic disease (see below). There may be a polymorphonuclear leucocytosis. The marrow shows erythroid hyperplasia. Megaloblastic change may occur and usually reflects depletion of folate reserves.

Increased erythropoietic turnover in the marrow is associated with increased levels of lactic dehydrogenase in the blood, which, in the absence of any dyserythropoietic state such as megaloblastic change, closely follows the severity of the haemolytic disorder.

If necessary red cell survival can be measured crudely using radioactive chromium (^{51}Cr). Surface counting done at the same time over liver and spleen may give an indication of where haemolysis is taking place. If transfusion has been given the patient's blood contains a mixed cell population which is not suitable for ^{51}Cr studies.

In these circumstances cross-matched donor cells should be used for labelling.

Classification. Haemolytic anaemia may be caused by:

1. *Intra-erythrocytic defects:*

   a. Hereditary: spherocytosis, disorders of glycolysis, haemoglobinopathies (abnormal haemoglobins and thalassaemias).

   b. Acquired: red cells produced by dyserythropoietic states, e.g. vitamin B_{12} and folate deficiency.

2. *Extra-erythrocytic abnormalities:*

   a. Antibodies (autoimmune and isoimmune).

   b. Physical trauma (prosthetic heart valve).

   c. Chemical trauma (drugs).

   d. Infections (malaria).

   e. Toxic factors associated with inflammatory or neoplastic disease and metabolic failure.

HAEMOLYTIC ANAEMIA DUE TO HEREDITARY ABNORMALITIES OF THE ERYTHROCYTE

The principal disorders are hereditary spherocytosis, G6PD deficiency, haemoglobinopathies, (e.g. sickle-cell disease) and thalassaemia. G6PD deficiency and haemoglobinopathies are most common in African blacks and thalassaemia in the Mediterranean area. There has been a rise in the incidence of these disorders in other countries including Britain because of immigration.

Hereditary spherocytosis

The exact abnormality is unknown but there are metabolic defects in the red cell membrane with increased leak of sodium ions into the cell, giving the sodium pump excessive work. Membrane loss occurs and this gradually compels the cell to lose its biconcave shape and become spherical. Spherocytes are destroyed by the spleen. The red cell life span is reduced giving rise to varying degrees of haemolytic disorder, often enough to cause anaemia. The haemolysis is extravascular.

Clinical features. Symptoms vary from none to those of fairly severe anaemia. Episodic jaundice may be noted. The spleen is often but not always palpably enlarged. The severity of the disorder tends to vary in any one patient with crises of haemolysis at times. The transient hypoplasia of red cell production, which can occur in normal persons in association with viral infections, presents as *aplastic crises* in these patients because of the greatly increased red cell turnover which has become their normal state. There is a liability to form gallstones composed of bile pigment and cholecystitis may be the presenting event. Leg ulcers sometimes occur.

Investigation. The diagnosis is made by demonstrating a haemolytic state together with spherocytes in the blood film, increased osmotic fragility due to the spherocytes and the demonstration of the same disorder in other members of the family. The Coomb's test (p. 517) is negative. There is an excessive loss of urobilinogen in the urine. Red cell survival studies with ^{51}Cr show destruction of red cells almost exclusively in the spleen. The differential diagnosis is from other causes of spherocytosis, particularly the various forms of immune haemolysis (p. 517). Loss of membrane due to trauma to red cells in the circulation usually gives rise to many more schistocytes (fragmented red cells) than are seen in hereditary spherocytosis.

Treatment. Splenectomy results in striking and usually permanent improvement both in the symptoms and in the anaemia. Operation should be advised when the anaemia causes persistent impairment of health, when severe haemolytic crises have occurred, when other members of the family have died from the disease, or where evidence of cholecystitis and cholelithiasis is present. Opinion differs as to the desirability of operation in mild cases with no resulting disability. The operation should be carried out during a period of remission, and in young children should be deferred until school age or older if possible. Following splenectomy, resistance to some infections may be impaired.

Severe haemolytic crises require treatment by blood transfusion. Blood must be matched very carefully and administered by very slow drip, as gross haemolytic transfusion reactions are common in this disease. Folic acid, 5 mg daily, may be prescribed to support the increased erythropoiesis. Iron is of no value unless a genuine deficiency is demonstrated.

Glucose 6-phosphate dehydrogenase deficiency

Glucose 6-phosphate dehydrogenase (G6PD) is the first enzyme in the hexose monophosphate shunt of the Embden-Meyerhof glycolytic pathway from which red cells derive most of their metabolic energy. The function of this shunt is to service the enzymes glutathione reductase and glutathione peroxidase which protect the red cells against damage due to oxidation. In the absence of G6PD this protective mechanism is impaired and certain drugs in sufficient concentration can seriously injure the red cell.

It is now known that the deficiency is inherited as a X-linked recessive disorder and has a high frequency among African blacks. In West and East Africa about 20% of males (hemizygotes) and about 4% of females (homozygous for the abnormal gene) are affected. A small number of heterozygous females are also deficient in G6PD. They have two populations of red cells, one deficient and the other normal. A similar deficiency occurs in Caucasian and Mongoloid races where it is usually more severe. Favism (haemolytic anaemia from the ingestion of the broad bean, Vicia faba) is due to deficiency of G6PD of the severe Caucasian variety. In black people the activity of the enzyme is about 15% of normal, whereas in the others it is often less than 1% resulting in greater clinical effects. Some cases of haemolytic disease of the newborn in Caucasians have been found to be due to the same defect. This problem is less common but important in the type found in black people. Other types of G6PD biochemically different from the above may be associated with congenital non-spherocytic haemolytic disease and have been found in persons of pure British ancestry. In these cases splenectomy is valueless.

Many drugs in common clinical use, e.g. some antimalarials and sulphonamides, are capable of precipitating haemolysis in individuals with G6PD deficiency. Infections may also potentiate the haemolytic action of drugs such as aspirin, chloramphenicol and chloroquine.

Clinical features. Persons with G6PD deficiency normally enjoy good health but are liable to haemolysis if any of the incriminated drugs or foods are ingested. However, the haemolytic effect is related to the dose and will not be clinically detectable if the amount does not exceed a critical level. It is often possible to employ doses which are not toxic. The anaemia, when it occurs, may be rapid in onset, becoming obvious between 2 and 10 days after exposure to the precipitating agent and may be sufficiently severe to cause haemoglobinuria as well as the other classical signs of haemolysis. In the type of deficiency prevalent in black people only older cells which have lost enzyme activity are involved so that the haemolysis is to some extent self-limiting even when the offending agent is continued. Young red cells have some G6PD activity and remain viable until their enzyme complement decays. Since in the Caucasian variety the enzyme deficiency is much more severe, destruction tends to be greater. Anuria is an infrequent but serious complication.

Investigation. Diagnosis can be confirmed by estimating the G6PD activity of the red cell but may not be entirely accurate if there is considerable reticulocytosis. A number of screening tests are also available, e.g. (1) the ascorbate cyanide test of Jacob and Jandl which monitors the whole glutathione regulating system of which G6PD is a fundamental part; (2) spot tests employing either the reduction of soluble tetrazolium compounds to insoluble purple formazan or the fluorescence of NADPH which is a bioproduct of G6PD activity. This last test can be performed on aged blood or blood collected on filter paper and dried. The Jacob and Jandl test has the advantage of being cheap. These tests should always be performed alongside normal controls.

Treatment is by removal of the toxic agent. Recovery is usually rapid but if the anaemia is severe, transfusion of red cells with a normal enzyme complement may be required. Thereafter the patient should be advised to avoid drugs which may precipitate the disorder.

The haemoglobinopathies

The haemoglobinopathies can be classified into three subgroups. In the first there is an alteration in the amino acid structure of the polypeptide chains of the globin fraction of haemoglobin, commonly called the abnormal haemoglobins. The best known example is sickle-cell anaemia.

Some 'abnormal' haemoglobins function as normal variants. In the second subgroup the amino acid sequence is normal but polypeptide chain production is impaired or absent for a variety of reasons; these are the thalassaemias. In the third subgroup there is the persistence of haemoglobin normally found in early life, namely haemoglobin F, into adult life. The hereditary persistence of high fetal haemoglobin is a benign condition and can be advantageous to persons carrying the haemoglobin S gene with which it is allelomorphic.

Sickle-cell anaemia

Abnormal haemoglobins are caused by amino acid substitutions in their polypeptide chains. These in turn reflect mutations in the structural genes controlling the production of these chains. There are four loci for these structural genes, all on autosomal chromosomes, active in postnatal life. They are designated alpha, gamma, beta and delta and are responsible for the production of the three main haemoglobins seen after birth, namely haemoglobins F, A and A2. Each of these haemoglobins contains, in common, two alpha chains and their differences reflect the possession of two gamma chains in the case of haemoglobin F, two beta chains in the case of haemoglobin A, and two delta chains in the case of haemoglobin A2 (Fig. 13.2). Thus the globin fraction of these three types of haemoglobin may be written $\alpha 2\gamma 2$ $\alpha 2\beta 2$ and $\alpha 2\delta 2$, respectively. Each globin chain carries one haem moiety in its folds. It is convenient and practical to represent normal adult haemoglobins by the capital letter A, fetal haemoglobin by the letter F, and the abnormal haemoglobins by S, C and E and so on. As there are now several hundred haemoglobin variants known, the letters of the alphabet do not suffice and for some years new variants have been given names, often of the towns or districts in which they were discovered. Sickle-cell haemoglobin is the most important but haemoglobin C, D and E are also significant in some parts of the world, particularly when inherited along with haemoglobin S or with β-thalassaemia (p. 516).

Modern nomenclature includes a statement of the site of the amino acid substitution. Thus sickle haemoglobin may be defined as:

$$\text{Hb S } \beta^{\text{6GLU-VAL}} \text{ or Hb S } \beta^{\text{A3GLU-VAL}}$$

The second method is more accurate since it defines the helix or bend in which the substitution occurs.

Control of haemoglobin synthesis is inherited from both parents. Thus a normal adult can be depicted as having the haemoglobin genotype AA, sickle-cell trait by AS and sickle-cell anaemia or homozygous S disease by SS. The inheritance when both parents have sickle-cell trait can be shown thus:

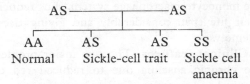

The patient with sickle-cell trait is relatively resistant to the lethal effects of falciparum malaria in early childhood. The high incidence of this deleterious gene in equatorial Africa is thus explained by the selective advantage for survival it confers in an environment of endemic falciparum malaria. Surprising, patients with sickle-cell anaemia do not have correspondingly greater resistance to falciparum malaria.

Sickle-cell anaemia has been recognised among black people and to a lesser extent in other races since the beginning of the century. It is caused by the presence of the abnormal haemoglobin, haemoglobin S.

Pathogenesis. When haemoglobin S is deoxygenated, the molecules of haemoglobin polymerise to form pseudo-crystalline structures known as 'tactoids'. These distort the red cell membrane and produce characteristic sickle-shaped cells. The polymerisation is reversible when reoxygenation occurs. The distortion of the red cell membrane, however, may become permanent and the red cell 'irreversibly sickled'. The greater the concentration of sickle-cell haemoglobin in the individual cell, the more easily tactoids are formed, but this process may be enhanced or retarded by the presence of other haemoglobins. Thus haemoglobin C participates in the polymerisation more readily than haemoglobin A, whereas haemoglobin F strongly inhibits polymerisation.

In sickle-cell anaemia most of the red cells contain haemoglobin S and little else and are very prone to sickle even in vivo under normal conditions. This happens particularly in those parts of the microvasculature which are sinusoidal and where the flow is sluggish. Sickle cells increase blood viscosity, traverse capillaries poorly and tend to obstruct flow, thereby increasing the sickling of other cells and eventually stopping the flow. Thrombosis may follow and an area of tissue infarction results causing severe pain, swelling and tenderness (infarction crises). In addition these cells are phagocytosed in large numbers by the monocyte-macrophage system, thus reducing their life span considerably and giving rise to haemolysis.

Clinical features. The two major problems are chronic anaemia due to reduced red cell survival and episodes of tissue infarction.

Anaemia. Problems do not arise until about the fourth month of life when haemoglobin F containing cells have given way to haemoglobin S containing cells. The anaemia is haemolytic in type and severe, the haemoglobin seldom rising above 10 g/dl and averaging approximately 8 g/dl. Secondary folate deficiency is common and exacerbates the anaemia. When anaemia is persistent, growth may be retarded and puberty delayed. Episodes of increased sequestration and destruction of red cells (*haemolytic crises*) occur, sometimes for no apparent reason and may lead to a swift fall in haemoglobin with rapidly enlarging spleen and liver. *Aplastic crises* occur in association with viral infections as in hereditary spherocytosis (p. 511) but the effect of the temporary cessation of erythropoiesis may be more dramatic as the haemolysis is severe.

The chronic anaemia is responsible for fatigue, reduced exercise tolerance, increased susceptibility to infection, cardiomegaly, leg ulcers and cholelithiasis. Hyperplasia of the marrow in the first year of life expands the marrow cavity producing bossing of the skull, prominent malar bones and protuberant teeth.

Infarction crises are characterised by episodes of severe pain and these punctuate the patients' lives. Commonly they occur in bones and spleen but no tissue is exempt. In the infant they classically affect the fingers and toes, producing large fusiform swellings (dactylitis). Metacarpal and tarsal bones may be affected and residual stigmata of shortening of digits due to epiphyseal involvement may occur. At any age mesenteric infarction may produce an acute abdominal emergency. The renal papilla is another site of trouble and infarction may give rise to painless haematuria. In adults aseptic necrosis of the head of the femur is a disabling complication.

Precipitating factors include dehydration, chilling and infection, but sometimes the attacks occur spontaneously. The onset is usually rapid and the pain excruciatingly severe (pain crisis) in the first 24 hours, thereafter abating over the next few days. Fever, increasing jaundice and malaise are common findings and, if persistent, may suggest the establishment of infection in the infarcted site. Salmonella osteomyelitis is common.

Pregnancy is hazardous unless careful antenatal care is provided and towards the end of pregnancy, infarction crises in the bones may liberate large amounts of fat and bone marrow emboli which cause diffuse microembolism of the lungs with pulmonary infarction, cor pulmonale and even death. These complications may also be seen in the less severe haemoglobin SC disease.

Sickle-cell anaemia should always be suspected in a patient who has had symptoms of anaemia since infancy and who belongs to a race which is often affected. In areas where sickle-cell anaemia is common, it should be considered in the differential diagnosis of many disorders. Patients must be adequately screened before major surgery and bloodless field surgery should never be employed, because infarction of the entire limb below the tourniquet may occur.

Investigation. Microscopic examination of the stained blood film will show some sickle-shaped red cells in patients with sickle-cell anaemia but these are not seen in patients with sickle-cell trait. The presence of haemoglobin S can be confirmed by the demonstration that the red cells will sickle within 20 minutes when mixed on a glass slide with a freshly prepared 2% solution of sodium metabisulphite under a cover slip. Positive and negative controls should be set up at the same time. Alternatively solubility tests may be employed. If neither of these is available, a small drop of blood diluted in saline may be incubated under a sealed cover slip overnight when sickling will occur. A positive result indicates the presence of haemoglobin S but does not distinguish between sickle-cell trait, sickle-cell anaemia, haemoglobin SC disease, sickle-cell thalassaemia, etc.

When suspected, the diagnosis should be confirmed by electrophoretic analysis of the haemoglobin and, if necessary, by a family study to demonstrate the inheritance. In this way true sickle-cell anaemia can be differentiated from other diseases in which haemoglobin S is combined with thalassaemia or some other abnormal haemoglobin such as C or D.

Antenatal diagnosis is discussed on page 17.

Treatment and prevention. There is as yet no reliable method of changing the genetic constitution of an individual and therefore no means of curing this disease. Management has to be aimed at alleviation of the symptomatology and the promotion of a way of life that will minimise the ill effects of the disorder. Regular folic acid supplements (5 mg daily) should be prescribed to support the greatly increased erythropoietic activity.

Exacerbation of the chronic haemolytic anaemia is commonly associated with infections and these should be treated promptly and prevented, e.g. life-long antimalarials taken where appropriate. Young patients with hyposplenism should be given phenoxymethylpenicillin and pneumococcal vaccine. Patients should avoid becoming chilled or dehydrated and exposure to hypoxia, e.g. at high altitudes.

An acute exacerbation may have no obvious precipitating cause. The spleen and liver may enlarge rapidly; serious depletion of blood volume may occur and the haemoglobin drop, sometimes with alarming speed (sequestration crisis). Transfusion is urgently required.

In less severe cases the patient should be adequately hydrated but transfusion with red cell concentrate used only if really necessary because of the risk of allo-antibody formation and subsequent reactions. Most patients are habituated to a haemoglobin level of about 8 g/dl and should be transfused only when the haemoglobin drops below 5 g/dl. Transfusion is used before planned surgery in order to raise the haemoglobin and reduce susceptibility to sickling. In acute cases, exchange transfusion is desirable to reduce haemoglobin S levels to 30%.

In pain crises, powerful, potentially addictive, analgesics may be necessary in the early stages; after 24–48 hours they should be replaced by milder non-addictive preparations. The prompt correction of dehydration often helps to relieve the pain. Antibiotics will be necessary if there are infective complications such as osteomyelitis.

Many lines of therapy to prevent in vivo sickling have been tried but even those with a theoretical hope of success have proved disappointing.

Prognosis. It is probable that in Africa, without medical attention, few children with sickle-cell anaemia survive to adult life. With full medical facilities and improved social and economic circumstances many patients survive and, although subject to recurrent ill-health, lead a fairly normal life but are unlikely to reach old age.

Other sickle-cell diseases

Sickle-cell trait. Most patients who are carriers of the sickle gene lead healthy lives. However, under certain circumstances they may be liable to sickling. These include bloodless field surgery and flying at altitudes over 15 000 feet (4575 m) if pressurisation is inadequate. In addition these patients are liable to attacks of painless haematuria due to infarction of the renal papillae.

Haemoglobin SC disease. This disorder behaves like a mild variety of sickle-cell anaemia. Episodes of infarction crises are less frequent and anaemia is either absent or less severe. Aseptic necrosis of the femoral head, retinal vein thrombosis and painless haematuria are not uncommon complications.

Pregnancy is the main hazard as the same complications occur as in sickle-cell anaemia, particularly fat and bone marrow embolisation of the lungs. Treatment should be by heparinisation and if necessary by premature induction of labour or delivery by caesarean section. Another risk is that the symptomatology may mimic closely other problems in pregnancy characterised by hypertension and proteinuria, but the treatment appropriate for these may be lethal. Sedatives should be avoided. Careful antenatal and postnatal care are required. Folic acid supplements will be needed and also iron if there is deficiency.

Haemoglobin C disease. This is a benign haemoglobinopathy which, in its homozygous form, is not associated with much morbidity. It may cause megaloblastic anaemia in pregnancy and considerable splenomegaly in adult life. No specific treatment is required other than folic acid supplements in pregnancy.

The thalassaemias

Thalassaemia is an inherited impairment of haemoglobin formation, in which there is partial or complete failure to synthesise a specific type of globin chain. The exact nature of the defect varies and it is probable that a number of different faults occur along the pathway which translates the genetic information into a polypeptide chain. The gene itself may be deleted. When the abnormality is heterozygous, synthesis of haemoglobin is only mildly affected and little disability occurs. When the patient is homozygous, synthesis is grossly impaired and severe anaemia results.

β-thalassaemia

Failure to synthesise beta chains (β-thalassaemia) is the commonest type and is seen in highest frequency in the Mediterranean area. Heterozygotes have thalassaemia minor, a condition in which there is usually mild anaemia and little or no clinical disability. Homozygotes (thalassaemia major) are either unable to synthesise haemoglobin A or at best produce very little and, after the neonatal period, have a profound hypochromic anaemia associated with much evidence of red cell dysplasia and increased red cell destruction. Haemoglobin F ($\alpha_2\gamma_2$) production normally ceases in the neonatal period, but because of the severe anaemia some production persists and provides much of the circulating haemoglobin. Thus these patients attempt to supply their requirements with haemoglobins that normally comprise only 3% of the total. At best they usually manage little more than 30 to 50% of the normal adult complement of haemoglobin.

Clinical features. The anaemia is crippling and the probability of survival for more than a few years without transfusion is low. Bone marrow hyperplasia early in life may produce head bossing and prominent malar eminences. The skull radiograph shows a 'hair on end' appearance and general widening of the medullary spaces which may interfere with the development of the paranasal sinuses. Development and growth are retarded and folate deficiency may occur. Splenomegaly is an early and prominent feature. Hepatomegaly is slower to develop but may become massive especially if splenectomy is undertaken. Transfusion therapy inevitably gives rise to haemosiderosis. Cardiac enlargement is common and cardiac failure, in which haemosiderosis may play a part, is a frequent terminal event.

There are several types of β-thalassaemia and a great variety of clinical manifestations which present a wide range of disease. For further study the reader is referred to publications dealing with this subject in greater detail (p. 553).

Diagnosis. Thalassaemia minor is often detected only when iron therapy for a mild hypochromic anaemia fails. The demonstration of microcytes, increased resistance of red cells to osmotic lysis and a raised haemoglobin A2 fraction (p. 513), together with evidence of the same abnormalities in other members of the family, establishes the diagnosis. In contrast haemoglobin A2 levels are diminished in iron deficiency states.

The diagnosis of thalassaemia major is made by the finding of profound hypochromic anaemia associated with evidence of severe red cell dysplasia, erythroblastosis, and the absence or gross reduction of the amount of haemoglobin A, raised levels of haemoglobin F and evidence that both parents have thalassaemia minor.

Treatment. Bone marrow transplantation from an HLA identical sibling donor offers the only hope of long-term survival. Otherwise transfusion is the mainstay in the management of homozygous β-thalassaemia and if possible the haemoglobin levels should be maintained between 10 and 12 g/dl. The intraperitoneal route may be used in young children to conserve veins. Iron therapy is strongly contraindicated but folic acid supplements should be given. Attempts to remove iron by the administration of chelating agents such as desferrioxamine should be employed but fail to keep pace with the iron deposition from transfusion therapy until the patient has been transfused with over 100 units of red cells when the level of iron overload becomes considerable and chelating agents more effective. Splenectomy may be required for mechanical reasons or for hypersplenism (p. 541). The later this can be done the better. Intercurrent infection must be treated vigorously with appropriate antibiotics.

Prevention. It is now possible to identify a fetus with homozygous β-thalassaemia by obtaining blood samples by fetoscopy sufficiently early in pregnancy to allow termination of pregnancy. This would be appropriate if both parents are known to be carriers (β-thalassaemia minor) and will accept such a termination.

α-thalassaemia

The reduction or absence of alpha chain synthesis is found mainly in S.E. Asia. There are probably at least two inherited abnormalities, one associated with severe, and the other with mild inhibition of alpha chain production. Heterozygotes of either abnormality are at little disadvantage since alpha chain production is adequate. A slight excess of gamma chain production at birth may form gamma-tetramers (haemoglobin Bart's) and this can be demonstrated by electrophoretic techniques. The combination in the patient of a mild and a severe α-thalassaemia disorder results in a deficiency of alpha chain production which is less than absolute, so that some normal haemoglobin is formed. There is an excess of beta chains and these form beta-tetramers (haemoglobin H) and this may explain the syndrome of haemoglobin H disease. The inheritance of the severe α-thalassaemia abnormality from both parents is incompatible with life and such offspring are stillborn.

AUTOIMMUNE HAEMOLYTIC DISEASE

In this disorder antibodies are formed against red cell antigens and cause inappropriate destruction of the cells (p. 27). There are two main types categorised on the basis of the thermal characteristics of their antibody. 'Warm' antibodies have a thermal optimum of 37°C, this being characteristic of most acquired antibodies. The majority are IgG. Warm type autoimmune haemolytic anaemia has antibodies of this type and these can almost always be shown to have Rhesus specificity. 'Cold' antibodies have a thermal optimum of 4°C, but sometimes a thermal range of up to 37°C. Naturally occurring antibodies tend to be of this type and most are IgM.

Warm type autoimmune haemolytic anaemia

Many cases are idiopathic but some occur in association with chronic lymphatic leukaemia, lymphoma and systemic lupus erythematosus.

Clinical features. Patients of all ages are affected. Symptoms vary with the severity of the disease and its cause and are mainly those of anaemia. In addition, in severe cases there may be fever, vomiting and prostration. Splenomegaly and sometimes hepatomegaly is present.

Investigation. The diagnosis is established by demonstrating evidence of antibody on the red cells by the direct antiglobulin test (Coomb's test). Antibody in the plasma may be shown by the indirect antiglobulin test. Elution of antibody from the red cells allows investigation of specificity against a panel of cells. The majority of these antibodies can be shown to have anti-Rhesus specificity (p. 518). Of these, anti-e is the commonest. Identification of specificity is useful as blood for transfusion which does not carry the specific antigen can be chosen. The blood film almost always shows polychromasia and spherocytosis.

Treatment should be with prednisolone, 60 mg daily for 3 to 4 weeks, the dose thereafter being slowly reduced. Response to treatment can be monitored with reticulocyte counts and haemoglobin estimation. If relapse occurs, the dosage should be raised and maintained for a further three weeks, when reduction may be tried again. If treatment fails from the beginning or, if after 6 months of steroid therapy the patient still has active haemolytic disease, splenectomy should be considered. If splenectomy fails, immune suppression with drugs such as azathioprine may be tried. However, disease which behaves in this way usually turns out to be chronic. Blood transfusion should be avoided unless an antibody has clearly been identified and antigen-free blood is available. In life threatening situations, the least incompatible blood available should be given, covered by high doses of prednisolone.

Cold agglutinin disease

Idiopathic cold agglutinin disease occurs mainly in the elderly and the symptoms reflect a tendency of the red cells to agglutinate and sludge in the microvasculature of the extremities where the blood is cooled. Raynaud's phenomenon is usually present and also acrocyanosis. A low grade chronic haemolytic anaemia occurs. All these problems are worse in cold weather. Investigations demonstrate an increased red cell turnover and a 'cold' antibody in enormously high titres. The antiglobulin test is almost always positive.

Treatment consists of keeping the extremities warm. Transfusion should be avoided if possible. Steroids and splenectomy are of little value but immunosuppressive therapy may decrease antibody levels in severe cases.

Cold agglutinin disease secondary to other disorders. Paroxysmal cold haemoglobinuria may be associated with syphilis or be idiopathic and have the Donath Landsteiner IgG antibody. Cold antibody-type disease may also occur in association with *Mycoplasma pneumoniae* infection and infectious mononucleosis when the haemolysis is usually self limiting. If found in lymphoma the haemolysis is usually more chronic.

ISOIMMUNE HAEMOLYTIC DISEASE

The term isoimmune is used to indicate that the antigen and the antibody come from different persons, although of the same species. This distinguishes it from autoimmune disease in which the antigen and the antibody are from the same individual.

Haemolytic disease of the newborn

This disease, previously called *erythroblastosis fetalis,* occurs in either sex at birth or within 2 to 3 days thereafter. In cases of Rhesus incompatibility the first-born in the family is usually healthy, but in successive children the severity of the disease increases and later children may be born dead. *Hydrops fetalis* is the most severe form, death occurring in utero; *icterus gravis neonatorum* is a dangerous illness but compatible with survival; haemolytic disease of the newborn is the mildest form. ABO incompatibility gives rise to a less severe form of the disease, but can affect first pregnancies. It occurs in Group O mothers carrying Group A or Group B infants.

It appears that in most cases the Rhesus (Rh) factor is the sensitising antigen. The majority (85%) of people, men and women, have red cells which contain the Rh antigen D. These people are said to be Rh-positive. Some of the children of an Rh-positive father and an Rh-negative mother are Rh-positive, since the factor is inherited as an autosomal dominant. The Rh-negative mother becomes sensitised by the Rh-positive antigen contained in the fetal red cells. The resultant maternal antibodies penetrate the placental barrier and cause haemolysis of the fetal erythrocytes. In about 1 pregnancy in 10 the mother is Rh-negative and the fetus Rh-positive. However, haemolytic disease of the newborn is very rare in first pregnancies provided the mother has not previously been sensitised by transfusion (see below). Furthermore, sensitisation does not occur as often as might be anticipated in subsequent pregnancies and the risk of an Rh-negative woman having a baby with haemolytic disease of the newborn in any pregnancy other than the first is about 1 in 22.

If a mother is Rh-negative and the father Rh-positive, the maternal serum must be tested for antibodies between the 32nd and 36th week of each pregnancy. If found, delivery should be carried out in hospital. If no antibodies are detected the infant will probably escape the disease, but nevertheless the cord blood should be tested for antibodies. If present, preventive treatment can be instituted.

An Rh-negative mother who has had an Rh-positive fetus may be sensitised to Rh-positive blood. If she receives a transfusion of Rh-positive blood a haemolytic reaction may occur. Consequently all women of child-bearing age or under and all pregnant women who may require transfusion must have their blood carefully typed for Rh factors as well as for the main blood groups.

Clinical features are those of severe haemolytic anaemia with oedema and enlargement of the liver and spleen. Clinical jaundice is usually absent for 24 hours after birth. Thereafter deep jaundice leading to kernicterus (p. 652) may occur. The severity of the jaundice is largely due to the immaturity of the fetal liver which is unable to conjugate the large amounts of bilirubin with which it has to deal. The blood picture is very striking. The haemoglobin level, which should normally be about 18 g per 100 ml at birth, falls rapidly. Enormous numbers of nucleated red cells and a reticulocytosis of 10 to 50% are found in the peripheral blood.

In severe cases the mortality rate is 70 to 80% without treatment, death occurring within 2 weeks, but with exchange transfusion the mortality is low. Spontaneous recovery occurs in mild cases.

Treatment. Exchange transfusion should be given to all severely affected infants, as this is the only method of treatment that will overcome heart failure in the very anaemic infant and prevent deep jaundice and kernicterus in others. Delay of even a day may prove fatal and hence early diagnosis is essential. Antenatal prediction from tests for antibodies in the maternal serum gives the infant the best chance. In mild cases simple transfusion will be sufficient, and in some instances no treatment is required.

Prevention. It is now believed that the most common cause of primary Rh immunisation may be transplacental haemorrhage during the third stage of labour. The likelihood of an Rh-negative women developing anti-Rh antibodies is related to the number of Rh-positive red cells present in her circulation immediately after delivery. These can be stained and quantitated. When they are found the mother should receive an injection of gamma globulin containing a high titre of anti-D immunoglobulin within 72 hours of delivery. This will destroy the infant cells that have leaked into the mother's circulation and will prevent the development of antibodies in the mother and haemolytic disease in later babies.

HAEMOLYTIC ANAEMIA DUE TO OTHER ABNORMALITIES

Physical trauma to red cells. Prosthetic heart valves, bacteria and intravascular fibrin formation associated with disseminated intravascular coagulation may all traumatise the red cells reducing their life span. Fragmented cells may be seen in the blood film.

Drugs, e.g. sulphasalazine or dapsone, may stress the metabolic processes of the red cells to the point of destruction even though the red cell is not enzyme deficient. Antigen-antibody reactions due to drugs acting as haptens may damage red cells directly or indirectly.

Malaria. Haemolysis always accompanies malaria and in severe or prolonged attacks very considerable anaemia may ensue (p. 772).

Inflammatory and neoplastic disease shortens the life span of the red cell. The mechanisms are complex and not completely understood. Excessive erythrophagocytosis by macrophages occurs. Red cells are damaged as they pass through affected tissue and drugs used in treatment may also harm them.

Paroxysmal nocturnal haemoglobinuria is a very rare disease in which an acquired clone of red cells is abnormally sensitive to lysis by complement in the blood causing intermittent haemolytic anaemia and haemoglobinuria. Thrombotic episodes are common. The disease is usually chronic but may progress to, or arise during, aplastic anaemia and may go on to acute leukaemia.

TRANSFUSION WITH INCOMPATIBLE BLOOD

Transfusion with incompatible blood may arise: (1) with clerical errors leading to the wrong blood being given; (2) when the infused red cells are of the wrong main blood group due to careless typing of the blood; (3) when the blood of recipient and donor are of compatible main groups but contain incompatible subgroups. Direct cross-matching of recipient's serum against donor's cells greatly reduces this risk; (4) from the transfusion of Rh-positive blood to a sensitised Rh-negative recipient.

Symptoms usually begin after only a few millilitres of blood have been given, and if the transfusion is immediately stopped there may be no serious consequences. In severe reactions the patient complains of shivering and restlessness, nausea and vomiting, precordial and lumbar pain. The pulse and respiration rates increase and the temperature rises. The blood pressure falls and the patient passes into a state of shock.

Jaundice appears after a few hours. There is

haemoglobinaemia, and possibly even haemoglobinuria; oliguria may occur with renal failure due to acute tubular necrosis. In severe cases anuria persists and uraemia develops, from which the patient may die. In others diuresis occurs even after several days and the patient recovers. In the majority the acute features subside in 24 to 48 hours. Delayed problems may arise from immune complexes causing renal damage.

Prophylaxis involves great care in the typing of blood and direct cross-matching before administration. The first 50–100 ml of any transfusion should be given very slowly and the transfusion stopped at once if any untoward symptoms develop. The patient should be under continuous observation during transfusion especially if unconscious.

Treatment of the established reaction involves giving hydrocortisone (100 mg i.v.), inducing a diuresis with mannitol and dealing with shock. If acute tubular necrosis occurs the measures recommended on page 403 must be instituted at once.

ERYTHROCYTOSIS AND POLYCYTHAEMIA

A raised haemoglobin level usually, but not always, indicates an absolute increase in the number of circulating red cells. In some patients it may be a spurious finding, the apparently high haemoglobin level being due to a reduction in plasma volume. This may occur because of dehydration or because of unknown mechanisms associated with stress (Fig. 13.3). A genuine increase in red cell numbers (erythrocytosis) occurs for a number of reasons which fall into three main groups:

1. When there is a physiological stimulus, as in hypoxia (p. 495) in which the production of erythropoietin is increased. Hypoxia may be due to altitude, pulmonary disease or congenital heart disease with cyanosis or where there are abnormal haemoglobins with a high oxygen affinity. The white cells and platelets are unaffected and there is no splenomegaly.

2. When there is a physiological response to a pathological stimulus. In this group the red cells are increased secondary to the production of abnormal amounts of substances with erythropoietin activity; this is occasionally found with certain benign and malignant tumours, e.g. of the kidney, liver, bronchus, uterus and cerebellum (haemangioblastoma) and with renal cysts. As in the first group the white cells and platelets are usually normal and there is no splenomegaly. However, the blood counts may be affected by the underlying disease.

3. When there is a pathological proliferation of red cells without erythropoietin stimulus. This is true or primary polycythaemia (polycythaemia vera, Fig. 13.3).

Stress or spurious erythrocytosis. Some patients with a high haemoglobin are found to have a red cell mass which is normal or even subnormal. The cause is a reduced plasma volume. This latter disorder tends to occur in middle-aged males who carry heavy responsibility or who are under stress for other reasons. It is often associated with hypertension and vascular disease. A more relaxed way of life or the use of tranquillisers sometimes has a beneficial effect with recovery of normal blood values.

Polycythaemia vera

Polycythaemia vera is one of a group of disorders of the pluripotential stem cells. These 'myeloproliferative disorders' (p. 521) have features in common and may progress from one form to another.

Clinical features. Polycythaemia vera occurs mainly in patients over the age of 40 and is more common in males than females. There may be no symptoms and the patient is diagnosed incidentally. Common symptoms are lassitude, loss of concentration, headaches, dizziness, blackouts, pruritus, epistaxis and 'indigestion'. Some present with manifestations of peripheral vascular disease. The patients often have a high colour, suffused conjunctivae, deep red palate and dusky red hands; retinal vein engorgement may be found. The spleen is palpable in 75% of cases at diagnosis. Thrombotic complications may occur and peptic ulceration is common, sometimes complicated by bleeding.

Investigation. The haemoglobin level is usually greater than 18 g/dl in males and 16 g/dl in

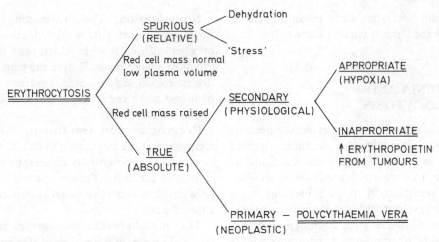

Fig. 13.3 Erythrocytosis and polycythaemia.

females. An associated elevation of white cell and platelet counts occurs in many cases. The bone marrow is hypercellular with erythroid hyperplasia, very active granulopoiesis and increased numbers of megakaryocytes. Iron depletion of the marrow is usual. The red cell mass is greatly increased and the plasma volume is often normal. The neutrophil alkaline phosphatase score (p. 528) is normal or elevated and urate levels are often high. Whole blood viscosity is increased. In some patients the above results may be marginal and the diagnosis uncertain. However, the presence of a raised red cell mass together with splenomegaly is virtually diagnostic.

Treatment. Venesection is the simplest therapeutic measure and the best to use if the diagnosis is in doubt; 500 ml of blood (less if the patient is elderly) may be removed and this venesection repeated within a day or two if necessary. Venesection should continue until the haematocrit reading is reduced to 45%. Clinical improvement occurs rapidly with the reduction of blood viscosity. Iron deficiency appears, if not already present, but generally iron is not prescribed as its deficiency curbs erythropoiesis. It may be given with other methods of treatment. Venesection should be used with caution when the platelet count is very high because of the risk of thrombosis.

Radioactive phosphorus (5 mCi of ^{32}P i.v.) is an excellent form of treatment when the diagnosis is certain. The full effect will not appear for 3 months but the white cell count and platelets respond more quickly. Further doses may be required.

Chemotherapy with busulphan (2–4 mg/d), or melphalan (2–4 mg/d) until the disease is brought under control is equally effective but requires more supervision and more frequent blood counts than with radioactive phosphorus. It carries a slightly greater risk of severe marrow depression. Pyrimethamine (p. 773) may be used if no other treatment is available but can be associated with drug-induced ill-health. Chlorambucil should not be used as it is associated with an increased incidence of acute leukaemia.

Prognosis. The average life span after diagnosis in treated cases exceeds 10 years. Some survive more than 20 years. Progress to a refractory state with anaemia, myelofibrosis or acute leukaemia eventually occurs if the patient does not succumb to intercurrent disease.

Other myeloproliferative disorders

In addition to polycythaemia vera there are other myeloproliferative disorders which are closely related and are either malignant or pre-malignant. These include myelofibrosis (p. 529) and essential thrombocythaemia (p. 546). There is a tendency for these disorders to terminate in an acute leukaemic phase.

DISEASES OF THE WHITE BLOOD CELLS AND THE MONOCYTE-MACROPHAGE SYSTEM

The term 'monocyte-macrophage' system is now replacing the widely used 'reticuloendothelial system' as the latter has little meaning and is inaccurate in the light of current knowledge.

NEUTROPENIA AND AGRANULOCYTOSIS

A reduction in the number of circulating neutrophil leucocytes (neutropenia) or their absence (agranulocytosis) is a potentially serious disorder.

Aetiology. In some cases the cause is an idiosyncrasy or sensitisation to, or poisoning by, a variety of drugs, notably amidopyrine, chlorothiazide, phenothiazines such as chlorpromazine, chlorpropamide, phenindione, troxidone, penicillin, various sulphonamides and the thiouracil derivatives. Exposure to insecticides should also be considered.

Neutropenia or agranulocytosis may follow excessive irradiation or the use of cytotoxic drugs or antimetabolites and is also found as an integral part of pancytopenia, leukaemia and some cases of hypersplenism. Rarely the disorder is inherited. In a few cases there is no discoverable cause — idiopathic agranulocytosis.

Pathology. In many cases the bone marrow shows a virtual disappearance of the granular cells and their precursors. In some the marrow contains early myelocytes, with few mature forms — an arrest of maturation, but such appearances may indicate early recovery. In others the appearances are those of the underlying blood disease.

Clinical features. There may be a history of exposure to one of the agents mentioned above. The onset may be either sudden or gradual. In acute and severe cases the condition begins with sore throat, fever and often rigors. There is rapidly advancing necrotic ulceration in the throat and mouth, with little evidence of pus formation. In fulminating cases the patient dies in a few days from toxaemia and septicaemia. In less acute cases there may be a preliminary period of malaise and weakness.

A chronic type has been described in which there is a persistence of neutropenia. Rarely the neutropenia occurs in cycles of 3 to 4 weeks (*cyclic neutropenia*). In such cases, the symptoms are chiefly recurrent malaise, low grade fever and sore throat.

Investigation. The outstanding and sometimes only abnormality is the reduction in absolute numbers of neutrophils which may be absent in the most severe cases. Where the cause is another disorder such as leukaemia, evidence of this may be found and a reduction in the haemoglobin and platelet count observed.

Prevention and treatment. All the drugs mentioned at the beginning of this section should be regarded as potentially dangerous and must be employed carefully. Patients taking them should be warned to report unusual symptoms, fever or a sore throat.

The most important measure in treatment is removal of the offending agent if it can be identified. The patient is at risk from septicaemia. Blood cultures should be done and the patient managed in the same way as those with the neutropenia and agranulocytosis that follows ablative chemotherapy used for acute myeloblastic leukaemia (p. 525). If the patient survives the acute phase, the outlook is fairly good, with recovery in many cases. In more chronic cases and where there is only neutropenia, infections should be dealt with as they arise.

INFECTIOUS MONONUCLEOSIS (GLANDULAR FEVER)

This is a benign, acute infective disease due to the Epstein Barr (EB) virus, a herpesvirus which also causes Burkitt's lymphoma and nasopharyngeal carcinoma. The EB virus infects, and replicates in, B lymphocytes. Infectious mononucleosis occurs chiefly in adolescents and young adults of either sex, sporadically or in epidemics. It is mildly infectious and often spread by direct oral contact — the 'kissing disease'. The incubation period is usually about a week to 10 days.

Clinical features. The most common presenting features are tiredness, malaise, headache, anorexia, fever and enlargement of superficial lymph nodes, particularly the posterior cervical. Petechial haemorrhages at the junction of the hard and soft palate may occur early and be followed by sore throat with or without exudate. A maculopapular rash often appears during the first 10 days in adults. Patients who have been given ampicillin for the sore throat develop a skin eruption due to the drug in over 90% of cases. Epigastric and right subcostal tenderness is common and reflects hepatitis. The spleen is often palpable. Pain in the right iliac fossa may result from mesenteric adenitis. Rarely there may be signs of meningitis or encephalitis.

Investigation. A mild neutrophil leucocytosis is often present in the first few days, thereafter being replaced by an increase in the characteristic atypical mononuclear cells. These are activated T lymphocytes. EB virus selectively infects B lymphocytes and may remain latent with reactivation especially in immunocompromised persons. The proportion of the atypical cells varies greatly from case to case. The total white cell count is commonly raised to between 10 and $20 \times 10^9/l$. Another herpesvirus infection, that due to cytomegalovirus (p. 730) and also toxoplasmosis (p. 781) may cause lymphadenopathy and changes in the blood similar to infectious mononucleosis.

Heterophil antibodies develop in the serum of patients with infectious mononucleosis. After the first week the Paul-Bunnel reaction becomes positive in titres of 1:200 or more in over 80% of cases and may remain positive for weeks. The 'Monospot test' is widely used as a screening procedure. It is a simple slide test which is quick and more sensitive than the Paul-Bunnell. The Wasserman reaction may be falsely positive. IgM directed against the viral capsid antigen and a positive heterophil antibody test are considered sufficient for a diagnosis of primary EB infection.

Treatment is symptomatic. The patient should be rested during the acute phase. Metronidazole may be useful in treating the oral lesions. Although recovery is invariable some patients have prolonged debility, with intermittent fever, sweating, inability to concentrate and depression. These symptoms may respond dramatically to corticosteroid therapy. Rarely thrombocytopenia or autoimmune haemolytic anaemia may occur; in most cases these also respond to corticosteroids.

THE LEUKAEMIAS

Leukaemias are a group of malignant disorders of the white blood cells characteristically associated with increased numbers of white cells in the blood.

Leukaemias are progressive and fatal conditions most often resulting in death from anaemia, haemorrhage or intermittent infection. The course may vary from a few weeks to several years depending on the type.

Aetiology. In the majority of cases the cause of the leukaemia is unknown. Several factors, however, now appear to be associated with the development of leukaemia. These are:

1. *Ionising radiation.* There was an undoubted increase in myeloid leukaemia following the atomic bombing of Japanese cities. A striking increase in leukaemia was also observed after the use of radiotherapy for ankylosing spondylitis.
2. *Cytoxic drugs.* These, particularly alkylating agents used in the treatment of cancer (p. 109), may induce myeloid leukaemia in some patients, usually after a latent period of several years.
3. *Exposure to benzene* in industrial situations.
4. *Retrovirus.* One rare form of T cell lymphocytic leukaemia appears to be associated with a retrovirus (p. 726) similar to the viruses causing leukaemia in cats and cattle.

Clinical and haematological features. The terms acute and chronic, when applied to leukaemias, refer to the clinical behaviour of the two main types of the disease. In acute leukaemia the history is usually brief and life expectancy, without treatment, short. In chronic leukaemias the patient may have been unwell for years and survival is measured in years. These differences are mirrored in the haematological findings. The general rule holds true that in malignant disease the more acute the clinical course, the more primitive or undifferentiated is the cell type. Thus in acute leukaemia primitive blast cells are characteristic whereas in the chronic forms differentiation to mature types of cell is seen.

Not all leukaemias are associated with an increased white cell count or even the appearance of abnormal cells in the blood. The term *subleukaemic* is used when the white cell count is within or below normal limits but abnormal cells are seen in the blood. *Aleukaemic* is used when there are no abnormal cells to be seen. In these cases the white cell count is usually subnormal. Almost all cases which present as subleukaemic or aleuk-aemic forms are acute leukaemias. The diagnosis is made from the marrow. Occasionally acute leukaemia presents as an aplastic anaemia and declares itself later.

Classification of Leukaemia:

Acute

1. Lymphoblastic
   a. T cell type
   b. B cell type
   c. Common type (cALL)
   d. Undifferentiated (null ALL)

2. Myeloblastic–French-American-British (FAB) classification:
   M1: Blasts without maturation
   M2: Blasts with some maturation
   M3: Hypergranular promyelocytic
   M4: Myelo-monocytic
   M5: Monocytic
   M6: Erythroleukaemic
   M7: Megakaryoblastic.

Chronic

1. Lymphocytic
2. Myeloid

Leukaemias are divided into lymphoid or myeloid varieties. Recent advances have shown, however, that this division may be rather artificial since in the acute leukaemias both types may coexist in the same patient. About 20% of blast transforma-tions of chronic myeloid leukaemias are lympho-blastic. Nevertheless, there is value in maintaining the division since the management of the two main types is substantially different.

Acute leukaemias of lymphoblastic and myeloblastic type can be subclassified as shown above. This is possibly of greater value in the lymphoblastic varieties since the subtype dictates greater variation in treatment.

Acute lymphoblastic leukaemia. The develop-ment of monoclonal antibodies has further advanced the identification and classification of these leukaemias. This subclassification is of major clinical significance since it is the common type, which constitutes 70% of all cases, that responds well to treatment and carries a very real chance of long-term remission. When immunological techniques are not available, acute lymphoblastic leukaemia may be recognised with some certainty on the basis of Romanowsky and special staining techniques using PAS and Sudan black.

Acute myeloblastic leukaemia is subclassified into seven varieties. This reflects the variable degree of maturation of the granulocyte series, the common involvement of the monocyte series with the granulocyte series and also the involvement of the erythroid and megakaryocyte elements. In M2 (p. 524), a degree of differentiation to the pro-myelocyte and even to the myelocyte stage can be seen and the latter may be associated with a more chronic course. In these cases the term 'subacute' has been used. Not all cases pursue an acute course even though the morphology of the disease would appear to indicate that they should; they may 'shoulder'. These merge with the myelo-dysplastic syndrome (p. 529).

Chronic leukaemias are divided into lymphocytic and myeloid. Chronic monocytic leukaemia is part of the myelodysplastic syndrome (p. 529) and usually terminates as acute myeloblastic leukaemia.

ACUTE LEUKAEMIAS

Acute leukaemias are disorders in which there is a failure of maturation. Proliferation of cells which do not mature leads to an ever increasing accumu-lation of useless cells which take up more and more marrow space. Eventually, this proliferation spills into the blood. The cells in acute leukaemia proliferate more slowly than normal haemopoietic tissue, a fact that is useful in treating these patients.

Acute myeloblastic leukaemia is the most com-mon type of acute leukaemia, except in young children in whom the lymphoblastic variety is more frequently found. In adults the incidence of acute leukaemia rises with age.

Clinical features. The disease may begin insidiously but the clinical onset is often abrupt with 'flu' like symptoms and fatigue. There may be fever, malaise and a rapidly advancing anaemia. Epistaxis, spongy bleeding gums or other haemor-rhagic manifestations including purpura are com-mon and are due largely to thrombocytopenia. Sore throat and ulcers in the mouth or pharynx are frequent, due to reduction in normal poly-morphonuclear leucocytes. Anorexia with weight loss is common. Hypertrophy of the gums is often noted in monoblastic (M4 and M5) leukaemias.

Muscle and joint pains may occur. The spleen and often the liver are enlarged in the later stages. There may be cervical lymphadenopathy secondary to pharyngeal sepsis but in the lymphoblastic form increase in the size of these and other lymph nodes is a common early feature.

Investigation. Blood examination usually shows a profound and increasing anaemia of normochromic type. The MCV is often raised. The white cell count may vary from a very low count of less than $1 \times 10^9/l$ to as high as $500 \times 10^9/l$ or more, but in the majority the count is less than $100 \times 10^9/l$. The blood film appearances are usually diagnostic of acute leukaemia since blast cells and other primitive cells are found. Sometimes marrow examination is required in aleukaemic forms before the nature of the disease is determined. Severe thrombocytopenia is usual but not invariable.

The marrow is involved in all cases and biopsy is the most important investigation. If it is impossible to obtain marrow by aspiration trephine biopsy should then be undertaken. The marrow is usually hypercellular with replacement of the normal elements by leukaemic blast cells in varying degrees. Special staining techniques and immunological tests are used to subclassify these diseases. The presence of Auer rods in the cytoplasm of the blast cells indicates a myeloblastic type of leukaemia.

Treatment. Accurate subclassification of acute leukaemias is of great importance as treatment of the lymphoblastic and myeloblastic varieties is very different. Chemotherapy (p. 109) is the major element in both, with radiotherapy (p. 107) being used in a minor role.

The first decision must be whether or not to give specific treatment. In the very elderly it may be unreasonable to subject the patient to unpleasant therapy which stands only a small chance of success for a brief period. In such cases supportive treatment should be given and this often alleviates distress. However, with the considerable improvement in the results of treatment, the view is taken that an attempt to achieve remission should be made in most patients.

SPECIFIC THERAPY is designed to eliminate the leukaemic tissue and allow the recovery of the normal haemopoietic cells. In *acute lymphoblastic leukaemia* it is fortunate that this can be achieved in the majority of patients using a regime based on vincristine and prednisolone, with other drugs such as anthracycline antibiotics and l-asparaginase sometimes added, a regime not so toxic to normal cell lines. Regrowth of the normal cells occurs as the leukaemic tissue regresses and the patient comes rapidly into remission. This is known as the *induction phase* of treatment. During it there is often massive cell lysis and allopurinol (300 mg/d) is prescribed to counteract excessive urate production.

A *consolidation phase* follows in which other drugs are used including daunorubicin, mercaptopurine, cytarabine and methotrexate. Using the last two drugs intrathecal therapy is also given together with irradiation of the cranium to eradicate disease in the central nervous system which may have survived the initial chemotherapy.

A *maintenance* phase of treatment follows in which the patient receives a repeating cycle of the above drugs until 2 or 3 years have been completed in remission. Active treatment is then withdrawn because the patient probably stands more chance of death as the result of treatment than from the disease itself. Unfortunately, patients with the T cell types of acute lymphoblastic leukaemia tend to respond but relapse more frequently and the few with B cell type respond poorly. If relapse occurs in any patient the chances of achieving long-term remission are greatly reduced.

Acute myeloblastic leukaemia must be managed rather differently. The three most useful drugs are daunorubicin, cytarabine, and thioguanine. All these are very toxic to normal as well as leukaemic cells. In addition daunorubicin is cardiotoxic. In order to eliminate the leukaemic tissue, a phase when the normal tissues are severely depressed must be accepted. During this *phase of ablation* the patient may be gravely at risk from infection and bleeding as there will be severe neutropenia and thrombocytopenia. Young patients tolerate this aggressive management better than old. Treatment is generally given in 'pulses'. A pulse of chemotherapy is a brief period of treatment between which there is an interval when no treatment is given. A number of pulses make up a course of therapy. Assessment of progress is made on blood and bone marrow findings. Once the marrow has been cleared of blast cells the normal haemopoietic tissue may be allowed to repopulate the marrow. The advantage of the more rapid proliferation of normal haemopoietic tissue is seen at this stage. As neutrophil production resumes, the patient rapidly feels better. Infections come under more effective control. Bleeding problems disappear as the platelet count rises.

At best only 50–60% of patients treated for acute myeloblastic leukaemia achieve a remission. In the others the disease is to a greater or lesser extent refractory to specific therapy. When it is evident that this is the case, chemotherapy is stopped, and the patient may have a few weeks of quite good life, with suitable support.

When remission is achieved and the bone marrow recovers the patient should receive maintenance therapy. There are many regimens but most employ the same drugs as are used for induction, except that daunorubacin must be used very frugally or not at all as its cardiotoxic effects are cumulative. Useful drugs are etoposide and cyclophosphamide.

Bone marrow transplantation is dealt with on page 509.

SUPPORTIVE THERAPY. The specific treatment of acute leukaemia, particularly the acute myeloblastic form, would be difficult, if not impossible, without intensive supportive therapy. *Anaemia* is the easiest problem to deal with; transfusions of red cell concentrate are given to maintain an adequate haemoglobin level, preferably above 10 g/dl. Bleeding is due mainly to thrombocytopenia and is exacerbated by infection. Platelet transfusions are required. Platelets are harvested from six freshly collected blood packs and pooled to provide one donation. Two or more donations may be required in a 24 hour period to control bleeding. Platelets may also be used for prophylaxis if bleeding is anticipated.

Infection, particularly septicaemia, is a serious and frequent problem. Unexplained fever over 38°C, lasting more than 6 hours, should be regarded as septicaemia until proven otherwise, if the patient is severely neutropenic (absolute neutrophil count less than $0.5 \times 10^9/l$). Parenteral antibiotic therapy should be administered (p. 48).

When antimicrobial therapy fails to control fever and there is severe neutropenia, white cell transfusion may be indicated. The preparation is usually obtained from a red cell compatible adult, whose white cells are harvested for 4 to 5 hours (*leucapheresis*), and irradiated to kill lymphocytes which might transplant to the recipient, and then administered. Patients with chronic granulocytic leukaemia and a high white cell count make excellent donors for these problems. The effect can be dramatic with rapid resolution of the fever. However, with improved antibiotic therapy and early treatment, white cell transfusions are now seldom used.

Management of infection other than septicaemia should be along standard lines, always keeping in mind, however, that any infection may give rise to septicaemia. Candidosis in the mouth, gastrointestinal tract and elsewhere tends to be intractable during periods of severe neutropenia, or if the patient is on steroid therapy; it requires treatment with antifungal agents (p. 46).

A reduction in the risk of infection may be achieved in several ways. The patient may be regularly bathed in antiseptic baths (povidone-iodine) and may be nursed in a protected environment, of which there are many kinds. The gut, which is a major source of infection, may be 'sterilised' using mainly unabsorbable antibiotics, and procedures such as brushing teeth or rectal examinations should be avoided.

Psychological support of the patient is of great importance. Most patients will rapidly discover their diagnosis if not told. It is preferable therefore to give the patients the opportunity to find out what they want to know and avoid telling them any untruths. In this way the patients' trust and confidence are retained and they understand why they must co-operate through an extremely stressful period of treatment. This is a delicate area of doctor-patient relationship and requires tact, sensitivity, and an understanding of the personality of the individual. The quality of the nursing service is also very important and a team of nurses familiar with the specialised management of leukaemia is required if the best results are to be obtained.

Isolation, which may be necessary because of the risk of infection, can be psychologically very disturbing to some patients. Others prefer it. Patients are at less risk of infection with resistant organisms at home that in hospital and should be discharged whenever possible if the home circumstances permit and they are sufficiently well. Often treatment can be given on an outpatient basis. Cranial irradiation causes almost total epilation. The prospect can be devastating, especially for women. Restyling of the hair, the choice of a good wig and the firm promise that the hair will grow in again go a long way to alleviate the patient's distress.

Prognosis. At the time of diagnosis it is difficult to give a prognosis other than to say that without treatment it is very poor. It is wise to explain that a clearer view of the outlook can be given after the effects of induction therapy have been observed. The prognosis for most cases of acute myeloblastic leukaemia is poor, the majority dying within a year. Patients with acute lymphoblastic leukaemia of the common (cALL) variety, can be encouraged to hope that they may have the prospect of long-term remission. For those who usually do not have a particularly good outlook, hope should always be maintained, as even in some of these cases the outcome of treatment may occasionally be better than anticipated.

CHRONIC LEUKAEMIAS

Chronic myeloid leukaemia

The disease occurs chiefly between the ages of 35 and 70 years. There is an extension of the marrow through the long bones. It is grey and gelatinous and is crowded with myelocytes and young polymorphonuclear leucocytes. Leukaemia infiltrations occur in the liver, spleen and lymph nodes and in most other organs.

Clinical features. The onset is insidious and the manifestations varied. Fatigue and lassitude are common. There may be slowly advancing anaemia with loss of weight, prominence of the abdomen and dragging discomfort in the left upper quadrant due to massive splenomegaly. Attacks of acute left upper abdominal pain may develop when infarction occurs in the spleen. Sternal tenderness and aching bones and arthralgia are common symptoms. Epistaxis or other haemorrhages may occur in the later stages. A hypermetabolic state may result in sweating, intolerance of heat and weight loss. Priapism is sometimes the presenting symptom. Secondary gout may also occur. However, sometimes at diagnosis the patient is asymptomatic.

The spleen is usually considerably enlarged and in occasional patients may reach the symphysis pubis. It is firm, smooth and painless but if infarction has occurred, it may be tender and a friction rub heard over it. There may be hepatomegaly but lymph nodes are not usually enlarged.

In some patients the chronic phase is followed by an accelerated phase in which control of the leucocyte count becomes difficult. Platelet counts often rise to high levels. Basophilia increases and the patient is less well. Eventually, in a variable period of time, transformation to an acute leukaemic phase occurs. In others the acute phase may appear without an intervening accelerated phase. In a few, no acute phase appears and the disease enters a chronic phase refractory to treatment. Acute transformation may be either lymphoblastic or myeloblastic. Unless it is the former, the outlook is extremely poor.

Investigation. Examination of the blood shows an anaemia, usually normochromic, normocytic in type which increases as the disease progresses. The white cell count is usually considerably increased to between 50 and 500 × 10^9/l. A blood film demonstrates the full range of granulocyte precursors from myeloblasts to mature neutrophils, the more mature forms being the most numerous. Myeloblasts usually number less than 10% of the total. There is also an increase in eosinophils and basophils and nucleated red cells are common. In the later stages, the appearance of an increasing number of myeloblasts may indicate the approach of a terminal acute phase and confirmation of this may be obtained from the bone marrow. The relative number of basophils also increases as the disease progresses. The platelet count is often high initially but with treatment usually comes down to normal levels.

The peripheral blood is more useful diagnostically than the bone marrow but the latter should be examined in order to exclude other conditions causing a leucoerythroblastic blood picture and to obtain material for chromosome analysis. In about 90% of cases chromosome analysis demonstrates the presence of the Philadelphia chromosome (p. 8).

The neutrophils of chronic myeloid leukaemia are usually deficient in alkaline phosphatase. Normal neutrophils stained for this enzyme can be crudely scored and usually give a result of between 20 and 100. In chronic myeloid leukaemia, the score is usually less than 5. However, a result within the normal range does not exclude the diagnosis. If initially low, the score often rises to normal with treatment.

Treatment. CHEMOTHERAPY. Effective palliative treatment can restore most patients to a period of symptom-free life. The method of choice is by chemotherapy using the alkylating agent busulphan (p. 109). It is given orally in a starting dose of 4 mg daily and can bring about a temporary but satisfactory clinical and haematological remission in a high proportion of cases, with marked reduction in splenomegaly. Generally no response is seen in the first 2 weeks. Thereafter the count falls and the results plotted on semilogarithmic paper against time give a straight line allowing prediction of the point at which the dose of busulphan may require reduction or withdrawal. On average, between 12 and 18 weeks are required to achieve a normal count, but rarely the count falls more rapidly and, unless dosage is stopped, severe and even lethal aplasia of the marrow may result. For this reason it is customary to stop the busulphan when the white cell count is between 10 and $20 \times 10^9/l$ and wait until it shows signs of rising before reintroducing the drug. Maintenance dosage of busulphan is generally 1–2 mg daily, but variation of the dose should be tailored to suit the individual patient, based on the regular blood counts which are of the utmost importance at this stage.

Alternatively a combination chemotherapy regimen employing a small dose of busulphan, 2 mg daily and either mercaptopurine 50 mg daily or thioguanine 80 mg daily may be used. Allopurinol influences the effective dose of mercaptopurine but not of thioguanine. If allopurinol is not being used the dose of mercaptopurine should be 100 mg daily. This regimen is given 5 days per week and results in a very much more rapid reduction in white cell count, taking on average 4–6 weeks, with correspondingly quicker induction of remission. Despite this, the regimen does not carry so great a risk of inducing severe aplasia as the count tends to plateau in the normal range of white cell counts. Dosage can be modified by varying the number of days per week on which the standard dose is given. The dose should be reduced when the count reaches normal levels.

Another satisfactory way of using busulphan is to give the drug in single doses of 50 mg at 3 or more weekly intervals. Remission is induced more quickly than by the single agent daily dose method and appears to be safe. Busulphan produces minor degrees of pulmonary fibrosis in most patients. In a few, however, this may assume serious proportions and then the drug should be stopped and never used again. Alternative drugs include hydroxyurea, melphalan, chlorambucil and dibromomanitol. Mercaptopurine and thioguanine are effective but when used alone are rather difficult to control. Radiotherapy to the spleen can also be given and is effective in inducing control of the disease. However, it has been shown to be inferior to busulphan therapy.

Interferon (p. 19) has now been shown to produce effective control of the disease, and in some cases reduce or even abolish the presence of the Philadelphia chromosome. Long-term therapy is required and is very expensive. It is not yet known whether cure can be achieved. Not all patients respond well and some tolerate interferon poorly. Initially, flu-like symptoms occur, which last up to 10 days, and then diminish. Somnolence, weight loss, dizziness, nausea, vomiting, diarrhoea, headaches, shortness of breath, constipation and loss of appetite may also occur. It is probably unwise to use interferon in patients over 70 years of age. However, despite the many possible side-effects, the majority of patients tolerate interferon therapy remarkably well.

SPLENECTOMY. Patients who present with massive splenomegaly and who run the risk of even more disabling enlargement in the terminal phase of the disease, may benefit from splenectomy, carried out when a good remission has been achieved.

Very high platelet counts, especially after splenectomy, appear to carry less danger of thrombotic complications than in other myeloproliferative disorders and may be well tolerated. The platelets are ineffective and may not be haemostatically adequate for major surgery, when platelet concentrations should be given postoperatively. If this is not done, there is a risk of intractable bleeding.

Prognosis. On average, patients with Philadelphia chromosome positive disease survive $3\frac{1}{2}$ years from the time of diagnosis. Philadelphia chromosome negative varieties, which are rare, carry a much poorer prognosis, the majority dying within one year. Long survival of up to 10 years or more occurs in a small proportion of patients.

In the majority the disease transforms sooner or later, either to an acute leukaemic phase, which may be either myeloblastic or lymphoblastic, or to a chronic refractory phase, with marrow fibrosis and an excess of basophils and blast cells. Unless the transformation is to acute lymphoblastic leukaemia, the outlook is extremely poor as the acute phase is very unresponsive to therapy. Sometimes the patient is diagnosed at the stage of transformation and this may account for some cases of acute leukaemia with the Philadelphia chromosome.

Eosinophilic leukaemia is a rare variant of chronic myeloid leukaemia and shows features of the hypereosinophilic syndrome in which cardiomyopathies and endomyocardial fibrosis occur, leading to severe cardiac failure. Treatment is difficult.

Erythaemic myelosis is a disorder of erythropoiesis analogous to acute or subacute leukaemia. It is closely related to and overlaps the M6 variety of acute myeloid leukaemia.

Myeloid metaplasia and myelofibrosis

Myeloid metaplasia is the appearance of precursors of red cells, granulocytes and platelets in abnormal sites such as the liver and spleen, and is usually associated with a leucoerythroblastic blood picture. This is not a phenomenon compensating for loss of marrow activity but is evidence of disordered behaviour by the precursor cell lines. Myeloid metaplasia is seen in myelofibrosis. Early in myelofibrosis the marrow may have little fibrous tissue and be hypercellular but as the disease progresses the fibrous tissue increases and may eventually fill most of the marrow space.

Clinical features are very variable. Most patients with myelofibrosis suffer lassitude, weight loss, night sweats and some intolerance of heat. The spleen may be greatly enlarged in myelofibrosis and splenic infarcts may occur. Rarely splenomegaly is absent. Peptic ulceration is common and there is increased incidence of gastrointestinal bleeding.

Investigation. Anaemia, sometimes macrocytic, is common. The white cell count varies with a diminution or increase of granulocytes and usually a leucoerythroblastic blood picture. The red blood cells show very characteristic tear drop poikilocytes. The platelet count may be very high, normal or low and giant forms are seen in the blood film. The neutrophil alkaline phosphatase score (p. 528) is frequently raised as are urate levels. The marrow is often difficult to aspirate and a trephine biopsy shows an excess of megakaryocytes and increased reticulin and fibrous tissue replacement. Folate deficiency is very common.

Treatment is largely supportive with blood transfusion, folic acid, and non-virilising androgen therapy. Corticosteroids may be helpful in some patients. Cytotoxic therapy should be used very cautiously. Splenectomy may be required if the grossly enlarged spleen is causing distress or because transfusion requirements are excessive but the outcome is unpredictable. Prognosis is generally rather poor. The disease is progressive with steady deterioration. Bone marrow transplantation should be considered for young patients.

Myelodysplastic syndrome. This is a group of uncommon disorders characterised by variable cytopenia, hypogranular neutrophils with hyper- or hyposegmentation, hypercellular marrow and megaloblastic-like changes in the erythroid precursors. Included in the syndrome are (1) refractory anaemia, (2) refractory anaemia with ring sideroblasts, (3) refractory anaemia with excess of blasts, (4) chronic myelomonocytic leukaemia, and (5) refractory anaemia with excess of blasts in transformation. All are relatively chronic disorders with a tendency to terminate as acute myeloid leukaemia. They occur mainly in the elderly. The marrow shows various dysplastic features.

Treatment is difficult. Transfusional support is often required. Some response has been obtained using low dose cytosine arabinoside therapy (20 mg b.d., s.c. for 3 weeks).

Chronic lymphatic leukaemia

This is the commonest variety of leukaemia. It occurs more frequently in males than in females and the majority of patients are over the age of 45. The disease is very rare in the Chinese and other mongoloid races.

Pathology. There is moderate enlargement of lymph nodes and other lymphoid tissues throughout the body, the normal structure being replaced by a mass of lymphocytes. The histology is that of diffuse well-differentiated lymphocytic disease, nodular histology being rare. The spleen and liver are moderately enlarged and show lymphocytic infiltration. The bone marrow becomes progressively infiltrated with lymphocytes which eventually replace the erythropoietic and myeloid tissue.

In this disease lymphocytes which would normally respond to antigens by transformation and antibody formation, fail to do so. An ever increasing mass of immuno-incompetent cells accumulate to the detriment of immune function and normal bone marrow haemopoiesis. The receptor profile of the lymphocytes almost always demonstrates a B cell type of disease. T cell disease occurs rarely. The light chains of immunoglobulins produced by these B cells tend to be either kappa or lambda in type (p. 21) indicating in the majority of cases, a monoclonal expansion of cells. The disease is closely related to and indeed overlaps with well-differentiated lymphocytic lymphoma (p. 537).

Clinical features. The onset is very insidious. Tiredness and vague ill-health are common although some patients are symptom free and the disorder is found incidentally. In contrast to chronic myeloid leukaemia the development of anaemia tends to be slower and the presenting feature is usually the finding of firm rubbery, discrete and painless lymph nodes in the cervical, axillary and inguinal regions. The spleen is usually palpable but smaller than in chronic myeloid leukaemia. The liver may also be enlarged. As a result of immunosuppression there is an increasing tendency to recurrent infections.

Investigation. Peripheral blood examination usually shows a mild but gradually increasing anaemia. Haemolytic anaemia may occur and is usually autoimmune in type. The white cell count may be greatly increased up to $1000 \times 10^9/l$ but in the majority of cases it is between $50-200 \times 10^9/l$. Of these cells about 95% or more are lymphocytes which are predominantly of the small variety. Lymphoblasts are rare but undifferentiated lymphocytes may increase in number in the terminal stages. The platelet count is either low normal or only mildly reduced.

Examination both by aspiration and trephine is required to assess the degree of marrow involvement. Dysplastic changes in the erythroblasts suggestive of folate deficiency may be noted and folate levels should be measured. Estimations of total proteins and immunoglobulin levels should be undertaken to establish the degree of immunosuppression which is common and progressive. In some patients immunoglobulin levels may be raised and there may be a monoclonal band. Urate levels are seldom raised because cell turnover is low.

STAGING. The disease may be staged according to the following criteria of the International Classification:

Clinical stage A: No anaemia or thrombocytopenia and less than three areas of lymphoid enlargement.
Clinical stage B: No anaemia or thrombocytopenia, with three or more involved areas.
Clinical stage C: Anaemia and/or thrombocytopenia regardless of the number of areas of lymphoid enlargement.

Treatment. Specific treatment may not be required until stage B or C of the disease is reached. The patient should be told that although the disorder is incurable it should be possible to live with it and that it may give little trouble for months or even years. Eventually specific treatment may be required and regular supervision by a haematologist becomes necessary. Patients with stage B and C disease will require specific and supportive therapy. Folate deficiency should be corrected. Anaemia may require transfusion with red cell concentrates. If the bone marrow is severely infiltrated, initial treatment with prednisolone 40 mg daily and oxymetholone 25–50 mg daily, for several weeks before starting cytotoxic drugs, may rescue the haemopoietic elements and allow more vigorous treatment.

There is disagreement about whether treatment should be by gentle single agent therapy employing chlorambucil, either continuously in doses between 2 and 5 mg daily, or intermittently at higher doses, or by more vigorous combination chemotherapy. The latter induces more convincing remissions judged by investigational findings, but has yet to be shown to improve the well-being or the survival of the patient in the long-term; the former method of treatment is therefore recommended. Combination therapy usually includes cyclophosphamide, doxorubicin, vincristine and prednisolone. Some believe doxorubicin is the most important of these drugs, but like daunorubicin it is cardiotoxic. Both are cytotoxic anthracycline antibiotics.

Alternatively radiotherapy may be used. Total body irradiation with a very small dose spread over 5 weeks in 10 treatments can be very effective and may induce satisfactory remission with a minimum of upset to the patient. Whichever treatment is used, dosage should be controlled by accurate blood counts, the absolute neutrophil count and the platelet count being the most important.

Infections must be treated with antibiotics. If there is severe depression of immunoglobulins, gammaglobulin intramuscularly may reduce the frequency and severity of infections. When the platelet count is low, the use of intramuscular immunoglobulin may not be possible and can be replaced by fresh frozen plasma given intravenously weekly. Gammaglobulin concentrate may be given intravenously if necessary. Splenectomy may be required for autoimmune haemolytic anaemia which has proved unresponsive to corticosteroid therapy.

Hairy cell leukaemia is a variant of chronic lymphatic leukaemia now recognised to be more common than was previously thought. It is a disease of adult life affecting males four times more frequently than females. The mean age is 50 years. Patients usually present with general ill health and troublesome infections especially in the skin and usually have considerable splenomegaly. Severe neutropenia, monocytopenia and the characteristic hairy cells in the blood and bone marrow are typical. These cells appear to be a cross between a B lymphocyte and a monocyte.

The diagnostic test is to show that the acid phosphatase staining reaction in the cells is resistant to the action of tartrate. The neutrophil alkaline phosphatase score is usually very high.

Splenectomy is the best treatment in the absence of interferon (p. 528) which, if tolerated, may reduce or eliminate the disease. Although many patients have a good outlook in others the disease progresses rapidly to death, usually from infections. It is in the latter group that interferon may prove particularly valuable. Corticosteroids may help but cytotoxic chemotherapy is seldom successful and is generally to be avoided.

Prolymphocytic leukaemia is another variant of chronic lymphatic leukaemia found mainly in males over the age of 60; 25% are of the T cell variety. There is massive splenomegaly with little lymphadenopathy and a very high white cell count, often in excess of $400 \times 10^9/l$. The characteristic cell is a large lymphocyte with a prominent nucleolus. Treatment is generally unsuccessful and the prognosis very poor. Leucapheresis for very high white counts, splenectomy and chemotherapy may be tried.

Exposure to ionising radiation

The use of nuclear radiation both for energy production and weapons raises the risk of a nuclear accident, either in peace, as at Chernobyl, or in war. There is much uninformed speculation about the effects of accidental exposure, some of it grossly exaggerated. No accident, however, can be treated lightly and the facts presented here, derived from the therapeutic use of ionising radiation and the effects of the atomic bombs dropped on Japanese cities, may provide some simple basic guidelines in the event of an accident.

Relatively high doses of radiation are tolerated when only part of the body is exposed but when the whole body is involved, tolerance is greatly reduced. Given time, the body is capable of repairing some of the damage done by radiation, provided it is not too severe. This forms the basis of the calculation of maximum permissible doses for workers employed in industrial projects in which radiation in one form or another is used. The therapeutic application of ionising radiation takes these factors carefully into account and also recognises the risk of inducing secondary malignancy. Since the majority of patients treated already has malignant disease, this risk is not generally regarded as a contraindication.

When an industrial nuclear accident occurs it is vital that all personnel leave the scene of radioactivity quickly to minimise exposure. If accidental exposure occurs, it is essential to obtain as accurate as possible an estimate of the radiation dose received and this will usually require the expertise of medical physicists. Workers who are likely to be exposed to radiation generally carry monitoring badges from which the doses can be calculated. If the accidental dose is relatively small, all that may be required is to remove the person from risk of further exposure. When the dose received approaches the limits of what the body can tolerate, the immediate risks are to the haemopoietic and gastrointestinal systems and can be monitored by general medical review and blood counts. Nausea and vomiting occurring under two hours from the time of exposure carry a very grave prognosis and treatment is generally useless. In patients whose symptoms develop at a later stage, support may be given in a similar way as for acute myeloid leukaemia receiving ablative therapy. Bone marrow transplantation from a sibling should be considered if facilities are available. The patient should have tissue typing performed at the earliest opportunity before his or her cells disappear.

The effects of a major atomic explosion, as from an atomic bomb, depend on where the human being is in relation to the explosion. Many are killed outright. Immediate survivors may die sooner or later from burns, both from flash exposure or the fire storm that follows, from blast and crush injuries or from radiation sickness. Radiation damage is due firstly to the intense burst of neutrons emitted at the time of the explosion and thereafter to radioactive fallout, although this is small in bombs in which the fireball does not hit the ground. Within 7 hours of such an explosion the radiation from the fallout drops to 10% of what it was 1 hour after the explosion and after 2 days the radioactivity has reduced to 1%.

Survival from the effects of the Hiroshima bombs was 95% of those more than 2000 metres from the explosion, despite exposure to immediate radiation. There was virtually no fallout as the fireball did not reach the ground. There was a small but definite increase in both acute and chronic myeloid leukaemia in survivors. Fetuses and young children exposed at the time of the bomb showed abnormalities in some cases but subsequent survivors had normal healthy children with no increase in deformity. The incidence of other tumours in the exposed population increased after a latent period of 10 to 15 years. These have occurred particularly in the thyroid, breast, lung, urinary tract and the haemopoietic systems.

The bombs used on the Japanese cities were small by modern standards. The scale of effects of the largest megaton bombs is not known but extrapolation from available evidence suggests that the population may be at risk up to 100 miles from the centre of the explosion in flat terrain. Hills and mountains may provide a degree of protection. Survivors who may benefit from medical treatment are likely to be so numerous as to overwhelm the medical and other services.

The need for prevention is obviously crucial and this responsibility involves every one of us.

THE LYMPHOMAS

This group of disorders is divided into two main types: Hodgkin's lymphoma and non-Hodgkin lymphoma.

Hodgkin's lymphoma

This disease is characterised by progressive painless enlargement of lymphoid tissues throughout the body. It occurs in both sexes, often in adolescence and early adult life, but it may be found also in older people. The pathogenesis is unknown and the condition is usually regarded as a form of malignant disease related to other neoplastic processes of haemopoietic tissue. It is distinguished from non-Hodgkin lymphoma by the presence of Reed-Sternberg cells, now thought to be the malignant cells.

Pathology. Microscopic examination of involved tissue, usually lymph nodes, shows variable obliteration of the normal architecture, with proliferation of lymphoid cells. Reed-Sternberg cells are giant cells with paired mirror imaged nuclei and prominent nucleoli; unless they are found it may be difficult to make a histological diagnosis. In addition there may be an increase in eosinophils, neutrophils, plasma cells and histiocytes in the tissue. The numbers of well-differentiated lymphocytes vary from many to few and the degree of lymphocytic depletion forms the basis for the main pathological classification of the disease. In some cases the fibrous stroma is increased. Caseation and necrosis are most unusual. Infiltration with areas of Hodgkin's tissue causes enlargement of the spleen and liver. The bone marrow, lungs, kidneys and alimentary tract may also be involved but deposits in the nervous system are rare.

The disease can be divided pathologically into sclerosing and non-sclerosing types. In the latter the degree of lymphocytic depletion correlates quite well with the aggressiveness of the disease and three types are seen, (1) lymphocyte predominant, (2) mixed cellularity in which neutrophils, eosinophils and plasma cells are common and (3) lymphocyte depleted, the most aggressive variety. In sclerosing disease, called nodular sclerosing, the cellular areas may also show variable lymphocytic depletion giving some clue about the aggressiveness of the disease. The nodular sclerosing variety is the most commonly encountered with the mixed cellularity type coming second, lymphocyte predominant third and lymphocyte depleted the least often seen.

Clinical features. The onset is insidious, usually with enlargement of one group of superficial nodes which may fluctuate in size. While the cervical nodes are often the first to be involved, the disease may also appear to start in the mediastinal and axillary nodes and more rarely in abdominal, pelvic and inguinal areas. Involved lymph nodes are usually painless, discrete and rubbery, though tenderness does occur in some cases, particularly when the nodes have enlarged rapidly. The overlying skin is freely mobile. Extension of the disease from the lymph nodes to adjacent tissues may occur, and is found particularly in the mediastinum. Pressure by node masses on neighbouring structures may cause a variety of problems, such as dysphagia, dyspnoea, venous obstruction, jaundice and paraplegia. Spleno-megaly is uncommon at the onset and even when present does not always signify involvement. Absence of splenomegaly does not exclude involvement of this organ. Rarely the disease may be limited to the spleen.

General features may include progressive weakness, loss of weight and drenching night sweats. Fever may be present and is very variable. In some there is a low-grade pyrexia and in others swinging fevers. The classical Pel-Ebstein intermittent fever is seldom seen now as the disease is modified by treatment. Pruritus is a troublesome symptom in about 10% of cases. Some patients experience discomfort at the site of a lesion shortly after an alcoholic drink.

Investigation. Anaemia is fairly common and progressive. It is usually normochromic and normocytic but occasionally there may be a haemolytic component. There is no diagnostic change in the white cells although a modest eosinophilia occurs in about 10–15% of cases. The total white cell count may be normal but is sometimes considerably raised and there is a neutrophil leucocytosis. Lymphopenia, when it occurs, is a bad sign and an indicator of lymphocyte depletion. In the terminal phase there may be leucopenia and thrombocytopenia which may be as much a reflection of treatment as of the disease. Bone marrow involvement is very uncommon at the outset but may be found later in the disease. The diagnosis can be established with certainty only by tissue biopsy, usually of a lymph node. Liver biopsy may provide the diagnosis in cases with hepatic enlargement.

STAGING. Hodgkin's disease is thought to arise in one area and spread from there to others. It is, therefore, important to establish the extent of the disease at the time of diagnosis because staging largely determines the therapeutic approach. To this end the patient requires intensive investigation including chest radiographs, bipedal lymphangiography, abdominal ultrasound, computed tomography, marrow trephine and aspirate. Gallium scanning and magnetic resonance imaging may also contribute, but are not yet widely available. A laparotomy for splenectomy and liver and lymph node biopsies should be carried out where possible if basic clinical staging reveals only IA or IIA disease.

There are four clinical stages based primarily on the extent of the disease (Ann Arbor classification):

Stage I: Involvement of a single lymph node region (I) or extra-lymphatic site (IE).

Stage II: Involvement of two or more lymph nodes regions (II) or an extra-lymphatic site and lymph node regions on the same side (above or below) the diaphragm (IIE).

Stage III: Involvement of lymph nodes regions on both sides of the diaphragm with (IIIE) or without (III) extra-lymphatic involvement or involvement of the spleen (IIIS) or both (IIISE).

Stage IV: Diffuse involvement of one or more extra-lymphatic tissues, e.g. liver or bone marrow. The lymphatic structures are defined as the lymph nodes, spleen, thymus, Waldeyer's ring, appendix and Peyer's patches.

Each stage is subdivided into 'A' or 'B' categories, according to whether they have systemic symptoms or not. The symptoms that place a patient in the 'B' category are: (1) unexplained weight loss of more than 10% of the body weight in the previous 6 months, (2) unexplained fever above 38°C and (3) night sweats.

Treatment. There are two main methods of treatment, radiotherapy and chemotherapy (p. 109). Megavoltage radiotherapy can eliminate the disease in a high proportion of patients provided the disease is localised. For this reason radiotherapy is chosen for most cases of stage I and II disease. Exceptions are when structures such as the lung are involved when chemotherapy may be used to shrink the lesion to dimensions suitable for radiotherapy. Moreover radiotherapy should not be used in stage II if three of more areas are involved, particularly if the patient has 'B' symptoms because such patients tend to relapse after this form of treatment; chemotherapy should be employed instead. As a generalisation patients with stage III or IV types of disease and any stage with 'B' symptoms are treated with chemotherapy. However, stage IIIA patients in whom only nodes in the upper abdomen are involved do well with radiotherapy. Conversely, patients with stage II disease involving three or more sites require chemotherapy.

RADIOTHERAPY consists of treatment of the node areas. For disease above the diaphragm a 'mantle' treatment is used and includes nodes in the neck, axillae and mediastinum. In some cases, if the mediastinum is involved this field is later extended downwards to include the para-aortic region. Disease below the diaphragm is given an 'inverted Y' distribution of irradiation which includes the coeliac, para-aortic, iliac and groin nodes and follows roughly the bifurcation of the aorta. If splenectomy has not been performed the spleen should also be irradiated. In female patients the 'inverted Y' irradiation causes severe damage to the ovaries and if a staging laparotomy has been done the opportunity is usually taken to place the ovaries behind the uterus where they may be more protected.

COMBINATION CHEMOTHERAPY (p. 111) has revolutionised the treatment of advanced Hodgkin's disease. The classical combination is nitrogen mustard, a vinca alkaloid such as vincristine or vinblastine, together with procarbazine and prednisolone, given in 2-week pulses (p. 525) at 4 weekly intervals. Five pulses are given after all objective evidence of disease has gone. The minimum number of pulses is six and it is seldom necessary to give more than 12. If the patient relapses during treatment, usually about the time of the third pulse, the disease is resistant to these drugs and treatment should be changed to an alternative combination.

Nitrogen mustard (p. 109) is very unpleasant for patients and must be given intravenously. In most patients nausea and vomiting occur and can be severe, usually starting 2 to 4 hours after the injection and lasting from 12 to 24 hours in some cases. Antiemetics can mitigate these side-effects significantly. Combinations of metoclopramide or domperidone with dexamethasone seem to give the best results.

Cyclophosphamide, which is a phosphorylated nitrogen mustard, may replace nitrogen mustard in the regimen. Little advantage is gained as regards adverse effects as it is a potent epilator and also may cause haemorrhagic cystitis.

Chlorambucil, also a nitrogen mustard analogue, has been used successfully in this regimen in place of nitrogen mustard and has the advantage that it can be given by mouth and is well tolerated. Patients can be managed easily on an out-patient basis. Nitrogen mustard and its analogues are all severely myelotoxic.

The vinca alkaloids, vincristine, vinblastine and vindesine are relatively less toxic to the bone marrow. In particular vincristine has this advantage but is more neurotoxic than vindesine which in turn is more neurotoxic than vinblastine (p. 113).

Procarbazine is a myelotoxic drug which is under suspicion as possibly the most oncogenic of the drugs in this combination.

Prednisolone is almost useless in this disease on its own but has been shown to play an essential role in combination with other agents. Antituberculous chemotherapy should be used if there is evidence of old untreated disease. Exacerbation of peptic ulceration can be controlled by cimetidine or ranitidine. Prednisolone should be withdrawn gradually over 3 days at the end of each pulse. In many instances prednisolone is a euphoriant and helps the patient to tolerate the side-effects of the other drugs.

Other combination chemotherapy regimes exist but none has been shown to be more effective than the one above. However, they do provide alternative chemotherapy when there is resistance to the classical combination. Useful drugs are etoposide, doxorubicin, ifosfamide, the nitrosoureas and bleomycin. A classification of cytotoxic drugs and the diseases in which they may be used is given in Table 13.1.

Chemotherapy carries a fairly high risk of inducing sterility in males (p. 113) and this may be permanent. To a lesser extent it is a risk in females, in whom evidence of premature menopause may also appear. Since many of these patients are young, the males in particular may require counselling about the effect of chemotherapy and be offered the possibility of sperm storage.

Prognosis. If the patient is not treated the disease is fatal. With stage IA disease, the 5-year survival rate in patients treated with radiotherapy exceeds 90%, and in stage IIA disease is greater than 70%. In more advanced disease the results of chemotherapy are very satisfactory and more than 50% of patients remain disease free after 5 years. Just how effective combination chemotherapy is, remains to be seen since many patients who were treated in this way are still alive. The prognosis so far as histological type is concerned seems to matter less when chemotherapy is used. The prognosis is relatively poor when evidence of resistance to treatment appears and very few of such patients survive thereafter for 5 years.

Table 13.1 Cytotoxic drugs and diseases in which they may be used.

Antimetabolite						
Methotrexate	ALL	NHL	Intrathecal			
Mercaptopurine	ALL	AML	CML			
Thioguanine	AML	CML	ALL			
Cytarabine	AML	MDS	ALL	NHL		
Asparaginase	ALL					
Alkylating agent						
Mustine	HD	NHL				
Cyclophosphamide	HD	NHL	AML	ALL	MY	PL
Chlorambucil	CLL	NHL	HD	WM		
Busulphan	CML	PV	ET	MF		
Melphalan	MY	CML	PV	ET		
Ifosfamide	NHL	HD				
Plant alkaloid						
Vincristine sulphate	ALL	AML	HD	NHL	CLL	PL MY
Vinblastine sulphate	HD	NHL				
Vindesine sulphate	HD	NHL				
Etoposide (VP-16)	HD	NHL	AML			
Nitrosoureas						
Carmustine (BCNU)	MY	HD	NHL			
Lomustine (CCNU)	MY	HD	NHL			
Antibiotic						
Daunorubicin	ALL	AML				
Doxorubicin	NHL	HD	PL			
Bleomycin sulphate	NHL	HD				
Mitoxantrone	ALL	AML	NHL			
Miscellaneous						
Hydroxyurea	CML	MF				
Dibromomannitol	CML					
Procarbazine	HD					
Deoxycoformycin	T-cell leukaemia/lymphoma					
Interferon	HCL	CML				
Glucocorticoids	ALL	NHL	CLL	MY	MF	

Key: ALL = acute lymphoblastic leukaemia; AML = acute myeloblastic leukaemia; CLL = chronic lymphocytic leukaemia; CML = chronic myeloid leukaemia; ET = essential thrombocythaemia; HCL = hairy cell leukaemia; HD = Hodgkin's disease; MDS = myelodysplastic syndrome; MF = myelofibrosis; MY = myeloma; NHL = non-Hodgkin's lymphoma; PL = prolymphocytic leukaemia; PV = polycythaemia vera; WM = Waldenström's macroglobulinaemia.

Non-Hodgkin lymphoma

In this group of disorders there is a malignant monoclonal proliferation of lymphoid cells, usually identifiable as B cells. Occasionally T cells are affected. Non-Hodgkin lymphomas merge with lymphoblastic and lymphocytic leukaemias with which they have many features in common.

Pathology and classification. In the past the most widely used classification was that of Rappaport which had the merit of simplicity. It drew attention to the division between lymphomas which retained a nodular structure (nodular or follicular) and those in which the architecture was lost (diffuse). Another classification, the Kiel, has also been widely adopted. More recently a 'Working Formulation' has been drawn up from these two classifications in which cases are allotted to one of three grades, low, intermediate or high. The criteria by which patients are allotted are complex but this grading provides a practical guide for the clinician and can be easily understood. Low grade lymphomas carry the best prognosis and high grade the worst. However, high grade lymphomas may respond better and patients can achieve long-term remission if treated properly.

Unlike Hodgkin's lymphoma the disease in non-Hodgkin lymphoma is frequently widespread at the time of diagnosis, often involving not only lymph nodes, but also bone marrow, spleen and other tissues. Early involvement of bone marrow is typical of nodular lymphoma. Extra-lymphatic tissue involvement at the time of presentation is more common and almost every organ or tissue may be the site of initial disease. In gastrointestinal lymphomas the stomach is most frequently and the rectum least frequently involved. Thyroid lymphomas tend to be associated with gastrointestinal involvement. Some skin lymphomas are T cell in type, e.g. mycosis fungoides. Most lymphomas involving extra-lymphatic tissues are of the diffuse variety and therefore have a rather poor prognosis unless well localised.

Clinical features. These lymphomas occur at all ages, are rare under 2 years and become more frequent with increasing age. Males are more often affected than females. Nodular lymphomas occur mainly in adults between the ages of 30 and 60.

Lymph node enlargement is the most common presenting finding, and is usually painless unless it has developed very quickly. The nodes are discrete and firm. The patient usually complains of tiredness, lassitude, loss of weight and occasionally fever and sweating. However, the patient may be symptom free. When the presentation is extra-lymphatic the symptoms will reflect the tissues involved. Quite often the diagnosis of lymphoma comes unexpectedly at laparotomy or during other investigative procedures. Weakness of the legs progressing to paraplegia may be due to an extra-dural lymphoma compressing the cord. Pressure effects in other areas may cause dysphagia, breathlessness, vomiting, intestinal obstruction or ascites and limb oedema. Pain is the main symptom of bone involvement which may present with a pathological fracture.

Physical examination often reveals more widespread node involvement than the patient has noticed. Unexplained lymphadenopathy which fails to resolve spontaneously within a few weeks should always be suspect. Moreover lymphomatous nodes may wax and wane in size and the shrinkage of nodes does not exclude a diagnosis of lymphoma. Splenomegaly usually indicates that the spleen is involved in the neoplastic process.

Investigation. Diagnosis is based primarily on histological findings from biopsy of a lymph node or other involved tissue. In some cases reactive hyperplasia is seen in the biopsy and a clinical suspicion of lymphoma is not confirmed initially. Further biopsies may eventually reveal a lymphoma.

The staging process is similar to that adopted for Hodgkin's disease except that laparotomy is seldom necessary although it may be required for diagnostic purposes when only retroperitoneal nodes are involved. Bone marrow aspiration and trephine biopsy should be done early in the investigation since marrow involvement is common and indicates stage IV disease. Blood counts usually show normal values unless there is splenomegaly with hypersplenism or a complicating autoimmune haemolytic anaemia when a reduced haemoglobin level, reticulocytosis and positive direct antiglobulin test (Coombs' test) will be found. In some cases a slight excess of lymphocytes may be present. Thrombocytopenia is uncommon. Moderate degrees of anaemia may be also present if there is considerable bone marrow involvement.

An evaluation of the cell membrane receptor characteristics of the peripheral blood and lymph node lymphocytes is helpful, particularly in cases in which the diagnosis is in doubt, but this has to be done in specialised laboratories. The demonstration of a monoclonal expansion of the B lymphocyte population is characteristic and other features may give a measure of the degree of differentiation of the cells. These techniques also assist in the identification of the less common cases of T cell lymphoma. For this a second biopsy of lymph nodes may be required. An assessment of immune competence is also important and immunoglobulin levels should be measured. In some cases a monoclonal band may be found.

Treatment. In the case of the more benign non-Hodgkin lymphomas, such as the nodular lymphocytic and even diffuse well-differentiated lymphocytic varieties, no specific therapy may be necessary if the disease is not advanced. Some patients can be observed for years before active measures are indicated.

RADIOTHERAPY. When treatment is required localised disease is best managed, as in Hodgkin's disease, with radiotherapy and this may be curative. However, non-Hodgkin lymphoma is often at stage III or IV when diagnosed and in these cases chemotherapy is generally the treatment of choice. Where there are pressure problems the local disease may be treated with radiotherapy in combination with chemotherapy. The more benign types of disease may also respond very well to total body irradiation, a form of radiotherapy that employs a very small dose of 150 centigrays over a period of 5 weeks in 10 doses of 15 centigrays each. This is very suitable for elderly patients as it is relatively free of side-effects.

CHEMOTHERAPY. Most cases of nodular lymphoma respond very well to gentle, single agent chemotherapy and chlorambucil is the drug usually chosen. More dramatic results in terms of induction of remission may be achieved with combination chemotherapy but there is as yet no evidence that this is of long-term benefit to the patient and it may cause considerably greater morbidity. Chlorambucil may be given as continuous therapy at a dose of 5 mg daily initially, reducing to 2 mg daily as indicated by leucocyte and platelet counts. This may be given over many months in order to control the disease. Alternatively the drug may be given intermittently in higher doses. Combination with prednisolone may be useful, especially at the start of treatment when the bone marrow may be heavily involved with lymphoma. The steroid therapy may be started before as described for chronic lymphatic leukaemia. Oxymetholone therapy may also help

to rescue the bone marrow. Long-term steroid therapy should be avoided.

Combination chemotherapy is indicated for the intermediate and high grade lymphomas. The latter should always receive the most aggressive chemotherapy as a number of cases can be rendered apparently disease free for long periods with this treatment. Radiotherapy does not appear to be able to achieve as good results. If these patients survive for a year without relapse after cessation of treatment they have a chance of long-term remission. There are a number of regimes but most physicians employ a combination of cyclophosphamide, an anthracycline antibiotic, a vinca alkaloid, bleomycin and steroid. The interpolation of high dose methotrexate therapy with folinic acid may improve the remission rate.

Rather less aggressive management has been used for the intermediate grade and accordingly cyclophosphamide, vincristine and prednisolone with or without doxorubicin is generally prescribed. All these combination regimens are given as pulses with variable periods of rest for bone marrow recovery between each pulse. The number of pulses is usually between six and 12 in any one course. Once the disease has become resistant to the standard drugs, second line chemotherapy usually produces only brief benefit and the value of achieving this at the expense of the patient's well-being has to be evaluated in each case. Useful drugs are etoposide, ifosfamide, the nitrosoureas, mitoxantrone and bleomycin. It may be better to deal with troublesome disease as it arises with short courses of radiotherapy. This palliative approach can be quite successful.

As a generalisation, patients over 70 years do not tolerate aggressive chemotherapy well. Adolescents who present with an undifferentiated lymphoma, which is often initially in the mediastinum, should be managed in the same way as patients with acute lymphoblastic leukaemia. Some patients with low-grade lymphocytic lymphoma progress to chronic lymphatic leukaemia and should be managed accordingly.

Chemotherapy for lymphoma has the problem of being toxic to the patient's normal blood-forming tissues. Successful treatment depends on greater sensitivity of the tumour and the quicker recovery of 'normal' cells after a pulse of treatment. The effect on the patient's normal tissues is usually monitored by watching the blood count. In this respect the white cell count, the absolute neutrophil count and the platelet count are the most useful. As the absolute neutrophil count drops below $0.5 \times 10^9/l$, infection with bacteria or fungi becomes an increasing risk. Similarly, bleeding is increasingly likely to occur as the platelet count drops below $50 \times 10^9/l$ although many patients tolerate very low levels for longer periods without serious bleeding. Dosage of myelotoxic drugs must be reduced once these figures are approached and some physicians would reduce the dose at higher levels. The effect of drugs may continue after they have been withdrawn and this should be kept in mind. Regular blood counts are absolutely essential for the satisfactory management of these patients.

SURGERY. In lymphomas of extra-lymphatic tissue, surgical excision may be employed and is usually supplemented with radiotherapy, with or without chemotherapy thereafter.

SUPPORTIVE THERAPY. General supportive measures such as blood transfusion with red cell concentrate should be used for anaemia when necessary. Infections should be treated promptly with antibiotics or other agents. A watch should be kept for the development of monilia infection in the mouth of patients who have developed neutropenia or are on steroids.

Prognosis. The mean survival of patients with intermediate grade lymphomas is in the region of 2 years and those with the high grade variety who do not respond well to treatment often survive less than 1 year. Patients with low grade lymphomas have a mean survival of 7 to 8 years. Patients with high grade lymphomas who obtain full remission on treatment have a 50% chance of long-term remission, possibly cure.

Burkitt's lymphoma

This form of lymphoblastic B cell non-Hodgkin lymphoma occurs predominantly in tropical Africa and New Guinea, although it also occurs less frequently in other parts of the world. There is strong evidence that the Epstein Barr (EB) virus plays an important aetiological role in its development. The majority of cases occur in children with a peak incidence between the ages of 4 and 8 years, although cases found outside the tropics show an older age distribution and a lower incidence of EB viral infection.

The disorder affects predominantly extranodal tissues with a marked predilection for the mandible and the maxillary bones. This may cause marked bone deformity, loosening of the teeth and, if the orbit is involved, extrusion of the eye with loss of sight. In the abdomen, involvement, often bilaterally, of the kidneys, adrenals, ovaries or lymph nodes may give rise to abdominal tumours. Extradural lesions of the spinal cord may cause sudden onset of paraplegia. Other sites which may be involved include long bones, the salivary glands, the thyroid, testes and the heart. Bilateral tumours of the breast may be seen in young adult women. In cases outside the tropics abdominal tumours are the most common finding and lymph nodes and marrow are more frequently involved.

The cytological appearance of Burkitt's lymphoma is characteristic with lymphoblast-type cells showing vacuolation in the cytoplasm and nucleus. Histologically the 'starry sky' appearance created by histiocytes scattered amongst sheets of primitive lymphoid cells is typical. Chromosome analysis shows an 8/14 translocation in a high proportion of cases and less often 2/8 or 8/22 translocation. Antibody to EB viral capsid antigen is found in most patients with the African variety.

Response to chemotherapy, particularly if the disease is localised, is very good. Cyclophosphamide is given intramuscularly, 40–60 mg/kg every 2 weeks for up to six doses. Since meningeal involvement often occurs later in the disease, prophylactic intrathecal methotrexate may also be given. The response to treatment is often dramatic with resolution of the disease following the first dose of cyclophosphamide. The prognosis is good especially for patients with localised disease.

MULTIPLE MYELOMA (MYELOMATOSIS)

This is a malignant disorder of plasma cells.

Immunopathology. Normal plasma cells are derived from B lymphocytes by transformation after exposure to antigenic stimuli; individual plasma cells manufacture immunoglobulins with only one type of light chain. The finding that in myeloma, and in other related malignant disorders of B lymphocytes, all the malignant cells produce the same immunoglobulin indicates that the tumour is derived originally from one cell by cloning; the disease is therefore monoclonal. The immunoglobulin is called a *paraprotein* and appears on electrophoretic strips as a clear-cut band. Each of the five normal types of immunoglobulin has light chains of either lambda or kappa varieties (Fig. 2.3). In myeloma the paraprotein produced belongs to one of these immunoglobulin types and has one or other of the two light chains. In some cases only part of the immunoglobulin molecule is produced by the tumour cells, most commonly the light chains. These appear in the urine as *Bence Jones proteinuria* and if myeloma is associated only with light chains it is known as Bence Jones myeloma.

In just over half of the patients with myeloma an IgG paraprotein is produced. About 20% are IgA producing and a similar percentage are of the Bence Jones variety. IgD, IgM and IgE myelomas are rare and together amount to only 2% of cases. Patients with myeloma which produces complete immunoglobulin molecules may excrete increased amounts of light chain in their urine. In some this appears as a new phenomenon and usually indicates an acceleration of the disease.

In the majority of patients the bone marrow is heavily infiltrated with atypical plasma cells which are usually larger and paler staining than normal plasma cells and contain nucleoli. Some cells may be multinucleated. Progressive replacement of the marrow occurs with eventual reduction of the normal cell lines, inducing anaemia, leucopenia and thrombocytopenia. Osteoclasts are stimulated and absorption of bone occurs, producing diffuse osteoporosis. Local tumour formation by the myeloma causes punched out translucencies in the bone radiograph. Rarely the disease may present as a solitary plasmacytoma either in bone or soft tissue.

Excessive production of the myeloma paraprotein is associated with progressive reduction in normal immunoglobulin levels and impairment of immune function.

Clinical features. The disease is very uncommon under the age of 30. It becomes increasingly frequent thereafter, having its peak incidence between 60 and 70 years. Males are affected rather more frequently than females and black people of Central African origin two to three times more often than Caucasians. There is a long preclinical phase, in some instances up to 25 years. The disorder may be discovered incidentally by laboratory tests during this phase and the patient may thereafter be observed for years before symptoms appear.

Symptoms usually reflect bone involvement, impairment of immune function, renal damage, anaemia or hyperviscosity. The diffuse osteoporosis and local erosion of bone by myeloma result in stress pain and eventual pathological fracture. The stress pain is often wandering, difficult to locate and described as 'rheumatics'. On the other hand the first intimation of trouble may be the sudden onset of acute pain due to pathological fracture. These symptoms arise mainly in weight bearing bones, the vertebrae, pelvis and femur being particularly susceptible. Collapse of vertebrae is common and produces nerve root pressure symptoms and shortening of stature. Patients are often severely crippled. Weight lifting may also cause pain in the arms whereas lesions in the skull seldom given rise to pain.

The progressive impairment of immune function due to the deficiencies of normal immunoglobulins and excess of abnormal immunoglobulins renders these patients susceptible to infections, particularly of the respiratory tract. Pneumonia is quite frequently the presenting illness and infection very often the cause of death.

The excessive production of light chains which are lost in the urine as Bence Jones protein, may damage tubular cells and block the tubular lumen. Renal failure may supervene. Light chains deposited elsewhere may result in amyloidosis (p. 391). Mobilisation of calcium from the skeleton may be excessive and cause hypercalcaemia, which may result in nephrocalcinosis. High calcium levels may also cause lethargy and drowsiness progressing to coma if untreated.

Patients often complain of tiredness which may be due to anaemia. Bleeding and bruising problems are seldom presenting features but they may be troublesome terminally and are due both to thrombocytopenia and hyperglobulinaemia.

Hyperviscosity is a problem in some patients with very high levels of paraprotein. It may impair the circulation, notably in the central nervous system, causing headaches, vertigo, dizziness, somnolence and stupor progressing to coma.

Clinical examination may reveal tender areas in the bones, kyphoscoliosis, muscle spasm and impaired mobility, particularly with vertebral involvement. Retinal haemorrhages, exudates and gross dilatation of the retinal veins, with periodic constrictions giving a 'string of sausages' appearance, suggest hyperviscosity.

Investigation. Assessment of myeloma is very dependent on laboratory findings. The degree of bone marrow involvement is reflected in the haemoglobin level, the white cell count and the platelet count and can be assessed directly with bone marrow examination. A high ESR is very characteristic but is not always present. Rarely myeloma cells appear in the blood as a plasma cell leukaemia.

The level of paraprotein production is evaluated using electrophoresis and measurement of the monoclonal band, the level being expressed in grams per litre. This measurement should be used to follow progress. Immune impairment can be assessed from the electrophoretic strip and the immunoglobulin levels. Renal function should be assessed by blood urea and by creatinine clearance. Plasma calcium should always be determined. Plasma alkaline phosphatase is usually within normal limits despite the bone involvement unless there has been a fracture when a transient rise may occur. Plasma urate levels should also be measured. β_2-microglobulin estimations provide useful prognostic information.

Diagnosis depends on finding at least two of the characteristic features of the disease. The bone marrow may be pathognomonic but is not always so. A firm diagnosis may depend on the demonstration of a monoclonal paraproteinaemia and punched-out lytic areas in bone radiographs together with osteoporosis. Reactive plasmacytosis in the marrow can mimic myeloma but the increased immunoglobulins are polyclonal. Paraprotein bands may be found in lymphomas, macroglobulinaemia and benign monoclonal gammopathy. In the last condition no other features of myeloma are present. Paraprotein bands may also be associated with a wide range of inflammatory, neoplastic and autoimmune disease. In such cases the level of paraprotein does not significantly increase with time and is usually less than 10 g/l.

Treatment. When treatment is required, cytotoxic therapy should be preceded by allopurinol to prevent gout and urate nephropathy. Local skeletal problems should be treated with radiotherapy and the general disease with chemotherapy. Melphalan is the drug of choice, although cyclophosphamide is probably as effective.

Patients in the preclinical phase generally do not require treatment. In the clinical phase melphalan may be given either alone as low dose continuous therapy, 2 mg daily or as high dose intermittent therapy ($7\,mg/m^2/d$ for 4 days) in combination with prednisolone, weaning off over the following 3 days. Such treatment should be administered in pulses every 4 to 6 weeks. The dosage of melphalan should be adjusted according to the white cell, absolute neutrophil and platelet counts. In most patients the disease is slowly brought under control. Progress should be evaluated by measuring the levels of paraprotein in the blood. When this has reached a plateau, chemotherapy may be stopped. A small proportion of patients are resistant to treatment and the disease is progressive.

In patients with the more rapidly advancing forms of myeloma more aggressive therapy may be required, using combination chemotherapy. Those who present with anaemia, hypercalcaemia and evidence of renal damage and in whom there is Bence Jones proteinuria require urgent management with high fluid intake and alkalinisation of the urine with oral bicarbonate. Corticosteroids and possibly mithramycin are given to reduce calcium levels. Careful transfusion with red cell concentrate is also required unless the haemoglobin is above 10 g/dl. Specific treatment under such circumstances should be with combination chemotherapy, bearing in mind that dose reductions may be required because of renal failure, the management of which is described on page 399. In this situation cyclophosphamide is contraindicated. BCNU and doxorubicin form a useful combination.

In younger patients extremely aggressive high dose melphelan ($140\,mg/m^2$ i.v.) may be given preceded by a conditioning dose of cyclophosphamide ($400\,mg/m^2$ i.v.) on day-7 together with the start of allopurinol therapy. Profound cytopenia and immunosuppression occur lasting several weeks and carry a major risk of serious infection and bleeding. In some cases, complete remission is achieved particularly in those with IgA type of disease. Such treatment requires provision of the highest quality of supportive care and should be undertaken only in those patients who have no other major problems.

Despite good control of the general disease, further episodes of bone pain and fracture may occur and require radiotherapy. Prophylactic irradiation of eroded vertebrae may be warranted before crush fracture has occurred. Fractures of femur and humerus require orthopaedic surgery with pinning of the bone, followed by radiotherapy. Bed-rest should be minimised to avoid further loss of calcium from the skeleton. Hyperviscosity problems may require plasmapheresis (p. 31). The use of anabolic steroids can be helpful in arresting further deterioration in the skeleton.

Maintaining the morale of the patients in the face of crippling and painful disease may be difficult but they should be encouraged to look forward to gradual improvement. Given time and good management many can return from a bed-ridden stage to active lives.

Prognosis. Without treatment the disease progresses relentlessly to death. With treatment the outlook for the majority of patients is considerably improved and a few may survive for many years. Bad signs at the time of diagnosis are a haemoglobin level of less than $7\,g/dl$, severe hypoalbuminaemia, intractable renal failure, thrombocytopenia, high β_2-microglobulin levels and plasma cell leukaemia. Prognosis should be guarded in any individual until the response to treatment has been assessed; this may take 6 months or more.

Waldenström's macroglobulinaemia is a rare disease of the elderly, more common in males than females. There is a monoclonal IgM paraproteinaemia and a tendency to develop a hyperviscosity syndrome. The marrow is infiltrated with neoplastic lymphocytes.

Untreated, the progress is often slow with eventual immune deficiency and susceptibility to infection. Chlorambucil on a long-term low dose basis, such as 2 mg daily, may control the lymphocyte proliferation and the advance of the disease. Some patients are unresponsive. Plasmapheresis may be required. The majority of patients survive 2 to 5 years and some live considerably longer.

Hypersplenism

This term is used to describe the depression of leucocyte and platelet counts in the peripheral blood which is often encountered in a wide variety of conditions in which splenomegaly is a prominent feature, such as portal hypertension. The cause of the leucopenia and the thrombocytopenia is not fully understood but may in part be due to excessive sequestration of leucocytes and platelets in the enlarged spleen.

Another important effect of splenomegaly is, for reasons unknown, an increase in total plasma volume. This dilutes the red cell mass which remains normal but the dilution gives a low haemoglobin reading, down to 8 g/dl in some patients. The spurious anaemia can be identified by measurement of the red cell mass and plasma volume and is corrected only by splenectomy which may also improve leucopenia and thrombocytopenia.

HAEMORRHAGIC DISEASE

Pathophysiology

The mechanism concerned in the arrest of haemorrhage can be divided into three stages. The first is spasm of damaged small blood vessels. The second is the aggregation of platelets forming plugs on the damaged areas of vascular endothelium. The third is the coagulation of blood which is the end product of a chain reaction involving many coagulation factors.

1. **The vascular reaction.** Spasm of small arterioles and capillary sphincters in response to injury constitutes an essential feature of natural haemostasis. It slows the blood loss and allows the other reactions to operate. Eventually the spasm relaxes and secondary bleeding develops if

the platelets and coagulation factors have not carried out their functions.

2. **The platelet.** Normal platelets do not adhere to vascular endothelium when it is intact. The natural anticoagulant, prostacyclin, produced by vascular endothelial cells from arachidonic acid, helps to prevent this. Platelets adhere readily to collagen under the vascular endothelium when it is exposed by injury. They also adhere to each other under the influence of adenosine diphosphate (ADP) released in damaged tissue. A primary platelet aggregate forms. At this stage it is possible for the platelets to break off into the circulation as small emboli which usually disintegrate rapidly. Primary aggregation probably occurs inside blood vessels when injury is minimal. When the injury is such that the full effect of the haemostatic mechanism is required, primary aggregation is followed by a change in the shape of the platelets. An irreversible phase of aggreg-

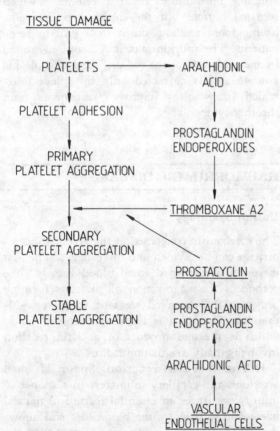

Fig. 13.4 Platelet aggregation, promoted by thromboxane A2, is inhibited by prostacyclin.

ation is reached, promoted by thromboxane A2 which is formed in platelets from arachidonic acid through prostaglandin endoperoxides (Fig. 13.4). Another factor involved in the irreversible phase of aggregation is ADP. Platelet granules release numerous substances including fibrinogen which participate in the formation of fibrin and in the establishment of a stable haemostasis.

Capillary bleeding can be stopped by platelet plug formation and does not require the coagulation mechanism. This is why the bleeding time is usually normal in haemophilia and why a lack of platelets gives rise to capillary bleeding (purpura). The platelet plug is inadequate for blood vessels larger than capillaries, because the blood pressure in them is too great and without the support of fibrin formation the platelet plug is expelled when vessel spasm relaxes. However, when injury is slight the full train of the haemostatic mechanism will not proceed as it will be inhibited by antithrombin III and other anticoagulant factors (p. 544). In this way blood flow can be maintained in blood vessels where the injury is not sufficient to require the cessation of flow.

3. **Coagulation of the blood.** The end point of the clotting mechanism is the formation of fibrin from fibrinogen. Haemostasis, initiated by vascular spasm and platelet plug formation, is strengthened by the laying down of a fibrin mesh. The fibrin then contracts and consolidates the initial repair by binding the tissues together. This can be achieved either (1) by an intrinsic system in the blood activated by contact with collagen exposed when the vascular endothelium is injured or (2) by an extrinsic system activated by tissue fluid. The intrinsic system is more potent but there appears to be interaction between the two.

The coagulation mechanism is a biological amplifier, a cascade of activated proenzymes (serine proteases) assisted by coenzymes. Precursor substances or factors circulating in the blood are activated and in turn activate other factors and so on. Ionised calcium is essential at several points in the mechanism.

Coagulation factors. Thirteen main coagulation factors have been named. It is now recognised that factor III (thromboplastin) and factor IV do not exist as distinct biochemical entities. Thrombo-

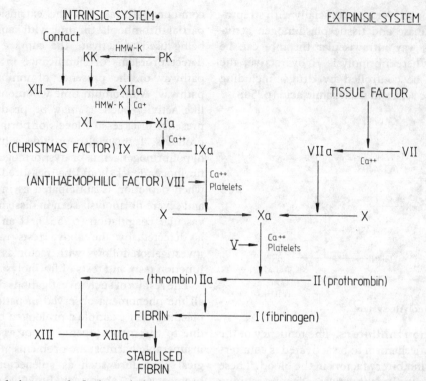

Fig. 13.5 Coagulation cascade. In the extrinsic system, tissue factors activate factor X in the presence of factor VII. In the intrinsic system, kallikrein (KK) and high molecular weight kininogen (HMW-K) interact with the contact factor XII at the contact surface. Prekallikrein (PK) is activated to kallikrein by activated factor XII with the assistance of the cofactor HMW-K which acts as an accelerator. In turn kallikrein activates further factor XII to factor XIIa. (Kallikrein also acts as a plasminogen activator and promotes fibrinolysis (Fig. 13.6).)

Activated factor IX (IXa) in the presence of cofactor VIII, platelet factor 3 (phospholipid) and calcium ions activates factor X. This is the point at which the intrinsic and extrinsic systems meet and is the start of the final common pathway in which activated factor X together with factor V, platelet factor 3 and calcium ions activate prothrombin to thrombin. Then conversion of fibrinogen to fibrin is almost instantaneous and fibrin is formed sufficiently quickly to prevent it being flushed away by further bleeding. Thrombin also activates factor XIII which stabilises the polymerised fibrin. Subsequent contraction of the fibrin depends on adequate numbers of platelets being involved in the clotting process.

plastin probably represents the co-operative activity of several factors. The term, factor VI, is no longer used. The factors involved in the blood coagulation cascade are shown in Figure 13.5.

Factor VIII (antihaemophilic globulin) is deficient in haemophilia. This molecule combines with von Willebrand's factor which is produced by endothelial cells and megakaryocytes and acts as a carrier for factor VIII in plasma. Deficiency of von Willebrand factor gives rise to von Willebrand disease. Factor VIII is measured by assay of its coagulant activity.

Factor XII is the only coagulation factor deficiency of which is not associated with a tendency to bleed. Such deficiency is more likely to be associated with a liability to thrombosis due to failure of activation of the fibrinolytic mechanism through the kallikrein system.

The fibrinolytic system (Fig. 13.6). This functions in much the same way as the coagulation mechanism. Plasminogen, an inert precursor, can be activated to form plasmin which digests fibrin to give fibrin degradation products. In excess, it will also digest fibrinogen and other coagulation factors. This system functions continuously to prevent the laying down of fibrin intravascularly and becomes very active when there is a threat of widespread intravascular coagulation. The activity of plasmin is controlled by the natural inhibitor, alpha$_1$-antiplasmin. When blood clots form, plasminogen closely bound to the deposited fibrin is slowly activated to digest the fibrin clot. This process can be accelerated artificially with strepto-kinase, urokinase and tissue plasminogen activ-ator. In this way intravascular thrombi can be dissolved. Where fibrinolysis is overactive, the process can be controlled by drugs, including aminocaproic acid and tranexamic acid (p. 548).

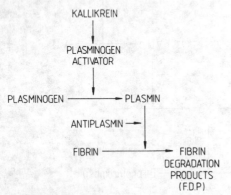

Fig. 13.6 Fibrinolytic system.

Coagulation inhibitors. The tendency of the coagulation mechanism to be activated is counter-balanced by inhibitory factors in the blood. These substances neutralise the activated factors rapidly. In circulating blood, activation of the coagulation mechanism is minimal and these inhibitors are effective. At the point of an injury, however, the activation of the coagulation mechanism is so powerful that the inhibitors are overwhelmed. One important inhibitor is antithrombin III which inactivates thrombin (factor II) and acti-vated factors IX, X, XI, and XII. It is required for the action of heparin. Patients who are deficient of antithrombin III are very liable to thrombosis.

Investigation of bleeding disorders

If there is suspicion that a patient has a bleeding disorder a basic screen of haemostatic function should be performed. Blood should be taken for a blood count, including platelet count and blood film and for basic coagulation investigations. A bleeding time should be done by the Ivy method which is an excellent test of capillary and platelet function and of von Willebrand factor levels.

Coagulation investigations should include a prothrombin time to evaluate the activity of factors II, VII and X and their function in the final common pathway and the extrinsic system. A partial thromboplastin time with kaolin (the latter being used to activate the contact factors) will detect problems of significance in the intrinsic pathway or the presence of inhibitors to this pathway. A thrombin time will monitor heparin-like activity such as may be produced by the presence of excessive levels of fibrin degradation products. It may also provide a hint of either hypofibrinogenaemia or dysfibrinogenaemia. The fibrinogen level should be measured, particularly when depletion is anticipated as in liver failure and severe fibrinolysis seen in disseminated intra-vascular coagulation (p. 551). If an abnormality is detected by the above tests more detailed investigation follows with factor assays, platelet function tests and tests of fibrinolysis.

The results of such investigations do not explain all the phenomena observed in patients who are bleeding. For example a prolonged bleeding time due to thrombocytopenia is not associated with insuperable haemostatic problems at a major sur-gical procedure such as splenectomy although haemostasis is abnormal. Equally, although the bleeding time may be normal in haemophilia, major surgery would be haemostatically impos-sible if special measures were not undertaken (p. 548). An intact extrinsic clotting system does not compensate for a defective intrinsic system as seen in haemophilia. The platelets are essential for controlling bleeding due to minor trauma and the coagulation mechanism for bleeding due to major trauma. Thus when platelets are deficient, capillary bleeding predominates and when the coagulation mechanism is faulty more serious bleeding occurs. These observations may partly explain anomalies in the clinical findings associ-ated with various defects in the haemostatic mech-anism.

Classification of haemorrhagic disorders

1. Defects of the blood vessels
a. The vascular purpuras.
   (i)   Infections, e.g. typhus, typhoid, menin-gococcal meningitis, measles, infective endocarditis, septicaemia.
   (ii) Chemical agents, e.g. aspirin, ergot, fru-semide, indomethacin, iodides, pheno-

barbitone, phenylbutazone, phenytoin, quinine and snake venom.

(iii) Anaphylactoid purpura (purpura simplex and Henoch-Schönlein purpura p. 570).

(iv) Metabolic purpura (uraemia p. 398, hepatic failure p 353).

(v) Scurvy (p. 69).

b. Hereditary haemorrhagic telangiectasia.

2. **Disorders of blood platelets**

a. Reduced numbers of platelets: idiopathic and secondary thrombocytopenic purpura.

b. Increased numbers of platelets: thrombocythaemia.

c. Defective platelets: hereditary and acquired thrombasthaenia.

3. **Defects of the clotting mechanism**

a. *Hereditary:*

(i) Haemophilia (factor VIII deficiency) or haemophilia A.

(ii) Christmas disease (factor IX deficiency) or haemophilia B.

(iii) von Willebrand's disease (also shows abnormalities of capillary and platelet function).

(iv) Deficiency of other clotting factors (all rare).

b. *Acquired:*

(i) Deficiency of certain coagulation factors due to vitamin K deficiency.

(ii) Oral anticoagulant therapy.

(iii) Advanced liver disease.

HAEMORRHAGIC DISORDERS DUE TO DEFECT OF THE BLOOD VESSELS

Most of these disorders are discussed with the primary cause noted above.

Hereditary haemorrhagic telangiectasia

This rare disease is transmitted as an autosomal dominant. It is characterised by bleeding from multiple telangiectases which consist of localised collections of non-contractile capillaries. The first and frequently the only symptom may be epistaxis but haematemesis, haemoptysis or bleeding elsewhere may occur. Telangiectases are not usually prominent till after the age of 20 and may be found on the face and hands, and in the mucous membrane of the nose, mouth and gastrointestinal tract.

Treatment of bleeding areas is sometimes difficult but cauterisation of the lesions in the nose may be helpful. Continuous oral iron therapy is usually required, sometimes with parenteral supplements. Oestrogens taken orally may reduce bleeding from mucous membranes in some patients.

HAEMORRHAGIC DISORDERS DUE TO ABNORMALITIES OF BLOOD PLATELETS

Thrombocytopenia occurs either because (1) platelets are consumed or destroyed almost as soon as they are made (consumption thrombocytopenia), or (2) because they are not being produced (production thrombocytopenia). In the first, megakaryocytes are found in normal or increased numbers in the marrow. In the second megakaryocytes are absent from the marrow or, if present, are incapable of platelet production because they are functionally abnormal, in which case they are usually part of a neoplastic process and are morphologically abnormal. In some diseases there is both a production and a consumption problem and it may prove difficult to know which is the greater.

Idiopathic thrombocytopenic purpura

This is a disease characterised by a severe reduction in the number of circulating platelets. In most cases it is thought to be due to an immunological attack on the platelets, the antibody being of IgG type. However, the demonstration of such an antibody is not always easy. Idiopathic thrombocytopenic purpura is seen in an acute and chronic form. The former is found mostly in young children equally in both sexes and is usually self limiting. The latter occurs at all ages and is more common in females. In the acute form a history of a recent acute respiratory tract illness is common.

Clinical features. There may be purpura and

bleeding from mucous membranes, haematuria and gastrointestinal bleeding. Intracranial haemorrhage is the greatest risk but is uncommon, particularly in children; headache, dizziness and confusion are symptoms that should warn of the risk of intracranial bleeding. In the chronic phase the severity is usually variable with remissions and relapses. Physical examination reveals varying amounts of purpura and bruising in skin and mucous membrane. The spleen is usually not palpable.

Diagnosis is established by finding severe thrombocytopenia with normal and increased numbers of megakaryocytes in the bone marrow in the absence of any overt cause. It is therefore mainly a consumption thrombocytopenia although production may be inhibited by antibody attack on the megakaryocytes. Demonstration of anti-platelet and anti-megakaryocyte antibodies is possible in some patients. There may be an associated iron deficiency anaemia.

Treatment. In young children acute thrombocytopenic purpura following viral infection seldom requires treatment unless there is evidence suggestive of intracranial bleeding.

In adults prednisolone (60 mg/d) should be given until the platelet count rises to normal levels when the dose should be cautiously reduced until the drug is withdrawn. Relapse may require reintroduction of a higher dose for a longer period but if this fails or if there has been no response to prednisolone in 3 to 4 weeks, splenectomy should be considered. The spleen should be removed under corticosteroid cover and platelet concentrates given, if required, only after the splenic artery has been clamped. Splenectomy is successful in about 50% of patients, giving lasting remission. Following splenectomy, resistance to infection is impaired, and therefore phenoxymethylpenicillin (250 mg b.d.) should be taken for 2–5 years, particularly by younger patients.

In others a chronic phase of the disorder occurs with remissions and exacerbations that may require periodic corticosteroid therapy. Elderly patients generally respond poorly to corticosteroids. Surprisingly, some patients survive chronic thrombocytopenia for years with remarkably little disability.

Recently intravenous IgG (0.4 g/kg/d for 5 days) has been used successfully. In some cases it can induce lasting remission. In others the rise in platelet count is short-lived but may be useful for covering splenectomy. It is very expensive. Immunosuppression with azathioprine or cyclophosphamide has also been used mainly for those in whom both steroids and splenectomy have failed.

Secondary thrombocytopenic purpura occurs in association with pancytopenia, leucopenia or hypersplenism. It may be caused by AIDS, multiple neoplastic deposits in the bone marrow or excessive exposure to X-rays or radioactive substances. It may be found in megaloblastic anaemia and in systemic lupus erythematosus and can follow massive blood transfusion.

Thrombocytopenia may occur as part of a general pancytopenia or alone because of sensitivity to drugs, such as chlordiazepoxide, chlorothiazide, chlorpropamide, frusemide, indomethacin, certain sulphonamides and tolbutamide. Here the prognosis is much better, provided the drug is withdrawn and transfusion given as required. Platelet concentrates are available in some centres.

Thrombocythaemia and thrombasthenia

In *thrombocythaemia* there is a raised number of platelets in the blood, usually in excess of $1000 \times 10^9/l$, with an excessive number of megakaryocytes in the marrow. In addition to thrombotic episodes there is also a tendency to bleed. Essential thrombocythaemia is a rare disease of the elderly which responds well to reducing the platelet count to normal with radioactive phosphorus or chemotherapy.

Thrombasthenia is a state in which the platelets, although normal in number, are defective in function. A group of very rare hereditary defects of platelets occur and are known as primary thrombasthenias. Acquired thrombasthenia is much more common and is seen in severe uraemia and after exposure to certain drugs, notably aspirin. The platelets in chronic myeloid leukaemia are ineffective and may not be adequate for major surgery.

HAEMORRHAGIC DISORDERS DUE TO DEFECTS IN THE CLOTTING MECHANISM

Haemophilia (haemophilia A)

Of the various factors in normal plasma concerned with the clotting mechanism the most important from a clinical point of view is the antihaemophilic factor (factor VIII), a deficiency of which leads to haemophilia. This factor is normally present in the globulin fraction of plasma; its site of production is unknown.

Haemophilia is characterised by a life-long tendency to excessive haemorrhage and a greatly prolonged coagulation time. The haemophilia gene is transmitted as an X-linked recessive character (p. 12). It follows that the sons of a haemophilic man do not suffer from haemophilia and do not transmit the trait to their descendants. The daughters of a haemophilic man all carry the trait. There is a 50% chance that sons of female carriers will suffer from haemophilia and a 50% chance that daughters will be carriers. In many instances no family history can be obtained and this may reflect the fact that the disorder has been handed down on the female side for several generations. Alternatively there may have been a genetic mutation.

Clinical features. The most common manifestation is haemorrhage into joints and in severe haemophiliacs these haemarthroses may occur frequently. They usually develop spontaneously and cause pain, which may be severe, with swelling, warmth and muscle spasm. With appropriate treatment the lesion settles in a few days as the blood is reabsorbed. Repeated episodes cause damage to the joint with wasting of the related muscles, leading to deformity and crippling. These effects can be minimised by proper management. The knee joints are most frequently affected but ankles, hips, shoulder, elbows and wrists are also involved. Haemorrhage into the musculature and soft tissues is a frequent and potentially disabling complication. Intra-abdominal bleeding may present diagnostic problems and haemorrhage from the gastrointestinal tract is relatively common and can be serious.

Superficial trauma gives rise to uncontrolled bleeding which will continue unless adequately treated. Intracranial haemorrhage may occur but is relatively uncommon unless related to trauma. Surgical procedures are not possible without replacement therapy. Tooth extraction will also promote prolonged bleeding.

The severity of haemophilia varies. In the worst cases the factor VIII coagulant activity is usually less than 2% of normal. Cases with activity of between 2–5% are usually only moderately affected while those with levels above 5% have problems only with major trauma. A small number of haemophiliacs, varying between 5–15% of all cases, have factor VIII inhibitors in the serum. This greatly complicates their management.

Investigation. Diagnosis is based on the sex of the patient, a family history if present, the clinical picture and the demonstration of deficiency of factor VIII coagulant activity in the absence of any other haemostatic defect. Female haemophiliacs are extremely rare, requiring the marriage of a haemophiliac to a carrier female. Haemophilia must be distinguished from Christmas disease (p. 548) and von Willebrand's disease (p. 548).

Efforts have been made to detect carriers by demonstrating a disparity between the levels of factor VIII coagulant activity and von Willebrand factor. The latter level is higher than would be expected from the coagulant activity. However, it is hoped that immunoradiometric assay used to determine the antigenic determinant of factor VIII will prove to be a more useful test for the carrier state.

Treatment is based on adequate replacement of the deficient factor. Factor VIII concentrate and cryoprecipitate (which contains factor VIII and is more easily prepared) are the main sources of material, both being obtained from freshly donated blood. Factor VIII concentrate may also be prepared from animal material but is strongly antigenic. Newer preparations appear to be less so. Unfortunately factor VIII has a short biological half-life of 8 hours so that repeated administration is necessary. The aim should be to maintain factor VIII activity above a level which is necessary to achieve haemostasis and the initiation of healing. For a haemarthrosis or for muscle and soft tissue bleeding a level of factor VIII above

30% of normal is usually adequate. Haematuria and retroperitoneal haemorrhage require levels above 50%, while tooth extraction and major surgery require levels approaching 100%.

In practice six or 12 packs of cryoprecipitate are usually given to the patient, with further administrations as required. Cryoprecipitate should always be of the correct blood group unless the patient is group O when cryoprecipitate from any donor can be given. The material should be prepared from donors known to be hepatitis B and HIV negative. Factor VIII concentrate is now treated by heat to kill the AIDS virus. Nevertheless, most patients receiving these preparations sooner or later develop hepatitis. In addition the frequent administration of foreign antigenic material appears to result in deterioration of immune function with altered T lymphocyte subset ratios. This may reflect the development of the acquired immunodeficiency syndrome (p. 726).

Teeth can be extracted under the cover of aminocaproic acid or tranexamic acid, both of which inhibit fibrinolysis, and this may greatly reduce the need for factor VIII. In mild haemophiliacs with the factor VIII levels above 7% the administration of the vasopressin analogue desmopressin (DDAVP) will cause a three to four-fold rise in factor VIII coagulant activity and may obviate the need to use cryoprecipitate or factor VIII concentrate. The dose of desmopressin is 0.3 μg/kg by infusion over 15 minutes and may be repeated once 6 to 8 hours later. Fluid intake should be restricted for 24 hours because of the antidiuretic effect of desmopressin. Dental extractions should always be done in hospital.

When inhibitors are present very large amounts of factor VIII may be required to overwhelm the inhibitor. Unfortunately this causes a very rapid rise in inhibitor levels and is likely to be useful for only a few days.

Blood transfusion may be given when there has been much blood loss. For open wounds, topical application of a thrombogenic agent, such as thrombin, is generally helpful but does not provide a satisfactory substitute for lack of factor VIII.

Haemarthroses and muscle bleeds require initial rest for the first 24–36 hours with splinting, followed by early mobilisation to minimise the risk of muscle wasting and deformity. Analgesics should be given when pain is severe but aspirin should be avoided as it may cause gastric bleeding. Addictive analgesics should be avoided. If aspiration is required for an extremely tense joint the procedure should be done before replacement therapy is started. Because haemophiliacs are repeatedly exposed to blood products, the incidence of hepatitis B and liver disease is relatively high and AIDS is also a hazard. The patients are also at risk of developing drug addiction as they require analgesics frequently.

Prevention. Severely affected patients should avoid trauma while at the same time leading as normal a life as possible. Home therapy, where patients have a supply of factor VIII and can inject themselves immediately bleeding occurs, has considerably improved the outlook for some patients. Regular administration to prevent bleeding in very severe haemophiliacs, although expensive in material, may be worthwhile. All haemophiliacs should be referred to a haemophilia centre for supervision and advice, not only in relation to their treatment, but also for help with the social and educational implications of their disorder.

Christmas disease (haemophilia B)

This disease, so-called after the first patient in whom it was recognised, is due to deficiency of factor IX and, like haemophilia A, is X-linked. It is 10 times less common than haemophilia. All that has been said about haemophilia applies to Christmas disease, except that replacement therapy is with factor IX concentrate. This has a longer half-life and requires to be given less frequently.

Von Willebrand's disease

This is a rare group of disorders which are usually inherited as autosomal dominant and are seen in both sexes equally. It is not dissimilar to haemophilia with which it may be confused and probably explains at least some of the cases of haemophilia reported in females. It is due to a variable reduction of the von Willebrand factor which is required for platelet adhesion to vessel walls and as a carrier for factor VIII in plasma. It is produced by endothelial cells and megakaryocytes.

Clinical features. There is excessive bleeding from cuts or other injuries. Patients who have very low factor VIII levels may develop bleeding episodes similar to those described for haemophilia although bruising and mucous membrane bleeding is commoner.

Investigation. The diagnosis is established by family studies, the finding of a prolonged bleeding time, a normal platelet count, failure of aggreation of platelets by ristocetin, impaired adherence of platelets to glass beads and reduced levels of factor VIII and von Willebrand factor. Lastly infusion of plasma or cryoprecipitate causes a prolonged rise in factor VIII levels in excess of that due to infused factor VIII, a phenomenon never seen in haemophilia and thought to be due to an increase in the von Willebrand factor. This also corrects the platelet defects.

Treatment. Fresh frozen plasma or cryoprecipitate should be given for troublesome bleeding or surgical procedures. Superficial bleeding will usually respond to simple pressure. Desmopressin may be used for patients with factor VIII levels above 7%.

Deficiency of the vitamin K dependent factors

Factor II (prothrombin) and factors VII, IX and X are synthesised by the liver. The fat-soluble vitamin K (p. 68) is required for this function. Deficient production of these factors occurs if there is biliary obstruction or other cause of malabsorption such as coeliac disease or severe liver disorder. When anticoagulation is required, drugs, particularly warfarin, are used to alter the synthesis of factors II, VII, IX and X; proteins are produced which are antigenically similar to these factors but do not have their procoagulant properties.

Clinical features. Patients with simple vitamin K deficiency or overdosage with oral anticoagulants are liable to excessive bruising, gastrointestinal haemorrhage, haematuria, epistaxis and excessive menstrual loss. When deficiency is associated with severe liver disease the clinical

and haemostatic problems are more complex because of the addition of other factor deficiencies, thrombocytopenia and toxic damage to the vasculature.

Treatment. In simple vitamin K deficiency, whatever the cause, phytomenadione (vitamin K_1 10 mg i.v.) corrects the factor deficiency within 6 hours. Treatment of anticoagulant overdosage is given on page 551.

The management of the bleeding problems in severe liver disease is complex and will depend on the identification of the coagulation factors involved, the platelet count and the degree to which fibrinolysis has been stimulated. Vitamin K is seldom deficient although it may be administered in the hope of producing some improvement. Fresh frozen plasma, platelets and blood transfusion may all be required. It is risky to use concentrates of factors II, VII, IX and X as these tend to induce disseminated intravascular coagulation (p. 551) unless the concentrates contain heparin. Generally, replacement therapy is best reserved for acute haemorrhage as its effects are short lived.

THROMBOSIS

In health, blood is kept in a fluid state by various mechanisms (p. 544) which may be upset in favour of thrombus formation in certain circumstances. A thrombus may be defined as an abnormal mass formed inside a blood vessel and consisting of various components of blood which have reacted together in ways similar to, but not identical to, the normal process of haemostasis.

There are two types of thrombus: (1) the white thrombus which occurs in arteries. It is formed by platelet adhesion and aggregation, with fibrin deposition in layers and may in time occlude the artery; (2) the red thrombus which consists of large amounts of fibrin and red cells and relatively few platelets. It forms mainly in veins or behind a white thrombus and is similar to the clot formed by blood in a tube. A red thrombus is soft and friable and in veins may easily be detached to cause pulmonary embolism.

Aetiology. The factors which predispose to the formation of thrombi in blood vessels fall into three main groups:

1. ABNORMALITIES OF BLOOD VESSEL WALLS due to:

a. Atherosclerosis.

b. trauma (e.g. needles, cannulas, irritant infusions and endothelial damage over a myocardial infarction).

c. Loss of venous tone, e.g. varicosities; and

d. Infiltration of the vessel wall by neoplastic disease.

2. ABNORMALITIES OF BLOOD FLOW due to:

a. Stasis occurring mainly in veins although it may develop in the auricles of the atria in atrial fibrillation. Stasis may also be due to lack of muscular activity as in general anaesthesia, to external pressure on veins (e.g. in pregnancy or neoplasia) or to venous pooling as occurs in cardiac failure.

b. Hyperviscosity either (i) because of an increase in the cellular components of blood as in polycythaemia vera or leukaemia or (ii) because of an increase in the protein levels as in myeloma or Waldenström's macro-globulinaemia.

c. Turbulence, caused for instance, by kinking of arteries forcing platelets on to the vessel walls.

3. ABNORMALITIES OF THE BLOOD due to:

a. Thrombocytosis occurring in disorders such as polycythaemia vera.

b. Hypercoagulable states from an increased activation of clotting factors during and after surgery, from decrease in the activity of the fibrinolytic mechanism as in factor XII deficiency and when there is a decrease in coagulation inhibitors in the blood, for instance antithrombin III deficiency.

c. Lack of prostacyclin (epoprostenol).

Prostacyclin. The vascular endothelium synthesises prostacyclin from prostaglandin endoperoxides produced from arachadonic acid by the enzyme cyclo-oxygenase (Fig. 13.4). Prostacyclin is an unstable compound with a half-life of 2 to 3 minutes; it inhibits platelet aggregation, promotes platelet disaggregation and causes vasodilation. These effects are the opposite of those caused by thromboxane A2 produced from the same precursors in platelets. It is thought that prostacyclin production is of major importance in inhibiting thrombus formation in blood vessels. Prostacyclin can also be produced in the lungs from which it perfuses the circulation. Levels of thromboxane A2 are low in people eating a seafood diet, e.g. Eskimos who have a low incidence of thrombosis. Aspirin inhibits cyclo-oxygenase and hence reduces the production of thromboxane A2 in platelets. However, by the same action, but in larger doses, it also probably reduces the production of prostacyclin by the cells of the vessel walls.

Clinical features. Thrombosis in both arteries and veins is a major cause of morbidity and mortality. In arteries the occlusion is often crippling, if not lethal, depending on the tissue affected and whether there is a good anastamotic circulation, e.g. in thrombosis of the coronary (p. 168), cerebral (p. 629), mesenteric (p. 321) and limb arteries (p. 191). On the venous side the local effects are usually less damaging to health but deep venous thrombosis producing pulmonary emboli can be lethal (p. 179). The effects of thrombosis of the cavernous and other venous sinuses (p. 637) or of the renal veins (p. 382), are often serious.

Treatment. The indications for the use of anticoagulant and other forms of therapy are discussed with the individual lesions.

HEPARIN THERAPY. Heparin is a natural, biologically produced anticoagulant which acts by accelerating the activity of antithrombin III (p. 544). The effect is virtually instantaneous. Heparin has a half-life of 60–90 minutes and disappears rapidly from the circulation. It is administered either by intermittent intravenous injection every 6 hours, by continuous intravenous infusion in a small volume or by intermittent (usually b.d.) subcutaneous injection. When given by continuous intravenous infusion the level of anticoagulation may be monitored by thrombin times or partial thromboplastin times with kaolin or, if necessary, by the whole blood clotting time. Heparin is seldom used for more than 2 weeks. Prolonged treatment can cause osteoporosis. It is often combined with oral anticoagulants, the heparin being used to initiate anticoagulation until the oral anticoagulants can exert their effect; heparin is then withdrawn. Overdosage may be treated either by stopping administration or, when there is haemorrhage, by giving protamine sulphate in a dose based on laboratory tests.

Heparin can be used either as an anticoagulant or as prophylaxis against thrombosis. The doses required for the latter are much smaller (low dose heparin) and do not alter coagulation tests. At this low dose intravascular thrombosis is discouraged but haemostasis is adequate for surgery.

ORAL ANTICOAGULATION. Warfarin is the drug of choice. Indandione derivatives such as phenindione are much more likely to produce hypersensitivity reactions. Anticoagulation should be initiated carefully as some patients require lower doses than others, and indeed the dose of 20 mg of warfarin on the first day and 10 mg on the following day, which is routinely given in many centres, will be excessive in a significant number of patients. It is better to give 10 mg of warfarin on the first day and then increase the dose in those who can tolerate the drug. The maintenance dose varies widely from 2–20 mg daily for 2–3 weeks if the thrombosis is uncomplicated or for 3 months or more if it is recurrent. Rarely, enormous doses are required in patients who metabolise the drug in an abnormal manner.

Therapy is usually monitored by the *prothrombin time,* preferably corrected to a standard ratio to make results comparable between centres. The therapeutic range is between ratios of 1:2 and 1:4. This test does not reflect factor IX deficiency. The *thrombotest* does and is regarded by some as preferable. Also the thrombotest can be done on finger prick blood.

Since many drugs interfere with the binding of warfarin to albumin or induce enzyme activity in the liver, thereby increasing warfarin metabolism, introduction or withdrawal of other drugs should be under medical supervision and the patient advised that such changes may have serious effects unless monitored. Transient illness also affects liver function and may require dosage alteration.

Patients should carry a card indicating that they are receiving warfarin. They should be advised specifically not to take aspirin or proprietary preparations containing aspirin, but to use paracetamol for headaches and other minor discomforts.

In the treatment of overdosage, withdrawal of the anticoagulant may be sufficient. If reversal of anticoagulation is required phytomenadione (vitamin K_1) should be used. The disadvantage is that unless dosage is small it will be difficult to re-establish oral anticoagulation for some time. Alternatively fresh frozen plasma or blood may be administered if there is a need to correct the defect quickly. Concentrates of factor II, VII, IX and X are seldom used, as preparations, certain to be free of hepatitis B and HIV infection, are difficult to produce.

FIBRINOLYTIC THERAPY. Thrombolysis by means of streptokinase or other agents (p. 195) is being used but is very expensive and potentially dangerous, especially postoperatively. Streptokinase is antigenic so that it can be given only for a limited period. This type of treatment is rarely used for longer than 2 days and is followed by anticoagulation.

Prevention. Low molecular weight dextrans have been used widely in surgical practice. Attempts to counteract the adhesive and aggregating properties of platelets with a variety of drugs such as aspirin and dipyridamole are being evaluated. Efforts are being made to produce a stable analogue of prostacyclin in the hope that it will prove to be a useful agent in the prevention of thrombosis.

Disseminated intravascular coagulation

This is a deranged state in which coagulation and lysis of fibrin produced by coagulation proceed simultaneously in the blood. It is a reflection of other problems, not a disease in itself.

Aetiology. The trigger is usually something that initiates intravascular coagulation. This may be transient or ongoing. Transient liberation of thrombogenic substances into the blood is seen classically in association with the end of pregnancy and parturition. Amniotic fluid embolism is potently thromboplastic and similar effects are seen in abruptio placentae, eclampsia and when there is a dead fetus in utero. Other triggers include malignancies, hepatic disease, severe trauma, anaphylaxis, hypoxia, venoms and sepsis. Bacterial endotoxins act indirectly through mediators such as granulocytes, platelets and damaged vascular endothelium.

Whatever the trigger, the effect is a threat to

the circulation and the fibrinolytic mechanism responds, sometimes dramatically, by lysing fibrin as it is formed. This response may overshoot, and excess plasmin produced by the fibrinolytic system digests fibrinogen and other factors as well as the fibrin, causing a severe haemorrhagic state. This occurs in addition to depletion of clotting factors and platelets by the coagulation process which initiated the problem. The result is a severe failure of the haemostatic mechanism (Fig. 13.7). The fibrin degradation products themselves have a 'heparin-like' effect which may exacerbate bleeding.

Clinical features. Specific clinical findings are present only in severe cases. Bleeding occurs at all venepuncture sites and from mouth, nose and other orifices. This is due to lysis of fibrin clots wherever they have been laid down. There is massive purpura with ecchymoses. The patient is usually gravely ill. Sometimes excessive fibrinolysis may occur locally at the site of a major operation, particularly on the brain or prostate. No evidence of this phenomenon is then seen systemically but local bleeding may be prolonged.

Diagnosis of disseminated intravascular coagulation is by laboratory investigation. It is necessary to show depletion of coagulation factors and platelets and evidence of an increase in the products of fibrin degradation products.

Treatment. When disseminated intravascular coagulation is severe, replacement of coagulation factors may be necessary. Heparin may be used when there is an ongoing stimulus to coagulation as in malignant disease. Antifibrinolytic drugs such as aminocaproic acid are given when fibrinolysis alone appears to be the major problem, usually for local haemostatic abnormalities.

In practice very severe disseminated intravascular coagulation is rare and in most cases the process is contained and excessive depletion of coagulation factors does not occur. In such cases the treatment is that of the underlying disorder.

PROSPECTS IN HAEMATOLOGY

For many years haematology has had a firm base in blood film and marrow morphology. This has determined the classification of many of the blood diseases. Electron microscopy has extended this base by demonstrating the ultrastructure of the cells. More recently immunological techniques have brought a new dimension to the subject. Dynamic concepts have appeared and resulted in new ideas about classification particularly in the field of lymphomas and leukaemias. Cells are now recognised to have characteristics not evident from light or electron microscopy. Antigens originally thought to be tumour related are now known to be characteristic of certain stages in the differentiation of cells. This is a rapidly expanding field of knowledge and further contributions to our understanding of the nature of these diseases will undoubtedly come.

The chemotherapy of acute lymphoblastic leukaemias of the common type has proved highly successful in obtaining long remissions, even in adults. The same degree of success has not been obtained in the myeloblastic leukaemias or in the lymphoblastic leukaemia of T and B cell type. Here there is room for improvement as new drugs become available. The use of bone marrow transplantation in the treatment of acute leukaemia holds out hope for younger patients who have disease that is unlikely to be eliminated by chemotherapy. Improvements in the management

DISSEMINATED INTRAVASCULAR COAGULATION

TRIGGER

INTRAVASCULAR COAGULATION

SEVERE / MILD

CONSUMPTION OF CLOTTING FACTORS AND PLATELETS

FIBRIN DEPOSITION

SPONTANEOUS RECOVERY

ACTIVATION OF FIBRINOLYSIS

MICROVASCULAR OCCLUSION

CLOTTING FACTOR DEPLETION THROMBOCYTOPENIA

DIGESTION OF FIBRIN AND FIBRINOGEN

FIBRIN DEGRADATION PRODUCTS

TISSUE NECROSIS

HAEMORRHAGE

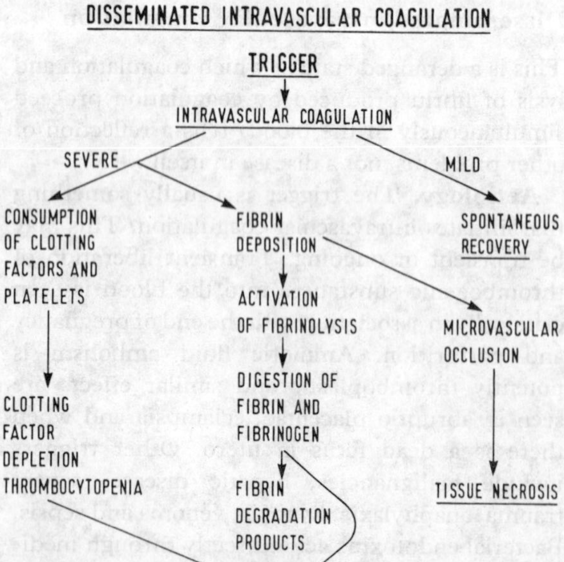

Fig. 13.7 Disseminated intravascular coagulation.

of the chronic leukaemias have been awaited for a long time and while no easy answers to the problems of these diseases can be foreseen it is now clear that bone marrow transplantation may have something to offer young adults and children.

Monoclonal antibodies from 'immortal' lines of mouse myeloma cells hybridised with human cells producing normal antibody are extremely specific, reacting with only one antigen. Monoclonal antibodies are used extensively for serological investigations; they can identify specific subsets of cells and stages of cell differentiation. In addition the use of monoclonal antibodies for therapeutic purposes is being explored, both to replace polyclonal preparations and as vehicles to carry drugs and other therapeutic weapons to specific cells. In this respect there is the possibility that human myeloma cells may be used instead of mouse myeloma cells to produce monoclonal antibodies, thus avoiding interspecies differences.

In the field of coagulation problems the understanding of the role of the prostaglandins in platelet and vascular endothelial function opens up the prospect of new therapeutic techniques to deal with the problems of intravascular thrombosis. The development of antisera to factor VIII will hopefully improve the measurement of that factor, assist in the identification of female carriers and enable the investigator to discover at the fetal stage whether a male offspring has the disease. Perhaps similar development will also occur in relation to factor IX deficiency.

The realisation that the therapeutic use of blood and blood products carries the risk of transmitting HIV infection and thereby the possibility of AIDS has increased the problems associated with this form of therapy. It has also increased the awareness of the risks to laboratory and other staff handling blood specimens and blood products.

N.C. ALLAN

FURTHER READING:

General haematology:

Thompson R B, Proctor S J 1984 A short textbook of haematology. Pitman, London. A comprehensive, readable account of haematology

Bangham A S, Hughes A S B, Patterson K G, Stirling L 1984 Manual of haematology. Churchill Livingstone, Edinburgh. Useful for clinical aspects

Practical haematology:

Allan N C 1986 In: Macleod J, Munro J (eds) Clinical examination, 7th edn. Churchill Livingstone, Edinburgh, pp 433–449. Describes basic haematological investigations and their interpretation

Dacie J V, Lewis S M 1984 Practical haematology, 6th edn. Churchill Livingstone, Edinburgh. For information regarding investigative procedures

Hirsh J, Brain E 1983 Haemostasis and thrombosis: a conceptual approach, 2nd edn. Churchill Livingstone, Edinburgh. An excellent and easily understood introduction to coagulation

Reference volumes:

Wintrobe M M 1981 Clinical haematology, 8th edn. Kimpton, London. Probably the best comprehensive reference volume

Hardisty R M, Weatherall D J 1982 Blood and its disorders, 2nd edn. Blackwell Scientific Publications, London. A reference volume particularly useful for its section on hemoglobinopathies and thalassaemias

Dacie J V 1985 The haemolytic anaemias. 1. The hereditary haemolytic anaemias, 3rd edn. Churchill Livingstone, Edinburgh. A very detailed review of these disorders

Biggs, R 1984 Human blood coagulation, haemostasis and thrombosis, 3rd edn. Blackwell Scientific Publications, Edinburgh

14

Diseases of connective tissues, joints and bones

Rheumatology deals with a heterogeneous group of disorders of connective tissues, joints and bones. The 'rheumatic diseases' are conditions in which pain and stiffness of some part of the musculoskeletal system are prominent. It is convenient, if rather arbitrary, to group these disorders according to whether the basis for the connective tissue pathology is primarily inflammatory, metabolic or degenerative.

Inflammatory diseases of connective tissue include rheumatoid arthritis and other types of inflammatory and infective arthritis, the spondarthritides and the diffuse connective tissue diseases characterised by multisystem organ pathology, systemic disturbance and evidence of immune dysregulation. Metabolic disorders include the crystal deposition diseases, gout and chondrocalcinosis, while the predominantly degenerative disorders are osteoarthrosis, spondylosis and a number of painful syndromes of the soft connective tissues.

Prevalence. Rheumatic diseases affect people of both sexes and all ethnic groups and ages. Their frequency increases with age so that as many as 40% of persons over the age of 65 years have some rheumatic complaint. In Britain 20 million people experience a rheumatic disorder each year. Five million suffer from osteoarthrosis, 500 000 have rheumatoid arthritis and there are 12 000 children with chronic juvenile arthritis. Eight million people consult their general practitioner annually with rheumatic complaints, amounting to 18% of all consultations in general practice. Rheumatic diseases are the commonest cause of

physical impairment in the community. The lives of more than one million persons are so impaired and one-fifth of these are severely disabled. No other group of diseases is responsible for greater loss of earnings. In 1978 the cost to the United States economy attributed to musculoskeletal disorders was 20 billion dollars.

DISEASES OF CONNECTIVE TISSUES AND JOINTS

INFLAMMATORY DISEASES

Rheumatoid arthritis; spondarthritis; juvenile chronic arthritis; infective and miscellaneous arthritis; systemic lupus erythematosus; progressive systemic sclerosis; polymyositis and dermatomyositis; arteritis.

RHEUMATOID ARTHRITIS

In its typical form rheumatoid arthritis is a chronic inflammatory, destructive and deforming polyarthritis associated with systemic disturbance, a variety of extra-articular lesions and the presence of circulating antiglobulin antibodies (rheumatoid factors). While the pattern of joint involvement is characteristically symmetrical and peripheral and its course prolonged, with exacerbations and remissions, atypical, asymmetrical and incomplete forms are not uncommon.

Epidemiology. Rheumatoid arthritis occurs throughout the world in all climates and all ethnic groups. The prevalence in developed countries is about 3% with a female to male ratio of 3:1. There is an annual incidence of 0.3% so that over the age of 65 years 16% of the female population and 5% of males are affected. The disease commences most commonly in the 3rd and 4th decades but the age of onset follows a normal distribution curve and no age group is exempted.

Incidence is five to sixfold higher than expected in twins and 1st degree relatives but not in spouses suggesting a fairly weak genetic predisposition. This has been confirmed by a modest but significant increase in HLA-D4 and HLA-DR4 in patients and their families associated with an approximately fivefold increase in relative risk in persons with these genetic markers. Higher incidence in urban than in rural Africans of the same ethnic origin suggests that environmental factors are important.

Aetiology and pathogenesis. Although the cause of rheumatoid arthritis remains obscure, progress has been made in identifying the cellular interactions and chemical mediators which lead to chronic inflammation in joints, local destruction of cartilage and bone and systemic manifestations of rheumatoid disease.

It is widely believed that an infection is the initiating factor, although no causative organisms have been identified. Current concepts suggest that the disease results from altered immune reactivity and persistent antigenic stimulation in genetically predisposed persons. Possible mechanisms for this which remain under continuing investigation include the persistence of elusive organisms or partially degraded bacterial cell wall peptidoglycans, cross-reactive immune responses between bacterial or viral antigens and articular components, viral induction of immune complexes or viral immunosuppression. Alternatively it is suggested that sensitisation to self antigens could be a consequence of enzymatic or free radical damage to proteins such as IgG or collagen. Whatever the mechanisms, there is much evidence for persistent immune overactivity, autoimmunity and the presence of immune complexes at sites of articular and extra-articular lesions, namely: (1) increased expression of DR antigen by synovial lining cells and dendritic cells; (2) sub-synovial foci of T helper cells in contact with antigen presenting dendritic cells; (3) increased numbers of plasma cells, lymphocytes and monocytes in the synovial membrane associated with local production of rheumatoid factors and lymphokines; (4) the presence of circulating IgM, IgG and IgA serum antiglobulins (rheumatoid factors) as well as anti-collagen and antinuclear antibodies; (5) the presence of self-associating IgG and IgG-IgM immune complexes within the phagocytic cells of synovial effusions; (6) depression of synovial fluid complement components in inflamed joints associated with activation of both the classical and alternative pathways; (7) the presence of serum factors which inhibit suppressor T lymphoctye activity; (8) amyloidosis complicating some cases of rheumatoid arthritis of long duration; (9) the importance of lymphocytes and cellular immunity in the pathogenesis of the disease is confirmed by the striking remission of activity which follows lymphocyte depletion by thoracic duct drainage, lymphocytophoresis or cytotoxic drug therapy.

Thus rheumatoid arthritis is considered to be both an extravascular immune complex disease and a disorder of cell-mediated immunity in which the following sequence of events leads to inflammation, granuloma formation and joint destruction: (1) localisation of unidentified antigen in joints and processing by antigen presenting cells; (2) release of immuno-potentiating factors such as interleukin 1; (3) interleukin 2 production and proliferation of T helper cells; (4) B lymphocyte proliferation and local synthesis of antiglobulin antibodies; (5) formation of immune complexes and activation of the complement pathway; (6) stimulation of neutrophil chemotaxis, cytolysis, lymphokine production and macrophage neutral protease secretion by biologically active complement components; (7) neutrophil and macrophage phagocytosis of immune complexes following IgG and C3 receptor recognition; (8) release of mediators of acute inflammation — vasoactive amines, proteases, polypeptides, oxygen radicals, prostaglandins and leukotrienes; (9) T lymphocyte infiltration and production of lymphokines; (10) macrophage and chondrocyte activation, pannus formation and enzymatic destruction of articular cartilage and bone by collagenase, neutral proteinases and interleukin 1; (11) stimulation of fever, acute phase response, bone marrow and muscle wasting by interleukin 1. The severity of erosive damage is related to joint movement and physical stress as well as the activity of the inflammatory disease, showing that mechanical factors are also important in the pathogenesis.

Pathology. The earliest change is swelling and congestion of the synovial membrane and the underlying connective tissue, which become infiltrated with lymphocytes (especially helper T cells), plasma cells and macrophages. Effusion of synovial fluid into the joint space takes place during active phases of the disease. Hypertrophy of the synovial membrane occurs with the formation of lymphoid follicles resembling an immunologically active lymph node. Inflammatory granulation tissue (pannus) is formed, spreading over and under the articular cartilage which is progressively eroded and destroyed. Later, fibrous adhesions may form between the layers of pannus across the joint space and fibrous or bony ankylosis may occur. Muscles adjacent to inflamed joints atrophy and there may be focal infiltration with lymphocytes.

Subcutaneous nodules have a characteristic histological appearance. There is a central area of fibrinoid material consisting of swollen and fragmented collagen fibres, fibrinous exudate and cellular debris, surrounded by a palisade of radially arranged proliferating mononuclear cells. The nodule has a loose capsule of fibrous tissue. Similar granulomatous lesions may occur in the pleura, lung, pericardium and sclera. Lymph nodes are often hyperplastic showing many lymphoid follicles with large germinal centres and numerous plasma cells in the sinuses and medullary cords. Immunofluorescence shows that the plasma cells in the synovium and lymph nodes synthesise rheumatoid factors.

Clinical features. ONSET. In the majority of patients the onset is insidious with joint pain, stiffness and symmetrical swelling of a number of peripheral joints. Initially pain may be experienced only on movement of joints, but rest pain and especially early morning stiffness are characteristic features of all kinds of active inflammatory arthritis.

In the typical case the small joints of the fingers and toes are the first to be affected. Swelling of the proximal, but not the distal, interphalangeal joints gives the fingers a 'spindled' appearance and swelling of the metatarsophalangeal joints results in 'broadening' of the forefoot. As the disease progresses, with or without intervening remissions, there is a tendency for it to spread to involve the wrists, elbows, shoulders, knees, ankles, subtalar and midtarsal joints. The hip joints are affected only in the more severe cases but neck pain and stiffness from cervical spine involvement is common. The mandibular, acromioclavicular and sternoclavicular joints are sometimes affected as indeed is every synovial joint.

In 10% of patients the disease starts as an acute polyarthritis with severe systemic symptoms, including fever, weight loss, profound fatigue and malaise. In some patients the onset is 'palindromic' with recurrent acute episodes of joint pain and stiffness in individual joints lasting only a few hours or days. In about a third of such cases the disease sooner or later evolves into a more typical poly-arthritis.

PROGRESSION. As the disease advances, pain, muscle spasm and joint destruction result in limitation of joint motion, joint instability, subluxation and deformities. At first deformities are correctable, but later permanent contractures develop and the joints may become completely disorganised.

Characteristic deformities include flexion contractures of the small joints of the hands and feet, the knees, hips and elbows. Anterior subluxation of the metacarpophalangeal joints is common with ulnar deviation of the fingers. Other finger deformities lead to more loss of function. These include the 'swan neck' deformity (hyperextension at the proximal interphalangeal joints and fixed flexion at the distal interphalangeal joints), the Boutonnière or 'button-hole' deformity (fixed flexion of the proximal interphalangeal joint and extension of the terminal interphalangeal joint) and a Z deformity of the thumb. Dorsal subluxation of the ulnar styloid at the wrist is common and may contribute to rupture of the fourth and fifth extensor tendons when these are already the site of tenosynovitis.

In the forefoot, subluxation of the metatarsophalangeal joints is followed by clawing of the toes, callosities over the exposed metatarsal heads and a painful sensation of 'walking on pebbles'. In the hind foot calcaneal erosions may develop at the insertions of the Achilles tendon or plantar fascia and eversion deformities at the subtalar joint are common.

EXTRA-ARTICULAR FEATURES. Rheumatoid arthritis is a systemic disease. Anorexia, weight loss, lethargy and myalgia occur commonly throughout its course and may precede the onset of articular symptoms by weeks or months.

Raynaud's phenomenon is common in the prodromal period and throughout the course of the disease.

Lymphadenopathy is particularly found in nodes draining actively inflamed joints but more generalised lymphadenopathy occurs and can give rise to diagnostic confusion when arthritis is minimal or quiescent. The nodes are discrete and not tender. Histology shows a reactive hyperplasia which can be confused with lymphoma.

Osteoporosis, muscle weakness and wasting occur adjacent to inflamed joints and more dif-fusely as part of the systemic disturbance. They are seen early in the course of the disease and often progress to become prominent features in very active or advanced cases.

Tenosynovitis and bursitis are frequent accompaniments of active arthritis as tendon sheaths and bursae are also lined with synovium. 'Triggering' of the fingers may be associated with nodules in the flexor tendon sheaths which can progress to permanent flexion contractures or tendon rupture if left untreated.

Popliteal cysts (Baker's cysts) communicate with the knee, but fluid is prevented from returning to the joint by a valve-like mechanism. The high pressure generated by flexion of the knee, especially when effusions are present, can result in gradual extension or sudden rupture of the cyst into the calf. Rupture is accompanied by calf pain, swelling, tenderness and pitting oedema. Diagnostic confusion with deep vein thrombosis can usually be avoided by careful consideration of the history but a venogram, or arthrogram is occasionally required to establish the correct diagnosis.

Subcutaneous nodules appear at some time in the course of the disease in about 20% of patients. They are usually seen at the sites of pressure or friction such as the extensor surfaces of the forearms below the elbow, the scalp, sacrum, scapula and Achilles tendon as well as on the fingers and toes. Ulceration and secondary infection are not uncommon. Nodules are almost invariably associated with positive tests for rheumatoid factor.

OCULAR MANIFESTATIONS. *Episcleritis* is a fairly common and benign feature in patients with nodular seropositive disease. The intermittent inflammation of the superficial sclera is usually painless. It is not associated with visual disturbance and requires no specific therapy.

Scleritis is a rarer but more serious condition. The eye is red and painful with inflammatory changes throughout the sclera and uveal tract. The pupil may be irregular from adhesions (synechiae) which can cause secondary glaucoma and visual impairment. Scleritis often requires systemic corticosteroid therapy as well as local measures.

Scleromalacia or thinning of the sclera may follow episodes of scleritis and is seen as a blue discolouration of the white of the eye. Perforation rarely occurs. *Scleromalacia perforans* follows necrosis of a scleral rheumatoid nodule and may require grafting or enucleation of the eye.

Keratoconjunctivitis sicca occurs in 10% of patients. Lack of lacrimal secretion results in grittiness, dryness, burning or itching associated with sticky mucous threads. The diagnosis can be confirmed by the Schirmer tear test.

Sjögren's syndrome and the sicca syndrome. The former is the association of xerostomia and keratoconjunctivitis sicca with a connective tissue disorder, usually rheumatoid arthritis. Sjögren's syndrome may also be associated with myasthenia gravis, autoimmune liver disease or thyroiditis.

Sicca syndrome is the term used when keratoconjunctivitis sicca and xerostomia occur in the absence of a connective tissue disorder. It is usually associated with HLA-DR3 rather than HLA-DR4 and patients with the sicca syndrome are more likely to have widespread and serious manifestations than those with Sjögren's syndrome. These include: salivary gland enlargement and malignancy; dysphagia and dyspareunia; severe dental caries; Raynaud's phenomenon and vasculitis; lymphadenopathy, leucopenia and hepatosplenomegaly; macroglobulinaemia; glomerulonephritis; and diffuse interstitial pulmonary fibrosis.

Patients with Sjögren's syndrome may have a wide range of organ-specific and non-organ-specific autoantibodies. An antibody to an extractable nuclear antigen, SS-B is characteristic of the sicca syndrome. The pathological feature which can be detected in the minor salivary glands on a simple lip biopsy is intense infiltration with lymphocytes and plasma cells.

Treatment is usually limited to scrupulous oral and ocular hygiene and the instillation of artificial tears (hypromellose eye drops). Drug hypersensitivity is sometimes a problem.

CARDIOVASCULAR MANIFESTATIONS. A-symptomatic pericarditis is a common and benign feature of seropositive rheumatoid arthritis while pericardial effusions and constrictive pericarditis occur infrequently. Rarely the formation of granulomatous lesions leads to heart block, cardiomyopathy, coronary artery occlusion or aortic regurgitation.

Vasculitis (p. 391). Diffuse necrotising vasculitis is relatively common in patients with nodules and positive tests for rheumatoid factor. Clinical manifestations vary with the size and site of the vessel involved. Small vessel disease of the terminal arterioles or capillaries is often associated with no more than nail fold infarcts, leg ulcers or purpura. Large areas of skin necrosis or digital gangrene have more sinister significance and may herald the onset of '*malignant*' *rheumatoid disease*. These patients are often febrile with severe systemic disturbance and multiple extra-articular manifestations. A larger vessel arteritis, histologically resembling polyarteritis nodosa, may result in catastrophic mesenteric, renal, cerebrovascular or coronary artery occlusion. Such patients frequently have evidence of circulating immune complexes, cryoglobulins and hypocomplementaemia.

PULMONARY MANIFESTATIONS. *Pleurisy or pleural effusions* occur in about 25% of men with rheumatoid arthritis. Diagnostic aspiration should be undertaken to exclude other causes (p. 261). *Caplan's syndrome* (p. 257) and *fibrosing alveolitis* (p. 256) are rare manifestations of rheumatoid arthritis.

NEUROLOGICAL MANIFESTATIONS. *Entrapment neuropathies* result from compression of peripheral nerves by hypertrophied synovium. Median nerve compression in the carpal tunnel is the most common and may be an early clinical manifestation of the disease. Others include ulnar nerve compression at the elbow, peroneal nerve palsy at the knee and posterior tibial nerve entrapment in the flexor retinaculum at the ankle (tarsal tunnel syndrome).

Peripheral neuropathy is usually symmetrical and limited to symptoms and signs of mild 'glove and stocking' sensory loss. *Mononeuritis multiplex* (p. 662) follows occlusion of vasa nervorum in patients with arteritis.

Cervical cord compression may result from subluxation of the cervical spine at the atlanto-axial joint or at a subaxial level. Atlanto-axial subluxation is a common finding in long-standing rheumatoid arthritis and can be diagnosed from lateral radiographs of the cervical spine taken in full flexion. Although usually associated with no more than neck pain radiating to the occiput, it can result in cord transection and sudden death if the neck is manipulated inadvertently under an anaesthetic. Less dramatic cases of progressive cervical myelopathy may present with limb weakness, difficulty in holding up the head and tetraparesis. These lesions occur more often at the subaxial level and may require operative decompression and fixation.

HAEMATOLOGICAL MANIFESTATIONS are very common in active rheumatoid disease. A normochromic normocytic anaemia of chronic disease (p. 503), which does not respond to oral iron, can often be complicated by true iron deficiency secondary to gastrointestinal blood loss from treatment with analgesic anti-inflammatory drugs. Much less frequently there may be a macrocytic anaemia associated with folate deficiency.

Felty's syndrome is the association of splenomegaly and neutropenia with rheumatoid arthritis; it tends to occur in patients with seropositive, long-standing, advanced but inactive arthritis. Other clinical features include anaemia, thrombocytopenia, lymphadenopathy, weight loss, skin pigmentation and vasculitic leg ulcers. Susceptibility to recurrent bacterial infections is common. A wide range of immunological abnormalities is present.

Treatment with corticosteroids is usually unsatisfactory. Splenectomy is reserved for patients with serious or life threatening recurrent infections and is followed by prolonged remission in about 60% of cases.

Complications. *Septic arthritis* (p. 571) may complicate rheumatoid arthritis usually in patients with long-standing nodular seropositive disease. In debilitated patients, fever and leucocytosis may be absent and signs limited to malaise and slight exacerbation of inflammation in one or more joints. *Staphylococcus aureus* is commonly implicated secondary to invasion from an ulcerated nodule or infected skin lesion.

Amyloidosis (p. 391) is a complication of prolonged active disease and is found in 25–50% of cases at autopsy making rheumatoid arthritis a leading cause of secondary amyloidosis.

Investigation. Active disease is associated with a raised ESR and C-reactive protein. The plasma protein profile shows increased globulin and fibrinogen and decreased albumin.

IMMUNOLOGICAL TESTS. IgM rheumatoid factors are detected by testing the ability of serum to agglutinate carrier particles coated with IgG. Polystyrene particles coated with human IgG are used in the latex slide test. Sheep or human erythrocytes coated with rabbit anti-erythrocyte antibody are used in the Rose Waaler sheep cell agglutination test (SCAT), the human erythrocyte agglutination test (HEAT) and the differential agglutination test (DAT). The latex fixation test is simple and sensitive but less specific so that it is frequently used as a screening test. The erythrocyte tests are less sensitive and more specific. Significant titres which exclude 95% of the normal population are: SCAT 1:32; DAT 1:16; latex 1:20.

The Rose Waaler test is positive in 70% of patients with rheumatoid arthritis but may not become so for a year or two. Positive tests are also found in Sjögren's syndrome (100%), other connective tissue diseases (15–30%), chronic liver disease, sarcoidosis, multiple myeloma and chronic infections. Up to 30% of patients with rheumatoid arthritis have positive tests for antinuclear factor.

RADIOLOGICAL EXAMINATION. In the early stages of the disease radiographs are normal or show no more than soft tissue swelling and periarticular osteoporosis. Progression to cartilage and bone destruction is seen as narrowing of the joint spaces and the development of marginal erosions often in the metatarsophalangeal joints. Very severe destructive changes ('*arthritis mutilans*') are associated with gross deformities and massive bone resorption. Marginal sclerosis and osteophyte formation are indications of secondary osteoarthrosis.

EXAMINATION OF SYNOVIAL FLUID can be of great value when the diagnosis is in doubt. Infection is excluded by microscopic examination of a Gram-stained smear, culture and gas liquid chromatography for bacterial products. In inflammatory joint disease the synovial fluid is of low viscosity, turbid, clots on standing and contains many cells. By contrast fluid from joints affected by traumatic or degenerative joint diseases is clear, viscid, does not clot and contains few cells. Examination of the spun sediment by polarising light microscopy will reveal crystals of monosodium urate or calcium pyrophosphate dihydrate in patients with acute gout or pseudogout. Measurement of synovial fluid total haemolytic complement activity can help to distinguish rheumatoid arthritis from other forms of inflammatory arthritis as its depression is seldom seen except in seropositive rheumatoid arthritis.

ARTHROSCOPY AND SYNOVIAL BIOPSY are occasionally required to exclude diseases such as tuberculosis and synovial tumours.

Treatment. Since the aetiology of rheumatoid arthritis is unknown treatment is empirically directed towards the relief of symptoms, the suppression of active disease and the conservation and restoration of function in affected joints. To a greater or lesser extent these aims can be achieved by combining treatment of the patient — by the judicious use of drugs, rest, physiotherapy and surgery — with the modification of the environment — by paying critical attention to housing, occupation, transport, the provision of aids and appliances, and statutory social benefits.

In a chronic and progressive disease which may have exacerbations and remissions over many years as well as systemic, psychiatric and social complications, both the general practitioner and rheumatologist have a special responsibility: (1)

to educate the patient to understand the nature of the disease and to develop a positive but realistic approach; (2) to create a relationship of continuing trust and support without undue dependence; (3) to co-ordinate a team of orthopaedic surgeons, occupational therapists, physiotherapists, nurses, social workers, and other allied health professionals in an integrated rehabilitation programme and (4) to improve the patient's general health.

In a disorder which is as complex and changeable as rheumatoid arthritis there is a need for repeated medical, functional and social reassessment if patients are to maintain their maximum physical, psychological, social and vocational potential.

GENERAL TREATMENT IN THE ACTIVE PHASE. Physical rest, anti-inflammatory drug therapy and maintenance physiotherapy are the cornerstones of treatment for exacerbations of rheumatoid disease. Admission to hospital may become necessary when widespread active polyarthritis is associated with signs of constitutional disturbance and there has been no response to rest at home and optimal doses of non-steroidal, analgesic, anti-inflammatory drugs (NSAID).

In most patients the rest from physical and emotional stress provided by 2 to 3 weeks in hospital is sufficient to induce a marked remission of symptoms without recourse to strict bedrest. The time in hospital allows for detailed assessments by all members of the arthritis team. It ensures that the programme of medical and physical treatment best suited to the individual's needs can be started under supervision and it provides an opportunity to plan the solution of outstanding functional and social problems with appropriate aids and social services.

In a few patients a period of complete bedrest may be required to induce a remission. In these circumstances it is essential to prevent the development of 'bed deformities'. The mattress should be firm or fracture boards inserted beneath it. A back rest with the minimum number of pillows should be in position during the day and only one firm pillow used at night. Pillows behind the knees must be avoided and a bed cage with padded footrest provided. The patient should spend an hour each day lying flat with a small pillow under the lumbar spine and two periods of 3 minutes lying prone will go a long way to prevent the development of flexion contractures of the hips. Foot and quadriceps exercises should be performed daily along with maintenance exercises for muscle groups in unaffected limbs and in the thoracic, gluteal and abdominal regions.

The anaemia of chronic disease (p. 503). responds best to induction of disease remission but iron is also indicated if it is deficient. Rarely folic acid is required for a macrocytic anaemia.

LOCAL MEASURES IN THE ACTIVE PHASE. *Corticosteroids*. Where one or more joints continue to be extremely painful and inflamed, intra-articular injection of a suspension of a corticosteroid such as triamcinalone hexacetonide will often bring symptomatic relief lasting weeks or months. The dose should be 2.5–40 mg according to joint size. Repeated injections at short intervals should be avoided, particularly in the case of weight-bearing joints. Local injection of a corticosteroid is also the treatment of choice for alleviating symptoms of median nerve compression in the carpal tunnel when this occurs during the course of an exacerbation of rheumatoid arthritis.

Rest splints can be very useful for stabilising a particularly painful joint, such as the knee or wrist, but are usually indicated only if general rest, non-steroidal anti-inflammatory drugs and intra-articular steroid injections fail to bring relief. Splints are also used to prevent or correct flexion deformity especially at the knee.

ANALGESIC AND ANTI-INFLAMMATORY DRUGS are the mainstay of therapy for active inflammatory arthritis. They can be very effective in relieving pain and stiffness in optimal anti-inflammatory doses but they do not alter the course of the disease and the margin between effective and toxic doses is often small.

Aspirin was formerly regarded as the drug of first choice but only 50% of patients are able to tolerate adequate doses. For anti-inflammatory, as opposed to simple analgesic, effect it needs to be given in doses of 4–6 g daily. It should be prescribed as soluble aspirin (the cheapest) or as enteric coated tablets when dyspepsia or occult gastrointestinal blood loss is a problem.

NSAID are listed in Table 14.1, with standard doses.

Table 14.1 Non-steroidal analgesic anti-inflammatory drugs (NSAID).

Drug	Usual dose
CARBOXYLIC ACIDS	
Salicylic acids	
Aspirin	600–900 mg × 6 d
Aloxiprin	1200 mg × 4/d
Benorylate	10 ml b.d.
Diflunisal	500 mg b.d.
Salsalate	1–1.5 g b.d.
Trilisate	1–1.5 g b.d.
Anthranilic acids	
Mefenamic acid	500 mg × 4/d
Propionic acids	
Fenbufen	300 mg mane
	600 mg nocte
Fenoprofen	600 mg × 4/d
Flurbiprofen	100 mg t.i.d.
Ibuprofen	400–800 mg × 4/d
Ketoprofen	100 mg t.i.d
Naproxen	500 mg b.d.
Tiaprofenic acid	200 mg t.i.d.
Acetic acids	
Diclofenac	50 mg t.i.d.
Fenclofenac	600 mg b.d.
Heterocyclic acetic acids	
Tolmetin	400 mg × 4/d
Indole acetic acids	
Indomethacin	25–50 mg t.i.d.
Sulindac	200 mg b.d.
ENOLIC ACIDS	
Pyrazolones	
Azapropazone	600 mg b.d.
Phenylbutazone	100 mg t.i.d.
(severe, active ankylosing spondylitis only)	
Oxicams	
Piroxicam	20 mg daily

Inhibition of prostaglandin synthesis appears to be a major pharmacological action of all these agents. Simultaneous inhibition of the protective effect of prostacyclin on gastric mucosa may, however, also be the basis for the common propensity of these drugs to cause gastrointestinal haemorrhage and perforation. NSAID should be avoided in patients with peptic ulceration.

NSAID with longer duration of action are convenient to use. However, cases of fatal hepatotoxicity following treatment with benoxaprofen have emphasised the potential danger of drugs with long half-lives in elderly patients with impaired renal function as well as re-emphasising the need for caution in prescribing any new NSAID preparation. Adverse effects have been reported on the blood, kidney and skin

For initial treatment it is advisable to use one of the established, less expensive NSAID, with a low incidence of side-effects, in moderate dosage, for a trial period of about 3 weeks. If the response is not satisfactory, another NSAID with which the clinician is familiar, can be used. The author's preference is to begin with a propionic acid derivative if aspirin is not tolerated. Ibuprofen appears to be the least toxic.

Paracetamol can also be given when pain relief is inadequate. Paracetamol dextropropoxyphene combinations are very widely used for this purpose. Although safe in moderate doses propoxyphene does have narcotic properties. In general, centrally acting narcotic analgesics have no place in the management of rheumatic diseases. A number of combinations of aspirin and paracetamol are marketed.

SLOW ACTING ANTIRHEUMATIC DRUGS. The use of a 'second line' or 'disease-modifying' drug should be considered in all patients where symptoms and signs of active inflammatory arthritis have persisted for 6 months despite adequate general measures and optimal doses of NSAID.

The antimalarials chloroquine phosphate (250 mg daily) or hydroxychloroquine sulphate (200 mg b.d.) may be used as an adjunct to basic therapy. Clinical benefit is noted in about half the patients in 4–12 weeks and the drug should be discontinued if there is no effect by 6 months. Occasional side-effects include nausea, diarrhoea, rashes, haemolytic anaemia, ototoxicity and neuromyopathy as well as a small risk of ocular toxicity after more than a year of therapy. Deposits of the drug in the cornea may produce disturbances of vision which tend to disappear when the drug is withdrawn. More rarely retinopathy can result in permanent visual impairment. If the drug is effective it is advisable to check the visual acuity and ophthalmoscopic appearance of the maculae after 1 year and at 6-monthly intervals thereafter. In order to reduce the risks of ocular toxicity the drug is given for only 10 months in each year. In some the dose can be halved without exacerbation of symptoms.

Penicillamine and gold are slow acting suppressive antirheumatic drugs which have been shown to decrease the progression of erosive changes as well as reduce the activity of the disease in 50–60% of patients. Because of a high incidence of toxic effects, treatment with these agents should be considered as an adjunct to basic therapy only in the following circumstances: (1) active progressive disease developing erosions and/or deformities; (2) nodules and/or high titres of rheumatoid factor with persistently active disease after 6 months treatment with optimal doses of anti-inflammatory drugs; (3) troublesome extra-articular features; (4) failure to respond to antimalarial drugs; (5) symptoms controllable only with unacceptably high doses of corticosteroids; (6) palindromic rheumatoid arthritis with frequent attacks or developing persistent inflammatory arthritis.

Penicillamine is marginally preferable to gold unless there is a previous history of severe dyspepsia because it can be given orally and because the side-effects, though numerous and potentially serious, are usually more predictable and manageable. Treatment is commenced with a single evening dose of 125 or 250 mg and dosage is increased by no more than 250 mg monthly to a maximum of 1g/d. Clinical benefit is noted several weeks after an effective dose has been achieved and reaches a maximum only after 4–6 months.

Early adverse effects include rashes, loss of taste, nausea, vomiting and a serious febrile reaction. Later side-effects include mouth ulcers, proteinuria and the nephrotic syndrome and more rarely diseases resembling systemic lupus erythematosus, myasthenia gravis, pemphigus and Goodpasture's syndrome. Thrombocytopenia and pancytopenia may occur at any time and are potentially the most serious toxic effects.

Patients must be monitored, initially at weekly intervals, by urinalysis and full blood counts including platelets. Proteinuria and mild thrombocytopenia are indications for cessation of therapy followed by reintroduction of the drug at lower dosage if the abnormalities disappear. It is advisable to withdraw penicillamine altogether if the side-effects recur. Febrile reactions and pancytopenia are absolute indications for drug withdrawal.

Chrysotherapy. After a test dose of 10 mg, weekly intramuscular injections of 50 mg sodium aurothiomalate are given until a response is obtained, usually at about 2–3 months. The intervals between injections are progressively increased provided the remission is maintained and the drug is continued indefinitely. The gold injections should be stopped if there has been no clinical benefit after 6 months.

Adverse effects include pruritic rashes, exfoliative dermatitis, mouth ulcers, enterocolitis, proteinuria and the nephrotic syndrome, thrombocytopaenia, agranulocytosis and aplastic anaemia, all of which are potentially serious and preclude further therapy. Patients who are HLA-DR3 positive are particularly at risk of developing a gold induced immune complex glomerulonephritis. Monitoring should include a routine urinalysis and full blood counts with platelets, initially prior to each injection.

Pruritus may respond to antihistamines and exfoliative dermatitis, thrombocytopenia, agranulocytosis and nephropathy to corticosteroids. Patients with agranulocytosis almost invariably recover if they can be protected from serious infection; those with aplastic anaemia have a more serious prognosis. Dimercaprol (BAL) combines with heavy metals to form a stable compound which is rapidly excreted in the urine; 3 mg/kg body weight should be administered intramuscularly 6 hourly for 3–4 days in patients with aplastic anaemia who have not responded to withdrawal of gold injections after 4–5 days. An oral gold compound is available which is less toxic but less effective than injected gold.

Other disease modifying antirheumatic drugs. Dapsone (50–100 mg/d, p. 759) is associated with slow clinical improvement and reduction of acute phase proteins, but haemolytic anaemia can be a troublesome side-effect, particularly in slow acetylators. Sulphasalazine (p. 315) is one of the safer second line agents. Nausea and vomiting can be troublesome, but are usually avoidable if treatment is started with 500 mg daily and increased gradually to a maximum of 500 mg qds over a period of 4 weeks. Other compounds which have been shown to have slow acting antirheumatic activity include the antibacterial agent rifampicin, the antihypertensive agent captopril and the penicillamine analogues 5-thiopyr-idoxine, pyrithioxine and thyopronine.

CORTICOSTEROIDS AND CORTICOTROPHIN have a very potent anti-inflammatory activity but do not possess the 'disease modifying' properties of the slow acting antirheumatic agents. Doses required to maintain adequate symptomatic relief on a long term basis are accompanied by an unacceptable level of side-effects so their use is justified only in exceptional circumstances.

The main indications for the use of corticosteroids are: (1) in exceptionally severe exacerbations which are not remitting with rest, intra-articular injections of corticosteroids and non-steroidal anti-inflammatory drugs; (2) when all other measures fail to control persistently disabling symptoms in breadwinners or young mothers who have to return to work; (3) in some elderly patients when acute disease is threatening to render them bedbound; (4) life or sight threatening visceral disease such as severe pericarditis, polyarteritis or scleritis. In each of these circumstances a slow acting antirheumatic agent is commenced simultaneously with a view to a gradual withdrawal of corticosteroid therapy when a remission has been obtained.

Prednisolone is the corticosteroid of choice. It should ideally be administered as a single morning dose of no more than 7.5 mg/d to minimise suppression of the hypothalamo-pituitary-adrenal axis. In practice an evening dose of 5 mg is sometimes more useful in overcoming intractable early morning stiffness. Enteric coated tablets or small doses of corticotrophin may be preferred in patients with a previous history of peptic ulceration. In other circumstances any possible advantages of corticotrophin seem to be outweighed by the disadvantages, namely the need for injections, the difficulty in knowing the dose of steroid being effectively administered and the high prevalence of mineralocorticoid side-effects.

IMMUNOMODULATION. Since rheumatoid arthritis is associated with evidence of both over-activity of humoral immunity and suppression of some facets of cell-mediated immunity both 'immunosuppressive' and 'immunostimulant' drugs have been considered for management of the disease. Increasing understanding of the complexity of regulation of the immune system and the 'immunopharmacology' of cytotoxic and immunostimulant drugs makes it clear that these agents may have variable and even opposing effects on the expression of immune responses depending on the dosage, the timing of administration and the subpopulation of cells predominantly affected. For example, immune stimulation may result from treatment with a drug which predominantly inhibits a suppressor cell population while functional immunosuppression can follow use of an immunostimulant which selectively activates these cells.

In practice a number of cytotoxic and immunostimulant agents have been found to have both symptomatic and slow acting 'disease modifying' activity in rheumatoid arthritis. The effects, which are empirical, may be mediated as much by 'anti-inflammatory' as by the 'immunoregulatory' activity and their usefulness is very strictly limited by immediate and potential long term toxicity.

The indications for the use of these agents are limited at the present time to: (1) life threatening extra-articular manifestations which have failed to respond to corticosteroids or second line agents; (2) severely active symptomatic and progressive joint disease that has failed to respond to all other forms of therapy; (3) patients receiving unacceptably high doses of corticosteroids in whom dose reduction has not been possible.

Azathioprine (p. 31) in both high dosage (2.5 mg/kg) and low dosage (1.25 mg/kg) has been shown to be effective. Adverse effects include vomiting, stomatitis, diarrhoea, hepatitis and particularly bone marrow suppression and susceptibility to infection. Monitoring is with fortnightly or monthly full blood counts.

Cyclophosphamide has a narrow therapeutic range (p. 534) but is effective in daily doses of 1–2 mg/kg. Adverse effects include alopecia, azoospermia, anovulation, cystitis, nausea and vomiting, susceptibility to infection, bone marrow suppression and teratogenesis. Monitoring is with fortnightly or monthly full blood counts and routine urinalysis.

Methotrexate (p. 109) is effective in low oral pulse doses of 7.5 or 15 mg/week. It is very rarely associated with bone marrow suppression; liver function must be monitored regularly and interstitial lung disease can be a rare complication.

Levamisole is an anthelmintic which has been shown to augment T lymphocyte responses as well as polymorph and macrophage chemotaxis and phagocytosis. It can be effective in patients with rheumatoid arthritis in doses of 150 mg once weekly. Adverse effects include febrile reactions, vomiting, urticarial and vasculitic rashes. A high risk of agranulocytosis even with weekly monitoring of blood counts precludes its use routinely.

MEDICAL SYNOVECTOMY. Synovial obliteration can be achieved with osmic acid or a variety of radiocolloids if pain, effusion and synovitis persist despite local corticosteroid injections, systemic drug therapy and physical measures. Yttrium-90 silicate is used for large joints such as the knee and Erbium-159 acetate for the small joints of the hands. Joints are immobilised for 72 hours to reduce spread to regional lymph nodes. Patients under the age of 45 should be excluded.

SURGICAL TREATMENT AND REHABILITATION. In the overall management of patients with severe and progressive rheumatoid arthritis there are many circumstances when orthopaedic surgical procedures are required to relieve pain and conserve or restore locomotor function.

Surgical decompression and synovectomy of the wrist and tendon sheaths of the hands are often needed when non-steroidal anti-inflammatory drugs, local injections of corticosteroids and simple physical measures have failed to relieve a carpal tunnel syndrome or flexion contractures of the fingers resulting from fibrosis and nodule formation. Flexor and extensor tendon synovectomy, the latter often accompanied by resection of a subluxated ulnar styloid, can be important measures in preventing tendon ruptures. Synovectomy of joints will not prevent disease progression but may be indicated for pain relief when drug therapy, local rest, intra-articular injections and radiocolloids have failed to provide symptomatic relief.

At a later stage, when tendons, cartilage and bone have been eroded and the mechanics of joints disturbed, reconstructive tendon surgery, osteotomy, arthrodesis and a variety of arthroplasties with or without prostheses play a major part in the rehabilitation of the patient. Forefoot pain resulting from subluxation of the metatarsophalangeal joints and clawing of the toes can be effectively relieved by excision of the heads and necks of the metatarsals if insoles and moulded shoes have failed to provide symptomatic relief. Hip arthroplasty can be remarkably effective in relieving incapacitating pain and restoring ambulation in patients with severely damaged joints. Total hip replacement is now the most frequent major elective operation undertaken in Britain where over 30 000 are performed annually. Resurfacing and total condylar arthroplasties of the knee are less consistently successful but nevertheless performed in preference to osteotomy and arthrodesis in rheumatoid patients with intractable pain and disability. Arthrodesis is, however, still the best solution when severe hind foot pain is associated with destruction and subluxation of the ankle and subtalar joints.

A number of 'salvage' and reconstructive operations are also available for relieving pain and restoring function in the upper limbs. Stabilisation or wrist arthrodesis, excision arthroplasty of the metacarpo-phalangeal joints with insertion of silastic spacers and arthrodesis of the PIP joints of the fingers are all procedures in appropriate circumstances to relieve pain and improve power grip. Pinch grip may be restored by arthrodesis of the interphalangeal joint of the thumb in patients with Z deformities. Radial head excision is a simple but effective procedure which will relieve the severe pain experienced on supination and pronation when the superior radio-ulnar joint is the major site of destructive change. Relief of pain and restoration of function to patients with advanced shoulder and elbow destruction is, however, still a major problem. Suitable prosthetic surgery for these joints is still very much in the developmental phase.

If surgical treatment is to be successful it is very important that the aims and consequences of each operation are carefully considered as part of an integrated programme of management and rehabilitation. This is often best achieved where physicians and surgeons with special experience work together in a combined rheumatology/orthopaedic clinic with other allied health professionals. Assessment of motivation, social support and environment are no less important than careful consideration of the patient's general health and detailed assessment of the extent of disease in other joints, the integrity of the cervical spine, the presence or absence of infection, arteritis or osteoporosis. In particular it must be appreciated that whereas many patients with slowly progressive disease can be maintained mobile and functionally independent by a series of major joint replacements carried out over a number of years, it is seldom possible to mobilise a patient, who has been chair- or bedbound for a long period, by multiple joint replacement during a single lengthy hospital admission. In these and other circumstances pain relief and functional independence are better served by provision of a suitable wheelchair, home adjustments, physical aids and social services.

When a patient cannot return to a former occupation it may be necessary to suggest a change of employment where less strain will be thrown on the damaged joints. Although disablement resettlement officers, industrial rehabilitation units and government retraining centres are sometimes helpful in such cases, it should be emphasised that patients have the best chance of returning to active work with their former employers. It cannot be stressed too strongly that adequate treatment in the early stages and throughout the course of the disease enables most patients to return to some form of wage earning activity. Disabilities of all kinds can be reduced even in the 25% of patients running a severe progressive course.

Prognosis. The course and prognosis in rheumatoid arthritis is very variable. In those patients with disease of such severity as to require admission to hospital, review after 10 years shows that: 25% will have a complete remission of symptoms and remain fit for all normal activities; 40% will have only moderate impairment of function despite exacerbations and remissions of disease; 25% will be more severely disabled; 10% will be severely crippled. If the many patients in the community are considered whose symptoms are never of such severity as to require admission to hospital the overall prognosis is much better.

A poor prognosis may be associated with: (1) high titres of rheumatoid factor; (2) insidious onset of disease; (3) more than a year of active disease without remission; (4) early development of nodules and erosions and (5) extra-articular manifestations.

SPONDARTHRITIS

This is a group of diseases in which an inflammatory arthritis, characterised by persistently negative tests for IgM rheumatoid factor, is variably associated with a number of other common articular, extra-articular and genetic features. These spondarthritides are: ankylosing spondylitis; Reiter's disease and reactive arthritis; psoriatic arthritis; enteropathic arthritis associated with ulcerative colitis and Crohn's disease; Behçet's syndrome; Whipple's disease and juvenile chronic arthritis.

The features held in common by the seronegative spondarthritides are: (1) an asymmetrical, inflammatory seronegative oligoarthritis; (2) sacroiliitis and/or spondylitis in some cases; (3) a tendency to develop inflammatory lesions of tendinous attachments to bone (enthesopathy); (4) anterior uveitis; (5) familial association and (6) a high prevalence of the histocompatibility antigen HLA-B27.

Current concepts of the aetiology of these disorders suggests that they may arise as an abnormal response to infection in genetically determined persons carrying the HLA-B27 antigen. In some, an inciting organism has been identified as in Reiter's disease which can follow bacterial dysentery or chlamydial urethritis, or in the reactive arthritis following infection with *Yersinia enterocolitica*. In the others the infectious agent remains obscure. It is uncertain whether possession of HLA-B27 predisposes towards disease because: (1) it is merely a marker for an immune response gene; (2) susceptibility to infection is increased as a result of cross-reactivity between an HLA-B27 determined host gene product and an antigen carried by the invading organism or (3) the inciting organism modifies HLA-B27 positive cellular receptors in such a way as to initiate an autoimmune reaction or render the cells more susceptible to cytotoxic lymphocytes.

Ankylosing spondylitis

In its typical form this is a chronic inflammatory arthritis with a predilection for the sacroiliac joints and spine and characterised by progressive stiffening and fusion of the axial skeleton.

Epidemiology. Typically ankylosing spondylitis is a disease with a peak onset in the second and third decades and a male to female ratio of about 4:1. More than 90% of affected persons carry the histocompatibility antigen HLA-B27. There is a greatly increased incidence in the 1st degree relatives of patients with ankylosing spondylitis, psoriatic arthritis, inflammatory bowel disease and Reiter's syndrome. Chronic prostatitis is more common than would be anticipated but it has not been possible to isolate organisms from prostatic fluid. Faecal carriage of some Klebsiella species is increased in ankylosing spondylitis and this may be related to exacerbations of the disease.

Pathology. Biopsy material from peripheral joints shows changes similar to those found in rheumatoid arthritis. Bony ankylosis, however, occurs more frequently. The characteristic *enthesopathy* comprises multiple foci of inflammation with lymphocytes and plasma cells at ligamentous attachments with adjacent erosion of bone. Healing of similar lesions at the junction of the vertebral bodies and annulus fibrosus of the intervertebral discs leads to the new bone formation (syndesmophytes) which is the hallmark of the disease.

Clinical features. The onset is usually insidious with recurring episodes of low back pain and stiffness sometimes radiating to the buttocks or thighs. Characteristically the symptoms are worse in the early morning and following inactivity. Occasionally the onset may be acute, resembling a lumbar disc protrusion. A few patients present with symptoms referable to the dorsal or cervical spine but such cases usually reveal evidence of previous sacroiliitis and lumbar spine involvement.

Chest pain aggravated by breathing results from involvement of the costovertebral joints. Plantar fasciitis, Achilles tendinitis and tenderness over bony prominences such as the iliac crest, ischial tuberosity and greater trochanter are typical. 25% of patients have an attack of acute anterior uveitis during the course of the disease and this may be the presenting feature in a few cases. In 10% a peripheral joint is first affected and in a further 10% symptoms begin in childhood as one variety of pauciarticular juvenile chronic arthritis (p. 569).

Early signs include failure to obliterate the lumbar lordosis on forward flexion, pain on sacro-iliac compression, and restriction of movements of the lumbar spine in all directions. As the disease progresses, stiffness increases throughout the spine, and chest expansion frequently becomes restricted. Severe spinal fusion and rigidity occurs in only a minority and in most of these is not associated with much deformity. A few develop kyphosis of the dorsal and cervical spine which can be incapacitating especially when associated with hip involvement.

Extra-articular features of ankylosing spondylitis include iritis, aortic regurgitation and conduction defects, apical pulmonary fibrosis, amyloidosis, osteoporosis and myelopathy associated with atlanto-axial subluxation.

Investigation. The ESR is usually raised but may be normal. Tests for rheumatoid factor and antinuclear factor are negative and synovial fluid complement levels are not depressed.

Radiological signs of sacroiliitis begin in the lower parts of the joints with irregularity and marginal sclerosis eventually progressing to fusion. In the lumbar spine there may be 'squaring' of the vertebrae owing to ossification of the anterior longitudinal ligament, syndesmophyte formation, erosion and sclerosis at the anterior corners of the vertebrae and facetal joint changes. Progressive ossification results in the typical 'bamboo spine'. Erosive changes may be seen in the symphysis pubis, the ischial tuberosities and peripheral joints. Osteoporosis and atlanto-axial dislocation can occur.

Radionuclide bone scanning may reveal evidence of sacroiliitis or spinal involvement when radiographs are negative but the increased uptake of the bone-seeking isotope is non-specific and reflects bone blood flow and turnover.

Treatment. The principles are to relieve pain and stiffness, maintain a maximal range of skeletal mobility and avoid the development of deformities. Early in the disease patients should be trained to do regular exercising at home and encouraged to take up active non-contact sports like swimming. Poor bed and chair postures must be avoided.

NSAID (p. 561) are used to relieve symptoms but do not themselves alter the course of the disease. A few patients with spondylitis find phenylbutazone the most effective drug; it can usually be given safely even over prolonged periods provided a daily dose of 300 mg is not exceeded.

Radiotherapy is occasionally indicated if the response to drug therapy is unsatisfactory. It does not affect the course of the disease and earlier regimes of treatment, when excessive radiation was employed, were associated with a tenfold increase in the risk of developing leukaemia.

Local corticosteroid injections can be helpful for plantar fasciitis and the management of other manifestations of enthesopathy. Systemic steroids are sometimes required for treatment of acute iritis.

Hip disease may require surgery and total hip arthroplasty has largely obviated the need for difficult spinal surgery in those with advanced deformity.

75% or more of patients with ankylosing spondylitis are able to remain in employment without significant loss of time from work. Restriction of chest movements does not predispose to pulmonary infection but systemic complications and especially hip involvement carry a worse prognosis.

Reiter's disease

Classically this is the triad of non-specific urethritis, conjunctivitis and arthritis that follows bacterial dysentery or exposure to the risk of sexually transmitted infection. Incomplete forms are frequent and include the commonest variety of inflammatory arthritis seen in young men. When arthritis alone follows sexual exposure or enteric infection with salmonella, shigella, yersinia or campylobacter the term *'reactive arthritis'* is frequently used.

Epidemiology. 1–2% of patients with non-specific urethritis seen at clinics for sexually transmitted diseases have Reiter's disease and there is a similar incidence following outbreaks of shigellosis. A male with HLA-B27 runs a 20% risk of getting the disease following an attack of shigella dysentery. Although predominantly a disease of young men, the apparent 50:1 male to female ratio is spuriously high as urethritis is frequently ignored in women and children.

Clinical features. The onset is typically acute with the simultaneous development of urethritis, conjunctivitis (in about 50%) and an inflammatory oligoarthritis affecting the large or small joints of the lower limbs, 1–3 weeks following sexual exposure or an attack of dysentery. There may be considerable associated systemic disturbance with fever, weight loss and vasomotor changes in the feet.

Often the onset is more insidious and many patients present with no more than monoarthritis of a knee or an asymmetrical inflammatory arthritis of some interphalangeal joints. Symptoms and signs of urethritis or conjunctivitis may have been minimal or forgotten. In such cases, heel pain, Achilles tendinitis or plantar fasciitis are valuable clues while the presence of circinate balanitis or the rash of keratoderma blenorrhagica can clinch the diagnosis even in the absence of the classical triad and without an overt history of sexual promiscuity or dysentery. The skin lesions can vary from mild macules, vesicles and pustules on the hands and feet to marked hyperkeratosis with plaque-like lesions spreading to the scalp and trunk. These may be associated with severe nail dystrophy and massive subungual hyperkeratosis.

Ocular involvement is normally limited to mild bilateral conjunctivitis which subsides spontaneously within a month. In 10% of patients acute iritis occurs at the outset. It is distinguished from simple conjunctivitis by injection of the ciliary vessels around the cornea, by a constricted, irregular or unreactive pupil and by cells in the anterior chamber on slit lamp examination. Unlike the conjunctivitis it requires urgent treatment. Chronic iritis may lead to glaucoma and blindness.

The urethritis is usually associated with minor dysuria and a clear sterile discharge. Sometimes it is asymptomatic and detected only by finding mucoid threads in the first voided specimen of early morning urine. Unusually there may be severe dysuria, haematuria and suprapubic discomfort from an associated acute haemorrhagic cystitis and prostatitis.

Usually the arthritis is self-limiting with spontaneous remission of symptoms within 2–3 months of onset. There is, however, a recurrence rate of about 15% per annum not necessarily related to further overt exposure to infection. Iritis occurs in 30% of patients with recurring arthritis. Low back pain and stiffness from sacroiliitis are common and 15–20% of patients develop spondylitis. Other rare extra-articular features include neurological and cardiological complications, e.g. meningo-encephalitis, peripheral neuropathy, pericarditis and pleurisy.

Investigation. The ESR is often greatly raised during the acute phase and may remain so for long after joint symptoms have settled. Polymorphonuclear leucocytosis and an anaemia of chronic disease (p. 503) are further indications of active systemic disturbance. The synovial fluid has the characteristics of a low viscosity inflammatory effusion with leucocyte counts as high as 50 000/ml but it is sterile on culture. Giant synovial macrophages can be seen but synovial fluid complement levels are not depressed as they are in seropositive rheumatoid arthritis. Serum tests for rheumatoid factor and antinuclear factor are negative. Tissue typing reveals HLA-B27 in more than 70% of cases.

Radiological examination. Periarticular osteoporosis, reduction of joint space and erosive changes can be seen when there is prolonged or recurrent inflammatory arthritis. The changes are often accompanied by marked periostitis especially in the metatarsals, phalanges and pelvis; there may be large and 'fluffy' calcaneal spurs. Sacroiliitis is indistinguishable from that seen in ankylosing spondylitis but the spinal changes include early isolated bony spurs and paravertebral ossification also found in psoriasis but not in ankylosing spondylitis.

Treatment is mainly symptomatic and supportive. Rest and NSAID (p. 560) are required during the acute phases together with judicious aspiration of joints and intra-articular or other local steroid injections. Systemic corticosteroids are very occasionally required. Iritis may be a medical emergency requiring topical, subconjunctival or systemic corticosteroids. Severe progressive arthritis and intractable keratoderma blenorrhagica very occasionally warrant cytotoxic drug therapy. The non-specific urethritis is usually treated with a short course of tetracycline but there is little evidence that it alters the course of the arthritis.

10% of patients have evidence of active disease 20 years after the onset. Spondylitis, chronic erosive arthritis, recurrent acute arthritis and uveitis are the major causes of long-term morbidity.

Psoriatic arthritis

This is a seronegative inflammatory arthritis found in patients with psoriasis, a past or family history of psoriasis or with characteristic changes in the nails.

Epidemiology. Psoriatic arthritis occurs in about 1 out of 1000 of the general population and in 7% of patients with psoriasis. 20% of all patients with seronegative polyarthritis have psoriasis while the prevalence of psoriasis in seropositive rheumatoid arthritis is no higher than that in the general population, suggesting that the association of the skin disease with seronegative arthritis does not arise by chance alone. The onset is usually between the ages of 25–40 years.

Clinical features. Five distinct clinical patterns of psoriatic arthritis are recognised:

1. An inflammatory arthritis involving the distal interphalangeal joints, not usually affected in rheumatoid arthritis, is seen in 15% of patients who almost invariably have associated nail changes (below).

2. An asymmetrical inflammatory oligoarthritis affecting the small joints of the hand and feet is the most common clinical pattern and accounts for 70% of all cases.

3. A symmetrical but persistently seronegative inflammatory polyarthritis clinically indistinguishable from 'seronegative rheumatoid arthritis' accounts for 15% of cases.

4. Arthritis mutilans with extensive bone resorption and telescoping digits occurs in less than 5% of cases.

5. Sacroiliitis and spondylitis indistinguishable from classical ankylosing spondylitis can occur alone or in association with any of the clinical patterns of peripheral arthritis.

Extra-articular features are limited to (1) skin lesions which may be widespread scaling lesions typically over extensor surfaces or insignificant and confined to such areas as the scalp, natal cleft and umbilicus where they are easily overlooked; (2) nail changes including pitting, onycholysis, subungual hyperkeratosis and horizontal ridging and (3) iritis.

Investigation. The ESR is usually only moderately raised and there may be a mild normochromic normocytic anaemia in active cases. Tests for rheumatoid factor and antinuclear factor are negative. Radiographs showing asymmetrical disease, terminal IP joint involvement and relatively little periarticular osteoporosis may help to distinguish psoriatic arthritis from rheumatoid arthritis. The changes in the axial skeleton resemble those in ankylosing spondylitis.

Treatment. NSAID are usually all that are required to control symptoms. Gold therapy can be used in persistently symptomatic progressive cases without exacerbation of the psoriasis but the antimalarials, chloroquine and hydroxychloroquine must be avoided. Immunosuppressive drugs are given very occasionally to try and control progressive arthritis mutilans or extensive incapacitating skin disease. Splints and prolonged rest are best avoided because of the increased tendency to fibrous and bony ankylosis but intra-articular steroid injections can be used with good effect in persistently active and symptomatic joints.

Prognosis is better than for rheumatoid arthritis with the exception of those rare cases with arthritis mutilans.

Other seronegative spondarthritides

Enteropathic arthritis. Two patterns of seronegative inflammatory arthritis are associated with ulcerative colitis and Crohn's disease.

Enteropathic synovitis. An acute, often migratory, non-erosive oligo-arthritis occurs in the course of the disorder in 12% of patients with ulcerative colitis and 20% of those with Crohn's disease. The knees, ankles and other weight-bearing joints are most commonly affected but the wrists and small joints of the fingers and toes can also be involved. The arthritis, which tends to follow exacerbations of the underlying bowel disease, sometimes in association with aphthous mouth ulcers, iritis and erythema nodosum, ceases to be a problem following total colectomy in cases of ulcerative colitis. The higher prevalence in Crohn's disease may reflect the greater difficulty in eradicating the bowel problem.

Sacroiliitis (16%) and *ankylosing spondylitis* (6%) are also seen in the course of these disorders, but they pursue an independent course and often precede the bowel disease.

Behçet's syndrome is rare in Western Europe but more common in Japan and Eastern Mediterranean countries; there is an association with HLA-B5.

Major criteria are recurrent aphthous stomatitis, skin lesions, iritis and genital ulceration. Minor criteria are inflammatory arthritis of large joints, intestinal ulceration, epididymitis and thrombophlebitis. In the presence of all four major criteria the syndrome is said to be 'complete'; in the presence of three, 'incomplete'. The arthritis is mono-articular or oligo-articular and non-erosive. It most frequently involves the knees, ankles, wrists and elbows. Occasionally the sacroiliac joints are affected.

Treatment is symptomatic with NSAID; corticosteroids and immunosuppressive therapy are reserved for the more serious systemic manifestations.

Whipple's disease is a rare disorder characterised by diarrhoea, abdominal pain, weight loss, pyrexia, skin pigmentation, malabsorption and arthritis. The pattern of the non-erosive arthritis can resemble the migratory oligo-articular enteropathic arthritis but sometimes it is symmetrical and polyarticular. Joint symptoms, most commonly affecting the knee or ankle, may precede other clinical manifestations by months or years and sacroiliitis and ankylosing spondylitis may occur. The diagnosis is confirmed by demonstrating the presence of PAS positive macrophages in a small intestinal biopsy. Treatment is with prolonged antibiotic therapy, usually tetracycline 1g daily for 1 year. Arthralgias and arthritis settle within a month of starting treatment.

JUVENILE CHRONIC ARTHRITIS

Four main patterns of chronic arthritis commence in childhood before the age of 16 years.

Systemic onset juvenile chronic arthritis (Still's disease) begins with a profound systemic disturbance in 10% of children with juvenile chronic arthritis. Lymphadenopathy, hepatosplenomegaly, pleurisy, pericarditis and a high intermittent fever are associated with myalgias, arthralgias and eventually polyarthritis. Weight loss and retardation of growth may be striking and there is often a characteristic evanescent macular rash which tends to appear when the temperature is raised. This pattern of disease is most common between the ages of 1 and 5 years. Remission of symptoms usually occurs within 6 months but half the children have recurrent attacks and one-quarter go on to develop a severe chronic polyarthritis.

Polyarticular juvenile chronic arthritis can occur at any age and accounts for 20% of all cases. Four or more large joints are commonly first affected acutely or insidiously. Inflammatory arthritis in the proximity of growing epiphyses may result in growth acceleration or arrest. Early fusion in the cervical spine and mandible give rise to the short stiff neck and receding chin very characteristic of adults who have had juvenile chronic arthritis. The overall prognosis is good and only 10–15% have severe destructive arthritis.

Seropositive polyarticular disease occurs in 10% of children with juvenile chronic arthritis and the onset is usually after the age of 8 years. The disease resembles severe adult onset rheumatoid arthritis with progressive erosive joint changes in more than half of those affected. Extra-articular features include nodules and vasculitis. Antinuclear factor tests are positive in 75%.

Pauci-articular juvenile chronic arthritis involves four or less joints in half or more of all children affected; at least two distinct subsets can be identified:

1. *Young girls* with mono- or pauci-articular arthritis but seldom any constitutional symptoms. HLA-DR5 and positive tests for antinuclear factor appear to be a marker for chronic iritis which can occur in up to half of this group. Three-monthly slit lamp examinations are required if this complication is to be detected and treated early enough to preserve normal vision.

2. *Older boys* with mono- or pauci-articular arthritis affecting hips, knees or ankles. Sacroiliitis is common and there is frequently a family history of iritis, ankylosing spondylitis or another spondarthritis. 75% of these boys are HLA-B27 positive and in some the disease gradually evolves into ankylosing spondylitis in early adult life.

Differential diagnosis of acute arthritis in childhood includes bacterial, viral and reactive arthritis as it does in adults and also rheumatic fever (p. 152) and osteomyelitis (p. 586).

Henoch-Schönlein (anaphylactoid) purpura is associated with abdominal pain and an acute arthritis affecting one or more joints for a few days at a time. The disease frequently follows an upper respiratory infection and usually lasts for less than 3 months. Intussusception, rectal bleeding and renal involvement (p. 391) are features of more severe cases.

Treatment. The principles of management in juvenile chronic arthritis do not differ from those in adult rheumatoid arthritis but special consideration has to be given to maintaining the child's education and helping parents to develop a sensible, vigilant but not overprotective approach to the child's disease. Bed-rest may be essential during acute phases but care must be taken to avoid development of flexion deformities of the hips and knees by regular prone lying and appropriate lightweight splints. Whenever possible the child should be kept mobile and ambulant and daily physiotherapy is given throughout to maintain a good range of joint movements and muscle strength. Hydrotherapy in a warm pool is particularly useful.

Aspirin is the drug of choice and its use here is an exception to the recommendation that aspirin should not be given to children aged under 12 years because of the risk of Reye's syndrome (p. 347). Naproxen (5 mg/kg) is safe and effective in children and experience is accumulating with other NSAID. Chloroquine, hydroxychloroquine, gold salts and penicillamine can be used with the same precautions as in adults.

Corticosteroids are reserved for children with severe systemic disease, those with chronic iritis not responding to local therapy and where very active joint disease does not respond to other measures. The use of corticotrophin or alternate day corticosteroids should·always be considered because daily doses of prednisolone as low as

3 mg/d can inhibit growth in children under age of 5 years. Older children can be taught to give their own injections of corticotrophin if this has to be continued for any length of time. Corticosteroids do not arrest the progression of disease. Immunosuppressive drugs are used only in persistently active disease.

Surgery is usually limited to the rehabilitation of children with deformities. Soft tissue release operations may be helpful in eliminating difficult flexion contractures and osteotomies may be required when joints have been allowed to fuse in poor positions. Total hip arthroplasty can be considered for severely destroyed joints as soon as growth has ceased.

INFECTIVE ARTHRITIS

Septic arthritis can accompany septicaemia at any age. *H. influenzae* is the common causative organism in infancy; staphylococcal and streptococcal infections are usually responsible in older children and adults. Other organisms which may be implicated are gonococci, pneumococci, meningococci, *Esch. coli*, *Pseudomonas* and *Proteus*. Important predisposing factors include debilitating illnesses, diabetes mellitus, immunodeficiency disorders and immunosuppression. Joint trauma, surgery, penetrating injury and intra-articular injections may lead to bacterial joint infections and may complicate rheumatoid arthritis and other established arthritides.

Clinical features. Characteristically septic arthritis has an abrupt onset with severe pain and swelling of a single joint associated with a swinging fever, severe malaise and a polymorphonuclear leucocytosis. Large joints are most frequently affected and the joint is hot, tender and swollen with an effusion; there is marked limitation of movement. The diagnosis may be missed when more than one joint is involved, in patients with rheumatoid arthritis or when the presentation is less acute in patients receiving corticosteroids or immunosuppressive drugs.

It is essential to try to establish the diagnosis early by joint aspiration and blood culture. The synovial fluid is typically turbid with a high polymorphonuclear cell count. Organisms may be easily and immediately identified on Gram stain of a film but special culture techniques may be required especially for gonococci and anaerobic organisms.

Radiographs show no more than soft tissue swelling initially. Later there may be periarticular osteoporosis, joint space narrowing, periostitis and articular erosions. In more long-standing infections the joint margins have a peculiar 'rubbed out' appearance.

Treatment. In all cases where bacterial infection is suspected treatment should be commenced with high parenteral doses of broad spectrum antibiotics as soon as joint aspiration and blood cultures have been completed and continued until the responsible organism and its sensitivity have been established. Appropriate antibiotics must then be administered for several weeks. Antibiotics readily cross the inflamed synovial membrane so that there is no need to inject them intra-articularly.

The joint should be rested and immobilised with a splint and daily joint aspiration undertaken until no more fluid reaccumulates. If the fluid becomes loculated or too thick for aspiration, surgical drainage is required.

The prognosis for recovery without joint damage should be excellent and is directly related to the speed with which antibiotic therapy is instituted.

Gonococcal arthritis is more common in females than males and not infrequently commences at the time of a menstrual period within 2–3 weeks of genital infection. Joint involvement is usually asymmetrical and polyarticular with an acute or subacute, migratory polyarthralgia or polyarthritis. Tenosynovitis, an 'additive' as opposed to 'flitting' pattern of joint involvement and a macular, vesicular or pustular rash are important diagnostic clues even in the absence of overt genital gonorrhoea. The diagnosis can be established by cultures of synovial fluid, blood, skin lesions or from the genital tract but organisms are identified in joints in only 20% of cases. Penicillin, 1 mega unit, is given daily for 2 weeks. There is a dramatic improvement in 3–4 days.

Meningococcal infection can be associated with (1) an acute transient polyarthritis that is seen simultaneously with the characteristic petechial rash, (2) a purulent monoarthritis which usually occurs after 5 days or (3) a flitting polyarthralgia in patients with chronic meningococcaemia. Penicillin is the treatment of choice.

Brucellosis (p. 748) is associated with polyarthralgia or transient polyarthritis. Much more rarely there may be a septic arthritis or spondylitis. Destructive lesions in one or more contiguous vertebrae lead to severe pain, disc narrowing, marginal proliferation of osteophytes with early bony fusion of vertebrae. Chronic bursitis and osteomyelitis may also occur. Diagnosis is established by blood and synovial fluid cultures coupled with rising serological titres of antibodies. Treatment is given on page 748.

Tuberculosis of joints is usually secondary to an established focus in the lungs or kidneys. Since the eradication of bovine tuberculosis in Britain, articular infection is rarely seen except in malnourished, socially deprived, elderly or immigrant groups. In more than three-quarters of all cases a single large joint is affected. Joint pain, stiffness, swelling and restriction of movements are associated with anorexia, weight loss and night sweats.

In the early stages radiographs show only peri articular osteoporosis and soft tissue swelling. Later there is narrowing of the joint space, bony erosion and collapse of subchondral bone with little associated periosteal reaction. The tuberculin skin test is strongly positive and diagnosis can sometimes be made by direct bacteriological examination and culture of synovial fluid. In other cases synovial biopsy is required. After antibiotic control has been established (p. 230), synovectomy may be required in those with extensive disease.

Leprosy (p. 756) can have a number of osteo-articular manifestations. Joint deformities of the hands and feet occur commonly as a sequel to peripheral nerve involvement and these may be complicated by neuropathic (Charcot) joints. Osteomyelitis may complicate digital ulceration and hypersensitivity reactions may resemble rheumatoid arthritis.

Syphilitic arthritis is now very uncommon. *Congenital* syphilis may be associated with painful para-articular swelling due to epiphyseal involvement soon after birth or painless effusions of the knees (Clutton's joints) in adolescents. *Acquired* secondary syphilis may be associated with a migrating polyarthralgia resembling rheumatic fever and Charcot joints are a feature of tabes dorsalis.

Lyme arthritis is an intermittent pauciarticular inflammatory arthritis which is preceded by a characteristic rash (erythema chronicum migrans). It is a tick borne spirochaetal disease which was first described in Lyme, Connecticut and which may respond to penicillin. Lyme disease may also cause chronic meningitis.

Fungal infections are rare. Blastomycosis, histoplasmosis and sporotrichosis can be associated with destructive lesions of bones and joints. Histoplasmosis and coccidiomycosis may also be associated with erythema nodosum and a benign polyarthritis.

Viral infections are commonly associated with arthralgia and transient polyarthritis, as in some cases of hepatitis B, mumps, chickenpox, infectious mononucleosis, adenoviral, enteroviral, parvoviral and arboviral infections.

Rubella. Arthritis follows 1–7 days after the rash or 2–6 weeks after vaccination in 30–40% of adults. A symmetrical inflammatory polyarthritis may be associated with symptoms of carpal tunnel compression or tenosynovitis. Joint pain, stiffness and swelling, which may be severe, usually settle in 1–4 weeks but the condition may persist with intermittent arthralgia for some months. Posterior cervical lymphadenopathy and a high lymphocyte count in the synovial fluid may be helpful in diagnosis.

MISCELLANEOUS DISORDERS OF SYNOVIAL JOINTS

Acromegaly is associated with a symmetrical arthropathy in 50% of cases. The small joints of the hands, wrists and knees are particularly affected as is the spine. Hypertrophy of synovium and articular cartilage are characteristically associated with periosteal new bone formation, osteophytosis, 'tufting' of the terminal phalanges and premature osteoarthrosis and hypertrophic spondylosis.

Amyloidosis (p. 391) can be associated with carpal tunnel compression and a polyarthritis

Table 14.2 SLE. Immunological abnormalities detectable in the blood.

Antinuclear antibodies	Lymphocytotoxins
Anti-DNA-histone (and LE cells)	Depression of CH_{50} and C3 and C4
Anti-DNA (single strand)	Antibodies against erythrocytes, leucocytes and
Anti-DNA (double strand)	platelets
Anti-RNA	Biological false positive tests for syphilis
Anti-Sm (named after a patient)	Circulating anticoagulants (anticardiolipin
Anti-Ul-RNP	antibodies)
Anti Ro/SS-A	Anti-thyroid (and other organ specific
Anti-La/SS-B	autoantibodies)
Anti-MA	Rheumatoid factors
Anti-PCNA	Cryoglobulins
	Circulating immune complexes

superficially resembling rheumatoid arthritis. The synovium is infiltrated with amyloid protein and the diagnosis can be made by finding fragments of amyloid tissue in the synovial fluid.

Hyperlipidaemia (p. 489). Type II can be associated with a migratory polyarthritis, and widespread xanthomas with tendon deposits. Type IV can be associated with arthralgia and morning stiffness and also hyperuricaemia and gout.

Sarcoidosis. Erythema nodosum and hilar lymphadenopathy are frequently associated with a symmetrical non-destructive inflammatory arthritis especially affecting the knees, ankles and wrists. A more specific asymmetrical destructive arthritis affects similar joints especially in black people. Biopsy of the synovium in such cases shows evidence of noncaseating granulomas. Radiologically there may be 'punched out' cystic bone lesions and also 'cortical erosions' and joint destruction.

SYSTEMIC LUPUS ERYTHEMATOSUS (SLE)

This is a multisystem connective tissue disease characterised by the presence of numerous autoantibodies, circulating immune complexes and widespread immunologically determined tissue damage.

Epidemiology. SLE affects individuals throughout the world but occurs more frequently in the United States and the Far East. American blacks are particularly susceptible, with a prevalence as high as 1 in 250 among females. The increasing use of sensitive tests for antinuclear antibodies suggest that mild and incomplete cases

frequently occur. The onset is most commonly in the 2nd and 3rd decades, with a female/male ratio of 9:1. In children and the elderly the sex incidence is more equal.

Aetiology and pathogenesis. Although the cause of SLE remains obscure, current concepts suggest that this is a multifactorial disorder in which there is profound *disturbance of immune regulation.* A defect of suppressor T lymphocytes is associated with polyclonal B lymphocyte activation and the uncontrolled production of autoantibodies and immune complexes (Table 14.2).

Evidence for *genetic factors* in the aetiology of the disease includes: (1) its occurrence in monozygotic twin pairs; (2) a higher than expected prevalence of SLE, other connective tissue diseases, antinuclear antibodies and immune complexes in related family members; (3) inherited deficiency of isolated complement components, notably C2 in some patients; (4) increased prevalence of the histocompatibility antigens HLA-B8 and DR3.

Evidence for the influence of *environmental factors* includes: (1) the provocative effect of sunlight; (2) the induction of lupus erythematosus by drugs (p. 575); (3) the importance of oestrogens as determinants of disease expression. Exacerbations commonly occur in pregnancy and the puerperium and prevalence is increased in fertile women, those using oral contraceptives and men with Klinefelter's syndrome.

Clear evidence of *viral infection* exists in animal models of SLE but in humans the findings are inconclusive.

Immunologically-mediated tissue damage results from at least two different mechanisms in SLE:

1. Direct antibody-mediated cytotoxicity. Brain

damage and abortion may be a consequence of cytotoxicity by cold reactive antibodies which cross-react with neural and trophoblast tissues.

2. Immune complex (and complement) mediated. The renal and vascular lesions of SLE appear to be a consequence of deposition of circulating DNA-Anti-DNA and other complexes in tissues.

Clinical features. *Arthritis*, arthralgia and fever are the commonest presenting features. Unlike other types of inflammatory arthritis, symptoms may begin during pregnancy and there may be a past history of spontaneous abortions. The arthritis can be transient and migratory or a more persistent seronegative poly-arthritis. Chronic inflammatory arthritis and teno-synovitis may lead to deformities and contractures but erosive changes are very uncommon.

Skin lesions are seen in more than two-thirds of patients. In addition to the classical, photosensitive erythematous 'butterfly' rash across the face, there may be lesions of discoid lupus or a vasculitic rash. The last may present as purpura or peri-ungual erythema with 'chilblain-like' lesions or digital infarcts. Livedo reticularis and Raynaud's phenomenon are common while bullous eruptions and panniculitis ('lupus profundus') occur more rarely. Alopecia can be a useful diagnostic pointer and is seen in more than 50% of patients. Painful oral or nasopharyngeal ulcers are rather less common.

Cardiopulmonary features include pericarditis, myocarditis and endocarditis, pleurisy, fibrosing alveolitis and acute lupus pneumonitis as well as a 'shrinking lung syndrome' with progressive elevation of the diaphragms and linear scars from recurrent pulmonary infarction. Lung function tests reveal impairment of ventilation and diffusion in these and many patients without overt clinical or radiological evidence of pulmonary involvement. Verrucous (Libman-Sachs) endocarditis may be demonstrated by echocardiography.

Renal involvement (p. 390) carries the worst prognosis. It may result in the nephrotic syndrome and renal failure or it may be limited to insignificant proteinuria or the presence of red cells or casts.

Central nervous system involvement is seen in

up to half the patients. In the majority this is limited to mild psychiatric disturbance or epilepsy but in a few there may be severe depression, dementia, organic psychosis, cranial nerve lesions, hemiplegia, transverse myelitis, chorea, cerebellar ataxia or peripheral neuropathy. The more severe manifestations are associated with a poor prognosis.

Other manifestations. Gastrointestinal symptoms are frequent but non-specific. Abdominal pain can be due to peritonitis, perisplenitis, pancreatitis or vasculitis. Gastric or duodenal perforation may be complications of corticosteroid therapy; colonic or gall bladder perforations are more likely to be a consequence of necrotising arteritis. Lymphadenopathy is found in half the patients and a moderately enlarged spleen in 20–30%. Ocular findings include kerato-conjunctivitis sicca, episcleritis and retinal vasculitis and soft exudates.

Investigation. The ESR is usually raised in active disease but the C reactive protein rarely so in the absence of infection. Haematological findings may include a normocytic normochromic anaemia of chronic disease, a Coombs' positive haemolytic anaemia, leucopenia, thrombocytopenia and immunological abnormalities.

IMMUNOLOGICAL FINDINGS. (Table 14.2) *Antinuclear antibodies* (ANF) can be detected in the serum of more than 90% of patients but positive tests are often found in rheumatoid arthritis, juvenile chronic arthritis, Sjögren's syndrome, fibrosing alveolitis, progressive systemic sclerosis and other connective tissue diseases. Chronic liver disease, thyroiditis, Addison's disease, myasthenia gravis and leukaemia can all be associated with a positive ANF as can therapy with a variety of drugs. Positive tests in low titre have no clinical significance and are frequently found in normal elderly people. The *LE cell test* is less sensitive, very time consuming and hardly more specific.

Anti-DNA antibodies and immune complexes. Antibodies to undenatured double stranded DNA have much greater specificity but are present in the serum in significant amounts in only about half the patients at any one time. High levels of anti-DNA antibodies coupled with depressed total haemolytic complement (CH_{50}) activity and low

C3 and C4 complement components suggest that there is activation of the classical complement pathway by active immune complex disease (Fig. 2.6, p. 26). Further evidence for circulating immune complexes may be obtained by finding a cryoprecipitate or by using one of a number of tests for CIq binding. Tissue evidence for immune complex deposition comes from detection of complement components and immunoglobulins by immunofluorescence at the dermoepidermal junction of normal skin or in organ biopsies.

The lupus anticoagulant is an anticardiolipin antibody which is also responsible for false positive biological tests for syphilis. High titres of anticardiolipin antibodies are associated with thrombocytopenia, thrombotic manifestations and some cases of recurrent abortion.

Treatment. Acute and life threatening manifestations of SLE require systemic corticosteroid therapy, often initially in doses of 40–80 mg prednisolone or equivalent daily. 'Pulse' therapy with methylprednisolone (1 g i.v. on 3 successive days) is occasionally required in patients with proliferative glomerulonephritis and rapidly deteriorating renal function. With remission of disease careful attempts are made to withdraw steroids or maintain patients on very low doses or alternate day regimes of steroid therapy. Articular symptoms and less severe inflammatory manifestations should be managed with NSAID therapy wherever possible. Anti-malarials are particularly useful in the management of patients with troublesome skin and joint lesions and they can reduce the frequency of severe exacerbations of disease.

Immunosuppressive drugs (p. 31) are reserved for patients with severe diffuse proliferative glomerulonephritis who are not responding adequately to corticosteroids and for those requiring maintenance steroid doses so high as to cause severe side-effects. The combination of plasma exchange and immunosuppressive drug therapy may be useful in some patients with serious steroid resistant exacerbations.

Prognosis for life has improved dramatically over the last 30 years so that the 5-year survival should now be better than 90%. Much of this improvement is, however, attributable to the detection of milder cases as a result of the availability of the sensitive ANF test for diagnostic purposes. Patients with severe renal, neurological or pulmonary involvement are at greatest risk. Renal biopsy can provide a guide to prognosis (p. 391). Infection is an important cause of morbidity and mortality particularly in patients receiving high doses of corticosteroids and immunosuppressives. Pregnancy is not contraindicated provided the disease is in reasonable remission and renal, cardiac and cerebral functions are intact.

Chronic discoid lupus erythematosus is probably more common than SLE. The skin lesions are characterised by photosensitivity, erythema, scaling, follicular plugging and telangiectasia. In the majority of patients the disease is limited to the skin. ANF tests are positive but anti-DNA antibodies are not usually found and complement levels are normal. SLE may occasionally supervene.

Drug-induced lupus. Positive tests for antinuclear factor are frequently encountered in patients receiving procainamide, hydralazine, anti-convulsants, oral contraceptives and phenothiazines. Much more rarely a syndrome resembling SLE develops. Fever, polyarthritis, skin lesions, lymphadenopathy, serositis and pulmonary infiltrates are frequent, but renal disease and neurological manifestations are rare. Complement levels are usually normal and antibodies to double stranded DNA absent. Slow acetylators of hydralazine and those with the HLA-DR4 histocompatibility antigen appear to be particularly at risk. Remission usually follows drug withdrawal. Occasionally a short course of corticosteroids is required.

Mixed connective tissue disease is characterised by clinical features resembling systemic lupus erythematosus, progressive systemic sclerosis (see below) and polymyositis (p. 577) in association with very high titres of a circulating antinuclear antibody with specificity for a ribonuclease sensitive extractable nuclear antigen (ENA) identified as a nuclear ribonucleoprotein (nRNP).

Women are affected four times more commonly than men. The onset is usually in the 3rd or 4th decade but may be at any age. Raynaud's phenomenon with 'sausage' swelling of the fingers, skin changes resembling dermatomyositis or scleroderma and a mild inflammatory polyarthritis are typically associated with proximal muscle weakness and tenderness and abnormal oesophageal motility. Diffuse interstitial pulmonary fibrosis is not uncommon but cardiac, renal and central nervous system involvement are very rare. The ESR and muscle enzymes are usually moderately raised. The condition is further characterised by an excellent prognosis and a good response to low dosage steroid therapy.

PROGRESSIVE SYSTEMIC SCLEROSIS

This is a generalised disorder of connective tissue characterised by fibrosis and degenerative changes in the skin (scleroderma) and many internal organs. Although its aetiology is unknown, it is believed to be at one end of the spectrum of diffuse connective tissue diseases where immunologically determined inflammation is followed by intimal thickening of small blood vessels and excessive production and cross-linking of collagen. Persons with the HLA haplotype A1 B8 DR3 appear to be genetically predisposed, and there is evidence of vascular hypersensitivity to cold and serotonin. Systemic sclerosis is less common than SLE but is seen throughout the world. Women are affected four times more frequently than men.

Clinical features. The onset is most frequently in the 30–50 year age group. Severe Raynaud's phenomenon is usually the presenting complaint and may precede other features by months or years.

Skin changes. Initially there is often well demarcated non-pitting oedema and induration associated with 'sausage' swelling and restriction of movement of the fingers. Later the skin becomes shiny with atrophy and ulceration of the finger tips with or without associated calcinosis. The skin of the face, limbs and trunk is variably affected and there may be striking pigmentation and telangiectasia. As scleroderma advances, the face may become taut and 'mask-like' with 'beaking' of the nose and difficulty in opening the mouth. Tightening of skin over bony prominences results in flexion contractures and liability to trauma.

Musculo-skeletal manifestations include arthralgia and a mild non-erosive inflammatory arthritis often characterised by 'leathery' crepitus in affected tendon sheaths or joints. Muscle weakness and wasting result from both disuse atrophy and low-grade myositis.

The gastrointestinal tract is involved in the majority of cases. Reflux oesophagitis associated with a sliding hiatus hernia is a common problem and loss of oesophageal peristalsis on recumbent barium swallow examination is often detected even in the absence of dysphagia. Dilatation of segments of large and small bowel occur less frequently, causing intermittent abdominal pain, constipation, distension and obstruction; there may be diarrhoea and malabsorption secondary to bacterial overgrowth. Systemic sclerosis may be associated with primary biliary cirrhosis and with Sjögren's syndrome.

Pulmonary fibrosis occurs in the majority of patients. In many it is limited to a symptomless defect in gaseous diffusion. In others progressive fibrosis is accompanied by increasing dyspnoea on exertion, a restrictive pattern of impaired lung function and reticulation and 'honeycomb' changes in the lower zones on a chest radiograph. Pulmonary involvement can be complicated by pulmonary hypertension and right ventricular failure, or by alveolar cell or bronchiolar carcinoma. Aspiration pneumonia may be a consequence of oesophageal involvement.

Other manifestations. Cardiac involvement is usually secondary to systemic rather than pulmonary hypertension but pericarditis, cardiomyopathy, heart block and aortic valve lesions can also occur. Renal involvement may develop at any stage of the disease and is an important cause of morbidity and mortality. Cranial or peripheral nerve lesions occur rarely.

Investigation. The ANF is positive in about 50% of patients with a nucleolar or speckled staining pattern. Antibodies to single stranded RNA and to an extractable nuclear antigen (anti-Scl-70) occur in 20% and may be a marker for pulmonary involvement. Anti-DNA antibodies are not detected and complement levels are normal.

Related syndromes. *The CRST or CREST syndrome* comprises a subset of patients whose disease is limited to Calcinosis, Raynaud's phenomenon, oesophageal (Esophageal) involvement, Sclerodactyly and Telangiectasia. An antinuclear antibody with specificity for a component of the chromosomal centromere is present in the serum.

Morphoea and linear scleroderma are localised forms of disease limited to characteristic, well demarcated, lesions of the skin and subcutaneous connective tissues. Serological findings are similar to those of systemic sclerosis and very occasionally systemic features do occur.

Eosinophilic fasciitis is a scleroderma-like condition characterised by pain, swelling and tenderness of the hands, forearms and feet where induration of the skin and subcutaneous tissues is not associated with Raynaud's phenomenon or systemic sclerosis. Carpal tunnel compression may be an early feature and the onset frequently follows abnormal exercise. Eosinophilia and hyperglobulinaemia are characteristic and the diagnosis is confirmed by finding an inflammatory cell infiltrate with prominent eosinophils in association with marked fibrosis of the subcutaneous fascia. Eosinophilic fasciitis responds to corticosteroids but is usually self-limiting.

Pseudo-scleroderma. Other conditions which may give rise to induration or brawny oedema of the skin that must be considered in the differential diagnosis of scleroderma include scleredema, scleromyxoedema, amyloidosis and acromegaly.

Treatment. No form of drug therapy has been proved to be effective in arresting the course of systemic sclerosis. Corticosteroids may produce some symptomatic benefit in early cases where inflammatory oedema or associated myositis and/or arthritis are prominent features. Nifedipine (p. 166) and prostacyclin infusions may occasionally be helpful in patients with severe Raynaud's phenomenon.

Attention should be paid to protecting the limbs from cold, the urgent treatment of chest infections and therapy for cardiac, respiratory and renal failure. Articular symptoms should be managed with NSAID. Episodes of steatorrhoea often respond to a short course of a broad spectrum antibiotic.

The outlook appears to be worse in those with late onset disease, widespread skin involvement of the trunk and renal, cardiac or respiratory disease. The overall 5-year survival is about 70%.

POLYMYOSITIS AND DERMATOMYOSITIS

These are diffuse connective tissue disorders in which muscle weakness and inflammatory changes in muscle and skin are the predominant features. They are relatively rare but occur throughout the world in all races and at all ages. The aetiology is obscure but persons with HLA-B8/DR3 appear to be genetically predisposed.

Viral infection (overt or latent) may be one of the factors which may stimulate or precipitate the autoimmune process responsible for the disease. Skeletal muscle cells appear to be destroyed by sensitised lymphocytes.

Clinical features. It is possible to define the following four rather arbitrary subsets:

1. *Adult polymyositis* occurs three times more frequently in women than men. The onset is usually insidious in the 3rd to 5th decade. The patient may experience difficulty in climbing stairs or rising from a low chair and on examination there is weakness of the pelvic and shoulder girdle muscles. Sometimes the onset is more abrupt with rapid progression of muscular weakness. Involvement of pharyngeal, laryngeal and respiratory muscles can lead to dysphagia, dysphonia and respiratory failure within a few days. In the majority of cases progression is less rapid and profound. Spontaneous remissions are followed by some return of muscle strength but there may be atrophy, calcinosis and fibrosis in damaged muscles leading to flexion contractures. Muscle pain and tenderness are unusual except in very acute cases. Mild arthralgia or inflammatory arthritis, Raynaud's phenomenon and erythematous rashes on the elbows and knuckles are frequent associated features.

2. *Adult dermatomyositis* is also more common in women. Acute or subacute muscle weakness is accompanied by periorbital oedema and a characteristic purple 'heliotrope' rash on the upper eyelids. In addition, there may be a photosensitive, erythematous, scaling rash on the face, shoulders, upper arms and chest with red patches over knuckles, elbows and knees. Muscle pain, tenderness and weight loss are common as are arthralgia and mild inflammatory polyarthritis.

3. *Inflammatory myositis associated with malignancy* is less common than was previously thought.

It is seen only after the age of 40. The onset of symptoms is usually insidious and the clinical picture does not differ from that of typical polymyositis or dermatomyositis. The associated carcinoma may not become apparent for 2–3 years. Its resection is sometimes associated with remission of the myositis.

4. *Childhood dermatomyositis* most commonly affects children between the ages of 4 and 10. Muscle weakness is usually accompanied by the typical rash of dermatomyositis. Muscle atrophy, contractures and subcutaneous calcification may be widespread and severe. Recurrent abdominal pain due to vasculitis is also a feature.

Investigation. Serum aminotransferases, aldolase and creatine phosphokinase are usually raised and can be useful guides to the activity of the disease. Tests for rheumatoid factor and ANF are often positive and there may be antibodies to an extractable nuclear antigen (PM-I, Jo-1, Mi). Electromyography may show characteristic changes which can be very helpful in distinguishing polymyositis from peripheral neuropathy. Muscle biopsy shows necrosis and regeneration in association with an inflammatory cell infiltrate.

Treatment. Prednisolone in doses of 40–60 mg daily is used initially to induce a remission. Muscle enzyme levels may fall before clinical improvement is noted. The steroid dose is then gradually reduced whilst continuing to monitor muscle strength and serum enzyme levels. Doses of 10–15 mg prednisolone daily are often needed to maintain the remission. Immunosuppressive therapy is occasionally used when there is no response to corticosteroids. The use of splints and physiotherapy to prevent contractures should not be neglected. Prognosis is closely related to the presence or absence of associated malignancy and to the age of onset, being poorer in older patients.

ARTERITIS

Vasculitis which occurs as part of rheumatoid arthritis, systemic lupus erythematosus, progressive systemic sclerosis and childhood dermatomyositis has been described in the relevant sections.

Polyarteritis nodosa (p. 193), Takayasu's arteritis (p. 193) and cranial arteritis (p. 193) are diffuse-connective tissue disorders in which immunologically determined vasculitis is the cause of the pathological changes. Polymyalgia rheumatica is related to cranial arteritis.

Polymyalgia rheumatica

This is a relatively common condition in elderly Caucasians, especially women.

Clinical features. The onset is often abrupt with severe pain and stiffness in the neck, back, shoulders, upper arms and thighs, often worse in the morning. There may also be fever, weight loss and depression. Physical signs are usually limited to slight tenderness of the acromio-clavicular or sterno-clavicular joints. Occasionally there may be evidence of a mild inflammatory arthritis in a more peripheral joint. The muscles themselves usually show no evidence of tenderness or atrophy and examination of the peripheral arteries is usually normal. However, up to one-third of patients at some time develop symptoms of cranial arteritis (p. 193) and are at risk of blindness from arteritic involvement of a branch of the ophthalmic artery.

The ESR is markedly raised in the majority of cases and there may be a normochromic normocytic anaemia of chronic disease. Temporal artery biopsy shows evidence of giant cell arteritis in about 40% of cases but the true frequency of arteritis is probably much higher.

Treatment. The response to corticosteroid therapy is dramatic. The diagnosis must be reviewed if there is no striking remission of symptoms within 4–5 days of starting prednisolone 15 mg once daily. Two to three weeks after starting therapy the dose of prednisolone is gradually reduced over several weeks. Most patients can be maintained in remission with 5–7.5 mg prednisolone daily. High dosage corticosteroids are given initially to patients with cranial arteritis (p. 193).

The natural history is for remission to occur in 6 months to 2 years although relapses are not uncommon and occasional patients have a more prolonged chronic disease. The need for maintenance corticosteroids should be reviewed by an attempt at gradual steroid withdrawal every 6 months.

METABOLIC AND DEGENERATIVE DISEASES OF CONNECTIVE TISSUES AND JOINTS

CRYSTAL DEPOSITION DISEASES

Gout

Gout is not a single disease. The term is used to describe a number of disorders in which crystals of monosodium urate monohydrate derived from hyperuricaemic body fluids give rise to inflammatory arthritis, tenosynovitis, bursitis or cellulitis, tophaceous deposits, urolithiasis and renal disease. Hyperuricaemia is a necessary but not a sufficient prerequisite for clinical manifestations of gout.

Epidemiology. Gouty arthritis is predominantly a problem of post-pubertal males and is seldom seen in women before the menopause. Asymptomatic hyperuricaemia is 10 times more common. Serum uric acid concentrations are distributed in the community as a continuous variable and are determined by a number of demographic factors of which age, sex, body bulk and genetic constitution are the most important. Serum uric acid levels are higher in urban than in rural communities and are positively correlated with intelligence, social class, weight, haemoglobin, serum proteins and a high protein diet.

Hyperuricaemia is arbitrarily defined as a serum uric acid level greater than two standard deviations from the mean, i.e. above 0.42 mmol/l in adult males and 0.36 mmol/l in adult females (p. 814).

Aetiology of gout and hyperuricaemia. Various genetic and environmental factors lead to hyperuricaemia and gout by decreasing the excretion of uric acid and/or increasing its production (Table 14.3).

DIMINISHED RENAL EXCRETION OF URIC ACID is the problem in more than 75% of patients with gout. In most of these there appears to be an as yet undefined genetically determined defect in fractional urate excretion.

INCREASED PRODUCTION OF URIC ACID is at least partly responsible for hyperuricaemia in 20–25% of gout patients. In the absence of significant renal impairment such patients are hyperexcretors of uric acid. Specific enzyme defects resulting in an increase in *de novo* purine synthesis should be suspected: (1) in the absence of disorders resulting in increased turnover of purines (Table 14.3); (2) if gout develops at an unusually early age; (3) if there is a family history of gout commencing at an early age; (4) if uric acid lithiasis is the first presenting feature.

Deficiency of hypoxanthine-guanine-phosphoribosyl transferase (HGPRT). The Lesch-Nyhan syndrome is a rare X-linked recessive error of metabolism in which gout and severe over-production of uric acid are associated with choreoathetosis, spasticity, a variable degree of mental deficiency and compulsive self-mutilation. The enzyme defect can be detected in red cell lysates; female carriers can be identified from skin fibroblast cultures or hair root analysis and pre-natal detection can be undertaken using amniotic fluid cells. The elucidation of the mechanism whereby this deficit in a purine salvage enzyme leads to primary purine overproduction has been a key to

Table 14.3 Factors predisposing to hyperuricaemia and gout.

Diminished renal excretion of uric acid		*Increased production of uric acid*
Renal failure	Lactic acidosis:	*Increased turnover of purines:*
Drugs	Alcohol	Myeloproliferative disorders,
Diuretics	Exercise	e.g. polycythaemia vera
Pyrazinamide	Starvation	Lymphoproliferative disorders
Low doses aspirin	Vomiting	e.g. chronic lymphatic
Lead poisoning	Toxaemia of pregnancy	leukaemia
Hyperparathyroidism	Type 1 glycogen storage	Psoriasis—severe, exfoliative
Myxoedema	disease	*Increased purine synthesis de novo:*
Down's syndrome	Unidentified	HGPRT deficiency
	inherited defect	PRPP synthetase overactivity
		Glucose-6-phosphatase
		deficiency
		Idiopathic

the understanding of purine metabolism and the development of allopurinol in the prevention of gout.

Phosphoribosyl pyrophosphate (PRPP) synthetase overactivity. Severe gouty arthritis and uric acid lithiasis is seen from an early age in families with inborn errors of metabolism resulting in increased activity in this enzyme. The defect can be detected in red cell lysates.

Glucose-6-phosphatase deficiency. Children with glycogen storage disease type 1 (von Gierke's disease) who survive to adult life develop severe gout and hyperuricaemia as a consequence of impaired uric acid excretion secondary to lactic acidosis and also of increased purine synthesis *de novo*. The enzyme defect can be detected only in the liver, kidney or intestine.

Idiopathic. The enzyme defect(s) responsible for most cases of gout with increased synthesis of purine *de novo* remain to be discovered.

Clinical features. *Acute gout.* The metatarsophalangeal joint of a great toe is the site of the first attack of acute gouty arthritis in 70% of patients; the ankle, the knee, the small joints of the feet and hands, the wrist and elbow follow in decreasing order of frequency. The onset may be insidious or explosively sudden, often waking the patient from sleep. The affected joint is hot, red and swollen with shiny overlying skin and dilated veins; it is excruciatingly painful and tender. Very acute attacks may be accompanied by fever, leucocytosis and a raised ESR and are occasionally preceded by prodromal symptoms such as anorexia, nausea or a change in mood. If untreated, the attack lasts days or weeks but it eventually subsides spontaneously. Resolution of the acute attack may be accompanied by local pruritus and desquamation.

Some patients have only a single attack, or suffer another only after an interval of many months or years. More often there is a tendency to have recurrent attacks. These increase in frequency and duration so that eventually one attack may merge into another and the patient remains in a prolonged state of subacute gout. Acute attacks are occasionally polyarticular and tenosynovitis, bursitis or cellulitis may be the presenting feature.

Acute attacks may be precipitated by sudden rises in serum urate following dietary excess, alcohol, severe dietary restriction or diuretic drugs or by sudden falls following initiation of therapy with allopurinol or uricosuric drugs. Acute attacks may also be provoked by trauma, unusual physical exercise, surgery or severe systemic illness.

Chronic gout. First attacks of gouty arthritis are seldom associated with residual disability but recurrent acute attacks are followed by progressive cartilage and bone erosion in association with deposition of tophi and secondary degenerative changes. Severe functional impairment and gross joint deformities may occur in chronic tophaceous gout. Tophi are frequently found in the cartilage of the ear, bursae and tendon sheaths.

Urate urolithiasis occurs in about 10% of patients with gout attending British hospital clinics. The incidence is much higher in hot climates. The formation of urate calculi is also favoured by: (1) hyperuricosuria; (2) purine overproduction; (3) excessive purine ingestion; (4) uricosuric drugs and defects in tubular reabsorption of uric acid and (5) low urine pH, e.g. in chronic diarrhoeal diseases or following ileostomy.

Chronic urate nephropathy results from a combination of renal tubular obstruction, uric acid calculi, hypertension, glomerulosclerosis and secondary pyelonephritis. It is rare in the absence of well-established chronic gouty arthritis.

Other manifestations. Gout and hyperuricaemia are frequently associated with obesity, type IV hyperlipoproteinaemia, diabetes mellitus, hypertension and ischaemic heart disease. Hyperuricaemia itself does not, however, appear to be a risk factor for vascular disease or diabetes.

Investigation. The serum urate level is usually raised but it is important to realise that this does not prove the diagnosis as asymptomatic hyperuricaemia is very common. Whenever possible synovial fluid should be aspirated and examined under polarising light. Acute attacks of gout can occur when the serum urate level is normal. This is usually seen in patients who have received treatment with allopurinol, a uricosuric agent or NSAID with uricosuric side-effects such as azapropazone (p. 561).

Joint radiographs are seldom useful in establishing the diagnosis. Although they may show characteristic punched-out erosions associated with the soft tissue swelling of urate tophi, occasionally flecked with calcium, the diagnosis will be clinically apparent in such cases and in others the erosions are indistinguishable from those seen in other forms of inflammatory arthritis.

Treatment. NSAID are the agents of choice. It is important to start treatment as early as possible, to use adequate doses and to avoid salicylates and diuretics. Patients known to have gout should keep a supply of NSAID with which they are familiar so that an acute attack can be aborted as soon as the first symptoms are noticed. Indomethacin (50 mg), azapropazone (600 mg 6-hourly) or naproxen (250 mg t.i.d.) are given until the acute attack subsides. Treatment is then continued with lower doses for 7–10 days. Colchicine is highly effective but causes vomiting and diarrhoea in many patients in the doses that need to be used (1 mg stat followed by 0.5 mg 2-hourly).

Prevention. Prolonged administration of drugs which lower the serum urate level should be considered following the resolution of the acute attack in patients with: (1) recurrent acute attacks of gouty arthritis; (2) tophi or evidence of chronic gouty arthritis; (3) associated renal disease; (4) gout and markedly raised serum urate.

Allopurinol is the drug of choice for long-term prophylaxis because of its convenience and low incidence of side-effects. It lowers the serum urate by inhibiting xanthine oxidase which is responsible for the conversion of xanthine and hypoxanthine to uric acid. Treatment is commenced with 300 mg once daily together with colchicine 0.5 mg b.d. to avert the acute attacks of gouty arthritis which frequently follow initiation of hypouricaemic drug therapy. It is important not to commence treatment with allopurinol until several weeks have elapsed after the last acute attack and to continue concurrent administration of colchicine for several months. The dose of allopurinol may have to be adjusted in the range of 300–900 mg daily to bring the serum urate within the normal range. If renal function is impaired lower doses (100 mg daily) should be used.

Uricosuric agents can also be very effective in lowering the serum urate level, reducing the frequency of acute attacks of gout and decreasing the size of tophi. Probenecid 0.5–1 g b.d. or sulphinpyrazone 100 mg t.d.s. are given with colchicine 0.5 mg b.d. Salicylates must be avoided as they antagonise the uricosuric effects of these drugs. Uricosuric drug therapy is contraindicated: (1) in gout with overproduction of uric acid and gross uricosuria; (2) in patients with renal failure (ineffective); (3) in patients with urate urolithiasis.

Diet. There is no need for severe dietary restrictions but grossly excessive purine intake and overindulgence in alcohol should be avoided. Gradual weight loss is encouraged in obese patients and is associated with a fall in serum urate. Severe calorie restriction must be avoided as it causes lactic acidosis and a rise in serum urate.

Surgery is occasionally required to deal with a large or ulcerating tophus.

Asymptomatic hyperuricaemia does not require prophylactic treatment in the absence of a history, family history or clinical evidence of gout. A search should be made for causes of secondary hyperuricaemia (Table 14.3). Obese subjects should be encouraged to lose weight gradually and blood pressure and renal function should be monitored annually.

Chondrocalcinosis and pseudo-gout

Pyrophosphate arthropathy: calcium pyrophosphate dihydrate (CPPD) deposition

In this variety of crystal deposition disorder, calcium pyrophosphate dihydrate (CPPD) crystals are deposited in fibrous and articular cartilage where they are associated with degenerative changes. Shedding of crystals into the joint space provokes an acute attack of synovitis — 'pseudo-gout'. Autopsy and radiological surveys indicate that chondrocalcinosis is a common age related finding often unassociated with symptoms of articular disease. The menisci and articular cartilage of the knee are the commonest sites.

Aetiology. Chondrocalcinosis and pseudo-gout are clearly not a single disease. The majority of cases are sporadic and no underlying cause can be found. Genetic factors are important in some families. A variety of metabolic disorders clearly predispose to chondrocalcinosis, namely hyperparathyroidism, haemochromatosis, hypothyroidism, gout, hypomagnesaemia and hypophosphatasia. No common determinant, comparable to the hyperuricaemia of gout has been identified but pyrophosphate concentrations are increased in synovial fluids. This, coupled with the association with hypophosphatasia, has suggested that the disease may be a consequence of defective pyrophosphatase activity.

Clinical features. Pyrophosphate arthropathy can mimic many other conditions. Six clinical patterns of disease are described.

Type A: Pseudo-gout. As with gout the affected joint becomes suddenly painful, warm, swollen and tender. The knee is the site of more than half of all attacks, the duration of which can vary from a few days to four weeks. Subacute or 'petite' attacks are not uncommon and there may be polyarticular clustering of acute attacks. Men are affected more frequently than women.

Type B: Pseudo-rheumatoid arthritis. In a few patients there is a subacute inflammatory polyarthritis which may last for several months.

Type C: Pseudo-osteoarthrosis with superimposed acute attacks.

Type D: Pseudo-osteoarthrosis without acute attacks. Types C and D account for nearly half the patients. Women are more frequently affected. Prominent involvement of the wrists and MCP joints clearly distinguishes pseudo osteoarthrotic chondrocalcinosis from primary generalised osteoarthrosis.

Type E: Asymptomatic is the most common.

Type F: Pseudo-neuropathic. Severe destructive changes resembling those of Charcot joints can occur in the knee and shoulder in the absence of any neurological defect.

Investigation. Radiographs show CPPD in articular cartilage, the menisci of the knees, the labrum of the acetabulum and glenoid cavity, the triangular cartilage of the wrist and the symphysis pubis. Examination of synovial fluid under polarising light microscopy allows CPPD crystals to be distinguished from monosodium urate crystals. X-ray diffraction techniques differentiate CPPD from calcium phosphate and calcium hydroxyapatite seen in synovial fluid in degenerative joint disease.

Treatment. Joint aspiration and intra-articular injection of corticosteroids are the most effective means for treating acute attacks of pseudogout. Colchicine and NSAID are less effective than in classical gout.

OSTEOARTHROSIS

Osteoarthrosis (OA, osteoarthritis, arthrosis or degenerative joint disease) is not a single disease. Rather it is the end-result of a variety of patterns of joint failure. To a greater or lesser extent it is always characterised by both degeneration of articular cartilage and simultaneous proliferation of new bone, cartilage and connective tissue. The proliferative response results in some degree of remodelling of the joint contour. Inflammatory changes in the synovium are usually minor and secondary.

Epidemiology. Radiological and autopsy surveys show a steady rise in degenerative changes in joints from the age of 30. By the age of 65, 80% of people have radiographic evidence of osteoarthrosis although only 25% may have symptoms. Males and females are both affected but OA is more generalised and more severe in older women. Geographical surveys show differences in both the prevalence of OA and the pattern of joint involvement. OA of the hips is much more frequent in Caucasians than in blacks or Chinese. Cold, damp climates are associated with more symptoms but not with greater radiological prevalence.

Aetiology and pathogenesis. OA is classified as primary if the aetiology is unknown and secondary when degenerative joint changes occur in response to a recognisable local or systemic factor (Table 14.4). Developmental abnormalities are believed to be of major importance in the aetiology of OA of the hip in the vast majority of cases. Abnormal surface contacts and weight bearing alignments lead to increased local mechanical stress and wear. Post-traumatic malalignment and incongruity of joints are well established as important predisposing causes of premature OA.

Metabolic diseases lead to degeneration of cartilage by very different mechanisms. In alkaptonuria (ochronosis) the genetically determined defect of homogentisic acid oxidase results in the accumulation of a pigmented polymer that binds to collagen

Table 14.4 Causes of secondary osteoarthrosis.

Developmental	Perthes' disease, slipped capital femoral epiphysis, epiphysiolysis, hip dysplasia, epiphysial dysplasias, intra-articular acetabular labrum
Traumatic	Intra-articular fracture, meniscectomy, occupational, e.g. elbows of pneumatic drill workers, hypermobility, e.g. Ehlers-Danlos syndrome, long leg arthropathy
Metabolic	Alkaptonuria (ochronosis), haemochromatosis, Wilson's disease, chondrocalcinosis
Endocrine	Acromegaly
Inflammatory	Rheumatoid arthritis, gout, septic arthritis, haemophilia
Aseptic necrosis	Corticosteroids, sickle-cell disease, caisson disease, SLE and other collagenoses
Neuropathic	Tabes dorsalis, syringomyelia, diabetes mellitus, peripheral nerve lesions
Miscellaneous	Paget's disease, Gaucher's disease

of cartilage, rendering it brittle and prone to mechanical degradation. There may be other inborn errors of metabolism where unknown colourless metabolites may induce changes in the biochemical composition of cartilagenous matrix in a similar way and so predispose to OA. Crystal deposition of calcium pyrophosphate dihydrate or hydroxyapatite may alter the properties of cartilage matrix directly and low-grade crystal inflammation may play a part in pathogenesis.

It is uncertain whether the degenerative joint disease seen in acromegaly (p. 429) is a consequence of joint incongruity following cartilage overgrowth or whether the endocrine disturbance results in a mechanically defective matrix. Paget's disease, Gaucher's disease and the various diseases associated with aseptic necrosis result in pathological changes in subchondral bone with consequent altered stresses on the overlying articular cartilage.

Current concepts of the pathogenesis of OA are based on the assumption that whatever the provoking cause, the final pathway of changes in articular cartilage will be identical. Two mechanical hypotheses merit consideration. The first suggests that the initiating event is fatigue fracture of the collagen fibre network. This is followed by increased hydration of the articular cartilage with unravelling of the proteoglycans and loss of proteoglycans into the synovial fluid. There is some tentative evidence of augmented neutral protease and collagenase activity but collagen may be lost simply as a result of mechanical attrition.

The alternative hypothesis suggests that the initial lesions are microfractures of the subchondral bone following repetitive loading. Healing of the microfracture leads to significant loss of resilience of the subchondral bone which in turn creates a shear stress gradient in the adjacent articular cartilage. As the process evolves, the cartilage surface becomes fibrillated and deep clefts appear with reduplication and proliferation of chondrocytes within them. Simultaneous proliferative changes commence at the joint margins with formation of osteophytes. Eventually articular cartilage is lost altogether in areas of maximum mechanical stress and the underlying bone becomes hardened and eburnated. Cysts may form but bony ankylosis does not occur.

Clinical features. The joints most frequently involved are those of the spine, hips and knees. In the majority of patients the disease is confined to one or only a few joints. The symptoms are gradual in onset. Pain is at first intermittent and aching. It is provoked by use of the joint and relieved by rest. As the disease progresses, movement in the affected joint becomes increasingly limited, initially as a result of pain and muscular spasm, but later because of capsular fibrosis, osteophyte formation and remodelling of bone. There may be repeated effusions into joints especially after minor twists or injuries. Crepitus may be felt or even heard. Associated muscle wasting is an important factor in the progress of the disease, as in the absence of normal muscular control the joint becomes more prone to injury. Pain arises from trabecular microfractures, traumatic lesions in the capsule and periarticular tissues, and a low grade synovitis. Nocturnal aching may be attributable to hyperaemia of the subchondral bone.

Nodal osteoarthrosis is a clinically distinct form of primary generalised OA which occurs predominantly in middle-aged women. Characteristically it affects the terminal IP joints of the fingers with the development of gelatinous cysts or bony outgrowths on the dorsal aspect of these joints (Heberden's nodes). The onset is sometimes acute with considerable pain, swelling and inflammation. Although these lesions may be associated with a good deal of deformity they seldom cause disability. Similar lesions may affect the proximal IP joints and the disorder also frequently involves the carpometacarpal joints of the thumbs, the spinal apophyseal joints, the hips and knees. A strong family history of Heberden's nodes is usual in such cases and though the existence of multigeneration families with the disorder appears to suggest a single autosomal dominant gene, careful family studies reveal polygenic inheritance in both nodal and non-nodal primary generalised osteoarthrosis. Patients with nodal primary generalised osteoarthrosis are probably also more susceptible to secondary OA, again emphasising the multifactorial aetiology of this disorder.

Investigation. The blood count and ESR are characteristically normal in osteoarthrosis. Synovial fluid is viscous and has a low cell count. Apatite crystals can be detected on rare occasions. Radiographs show loss of joint space and formation of marginal osteophytes. Subchondral bone sclerosis, bony remodelling and cyst formation are seen in more advanced cases.

Treatment. Although the pathological changes of osteoarthrosis are irreversible much can be done to alleviate symptoms particularly in the early stages. Periods of rest and avoidance of undue trauma and physical stress to affected joints are essential. This may involve such measures as the fitting of rubber heels to reduce jarring and minimise the risk of slipping, the provision of built-up shoes to equalise leg lengths, weight loss in obese patients with OA of the knee or hip and the provision of a suitable walking stick. Occasionally patients may have to be advised to change their occupation, transfer to lighter work or give up unduly strenuous hobbies.

NSAID can be used to relieve pain and stiffness but are often disappointingly ineffective in osteoarthrosis.

Occasional intra-articular or periarticular corticosteroid injections can be very helpful especially in the knee. Hydrotherapy may be useful for patients with OA of the hip associated with pain and muscle spasm. Hip or knee arthroplasty may be necessary in advanced cases (p. 564). Arthrodesis is occasionally considered if the knee is the only joint involved.

MISCELLANEOUS LESIONS OF CONNECTIVE TISSUE

General aspects. Musculo-skeletal aches and pains are extremely common and become more frequent with increasing age. More than one-third of all 'rheumatic' complaints cannot be attributed to defined diseases of the spine, peripheral joints or connective tissues. Many are trivial, self-limiting and cause little disability. Others can be more troublesome. The neck, shoulder girdle, back and gluteal regions are the common sites for many of these complaints. Muscular spasm of reflex origin is a prominent feature and must be differentiated from limitation of movement due to structural damage. Absence of signs of systemic illness and a normal ESR will help to distinguish these *regional rheumatic disorders* from the inflammatory connective tissue diseases.

Certain factors may be of importance in precipitating attacks in susceptible individuals. Exposure to cold and damp has always been suspected as a cause of nonarticular 'rheumatic' complaints. Unaccustomed physical effort, undue fatigue, minor injuries and poor posture have also been incriminated. Any reduction in muscular efficiency will render an individual more prone to sprains of tendons, ligaments and extra-articular soft tissue structures. Loss of resilience and elasticity of the intervertebral discs can occur long before radiological evidence of disc degeneration becomes apparent and the interfacetal joints of the spine may be more exposed to strains and sprains.

Pain arising from such deep structures is poorly located and referred diffusely to the overlying skin. Pain may be referred from the cervical intervertebral joints to the occipital region, shoulder girdle and arm. 'Lumbago' and 'sciatic pain' (p. 660) without signs of root pressure may be caused by minor disc injury. More often they appear to be associated with acute or chronic 'sprain syndromes'. Although poor posture, flabby muscles and obesity may be predisposing causes, occupational factors may be of great importance. Absence from work due to 'rheumatic' complaints is much higher among miners, dockers and foundry workers than it is among clerks or employees in light industry. Up to 10% of the population may have abnormally lax joints and ligaments without the stigmata of inherited connective tissue disorders such as the Marfan or Ehlers-Danlos syndrome. Such persons are particularly prone to recurrent sprains, dislocations and arthralgia—

the '*hypermobility syndrome*'.

Diffuse muscular pain and stiffness is common in certain infections, particularly of viral origin, such as influenza, rubella and measles. Localised pain occurs in epidemic myalgia (Bornholm disease p. 261). Many anxious and depressed people complain of aches and pains, particularly in the region of the neck, shoulders or lower back.

Specific lesions. *Shoulder pain* is frequently a consequence of extra-articular traumatic, degenerative or inflammatory lesions of the capsule or 'rotator cuff' of tendons. *Supraspinatus tendinitis* is characterised by a 'painful arc' on arm abduction which can be abolished by external rotation. There is localised tenderness over the greater tuberosity of the humerus and a radiograph may show calcification in the supraspinatus tendon. Rupture of calcific material into the subacromial bursa occasionally results in acutely painful 'gout-like' attacks of inflammatory *subacromial bursitis*. Fluid aspirated from the bursa beneath the acromion contains crystals of calcium hydroxyapatite. Local injection of hydrocortisone is used to give symptomatic relief. *Bicipital tendinitis* can be recognised by pain and tenderness over the bicipital groove aggravated by resisted flexion of the elbow.

'*Frozen shoulder*' is the name given to a common and disabling condition in which severe spontaneous shoulder pain is associated initially with capsular tenderness and painful restriction of all shoulder movements and later with painless restriction of movements alone. A frozen shoulder may be a late consequence of a rotator cuff lesion and sometimes follows myocardial infarction, hemiplegia, herpes zoster, breast or thoracic surgery. Treatment is with analgesics and local corticosteroid injection in the early phase and mobilising exercises after the pain has resolved. The natural history is for slow but complete recovery, the complete cycle sometimes taking as long as two years.

In the *shoulder-hand syndrome* restricted shoulder movements are associated with a painful swollen hand. The condition is characterised by burning pain, vasomotor changes and severe limitation of movements of the hand. A radiograph of the hand shows patchy osteoporosis after some weeks or months. It may be a sequel to the same disorders that precede a frozen shoulder but epilepsy, barbiturates and antituberculous drugs can also be predisposing factors. Not infrequently these patients have an hysterical personality. Treatment is aimed at mobilising the affected limb. Analgesics, a short course of systemic corticosteroids, sympathetic nerve block and physiotherapy each have their advocates in this difficult situation. The prognosis for complete recovery is less certain than in frozen shoulder.

'*Tennis elbow*' appears to follow partial tears of the origin of the extensor muscles at the lateral epicondyle. Local tenderness and pain on active wrist extension are characteristic. '*Golfer's elbow*' results from similar lesions in the origin of the common flexor tendon at the medial epicondyle. Local corticosteroid injections relieve both conditions.

DISEASES OF BONE

PHYSIOLOGY

Bone is a specialised form of metabolically active, mineralised, connective tissue. It consists of cells of monocyte-macrophage origin (bone forming osteoblasts, bone resorbing osteoclasts, resting osteocytes) and an organic matrix of type I collagen, proteoglycan and some bone specific glycoproteins. The skeleton contains more than 99% of the body calcium in the form of a crystalline calcium phosphate complex (hydroxyapatite). The tubular mid-sections of long bones (diaphyses), which make up 80% of the skeletal mass, are composed of circumferential lamellae of compact, cortical bone consisting of longitudinally orientated osteons surrounding central Haversian canals which carry the capillaries. Extracellular fluid reaches the bone osteocytes by a radial system of canaliculi and there are lateral vascular communications with the periosteal vessels through Volkmann's canals. The distal ends of the long bones (metaphyses), the vertebrae and the flat bones are composed of more loosely packed cancellous bone. Although it accounts for only 20% of the skeletal mass, the trabecular surface area of this cancellous bone is as large as that of compact bone, rendering it relatively more susceptible to metabolic diseases. From the physiological point of view it is important to realise that bone is bounded by a number of distinct cellular surfaces—the endosteal, periosteal, Haversian and trabecular envelopes.

In the growing phase of infancy and childhood the size and shape of bones changes rapidly as part of the modelling process. The marrow cavity and outer cortex expand due to endosteal resorption and periosteal accretion of bone and bone turnover may be as high as 200% per annum. Following skeletal maturity this is reduced to less than 5% but the rate of endosteal resorption is reduced less than that of periosteal accretion. Thus while the outer diameter of normal older bones is greater than that of younger ones, the cortex is progressively thinned with advancing years. Deformities and short stature may be a consequence of diseases interfering with the modelling process during the growing period. Examples include metabolic diseases such as rickets, inflammatory diseases such as polyarticular juvenile chronic arthritis, and bone dysplasias such as osteopetrosis.

Modern methods of bone histomorphometry, in which iliac biopsies are taken following double tetracycline labelling, have revealed a second form of bone turnover or remodelling. This occurs throughout life and accounts for more than 95% of turnover in the mature skeleton. Remodelling occurs in 'programmed packages'; the sequence of cellular events is invariably one of activation followed by a period of osteoclastic resorption and then a period of osteoblastic formation along the freshly resorbed trabecular surface. The whole sequence is completed in 4–6 months in healthy adults. Trauma and hyperthyroidism are two of the numerous factors that can activate the remodelling process, while oestrogens suppress it. Fluoride uncouples the remodelling sequence and stimulates osteoblastic activity.

Increased turnover of bone, whatever the cause, is associated with a rise in the plasma alkaline phosphatase and an increase in the urinary excretion of hydroxyproline and the bone specific glycoprotein, osteocalcin.

CLASSIFICATION OF DISEASES OF BONE

1. Infections.
2. Metabolic and endocrine diseases:

   a. Rickets and osteomalacia (p. 64),
   b. Nutritional deficiency, e.g. of calcium,
   c. Osteoporosis (p. 67),
     (i) Post-menopausal,
     (ii) Associated with endocrine disease, e.g. in hypogonadism, hyperthyroidism, Cushing's syndrome and hypopituitarism,
     (iii) Iatrogenic, e.g. corticosteroid therapy,
     (iv) Chronic wasting diseases, e.g. rheumatoid arthritis or malignancy,
     (v) Hereditary diseases, e.g. osteogenesis imperfecta (p. 10),
     (vi) Idiopathic juvenile osteoporosis.
   d. Hyperparathyroidism (p. 445).
3. Paget's disease.
4. Disorders of collagen, e.g. Marfan's syndrome (p. 192).
5. Mucopolysaccharidoses, e.g. Hurler syndrome (p. 15) and Hunter's syndrome (p. 15).
6. Skeletal dysplasias.
7. Neoplastic disease:
   Primary, benign or malignant.
   Secondary malignant.

Infections, Paget's disease, neoplasia and skeletal dysplasias are discussed in this chapter and other diseases of bone where indicated by the page references.

INFECTIONS

Osteomyelitis is most commonly encountered in children under the age of 12. The onset is abrupt with fever, malaise and severe pain at the site of bone infection. When this is close to a joint there may be a 'sympathetic' effusion and diagnostic confusion with septic arthritis. Isotope scanning and careful delineation of the site of bone tenderness can be helpful in establishing the correct diagnosis but radiographic changes do not occur for some days or weeks.

Staphylococci are the most frequent organisms responsible and in about half the cases haematogenous spread has occurred from a boil or superficial infection. Hypogammaglobulinaemia, malnutrition or debilitating illness may all be predisposing factors. Salmonella can also cause osteomyelitis and this infection is a common complication of sickle-cell anaemia (p. 514).

An antibiotic, e.g. sodium fusidate (p. 44) must be commenced after taking blood for culture as soon as the diagnosis is suspected, and continued in adequate doses for long enough to eliminate the infection. Delay in starting treatment or inadequate therapy may result in chronic indolent bone infection (*Brodie's abscess*) with sequestrum formation. Surgical exploration and decompression are required if there is not an immediate response to antibiotics.

Tuberculous osteomyelitis has become much less common in Britain since the elimination of bovine tuberculosis but there is some evidence of a recent increase in the elderly population and immigrant communities. In 50% of cases the spine is affected. Typically the infection starts at the margins of vertebral bodies with subsequent invasion of the disc space. Destruction of bone leads to angular kyphosis. A paravertebral 'cold' abscess may form and track to the thigh, chest wall or neck. The hip, knee, ankle or wrist joint may be affected by spread from adjacent bone. Tuberculous dactylitis and sacroiliitis are unusual but characteristic lesions. The treatment of tuberculosis is described on pages 230 to 233.

PAGET'S DISEASE (OSTEITIS DEFORMANS)

This disease which is characterised by softening, enlargement and bowing of bones is uncommon before the age of 40 years but increasingly frequent thereafter. There is increased flow through affected bones with resorption followed by excessive osteoblastic bone formation resulting in a high rate of bone turnover, raised levels of plasma alkaline phosphatase and increased urinary excretion of hydroxyproline. This activity is reflected in abnormal isotope bone scans and radiological evidence of localised bone enlargement, altered trabecular pattern and alternating areas of rarefaction and increased density. Recent evidence suggests that Paget's disease may be associated with a paramyxovirus infection of osteoclasts.

Clinical features. Men are more commonly affected and there may be a family history of the disease. Often the condition is symptomless and detected only when radiological examination is made for some other reason. In others there is pain of a deep aching character often aggravated by weight bearing. The pelvis, femur, tibia, lumbar spine and skull are common sites of bone involvement. The increased vascularity may cause warmth of the affected part on palpation; rarely widespread arteriovenous shunting causes high output cardiac failure. Enlargement and deformity of bones develops when the condition is advanced. Bowing of the femur and tibia is characteristic and Paget's disease may predispose to secondary osteoarthrosis of the hip. Fractures may occur spontaneously or after minor trauma but they usually heal normally. Skull involvement may result in headache, progressive enlargement of the cranium and deafness from compression of the auditory nerves. Paraplegia can follow vertebral involvement. Osteogenic sarcoma is an uncommon late complication. The serum calcium and phosphate are usually normal with high levels of alkaline phosphatase and increased hydroxyproline excretion during phases of active disease.

Treatment. Calcitonin (p. 445) is used for severe bone pain not controlled by analgesics. Subcutaneous injection of 100 MRC units of salmon calcitonin three times weekly can be continued for 6 months and recommenced if pain recurs. Mithramycin and diphosphonates, which reduce bone turnover, are less satisfactory alternatives.

Confinement to bed may be followed by rapid mobilisation of calcium with hypercalcaemia, hypercalciuria and formation of renal calculi. Such patients should be given a high fluid intake and measures must be taken to lower the serum calcium if it becomes dangerously high. Pain due to secondary degenerative joint disease is treated with NSAID. Hip arthroplasty is occasionally required. Osteogenic sarcoma is treated with early surgery but has a poor prognosis.

NEOPLASTIC DISEASE

Malignant neoplasms of bone can cause diffuse skeletal aches and pains that are not infrequently dismissed as being 'rheumatic'.

Metastases from carcinomas of the bronchus,

breast or prostate, are the commonest tumours of bone. Secondary deposits from most primary tumours appear typically as osteolytic areas on radiological examination and are frequently associated with a rise in serum alkaline phosphatase. Only prostatic metastases are commonly osteosclerotic and associated with a rise in serum acid phosphatase. Metastatic deposits can often be localised by skeletal isotope scans before radiological changes are apparent and widespread bone metastases can occur even in the absence of symptoms. A number of malignancies are hormone dependent and useful remissions can sometimes be obtained following hypophysectomy or administration of androgens to patients with metastatic breast cancer, or dienoestrol to those with prostatic metastases (p. 414). Local radiotherapy and cytotoxic chemotherapy can occasionally be helpful in symptomatic management.

Multiple myeloma (p. 538) may also present with skeletal aches and pains associated with 'punched-out' osteolytic lesions on radiological examination. Unlike metastatic carcinoma these deposits usually fail to take up bone seeking isotopes and the serum alkaline phosphatase is normal.

Primary bone tumours are less common. Ivory *osteomas* are benign tumours which occur most frequently in the vault of the skull and are not usually associated with symptoms. Cancellous osteomas (osteochondromas or exostoses) are slender out-growths of bone which arise from the metaphyses of long bones or from the flat bones of the pelvis and scapulae. They may give rise to pressure symptoms and most frequently present during adolescence. Diaphyseal aclasis (multiple exostosis) is a rarer disorder inherited as an autosomal dominant and seen in younger children.

Primary osteosarcomas occur most frequently in the lower end of the femur, the upper end of the tibia or the upper end of the humerus. These are tumours of young people rarely seen after the age of 20. Swelling with or without vague aching are the presenting symptoms and the bone may be tender and warm. Radiographs show a characteristic increase in radiolucency associated with bone expansion, triangular areas of new bone formation at the periosteal margin and a 'sun-ray' appearance due to new bone formation. Early blood-borne metastases to the lungs are common and the 5-year survival is less than 10% despite treatment with radiotherapy and amputation.

Fibrosarcomas are of two types. Endosteal fibrosarcomas arise within bones and give rise to destructive lesions as they grow out. They metastasise to both the local lymph nodes and the lungs and are associated with a poor prognosis despite treatment with radiotherapy or amputation. In contrast periosteal fibrosarcomas seldom invade bone or metastasise to distant sites. Treatment is with local excision, repeated in the event of recurrence.

Benign chondromas arise from cartilage within the long bones or small bones of the fingers. Multiple enchondromatosis is an unusual disorder of childhood in which multiple chondromas give rise to unsightly swellings attached to bones. Malignant change is very rare in chondromas.

Chondrosarcomas occur in the long bones, pelvis or scapulae of adults. Pain and swelling are the presenting features and bone radiographs show only loss of bone density associated with some speckled calcification. Amputation is the treatment of choice and the 5-year survival is better than 50%.

Ewing's tumour is a highly malignant bone neoplasm which affects children between the ages of 5 and 15. It probably arises from the marrow endothelium and has characteristic radiographic features. Areas of osteolytic bone destruction are surrounded by layers of periosteal new bone formation giving the lesions an 'onion skin' appearance. Pain, swelling and tenderness may be associated with fever and leucocytosis so that these tumours can easily be mistaken for osteomyelitis. The 5-year survival is virtually nil despite radiotherapy and amputation.

Giant cell tumours of bone may be benign or malignant. They usually occur in young adults and present with pain and swelling of a long bone in the neighbourhood of a joint. Radiographs show a typically eccentric tumour with a 'soap-bubble' appearance. With local excision the prognosis is relatively good even for malignant tumours.

Osteoid osteoma is a rare cause of severe bone pain which is characteristically worse at night and relieved by NSAID. The condition occurs between the ages of 10 and 30 in any bone except the skull. There may be warmth, swelling and tenderness on palpation and radiographs show some increase in sclerosis with a characteristic area of translucency surrounding a central nidus. Excision of the nidus cures the symptoms and these lesions do not recur.

SKELETAL DYSPLASIA

The skeletal dysplasias form a large and heterogeneous group of conditions which cause bone and joint deformity. Those with predominant epiphyseal involvement such as multiple epiphyseal dysplasia may be associated with premature osteoarthrosis. Those with predominant metaphyseal involvement such as achondroplasia are associated with short-limbed dwarfism (p. 432). There are disorders such as osteogenesis imperfecta, idiopathic juvenile osteoporosis and the hereditary osteolyses in which decreased bone density, fractures and bone loss are prominent features and others, such as osteopetrosis and sclerosteosis where increased bone density occurs.

Skeletal abnormalities are prominent in a number of hereditary disorders of connective tissue such as the Marfan syndrome or neurofibromatosis as well as in inborn errors of metabolism such as the mucolipidoses, and homocystinuria. The reader is referred to Fairbank and McKusick's books (p. 590) for details of all these groups of conditions.

PROSPECTS IN RHEUMATOLOGY

There have been no dramatic 'breakthroughs' in the understanding or treatment of the rheumatic diseases since the 14th edition of this textbook was published in 1984.

Nevertheless, our knowledge of the genetic, cellular and biochemical basis for regulation of immune responses is progressing apace with the widespread application of molecular biological probes and monoclonal antibodies. Parallel progress has been made in understanding the biochemical basis of receptor activation, intercellular co-operation and the complex networks of immunological and inflammatory mediators, as well as the organisation and regulation of the macromolecules of bone and cartilage.

Hopes that a new 'generation' of safe and effective anti-inflammatory drugs would emerge have proved to be premature, but research on inhibitors of the leukotriene pathways and selective prostaglandin inhibitors continues. Small advances have been made in understanding the mode of action of gold salts, antimalarials, penicillamine and the immunomodulating drugs, all of which have been shown to have significant practical value in slowing the progress of inflammatory joint diseases such as rheumatoid arthritis, but there is still a very real need for similar 'disease remitting' drugs with less formidable toxicity. Some progress in this direction has come from the use of a new oral gold compound and the rediscovery that sulphasalazine is an effective disease-modifying antirheumatic agent.

Advances in diagnostic immunological tests continue to improve the definition of subsets of patients with diffuse connective tissue disorders. For example there is the identification of the lupus anticoagulant and its association with thrombotic disease and fetal loss. The identification of the Jo-1 antigen as histidyl-tRNA and its association with myositis and interstitial lung disease have begun to lead to new approaches to the understanding and treatment of subsets of patients with SLE and polymyositis. Continuing progress can be anticipated in the diagnosis, treatment and prognosis of these systemic rheumatic diseases.

Overall, the outlook for patients with rheumatic diseases has substantially improved over the last 30 years. In particular, the remarkable developments in prosthetic surgery have transformed the lives of patients with advanced and crippling rheumatoid arthritis and osteoarthrosis of the hip. Continuing collaboration between bioengineers and orthopaedic surgeons is gradually overcoming the technical problems involved in developing suitable prostheses for severely damaged knees, elbows, ankles, shoulders and hands, so that some practical advances can be expected. Progress along these lines is, however, likely to be progress with diminishing returns. In many ways, the anatomy of the hip joint makes it uniquely suitable for total joint replacement; a similar degree of success is unlikely in other joints. Already waiting lists for hip arthroplasty are many years in length, and it is calculated that Britain would require one new 300-bedded hospital annually just to cope with this single operation. As numbers of patients with replaced joints increases, so do the problems of loosening and infection of prostheses, particularly in those with multiple joint replacement. Future efforts must clearly be directed towards preventing and curing, or at least controlling these disorders rather than simply improving salvage surgery.

GEORGE NUKI

FURTHER READING:

Scott J H S 1986 In: Macleod J, Munro J (eds) Clinical examination, 7th edn. Churchill Livingstone, Edinburgh. Gives an account of the examination of the locomotor system

Scott J T 1986 Copeman's Textbook of the rheumatic diseases, 6th edn. Churchill Livingstone, Edinburgh. Standard British textbook. Excellent and comprehensive source of information on all aspects of clinical rheumatology

Kelley W N, Harris E D Jr, Ruddy S, Sledge C B (eds) 1985 Textbook of rheumatology. Saunders, Philadelphia. Major international textbook with comprehensive basic science and clinical coverage

Dieppe P A, Docherty M, Macfarlane D G, Maddison P J 1985 Rheumatological medicine. Churchill Livingstone, Edinburgh. Concise British text book

Hughes G R V 1986 Connective tissue diseases, 3rd edn. Blackwell Scientific Publications, Oxford. Concise clinical monograph on the diffuse connective tissue diseases. Includes information on clinical applications of immunological tests

Panayi G S 1982 Scientific basis of rheumatology. Churchill Livingstone, Edinburgh. Sixteen comprehensive reviews covering genetics, immunology, inflammation, connective tissue degradation, mechanism of drug action and the biomechanical basis of joint actions and replacement

Hart F D 1982 Drug treatment of the rheumatic diseases, 2nd edn. ADIS Press, Sydney. Multi-author monograph covering all aspects of clinical pharmacology and therapeutics

Lawrence J S 1971 Rheumatism in populations. Heinemann, London. Source book of information on epidemiology of rheumatic diseases

Emmerson B T 1983 Hyperuricaemia and gout in clinical practice. ADIS Press, Sydney

Nuki G 1980 The aetiopathogenesis of osteoarthrosis. Pitman Medical, London. Research reviews

Hadler N H 1984 Medical management of the regional musculoskeletal diseases. Grune and Stratton, New York

Wynne-Davis R, Fairbank T G 1976 Fairbank's Atlas of general affections of the skeleton, 2nd edn. Churchill Livingstone, Edinburgh. Concise and beautifully illustrated introduction to skeletal dysplasias and other general disorders of bone

McKusick V A 1979 Heritable disorders of connective tissue, 5th edn. Mosby, St Louis. Classical monograph

15

Diseases of the nervous system

The approach to patients presenting neurological problems must follow a logical course starting with the history and followed by the physical examination. The latter reveals neurological signs which reflect disordered neural function. The nature and distribution of these signs depend on the anatomical localisation of lesions within the central nervous system. It is a fundamental error to relate particular signs to specific pathological processes. Paralysis of one side of the body, hemiplegia, may equally well arise from a stroke or from a cerebral tumour since both lesions may similarly interrupt motor pathways. It is the history of the neurological illness which indicates the nature of the pathological process involved. A careful chronological assessment of the way in which a neurological disability has developed is essential if a diagnosis is to be made. Attention to the symptoms and signs which indicate loss of function of particular parts of the nervous system then follows for purposes of localisation.

Lesions which suddenly affect the nervous system, cause maximal disability within a few hours and after a static period of days or weeks then show a tendency to improve are usually due to vascular disturbances and sometimes to trauma. Disabilities of insidious onset and slow but inexorable progression are often due to degenerative disorders or to tumours of the central nervous system. A remittent history, wherein episodes of disability are followed by periods of improvement, with later recurrence of symptoms elsewhere in the nervous system, is characteristic of multiple sclerosis. Inflammatory lesions such as infections often develop rapidly, but less acutely than trau-

matic or vascular catastrophes and the recovery phase is also usually rapid. Some conditions are characterised by paroxysmal short-lived disorders of function, followed by rapid and complete recovery. A history of this type may be due to epilepsy or migraine or to transient ischaemic attacks.

These general principles are a useful guide but atypical presentations occur. Sometimes a neoplasm may produce very rapid deterioration and occasionally repetitive, minor vascular lesions give rise to a progressive, 'step-wise' deterioration of function.

Some diseases cause systematised affection of cells or fibres of similar type; these conditions, of which motor neurone disease is a good example, usually result in bilateral and symmetrical dysfunction. Tumours produce progressive involvement of adjacent neural structures causing clinical disabilities which may later be accompanied by symptoms resulting from the occupation of space by the tumour within the confines of the skull or the spinal canal.

A neurological diagnosis is achieved by the integration of all the information gained from the patient's history, the general medical examination and the neurological examination.

ANATOMY AND PHYSIOLOGY

The motor system

Movements, whether voluntary or involuntary, are the result of the contraction or controlled relaxation of groups of muscles and never of only a single muscle. They are effected by contraction of muscles which act as prime movers and reciprocal relaxation of their antagonists. The action of the prime movers is provided with a firm base by contraction of synergists which stabilise the joints, and by appropriate adjustments of posture. The postural adjustments are largely under the control of the extrapyramidal motor system and the vestibular and spinal reflexes.

Voluntary movements require the participation of the precentral gyrus of the cerebral cortex ('motor area') and the timing and degree of contraction or relaxation of the muscles of the synergy are co-ordinated by the cerebellum, especially when a movement involves more than one segment of a limb.

The activities of the upper motor neurones from the motor area of the cortex, the extrapyramidal motor system and the cerebellum influence, directly or indirectly, the cells of the anterior horn of spinal grey matter or motor cranial nuclei from each of which a lower neurone runs to a group of muscle fibres. Thus the lower motor neurone is the 'final common path' for all efferent impulses directed at the muscle and the groups of anterior

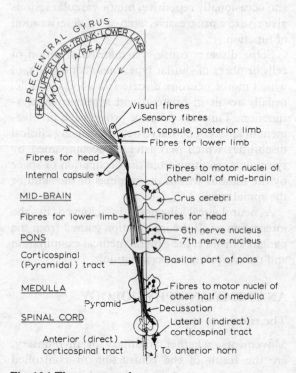

Fig. 15.1 The motor pathways.

horn cells may be considered to 'represent a muscle' in the same sense as the cells of the motor cortex 'represent a movement'. This distinction is vital to an understanding of the signs and disorders of the motor system.

Upper motor neurone. The fibres arise from the cells in the precentral gyrus ('motor area'). These initiate movements of different parts of the opposite side of the body, the parts being represented in the following order from below upwards — tongue, face, hand, forearm, arm, trunk, thigh, leg, foot and perineal areas with considerable overlap. The cortical area representing movements of each of these parts is proportional to its functional importance rather than to its anatomical size. The projections of the upper motor neurones through the corticospinal (pyramidal) tracts to the contralateral motor nuclei of the brain stem and anterior horn of the spinal cord are shown in Figure 15.1.

A destructive lesion of the lateral corticospinal tract above its decussation causes a loss of some voluntary movements of part of the opposite side of the body, according to the fibres involved. In the upper limb, shoulder abduction, elbow, wrist and finger extension and the small hand muscles tend to be more severely affected; in the lower limb, hip and knee flexion and dorsiflexion of the foot bear the brunt. Automatic associated movements, such as the stretching of a paralysed arm when yawning, may persist and other voluntary or reflex movements using the same lower motor neurones and muscles may be preserved. This is the essential difference between paralysis of upper motor neurone type and that due to a lower motor neurone lesion.

For the same reason stretch reflexes (p. 598) are retained but these are usually of heightened activity. This indicates that the corticospinal tract normally carries fibres which are inhibitory to the stretch reflex. The pattern of cutaneous protective reflexes also changes, causing the emergence of an extensor plantar reflex.

There are thus two types of disturbance, a negative one due to loss of a particular activity, and a positive one due to the release of lower levels from control. This is a principle of general application in the nervous system and the concept is important in understanding the signs of upper motor neurone disease. Another type of positive symptom results from irritative lesions (usually incomplete damage to a nerve cell or its fibre) which causes spontaneous activity of the affected neurones. Spontaneous activity in upper motor neurones causes involuntary movements as in focal epilepsy (p. 617).

SIGNS OF A LESION OF THE UPPER MOTOR NEURONE are:

1. Weakness or paralysis of movements of part of one side of the body.

2. Increase of tone of spastic type. This is characterised by an increased resistance to passive movement, which is maximal at the beginning of movement, smoothly sustained, and suddenly lapses as passive movement is continued ('clasp-knife' response). It occurs predominantly in flexor muscles in upper limbs and extensor muscles in the lower limbs (the antigravity muscles).

3. Increase in amplitude of tendon reflexes: clonus may be present.

4. Loss of the abdominal reflexes.

5. An extensor plantar response (Babinski reflex).

6. No muscle atrophy apart from slight wasting which may occur as a result of disuse.

7. Normal electrical excitability of the involved muscles (p. 608).

These signs occur with disease involving any part of the upper motor neurone, but the exact level at which the lesion lies may be determined by the upper level of increased reflexes and by associated features.

Cortex. Localised paralyses affecting, for example, one limb only, are characteristic of lesions at the cortical level. The upper motor neurones are spread over a wide area in the precentral gyrus and only very large lesions could cause a hemiplegia. There may be associated evidence of cortical dysfunction such as dysphasia and focal epileptic fits sometimes occur.

Internal capsule. As the fibres here are closely packed, a hemiplegia is likely. There may be hemihypoaesthesia and hemianopia from damage to adjacent sensory and visual fibres respectively.

Brain stem. Lesions here are rarely confined to the corticospinal tract. One presentation comprises affection of one or more cranial nerves on the side of the lesion and signs of an upper motor neurone lesion on the opposite side.

Spinal cord. The corticospinal tracts may be affected bilaterally. The level of the lesion in the cord is often delineated by accompanying lower motor neurone signs, sensory disturbance or loss of tendon reflexes.

Lower motor neurone. Axons emerge from the nuclei of the motor cranial nerves and from the cells of the anterior horns of the spinal cord. They pass through the anterior nerve roots to enter a mixed peripheral nerve in which they run to the muscles which they supply. Each lower motor neurone axon has terminal branching so that it is distributed to the motor end-plates of a group of muscle fibres. The anterior horn cell, the axon and a group of muscle fibres comprise the motor-unit and each muscle contains a large number of such units.

The anterior horn cell is activated by impulses from the corticospinal tracts, from the extrapyramidal tracts, and from some afferent fibres of the posterior nerve root responsible for spinal reflexes. The lower motor neurone is thus an integral part of the spinal reflex arc and is the final common pathway for all motor impulses, involuntary or voluntary, directed to a muscle.

Normal nutrition of a muscle appears to depend on its contact with the spinal cord through the lower motor neurone since, if it is interrupted, the muscle rapidly wastes.

SIGNS OF A LESION OF THE LOWER MOTOR NEURONE. The following signs will be present only in those muscles supplied by the particular neurones affected:

1. Weakness or paralysis of muscles. This affects all movements in which they take part whether as prime movers or synergists, voluntary or involuntary, or in reflex contractions.

2. Loss of tone on passive movement (flaccidity).

3. Wasting of the affected muscles which appears within 2 or 3 weeks of an acute lesion (atrophy).

4. Absence of reflexes subserved by the affected neurones. Abdominal and plantar reflexes remain normal unless the neurones to the appropriate muscles are damaged and then these reflexes cannot be elicited.

5. Single muscle fibres contract spontaneously when they are no longer influenced by their

associated lower motor neurone. This phenomenon, called fibrillation, is detectable by electromyography but is invisible through the skin. Lower motor neurones which are damaged but still able to conduct impulses may give rise to spontaneous contractions of bundles of fibres in the muscles supplied. Such contractions of motor units (fasciculation) may be visible, e.g. in motor neurone disease.

6. Contractures of muscles develop due to replacement of fibrous tissue and 'trophic' changes such as dryness and cyanosis of the skin, and brittleness of the nails appear partly due to impaired circulation.

7. The electrical excitability of the peripheral nerves and muscles is altered. These tests may be combined with electromyography to confirm that a weak and wasted muscle is denervated. Lesions of peripheral nerves short of complete interruption may cause slowing of conduction.

If lower motor neurones are damaged in the cord or nerve roots the muscles and reflexes affected in the ways described above will be those supplied by one or more segments of the spinal cord. If the neurones are damaged more peripherally after they have been redistributed in the nerve plexuses, the paralysis will occur in the territory supplied by the appropriate peripheral nerve and it is probable that there will be similar damage to sensory fibres with which the motor fibres are associated in the mixed nerve.

Extrapyramidal system. This is a complex neuronal network, extending from the cortex to the medulla, from which emerge descending spinal pathways and cortical connections whose influence initiates and modifies motor activity. Interspersed in this latticework of fibres are areas of grey matter. Some of these are only loose aggregations of nuclei in the reticular formation of the brain stem, but there are also several well defined nuclear masses called the basal nuclei (ganglia), which include the caudate nucleus, the lentiform nucleus (globus pallidus and putamen), the substantia nigra and the subthalamic nucleus.

There are rich interconnections between the constituents of the basal nuclei and thence via the ventrolateral nucleus of the thalamus to the extrapyramidal areas of the cortex and to the medullary reticular formation. The normal functions of the extrapyramidal system are ill-understood, but appear to be important for initiating voluntary movements and adjusting posture.

SIGNS OF AN EXTRAPYRAMIDAL LESION. *Disturbance of voluntary movements*. There is not true paralysis in extrapyramidal disease, but rather slowness of movement and poverty of movement in that spontaneous gestures, changes in facial expression, and associated movements for postural adjustment, such as swinging the arm when walking, are lost on the side opposite to the lesion.

Disturbance of tone. Tone may be increased as in parkinsonism or decreased as in chorea. Increase in tone, extrapyramidal type, has characteristic features. It is present throughout the whole range of passive movement; it affects opposing muscle groups equally; it may be smooth and plastic ('lead-pipe rigidity') or intermittent ('cogwheel rigidity') which is more common.

Involuntary movements. There are many varieties, notably the tremor of parkinsonism (p. 648), choreiform movements (p. 652) and athetosis (p. 652).

Cerebellum. This is the most important part of the nervous system for the co-ordination of movement and the muscular contractions required to maintain posture.

The cerebellum receives impulses from many sources — principally the proprioceptive end-organs, the skin, the vestibular nuclei and the cerebral cortex. The pontine nuclei and the inferior olive relay fibres from the cerebral motor cortex and basal nuclei respectively to the cerebellar cortex of the opposite side. The cerebellar cortex integrates this information about body posture, limb position and motor intention and sends efferent fibres via the cerebellar nuclei to the reticular formation, red nucleus and vestibular nucleus of the opposite side, whence fibres descend to influence motor cells in the anterior horns of the spinal cord; as these descending fibres cross again each cerebellar hemisphere controls the ipsilateral side of the body. Efferent fibres from the cerebellum also ascend to the contralateral thalamus through which the cerebral cortex is influenced. The cerebellum is thus a great co-ordinating centre controlling the synergistic action of muscles during voluntary and automatic movements as well as adjusting posture.

SIGNS OF A CEREBELLAR LESION. The effects of disease of the cerebellum are best seen in acute lesions, for in chronic conditions considerable compensation occurs so that the deficit is less than might be expected. A lesion of the cerebellar hemisphere produces all its effects on the ipsilateral side of the body. The principal signs are:

Hypotonia. The muscles show diminished resistance to passive movement and, when an outstretched limb is suddenly displaced, it makes a greater excursion than usual and oscillates before resuming its posture.

Disturbance of tendon reflexes. The reflexes are diminished or pendular as when the knee jerk is followed by a series of diminishing oscillations.

Disturbance of posture and of gait. The head may be tilted towards the side of the lesion and the patient leans or may even fall towards that side. The gait is reeling and broad-based with a tendency to stagger to the side of the lesion.

Disorders of movement. Inco-ordination, hypotonia and the fact that muscular contraction is unregulated by the muscle spindles causes ataxia which manifests itself in different ways:

1. Dysmetria. Movements are not accurately adjusted to their object, so that the finger may overshoot or fall short of the object it is required to touch. If a movement is attempted with the eyes closed the finger overshoots towards the side of the cerebellar lesion ('past-pointing').

2. Dyssynergia. Movements which involve more than one joint are broken up into their component parts. When severe this leads to a decomposition of movement which resembles the jerky movements of a marionette.

3. Intention tremor. A combination of dyssynergia and dysmetria causes faulty correction of the badly directed limb movement so that it approaches the target in a zig-zag manner. The coarse irregular tremor increases as the target is approached. It is not more marked when the eyes are closed. The contraction of muscles necessary to maintain a posture may be similarly affected so that tremor at rest occasionally occurs in cerebellar disorders.

4. Dysdiadochokinesis. The arrest of one movement and its immediate replacement with the opposite movement requires accurate co-ordination of the various muscles of the synergy. Rapidly alternating movements are therefore disturbed and carried out in a clumsy, irregular, jerky fashion.

5. Rebound phenomenon. For the same reason a strong contraction cannot be arrested when resistance is suddenly removed, whereupon the limb shoots beyond the normal range.

6. Disorders of articulation and phonation. Articulation is irregular, slurred and explosive as the volume of sound is poorly controlled. A rarer form of dysarthria is 'scanning-speech' in which the syllables tend to be separated from each other.

7. Disturbance of eye movement. Jerking nystagmus in the horizontal plane is commonly seen. It is a defect of postural fixation involving conjugate gaze (p. 610). In a unilateral cerebellar lesion the movements are greater in amplitude and slower in rate when the eyes are deviated to the side of the lesion.

The sensory system

Superficial sensation which arises from the skin has four primary components, touch, pain, warmth and cold. *Deep sensations* arising from subcutaneous structures are deep pain, pressure and proprioception which enables the recognition of movements of joints and the position of the parts of the body relative to one another. Vibration is a sensation due to rhythmical stimulation of groups of deep and superficial touch receptors.

Some of the afferent impulses carried in 'sensory' nerve fibres do not reach consciousness but convey impulses directly or indirectly to motor neurones for reflex functions or to the cerebellum for purposes of co-ordination, e.g. many impulses from muscle and tendon receptors.

All sensory impulses arise in the sensory receptors or end-organs which are widely distributed throughout the body. It is probable, though debatable, that specialised receptors respond to specific types of stimuli. Stimulation of an end-organ causes impulses to pass along the first sensory neurone to the spinal cord. This neurone has its cell body in a dorsal root ganglion but does not synapse until it reaches a second order neurone in the spinal cord or brain stem.

On entering the cord by the posterior nerve root, fibres subserving proprioception, vibration

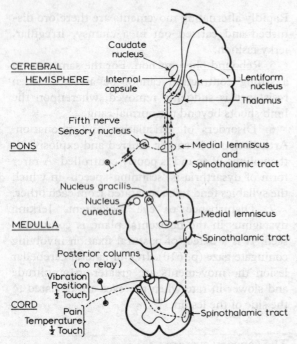

Fig. 15.2 The sensory pathways.

and a proportion of touch sensation turn medially and ascend in the posterior column of the same side to the lower part of the medulla oblongata to synapse with cells in the gracile and cuneate nuclei (Fig. 15.2). From there, the second order neurone crosses to the other side of the medulla and ascends in the medial lemniscus to the main sensory nucleus of the thalamus.

Fibres subserving pain, warmth, cold and the remainder of touch sensation synapse in the posterior horn of the spinal cord soon after entering it. Most of the second order neurones cross at the same level, or one or two segments higher, to reach the anterolateral column where they ascend to the thalamus as the spinothalamic tract. Some of these fibres do not cross but enter the ipsilateral spinothalamic tract.

As it ascends through the brain stem the tract gradually intermingles with the medial lemniscus and terminates along with it in the main sensory nucleus of the thalamus. Third order neurones, maintaining their functional specificity, are then relayed from the thalamus to the sensory area of the cortex which is situated in the postcentral gyrus.

Areas of the sensory cortex representing the different parts of the body are arranged in a similar manner to the motor cortex. Some appreciation of sensation is possible at the thalamic level but the cortical projection is necessary to allow discrimination of the intensity and pattern of stimulation. From the postcentral gyrus further connections are made with other parts of the cortex, particularly in the parietal lobe where the information derived from superficial and deep sensation is integrated so that judgement of the size, shape, weight, texture and pattern of objects is possible. This sensory information is also integrated with information derived from the special senses to provide a mental picture of the body (body image).

This synthesis is mainly carried out in the nondominant (right) parietal lobe. The corresponding part of the left cerebral hemisphere is important for other mental functions in which recurrent patterns of stimulation achieve the status of symbols and so are used for the receptive and interpretative aspects of speech functions. For this reason it is usually called the dominant or major hemisphere (in some left-handed people speech is mainly represented in the right hemisphere). This important part of the parietal lobe is connected with the lower part of the motor cortex of the same side so that patterns of lip, tongue, respiratory and finger movements may be used to convert ideas into motor symbols, the motor side of speech. An understanding of the link between symbol and meaning requires a knowledge of the physiological basis of the mind which we do not have at present.

Most of the afferent signals entering the central nervous system never reach consciousness. Some are used for spinal reflexes and make contact directly or through interneurones with motor neurones. Other fibres which originate in muscle receptors end at the base of the posterior horn in contact with second order neurones. These neurones turn laterally to the periphery of the cord to ascend in the anterior and posterior spinocerebellar tracts to the cerebellar cortex. Most of these ascend without crossing but some second order neurones cross to the opposite anterior spinocerebellar tract. These fibres carry some of the proprioceptive information required to enable the cerebellum to co-ordinate limb movements.

Still other sensory fibres, which do not carry 'sensation' in the ordinary sense, are extremely important for the maintenance of consciousness. These are collateral branches of the main spinothalamic pathways and of the special sensory tracts which turn medially into the upper part of the reticular formation in the midbrain. Here there is a chain of short neurones with intimate interconnections which also receives neurones from most parts of the cerebral cortex. It is therefore an important integrating centre. At its upper end it communicates with the non-specific nuclei of the thalamus which relay impulses to all areas of the cortex. Activity in this system is considered to be essential for the conscious state and may be important in some mental functions in collaboration with the cerebral cortex.

Disease of the sensory system may be accompanied by positive phenomena such as pain or paraesthesiae due to spontaneous activity or irritation of sensory neurones, or by negative phenomena in which there is loss of the ability to appreciate some modality of sensation (anaesthesia and analgesia). These symptoms occur only with disorders of the first or second order neurones, i.e. from the end-organs to the thalamus.

Suprathalamic lesions show certain differences. Paraesthesiae may occur with irritative lesions of the sensory cortex but anaesthesia does not. Instead there is a loss of sensory discrimination and of spatial and quantitative aspects of sensation.

SIGNS OF SENSORY LESIONS. *Peripheral nerve.* With a complete lesion all forms of sensation are lost in the area supplied by the affected nerve, but the zone of anaesthesia may be limited by the fact that neighbouring nerves overlap into its territory, the extent varying from person to person. The resistance of different types of fibres to disease need not be the same so that it is common for one type of cutaneous or deep sensation to be more affected than another and indeed some may be spared. If the afferent fibres of a reflex arc are affected, as for instance in the sciatic nerve in the ankle jerk, the reflex concerned is lost.

Some neuropathies do not affect individual nerves but rather damage fibres selectively. As a general rule the longest fibres are most susceptible and so the sensory and motor disturbance is first

noticed at the tips of all the toes and fingers, irrespective of nerve supply, and spreads proximally as the advancing disease involves progressively shorter fibres. This produces a 'glove and stocking' distribution of sensory loss.

Posterior root. The different forms of sensation are affected by a posterior root lesion in the same way as for a peripheral nerve but the distribution of the loss follows a dermatomal pattern. The overlap from adjacent roots may be so great that no anaesthesia can be detected. When the root is irritated, pain and paraesthesiae are experienced in the full dermatomal distribution of the root; pain may also be experienced in the deep structures such as muscles and ligaments which are supplied by the root. These structures do not necessarily underlie the dermatome. Any reflex subserved by the involved root is also lost, e.g. the ankle jerk where the S1 posterior root is damaged by a prolapsed intervertebral disc.

Posterior column. A lesion confined to the posterior column of the spinal cord will cause loss of position and vibration sense on the same side, but the sensations of pain, touch, warmth and cold will be preserved (Fig. 15.3).

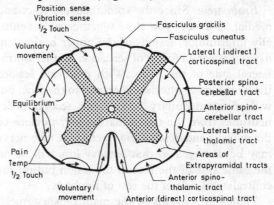

Fig. 15.3 Cross-section of spinal cord.

The loss of the sense of position causes sensory ataxia since the patient is unable to control movements by awareness of the position achieved at each instant. Sensory ataxia differs from cerebellar ataxia in that it is more marked when the eyes are closed, because vision can compensate to a certain extent for loss of proprioceptive information. Thus there is unsteadiness in the finger-nose test which is greater when the eyes are closed but without the marked tremor of cerebellar ataxia. The gait is ataxic and the patient walks with a broad base to provide a firmer foundation and steps high to make sure that the feet clear the ground which cannot be felt with certainty. If the eyes are closed it is not possible to stand with the feet close together without swaying (Romberg's test). Vibration sense is abolished below the level of the lesion ipsilaterally.

The same symptoms will be found if the first order neurones of the proprioceptive nerve fibres are damaged peripherally but they will then be associated with other signs of peripheral nerve disease.

Spinothalamic tract. Lesions of the anterior and lateral spinothalamic tracts in the anterolateral columns of the cord or their continuation through the brain stem cause impairment of the ability to appreciate pain, warmth and cold on the contralateral side of the body below the level of the lesion. Touch is usually modified (it feels 'different') but not abolished because of its alternative pathway in the posterior columns. This is the situation produced by the operation of anterolateral cordotomy for the relief of intractable pain.

Brain stem. Since the spinothalamic tract and medial lemniscus run close together and eventually intermingle, lesions of the upper brain stem usually affect all forms of sensation on the contralateral side of the body. With midbrain lesions the hemihypoaesthesia will extend to the face, but with pontomedullary lesions the second order neurones from the trigeminal sensory nucleus or the nucleus and descending tract of the fifth nerve may be damaged so that sensory loss will be on the same side of the face as the lesion but on the contralateral side of the rest of the body.

Thalamus. Lesions of the main sensory nuclei in the lateral part of the thalamus may cause spontaneous pain of most unpleasant quality in the opposite side of the body. The threshold for pain is raised on the opposite side of the body but when it is exceeded the resulting pain is exquisite and has the same unpleasant quality which often causes considerable emotional reaction.

Loss of other modalities of sensation occurs on the opposite side of the body.

Sensory cortex. Lesions above the thalamus do not abolish any form of sensation though the threshold may be raised. There is impairment of position sense, of two-point discrimination, of the ability to localise touch and to recognise objects in the palm of the hand (astereognosis) since shape and texture cannot be identified though the patient is able to feel the object.

Disturbance of the spatial aspects of sensation is greatest when the parietal lobe is involved, and especially in lesions of the 'minor' hemisphere this may cause disturbance of the body image and of spatial orientation. For instance the patient may be unable to recognise part of the body on the side opposite to the lesion or may feel that it is distorted. One side of external space or of the body may be ignored and this is most evident if the unaffected side of the body, or visual field, is stimulated simultaneously. When presented with this 'perceptual rivalry' the brain 'ignores' the stimulus on the side contralateral to the affected parietal lobe ('sensory inattention') though a stimulus applied to that part alone would be recognised immediately.

Lesions of the dominant hemisphere in the region where parietal, temporal and occipital lobes meet (angular and supramarginal gyri) are associated with receptive dysphasia (p. 601). This is a special case of the failure to analyse the temporal and spatial aspects of sensory stimuli.

The reflexes

Certain functions are economically catered for by the nervous system by means of reflexes, which are short chains of neurones (the reflex arc) connecting a receptor to an effector organ such as muscle or gland, so that an appropriate stimulus invariably leads to a specific response. The quantity but not the nature of the response may be modified by other stimuli or by supraspinal influences from the cortex, extrapyramidal system or the cerebellum.

There are two main categories of reflex — postural and protective. The appropriate stimuli for postural reflexes are muscle stretch and vestibular impulses. Protective reflexes are evoked by stimuli to pain receptors. They are usually superficial (cutaneous or corneal); the protective 'spasm' of muscles around a painful lesion is similar in nature.

Tendon (stretch) reflexes. A basic postural reflex depends on the stimulation of muscle spindles when a skeletal muscle is stretched. The afferent fibre enters the cord by a posterior nerve root and communicates directly or via a chain of interneurones with the anterior horn cells which control the stretched muscle, thus causing it to contract and so resist the displacement. A sudden tap to a tendon results in a sharp but brief contraction of the muscle. This activity may be increased by certain manoeuvres such as clenching the teeth or pulling the interlocked hands apart. This is termed *reinforcement* of the reflex and tendon jerk should not be declared absent until reinforcement has failed to make it visible.

The stretch reflex is inhibited by receptors in the tendon if muscle tension rises too high, thus risking the integrity of its fibres. This may happen when the reflex is exaggerated by withdrawal of a normal inhibitor effect of the corticospinal tract so that the contraction is abruptly stopped. This is the mechanism of the 'clasp-knife' response.

There are also supraspinal facilitatory and inhibitory influences from the extrapyramidal system and cerebellum so lesions of these systems may abolish the reflexes.

An example of a monosynaptic stretch reflex is a knee jerk. A tap on the patellar tendon activates stretch receptors in the quadriceps muscle giving rise to impulses in first order sensory neurones which pass directly to the lower motor neurones to the quadriceps muscle making it contract. A lesion anywhere along this path will cause loss of the reflex; hence it is important in the localisation of disease to know through which spinal segment each reflex passes.

The common tendon reflexes are the brachioradialis (C 5–6), the biceps (C 5–6), the triceps (C 7), the knee (L 3–4) and the ankle (S 1).

Superficial reflexes. These are polysynaptic reflexes originating from stimuli to superficial structures. The interneurones may connect with motor neurones at several segmental levels and so the response may be a co-ordinated movement, usually designed to withdraw the stimulated part from a potentially dangerous stimulus.

There are very many of these reflexes, some of which are conflicting. For example, stimulation of the sole of the foot evokes both flexion and extension reflexes. Which reflex will predominate is determined by higher influences. The nature of this influence is unknown but is believed to require the corticospinal (pyramidal) tract and damage to this tract will cause a change in the predominant reflex pattern.

PLANTAR REFLEX. When the outer border of the sole of the foot is stroked in normal people after infancy, there is plantar flexion of the great toe. In 1896 Babinski pointed out that when the upper motor neurone was damaged the same stimulus caused dorsiflexion of the toe. (Anatomically this is described as an extensor plantar response though physiologically it is part of the flexion withdrawal reflex.)

When the reflex is well developed it can be elicited from the medial side of the sole of the foot or even from the lower part of the leg and the hallux response is accompanied by dorsiflexion and abduction or fanning of the other toes and even withdrawal of the limb.

The fundamental importance of the extensor plantar or Babinski response as a sign of loss of function of the upper motor neurone is widely accepted but it may occur in transient form during temporary states such as coma or after an epileptic fit and need not indicate permanent damage. It is often extensor in normal infants during the first year of life.

ABDOMINAL REFLEXES. When the skin on one side of the abdomen is stroked with an orangestick, there is a reflex contraction of the underlying muscles, a reflex for protection of the viscera. This may be lost on the affected side in disease of the upper motor neurone though the sign is less reliable than the plantar reflex. For instance the abdominal reflexes may be lost early in multiple sclerosis yet retained despite severe pyramidal tract damage in motor neurone disease. These reflexes may not be obtained on either side in elderly, obese or multiparous patients and may be lost where operative incisions have severed the nerves concerned. The abdominal reflexes are served in their peripheral course by the intercostal nerves arising from segments T 8 to 12.

CORNEAL REFLEX. A light touch on the cornea provokes a blink of the eyelids on both sides. The afferent path for this reflex is the first division of the trigeminal nerve and the efferent path is the facial nerve. Loss of both corneal reflexes is a valuable indication of a deepening level of unconsciousness from any cause but should be elicited with discretion to avoid accidental damage to the cornea.

Nervous control of the bladder and rectum

Bladder. The nerve supply to the bladder is derived from three sources:

1. Sympathetic, from the first and second lumbar segments via the inferior hypogastric plexus and hypogastric nerves, which relax the bladder wall and contract the sphincters.

2. Parasympathetic, from segments S 2, 3, 4 via the pelvic nerves (nervi erigentes) which contract the bladder wall and relax the internal sphincter.

3. Somatic, from segments S 2, 3, 4 via the pudendal nerves, which contract the external sphincter of the urethra.

Afferent impulses from the bladder wall travel via the pelvic nerves and from the sphincters via the pudendal nerves. Distension of the bladder activates stretch receptors in the bladder wall and stimulates the parasympathetic fibres by means of a reflex arc through the upper sacral segments of the spinal cord; for example in the infant the bladder empties automatically when distension reaches a certain degree. Subsequently two descending pathways from higher levels assume control, one which inhibits the automatic reflex emptying, and the other which relaxes the inhibition when appropriate. The expression of urine is then promoted by contracting the abdominal and relaxing the pelvic muscles.

Interruption of the sacral reflex leads to retention of urine. This is accompanied by loss of bladder sensation if the lesion is on the afferent side of the arc, as in tabes dorsalis.

Damage to the anterior sacral nerve roots causes an atonic bladder without loss of sensation ('lower motor neurone paralysis'). Lesions in the spinal cord above the sacral segments may damage the inhibitory fibres, causing urgency, precipitancy or incontinence of urine, or damage to the facilitatory fibres may cause hesitancy or retention. If the higher control is completely lost there is a period of retention with overflow from a passively dilating atonic bladder until the sacral reflex begins to function as in infancy, restoring automatic bladder emptying. The bladder becomes hypertonic ('upper motor neurone paralysis') and may shrink if this is not prevented.

Cerebral lesions at the vertex near the motor or sensory areas may also give rise to incontinence or retention, and with frontal lobe lesions the intellectual disturbance may be associated with failure to inhibit reflex emptying.

Rectum. This has a dual nerve supply from the sympathetic (inhibitory) and the parasympathetic (facilitatory) systems. Disturbances of function similar to those in the bladder occur, but are less severe and more transient (p. 320).

Speech

Speech employs verbal symbols to communicate thoughts and information. Coherent speech requires the formulation of propositions, which are translated into conventional symbols, earlier acquired and readily accessible, which then reach external expression by means of an efficient vocalising apparatus. Disease processes may interrupt this sequence at various levels to produce different types of speech defects.

INTELLECTUAL IMPAIRMENT. Speech is deranged as a result of a generalised deficit of intellectual function which prevents the organisation of meaningful propositions. Such a disturbance reflects a diffuse impairment of cortical function which may be a temporary phenomenon in toxic confusional states (delirium) or permanent in dementia.

DYSPHASIA. This comprises disturbances of the symbolic aspects of language and these arise as a result of damage in or near the cortex of the dominant hemisphere.

The nature of the defect varies with the site of the lesion. In *expressive, motor or non-fluent dysphasia* the patient can formulate thoughts in appropriate words (i.e. internal speech is preserved) but is unable to translate them into corresponding sounds. This occurs despite an intact articulatory system and represents a specialised form of apraxia (p. 603) which results from lesions in the posterior part of the inferior (3rd) frontal convolution (Broca's area). The resulting non-fluent speech (Broca's dysphasia) is characterised by a reduced output of words, errors of articulation and grammar and may have a 'telegraphic' quality.

Impaired comprehension of language is called *receptive, sensory or fluent dysphasia*. The patient fails to understand or carry out spoken instructions. Internal speech is disturbed and hence there is also impairment of the patient's external speech. This is an agnosic deficit (p. 603) and results from lesions of the posterior part of the upper temporal convolutions and the angular gyrus of the parietal lobe (Wernicke's area). Although patients with Wernicke's dysphasia may have a normal or increased output of fluent and well-articulated speech, much of its content is irrelevant and may contain incorrectly substituted words (verbal paraphasia) or letters (literal paraphasia), or entirely new words (neologisms).

Conduction dysphasia may contain elements of both Broca's and Wernicke's dysphasia, but is characterised by a marked inability to repeat words or phrases spoken by the examiner. The lesion responsible lies between Wernicke's and Broca's areas in the perisylvian region.

Global dysphasia. In clinical circumstances all the speech areas of the major hemisphere are often injured together, which results in severe combined receptive and expressive dysfunctions. This picture, called *'global or central dysphasia'*, is usually due to occlusion of the internal carotid or middle cerebral artery which supply all the regions concerned with speech and their connections.

DYSARTHRIA. This is imperfect articulation of speech. Precise enunciation of words requires normal function and co-ordination of lips, tongue and palate. Any abnormality thereof results in slurring and distortion of speech. Dysarthria may be due to mechanical derangements such as cleft palate or ill-fitting false teeth. Lesions of muscles, myoneural junctions, or lower motor neurones of lips, tongue or palate will also result in dysarthria as will upper motor neurone and extrapyramidal affections of these structures.

When normal monitoring of speech is disturbed by deafness, dysarthria may ensue. This is particularly liable to occur when auditory feedback is distorted by impaired hearing in early childhood.

DYSPHONIA. Reduced volume of speech, often accompanied by hoarseness, results from dysfunction of the phonating mechanism. This may be due to weakness of respiratory movements so that air flow across the vocal cords is reduced or to malfunction of the vocal cords. The causative lesion may be in the respiratory musculature, in the peripheral nerves, or in central structures. Thus, for example, bilateral palsies of the recurrent laryngeal nerves cause aphonia. Dysphonia may occur in bulbar palsy or it may result from extrapyramidal disease, such as parkinsonism. Complete aphonia is usually hysterical.

The visual pathway

The optic nerve carries second order neurones, the first order neurones being very short fibres within the retina. For much of its length the optic nerve is surrounded by a protrusion of the meningeal membranes into which cerebrospinal fluid can pass, especially if intracranial pressure is raised. For these reasons the optic nerve is liable to suffer from different pathological states than other nerves.

The visual pathway is illustrated in Figure 15.4. Sensory impulses from the retinae pass along the optic nerves to the optic chiasma where the fibres from the temporal half of the retina continue posteriorly in the lateral angle of the chiasma into the optic tract on the same side. Fibres from the nasal halves of the retinae decussate so that the optic tract carries fibres from that part of each retina which receives light from the contralateral half of the visual field of each eye (the light rays crossing in the refractory media of the eyes). In the same way the light rays from the upper part of the visual field stimulate the lower part of each retina and the fibres arising there remain inferior throughout their further path to the cortex.

The optic tracts continue to the lateral geniculate bodies where the fibres concerned with vision synapse and the impulses are relayed along the optic radiations to the occipital cortex. The uppermost fibres which carry impulses derived from the superior quadrants of each retina (lower quadrants of visual fields) pass directly through the parietal lobe, whereas the lowermost fibres which relay impulses from the lower quadrants of the retina (upper quadrants of visual fields) sweep downwards and forwards round the temporal horn

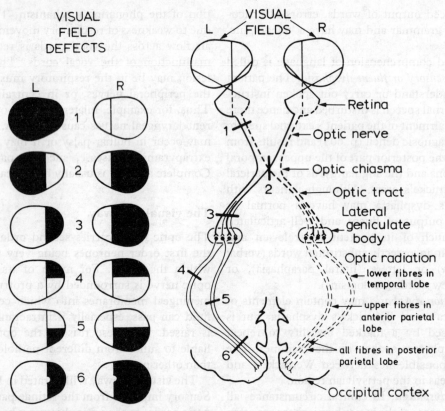

Fig. 15.4 Visual pathways and field defects.

of the lateral ventricle in the temporal lobe before passing to the occipital cortex.

Throughout the whole of the visual pathway fibres from the various parts of each retina maintain approximately the same relationship with each other.

Some fibres originating in the retina and passing centrally in the optic nerve form the afferent limb of the light reflex arc of the pupils. These bypass the lateral geniculate bodies and pass medially to the superior colliculi of the midbrain where they synapse with neurones which pass to the nuclei of the third cranial nerves on each side. From these nuclei arise the efferent limbs of the light reflex (direct and consensual) to the sphincter muscles of the irises.

No visual stimulus is required for the accommodation 'reflex' of the pupil which is more properly an associated contraction related to the movement of convergence of the eyes. This is believed to involve an unidentified cerebral path and a midbrain nucleus which controls the pupillomotor

cells of both third nerve nuclei. This explains the dissociation between the light reflex and the convergence reflex which may occur in neurosyphilis and other diseases.

Clinical manifestations of lesions of the visual pathway. THE OPTIC NERVE. A complete lesion of the optic nerve produces total loss of vision in the affected eye. There is no light reflex, direct or consensual, when that eye is illuminated but both pupils contract normally when the unaffected eye is illuminated. The pupil may be slightly larger in the blind eye. If the lesion is only partial, islands of loss of vision (*scotomas*) of various shapes occur in the field of the affected eye. When the fibres originating in the macular area are damaged there is a loss of visual acuity which cannot be corrected by lenses. Direct and consensual light reflexes are depressed or absent when the abnormal eye is stimulated but the convergence pupil response is unaffected.

THE OPTIC CHIASMA. A lesion of the central portion of the chiasma involves the decussating fibres from the nasal halves of both retinae and so gives rise to bitemporal hemianopia. In practice such lesions are rarely symmetrical and hence the degree of involvement of the visual fields of each eye is often unequal. A pituitary tumour first compresses the lower fibres and so the bitemporal hemianopia begins in the superior quadrants, whereas a suprasellar cyst compresses the chiasma from above so that field loss starts in the lower quadrants.

THE OPTIC TRACTS. A lesion of an optic tract gives rise to a homonymous hemianopia, the lost half of the field of vision of each eye being on the side opposite to the lesion. The involvement of the two fields is often unequal ('incongruous'), being slightly greater in the field of the eye on the side of the lesion.

THE OPTIC RADIATION. The effects of a lesion of the optic radiation depend on its exact site. A lesion of the temporal lobe involves the lower fibres only and gives rise to a homonymous defect involving mainly the upper quadrants of the visual fields (Fig. 15.4). A lesion in the anterior part of the parietal lobe causes a homonymous hemi-anopia mainly affecting the lower quadrants as it affects fibres from the upper part of the retinae. A lesion at the posterior part of the parietal lobe, where both groups of fibres are again adjacent, gives rise to a total homonymous hemianopia.

THE OCCIPITAL CORTEX. A destructive lesion of one occipital cortex gives rise to a complete (and congruous) homonymous hemianopia if it is extensive, or to a scotoma which is present in the fields of both eyes. Irritative lesions, as in the ischaemia caused by migraine, cause halluci-nations of flashing lights which are referred to the contralateral field of both eyes.

The localising signs of cerebral disease

The prefrontal lobe. This comprises the frontal lobe anterior to the precentral gyrus. It is concerned with some aspects of psychological reactions, notably the ability to make intelligent anticipations of the future, and the emotional correlations of thought.

Disturbances of these functions cause vague psychiatric disorders which are difficult to diag-nose in the early stages. The patient loses appreci-ation of the consequences of actions, fails to take forethought and becomes apathetic or morbidly facetious. With progressing dementia, memory and intellect become impaired and social sense is also affected. The patient becomes careless about dress and appearance and may micturate in public or become incontinent without seeming to care.

Physical signs are few but there may be general-ised convulsions and a grasp reflex may be found in the contralateral hand. With this reflex, the patient involuntarily clutches at an object which is drawn lightly over the palm between the index finger and the thumb. The contralateral arm may be ataxic if the frontopontine fibres connecting with the cerebellum are interrupted. Expanding lesions of a frontal lobe may compress the under-lying olfactory nerve causing unilateral loss of the sense of smell.

These signs may be missed in a routine examin-ation. It is important, therefore, to search for them when confronted with a patient with early mental changes.

The precentral gyrus. Lesions in this region give rise to unequivocal signs. Jacksonian epilepsy (p. 617) occurs and monoplegia readily develops. A lesion such as a meningioma arising from the falx cerebri involving the superior ends of both 'motor areas' may give rise to signs of an upper motor neurone lesion in both lower limbs, the upper limbs being spared. When a lesion in the dominant hemisphere extends forwards from the inferior end of the precentral gyrus it gives rise to dysphasia of expressive type.

The parietal lobe. Lesions of this area may also present with Jacksonian epilepsy, but of sensory type, and in addition there is disturbance of the integrative and localising aspects of sen-sation on the opposite side of the body.

Lesions situated more posteriorly in the parietal lobe may cause:

1. Spatial disorientation — lack of the patient's ability to find the way from one place to another.

2. Apraxia — loss of the ability to perform a pattern of movements though the patient under-stands its purpose and has no motor or sensory deficit.

3. Agnosia — loss of the ability to recognise a previously familiar object though the patient has good vision and sensation.

4. 'Perceptual rivalry' (p. 598).

5. Receptive dysphasia — lesions of the dominant angular and marginal gyri or the posterior temporo-parietal junction cause receptive dysphasia which may be predominantly for written or spoken speech. There may be specialised types of dysfunction such as the loss of ability to count or to recognise parts of the body such as a particular finger.

6. Homonymous hemianopia — deep posterior lesions in the parietal lobe may involve the optic radiation and so cause a contralateral homonymous hemianopia (Fig. 15.4).

The occipital lobe. Irritative lesions cause crude visual hallucinations such as flashing lights, while destructive lesions cause a contralateral homonymous hemianopia.

The temporal lobe. Irritative lesions in the posterior temporal lobe may cause visual sensations which are more elaborate than with occipital lobe irritation. Patterns of moving colours or hallucinatory pictures may be experienced by the patient.

A similar lesion of the anterior part of the temporal lobe may cause auditory hallucinations (superior temporal gyrus), gustatory and olfactory hallucinations (uncus) or misinterpretations (illusions) of auditory and visual sensations. These are often associated with altered states of consciousness such as dreamy states, automatic behaviour, temporary upsets of memory (*déjà vu*, p. 618) or brief amnesia.

In affections of the dominant hemisphere there may be dysphasia of receptive type.

An important sign easily overlooked is a homonymous upper quadrantanopia due to destruction of the lower fibres of the optic radiation which sweep down into the temporal lobe (Fig. 15.4).

INVESTIGATION

The selection of appropriate investigations is based on the clinical picture and should always take account of the discomforts and dangers attendant upon the techniques employed. In a few cases extreme clinical urgency will demand that the definitive test, even if invasive, be performed immediately. In most instances, however, it is wise to start with those investigations which are least disturbing and only later to proceed to uncomfortable or hazardous tests.

Radiological examination

Plain radiographs are important preliminary investigations in many neurological problems. A chest radiograph may reveal a bronchial carcinoma and hence explain a wide variety of metastatic and non-metastatic neural complications. Plain radiographs of the skull are indicated when the clinical picture is suggestive of an intracranial lesion. They may show erosions caused by tumours; thickening of the vault of the skull may be provoked by a subjacent meningioma. Lesions such as gliomas, tuberculomas and arteriovenous malformations may be delineated by abnormal calcification. Enlargement of the pituitary fossa due to a tumour within it may be detected, while erosion of the clinoid processes can be due to chronically raised intracerebral pressure from any cause.

Radiographs of the spine should be performed whenever a lesion of the cord or nerve roots is suspected. The vertebral bodies, the pedicles and the disc spaces may display abnormalities which would localise the site and suggest the cause of compression of the spinal cord.

More complex radiological investigation is discussed on pages 607–608.

The cerebrospinal fluid

The cerebrospinal fluid (CSF) is secreted by the choroid plexuses in the lateral, third and fourth ventricles. It leaves the ventricular system through apertures in the roof of the fourth ventricle and flows through the cerebral and spinal subarachnoid spaces. It is returned into the venous sinuses by the arachnoid villi.

An examination of the CSF used to be almost a routine procedure in the investigation of neurological disorders. It still often provides information of value, but with the development of non-invasive methods of investigation the indications for its use are fewer. A lumbar puncture is essential when acute or chronic infection of the brain or meninges is suspected. If subarachnoid haemorrhage is a possibility and CT scanning is either normal or unavailable, lumbar puncture should always be carried out. It should usually be performed in patients suffering from multiple sclerosis or the Guillain-Barré syndrome. It is seldom of primary importance in the diagnosis of cerebral tumours or in the investigation of epilepsy. Lumbar puncture should not be carried out if there is a suspicion of raised intracranial pressure unless there is a strong possibility of meningitis.

In health, the pressure in the lumbar subarachnoid space with the patient lying on one side is 5–15 cm of CSF. Other adult reference values are given in Table 21.4 (p. 816). Note should be made of the appearance of the fluid. Normally clear and colourless, the CSF becomes turbid if it contains many cells. If blood-stained, the fluid should be collected in three successive tubes to differentiate between a traumatic puncture in which the later collections will be less contaminated, and a subarachnoid haemorrhage in which successive tubes will be uniformly red. Blood-stained fluid should also be centrifuged to see whether the supernatant fluid has a yellow tinge (xanthochromia). The CSF may also sometimes be yellowish in deeply jaundiced patients or when its protein content is much increased.

Laboratory examination of the CSF should include a cell count, estimation of the protein and glucose content and serological examination for syphilis. In appropriate circumstances microbiological studies, bacterial or viral, should be carried out.

Cell count. The total number of cells and the different cellular components should be counted in a fresh specimen. Normal CSF contains less than five lymphocytes per cubic millimetre. In bacterial meningitis the cell count may rise to many hundreds or several thousands per cubic millimetre with a marked predominance of polymorphs. Lymphocytosis of moderate degree is found in tuberculous meningitis and viral meningitis, though in the initial stages of these conditions there also may be an increase in polymorphs. A slight to moderate rise in the lymphocyte count may be found in viral encephalitis, sarcoidosis, active neurosyphilis and sometimes in multiple sclerosis. Atypical mononuclear cells may be found when the meninges are invaded by metastatic tumour or lymphoma.

Protein. A moderate elevation may be found in many intracranial diseases including acute infections, neurosyphilis, vascular lesions and many cases of cerebral tumour. Very high protein contents are found in the Guillain-Barré syndrome and when compression of the spinal canal blocks the CSF flow. A few systemic diseases, notably diabetes and hypothyroidism, may also be accompanied by a rise in CSF protein.

The total protein in most cases of multiple sclerosis is within normal limits, but the IgG level (normally 6 to 12% of the total protein) is significantly raised (greater than 20%) in approximately two-thirds of patients with multiple sclerosis whether or not the disease is active. IgG is formed by lymphocytes (oligoclonal) within the central nervous system and not by passive transfer from the blood.

Local synthesis of IgG within the CNS can be inferred with more certainty if the CSF IgG concentration is compared with that in blood, and corrected for the CSF/blood albumin ratio (CSF IgG index). The abnormality most characteristic of multiple sclerosis is the presence of oligoclonal bands in the gamma globulin region when concentrated CSF is subjected to electrophoresis on a gel with a pH gradient (iso-electric focusing). Similar bands may be seen in other disorders, e.g. neurosyphilis and SLE.

Glucose. The CSF glucose is related to blood glucose, being approximately 1.7 mmol per litre below the blood level. A high glucose content, therefore, may be found in diabetes and it is always wise to measure the blood glucose concentration at the same time as CSF examination. A marked reduction in CSF glucose is a feature of bacterial meningitis; in severe cases glucose may be absent. A moderate reduction in glucose is found in tuberculous and carcinomatous meningitis and CNS sarcoidosis. The glucose content is usually normal in viral meningitis.

Serology. Tests for syphilis are described on page 416.

Microbiological investigation. Whenever infection is suspected the CSF should be centrifuged and the deposit examined microscopically after Gram staining, and, if tuberculous meningitis is suspected, after Ziehl-Neelsen staining. Cultures should also be prepared from the CSF in cases of suspected infection and antibiotic sensitivities determined. In certain instances viruses may be cultured from the CSF, but usually the diagnosis of viral infection depends on rising antibody titres found in paired sera rather than by isolation of the virus in the CSF.

Miscellaneous tests. In certain situations, more specialised and refined examinations of the CSF may be carried out. For example in carcinomatous meningitis examination of a fresh CSF specimen after cyto-centrifugation may reveal malignant cells. In cases of severe meningitis antibiotic levels may be measured in the CSF as a guide to treatment.

INVESTIGATION IN RELATION TO SITE OF LESIONS

The choice of more sophisticated and specific tests is determined by the site of neurological lesions. Such investigations include clinical neurophysiology (electroencephalography, evoked potentials and electromyography), radionuclide scanning, computed tomography and other imaging techniques including cerebral angiography.

Investigation of intracranial disease

A wide variety of techniques is available for investigation of intracranial lesions; harmless, non-invasive tests should be employed first.

The electroencephalogram (EEG). This records the electrical potentials of the brain after they are attenuated by passing through the skull and scalp. Potential changes are recorded simultaneously over several areas. Intracranial disease may cause normal electrical rhythms to be suppressed, or, more commonly, abnormal wave forms may be engendered. Such abnormalities may be generalised or localised. The EEG is the most valuable non-invasive test to confirm encephalitis.

EEG abnormalities are more marked with acute lesions such as cerebral abscess than those which are slowly progressive or chronic. Lesions within the substance of the brain such as gliomas produce more marked and earlier abnormalities than lesions such as meningiomas or angiomas lying outside the brain tissue. The potential changes indicate the locus of a lesion but not its pathology.

The EEG is more precise in its definition of lesions lying in the cerebral hemispheres than it is in lesions lying within the posterior fossa. The EEG is of prime diagnostic value in functional disorders, especially epilepsy. Generalised or localised paroxysmal activity in the form of spikes or sharp waves may be detected between seizures, and may be induced by hyperventilation, photic flicker stimulation, sleep or drugs. It is now possible to record EEGs from ambulant patients for 24 hours or longer, and this may provide diagnostic information in selected cases. A normal EEG does not exclude the diagnosis of epilepsy; likewise, the presence of paroxysmal activity is not in itself diagnostic without an appropriate history.

Evoked potential recording. Over the past decade, the development of digital signal averaging has permitted the measurement of small cerebral and spinal potential changes evoked by visual, auditory and peripheral nerve stimuli. An averaged response, relatively free of muscle and AC interference, is built up by storing responses to 100–1000 sequential stimuli. Visually evoked potentials (VEP) are the most useful clinically, and are recorded with an array of scalp electrodes over the occipital region. Stimulation is usually with a reversing chequer-board pattern which is either projected on to a screen or displayed on a television set. The dominant response from a normal eye is a positive wave with a peak at about 100 milliseconds. Lesions of the retina, optic nerve, chiasma, tract, radiation or occipital cortex may all disrupt or delay the response, but demyelinating lesions of the optic nerve often cause marked delay with relatively good preservation of the wave form. A delayed VEP in a patient with clinically normal vision can therefore be of much diagnostic help in multiple sclerosis.

Somatosensory evoked potentials (SSEP), recorded from the brachial plexus, cervical spine and contralateral parietal area when the median or ulnar nerve is stimulated electrically, many similarly help detect lesions in the ascending sensory pathways. Auditory evoked potentials (AEP) in response to click stimuli arise largely from the brain stem and may give evidence of cochlear, acoustic nerve or brain stem disorders.

Radionuclide cerebral scanning. This is an innocuous and useful investigation. An injected radioisotope (such as technetium) is often taken up differentially by diseased intracranial tissue compared to normal brain substance. Differing intensities of radio activities are recorded through the skull and abnormal areas mapped. In this way tumours, particularly meningiomas, can be localised and areas of infarction defined. The technique is in general much less sensitive or specific than CT scanning.

Computed tomography (CT scan). This is an accurate and sensitive tool and, with contrast enhancement, will reveal the vast majority of cerebral tumours, cerebral haemorrhages, and abscesses and also cerebral atrophy. The technique can also be applied to scan the spinal cord and roots. It has reduced the need for arteriography and markedly reduced the demand for pneumoencephalography. A CT scan will demonstrate the size and position of the cerebral ventricles and will detect the majority of supratentorial tumours, infarcts and haematomas. The posterior fossa is less well visualised because of artefacts produced by the petrous bones. Small low-density lesions such as infarcts and some gliomas may be missed. Arteriovenous malformations, small subdural haematomas and intrinsic lesions in the brain stem may also be undetected.

Emission computed tomography. This is a technique of imaging in which radio-labelled tracers are injected intravenously and the emitted radiation from the brain is recorded by scintillation detectors. As with CT scanning, a computer is used in order to construct a two dimensional image of the brain. Spatial resolution is less good than conventional CT but functional changes such as oxygen uptake and neurotransmitter storage can be studied. The equipment is costly and is used primarily for research.

Magnetic resonance imaging. This procedure utilises the magnetic properties of hydrogen nuclei within the brain. The brain is exposed to a magnetic field and the hydrogen nuclei within it are excited by radio frequency radiation and the signals thus produced are detected and computed. The brain is scanned to produce images of brain slices similar to those of conventional CT scanning.

Since grey matter contains much more water (and hydrogen nuclei) than white matter this technique vividly differentiates grey and white matter. It produces imaging of the posterior fossa which is superior to that of conventional CT scanning. The facility to construct a midline sagittal image of the brain and upper cervical cord is particularly valuable for the investigation of disorders at the cranio-vertebral junction. As well as revealing space-occupying lesions it will demonstrate small lesions within white matter such as those in multiple sclerosis. It is particularly valuable in the diagnosis of demyelinating diseases and in those metabolic and toxic conditions where demyelination is a feature but small infarcts may be indistinguishable from plaques of demyelination.

Cerebral angiography. With the advent of the CT scan, angiography is rarely the primary investigation in cases of cerebral tumour. However, it still has a place in defining precise anatomy when a mass has been demonstrated on the CT scan and operation is contemplated. It is also the appropriate investigation when clinical signs point to a lesion of a blood vessel such as an aneurysm or stenosis. Carotid and vertebral arteriography are uncomfortable and potentially hazardous and should be used only if there are appropriate indications.

Digital subtraction angiography employs computer enhancement to subtract soft tissue and bone images from vascular outlines. Using a venous bolus injection of contrast medium, it is possible to obtain reasonable images of extracranial arteries, but good quality views of intracerebral vessels require arterial injection. With a venous injection it is possible to perform angiographic studies at low risk, but at present the image quality is inferior to conventional arteriography.

Pneumoencephalography. The injection of air into the lumbar subarachnoid space to outline the cerebral ventricles and CSF spaces is now rarely performed. *Air-CT meatography* is a modern refinement in which small volumes of air are manoeuvred into the cerebello-pontine angle and CT images taken to outline the internal auditory meatus and its contents. The technique is used mainly for the detection of small acoustic neuromas.

Investigation of the spinal cord

Myelography may be required for the investigation of localised damage to the spinal cord and radiculography is used to outline abnormalities of the nerve roots. The contrast media used are not harmless. These procedures should be reserved for patients in whom the radiological findings will significantly affect management.

Investigation of muscles and peripheral nerves

The investigation of primary diseases of muscle may require extensive biochemical testing. Of general applicability is the estimation of serum enzymes such as aldolase, lactic dehydrogenase and, most specifically, creatine phosphokinase whose concentrations reflect the rate and extent of muscle fibre disintegration.

Peripheral nerve disorders may also require a range of biochemical investigations such as vitamin assays, blood urea, plasma protein electrophoresis, urinary porphobilinogen and glucose tolerance tests to determine the primary cause.

Electromyography (EMG). This is useful in the investigation of peripheral nerve and muscle disorders. Muscle or nerve action potentials are detected by surface or needle electrodes. The signals are amplified and displayed on an oscilloscope so that their latency, amplitude and duration can be measured. Needle electrode study of muscles during voluntary contraction helps identify denervation and differentiates it from myopathic disorders. Many peripheral nerves can be stimulated electrically and conduction velocities in motor and sensory fibres can be measured separately. Velocity and amplitude measurements help gauge the type and severity of polyneuropathies and may define the site of localised nerve compression, as in the carpal tunnel syndrome. Disorders of peripheral nerve which are due to demyelination cause marked reduction in conduction velocity, whereas primary axonal degeneration is characterised by reduced amplitude of sensory and motor potentials.

Tests of the autonomic nervous system, dependent on measuring cardiovascular responses to the Valsalva manoeuvre, deep breathing and sustained hand grip, can be performed in selected cases. Abnormalities are seen particularly in polyneuropathy due to diabetes mellitus, alcoholism and amyloidosis.

DISEASES OF THE CRANIAL NERVES

The cranial nerves are frequently involved in generalised disease of the nervous system. In addition, there are specific conditions affecting a single cranial nerve.

THE FIRST CRANIAL NERVE

The olfactory nerve arises from olfactory receptors in the nasal mucosa. The fine first order fibres pass through the cribriform plate in the floor of the anterior fossa of the skull. They synapse in the olfactory bulb, and second order neurones run to the olfactory area of the brain (the anteromedial part of the temporal lobe) and to higher autonomic centres via the olfactory tract which lies under the orbital surface of the frontal lobe.

Lesions of this tract (e.g. due to a frontal lobe tumour) may cause ipsilateral loss of the sense of smell (anosmia). More commonly anosmia is due to nasal or sinus disease impeding air flow or to infective damage to the olfactory nerve endings. Post-traumatic anosmia is due to damage to these fragile fibres as they pass through the cribriform plate.

THE SECOND CRANIAL NERVE

The anatomy and central connections of the optic nerve are described on page 601 and the visual field defect caused by a lesion of the nerve on page 602.

Papilloedema means swelling of the optic nerve head (optic disc). The main disorders causing papilloedema are:

1. Increased intracranial pressure due to lesions within the cranial cavity such as cerebral tumour, cerebral abscess, or meningitis. The rise in pressure of the cerebrospinal fluid causes distension of the subarachnoid space round the optic nerve and compresses the venous drainage of the retina.

2. Obstruction of the venous drainage from the orbit by thrombosis of the central vein of the

retina, cavernous sinus thrombosis or, rarely, an orbital neoplasm.

3. Lesions of the optic nerve itself, some of them inflammatory, may also cause swelling of the optic disc which is usually then referred to as *papillitis*.

4. Diseases of the retinal arteries such as cranial arteritis.

5. Extracerebral conditions such as malignant hypertension and severe chronic respiratory failure.

The earliest manifestation of papilloedema is engorgement of the retinal veins, followed by an intensified pink colouration of the optic disc and blurring of its margin which usually begins on the nasal side. As swelling proceeds the physiological cup is obliterated and the whole optic disc may be elevated. If the papilloedema is severe and particularly when it is of rapid development, there may be accompanying haemorrhages abutting on to the disc (Plate II). If papilloedema is of long standing the disc becomes progressively paler as optic atrophy develops.

Often it is of clinical importance to differentiate the swelling due to raised intracranial pressure from that due to lesions of the optic nerve which present indistinguishable ophthalmoscopic appearances. The visual acuity is usually well preserved when papilloedema is due to raised intracranial pressure whilst optic neuritis usually causes marked loss of visual acuity. Papilloedema due to raised pressure gives rise to early enlargement of the blind spot. Chronic severe papilloedema may be accompanied by peripheral constriction of the visual field. Optic neuritis causes a central scotoma.

Optic neuritis encompasses inflammatory, demyelinating and some vascular diseases of the optic nerve which, in common, cause loss of vision. In many cases pain in the eye aggravated by movement, and tenderness over the eye precede or accompany the visual disturbance. There is a loss of central vision and the direct reaction to light is impaired whilst the consensual light reflex is preserved. When the lesion lies anteriorly in the nerve there may be *papillitis* (swelling of the optic disc). Where the ophthalmoscopic appearances are normal, the lesion lies posteriorly and is called a *retrobulbar neuritis*. The visual evoked potential from the affected eye is often absent or very diminished and delayed during the acute phase. As recovery takes place, the VEP usually returns but tends to be delayed in onset and may show an altered wave-form.

Optic neuritis is most commonly due to demyelination, itself usually a manifestation of multiple sclerosis, and in this condition recovery of vision within 4 to 6 weeks is usual. Rarer causes include excessive smoking of strong pipe tobacco, vitamin deficiencies, syphilis and toxins such as methyl alcohol.

Nutritional amblyopia is a progressive failure of vision due to a retrobulbar neuropathy which may occur in severe malnutrition. Sometimes in West Africans and West Indians the visual failure is associated with lesions of the spinal cord (p. 657).

Optic atrophy. Loss of fibres in the optic nerve is followed by reactive gliosis and reduced vascularisation. These pathological changes are manifest clinically by pallor of the optic disc and may result from many causes including (1) optic neuritis from the various causes listed above; (2) pressure on the optic nerve by glaucoma, tumours, aneurysms, etc.; (3) long-standing papilloedema; (4) thrombosis of the central retinal artery; (5) trauma.

THE THIRD, FOURTH AND SIXTH CRANIAL NERVES

The *third nerve (oculomotor)* supplies all the external ocular muscles except the lateral rectus and the superior oblique. It also supplies the levator palpebrae superioris, the constrictor of the pupil, and the ciliary muscle. It may be involved in multiple sclerosis, meningovascular syphilis, diabetes mellitus, and cerebral aneurysms which may compress the nerve at several sites.

The manifestations of a third nerve palsy are ptosis, diplopia, external deviation of the eye (divergent strabismus, due to the action of the unopposed lateral rectus muscle) and defective ocular movement in the directions in which the muscles supplied by the third nerve move the eye. The patient complains of double vision but in a long-standing lesion one of the images is suppressed. A complete lesion of the third nerve also paralyses the constrictor of the pupil; consequently the pupil is large and fails to react to light (by the direct or consensual path) or on convergence.

The *fourth nerve (trochlear)* supplies the superior oblique muscle. A lesion of this nerve gives rise to defective movement and diplopia which is maximal when the patient attempts to look down with the eye turned inwards. The pupils are not affected. An isolated lesion of the nerve is rarely encountered, as usually there is also involvement of either the third or sixth nerve.

The *sixth nerve (abducent)* supplies the lateral rectus muscle of the eye. A lesion of this nerve causes diplopia due to inability to abduct the eye, and deviation of the eye medially (convergent strabismus) due to the unopposed action of the medial rectus muscle. The sixth nerve may be involved by pressure from an aneurysm in the cavernous sinus.

Both the third and the sixth nerves may be involved indirectly by disorders which raise intracranial pressure or displace the brain stem. The nerves are stretched or compressed as secondary events, and their dysfunction may thus represent *'false localising signs'* of cerebral tumour, haematoma, hydrocephalus or oedema.

Squint

Squint (strabismus) may be paralytic or concomitant.

Paralytic squint is due to weakness of one or more of the extraocular muscles. Defective movement of the eye can be seen when the patient uses the weak muscle to move the eye, and this usually causes diplopia. The rules for identifying the paretic muscles causing diplopia or squint are:

1. The separation of the images is greatest when the patient attempts to look in the direction to which the paretic muscle should move the eye.

2. In this position, the most peripheral image is the 'false image' from the affected eye. It is identified by covering one eye with a green glass and the other with a red one.

Concomitant squint ('lazy eye') is due to failure to maintain the correct posture of an eye which is so defective in vision that its image is suppressed by the brain. There is no muscle paresis and both eyes are capable of full movements in all directions. The most common cause is an error of refraction during childhood. If recognised and properly treated with suitable spectacles the squint can be prevented, though a 'latent squint' often remains.

Nystagmus

Nystagmus is a series of involuntary, rhythmic oscillations of one or both eyes. It may be manifest in horizontal or vertical planes or as a series of rotations of the eye about its central axis (rotary nystagmus). The oscillations may be equal in speed and amplitude in both directions of movement (pendular nystagmus) or movement in one direction may be faster than in the other (phasic nystagmus). When there are fast and slow components, the direction of the nystagmus is arbitrarily defined by the direction of the fast component. When severe, nystagmus may be present on looking to the side opposite to the fast component — this is a measure of severity, not an indication of nystagmus to both sides. It may occur spontaneously or be induced in response to a stimulus such as rotation of the head. When testing for nystagmus it is important to keep the visual fixation point within the field of binocular vision. Some normal people show sustained fine jerking nystagmus at the extremes of lateral gaze, especially when fatigued.

Types and causes of nystagmus. PHASIC (JERK) NYSTAGMUS. This is often seen in the horizontal plane and is evoked by lateral gaze to one or both sides. When the amplitude of the nystagmus is equal in both eyes the causative lesion may be in the cerebellum, the vestibular apparatus or nerve, or the cerebellar and vestibular connections in the brain stem. With cerebellar and brain stem lesions the nystagmus is maximal when gaze is directed towards the side of the lesion. Lesions of the vestibular apparatus or nerve can cause either horizontal or rotatory nystagmus maximal on looking away from the lesion. Vertical nystagmus with a fast upward component on up-gaze may be seen with lesions at the superior colliculus, but occurs also in conjunction with dysfunction of the medial longitudinal fasciculus (see below). Down-beating vertical nystagmus on lateral or downward gaze is characteristic of lesions at the foramen magnum involving the medulla and cerebellar tonsils.

INTERNUCLEAR OPHTHALMOPLEGIA. Conjugate lateral gaze is initiated from the contralateral frontal lobe via the paracentral pontine centre for lateral gaze, and is effected by simultaneous activation of the sixth nerve nucleus on one side and the medial rectus portion of the third nerve nucleus on the other. The medial longitudinal fasciculus (MLF) links these two nuclei and is responsible for smooth co-ordination of conjugate eye movements. Lesions of the MLF cause a form of eye movement disorder called internuclear ophthalmoplegia, in which the two eyes fail to co-ordinate on lateral gaze resulting usually in sluggish adduction of one eye and irregular coarse phasic nystagmus in the abducting eye (ataxic nystagmus). The defect is most striking when the patient makes rapid lateral eye movements. The abnormality is often bilateral in multiple sclerosis, brain stem tumour and Wernicke's encephalopathy, but may be unilateral when due to vascular disease.

OCULAR (FIXATION) NYSTAGMUS. Reflex mechanisms enable a visual target to be viewed by the macular area of each eye even when the target is moving. These reflexes are mediated through pathways which run from the eye to the occipital cortex and parietal lobe and thence to the pretectal area of the midbrain.

Optokinetic nystagmus is a physiological phenomenon which can be observed when a series of targets move past the visual field (e.g. when sitting on a moving train passing telegraph poles). The fixation reflex tracks the target as far as possible (slow component) and then the eyes jerk back (fast component) to pick up the next target.

When central vision is poor (e.g. because of severe refractive error or macular disease) ocular nystagmus of pendular type may be seen on central gaze. In some patients this becomes coarser or phasic on lateral gaze. Ocular nystagmus is often congenital. Pendular nystagmus of similar type is sometimes seen in diffuse brain stem lesions due to multiple sclerosis or tumours.

POSITIONAL NYSTAGMUS. Some patients develop nystagmus only when the head is placed in certain positions. Two main types of disorder are recognised:

Peripheral type. Here nystagmus and vertigo occur usually a few seconds after the head is tilted backwards below the horizontal and with the affected ear lowermost. The vertigo is often profound and the nystagmus usually rotatory, but they tend to settle if the position is maintained. The disorder — benign positional vertigo — is probably due to calcific degeneration of the otolith organ causing small particles to fall on to the cupola of the semicircular canals. Patients may give a history of ear infection or head trauma. The condition usually remits within a few months.

Central type. Lesions of the cerebellum and brain stem vestibular connections may cause nystagmus when the head is turned backwards and to one or both sides. Vertigo is not usually marked and the nystagmus begins immediately and continues as long as the posture is maintained. Causes include multiple sclerosis, tumours, vascular lesions, syringobulbia, encephalitis and alcoholism.

THE FIFTH CRANIAL NERVE

The trigeminal nerve has an extensive sensory distribution though its three branches, the ophthalmic, maxillary and mandibular divisions. It supplies the skin of the face (excluding the angle of the jaw), the cornea, the sinuses, the mucous membrane of the nose, the teeth, the tympanic membrane and common sensation (but not taste) to the anterior two-thirds of the tongue. The motor division of the nerve innervates the temporal, masseter and pterygoid muscles which are responsible for the movements of the jaw.

The nerve fibres and nuclei may be involved within the brain stem by conditions such as syringobulbia and thrombotic lesions, and the peripheral nerve by localised pressure such as occurs in cerebral aneurysms in the region of the cavernous sinus, and by tumours of the cerebellopontine angle. The ganglion of the nerve may also be involved by herpes zoster, giving rise to the characteristic shingles lesion over the skin of the face and causing ulceration of the cornea when the ophthalmic division is involved.

Tumours in the maxillary sinus cause symptoms and signs in the distribution of the second trigeminal division. A lesion in the infratemporal fossa may involve the mandibular branch.

Trigeminal neuralgia

This condition, which usually affects elderly people, is of unknown aetiology and without recognised histopathology.

Clinical features. Pain, usually paroxysmal and sharp, is the characteristic feature. It is confined to the distribution of the fifth nerve. The maxillary or mandibular divisions of the nerve are usually first involved and spread from one to the other is common but the ophthalmic division is rarely affected.

Each paroxysm lasts for only a few seconds but the stab of pain may be followed by a dull ache, or frequent attacks following one another may make the pain appear to be of longer duration. The pain is precipitated by touching localised 'trigger zones' on the affected side of the face. A cold wind blowing on the face, washing the face, chewing or even talking may be sufficient to bring on an attack. Paroxysms may continue for days or weeks, after which a remission of equal or longer duration may follow, but remissions become shorter and less frequent as the disease progresses. The agonising pain commands the patient's full attention. It may provoke a spasm of the facial muscles. No abnormalities of fifth nerve function can be detected on examination.

When a typical history is volunteered by an elderly patient the diagnosis is obvious. If similar symptoms occur in a young person the possibility of multiple sclerosis needs to be considered. Facial pain, mimicking trigeminal neuralgia, may rarely be a manifestation of a basilar aneurysm or cerebral tumour, particularly of a neurofibroma of the fifth nerve itself. When the fifth nerve is implicated in disease processes, the pain is often continuous and there are usually signs of fifth nerve dysfunction; there may be associated disturbances of other cranial nerves or neural pathways.

Treatment. Carbamazepine is the most effective drug. It is important to start with a small dose (100–200 mg/d) and gradually to increase the dose over 2–3 weeks to 200–400 mg t.i.d., aiming for a plasma level of 30–50 μmol/l. Phenytoin (200–400 mg/d) or clonazepam 1–2 mg t.i.d. are alternatives worthy of trial.

Long remissions may occur. If pain persists and remissions are rare or of short duration it is necessary to interrupt the central passage of pain impulses by injection of phenol or alcohol into a branch of the nerve, if neuralgia is localised, or into the Gasserian ganglion.

Section of the sensory part of the fifth nerve or its descending root in the medulla has the disadvantage of requiring intracranial operation but permits sparing of corneal sensation which is difficult to achieve with injection of the ganglion. These procedures secure permanent relief but the face becomes anaesthetic. Loss of sensibility from the cornea demands that special care must be taken to avoid trauma with its danger of subsequent corneal ulceration.

Radiofrequency coagulation of the trigeminal root is also effective, but its beneficial effect tends to wear off after weeks or months. Posterior fossa microvascular procedures to identify arterial loops and separate them from the trigeminal rootlets have been reported to be successful. The need for these more invasive treatments needs to be weighed against the patient's age, condition and response to medical therapy.

THE SEVENTH CRANIAL NERVE

The facial nerve innervates the muscles of expression of the face and, through its chorda tympani branch, carries taste fibres from the anterior two-thirds of the tongue. Paralysis of the facial muscles may be due to: (1) lesion of the fibres of the upper motor neurones concerned with voluntary movement; (2) lesion of the fibres of the upper motor neurones concerned with emotional movement; (3) lesion of the lower motor neurones.

1. Upper motor neurone fibres originating in the lower part of the precentral gyrus are distributed to the part of the opposite facial nucleus subserving the muscles of the lower part of the face, and to the parts of the facial nuclei on both sides of the pons which supply the upper parts of the face. Accordingly, a lesion of the upper motor neurones affects more severely the voluntary movement of the lower part of the face, contralat-

erally. Weakness of the upper part (the orbicularis oculi and frontalis muscles) may occur transiently but is often absent because the lower motor neurones to the upper facial muscles are supplied by upper motor neurones from both hemispheres. The patient is unable to retract the angle of the mouth on command, but in smiling and talking the mouth may move well because emotional movement is controlled by upper motor neurones which are not those concerned with voluntary movement of the face.

2. Upper motor neurones concerned with emotional movement of the face take origin further forward in the frontal lobe and so may be damaged by a lesion which spares the fibres for voluntary movement of the face. Involvement of these fibres is revealed by defective movement of the angle of the mouth when the patient smiles, with preservation of the ability to retract the angle of the mouth on command.

3. Since the lower motor neurone is the final common pathway, complete damage to the facial nucleus or nerve abolishes both voluntary and emotional movements equally in upper and lower parts of the face. Lower motor neurone paralysis restricted to part of the facial muscles can occur only when the lesion is distal to the branching of the nerve, e.g. with disease of the parotid gland, through which the nerve passes, or in leprosy.

The most common cause of damage to the nerve proximal to its branching in the parotid gland is Bell's palsy but the nerve may also be damaged by disease of the brain stem, by an acoustic neuroma, or by inflammation during its passage through the middle ear.

Bell's palsy

This term should be restricted to cases of isolated facial paralysis of unknown cause. Bell's palsy is accompanied by oedema of the facial nerve within the facial canal. It is more common in arterial hypertension. Exposure to cold wind appears to be a trigger in some cases. It has been suggested that the swelling may be due to a viral infection since minor epidemics of the condition occasionally occur. Swelling within the rigid facial canal results in pressure on the nerve causing paralysis of function. The degree of nerve damage varies from conduction block, through demyelination, to axonal disintegration and Wallerian degeneration.

Clinical features. The condition occurs in both sexes at any age. The first symptom is often an ache in the region of the stylomastoid foramen which may persist for a few hours or 1 or 2 days. A unilateral facial paralysis then develops. The eye on the affected side cannot be closed and the mouth is drawn over to the opposite side so that often it may appear to the patient that there is a spasm of the normal side. Saliva and fluids may escape from the angle of the mouth. Food may collect between the teeth and the paralysed cheek when the patient is eating. The patient often complains that the affected side feels 'numb', but there is no objective impairment of sensation of the skin.

In most instances the lesion is distal to the chorda tympani and facial paralysis is the only feature. In a minority of cases when the lesion lies proximal to the chorda tympani there will be loss of taste on the anterior two-thirds of the tongue and diminished salivation. When the lesion is proximal to the nerve to the stapedius, hyperacusis on the affected side is an additional complaint.

Physical examination reveals paralysis of the upper and lower parts of the affected side of the face. The lines of expression are flattened, the patient is unable to wrinkle the brow or whistle or retract the angle of the mouth. The eye on the affected side cannot be closed, and on attempting to do so the eyeball rolls upwards (Bell's sign).

Treatment and prognosis. ACTH or oral corticosteroids, if started early, may increase the rate of recovery, maximum benefit being obtained if they are given within 48 hours of the onset of the palsy. Dexamethasone (2 mg t.i.d.) for 5 days is a suitable treatment.

Recovery occurs in over 90% of patients, usually after 2 or 3 weeks and is complete after 2 to 3 months. Approximately 5% of patients have permanent loss of function and develop facial contractures and involuntary spasms of the facial muscles. Complete recovery is virtually certain if there is any return of voluntary movement within a week after the onset and is probable if recovery of function begins within a month.

A guide to the prognosis is given by electrodiagnostic studies. Direct facial nerve conduction measured across the face may be normal in the early stages, even with a severe lesion. If Wallerian degeneration occurs the evoked muscle action potential amplitude decreases progressively and indicates a poorer prognosis. Early preservation of the electrically elicited blink reflex is a good prognostic sign.

Some authorities advocate early surgical decompression of the facial canal in severe cases, but since the majority of patients will recover spontaneously, it is difficult to judge the necessity of operation until it is too late to prevent axonal degeneration.

THE EIGHTH CRANIAL NERVE

The auditory nerve has two components, the cochlear nerve which is concerned with hearing and the vestibular nerve which is concerned with the appreciation of the position of the head and its movement in space. It is impossible without special tests to differentiate lesions involving these nerves from lesions confined to their endorgans in the inner ear. Irritative lesions of the inner ear or of the cochlear nerve cause *tinnitus,* and destructive lesions *deafness.* Thus, tinnitus is often due to aural causes but it may be an early symptom of a neuroma of the eighth nerve (acoustic neuroma) which is the most important destructive lesion of the eighth nerve. It may also be damaged in meningitis, and by the toxic effects of streptomycin or kanamycin.

Irritative lesions of the vestibular part of the eighth nerve cause *vertigo* which is a subjective feeling of movement of the external environment or of the head. The movement may be rotatory or a feeling of displacement in one direction. Vertigo is accompanied by a disturbance of balance which usually causes the patient to seek support and, if sudden and severe, may throw the patient to the ground.

The most important causes of vertigo are:

1. *Cerebellar lesions.* Vertigo may occur when the cerebello-vestibular connections are involved but this symptom is not invariable.

2. *Brain stem lesions.* Atherosclerosis of the basilar artery, medullary infarction or syringobulbia may cause severe vertigo when they involve the vestibular nuclei. The vertigo may be produced by particular positions of the head.

3. *Lesions of the vestibular nerve.* An acoustic neuroma may damage the nerve and cause vertigo. Vestibular neuronitis is a more common cause; it is a benign short-lasting condition of unknown aetiology which may occur in epidemics. It is presumed to have a viral basis, and often accompanies an acute febrile illness. The acute symptoms usually last only a few days, but positional vertigo of the peripheral type (p. 611) may persist for weeks or months.

4. *Aural lesions* of many kinds, including otitis media and Ménière's syndrome, cause vertigo. The labyrinth may be damaged in a head injury and the vertigo may then be positional of the peripheral type. It is a benign condition which may disappear after a few months. The labyrinth may be damaged by mumps and by drugs such as streptomycin, quinine and salicylates. Hearing is almost invariably affected when the lesion is labyrinthine rather than in the nerve or its central connections.

5. *Ocular lesions.* Diplopia may be accompanied by vertigo because the false projection of one image causes confusion regarding position in space.

Ménière's syndrome

Ménière's syndrome is characterised by recurrent paroxysms of vertigo associated with tinnitus and progressive nerve deafness. The cause is unknown but the condition is associated with dilatation of the endolymphatic system due to increase in the amount of endolymph. Many patients also give a history of migraine and the syndrome may have a vascular basis.

Clinical features. The most common initial symptoms are progressive deafness and tinnitus which are frequently slight at the onset. Sooner or later vertigo occurs and is characterised by suddeness of onset and severity. It may develop so abruptly that the patient may fall, and at the height of the attack may be unable to stand. There is often accompanying nausea and vomiting, and there may be sweating, weakness and faintness. Deafness and tinnitus may be intensified during the attack, which may last for a few minutes to several hours. Examination during an attack shows rotatory nystagmus and unsteadiness of stance and gait. Between attacks there is only nerve deafness with impaired vestibular function as shown by caloric tests. Audiometry shows mid-low frequency sensorineural deafness. The frequency of attacks tends to decrease as deafness increases but the disease may last many years.

Treatment. No treatment will abort an episode of vertigo; during severe attacks the patient should lie still and may be helped by an intramuscular injection of 50 mg of chlorpromazine or prochlorperazine (12.5 mg). Treatment is aimed at preventing or reducing the number of attacks and includes cinnarizine (15 mg t.i.d.), betahistine (8 mg t.i.d.), and prochlorperazine (5 mg t.i.d.). If attacks continue to be disabling or deafness is worsening, surgical procedures to improve drainage of endolymph need consideration.

Acoustic neuroma (neurilemmoma)

This is a benign tumour arising from the covering tissues of the eighth nerve. It usually occurs within the internal auditory meatus, and expands towards the cerebello-pontine angle where it may involve the fifth and seventh nerves, and eventually, the cerebellum and brain stem. The tumour is more common in people with neurofibromatosis, when it may be bilateral. Early symptoms are unilateral deafness and tinnitus, together with insidious vertigo. When the tumour reaches large size, signs of cerebellar dysfunction and features of raised intracranial pressure ensue.

Clinical assessment reveals unilateral sensorineural deafness, and there may be phasic nystagmus initially on looking away from the lesion, and eventually, as the cerebellum is involved, on looking towards the lesion. There may be signs of impaired trigeminal sensation, depression of the corneal reflex, facial weakness and, later, cerebellar signs, pyramidal tract involvement and papilloedema.

Diagnosis rests on finding unilateral neural deafness, depressed caloric vestibular function on the same side, and delayed auditory evoked potentials. Plain X-rays or tomograms of the internal auditory meati may show enlargement on the affected side, and large tumours can be seen on CT scan. The definitive procedure to delineate a small tumour is air-CT meatography (p. 607).

Treatment is surgical, and best results are obtained if this is undertaken early. Unfortunately, deafness and facial weakness often result, but with early treatment, long-term prognosis is good.

THE NINTH, TENTH AND ELEVENTH CRANIAL NERVES

These nerves are grouped together because isolated lesions of one nerve are rarely encountered. The *glossopharyngeal nerve* (IX) transmits taste and common sensation from the posterior one-third of the tongue and motor fibres to the pharynx; the *vagus nerve* (X) is the parasympathetic nerve for the viscera of the thorax and upper part of the abdomen and also supplies somatic motor fibres to the soft palate and the larynx; the *spinal accessory nerve* (XI) supplies the trapezius and sternomastoid muscles. Unilateral lesions disturb their somatic functions but do not appreciably affect visceral function.

These nerves or their nuclei may be involved by disease of the medulla such as syringobulbia or in their course across the posterior fossa by neoplasms and basal meningitis. Lesions at the jugular foramen, such as thrombophlebitis of the internal jugular vein following suppuration in the skull or neck, may involve all three nerves as they emerge from the skull. Glossopharyngeal neuralgia is described on page 625 and laryngeal paralysis on page 242.

THE TWELFTH CRANIAL NERVE

The hypoglossal nerve supplies motor fibres to the muscles of one side of the tongue. Upper motor neurone lesions cause spastic contraction of the muscle fibres. The tongue is small and pointed but not atrophic. Articulation is defective (spastic dysarthria) especially for the lingual sounds. There is rapid recovery of function after a unilateral lesion of upper motor neurone type, but bilateral lesions cause permanent dysarthria. This may occur in motor neurone disease or in pseudobulbar palsy (p. 630). Lower motor neurone lesions cause wasting and fasciculation of the affected part of the tongue and, when protruded, the tongue deviates to the side of the lesion. These changes may be seen in motor neurone disease.

The lower cranial nerves may be involved by carcinoma of the nasopharynx spreading to the base of the skull so otolaryngological examination is necessary. All cranial nerves, but particularly those emerging from the base of the skull, may be affected by bone disease in that area, particularly by Paget's disease.

THE CERVICAL SYMPATHETIC NERVES

The higher centres for autonomic functions in the hypothalamus are connected with some areas of the cortex, notably the orbital surface of the frontal lobe and insula. From the hypothalamus sympathetic fibres descend through the brain stem and spinal cord to their lower neurones in the small lateral horn of the thoracic region of the spinal cord from which they pass into the anterior spinal roots from T1 to L2. Fibres destined for the head and neck emerge mainly through the first thoracic anterior root, and ascend in the cervical sympathetic chain, reaching their final destination by means of the plexuses in the walls of blood vessels.

Stimulation of the cervical sympathetic fibres causes dilatation of the pupil, protrusion of the eyeball and elevation of the upper eyelid; conversely paralysis of these fibres results in pupillary constriction, enophthalmos and ptosis (*Horner's syndrome*). In addition, sweating is impaired on that side of the face. These signs may occur in lesions of the brain stem such as syringobulbia and thrombosis of the posterior inferior cerebellar artery, in lesions of the cervical part of the spinal cord such as syringomyelia, and in lesions at the thoracic outlet such as bronchial carcinoma at the apex of the lung.

THE EPILEPSIES

An epileptic fit may be defined as a brief disorder of cerebral function, usually associated with a disturbance of consciousness, and accompanied by a sudden, excessive, electrical discharge of cerebral neurones. The electrical activity recorded by the electroencephalogram (EEG) is of high voltage relative to the background and results from an unphysiological, synchronous discharge of an aggregation of neurones.

The basic mechanism of epilepsy depends on a population of abnormal, hyperexcitable nerve cells. Such susceptible neurones are subject to excitatory and inhibitory influences from other sources. Excitatory chemical transmitters released from connecting nerve terminals tend to depolarise epileptic neuronal membranes; inhibitor transmitters lead to hyperpolarisation of membranes. The discharge of the abnormal group of cells is governed by the balance at a given time between these two opposing factors. Acetylcholine is an excitatory transmitter. Gamma-aminobutyric acid (GABA) is an inhibitory transmitter and hence has anticonvulsant properties.

Classification. Epilepsy may be generalised or partial (focal). Generalised seizures may be tonic-clonic (grand mal) or absences (petit mal).

In *generalised seizures* loss of consciousness is accompanied by symmetrically synchronous EEG discharges. It has been suggested that generalised fits originate in midline diencephalic areas. The site of the abnormal discharge could be in the cortex and the generalised manifestations occur because of rapid spread to brain stem structures leading to loss of consciousness and then to the secondary evocation of bilateral discharges over the hemispheres.

In *partial (focal) seizures* epileptic activity may remain localised to one part of one cerebral hemisphere, and consciousness may be preserved (simple partial seizure). If the epileptic discharge spreads to the opposite hemisphere via the midline structures, then consciousness is impaired (complex partial seizure). Sometimes partial seizures evolve to affect the whole cortex and a tonic-clonic seizure results (secondary generalisation).

Aetiology. In many, perhaps the majority, of cases, epilepsy arises from causes which at present cannot be identified. This large category of cryptogenic or idiopathic epilepsy includes many cases in which generalised fits first occur in children whose relatives are similarly affected but also includes many other patients without a family history or with atypical fits.

Any intracranial disease may give rise to epilepsy, either as a manifestation of an active pathological process or as a sequel thereof.

Important causes of 'symptomatic' epilepsy include cerebral tumours, head injuries and cerebrovascular disease.

Fits may occur as a result of disease elsewhere than in the brain. Hypoglycaemia, hyperglycaemia, uraemia, heart block, ingestion or sudden withdrawal of alcohol or drugs are but a few of the conditions which may evoke seizures. About 5% of patients with epilepsy are sensitive to light, e.g. flicker, and, in many of these, attacks are induced by watching television.

Clinical features. TONIC-CLONIC SEIZURES (grand mal). These fits conform to a stereotyped clinical pattern in which several stages may be recognised: (1) a *prodromal phase,* lasting hours or days, may warn the patient that an attack is impending. This is an occasional phenomenon and usually takes the form of a change of mood. (2) An *aura,* which is uncommon in grand mal fits. When it does occur, it is brief, usually being no more than an apprehension that a fit is about to happen or a 'feeling' in the epigastrium. An aura occurs if the seizure starts in one part of the cortex and then spreads; it is therefore an indication of secondary generalisation. (3) The *tonic stage,* which is an invariable part of a grand mal attack. At the onset of this stage the patient loses consciousness and, if upright, falls to the ground. A sustained, tonic spasm of all the musculature occurs and involves the respiratory muscles, so that air is forcibly expired through the partially closed glottis giving rise to a sound or 'cry'. This phase lasts 20 to 30 seconds and during this time respiratory movements are suspended so that cyanosis occurs. (4) A *clonic phase* in which the sustained tonic spasm gives place to interrupted powerful jerking movements of face, body and limbs. The movements of jaw and tongue cause saliva to froth in the mouth. This stage, also, lasts about half a minute. During the tonic and clonic stages the patient may bite and chew the tongue and may be incontinent of urine and, less often, of faeces. (5) The *stage of relaxation.* After movements cease, the patient lies in a flaccid comatose state which evolves into normal sleep. This phase often lasts only a few minutes but may be prolonged for half an hour or more. After regaining consciousness there is often a phase of variable duration wherein the patient is confused and may suffer from headache. Examination in the immediate postictal period often reveals extensor plantar responses.

ABSENCE SEIZURES (petit mal). The term petit mal is often used imprecisely. It is best restricted to those cases showing a characteristic EEG pattern, namely bilaterally synchronous spike and slow wave complexes occurring at a frequency of three per second. This pattern occurs with three types of clinical manifestation:

1. The most common variety of attack takes the form of a transient loss of consciousness. The patient interrupts current activity and may stare blankly ahead. The whole episode usually lasts only 10 to 15 seconds, and is so brief and undramatic that it may pass unnoticed. Such 'absences' may occur very frequently in childhood. Petit mal invariably starts in childhood but may persist into adult life. Sometimes the attacks cease during adolescence or give place to grand mal fits.

2. Less commonly the brief loss of consciousness is accompanied by myoclonic jerking of the arms.

3. The least common type of attack is the akinetic seizure in which the patient falls to the ground unconscious but recovers consciousness, and is able to rise again, almost immediately.

PARTIAL SEIZURES (focal epilepsy). Since there are many neuronal regions from which epileptic discharges may originate there are many clinical variations of focal fits. Any focal discharge may spread to become generalised, and initially localised clinical disturbances may progress to a grand mal fit. It is important, therefore, to establish the nature of the phenomena which occur at the onset of any form of seizure since these indicate the site of origin.

1. The *temporal lobe* is the commonest site of partial epilepsy. Most characteristic of the clinical manifestations are hallucinations of smell though these are uncommon; hallucinations of taste, hearing or sight also occur. Also indicative of temporal lobe fits are disturbances of memory including the *déjà vu* phenomenon. This refers to the patient's sensation of reliving an experience or a feeling of great familiarity with the environment. Sometimes these features are associated with intense emotional or mood changes.

Simple temporal lobe seizures consist of hallucination or *déjà vu* feelings without full loss of awareness. More often a complex partial seizure occurs and awareness is lost. Such attacks are usually more prolonged than absence seizures, and typically last 1–3 minutes. Occasionally the patient during this state will carry out well-coordinated and apparently purposeful motor acts, even of a violent or antisocial nature, without any memory of such activity thereafter (*automatism*). Temporal lobe discharges do not always give rise to such distinctive clinical features and an EEG may be required in order to reveal the temporal lobe origin of seizures.

2. *Jacksonian epilepsy* is a term best restricted to fits in which clinical disturbance of function, initially confined to a circumscribed part of the body, spreads to involve adjacent areas. There is a relatively slow 'march' of clinical events which reflects the spread of the electrical discharge to nearby cortical areas. Motor seizures usually take the form of involuntary twitching or clonic movements which begin in part of a limb, spread to involve the whole limb, then perhaps the whole of one side of the body or the involvement may even eventually become bilateral. The extent of the spread is highly variable. Consciousness may or may not be lost.

Sometimes after recovery from a Jacksonian fit, the parts affected remain paralysed. This is called a *Todd's palsy* and if prolonged for more than an hour or two suggests that there is a structural lesion in or near the cortical representation of the paralysed part.

Diagnosis. Observation of an episode by a trained person is the best and most certain method of diagnosis, but is rarely possible. A good description by, and cross-examination of, an eyewitness furnishes useful, and often conclusive evidence. The patient's own account of the attacks and the circumstances attendant upon them will sometimes give diagnostic information. The EEG is not a substitute for this type of clinical assessment nor can an EEG, recorded between attacks, alone establish or refute a diagnosis of epilepsy. The EEG may be helpful in supporting a clinical diagnosis and may be of great value in localising a cerebral cause of symptomatic epilepsy.

The yield of diagnostic EEG abnormalities can be increased with a prolonged recording time and inclusion of a period of natural or drug-induced sleep. In difficult cases with frequent clinical symptoms, prolonged simultaneous EEG and video monitoring or ambulatory EEG recording may establish the diagnosis.

After the diagnosis of epilepsy has been established the next stage is to attempt to determine its cause. In practice the most important aspect of this process is to recognise patients whose epilepsy is due to a structural or progressive lesion. Fits of recent onset, of focal nature, occurring in patients of middle age, would obviously suggest an underlying lesion, perhaps a tumour. Accompanying headache and neurological signs would strengthen such a suspicion. Fits occurring for the first time in the elderly are often due to cerebrovascular disease. They may be the result of infarction, but some are due to cerebral ischaemia secondary to cardiac arrhythmias in such conditions as the sick sinus syndrome (p. 130).

The history and examination will often furnish pointers to the aetiology of fits and hence to the need for special investigations. Blood tests to exclude syphilis, hypocalcaemia, hypoglycaemia and polycythaemia are worthwhile and an ECG should always be performed. Specialised radiological techniques such as CT scanning should be considered if the epilepsy presents after adolescence or if the history or EEG suggests a focal onset. Before embarking on more traumatic investigations, the need for such tests should be appraised in the light of the clinical features. In many instances observation of a patient over a period is the most valuable and least distressing course of action.

Treatment. The care of the patient comprises social and psychological as well as pharmacological aspects. Patients and their relatives and too many of the general public believe that epilepsy bears a stigma. Many patients are more socially disabled by feelings of bitterness and aggression engendered by society's rejection than by their fits. Simple, rational explanations of the nature and causes of seizures should be given.

Restrictions should be kept to a necessary minimum. Children, in particular, are often in danger of being overprotected by their parents, but until fits are well controlled it is unwise for children to cycle on public roads, nor should they swim alone.

An epileptic child should be educated at a normal school unless there is an intellectual deficit.

An adult should be guided into an occupation at which neither the patient nor the community is put at risk by a propensity to fits. Exposure to moving machinery and work at heights should be avoided. The legal restrictions about driving should be explained to patients. In Britain no one who has suffered from fits may drive a motor vehicle until free of attacks during waking hours for 2 years. If seizures have occurred exclusively during sleep for 3 years, driving may also be resumed. Continued treatment with antiepileptic drugs does not debar the patient from driving.

Note should be made of factors which precipitate attacks. Deprivation of sleep is an important factor. Some patients have fits only during sleep, or when they are pyrexial. Others recognise that certain sensory stimuli, such as flickering light or emotional disturbances, trigger their seizures.

During a fit the patient should be protected from injury. It will rarely be possible to break the fall during a grand mal attack because the warning is too short. The patient should be moved away from fires and sharp and hard objects. A padded gag should be inserted between the teeth if this can be accomplished without force. The incident should be treated with a minimum of fuss. Embarrassment because of public attention is usually the most distressing aspect of a fit from the patient's viewpoint.

ANTIEPILEPTIC DRUGS. These will usually be needed to control fits but a first seizure requires only investigation initially. Phenytoin, carbamazepine, sodium valproate, primidone and phenobarbitone are all effective in *tonic-clonic seizures,* and good control can be expected in more than 80% of cases. *Partial seizures* respond less well to any drug, but carbamazepine and phenytoin are probably best. The dosage needs to be tailored to the individual needs and responses of patients. Phenytoin and phenobarbitone have half-lives which are greater than 24 hours and can be given once daily. Carbamazepine and primidone should be given in divided doses twice or thrice daily. An average daily dose, for an adult, of phenytoin is 200 to 400 mg, and of phenobarbitone 60 to 120 mg daily. Primidone is given in a dosage between 750 and 1500 mg daily and carbamazepine between 600 and 1800 mg daily. Sodium valproate (400–3000 mg/d) can adequately be given twice a day.

Hepatic metabolism of antiepileptic drugs varies because of genetic differences, and when possible, their levels in the blood should be monitored (Table 21.7, p. 818) so that the patients can be adequately treated and toxic effects avoided. It is better to use one drug, rather than a combination; if a single drug does not control fits a different agent should be substituted and at least three single drugs tried before combinations are used. Phenytoin may be combined with phenobarbitone or carbamazepine, though, because of induced hepatic enzymes, the serum level of phenytoin may be reduced when it is given concurrently with carbamazepine. Primidone and phenobarbitone should not be given together, since primidone is partially converted into phenobarbitone.

All of these drugs may cause drowsiness; they may also cause rickets or osteomalacia (p. 65) and folate deficiency resulting in megaloblastic anaemia. Phenytoin also gives rise to gingival hyperplasia in children and coarsening of features in adults. Rarer toxic effects of phenytoin include lymphadenopathy and a syndrome mimicking systemic lupus erythematosus.

All of these drugs have some teratogenic effect which is probably most marked with phenytoin. Until more is known about the teratogenic risks of antiepileptic drugs, carbamazepine or sodium valproate are preferable to phenytoin or phenobarbitone for the treatment of epilepsy in women in the reproductive years. The risk to the fetus is less than from uncontrolled seizures, so it is advisable not to change anticonvulsants during pregnancy.

After the patient has been free from epilepsy for at least 2 years, antiepileptic therapy can be gradually withdrawn in many cases.

Absence seizures (petit mal). Ethosuximide and sodium valproate are the most useful drugs in this condition. Ethosuximide (500–1500 mg/d) can be given twice a day. It has no effect on tonic-clonic seizures, so if these are also present, sodium valproate is the drug of choice. Ethosuximide occasionally causes nausea, drowsiness and, rarely, leucopenia. Sodium valproate may act partly by inhibiting breakdown of gamma-aminobutyric acid (GABA), thereby increasing neuronal inhibition. Valproate usually causes little sedation, but tremor, hair loss, anorexia, nausea and weight gain are fairly common. Very rarely, fatal hepatic necrosis has occurred, usually within the first 6 months of therapy. It is wise to check liver function tests regularly over this period.

Status epilepticus. This refers to a continuous succession of fits occurring without any period of recovery of consciousness. Status epilepticus may be fatal if not rapidly controlled. It is commoner in childhood and in patients who have intracranial lesions but it may occur in all types of epilepsy if medication is irregular or is suddenly withdrawn.

Treatment should be prompt and energetic since status epilepticus constitutes a grave emergency. Adequate respiration must be maintained and the fits suppressed. Intravenous diazepam is probably the most useful drug for the control of status epilepticus. Initially 10 mg should be injected intravenously and this should be repeated at 5-minute intervals until the fits are controlled; thereafter the drug is given by slow intravenous infusion (no faster than 2 mg/min). Intravenous diazepam may impair respiration and cause hypotension; it should be used only when facilities for cardiopulmonary resuscitation are available.

If diazepam fails to control seizures, intravenous chlormethiazole (0.5–1.2 g/h) or phenytoin (intravenously no faster than 50 mg/min up to a total loading dose of 18 mg/kg) should be tried. In resistant cases an intravenous infusion of thiopentone is usually effective, but this often brings with it the need for artificial ventilation. Bedside EEG and ECG monitoring greatly facilitate the management of this dangerous condition.

Narcolepsy

This is characterised by irresistible attacks of sleep from which, however, the patient can be aroused immediately. Several attacks may occur in a day. Narcolepsy is associated with three other phenomena; (1) *cataplexy,* in which, as a result of a sudden emotion, power is lost from the limbs, though consciousness is preserved; (2) *sleep paralysis,* in which on waking or falling asleep the patient is unable to move though mentally wide awake; (3) *hallucinatory states,* in which vivid and terrifying hallucinations occur, often just as the patient is falling asleep. This related group of symptoms is believed to be due to a disorder of that part of the brain stem reticular formation responsible for REM sleep. A characteristic feature is for the sufferer to pass directly from waking into rapid eye movement sleep (REM-onset sleep). In most cases no abnormality can be demonstrated in the nervous system. The disorder is strongly associated with HLA-DR2, and also occasionally with multiple sclerosis. An autoimmune mechanism has been postulated, but is unproven.

Dexamphetamine sulphate (5–10 mg b.d.) or methylphenidate hydrochloride (10 mg b.d.) reduces the frequency and intensity of narcolepsy. Cataplexy often responds dramatically to treatment with a tricyclic antidepressant such as clomipramine (25–50 mg t.i.d.).

CEREBRAL TUMOURS

Intracranial tumours account for 2% of deaths at all ages. Neoplasms classified histologically as malignant and benign occur but the implications of these categories differ from those in other sites. Since they grow within the rigid confines of the skull all types of neoplasm may cause disability and death by impinging on and displacing the cranial contents. The clinical features produced by an intracranial tumour depend primarily on its site of origin and its rate of growth. The histological characteristics of tumours offer a guide to rapidity of growth and to the possibility of complete removal.

Pathology. Malignant cerebral tumours rarely give rise to extracerebral metastases, but approximately a half of all brain tumours are secondary deposits from carcinoma elsewhere, particularly in bronchus and breast.

Gliomas. Of primary cerebral tumours those derived from glial cells are the commonest, accounting for a quarter of all cerebral tumours. Gliomas vary in cellular type, in degrees of malignancy and in rates of growth. An astrocytoma Grade 1 is a slow-growing, infiltrative tumour which may spread widely throughout the brain, sometimes for years, before causing serious disability. A Grade 4 astrocytoma (also called a glioblastoma multiforme) is a highly malignant, fast-growing tumour causing rapid clinical deterioration. Other glial tumours such as oligo-dendroglioma and ependymoma are graded from 1 to 4 as the degree of malignancy increases. Medulloblastoma occurs most commonly in children, arises usually in the cerebellar vermis, and is almost always highly malignant. Gliomas can rarely be completed excised.

Meningiomas comprise approximately one-fifth of intracranial tumours. They are almost always benign, encapsulated, attached to the dura mater and, in the majority of instances, completely removable. Their common sites of origin are the convexities of the hemispheres, the sphenoidal ridges, the suprasellar region and the olfactory groove.

Less common tumours. Craniopharyngiomas (p. 428), adenomas of the pituitary gland (p. 427) and neuromas from the sheaths of the eighth and fifth cranial nerves are benign and potentially curable. Cerebral lesions resembling tumours also occur in sarcoidosis, cysticercosis, echinococcosis (as hydatid cysts), and in schistosomiasis. Tuberculoma is still common in underdeveloped countries.

Intraventricular tumours are rare but colloid cysts of the third ventricle and papillomas of the choroid plexus can cause raised intracranial pressure and are removable.

Clinical features. Primary brain tumours occur at all ages with a maximal incidence in the fifth decade. Medulloblastomas are commonest in children. Acoustic neuromas usually present in the third and fourth decades. Glioblastomas and meningiomas are commonest in middle life. In general brain tumours in children are situated in the posterior fossa and in those over 30, supratentorial tumours account for 85% of cerebral neoplasms.

Cerebral tumours produce symptoms and signs by their local effects and by causing alterations in intracranial pressure and hydrodynamics.

FEATURES DUE TO LOCAL INVOLVEMENT. The local effects of a tumour on adjacent cerebral tissue may cause paralysis of function and/or excitatory effects. The neural deficits produced by a neoplasm are dependent on the site of origin of the tumour. Lesions in the various lobes of the brain can cause the types of dysfunction outlined on pages 603–604. Vascular lesions affecting these structures cause similar disturbances but differ in the rapidity of their development.

In general the focal disabilities produced by a tumour are of slow onset and are progressive. The rate of this progression is highly variable and depends on the rate of growth of the tumour and its nearness to neural structures whose interruption evokes clinical signs. Occasionally localised oedema in the brain tissue surrounding a tumour will cause a rapid progression of paralytic symptoms and the picture thus produced may mimic a cerebrovascular lesion. Sometimes, too, the initial manifestations of a metastatic tumour are of sudden onset, followed by a period of improvement. Rarely, haemorrhage into a tumour causes an acute presentation resembling a stroke.

In addition to local paralytic effects the infiltration by tumour cells of an area of cerebral cortex often evokes excitatory responses in neighbouring neurones. Thus a discharging epileptic focus may be a manifestation of a cerebral tumour. The nature of the seizure depends on the site of origin of the epileptic discharge and the extent of its propagation. Focal epilepsy beginning in adult life should always suggest the possibility of a tumour.

Headache is a common, but not invariable manifestation of cerebral tumour. The tumour mass tends to distort and exert traction on nearby arteries, venous sinuses or meninges which are pain sensitive structures. Headache is often localised to one area of the cranium and its site offers a rough guide to the location of the tumour. In general headache is felt on the same side as the neoplasm. Tumours which lie in the anterior and middle cranial fossae are often attended by headaches situated in front of a line joining the ears. Posterior fossa tumours usually cause headaches which are felt over the occiput or nuchal area. There are many exceptions to these generalisations. Headache also commonly accompanies an increase in intracranial pressure; its features are discussed below.

FEATURES DUE TO INCREASED INTRACRANIAL PRESSURE. Since cerebral tumours occupy space within the rigid skull they may cause an increase in pressure within the cranium. The liability of tumours to do this varies and several mechanisms may be involved. The mass of the tumour itself, if large enough, will cause a rise in pressure due to relative incompressibility of the brain. Slowly growing tumours may achieve large size before there is any rise in pressure whereas a highly malignant and rapidly growing tumour, though relatively small, may cause early changes.

Raised intracranial pressure may also result from obstruction to the flow of cerebrospinal fluid. Subtentorial tumours are particularly liable to do this but even supratentorial lesions may cause obstruction between the third and fourth ventricles. Tumours of the temporal lobe may compress the third ventricle.

Tumours lying within the ventricles themselves may cause a sudden rise in intracranial pressure in the absence of focal neurological abnormalities. Increased pressure may also occur as a result of cerebral oedema or from obstruction of the cerebral venous system by malignant tissue impairing the absorption of CSF. Whichever of these mechanisms is operative the end result is a rise in pressure within the skull causing similar clinical features.

Headache is an almost invariable accompaniment of increased intracranial pressure; the pain is felt diffusely over the head and is aggravated by manoeuvres which cause a further rise in intracranial pressure. Thus headache is intensified by bending, coughing and straining at stool. Such headaches often tend to be particularly troublesome on waking in the morning when the patient is lying flat and to be relieved to some extent by standing upright and moving about, since this causes a fall in intracranial pressure.

Clouding of consciousness occurs, varying in degree from listlessness and drowsiness to near coma, depending on the level of the raised pressure and the rapidity of its attainment. During the early stages there may be behavioural and personality changes with apathy and irritability, or withdrawal and inattention, predominating.

Generalised epileptic fits are commonly produced by raised intracranial pressure from tumours at any site.

Dizziness is complained of by many patients with increased intracranial pressure. This may take the form of true rotatory vertigo or of sensations of light-headedness or unsteadiness. Such feelings of instability are often produced or aggravated by head movement.

Papilloedema is one of the most significant signs of raised intracranial pressure. It may be of insidious onset and slow progression but often a sudden rise in pressure due to cerebral oedema or obstructive hydrocephalus causes the rapid development of papilloedema attended by haemorrhages radiating out from the optic disc.

The amount of visual disturbance produced by papilloedema is variable. Often there is little change in the visual acuity but the production of transient blurring of vision when the patient stoops or bends is characteristic. Such episodes (visual obscurations) may also cause transient loss of colour vision and are a symptom of seriously raised intracranial pressure which may damage the optic nerve permanently if not treated urgently.

Swelling of the optic nerve head is usually bilateral but may be unilateral in the early stages. When the underlying lesion has caused optic atrophy in one eye papilloedema occurs only in the other eye. Such is the case sometimes with tumours of the inferior surface of a frontal lobe which compress the adjacent optic nerve causing optic atrophy; as the tumour grows in size raised intracranial pressure supervenes and papilloedema occurs in the other eye. This is known as the *Foster Kennedy syndrome*.

Vomiting, progressive *bradycardia* and arterial *hypertension* occur as the intracranial pressure continues to rise.

Brain displacements. The rise in intracranial pressure does not necessarily occur evenly over the whole of the cerebral contents and sudden alterations in pressure relationships within the skull may lead to displacement of parts of the brain. Large supratentorial lesions may cause herniation of the hippocampal gyrus and the upper brain stem downwards through the incisura of the tentorium. This not only causes damage to the hippocampal gyrus itself but may also lead to compression of the cerebral peduncles, occlusion of the posterior cerebral artery and stretching of cranial nerves, particularly the sixth.

These developments can cause *false localising signs* which may lead to erroneous localisation of the tumour. Commonest of these is the sixth nerve palsy occurring on the side of the lesion or bilaterally. The third nerve may similarly be involved and occasionally the fourth nerve is also implicated. The cerebral peduncle on the side opposite the tumour may be compressed giving rise to upper motor neurone signs on the side of the lesion. Compression of the posterior cerebral artery may lead to a homonymous hemianopia or quadrantanopia (Fig. 15.4).

Very rapid downward movement of the brain stem may lead to haemorrhage in the midbrain with coma and death. Another form of herniation or 'pressure cone' is the downward movement of the cerebellar tonsils so that they impact within the foramen magnum thus compressing the medulla. This may lead to further aggravation of raised intracranial pressure since the onward passage of cerebrospinal fluid into the spinal subarachnoid space is blocked. Such an event is often manifest by loss of consciousness and the rapid development of palsies of the sixth and third nerves with dilatation of the pupil on the side of the lesion being followed by dilatation on the opposite side. Frequently when a medullary pressure cone has occurred the patient takes up a decerebrate posture, at first intermittently. These developments almost invariably lead to death.

Such brain displacements and pressure cones may occur spontaneously because of increased cerebral oedema or some other alteration in cerebral haemodynamics caused by the tumour's growth but are particularly liable to be produced if the closed CSF system is disturbed by lumbar puncture.

Investigation of cerebral tumours should, in most instances, begin with simple and non-traumatic procedures including radiography of the skull and chest followed by one of the imaging methods described on page 607. Some tumours will be demonstrable by radionuclide scanning, but CT and MRI scanners are considerably more sensitive for the detection of small lesions, and in addition provide information on the cerebral ventricular system. Cerebral angiography is often performed to define the tumour circulation.

Treatment. MEDICAL MANAGEMENT of tumours can never be anything more than temporary or palliative. Relief of raised intracranial pressure is often required when surgery is not available or when life is threatened before investigation has revealed the diagnosis. This can best be achieved by the administration of dexamethasone 4 mg four times daily, initially given by injection and later by mouth; striking improvement in a patient's conscious level is often produced and sometimes regression of focal disabilities. In severe and acutely raised intracerebral pressure, a larger dose of dexamethasone (e.g. 16–20 mg) may be given intravenously. In such a situation, a rapid but transient reduction in intracranial pressure may be achieved with an intravenous infusion of 200 ml of a 20% solution of the osmotic agent mannitol. Both methods are often used simultaneously.

Cytotoxic drugs, such as cyclophosphamide, administered either systemically or through a carotid artery, offer little more than temporary palliation.

SURGERY is the definitive treatment of intracranial tumours. When possible the whole of a tumour should be excised but complete removal of the tumour depends on a number of factors. The tumour may be inaccessible and thus its exposure may be attended by unacceptable brain damage. It may invade areas where excision of small amounts of tissue may cause major disability as is particularly likely to happen in the brain stem or in areas of the dominant hemisphere.

Meningiomas and neuromas offer the best prospects for complete removal without unacceptable damage to vital structures. Meningiomas can usually be totally excised and rarely is there any recurrence. Meningiomas of the olfactory groove, those in the suprasellar area and those over the convexity of the hemispheres have a particularly favourable prognosis. Often, meningiomas of the inner part of the sphenoidal ridge and within the cerebello-pontine angles cannot be completely removed but their partial excision results in long continued improvement. Even after a successful removal of a meningioma, a number of patients may develop recurrent fits.

Craniopharyngiomas can sometimes be completely removed but often the proximity of the hypothalamus prevents this. Pituitary adenomas can usually be extirpated and, even when only incomplete excision is possible, further visual loss is prevented.

Colloid cysts of the third ventricle and other intraventricular neoplasms can often be removed but sometimes their complete excision is technically very difficult.

Gliomas. Malignant gliomas cannot be removed completely, though favourably situated tumours may benefit markedly for a time from partial removal. Less malignant, slow growing tumours such as Grade 2 astrocytomas and oligodendrogliomas, though they can rarely be completely excised, may benefit for many years from partial removal. The prognosis for cystic astrocytoma is particularly good if the cyst is drained and as much as possible of the tumour removed. Medulloblastoma of the cerebellar vermis, found in childhood, cannot be excised completely and surgery produces little improvement.

Palliative surgery may have a place when complete excision of a tumour cannot be attempted. Partial removal or drainage of a cyst is often of benefit. Decompression and hence relief of raised intracranial pressure may be produced by removing part of the tumour, or even by excising normal brain tissue in the frontal or temporal lobes. Removal of part of the skull vault is also effective in reducing pressure. Internal hydrocephalus may be relieved by a short-circuiting procedure in which a drain is placed in one of the lateral ventricles and led into the cisterna magna or peritoneal cavity.

RADIOTHERAPY may improve survival in cases where total surgical removal of the tumour is not feasible. Some tumours (e.g. medulloblastoma and microglioma) are very radio-sensitive. However, radiation damage, both acute and late, may ensue and cause further disability.

Prognosis. The precise surgical approach and the prognosis for a cerebral tumour can be assessed only in the light of its site, its pathological nature, its blood supply and the degree of disability it causes. Early treatment is particularly important for those tumours which are susceptible to complete removal and which menace life or sight. Early diagnosis of acoustic neuromas and pituitary tumours markedly improves the outlook for their treatment.

Death is inevitable if a malignant tumour can not be removed, though it may be postponed by palliative decompression; even so, the average expectation of life is less than 6 months in the case of the more malignant growths. Benign tumours can be removed completely if they grow in an accessible part of the brain, as can gliomas, or even a solitary metastatic tumour, when they are in a part of the brain such as the frontal lobe or cerebellum which can be sacrificed with relative impunity. Some very low-grade gliomas grow so slowly and permeate the brain so widely that surgical intervention will not improve the duration or quality of survival.

HYDROCEPHALUS

Hydrocephalus denotes an excessive amount of CSF within the cranial cavity. It may be a consequence of atrophy of the brain parenchyma, which results in passive dilatation of the ventricles; it is then called compensatory hydrocephalus. Rarely hydrocephalus may result from oversecretion of CSF by a papilloma of the choroid plexus.

Much more commonly hydrocephalus is caused by obstruction to the CSF circulation or to a failure of absorption. Obstruction may occur anywhere within the ventricular system due to an intraventricular tumour or from extrinsic compression by a space-occupying lesion or oedema. The narrow channels in the third ventricle, aqueduct and fourth ventricle are particularly likely to be occluded. Inflammatory exudate may block the foramina in the fourth ventricular roof or occlude the subarachnoid space. Absorption through the arachnoid villi may be prevented by thrombosis of the sagittal sinus.

In normal-pressure hydrocephalus the ventricular system is dilated, initially from an obstruction to flow due to trauma, meningitis, or other cause. The initial lesion subsides. It is postulated that the force exerted outwards on the brain is proportional to the surface area of the ventricles. These having been dilated, the force exerted on the brain, by fluid at normally innocuous pressure, is increased. The brain atrophies and the conditions for progressive centricular dilatation and cerebral atrophy are established. Dementia and ataxia result. An operation which reduces CSF pressure by a shunt from a lateral ventricle to the superior vena cava sometimes improves the patient's dementia and ataxia.

HEADACHE

Headache is a term which literally describes pain felt anywhere in the head. Custom usually restricts its usage to pains in the region of the cranial vault; facial pain and nuchal pains are excluded, but the lines of demarcation are vague and overlapping.

Headache poses certainly the commonest, probably the most ambiguous and sometimes the most difficult clinical problem in medicine. It has a multiplicity of causes but is produced by relatively few mechanisms. In the vast majority of cases the cause is trivial and reversible but in a few patients headache presages sinister intracranial disease.

The extracranial coverings and arteries are sensitive to pain. Within the cranial cavity there are few pain sensitive structures. The brain parenchyma, pia-arachnoid, ventricular linings and choroid plexuses are insensitive. Pain can be evoked from the venous sinuses, the arteries and the dura mater at the base of the brain. Displacement and distortion of these structures, particularly if rapid, cause headache. The fifth, ninth and tenth cranial nerves contain pain fibres and direct compression of these nerves produces pain.

Clinical features. Pain in the head may be due to lesions in nearby structures, such as the eye and ear, causing referred headache; it may be due to the cranial neuralgias, meningeal irritation, vascular disturbances, traction and distortion of intracranial structures, or to psychogenic causes.

REFERRED HEADACHES. Eye diseases such as glaucoma and iritis cause frontal headache. Ciliary spasm induced by some errors of refraction may cause pain but 'eye strain' is certainly not a common cause of headache. Nasal and sinus disease causes pain in the malar, nasal and frontal areas which responds to vasoconstriction in the form of nasal drops. Dental and aural conditions may cause pain spreading far beyond the area of primary pain. Occipital headaches occasionally result from severe cervical spondylosis. A cold stimulus on the soft palate in some people evokes a dull, frontal headache (ice-cream headache).

CRANIAL NEURALGIAS. The episodic, lancinating pain of trigeminal neuralgia (p. 611) and the continuous, burning pain of postherpetic neuralgia (p. 645), both occurring within the distribution of the fifth cranial nerve, present well-defined and usually easily-recognised entities.

Glossopharyngeal neuralgia is less common and is characterised by pain, usually of a stabbing character, felt in the pharynx and deep in the ear. The pain occurs in bouts and may be triggered by swallowing or talking. It responds to treatment similar to that given for trigeminal neuralgia.

Temporomandibular neuralgia arises as a result of derangement of the temporomandibular joint secondary to an alteration of the bite caused by loss of teeth, ill-fitting dentures or habitual overclosure of the jaws because of tension. Pain which varies from a dull ache to intense stabs may radiate from the region of the affected joint to the temporal and frontal areas, the cheek, lower jaw and occasionally the neck. In malocclusion, a prosthetic device to prevent overclosure of the jaw is a simple and usually effective treatment.

MENINGEAL IRRITATION. Headache is an almost invariable accompaniment of encephalitis and meningitis. It is probable that meningeal inflammation lowers the pain threshold of the pain-sensitive structures at the base of the brain so that minor mechanical stimuli produce headache. The headache is usually generalised though it may be more intense in the occipital region, is of a continuous aching or boring character and is frequently associated with photophobia and drowsiness. The pain is increased by exertion and even by minor movements of the head; the accompanying pyrexia and neck stiffness usually make the diagnosis obvious.

Blood in the CSF due to subarachnoid haemorrhage produces headaches and neck rigidity similar to those of meningitis, but the pain in this condition is characteristically of abrupt and even explosive onset and may be accompanied by loss of consciousness.

VASCULAR HEADACHES. These are almost always described as throbbing in character and are aggravated by head movements. They may arise from dilatation of the intracranial or extracranial arteries after overindulgence in alcohol, in fever and in the hypercapnia of respiratory failure. Severe arterial hypertension may cause headaches in the early morning. In the elderly, localised temporal headache may be due to cranial arteritis.

Migraine (see below) is the commonest form of vascular headache. A migranous variant, '*cluster*' *headache* (migrainous neuralgia), presents a distinctive picture, which is unilateral, intense and brief. Attacks last usually 20–60 minutes, but recur one or more times daily for a period of days or weeks, and then there is often a prolonged period of freedom, hence the name 'cluster'. The pain is usually severe and burning, primarily involves the frontal region and the eye but often spreads to the face and sometimes to the neck. It occurs most commonly in young males, characteristically wakes patients from sleep and is often accompanied by flushing of the skin, nasal congestion, epiphora and injection of the conjunctival vessels. The attacks are too brief to respond to acute treatment, and management is based on prevention. Alcohol and vasodilating drugs should be avoided. Ergotamine tartrate may prevent attacks if given rectally or by inhalation, but is not effective by mouth. Propranolol and pizotifen (see below) are sometimes helpful, but lithium carbonate (250–500 mg t.i.d.) is particularly useful in resistant cases.

Rare causes of vascular headaches include saccular aneurysms and arteriovenous malformations (p. 633).

HEADACHES DUE TO TRACTION ON INTRACRANIAL STRUCTURES. Headaches may occur in the presence of an expanding intracranial lesion such as cerebral tumour or subdural haematoma whether or not there is a generalised rise in intracranial pressure (p. 621).

Traction headache due to reduced CSF pressure may occur after lumbar puncture; patients tend to develop their symptoms when standing or sitting and a recumbent posture produces rapid relief. Traction headaches, whether produced by raised or lowered intracranial pressure, are usually aggravated by bending, straining at stool and coughing.

Benign intracranial hypertension is a rare condition usually occurring in obese women. It causes traction headaches unassociated with any space-occupying lesion. Restoration of normal weight may be curative.

TENSION HEADACHE. This is probably the commonest cause. The pain is variable in severity and site. Its quality may be described as 'dull', 'pressing', 'tight' and 'stabbing'. The site may be frontal, bitemporal, parietal or occipital and the pain tends to get worse towards the end of the day or during periods of stress. Although muscle contraction may be responsible, it is likely that vasoconstriction in muscle is also involved. Many sufferers can identify psychological or physical stress factors and some are suffering from an anxiety state or depression. Simple analgesics are often ineffective and muscle relaxation by anxiolytic or antidepressant drugs or psychological methods of stress management are more helpful.

Investigation and treatment. The extent and nature of investigations to be employed are determined by the history. Non-traumatic procedures such as radiographs of chest and skull and computed tomography should precede more traumatic investigations. A detailed history followed by a meticulous examination will help not only to clarify the diagnosis but will also be therapeutic in patients suffering from psychogenic headache. Reassurance and explanation after careful clinical assessment of these patients is often more effective than analgesics.

Migraine

Migraine is characterised by periodic headaches which are typically unilateral and are often associated with visual disturbance and vomiting. A classification is given in Table 15.1.

Table 15.1 Classification of principal forms of migraine.

Classical migraine	Visual or sensory symptoms precede or accompany the headache.
Common migraine	No visual or sensory features. Headache, nausea, vomiting, photophobia
Basilar artery migraine	Occipital headache preceded by vertigo, diplopia, dysarthria, ± visual and sensory symptoms. Sometimes loss of consciousness
Hemiplegic migraine	Prolonged headache lasting hours or days, followed by hemiparesis which recovers slowly over several days

Pathogenesis. There is now good evidence that, in classical migraine, there is focal cerebral oligaemia at the onset of the attack. This is often occipital in site, but may spread to the parietal and temporal lobes. Oligaemia may be secondary to some primary cortical dysfunction, since attacks can be set of by neural stimuli (e.g. bright light or strong odours). Others believe that vasospasm is responsible for the initial dysfunction. During the headache phase, there is dilatation and oedema of extracranial arteries, and probably some alteration in pain sensitivity in their walls. These vascular changes may be due to fluctuations in blood 5-hydroxytryptamine levels.

There is a genetic predisposition; approximately three-quarters of patients who suffer from migraine have close relatives similarly affected.

Migrainous attacks may be precipitated by a variety of factors such as menstruation, flashing lights, stress and anxiety. Cheese, chocolate, sherry and red wine are common precipitants and are all rich in tyramine, experimental ingestion of which will often promote an attack. Reserpine, which liberates 5-hydroxytryptamine (serotinin) in the brain, can also cause migraine. It is of interest that some serotonin antagonists are helpful in treatment. The significance of these findings is not clear but it seems likely that, in some and perhaps many instances, migraine is mediated by one or more biochemical disturbances.

Clinical features. The condition usually starts after puberty and continues until late middle life. Attacks occur at intervals which vary from a few days to several months. They last from a few hours to several days and leave the patient weak and exhausted.

In classical migraine premonitory symptoms are associated with focal cerebral oligaemia. There is commonly a sensation of white or coloured lights, scintillating spots, wavy lines, or defects in the visual fields. Paraesthesiae or weakness of one half of the body may be experienced or there may be numbness of both hands and around the mouth. These symptoms may last up to half an hour, and are followed by headache which usually begins in one spot and subsequently involves the whole of one side of the head; this may be the same or the side opposite to the visual or sensory symptoms. The side affected is not constant with each attack and the headache often becomes bilateral. The pain is usually severe and throbbing and is associated with vomiting, photophobia, pallor, sweating and prostration which may necessitate the patient taking to bed in a darkened room.

Variants are shown in Table 15.1 and cluster headache is described on page 625. Rare cases of headache resembling migraine are caused by a cerebral aneurysm or angioma ('symptomatic migraine'). In these cases the pain is unilateral and usually associated with focal signs.

Treatment. An attentive physician, a carefully recorded history and a meticulous examination followed by a full explanation of the nature and phenomena of migraine often relieves the patient's anxiety about the possibly sinister significance of the headache. These simple measures are themselves effective therapy as is the physician's continuing interest in the patient's well-being. Neither the patient's personality nor the stresses and strains of life can be altered, but such trigger factors as bright lights, oral contraception and dietary precipitants can be avoided.

Acute attacks of common migraine usually respond to soluble aspirin (600–900 mg) or paracetamol (1 g) with or without an antinauseant such as metaclopramide or prochlorperazine. In classical migraine, ergotamine tartrate, 0.5–1.0 mg sublingually, rectally or by inhaler, may abort the headache phase if taken as soon as visual or sensory symptoms are felt. Ergotamine itself causes nausea and vomiting, and many patients cannot tolerate it. Excessive use may lead to vasospasm and, paradoxically, headache. No more than 12 mg should be given in a week, and it is contraindicated in pregnancy, ischaemic heart disease and peripheral vascular disorders.

If migraine attacks occur frequently enough to disrupt work and social life (e.g. weekly), then drug prophylaxis is justified. Useful agents are propranolol (40–80 mg t.i.d.), and pizotifen (1.5–3 mg nocte). Antidepressants such as amitriptyline (25–100 mg nocte) may also be helpful. All these agents have some blocking activity on 5-HT receptors, and in resistant cases methysergide (1–2 mg t.i.d.) is often effective. This is a potent 5-HT antagonist and can cause retroperitoneal fibrosis with prolonged use; it should be given for courses of only 3 months and renal function should be carefully monitored.

CEREBROVASCULAR DISEASES

Intracranial vascular lesions are the third commonest cause of death in Western countries. The pithy and commonly used term 'stroke' describes the sudden neurological defect that often ensues. The annual incidence of strokes of various types is more than 1% in those over 65 years old. In every 1000 of the population in any one year, two people will suffer an initial stroke and one will die from a stroke. The high morbidity caused by cerebrovascular disease in the elderly is reflected in the large number of hospital beds occupied by such patients.

Despite the prevalence of the problem and its high cost in economic terms as well as human disability, cerebrovascular disease claimed, until recently, less attention and study than some rarer conditions. Diagnoses of 'cerebrovascular accident' or 'stroke' without specification are still common. Such imprecision in assessment leads to vagueness about prognosis and apathy in treatment. Conversely, attempts rigidly to link patterns of clinical disability to blockage of individual cerebral arterial branches have been shown to be simplistic and often misleading as well as therapeutically unrewarding.

Knowledge of the natural history of intracranial vascular disease is still incomplete. Cerebrovascular disease may be due to lesions of veins and capillaries as well as arteries but the latter are much the commonest. Arterial lesions can logically be divided into two main groups: (1) ischaemic cerebral lesions due to reduced perfusion of brain tissue by blood and often resulting in infarction; (2) haemorrhagic lesions in the brain or in the spaces between the brain and skull. Pathological studies indicate that 80–85% of acute strokes are due to cerebral infarction. This division into ischaemic and haemorrhagic lesions is pathologically clear and although clinical differentiation is often difficult the two processes should be discussed separately.

1. ISCHAEMIC CEREBRAL LESIONS

Cerebral ischaemia may be caused by atherosclerosis, embolism, arteritis, arteriospasm or hypotension, alone or in combination, and result in infarction manifest clinically as a stroke, transient ischaemic attacks or dementia.

General considerations. Approximately a fifth of the cardiac output at rest normally passes through the carotid and vertebral arteries to supply intracranial structures. A reduction in total cerebral blood flow to less than half of normal will impair cerebral function.

Occlusion of a cerebral artery usually, but not necessarily, leads to infarction in the tissue it supplies. A system of anastomoses and collateral channels affords a safety mechanism. The circle of Willis (Fig. 15.5) usually provides wide connecting channels between the two carotid arteries and the vertebrobasilar system. Perforating branches from the major cerebral arteries and from the circle of Willis pass through the brain to anastomose with capillaries derived from other branches of the anterior, middle and posterior cerebral arteries which ramify over the surface of the hemispheres and penetrate through the cortex. A similar anastomosis between centrifugal and centripetal twigs is found in the brain stem where the vertebral and basilar arteries give off penetrating and circumferential branches. At the junctions between their areas of supply the anterior cerebral artery anastomoses with the middle cerebral artery which in turn anastomoses with posterior cerebral branches. There are also collateral channels between the internal and external carotid circulations through their orbital branches.

These alternative routes of blood supply to the brain mean that the effects of impaired cerebral flow are determined by complex factors. Systemic hypotension tends first to produce ischaemia in the border zones between the anterior, middle and posterior cerebral arteries. Variations in this pattern occur if, in addition to generally reduced brain perfusion, there is a local blockage in one of the branches of the three major vessels.

If one internal carotid artery is occluded in the neck there is an immediate increase in flow through the other carotid artery. Young adults who sustain a blockage within one of the four major arterial trunks may manifest no ill-effects. However, the occlusion of one of these arteries in the neck in the presence of widespread arterial disease (a likely accompaniment in the elderly) may give rise to extensive infarction. The compensatory mechanisms are less effective more distally and occlusion of one of the deep penetrating branches arising from the circle of Willis often produces infarction of predictable extent.

The effects of any arterial obstruction depend, in part, upon the rate of its development. Sudden blockage is more likely to produce infarction than is the gradual reduction of an arterial lumen which allows time for collateral channels to open.

Reduced blood flow is often attributed to arterial spasm. Cerebral vasoconstriction occurs in young people and is responsible for transient cerebral dysfunction in migraine and may, in this condition, rarely lead to infarction. Spasm also occurs if cerebral arteries are manipulated during craniotomy and as a result of irritation after a subarachnoid haemorrhage or during angiography. There is, however, no evidence that arterial spasm plays any significant part in the production of ischaemia in elderly patients suffering from cerebrovascular disease.

Atherosclerosis is by far the commonest cause of reduced blood flow, thrombosis, embolism and arterial occlusion. Other causes are embolism from the heart and arteritis due to syphilis, SLE or giant cell inflammation.

Cerebral atherosclerosis

Atheromatous changes in cerebral arteries are almost invariable findings in people over 60 years old, but even quite extensive atheroma is commonly symptomless. Atheromatous plaques may cause narrowing (stenosis) or may lead to thrombosis and occlusion of arteries. Fibrin, platelet and lipid emboli may arise from such plaques in the proximal vessels including the aorta and be carried distally in the cerebral circulation eventually to impact in small vessels. These mechanisms can cause localised ischaemia or infarction or a generalised, progressive loss of brain tissue.

Aetiology. There is an association between cerebrovascular disease and ischaemic heart disease. In those patients who suffer an attack of transient cerebral ischaemia more people die from myocardial infarction than from cerebral infarction. Atheroma and thrombosis are related to both conditions. Despite this association the risk factors of cerebrovascular disease are not as well understood as those in myocardial ischaemia and there are notable discrepancies between the two. Genetic predisposition, hyperlipidaemia and diabetes seem to be much less important factors in

cerebral than in myocardial infarction. Cigarette smoking and obesity have been clearly linked to an increased incidence of coronary arterial disease but not to liability to strokes. Hypertension is a factor which seems strongly to predispose to both. Polycythaemia also increases the risk of stroke.

Clinical features. Symptoms are rare before the age of 40 years, and uncommon before 50. The clinical presentations comprise (1) completed stroke, i.e. rapid onset of focal cerebral dysfunction, with symptoms persisting more than 24 hours, (2) developing stroke, i.e. a relatively slow, or step-wise, extension of an infarct — sometimes called a stroke-in-evolution, (3) transient ischaemic attacks, i.e. acute onset of focal cerebral dysfunction, with symptoms lasting less than 24 hours, (4) progressive, diffuse loss of cerebral functions. More than one of these patterns may be manifest in a single patient.

This classification is crude, but useful clinically. Although patients with symptoms of transient ischaemic attacks might be thought to have recovered fully, in many cases subtle signs may persist, indicating that some infarction has occurred. After a series of transient ischaemic attacks a patient may present with a completed stroke which may also supervene during the course of progressive, diffuse cerebral atherosclerosis.

1. COMPLETED STROKE. Haemorrhage and occasionally cerebral tumour, as well as infarction, may sometimes be the cause. When due to infarction, there are often premonitory features such as headache during the few days preceding a stroke.

The onset of focal disability may occur at any time. The patient may awake with an established lesion. Very frequently the deficit evolves during a period of 1 or 2 hours. Rarely the maximal level of disability will be attained within a few minutes and occasionally impairment will progress for 1 or 2 days. Loss of consciousness at the onset occurs in a minority of cases though drowsiness is common. Severe headache is unusual. Epileptic fits, sometimes of the focal type, occasionally occur at the beginning or during the extension of a stroke, especially if it is due to an embolus.

The neurological picture depends on the site of infarction. The area supplied by the middle cerebral artery is most commonly involved so that a hemiplegia involving particularly the face but also the arm and leg on the side opposite the lesion is a frequent presentation.

If the paralysis develops very rapidly it may initially be of flaccid type, but spasticity and hyperreflexia are soon manifest and usually are detected from the onset. There may be hemianopia and hemianaesthesia on the side of the hemiplegia. If the infarct lies in the dominant hemisphere dysphasia may supervene. This familiar stroke pattern reflects the frequency of infarcts in the brain territory supplied by the middle cerebral artery but it should not be assumed that the causal lesion lies within this artery. In more than half of cases presenting this picture the primary lesion lies in the internal carotid artery or in more proximal vessels.

Other clinical presentations occur. An infarct within the area normally supplied by the anterior cerebral artery often causes a hemiplegia in which the leg is weaker than the arm and which may be accompanied by disturbance of micturition, apraxia or motor dysphasia. Lesions in the posterior cerebral territory usually lead to contralateral homonymous hemianopia with macular sparing and occasionally, if the thalamus is involved, diffuse, burning pain on the opposite side of the body. This thalamic syndrome may also result from infarcts in the area served by the anterior choroidal artery.

Approximately a tenth of infarcts involve the brain stem where they are more commonly accompanied by severe headaches than are those within the hemispheres. Vertigo, ataxia and vomiting, double vision and nystagmus are common features. A crossed paralysis, with ipsilateral affection of one or more cranial nerves and contralateral long tract (usually pyramidal) signs are characteristic of brain stem infarction.

2. STROKE-IN-EVOLUTION. The temporal pattern of a stroke is sometimes extended. Disability may increase by step-wise progression; sudden deteriorations are interspersed with static intervals. Less commonly there is slow uninterrupted progression; the deficit spreads and intensifies. The full extent of the patient's lesion may not be exhibited for 3 or 4 days; occasionally the disability may extend for 1 to 2 weeks. This type of clinical presentation, which suggests the diagnosis of a cerebral tumour, may be associated with occlusion of an internal carotid artery.

3. A TRANSIENT ISCHAEMIC ATTACK is a sudden deficit followed, within 24 hours, by complete recovery of function. Most such episodes last only a few minutes but should be regarded as possible harbingers of a more severe stroke in the next 6 months. If symptoms persist for more than 1 hour infarction has probably occurred. Symptoms depend on the site of ischaemia. Transient loss of vision in one eye (*amaurosis fugax*) and a hemiparesis or sensory disturbance affecting the contralateral half of the body are due to ischaemia in the carotid territory. Ischaemia affecting the area supplied by the vertebral and basilar arteries may cause vertigo, diplopia, hemiparesis or loss of consciousness.

The duration and frequency of transient ischaemic attacks are variable. Some patients suffer many attacks daily for periods of a week or more; attacks then cease and may not recur for months or years. Other patients have only occasional episodes at intervals of months. The attacks in an individual are usually stereotyped, the pattern and duration of dysfunction being repeated.

Frequently transient ischaemic attacks are due to emboli which arise from atheromatous plaques, are carried distally, lodge in and block small arteries and then break and disperse. In other cases flow through a stenotic artery may be reduced because of hypotension and may cause transient cerebral ischaemia. Occasionally, in cervical spondylosis, neck rotation leads to pressure on, and reduced flow through, a vertebral artery causing ischaemia in the brain stem. Some transient strokes may be due to small intracerebral haemorrhages.

4. PROGRESSIVE DIFFUSE LOSS OF CEREBRAL FUNCTIONS. Gradual reduction in cerebral blood flow leads to progressive brain atrophy which is reflected in a clinical picture of blunted intellectual function and multiple motor deficits. This type of pattern is often associated with hypertensive changes in the small cerebral vessels, and causes multiple small lacunar infarcts rather than large cortical lesions. Increasing dementia (*multi-infarct dementia*) may predominate but is usually accompanied by features of bilateral lesions of the pyramidal tracts, notably supranuclear bulbar

palsy (*pseudobulbar palsy*). These defects cause lability of emotional expression, dysarthria and dysphagia as well as a reduction in spontaneity, drive and movement which mimics parkinsonism. Sudden accelerations of disability, or transient episodes of neural deficit, usually differentiate this type of vascular disease from other causes of progressive cerebral atrophy and dementia.

Diagnosis and treatment are discussed on pages 633 and 635.

Cerebral embolism

The role of cerebral embolism in the production of cerebral ischaemia and infarction is consistently underestimated. Post-mortem studies have shown that at least half of cerebral infarcts can be attributed to embolisation from the heart or from atheromatous plaques in the large arteries in the neck and thorax. Transient ischaemic attacks are frequently the result of emboli from these same sources.

The disability produced by the lodgement of an embolus in a cerebral artery may be of very sudden onset. However, in many instances the pictures produced by cerebral infarction due to thrombosis and those due to cerebral embolism are indistinguishable in terms of the time, course and nature of the neural findings. A firm diagnosis of embolism demands evidence of a source of emboli and the presence of multiple sites of impaction. In many cases of cerebral embolism both criteria — and particularly the latter requirement — are absent. Arrhythmia, particularly atrial fibrillation associated with rheumatic or ischaemic heart disease, may lead to the presumptive diagnosis of cerebral embolism. In contrast evidence of an embolic source within large proximal arteries is often difficult to obtain.

Direct evidence of embolisation is occasionally provided by ophthalmoscopy. Emboli, composed mainly of platelet aggregations, can sometimes be seen in the retinal vessels of the affected eye during an attack of transient monocular blindness. The likelihood of embolic infarction may be inferred if there is a history of earlier transient ischaemic attacks. The presence of an embolic site is suggested by a bruit localised to the region of the carotid bifurcation.

More cerebral emboli arise in the heart than in any other site. Thrombus following myocardial infarction is the commonest source of emboli; rheumatic valvular lesions, infective endocarditis and atrial myxoma are other potential causes of cerebral embolism. A large embolus of cardiac origin may block the internal carotid artery at its origin. Smaller emboli often lodge at the trifurcation of the middle cerebral artery. Embolism at these sites is usually followed by thrombosis and complete occlusion.

A meticulous exploration of the possibility of embolic ischaemia should be made in all cases of occlusive cerebrovascular disease since the patient's management may thus be significantly influenced (p. 636).

Arteritis

A completed stroke or multifocal, minor cerebral lesions or a toxic confusional state may be a manifestation of arteritis due to systemic lupus erythematosus or polyarteritis nodosa. Associated systemic features will usually suggest the diagnosis. Cranial arteritis is a frequent cause of arterial inflammation in the elderly and occasionally the disease causes cerebral infarction.

Cerebral infarction may be the presenting feature of meningovascular syphilis and the possibility should always be considered when a stroke occurs in a relatively young person. Occasionally tuberculous arteritis, associated with meningitis, may cause cerebral infarction.

2. HAEMORRHAGIC CEREBRAL LESIONS

These may be the result of (1) primary intra-cerebral haemorrhage associated with hypertension, (2) subarachnoid haemorrhage usually from a saccular aneurysm or (3) trauma causing extra-dural or subdural haematomas.

Primary intracerebral haemorrhage

Intracerebral haemorrhage is strongly associated with hypertension. In malignant hypertension there is fibrinoid necrosis of arterioles, and vessels so affected rupture to cause bleeding into the brain. Patients with long-standing hypertension develop hyaline changes in the muscular and elastic arterial layers which give rise to small aneurysms that are also liable to rupture. The penetrating branches of the middle cerebral artery, notably the lenticulostriate arteries, are particularly prone to develop such microaneurysms and the majority of intracerebral haemorrhages occur in the region of the internal capsule.

An intracerebral haemorrhage usually presents abruptly when the patient is awake and is prone to occur whilst he or she is engaged in physical exertion. There may be premonitory severe headache and in over half of patients there is loss of consciousness, sometimes accompanied by an epileptic fit. Since the internal capsule is so frequently involved, a hemiplegia commonly supervenes and initially may be of the flaccid type. When the haemorrhage is massive and bleeding persists, intracranial pressure is raised; coma deepens and papilloedema develops. Haemorrhages frequently extend into the lateral or third ventricles and sometimes there is rupture through the surface of the brain into the subarachnoid space so that in many cases of initially intracerebral haemorrhage, blood is found in the cerebrospinal fluid.

A massive haemorrhage accompanied by loss of consciousness has a grave prognosis; approximately a half die within a few days. Smaller haemorrhages occurring in any part of the brain may present a clinical picture indistinguishable from infarction. The severity of paralysis, presence of headache or loss of consciousness are not reliable guides in the differentiation of cerebral haemorrhage from infarction. Vomiting is more common after a haemorrhage, but the only reliable test is a CT scan carried out early in the illness.

Haemorrhage into the pons usually produces rapid loss of consciousness, pinpoint pupils and periodic respiration; often there is bilateral involvement of cranial nerves and pyramidal pathways. Hyperpyrexia is sometimes a feature.

Cerebellar haemorrhage is frequently of abrupt onset and is usually ushered in by occipital headache, vomiting, vertigo and ataxia. Consciousness is often lost after a few hours at which time the patient frequently develops pupillary constriction and a contralateral hemiplegia from involvement of the brain stem.

Subarachnoid haemorrhage

Haemorrhage into the subarachnoid space is the result of rupture of an aneurysm in over 50% of cases. In about 5% the source of bleeding is an arteriovenous malformation. In older patients subarachnoid haemorrhage is usually the result of diffuse cerebrovascular disease. Other causes are trauma, extension of an intracerebral haemorrhage or a bleeding cerebral tumour.

The onset of subarachnoid haemorrhage is often marked by severe and sudden headache, which is sometimes followed by impairment or loss of consciousness. There may be focal features whose nature depends on the site of the lesion; diplopia or other cranial nerve lesions, hemiparesis and aphasia occur. Signs of meningeal irritation, i.e. neck stiffness and a positive Kernig's sign, develop. Ophthalmoscopy may reveal unilateral or bilateral haemorrhages between the retina and the hyaloid membrane. The shape of these subhyaloid haemorrhages is determined by gravity so that the upper border is horizontal if the patient is sitting upright. If the subarachnoid haemorrhage is extensive and continuous, papilloedema may occur.

The outlook for subarachnoid haemorrhage due to an extension of intracerebral bleeding is similar to that of the primary condition. If subarachnoid haemorrhage is due to the rupture of a saccular aneurysm bleeding is liable to recur within 6 to 8 weeks.

Saccular aneurysm. The first manifestation of an intracranial aneurysm is often a subarachnoid haemorrhage, but sometimes aneurysms present focal features before rupture. The nature of these depends on the site of the aneurysm (Fig. 15.5). An aneurysm of the internal carotid artery within the cavernous sinus usually causes pain or paraesthesiae in the distribution of the ophthalmic division of the fifth nerve, and a third nerve palsy, sometimes accompanied by palsies of the fourth and sixth nerves. Rarely, an aneurysm of the internal carotid artery will rupture into the cavernous sinus, forming a caroticocavernous fistula. This causes severe pain in and around the eye, pulsatile exophthalmos, papilloedema and complete ophthalmoplegia. A loud bruit can usually be heard over the affected eye.

Aneurysm of the supraclinoid part of the internal carotid artery may compress the optic nerve, chiasma or tract leading to impaired visual acuity and a variety of scotomata and visual field defects. These disturbances may be accompanied by paralysis of the third nerve.

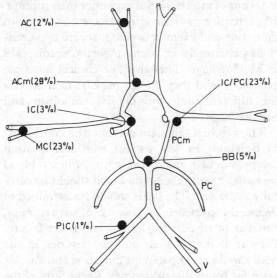

Fig. 15.5 Arteries contributing to the circle of Willis, their major branches and the commonest sites of aneurysm with frequency of occurrence in brackets. AC = anterior cerebral artery; ACm = anterior communicating artery; B = basilar artery; BB = basilar bifurcation; IC = internal carotid artery; IC/PC = internal carotid/posterior communicating artery; MC = middle cerebral artery; PC = posterior cerebral artery; PCm = posterior communicating artery; PIC = posterior inferior cerebellar artery; V = vertebral artery.

Aneurysms of the middle cerebral artery tend to present with bleeding, but occasionally their presence will be heralded by focal epilepsy or by a progressive hemiparesis. Anterior communicating and anterior cerebral aneurysms may compress the optic chiasma from above, resulting in bilateral loss of the inferior part of the visual fields.

Posterior communicating aneurysms often lead to an isolated third nerve palsy. Aneurysms of the posterior cerebral artery may compress the cerebral peduncle and the adjacent third nerve causing an ipsilateral third nerve palsy and contralateral pyramidal tract signs.

Arteriovenous malformation. A subarachnoid haemorrhage without antecedent clinical features is the commonest presentation of an arteriovenous malformation. Some present with epilepsy accompanied later by progressive focal signs and others cause recurrent localised headaches of throbbing character which superficially may resemble migraine. A bruit may be heard over an eyeball or through the skull overlying a large arteriovenous malformation.

Extradural and subdural haematoma

Extradural haematomas are produced by skull fractures involving the branches of the middle meningeal artery. Symptoms usually develop a few hours after the injury. Coma rapidly ensues with an obvious hemiparesis. Later tentorial herniation often rapidly causes death so that operation should be undertaken urgently.

Subdural haematoma may occur as an acute complication of a head injury from venous haemorrhage into the subdural space. The picture then resembles that of an extradural haematoma.

A *chronic subdural haematoma* may follow a minor head injury especially in an elderly patient. Often the injury is so slight that it is forgotten. After an interval of weeks or months the patient may present with headache, a confusional state, or the development of focal neurological signs such as hemiparesis. Characteristically, as the subdural haematoma increases in size, there is fluctuation in the level of consciousness, and, later, signs of raised intracranial pressure may be manifest. The progressive changes may closely mimic a cerebral tumour and require investigation along similar lines. Exploratory burr holes in the skull may confirm the diagnosis and produce dramatic benefit in the case of a haematoma.

Diagnosis of cerebrovascular disease

Clinical features. The diagnosis and assessment of a patient suffering from cerebrovascular disease ideally comprises four stages. Firstly, the nature of the patient's disabilities are defined and the site and extent of the lesion inferred. Secondly, other possible causes of the disturbance of function are excluded. Thirdly, the nature of the vascular pathology is determined. Fourthly, the state of the systemic circulation is investigated and associated diseases delineated.

The time course of a completed stroke will usually suggest the correct diagnosis. Occasionally patients suffering from a cerebral tumour will present with a rapidly developing disability. Multiple sclerosis and demyelinating encephalopathies present acutely but in most instances the age of onset, multiple lesions affecting the spinal cord as well as the brain and a characteristic earlier history will distinguish these conditions from cerebrovascular disease. The progression of a stroke-in-evolution may closely imitate the features of a rapidly growing tumour.

Transient ischaemic attacks (TIA) may need to be distinguished from epilepsy and migraine. Consciousness is unimpaired in most transient ischaemic attacks. Migraine rarely presents after the age of 50 years whilst transient ischaemic attacks usually occur after this age. TIAs are rarely accompanied or followed by headaches. The neurological symptoms of migraine tend to develop slowly over several minutes, and often migrate between vascular territories; symptoms of TIAs are abrupt in onset and remain within the province of a single vessel.

Progressive, diffuse, cerebral atherosclerosis may be difficult to distinguish from other forms of dementia; differentiating features are given on page 681.

The elucidation of the type of cerebrovascular disease is sometimes difficult. It is important rapidly to define those conditions which require life-saving, urgent or specific treatment. The history of trauma and the clinical features are distinctive in extradural and acute subdural haematoma. The diagnosis of chronic subdural haematoma can occasionally be made with confidence on clinical grounds but the possibility of this condition should be considered and investigated particularly in an elderly patient manifesting a progressive cerebral deficit accompanied by headache. Signs of meningeal irritation indicate a subarachnoid bleed which can be confirmed by CT scan or lumbar puncture. Arteritis may be recognised because of accompanying systemic clinical features and by the results of simple investigations such as a raised ESR, positive ANF or positive serology for syphilis.

An attempt should be made to distinguish between patients with cerebral infarction and those who have bled into the brain. A history of transient ischaemic attacks favours a diagnosis of infarction rather than haemorrhage. The development of neural disability during sleep is likely to be due to infarction; onset during exertion suggests a haemorrhage. Blood in the CSF obviously indicates intracranial bleeding. A source of emboli is in favour of arterial occlusion rather than rupture. Hypertension is frequently associated with both infarction and haemorrhage but severe hypertension, particularly in young patients, predisposes to haemorrhage. Though these clinical hints are generally valid they do not provide firm criteria for differentiating thrombosis, embolism and haemorrhage.

The cerebral circulation cannot be considered in isolation. In any patient who suffers from cerebrovascular disease the status of heart, blood pressure, blood vessels and blood should be carefully appraised. The heart should be examined to define the presence or absence of arrhythmias, valvular or myocardial lesions and heart failure. Peripheral limb vessels and the arteries in the neck should be palpated for pulsation and auscultated for bruits due to stenoses. Recordings of the blood pressure are mandatory. Abnormalities of the blood, particularly anaemia, polycythaemia and thrombocytopenia should be sought.

Investigation. The extent to which diagnostic investigations should be pursued depends on individual circumstances.

Computed tomography will not only reveal tumours but in many instances will define the nature of cerebrovascular lesions. Intracerebral bleeding gives high density abnormalities so that even very small haemorrhages are detected. Intraventricular, subarachnoid and subdural haemorrhages are readily distinguished and sequential scanning will monitor the subsequent organisation and resolution of intracerebral haematomas. Ruptured aneurysms can be differentiated from primary intracerebral haemorrhage in almost all instances and the site of the aneurysms predicted with fair accuracy. A normal CT scan does not exclude subarachnoid haemorrhage, and if this is suspected, lumbar puncture should be the next investigation.

Cerebral infarction leads to low density abnormalities which may be detectable within a few hours of onset. Some infarcts are not revealed by computed tomography but even in these cases the confident exclusion of tumours and haemorrhage enables a firm presumptive diagnosis to be made.

Other investigations are less informative. The EEG usually shows marked abnormalities after infarction or haemorrhage and serial recordings demonstrate progressive improvement. Similar EEG abnormalities due to tumour persist and become more marked. Cerebral angiography should be undertaken only if surgery is likely to be required. It should be performed if there is evidence of a tumour, vascular malformation, or extracranial vascular disease in a young patient which might be amenable to surgical treatment.

Treatment of cerebrovascular disease

The management of patients suffering from cerebrovascular disease should be approached in a logical sequence. Initially patients may need to be protected from the dangers of unconsciousness and immobility. The causal lesion should be treated if possible and measures to improve functional recovery instituted. Patients who survive but are left with residual disability need support and rehabilitation. Finally, progression and recurrence of cerebrovascular lesions should, as far as possible, be prevented.

General measures. An adequate airway should be established in those patients whose consciousness is impaired. The patient's fluid and nutritional intake should be maintained, employing a nasogastric tube or intravenous infusion if necessary. Pressure sores should be prevented by frequent alteration of the patient's posture, the use of pads and massage of vulnerable areas of skin. Catheterisation may be needed because of urinary incontinence. Rapid cleaning is required for the patient who is incontinent of faeces. Passive movement of limbs should be started early and the patient should be moved from bed and sat in a chair for periods during the day as soon as possible. Intercurrent urinary or respiratory infections should be treated with appropriate antimicrobial agents.

Specific medical treatment. A minority of patients have treatable underlying conditions. Severe hypertension should be controlled but too rapid reduction of blood pressure may exacerbate the area of cerebral infarction; hypotensive drugs

must therefore by used sparingly and with caution. Those with meningovascular syphilis should be given a course of penicillin. Those suffering from temporal arteritis or a connective tissue disease may need corticosteroids. Polycythaemia or anaemia should be treated appropriately.

Neurosurgery. Early referral (within 24 hours) to a neurosurgeon with a view to operation is required for patients who have bled from a ruptured aneurysm. The neck of the aneurysm should be clipped if this is technically possible. The wall of the aneurysm may be reinforced by plastic or muscle. If such a direct attack is impracticable carotid ligation may reduce the liability to further bleeding from the aneurysm. Surgical drainage of extradural and subdural haematomas usually produces dramatic and rapid improvement.

Stroke. Little can be done to reverse the effects of infarction or haemorrhage. In a very few instances blood flow has rapidly been restored through an occluded carotid artery by surgical removal of thrombus. This is effective only when the affected artery is accessible and when the operation is carried out within a few hours of the onset of the symptoms. These conditions very rarely pertain.

Treatment is aimed at minimising the extent of brain death. Around the margins of an infarct or haemorrhage there is potentially viable tissue whose function can be restored if an alternative supply of blood is available. Attempts to provoke cerebral vasodilation have not been effective and it is likely that the promotion of generalised cerebral vasodilation could be harmful by 'stealing' blood from the damaged area.

Low-molecular-weight dextran has been employed in the expectation that its effects in decreasing the aggregation of platelets and blood viscosity would improve cerebral circulation. High doses of corticosteroids (e.g. dexamethasone) have also been used in acute stroke, but although there is evidence that these treatments reduce the early death rate from severe strokes, there is no long-lasting benefit.

Anticoagulants have no place in the treatment of an established stroke. Thrombolytic agents such as streptokinase are ineffective. There is thus as yet no specific medical treatment available which significantly and consistently improves the outlook for patients who have suffered a stroke.

Stroke-in-evolution. The early use of anticoagulants has been advocated to halt progression in an evolving stroke. There is some evidence that this treatment does help but there is a danger that anticoagulants may cause haemorrhage and before they are used in this situation an intracerebral haemorrhage must be excluded by investigation. There may be a place for the use of low-molecular-weight dextran in the treatment of a stroke of gradual development.

Transient ischaemic attacks. Anticoagulants (p. 550) seem to reduce the incidence of future strokes. Inhibitors of platelet aggregation have also been employed. Aspirin (75–300 mg/d) reduces subsequent strokes in patients who have suffered a TIA. Dipyridamole (100 mg t.i.d.) is less effective, but may be given when aspirin is contraindicated.

Cerebral embolism. Anticoagulants should be given, provided other conditions do not contraindicate their use.

Rehabilitation. A large number of patients are left with residual deficits as a result of cerebrovascular lesions. Much can be done to mitigate disabilities so that patients can live a largely independent life in the community. Early institution of treatment is essential. In the period immediately following a stroke, passive movements of limbs should be practised. Supervised exercises and encouragement should later aim at the development of mobility. Few patients, no matter how severe their original hemiplegia, cannot be taught to walk again. Later the patient should be guided in the performance of the activities of everyday life. Modifications of dress, housing, baths, lavatories and kitchen equipment may enable the patient to cope at home.

Throughout the period of rehabilitation communication should be encouraged, using, if appropriate, the skills of the speech therapist. The degree and extent of paralysis is less of a bar to successful rehabilitation than are disorders of perception, spatial disorientation, dysphasia and, particularly, dementia. Co-operation between physicians, nurses, physiotherapists, occupational therapists, speech therapists and social workers improves the end result of the physical and social rehabilitation of patients who have had a stroke.

The recruitment and education of relatives enables them to continue rehabilitation at home.

Prevention of recurrence. Some of the treatments outlined above, such as anticoagulant therapy and inhibitors of platelet aggregation, are preventive measures. The most important prophylactic factor is the control of hypertension by appropriate drugs. It has been shown conclusively that early, effective and continued reduction of high blood pressure significantly improves the outlook for both occlusive and haemorrhagic cerebrovascular disease. Cigarette smoking should be stopped, diabetes and hyperlipidaemia treated, and polycythaemia controlled by venesection or radioisotope therapy.

If an otherwise fit patient has had recurrent carotid territory TIAs, and a significant carotid artery stenosis is shown in the neck, then carotid endarterectomy may prevent a subsequent stroke. However, both investigation with angiography and the surgery carry risks of causing a stroke. As yet, no good data allows us to balance these risks with certainty.

Prognosis for an individual suffering from a cerebrovascular lesion depends on complex factors. There are some general guidelines. In one well-studied series of strokes the mortality within the first month after infarction was roughly 30%. From proven intracerebral haemorrhage the mortality in the same period was 80%. After a subarachnoid haemorrhage 65% died within 1 month. This investigation emphasised the poor prognosis after large haemorrhagic lesions.

Signs of a poor outlook for a stroke, whether due to infarction or haemorrhage, are impairment of consciousness, defects in conjugate gaze and a severe hemiplegia. Of those who survive an initial stroke, life expectancy is roughly halved. Approximately 10% suffer a second stroke within 1 year of the first and 20% within 5 years. Many patients who initially present with stroke die from myocardial infarction.

The prognosis in patients who suffer transient ischaemic attacks is difficult to ascertain because of difficulties of definition. A subsequent stroke is to be expected in approximately one-third of patients who have transient ischaemic attacks and is most likely to occur within 3 years of the first attack. In 50% of patients attacks cease within 1 to 3 years of their onset. Transient ischaemic attacks are attended by a worse prognosis (in terms of survival) in people below the age of 65 than in those over that age when compared with the rest of the population.

Much further work is needed to define the factors which influence the prognosis of cerebrovascular disease.

Thrombosis of intracranial veins and venous sinuses

Intracerebral venous thrombosis may be infected or aseptic; both are relatively uncommon. Infection may spread to the veins or sinuses from the face, dental roots or middle ear; it may also follow fracture of the skull, meningitis or septicaemia. Complications such as meningitis, suppurative encephalitis or brain abscess may ensue.

Aseptic thrombosis may occur in water and salt depletion, polycythaemia, malaria and marasmus, and occasionally in the puerperium or in users of oral contraceptives.

Clinical features. *Cavernous sinus thrombosis* nearly always follows an infection such as a boil on the face. Usually the patient is gravely ill, and before antibiotics were available few patients survived. Headache and fever are marked and there is a neutrophil leucocytosis. Occlusion of the ophthalmic veins causes proptosis, chemosis and oedema of the eyelids. There are almost always complete palsies of the third, fourth and sixth nerves as well as pain in and above the eye and diminished sensation over the forehead. Papilloedema in the affected eye is common. The condition is usually initially unilateral but often becomes bilateral within 2 to 3 days.

Superior sagittal sinus thrombosis. Severe headache, papilloedema, and a generalised epileptic seizure are followed by signs of spreading thrombophlebitis of cortical veins, including motor, sensory or visual disorders on one or both sides according to the areas of cortex affected.

Transverse sinus thrombosis. The onset is similar to superior sagittal thrombosis but extension to the superior petrosal sinus and lower cortical veins causes unilateral syndromes of local infarction. Spread to the jugular veins may cause palsies of lower cranial nerves.

Investigation. CT scan may be relatively normal, but there may be evidence of brain oedema, narrowed ventricles and low density changes. Angiography provides more direct evidence of venous occlusion. The CSF is under increased pressure and often xanthochromic. Increased numbers of both red and white blood cells are present in the fluid, and its protein content is usually elevated.

Treatment. The administration of antibiotics has markedly improved the outlook for infected thromboses. Surgical drainage of an abscess may be necessary. Anticoagulants are unhelpful but dexamethasone (4 mg t.i.d.) reduces the cerebral oedema.

INFECTIONS OF BRAIN, MENINGES AND SPINAL CORD

SUPPURATIVE ENCEPHALITIS AND INTRACEREBRAL ABSCESS

Aetiology and pathology. Direct infection may occur following a compound fracture of the skull or there may be local spread by suppurative thrombophlebitis from an infected ear, paranasal sinus or scalp. Metastatic infections may occur from the lungs or from infective endocarditis.

The initial infection causes a suppurative encephalitis. The pus is slowly localised by a surrounding wall of gliosis which in a chronic abscess may form a tough capsule. Multiple abscesses, communicating or discrete, occur, particularly with metastatic spread.

Clinical features. There are three main types of presentation:

Acute encephalitis. Soon after head injury or otitis media the patient develops headache, fever, vomiting and drowsiness progressing to coma. Focal cerebral signs may be present.

Subacute or delayed encephalitis. Head injury, cranial infection or infected embolism may be followed after weeks or months of apparent recovery by symptoms of encephalitis or of a chronic space-occupying lesion. During the latent interval there may be minor headache, irritability, malaise and intermittent pyrexia. These features should lead to a search for a focal cerebral lesion in patients with infections such as otitis media or bronchiectasis.

Chronic abscess. This may follow one of the previous types of onset or there may be nothing to suggest that the lesion is infective. The chronic abscess causes focal symptoms of a cerebral lesion (p. 603) and those of raised intracranial pressure which are indistinguishable from those of cerebral tumours. The temperature is usually normal.

Diagnosis. The possibility of an abscess should be considered if there is a progressive, focal, intracranial lesion, especially if associated with congenital heart disease. The likelihood is increased if there are signs of infection, such as pyrexia, leucocytosis or a raised ESR but these may be absent if there is a chronic abscess. The EEG may show focal abnormalities. The CSF may show a pleocytosis or a raised protein but often is normal and should not be examined if there are signs of raised intracranial pressure. Contrast enhanced CT scanning will define the vast majority of intracranial abscesses.

Treatment. High dosage antibiotics are given as for pyogenic meningitis (p. 639). Metronidazole (500 mg t.i.d. i.v.) should be included to combat the anaerobic organisms frequently present. When a collection of pus has been demonstrated it should be aspirated and appropriate antibiotics instilled into the cavity. This procedure may need to be repeated. After the infection has been controlled excision of the abscess may be necessary. It is important to treat the underlying cause if possible.

Spinal epidural abscess

This condition usually arises as a metastasis from infection elsewhere, often a boil, which may be so trivial as to be easily overlooked. Pain of root distribution is severe. It develops acutely and is followed by progressive loss of sensation and power in the lower limbs with sphincter disturbance. The signs are those of transverse myelitis (p. 657) but the local root irritation is the clue to the true cause. The temperature may be only slightly raised, but a polymorphonuclear leucocytosis is found in the blood. There may be radiological evidence of localised osteomyelitis of the spine. Paraplegia will become complete and irreversible if treatment is delayed. Large doses

of antibiotics such as benzylpenicillin 600 mg 4-hourly should be given immediately and the patient transferred to the care of a neurosurgeon without delay.

MENINGITIS

Viral infection (p. 641) is now the commonest cause of meningitis. Bacterial infection has become rare since the introduction of the antibiotics, and, for similar reasons, tuberculous meningitis (p. 639) is now seldom seen in Britain. In some areas meningitis may be caused by spirochaetes (leptospirosis, p. 761; Lyme disease, p. 572; syphilis p. 640), Rickettsia (typhus fever, p. 738), protozoa (amoebiasis, p. 774) or fungi (cryptococcosis, p. 777).

Inflammation of the meninges can also be due to causes other than infection, for example blood in the CSF in subarachnoid haemorrhage (p. 632). Meningeal irritation ('*meningism*') without inflammatory reaction occurs in acute specific fevers, otitis media and pneumonia in childhood. Cellular reaction (lymphocytic) may be associated with symptoms and signs of meningeal irritation in poliomyelitis (p. 644) and acute encephalomyelitis (p. 637). Sarcoidosis and malignant disease are rare causes of meningitis.

Bacterial meningitis

The most common organisms are *Neisseria meningitidis, Streptococcus pneumoniae* and *Haemophilus influenzae.*

Pathology. The pia-arachnoid is congested and infiltrated with inflammatory cells. A thin layer of pus forms and this may later organise to form adhesions. These may cause obstruction to the free flow of CSF leading to hydrocephalus, or may damage the cranial nerves at the base of the brain. The CSF pressure rises rapidly, the protein content increases and there is a cellular reaction which varies in type and severity according to the nature of the inflammation and the causative organism. The sugar content of the CSF is decreased in bacterial infections and in carcinomatosis of the meninges. If the patient is not kept in electrolyte balance the chloride content may be reduced due to loss by sweating and vomiting.

Clinical features. Signs of meningeal irritation are present:

Neck rigidity. The patient complains of neck stiffness and the examiner is unable to put the patient's chin on the chest by passive flexion of the neck. Spasm may be so severe, particularly in children, as to cause head retraction.

Kernig's sign. If the patient's thigh is flexed to 90 degrees from the abdomen, it is then impossible to straighten the knee passively owing to spasm of the hamstring muscles. This manoeuvre stretches the roots of the sciatic nerve which are inflamed at their exits from the spinal theca.

Other features of meningococcal infection are described on page 746.

Investigation. Microbiological examination of the CSF (p. 605) usually determines the nature of the infection. In cases of pyogenic meningitis in which Gram stain and/or culture of CSF is negative, counter current immunoelectrophoresis of the CSF is useful for the detection of bacterial antigens.

Treatment. Meningococcal and pneumococcal meningitis should be treated initially with large doses of benzylpenicillin intravenously — 1.2–2.4 g 4-hourly for adults and 150 mg/kg/d given 4-hourly for children.

For meningitis due to *H. influenzae* chloramphenicol (p. 42) is effective given intravenously initially, and orally when the patient can swallow. Chloramphenicol is also a useful alternative to penicillin if the patient is known to be allergic to the latter.

Pending the identification of the bacteria causing pyogenic meningitis, treatment of adults can be commenced with benzylpenicillin and of children with chloramphenicol. Single doses of long-acting chloramphenicol are also useful in areas where medical facilities are limited.

Tuberculous meningitis

Aetiology and pathology. The condition occurs most commonly shortly after a primary infection in childhood or as part of miliary tuberculosis. The usual local source of infection is a caseous focus in the meninges or brain substance adjacent to the cerebrospinal fluid pathway.

The brain is covered by a greenish, gelatinous exudate especially around the base, and numerous scattered tubercles are found on the meninges.

Clinical features. In children the onset of tuberculous meningitis is so insidious that it may be weeks before the parents realise that the illness is serious. At first there is merely lassitude, loss of interest in toys and in play, unwillingness to talk, anorexia and constipation. Headache, at first slight, gradually becomes worse but meningeal signs may not appear for days or weeks.

In adults the malaise, headache and meningeal signs usually progress more rapidly. There may be vomiting. The temperature is intermittently raised initially but remains raised, though rarely to high levels, once meningeal signs appear. The condition then progresses more rapidly, and in untreated cases cranial nerve palsies, hemiparesis or other signs of cerebral damage, hydrocephalus with drowsiness, coma and moderate papilloedema may occur. In miliary tuberculosis choroidal tubercles may be seen in the fundi.

The CSF is under increased pressure. It is usually clear but, when allowed to stand, a fine clot may form. The fluid contains up to 400 cells/mm³, predominantly lymphocytes; the count must be made on a fresh specimen before it forms a clot. There is a rise in protein and a marked fall in glucose. Detection of the tubercle bacillus in a smear of the centrifuged deposit from the CSF may be difficult, the clot being the most likely place to find it. Inoculation of CSF into a guinea-pig is valuable for confirming the diagnosis if this cannot be done from smears or cultures of the CSF, but as the outcome will not be known for 6 weeks, treatment must be started without waiting for confirmation.

Treatment and prognosis. Chemotherapy should be started as soon as the diagnosis is made using one of the regimens described on page 230, together with pyrazinamide (p. 230). All patients should also receive prednisolone, 10 mg four times daily. If subsequent lumbar punctures suggest the development of a spinal subarachnoid block, then hydrocortisone hemisuccinate should be injected intrathecally each day in a dose of 1 mg/kg. If obstructive hydrocephalus develops in spite of treatment with corticosteroids, surgical methods for ensuring continuous ventricular drainage must be adopted. During the acute stage of the illness skilled nursing is essential and measures must be taken to maintain adequate hydration and nutrition.

The intensive regime of drug treatment should be continued for 8 weeks and be followed by a continuation phase (p. 231). Prednisolone is then reduced to 20 mg daily and stopped after about 3 months.

Untreated tuberculous meningitis is fatal in a few weeks but complete recovery is the rule with modern treatment if it is started before the appearance of focal signs or stupor. When treatment is started at a later stage the recovery rate is 60% or less and the survivors may be mentally deficient, epileptic, deaf, blind or show some other permanent deficit.

Viral meninigitis

Acute lymphocytic choriomeningitis and other forms of viral meningitis are described on page 642.

NEUROSYPHILIS

An old neurological aphorism states that neurosyphilis may mimic any neurological disease. Neurosyphilis may present as an acute or chronic process. It may involve, singly or in combination, the meninges, blood vessels and parenchyma of brain and spinal cord and cause meningovascular syphilis, general paralysis of the insane, tabes dorsalis and combined lesions. Though the clinical manifestations produced are diverse, certain general observations are pertinent.

Pupillary abnormalities, described by Argyll Robertson, may accompany any neurosyphilitic clinical syndrome. The pupils are small, irregular and unequal. They do not react to light but respond to convergence and show an impaired response to mydriatics. The irises may be atrophied. In relatively few instances will all of these features be present. The complete picture of Argyll Robertson pupils is most frequently seen in tabes dorsalis.

Examination of the CSF reveals abnormalities in the vast majority of cases of neurosyphilis. An increase in the cell count, usually lymphocytic and of moderate degree is almost invariably present when the disease is active. A moderate rise in the protein content is usual and the gamma globulin fraction thereof is often increased. Serological tests for syphilis (p. 416) are usually positive.

Meningovascular syphilis

The essential lesion is endarteritis obliterans which may lead to arterial thrombosis and to the formation of a granuloma or gumma. The meninges may be covered by an exudate which damages cranial nerves. Lesions may predominantly affect arteries or meninges or both structures may be involved.

Clinical features. These usually occur within 5 years of the primary infection.

Intracranial lesions. Occlusion of a cerebral artery may be due to syphilis which should be considered as a possibility in cases of stroke, particularly when cerebral infarcts occur in young people.

Basal gummatous meningitis may present with cranial nerve palsies. Meningitis over the surface of the hemispheres may give rise to headaches and fits in addition to focal signs of cortical dysfunction. Rarely, a single large gumma may present as a slow growing cerebral tumour.

Spinal lesions. Thrombosis of the anterior spinal artery gives rise to lower motor neurone signs at the level of the lesion. Below the affected segments, upper motor neurone disturbance is usually manifest and there may also be impairment of pain and temperature sensation.

General paralysis of the insane

The principal pathological changes are seen in the cortex. There is degeneration of cortical neurones giving rise to atrophy, particularly marked over the anterior part of the hemispheres. The meninges are thickened and infiltrated with lymphocytes. General paralysis of the insane usually presents 5 to 15 years after the primary infection. Men are much more often affected than women.

Clinical features. The initial and most characteristic feature is dementia (p. 680), often of insidious onset and slow progression. Signs of upper motor neurone lesions, usually bilateral and initially mild, are usually present and tremors of the head and lips are often manifest. Less common features include epileptic fits and transient episodes of focal cerebral disturbance such as hemiplegia, hemianopia or dysphasia.

Tabes dorsalis

The primary lesion is a degeneration of first order sensory neurones, central to the dorsal root ganglia, in the lower thoracic and lumbar nerve roots. Obvious macroscopic wasting affects the dorsal columns but all modalities of sensation may be impaired. Males are more often affected than females, usually 5 to 20 years after the primary infection.

Clinical features. Sensory disturbances are the most common initial symptoms. 'Lightning' pains of severe, lancinating nature occur in paroxysms. They are most common in the legs. Pains radiating around the trunk in a 'girdle' distribution also occur.

Other disabilities may accompany these sensory manifestations or may be presenting features. Ataxia, of sensory type, due to proprioceptive loss is often prominent. Sensory loss may cause retention of urine with overflow incontinence. Failing vision or diplopia may be symptoms. Perforating, painless ulcers of the feet and swollen, unstable joints (Charcot's joints) are sometimes found. Visceral crises may cause acute symptoms and the disturbance in function may point to disease in the affected organ rather than in its innervation. Most typical are gastric crises which give rise to abdominal pain and vomiting.

The signs of tabes are most explicable on the basis of posterior root lesions. Tendon reflexes are lost, due to interruption of the reflex arcs, first at the ankles, then at the knees and later in the upper limbs. Hypotonia with resultant hyper-extensibility of the joints appears. The pain fibres are affected early with delay in or impairment of the response to pin prick over a characteristic distribution e.g. the nose, the perineum and the distal part of the lower limbs. Deep pain appreciation is also impaired so that the tendo calcaneus, calf muscles and testes become insensitive to pressure. Vibration and position sense in the feet are also lost early, but light touch is not affected until a later stage. The combination of loss of position sense and hypotonia gives rise to severe ataxia, so that the patient walks on a wide base lifting the feet high and stamping them down in an irregular and forceful manner. Romberg's test (p. 598) is positive. The plantar responses remain flexor, but may be absent as a result of sensory loss. Bilateral ptosis with compensatory wrinkling of the forehead and Argyll Robertson pupils constitute a typical tabetic facies.

Combined neurosyphilitic lesions

It is emphasised that the clinical syndromes outlined above represent only the commoner presentations of neursyphilis. Combinations of pathological lesions also occur and give rise to mixed clinical pictures. Tabetic manifestations sometimes accompany those of general paralysis of the insane (*taboparesis*) and may lead to cases of dementia accompanied by ataxia, lightning pains or areflexia; patients presenting with visceral crises may be found to have extensor plantar responses.

Treatment of neurosyphilis. The essential part of the treatment of neurosyphilis of all types is the injection of procaine penicillin 600 mg –1.2 g daily for 3 weeks (p. 417). The aim of treatment is to arrest the disease and restore the blood and CSF to normal. Further courses of penicillin must be given if symptoms are not relieved, the condition continues to advance, or the CSF continues to show signs of active disease. The first abnormality to regress is the increase in cells but these may not return to normal until 3 months after treatment has been completed. The elevated protein takes longer to subside and the Wassermann reaction may never revert to normal. Lumbar puncture should be repeated at 6-monthly intervals for 2 years and further courses of penicillin given so long as signs of activity remain. Evidence of clinical progression at any time is an indication for renewed treatment.

VIRAL INFECTIONS

A classification of viruses is given on page 726.

Some viruses have a propensity for invasion of nerve cells and are called 'neurotropic'. The affinity may be specially marked for one type of nerve cell; varicella-zoster virus particularly involves sensory neurones and the anterior horn cells are vulnerable to an enterovirus in poliomyelitis. Though these viruses most commonly invade their sites of predilection they may also sometimes involve the nervous system more widely; the virus of poliomyelitis often gives rise to a meningo-encephalitis and the varicella-zoster virus may rarely cause motor disability.

Many viruses which usually cause diseases of other systems may sometimes implicate the nervous system. The many varieties of echo and Coxsackie viruses, which are common enteric pathogens, fairly often cause neurological disease as well as more widespread manifestations in other systems. The viruses of herpes simplex and mumps, among many others, may occasionally invade the nervous system. Congenital cytomegalovirus infection can cause brain damage.

Some neurological diseases, of which encephalitis lethargica is one, are presumed to be of viral origin because of their epidemiological, clinical and pathological features though the causal agent has not been identified.

Neurological disorders are sometimes indirectly associated with viral diseases. In these instances abnormal immunological responses, evoked by the virus, cause damage to neural tissue without any viral invasion of neurones. The demyelinating encephalomyelitis (p. 648) which may follow any of the exanthemata is such an entity.

Slow (prion) viral infections may cause chronic or relapsing neurological disease. These conditions exhibit a latent period of many months or years between the initial infection and the subsequent clinical illness which, once manifest, tends to run a protracted course.

Kuru is a disease which occurs only in the members of one cannibalistic New Guinea tribe. It can, however, be transmitted to chimpanzees and there is much evidence to suggest that kuru is a slow viral infection transmitted by the eating of the infected brains of dead tribal members. There is degeneration of grey matter, most marked in the cerebellum, causing a progressive ataxia.

Creutzfeldt-Jakob disease is a subacute encephalopathy characterised by presenile dementia, epilepsy, myoclonus, extrapyramidal and motor neurone signs and can also be transmitted from man to chimpanzees.

A low viral infection has been adduced as a possible cause of a number of chronic neurological diseases, including motor neurone disease and multiple sclerosis.

Viral meningitis

Viral infections of the central nervous system such as encephalitis and poliomyelitis may be associated with meningitis. Viral meningitis can also occur alone, without clinical manifestation of parenchymal involvement of the nervous system, in acute lymphocytic choriomeningitis and infection by echo or Coxsackie viruses. Thirdly, meningitis may develop as a complication of viral infections primarily involving other organs, e.g. mumps, measles, infectious mononucleosis, herpes zoster, hepatitis and HIV infection.

Acute lymphocytic choriomeningitis is caused by an arenavirus, endemic in house mice and pet hamsters. The condition occurs mainly in children and young adults. The onset is acute and evidence of meningeal irritation develops rapidly. Focal neurological signs are usually absent. There may be a high pyrexia which gradually reverts to normal in 5 to 7 days. The CSF is under increased pressure. It is usually clear but may be turbid as there is an excess of lymphocytes which may persist long after clinical cure. There may be a slight increase in the protein but the sugar and chloride levels are normal.

Lymphocytic choriomeningitis has to be differentiated from pyogenic meningitis in which the turbid CSF contains an excess of polymorphonuclear leucocytes and the causative organism can be isolated. Tuberculous meningitis may be difficult to distinguish owing to the technical difficulties of isolating the tubercle bacillus. A normal level of sugar in the CSF is in favour of a diagnosis of acute lymphocytic choriomeningitis. If there is any serious doubt as to the diagnosis, it is better to start treatment for tuberculous meningitis while awaiting further bacteriological reports.

There is no specific treatment for lymphocytic choriomeningitis. The patient is kept at rest in bed on symptomatic measures until the temperature has returned to normal. Complete recovery is the rule.

Viral encephalitis

All of the viruses which cause meningitis may also give rise to an encephalitis. Encephalitic features may predominate or a combined picture of meningoencephalitis may occur. More specific types of viral encephalitis occur in epidemic forms, such as Japanese B encephalitis (p. 736). Sporadic cases occur from influenzal, herpes simplex and arboviral infection but often the causative virus is not isolated.

Pathology. The distribution and extent of lesions vary to some extent with the type of infecting virus. There is usually diffuse damage to cells in the cortex, basal ganglia and brain stem. Inclusion bodies are often present in neurones and glial cells. There is usually infiltration between neurones and the perivascular spaces by polymorphonuclear cells initially and later by lymphocytes and monocytes. There is accompanying neuroglial proliferation. Herpes simplex encephalitis tends particularly to affect the temporal lobes and in encephalitis lethargica the substantia nigra, midbrain and basal ganglia are most prominently involved.

Clinical features. An acute onset of headache, often accompanied by fever, is the usual clinical presentation common to all types of viral encephalitis. Disturbance of consciousness, varying from mild drowsiness to deep coma, usually supervenes early and may sometimes advance dramatically. Epilepsy of focal or generalised type is common. A variety of focal signs such as aphasia, hemiplegia or tetraplegia, cranial nerve palsies and sensory disturbances may occur but sometimes there are none. The clinical features usually do not enable a firm diagnosis of the causal agent to be made but some types of encephalitis present distinctive manifestations as follows:

Herpes simplex encephalitis. This is the most common type in Britain. The onset is usually acute and commonly is marked by behavioural disturbance and a confusional state resembling a psychosis. This often lasts 2 or 3 days before other features develop. Myoclonus and seizures are very common; the EEG often shows periodic lateralised epileptiform discharges. Papilloedema and variable focal neurological signs may be present, commonly of temporal lobe dysfunction. Progression over a few days to coma is frequent.

Brain stem encephalitis is presumed to be of viral origin but the causal agent has not been defined. There is usually an antecedent history of mild upper respiratory infection. The onset, attended by headache, is often marked by double vision and dysarthria. Later there is increasing drowsiness and progressive cranial nerve involvement.

Encephalitis lethargica occurred in epidemic form during the 1920s and sporadic cases still appear. The illness varies markedly in severity. Headache and double vision may be the only features but sleep disturbances, upper motor neurone and extrapyramidal signs may be manifest. Oculogyric crises or parkinsonism may develop during the early stages of the illness or may be a sequel.

Epidemic myalgic encephalomyelitis is a condition which is presumed, though not proven, to be of viral origin. Coxsackie viruses have been implicated in some cases and Epstein Barr virus may cause a similar syndrome. It occurs in closed communities such as schools and hospitals. Common features are headaches, diffuse muscle pains, exhaustion, low grade pyrexia, lymphadenopathy, paraesthesiae and marked mood disturbances which may recur over long periods — the postviral fatigue syndrome.

Subacute sclerosing panencephalitis is thought to be due to infection by a myxovirus which is either measles virus or a closely related agent. It occurs in children and adolescents. The onset is usually an insidious intellectual deterioration, apathy and clumsiness accompanied later by myoclonic jerks and other involuntary movements. The EEG is distinctive, showing bursts of triphasic slow waves. As the disease progresses, rigidity and dementia supervene.

Rabies presents a distinctive clinical picture described on page 731.

Progressive multifocal leucoencephalopathy is a rare condition occurring late in the course of an antecedent disease, e.g. lymphoma or carcinoma. The pathological findings comprise widely disseminated demyelinating lesions in the brain together with distinctive changes in the glial cells suggestive of invasion by one of the papova group of viruses. It is a condition of rapid and progressive nature usually leading to death within a few weeks or months of its being manifest. The clinical picture varies widely. Hemiparesis is the commonest disability but dysphasia, dysarthria and hemianopia are also frequent. Dementia may occur, as may convulsions.

Acquired immunodeficiency syndrome. Chronic encephalitis may be one of the cerebral manifestations of AIDS (p. 726).

Diagnosis. These various forms of viral encephalitis should first be distinguished from other intracranial diseases such as cerebral tumour or abscess, from encephalopathies, from demyelinating encephalomyelitis (p. 648) and from trypanosomiasis (p. 779). Thereafter the type of viral infection should, if possible, be determined.

The differential diagnosis depends on the nature of the clinical features and the attendant circumstances. When the predominant features are progressive focal affection of one hemisphere accompanied by headache and drowsiness, the picture may strongly suggest a space-occupying lesion and intensive investigation may be needed to exclude such conditions as cerebral abscess. When the illness is mild, neurological signs indefinite and there are attendant general signs of viral infection the diagnosis will often be made presumptively after the patient improves.

Investigations are more helpful in excluding other lesions than in confirming the diagnosis of viral encephalitis. If consciousness is depressed or focal signs are present, lumbar puncture may be hazardous and should be deferred until CT scanning has excluded a tumour or hydrocephalus. In a minority of instances the CSF is normal. Usually the CSF pressure and protein content are moderately raised and there is pleocytosis. This is usually lymphocytic, but polymorphs may predominate in the early stages. The sugar content is normal. The EEG is usually altered. There is a diffuse slowing of the rhythms but the findings are non-specific except in subacute sclerosing panencephalitis. Periodic epileptiform discharges are typical of, but not confined to *herpes simplex* encephalitis.

Occasionally in herpes simplex encephalitis a radionuclide scan will show areas of increased uptake in one or both temporal lobes. This condition is potentially treatable so that it is important to establish the diagnosis when the patient's illness is severe and progressive. In such circumstances a biopsy of the temporal lobe may be justified but urgent virological and immunological study of the CSF may provide positive evidence of *H. simplex* virus, and should be performed first.

Serological tests and culture may identify the infecting virus but the results of such tests are usually available too late to guide treatment.

Treatment and prognosis. The management of most cases of viral encephalitis consists of nursing care and the prevention of intercurrent infections. When a positive diagnosis of herpes simplex encephalitis has been made, an antiviral agent such as acyclovir (p. 46) may be used together with dexamethasone (4 mg t.i.d.).

Most patients survive and may recover completely but persisting focal defects are frequent. A significant number (perhaps 10–30%) die. The outlook is particularly poor in herpes simplex encephalitis and in subacute sclerosing panencephalitis. Brain stem encephalitis has a good prognosis; complete, if sometimes slow, recovery is almost invariable.

Poliomyelitis

Aetiology and pathology. The disease is caused by one of three related polio viruses which comprise a subdivision of the group of enteroviruses. It is much less common following the widespread use of oral vaccines but is still a major problem in developing countries. Infection usually occurs through the nasopharynx.

The virus is liable to affect the grey matter of spinal cord, brain stem and cortex and has a particular propensity to damage anterior horn cells especially those within the lumbar segments. There is often accompanying infiltration of the meninges with lymphocytes.

Clinical features. The incubation period is 7–14 days. At the onset there is usually mild fever and headache which improves after a few days. Many cases do not progress beyond this stage. In other instances, after a period of well-being lasting approximately a week, there is a recurrence of pyrexia and headache accompanied by neck stiffness and signs of meningeal irritation. Paralysis may occur later. The extent is variable. Weakness of one muscle group may progress to widespread paresis. Respiratory failure may supervene if intercostal muscles are paralysed or the medullary motor nuclei are involved.

The CSF shows a lymphocytic pleocytosis, a rise in protein and a normal sugar content.

Treatment and prognosis. In the early stages bed-rest is imperative. At the onset of respiratory difficulties a tracheostomy and intermittent positive pressure respiration are required. Subsequent treatment is by physiotherapy and orthopaedic measures.

Epidemics vary widely in their incidence of abortive and nonparalytic cases and in mortality rate. Death occurs from respiratory paralysis. Paralysis is greatest at the end of the first week of the major illness. Gradual recovery may then take place for several months but any muscle showing no signs of recovery by the end of a month will not regain useful function. It is difficult to make a more definite prediction about the extent of permanent disability until 3 to 6 months after the onset. Second attacks are very rare but occasional patients show late deterioration in muscle bulk and power many years after the initial infection.

Prevention is by oral vaccination (p. 38).

Herpes zoster (shingles)

Invasion of posterior root ganglia by the varicella-zoster virus causes pain followed by a rash over the cutaneous distribution of the affected nerve. Zoster is believed to be due to reactivation of a previous infection by the varicella-zoster virus which has lain dormant in the body. The frequency and severity of zoster increases with age and in immunocompromised patients. Chickenpox may be contracted from a patient with zoster.

Clinical features. The first symptom is usually severe continuous pain in the distribution of the affected nerve root. After 3 or 4 days the skin in the painful area becomes reddened and vesicles appear which dry up over the course of 5 or 6 days, leaving small scars. The pain of zoster usually subsides as the eruption fades, but occasionally, especially in old people, it may be followed by a persistent and intractable neuralgia which may last for months.

Any dorsal root ganglion may be infected, most commonly those supplying the trunk where two or three adjacent dermatomes on one side only are often involved. Infection of the trigeminal ganglion usually involves the ophthalmic division; the vesicles appear on the cornea and may lead to corneal ulceration with the danger of scarring and impairment of vision (*ophthalmic herpes*).

Segmental muscle wasting may occur sometimes from involvement of the motor root. The virus occasionally invades the spinal cord or the brain giving rise to myelitis or encephalitis.

Treatment. Idoxuridine (p. 46) may be applied to the skin in a 5% solution in the early stages of the evolution of the rash; 0.1% drops are used for corneal infections. Systemic acyclovir is indicated for immunocompromised patients or when the infection is especially severe. The treatment of postherpetic neuralgia is difficult. Analgesics should be continued, but addictive ones, such as morphine must be avoided. Amitriptyline (25–100 mg/d) may help, and transcutaneous nerve stimulation is sometimes effective.

DEMYELINATING DISEASES

Loss of myelin sheaths occurs with many disorders of the central and peripheral nervous systems but there is a particular category with certain clinical and pathological features in common in which loss of myelin is considered to be the primary change and the axis cylinders may be spared or, if affected, are damaged secondarily. The lesions are almost entirely confined to the white matter of the central nervous system. They are initially inflammatory in type but differ from lesions caused by direct viral infection and so they are grouped separately from viral encephalitis.

MULTIPLE SCLEROSIS

Multiple sclerosis, also known as *disseminated sclerosis,* is the commonest of the demyelinating diseases. It affects about 1 in 2000 of the population in Britain.

Aetiology. The cause of the disease is unknown but there is much information about its prevalence and about the factors associated with its development. Incidence varies widely in different geographical areas. It is very low in the tropics and high in the temperate zones of both northern and southern hemispheres. Migrants from a high to a low prevalence area have a reduced risk of developing multiple sclerosis. Those who migrate from a low to a high prevalence area are at greater risk than had they remained in their original environment. These effects apply only to those who move before the age of 15 years.

A genetic susceptibility is suggested by an increased frequency of HLA-A3, B7 and Dw2/DRw2 in European patients with multiple sclerosis. There is also a greater occurrence of the disease in close relatives of sufferers than in the general population.

The part played by an autoimmune mechanism, possibly induced by a slow viral or a persistent measles infection, is also being studied but the results are inconclusive. One theory is that in genetically susceptible individuals the disease follows a dormant viral infection, either directly or via an immunological mechanism.

Pathology. The acute lesion consists of a circumscribed area in which the myelin sheaths have undergone destruction while the axis cylinders show only irregular swelling. The plaque has a swollen pinkish appearance because blood vessels are dilated, but there is little infiltration with inflammatory cells. Gliosis follows, so that the chronic lesion is a scar with a shrunken greyish appearance. The lesions are widely scattered in the white matter of the brain, especially round the ventricles, in the spinal cord and in the optic nerves. Despite the disseminated distribution there is a tendency for spinal cord and brain stem lesions to occur in symmetrical situations.

Clinical features are diverse. It is impossible to outline a 'typical' history. Characteristic features are a relapsing and remittent course and widespread lesions which result in varied symptomatology. The first manifestation may occur at any age but onset before puberty or after the age of 60 is rare. Initial symptoms present between 20 and 40 years of age in the majority of cases. Women are affected about one-and-a-half times as often as men.

Weakness of one or more limbs developing acutely is probably the commonest presentation. Unilateral retrobulbar neuritis is also a frequent mode of onset as are paraesthesiae affecting a limb or felt in a girdle distribution around the trunk. Diplopia, vertigo and ataxia are also common initial features. Less frequent are epilepsy, aphasia, hemiplegia, facial palsy and bouts of facial pain resembling trigeminal neuralgia.

In most instances the symptoms and signs of the initial manifestation recover completely within 1 to 3 months of the onset. A period of well-being follows and after a very variable interval there is a recurrence in many cases within 2 years. In a few instances there is no remission; the initial disability progresses and more widespread deficits develop. A minority of patients suffer three or four further exacerbations during the year following the onset. Another small group remains well for more than 10 years after the first disturbance.

The outlook for the second and subsequent manifestations is variable. Some patients continue to show exacerbations with virtually complete recovery for many years. In other instances successive relapses are attended by diminishing degrees of improvement. Eventually half of the sufferers enter a chronically progressive stage with persisting and increasing disability.

The signs depend on the site of the demyelinating lesion. Pallor of one or both optic nerve heads is common and is particularly prominent over the temporal halves of the discs even in patients who give no history of an earlier retrobulbar neuritis. Many patients develop diplopia from involvement of the midbrain. Nystagmus is often found.

Signs of motor dysfunction are usually present at some stage, particularly involving the upper motor neurone. The abdominal reflexes are often absent early and remain so. Later upper motor neurone signs in both legs and arms become more marked. Spasticity and paraplegia in flexion and flexor spasms ensue. In people who develop the disease in middle age the only manifestation is often a slowly progressive, moderate paraparesis without remission but without severe exacerbations. Motor and visual deficits are often temporarily but strikingly aggravated after a hot bath.

Cerebellar signs include the staccato, interrupted rhythm of scanning speech, ataxia and intention tremor; they are usually found during the progressive stage of the disease and are especially disabling.

Sensory symptoms are almost invariable at some time during the course of the disease. Paraesthesiae of varying type and distribution occur. Objective impairment of superficial sensation is usually less prominent than would be anticipated from the intensity of symptoms. A distinctive symptom is a tingling or 'electric shock-like' sensation which radiates into the arms, down the back, or into the legs when the patient flexes the neck. This is sometimes called the 'barber's chair' sign. It is most commonly due to multiple sclerosis but is not diagnostic thereof since it may occur in other diseases of the cervical cord such as compression or syringomyelia.

Localised muscle wasting, parkinsonian tremor and choreoathetotic movements are rare and it is unusual for the spinothalamic tracts to be involved to such an extent as to cause painless burns and trophic lesions. As the disease progresses sphincter disturbances occur, notably frequency and urgency of micturition or hesitancy and retention.

Some patients exhibit a sustained euphoria; others are fully aware of their disabilities and may become depressed. Late in the course of the disease there is often significant intellectual impairment.

Investigation. The diagnosis of multiple sclerosis depends clinically on the demonstration of lesions occurring at different times and at different sites in the central nervous system. Sometimes the occurrence of multiple lesions may not be apparent clinically but delayed evoked potentials after visual, auditory or somatosensory stimulation may indicate the presence of earlier lesions. Disseminated lesions in the white matter can be detected by CT and magnetic resonance imaging.

There is no specific test which will confirm the diagnosis. A raised proportion of gammaglobulin in the CSF in the presence of a normal total protein is present in approximately 70% of patients suffering from multiple sclerosis. Oligoclonal bands of IgG are present in over 90% of patients with multiple sclerosis but they are also found in other diseases (p. 605).

In some cases the diagnosis of multiple sclerosis has to be achieved by a process of exclusion. It is important in all patients to eliminate potentially curable conditions such as syphilis, vitamin B_{12} deficiency and spinal cord compression.

Treatment. There is no curative treatment but much can be done to support the patient during the course of the illness. Corticosteroids promote more rapid and complete recovery during acute exacerbations; 2 mg of dexamethasone given orally three times daily, for 5–10 days, is an adequate course of treatment. There is no evidence that prolonged administration of corticosteroids significantly alters long-term prognosis. Azathioprine may possibly reduce the relapse rate and is currently under trial.

Spasticity may become severe in multiple sclerosis and baclofen in a dose of 20 to 60 mg daily is sometimes helpful but too high a dose causes muscle weakness. Diazepam (2–10 mg t.i.d.) is also used to relieve spasticity. Severe, painful flexor spasms may be relieved by the intrathecal injection of phenol in glycerine.

Of prime importance in the management is encouragement and support of patients and their relatives. Regular medical supervision contributes to this end. Patients with motor disabilities should avoid any gain in weight. Periods of physiotherapy help the disabled patient. Assisted and passive movements and walking exercises improve gait as well as the patient's morale. In general the patient should be advised to avoid long periods in bed during intercurrent infections. Pressure sores should be prevented by advice about changes in posture and skin care; should they occur they must be treated early and vigorously in hospital.

Walking aids such as tripod supports or frames and the provision of wheel-chairs and motor vehicles together with the advice of an occupational therapist may enable the patient to function more easily at home and at work and to enjoy some form of social life. Nurses and social workers should regularly visit patients at home to assist in their care and to ensure that all the help which the community can provide is made available.

The care of the bladder is particularly important. Infections should be treated with an appropriate antibiotic. Male patients suffering from incontinence, urgency and frequency can be relieved by continuous drainage, through a tube attached to the penis, into a portable urinal strapped to the thigh. In some patients bladder neck resection is helpful. Various appliances are now available which help incontinent female patients. A permanent in-dwelling catheter, changed at intervals of a month or two, often makes life more comfortable and helps to prevent pressure sores but infection and leakage are problems, especially in female patients. For these reasons, urinary diversion via a urostomy is sometimes performed.

Prognosis is variable. Multiple sclerosis does not inevitably lead to immobility and a chairbound or bedridden existence. Approximately 5% of patients die within 5 years of the onset of the disease but a rather larger proportion remain well and retain unrestricted mobility for 20 years. The disease may run a progressive, disabling course, or may be relatively benign. It is not possible to predict the outlook with confidence in any individual patient though there are some useful indicators.

A favourable course often follows when retrobulbar neuritis is the initial manifestation, particularly when it occurs unaccompanied by any other neural deficit. A long gap between the presentation and the next recurrence often presages a fairly good prognosis, and particularly so if both manifestations recovery completely. If motor function is only slightly impaired during the early years of the disease, crippling disability is usually long delayed. Repeated episodes of purely sensory deficit with complete recovery point to a benign course. Those whose initial manifestation is relatively late have usually a better prognosis. An onset in the late teens or early twenties is often attended by a bad prognosis. Incomplete recovery from the initial attack is a sinister feature. Early recurrence, within 6 months of the initial manifestation, also suggests that relapses are likely to be frequent and disability rapidly progressive. However, at any stage of the disease striking improvement may follow sudden deterioration.

Acute demyelinating encephalomyelitis

This is a group of related acute disorders occurring without obvious cause about a week after diseases such as measles and chickenpox or following vaccination. There are areas of perivenous demyelination widely disseminated throughout the brain and spinal cord probably due to an immunological reaction.

Headache, vomiting, pyrexia, delirium and signs of meningeal irritation are presenting features. Fits or coma may occur. Flaccid paralysis and extensor plantar responses are common but sensory loss is unusual. Cerebellar signs may be present especially when the disorder follows chickenpox. The CSF may be normal or show a small increase of mononuclear cells and protein.

Neuromyelitis optica is a restricted form of the disease characterised by massive demyelination of the spinal cord and both optic nerves.

ACTH 80–120 units by injection or prednisone 60 mg by mouth daily for several days followed by a maintenance dose for 2 to 3 weeks is beneficial. These drugs must be used with caution in chickenpox if encephalitis develops before the rash has subsided as it may become confluent and haemorrhagic. The usual care of the paralysed and incontinent patient is required.

The mortality rate is high in neuromyelitis optica and in postvaccinal encephalomyelitis but is low in the postexanthematous cases. If the patient survives, the recovery may be remarkably complete and second attacks are very rare.

DISEASES OF THE EXTRAPYRAMIDAL SYSTEM

In diseases of this system voluntary movement is disturbed, involuntary movements appear and muscle tone is altered.

PARKINSONISM

Parkinsonism is the name given to a clinical syndrome comprising impairment of voluntary movement (hypokinesis), rigidity and tremor. Its incidence is approximately 1 in every 1000 of the population rising to about 1% in those over 60 years.

Aetiology. Parkinsonism is caused by lesions in the basal nuclei and is associated particularly with damage to the interconnecting system between the substantia nigra and the corpus striatum. The nigrostriatal pathways utilise dopamine as a neurotransmitter, and parkinsonism is associated with dopamine deficiency. The precise pathophysiology and the interdependent biochemical abnormalities in parkinsonism are incompletely defined.

The commonest entity, accounting for perhaps

three-quarters of cases, is *paralysis agitans* (also called idiopathic parkinsonism or Parkinson's disease) which is of unknown origin. Parkinsonism is a recognised sequel of encephalitis lethargica and rarely results from other encephalitides caused by such viruses as Coxsackie type B and Japanese B but no convincing evidence exists to implicate viral infection as a cause of Parkinson's disease. Hereditary factors are not important in typical cases, since concordance between pairs of identical twins is low. Parkinsonism is frequently — and usually wrongly — attributed to cerebral atherosclerosis. Many patients suffering from parkinsonism also show signs of cerebral atherosclerosis, but it is probable, in most instances, that the two conditions — both common in the elderly — occur coincidentally. Discrete cerebrovascular lesions affecting the substantia nigra may, very occasionally, cause parkinsonism.

Of the known causes of parkinsonism, drugs which block postsynaptic dopamine receptors (phenothiazines and butyrophenones) or deplete dopamine stores (reserpine and tetrabenazine) are the best known. Parkinsonism may occasionally follow a single head injury and is often a sequel of repeated head trauma in the 'punch-drunk' syndrome. There are other infrequent causes of parkinsonism, namely cerebral tumours, notably those causing midbrain compression, parasagittal and sphenoidal ridge meningiomas, meningovascular syphilis, carbon monoxide poisoning, manganese poisoning and copper deposition in Wilson's disease. Severe parkinsonism has occurred in drug addicts exposed to methyl-phenyl-tetrahydro-pyridine (MPTP). The active toxin appears virtually selective for the substantia nigra neurones, and has some chemical similarity to paraquat and other herbicides.

Pathology. In parkinsonism the most consistent histological change is cellular loss and depigmentation of the substantia nigra. In paralysis agitans the characteristic pathological changes accompanying loss of cells are Lewy bodies (hyaline masses of cytoplasm and sphingomyelin) in the central areas of the substantia nigra. In postencephalitic parkinsonism the cell depletion affects the whole substantia nigra and is usually more severe than in paralysis agitans. Other changes, such as atrophy of the globus pallidus

and patchy cortical atrophy, are inconstant.

Clinical features. Two-thirds of patients first develop symptoms in the fifth or sixth decades. Initial manifestations are usually so slight and develop so insidiously that a gap of 2 or 3 years may elapse between the onset of the condition and its diagnosis. Occasionally the presentation is acute and progression is rapid; this is particularly likely in postencephalitic or drug-induced cases.

Tremor is usually the feature which causes the patient to seek advice. It first involves the fingers and spreads to proximal parts of the arms; it may later extend to the tongue and legs. The tremor is slow and in the earliest stages involves rhythmical movement of the thumb towards the fingers. The fully developed movement comprises a combination of adduction and abduction of the thumb, flexion and extension of the interphalangeal and metacarpophalangeal joints as well as pronation and supination of the wrists. Tremor is present at rest and often is lessened during purposive activity. Stress and embarrassment aggravate the tremor's amplitude. These factors are operative during clinical testing so that requested movements may be accompanied by increased, rather than reduced tremor. Head tremors are rare in parkinsonism. Tremor may never be present during the course of the condition and often diminishes as rigidity progresses.

Rigidity is usually detectable early. Resistance to passive movement is increased throughout the range of movement of a joint. Concurrent tremor may lead to the 'cog-wheel' phenomenon — a superimposed jerky sensation. Profound rigidity is accompanied by fixed abnormalities of posture. The patient is flexed at neck, hips, elbows and knees. The hands are flexed at the metacarpophalangeal joints and hyperextended at the interphalangeal joints; these deformities, accompanied by adduction of the thumb across the palm, present a characteristic picture.

Hypokinesis, comprising delay in initiation of movements together with paucity, slowness and lack of precision of movements, is the most disabling feature. Of insidious onset it may first be manifest by a gradual reduction in size and legibility of a patient's handwriting. Other fine movements, such as fastening buttons and laces, are impaired, and later feeding and even turning over in bed become difficult. There is often difficulty in rising from a chair and in starting to walk. Loss of normal arm swinging when the patient walks is a very early sign of hypokinesis.

Later the gait displays characteristic features. Steps are short and shuffling. Walking is usually slow but is sometimes accompanied by periods of uncontrolled acceleration when walking downhill. This phenomenon, called festination, causes patients to take ever more rapid, smaller and smaller steps as they chase their own centre of gravity. Falls often result and are due mainly to loss of normal postural reflexes necessary for standing and turning.

Normally pliant emotional movements of the face are slow in starting, reduced in amplitude and prolonged in their accomplishment. Blinking is usually reduced but spontaneous blepharo-spasm is an occasional feature, particularly in postencephalitic parkinsonism. Blinking provoked by tapping the glabella does not show the normal habituation.

Impaired pupillary accommodation is a common finding in all types of parkinsonism. Sustained, involuntary, conjugate deviation of the eyes, usually upwards, called oculogyric crises, may last for minutes or hours; they occur in postencephalitic and drug-induced parkinsonism.

Speech is often affected. Some loss of voice volume is almost invariable. Delayed initiation and dysarthria are common. The cadence is slow; inflection is restricted so that speech becomes monotonous.

Hypokinesis may be overcome for short periods under the influence of a strong emotional drive such as fear or anger. Though the defects in voluntary movement are often striking and disabling, power is well preserved.

Signs of upper motor neurone involvement are not found in uncomplicated paralysis agitans, but they may be detected if there is accompanying cerebral atherosclerosis; they commonly occur in postencephalitic and post-traumatic parkinsonism and are found in those rare instances where parkinsonism is due to a cerebral tumour.

Differential diagnosis. Physiological tremor often is exaggerated in the elderly and by anxiety, alcoholism and thyrotoxicosis. It is much faster than parkinsonian tremor, tends to occur only in one plane and lacks the abduction/adduction movement of the thumb. Exaggerated physiological tremor present on holding out the hands or on movement may occur sporadically or have a genetic basis (essential or familial tremor). Symptoms tend to start early in adult life, and are markedly improved by drinking a small quantity of alcohol.

Cerebellar atrophy is of fairly frequent occurrence in elderly patients who manifest intention tremor. Such a tremor is relieved when an affected limb is supported and relaxed and increases as the limb approaches a target.

Depressed and hypothyroid patients are often apathetic and lack normal facial expressiveness so that their appearance may suggest a diagnosis of parkinsonism.

Atherosclerotic dementia, with its attendant apathy, is often associated with increased tone due to bilateral upper motor neurone signs and may mimic parkinsonism. Other clinical features such as an exaggerated jaw jerk, increased tendon reflexes and spasticity rather than rigidity differentiate this condition from parkinsonism.

Treatment. Ideally, this should be aimed at the cause. The drug-induced condition is the only type which is both relatively common and curable if the offending drug is discontinued. In the majority of parkinsonian patients the cause is not known and treatment is designed to ameliorate disability. The most generally effective therapy for established cases is a combination of an anticholinergic preparation together with levodopa and a dopadecarboxylase inhibitor.

Anticholinergic drugs produce modest improvement in early tremor and rigidity but have little effect on hypokinesis. They cause confusion and hallucination in the elderly and should be avoided in patients older than 65. There are a number of synthetic preparations, such as benzhexol hydrochloride (2 mg or 5 mg), benztropine (2 mg) and orphenadrine (50 mg). One of these drugs is introduced in small amounts, such as one tablet twice daily, and the dose is increased until dryness of the mouth or blurring of vision supervenes. The dose is then reduced slightly to obviate these effects.

Dopamine replacement. Levodopa has strikingly improved the treatment of parkinsonism. Given by mouth in doses varying from 2 to 8 g (average 5 g daily) levodopa reduces disability in more than two-thirds of patients and is particularly effective in relieving hypokinesis. The drug causes many side-effects, some of which develop early, e.g. nausea, vomiting, and cardiac arrhythmias; these are reduced if the drug is given together with a dopadecarboxylase inhibitor.

More than 90% of an orally ingested dose of levodopa is metabolised in extracerebral tissues and does not reach the brain. Selective inhibition of extracerebral dopadecarboxylase reduces the amount of levodopa required to produce a therapeutic effect and also diminishes the side-effects caused by peripheral breakdown of levodopa. Preparations are available which combine levodopa with extracerebral dopadecarboxylase inhibitors, e.g. 250 mg of levodopa and 25 mg of carbidopa or 50 mg of benserazide. One such tablet is equivalent in its therapeutic effect to 1 g of levodopa. This combined therapy, like levodopa itself, must be introduced in small amounts (50 mg levodopa b.d.) and the dose increased gradually over the first month. Nausea, vomiting and postural hypotension occur less frequently than with levodopa used alone. Dose-related side-effects are commonly dyskinesias, particularly of the face, dystonic postures and psychiatric disturbance including hallucination and delusions.

After at least 3 years of good control with levodopa, some patients develop fluctuations in their abilities during each day. This phenomenon has been called the 'on-off' effect, since the patient may alternate quite abruptly between periods of good mobility and spells of hypokinesis, dyskinesia and tremor. In its simplest form, the 'on-off' effect is due to fluctuation in blood and brain levodopa levels. As the disease progresses and more nigro-striatal neurones are lost, levodopa is stored less effectively and individual doses are beneficial for shorter periods. End of dose deterioration of this type can often be improved by giving the levodopa in frequent (1.5–3 hourly) small doses. Another approach is to add the selective type B monoaminoxidase inhibitor selegiline (5–10 mg/d) which may slow the breakdown of dopamine. In more complex cases, 'on-off' phenomena occur unpredictably and may be due to other mechanisms such as receptor blockade by dopa metabolites. In addition to giving frequent small doses of levodopa combination therapy, some patients are helped by adding bromocriptine (see below).

Dopamine receptor agonists. These drugs act principally by stimulating striatal dopamine receptors on postsynaptic sites, but probably also modulate presynaptic function. The best known is bromocriptine but other agents such as lisuride and pergolide have similar effects. Bromocriptine may be used alone or in combination with levodopa. An initial dose of 2.5 mg is given, and then the daily dose increased slowly over several weeks to 30–60 mg. Nausea and psychiatric side-effects are common, but dyskinesias are rather less frequent than with levodopa. Used alone, these agents are less impressive and more expensive than levodopa, but may have long-term benefits of fewer dyskinetic and 'on-off' problems.

Amantidine (100 mg b.d. or t.i.d.) potentiates endogenous dopamine and has a weak and usually short-lived effect on tremor and hypokinesis. It commonly causes vasodilation with livedo reticularis and oedema, and may also cause confusion and seizures in some cases.

Therapeutic strategy. Patients with early Parkinson's disease, with mainly tremor and little hypokinesis can be treated sometimes for years with anticholinergic agents alone. Amantidine may be used with benefit if hypokinesis is mild. Moderate or severe hypokinesis responds best to levodopa plus a decarboxylase inhibitor. Dopamine agonists have a less well-defined role, and tend to be used later as adjunctive agents.

Stereotactic thalamotomy is now rarely employed; however, it may be helpful in occasional patients whose disability is unilateral tremor unresponsive to medical treatment.

Prognosis. There are extreme variations in the rate of progression and the degree of disability produced. 20% of patients suffering from parkinsonism at any given time cannot cope independently with the normal activities of living. The mortality of patients suffering from parkinsonism is three times that of the general population of similar age. Levodopa, though it ameliorates disability, does not slow the progress of the basic pathology. There is some evidence that the rate of progression may be accelerated by levodopa and therefore a case can be made for withholding its use until symptoms become disabling.

Other disorders of the extrapyramidal system

Wilson's disease (hepatolenticular degeneration) is described on page 359. In the cerebral type necrosis and sclerosis of the corpus striatum cause basal ganglion syndromes in adolescence. Most common is choreoathetosis, but parkinsonism may be caused according to the site mainly affected. There is usually cortical involvement leading to progressive dementia in which loss of emotional control is a feature.

Kernicterus is a disorder of the basal ganglia and auditory nuclei occurring in association with neonatal haemolysis, particularly in premature infants. It may be caused by haemolytic disease of the newborn (p. 518), but prematurity is more important than Rh incompatibility.

Premature babies have a functional immaturity of the glucuronyl transferase enzyme system of the liver, and, as a result, unconjugated bilirubin formed by haemolysis is not conjugated. Unconjugated bilirubin rapidly rises to toxic levels which depress oxidative metabolism of brain cells, and in particular those of the basal ganglia. The danger decreases rapidly about 10 days after the birth in normal full-term infants when the liver enzyme system matures, but the premature baby is in danger for a longer period.

Convulsions, coma, opisthotonos and rigidity may be early manifestations but athetoid movements or spastic paralysis, deafness of nuclear type, and mental deficiency may not appear until the baby is several months old.

Prevention depends on the early detection of haemolytic jaundice, especially in the premature child, and its prompt treatment by exchange transfusion (p. 519). There is no treatment for established kernicterus and the future management is that of the child with cerebral palsy.

Chorea. Choreiform movements are irregular, jerking, ill-sustained and unpredictable, easily recognised when fully developed. In milder forms the condition may seem to be no more than restlessness or fidgeting. Often chorea is accom-panied by athetoid movements. Chorea may be the sole neurological manifestation of systemic lupus erythematosus, idiopathic hypoparathyroidism or polycythaemia vera.

Sydenham's chorea (St Vitus' dance) occurs in adolescents and is commoner in girls. It often follows a streptococcal throat infection. The onset may be abrupt or insidious. Choreiform movements are usually generalised and are accompanied by emotional lability so that often the condition is thought initially to be psychogenic. Pregnancy may precipitate a recurrence of chorea.

Because of the agitation, the patient, in all but the mildest cases, should be admitted to hospital and preferably be nursed in isolation. Diazepam or haloperidol should be prescribed. An initial course of penicillin should be given.

Most patients recover within a month, though more prolonged illnesses occur and relapses are common. Since many patients later develop valvular heart disease their future observation and management should be as for rheumatic fever.

Huntington's chorea is of autosomal dominant inheritance and usually first presents in the thirties. Choreiform movements, often particularly prominent in the face, are accompanied by progressive dementia. The movements may be well controlled by tetrabenazine (50–200 mg/d) which is usually tolerated in this condition. The mental deterioration is untreatable and institutional care may be needed as the disease progresses. Because the disorder may not present until the fourth or fifth decade, people with an affected relative often seek genetic advice before the disease can be excluded. It is hoped that new gene mapping techniques will allow the detection of potential sufferers early in life.

Ballism and athetosis. Flinging limb movements of wide amplitude are called *ballismic movements*. They resemble chorea but are much more violent and affect more proximal muscle groups. It is sometimes an arbitrary decision whether one calls movements severe chorea or ballism. Usually they suddenly affect one side of the body (hemiballism or, if less dramatic, hemichorea) as a result of a subthalamic vascular lesion in elderly patients. Spontaneous improvement usually occurs over a period of weeks and during this time tetrabenazine may decrease the disability. When hemiballism persists it can be treated by stereotactic thalamotomy.

Athetoid movements are relatively slow, confluent, writhing and usually most prominent at the periphery of the limbs. They are often accompanied by choreiform movements and by forced axial rotations of the trunk and neck (torsion dystonia). Athetosis usually results from cerebral hypoxia or trauma at birth or during the neonatal period and from kernicterus. Drug treatment is usually ineffective, though tetrabenazine, haloperidol or diazepam occasionally produce improvement in mild cases. Stereotactic procedures, indicated only in severe disability, sometimes help.

DIFFERENTIAL DIAGNOSIS. The involuntary movements of chorea, athetosis and ballism must be distinguished from *tics* which in most cases are not due to organic disease. Tics are usually rapid, repetitive, co-ordinated and stereotyped movements, most of which can be mimicked. Their pattern varies widely but an individual's tic tends to be reproduced faithfully. Common mild tics, including blepharospasm, sniffing, and shrugging movements, may be irritating but rarely need treatment. When well established in an adult they are virtually irremediable. In contrast, many children develop tics, often elaborate facial movements which cause much parental concern but which almost always disappear.

In adults, involuntary movements may be induced by drugs. Amphetamine addiction leads to repeated, rapid chewing movements of the jaws. Complex tongue, mouth, and cheek movements may result from taking phenothiazines or levodopa. Withdrawal of the causal drug usually leads to improvement in the case of levodopa; but if phenothiazines are the cause, dyskinesia may persist or worsen after drug withdrawal. This problem is usually seen in the elderly after years of phenothiazine therapy (*tardive dyskinesia*); it is difficult to treat but may respond to a more selective dopamine receptor blocking drug such as pimozide or sulpiride. Tetrabenazine reduces dopamine release and is also helpful.

Spasmodic torticollis is a form of involuntary movement which comprises turning of the head to one side and starts most commonly in the thirties. Initially rapid and correctable rotating movements may give place to long-sustained and later to fixed deviation of the neck.

DEGENERATIVE AND CONGENITAL DISEASE

In many diseases of unknown cause, there is clinical and pathological evidence of damage which is confined to a special type of neurone, e.g. motor neurone disease. Although no causative factors have been identified, it seems probable that many of the following disorders will ultimately be classified together as being due to 'biochemical lesions'. The metabolic functions of the neurone are controlled by its cell body but when any gradual failure of any of these processes occurs the effect is first seen at the end of its axon, so that there occurs a progressive 'dying back' of the neurone from its termination towards the cell body, associated with loss of nucleo-protein in the cell (chromatolysis). This is the typical feature of the pathology of the degenerative and congenital disorders.

Motor neurone disease

This rare disorder of unknown cause is the paradigm of a systematised neurological disease.

Loss of motor neurones and gliosis can be demonstrated in the motor cortex, in the motor nuclei of the brain stem and in anterior horn cells of the spinal cord. In the cord, there is also loss of myelinated corticospinal fibres.

Clinical features. Motor neurone disease is characterised by the insidious onset and uninterrupted progression of combinations of lesions of upper and/or lower motor neurones. Fasciculation (p. 594) is common. Motor neurone disease is twice as frequent in males and is rare before 40 years of age. The commonest age of onset is in the sixth decade. Some patterns of evolution are frequently manifest and are usefully categorised because they offer a guide to prognosis.

PROGRESSIVE BULBAR PALSY comprises dysarthria, dysphonia and dysphagia. Impaired articulation is usually the earliest feature but difficulty in swallowing, hoarseness and loss of voice volume supervene. There are signs of true, as well as supranuclear, bulbar palsy. Wasting and fasciculation of the tongue are accompanied by spasticity thereof and a pathologically brisk jaw jerk.

Features of bulbar palsy eventually develop in the later stages of the other types listed below.

AMYOTROPHIC LATERAL SCLEROSIS is probably the commonest mode of presentation and is characterised by lower motor neurone signs in the upper limbs and upper motor neurone signs in the legs. Wasting and weakness of the small muscles of the hands, usually the earliest manifestation, are accompanied by spasticity of the legs and extensor plantar responses. Wasting and fasciculation spread to the proximal arm muscles and the leg musculature; increased tendon reflexes in the arms may later indicate involvement of the upper motor neurones.

PROGRESSIVE MUSCULAR ATROPHY implicates only lower motor neurones for long periods. It usually presents with foot drop, which is often initially unilateral but eventually becomes symmetrical. Wasting and weakness of the hands, proximal spread of lower motor neurone affection in the limbs and the addition of upper motor neurone involvement occur after an interval of years.

COURSE. These labelled entities are frequently recognised but variant patterns are common. As the disease progresses the pictures of the different categories merge so that the final picture usually includes severe bulbar palsy as well as upper and lower motor neurone signs in all four limbs. Full awareness and normal intellectual abilities are usually preserved intact throughout the course of the illness. The CSF is almost always normal.

Differential diagnosis. Four pathological processes which are potentially treatable may closely mimic motor neurone disease and should always be excluded. (1) An occult carcinoma (particularly of the bronchus) may produce systematised motor neurone lesions. A chest radiograph should always be obtained in patients presenting the features of motor neurone disease, and if there are indicative clinical features further investigations should be performed. (2) Diabetic amyotrophy (p. 484) may resemble motor neurone disease and accordingly diabetes mellitus must be excluded. (3) Meningovascular syphilis can present a picture similar to that of motor neurone disease and syphilitic serology is therefore an essential investigation. (4) Cervical spondylosis which can cause lower motor lesions in the arms

and upper motor neurone lesions in the legs, can be excluded by radiological examination.

Treatment and prognosis. No medical treatment improves the outlook in motor neurone disease. Management includes the provision of walking aids and wheel-chairs and the maintenance of morale. Physicians have a duty to support patients and their relatives and to relieve distress in the disease's terminal stages.

Motor neurone disease is inexorably progressive and invariably fatal. Death usually results from pneumonia and respiratory failure and within 2 years of the onset of bulbar palsy. Amyotrophic lateral sclerosis is compatible with 4 or 5 years of life from the initial manifestation. Progressive muscular atrophy runs the most prolonged course; death usually occurs in 8 to 10 years from the onset.

The final state, of anarthria, aphagia and widespread limb weakness, in a person fully aware of the position, is extremely distressing for the patient and the family.

Spinal muscular atrophies

These are a group of genetically determined disorders of the anterior horn cell which present with weakness and wasting usually of proximal muscles. They may be confused with primary myopathies (p. 666) but can be distinguished from them by electromyography and muscle biopsy. A distal form, affecting muscles of the hands and feet, is one of the causes of *peroneal muscular atrophy* (Charcot-Marie-Tooth syndrome). Various proximal forms are classified according to the age of onset. The *Werdnig-Hoffman type,* of infantile onset, is severe and rapidly progressive, whereas the adult-onset spinal muscular atrophy often progresses slowly. The lower motor neurone palsies with fasciculation may be mistaken for the graver motor neurone disease. Treatment is confined to orthopaedic management but specialised investigation is required to determine the prognosis and for genetic counselling.

The hereditary ataxias

This is a group of related hereditary or familial disorders in which the systems of neurones which 'die back' are mainly the spinal and brain stem tracts leading to the cerebellum, the corticospinal tracts, and the optic nerves. Different combinations of these form recognisable clinical pictures, which usually 'breed true' in a family. The group forms a link with hereditary disorders of the peripheral nerves such as peroneal muscular atrophy and with neurofibromatosis (p. 656) and these may occur in association with the hereditary ataxias either in one individual or in the same family. Congenital deformities, particularly pes cavus, are also commonly present.

Clinical features. The onset may be any time from infancy to middle life. Symptoms are slowly progressive. Where cerebellar or spinocerebellar neurones are involved there is progressive ataxia of gait, followed by intention tremor of the arms, dysarthria of explosive type and, in some types, nystagmus. Where the main lesion is in corticospinal tracts there is a hereditary spastic paraplegia. Optic atrophy and loss of bladder reflexes may occur.

Friedreich's ataxia is the most common type, usually familial but occasionally sporadic. There is degeneration of the spinocerebellar and corticospinal tracts, and of the posterior columns. There is therefore very severe ataxia. Tendon jerks are lost at an early stage, muscle tone is decreased and the plantar reflexes are extensor. Muscle, joint and vibration senses are impaired as the posterior column degeneration progresses. Scoliosis and pes cavus are almost invariable and other congenital abnormalities such as spina bifida are common. There may be associated hypertrophic cardiomyopathy, diabetes mellitus or deafness.

Treatment and prognosis. There is no specific treatment. Co-ordination exercises and occupational therapy will help the patient to overcome the disability in the early stages but a wheel-chair life becomes inevitable later. Scoliosis and pes cavus may require appropriate appliances or orthopaedic surgery. All diseases of this group are progressive but compatible with a long life.

Syringomyelia

Cavities, filled with fluid and surrounded by glial tissue, lying near to the centre of the spinal cord, are the characteristic pathological lesions.

Aetiology. The most important factor is failure of development of the foramina of Magendie and Luschka. Cerebrospinal fluid cannot escape into the subarachnoid space from the fourth ventricle since its roof is imperforate. Pressure rises within the closed ventricular system and is communicated to the central canal of the cord which expands along irregular paths of least resistance.

The expanding cavity usually disrupts second order spinothalamic neurones, often interrupts the lateral columns, and may extend laterally to damage anterior horn cells (Figs. 15.2 and 15.3). Clinical signs predictably reflect the interruption of function of these neural structures; this is usually maximal in the lower cervical region.

Dilatation of the central canal of the cord may also result from increased pressure in the canal associated with congenital malformations of the brain in the region of the foramen magnum, e.g. herniation of parts of the cerebellum through the foramen magnum (*Arnold-Chiari syndrome*).

Clinical features. Symptoms are of insidious onset, and slow progression. Patients usually present in the third or fourth decade but signs may be detectable much earlier. A most characteristic sensory feature is 'dissociated' sensory loss, i.e. loss or depression of pain and temperature sensation with preservation of the modalities of touch, vibration and position. The patient often recognises this sensory loss and seeks advice because of it. Less commonly, when pain fibres are irritated, pain in the arms is a presenting feature. Loss of protective sensory functions leads to trophic lesions such as painless burns and ulcers on the hands and sometimes painless, disorganised joints (Charcot's joints) in the upper limbs.

Wasting of the small muscles of one or other hand is often manifest early. Loss of one or more reflexes in the arms is almost invariable. Characteristically there are upper motor neurone signs in the legs. Hyperreflexia in the legs and extensor plantar responses are common.

Upward extension of the cavities to involve the lower brain stem (*syringobulbia*) leads to dissociated sensory loss on the face, palatal palsy, Horner's syndrome and nystagmus. Kyphoscoliosis, pes cavus and spina bifida are often found.

Investigations should be aimed at defining

potentially treatable anomalies around the foramen magnum. Radiographs of this area may
show bony malformations. CT scanning or myelography demonstrates cysts or malformations of
the medulla. The most sensitive and least invasive
method for the investigation of syringomyelia is
magnetic resonance imaging.

Treatment and prognosis. Where causative
congenital lesions are demonstrated early, surgical
treatment is indicated. Decompression of the
foramen magnum, opening the roof of the fourth
ventricle, aspiration of the cavity in the cord and
occlusion, by muscle, of the upper end of the
central canal, may prevent progression of the
disease. If surgical treatment is not feasible, management is directed towards preventing injury. In
the rarer cases where pain is a problem, it may be
relieved by radiotherapy aimed at the cavity. If
untreated the condition is slowly progressive, and
worsens if the brain stem is involved.

Neurofibromatosis (von Recklinghausen's disease)

This is an autosomal dominant disorder in which
fibromas are derived from the neurilemmal sheath
of the peripheral nerves, nerve roots or cranial
nerves. Tumours such as gliomas, meningiomas
and phaeochromocytomas may be associated with
neurofibromatosis.

Clinical features. A patient may show only
one or many of a wide range of cutaneous or of
peripheral or central neurological abnormalities.
Some of the more common are *café-au-lait* patches
of skin pigmentation, cutaneous fibromas and
benign tumours of peripheral nerves which are
discrete, movable lumps arranged along the course
of nerves. The nerve trunks may be thickened or
there may be a diffuse plexiform growth.

Solitary neurofibromas may occur on a spinal
nerve root or on a cranial nerve, especially the
eighth. The tumours may also occur within body
cavities, in the eyes and within the bones where
they cause cystic change or kyphoscoliosis. New
tumours gradually appear throughout life but
the progress is slow. Any tumour may become
malignant but the chances of it doing so are small.

Biopsy of a tumour is rarely necessary. With
intracranial and intraspinal types the protein level
of the CSF is very high. Radiological examination
may show that an internal auditory meatus or
intervertebral foramen is widened if it contains a
neurofibroma.

Treatment. No treatment is required unless
there is cerebral or spinal compression, or sarcomatous change, when removal of the tumour is
necessary.

NUTRITIONAL NEUROLOGICAL DISEASES

Malnutrition may cause lesions in a number of
sites in the nervous system. Deficiencies, particularly of the B vitamin group, are important causes
but there are often multiple contributary factors
and vitamin deficiencies may be combined with
protein deficiency and toxins, notably alcohol.
The various neurological syndromes that ensue
are best considered on an anatomical basis.

Lesions of the cerebral cortex. Vitamin B_{12}
or folate deficiency may cause a toxic confusional
state and, if the deficiency is prolonged, may result
in dementia. Pellagra (p. 72) gives rise to marked
impairment of higher cerebral function, delirium
and dementia. An isolated deficiency of pyridoxine
(p. 74) occasionally occurs in infants and causes
irritability and epileptic fits.

Alcoholics may develop a slowly progressive
dementia with cerebral atrophy due in part to a
direct toxic effect of alcohol but associated
multiple vitamin deficiencies also contribute.

Brain stem lesions. Rapidly developing,
severe deficiency of thiamin may cause *Wernicke's
encephalopathy* (p. 71). Pathologically there are
petechial haemorrhages in the brain stem and
widespread patchy necrosis of neurones. Clinically
there are disorders of ocular movement with
nystagmus often accompanied by memory defect
and confabulation (*Korsakoff's psychosis*, p. 71).
The condition, if untreated, may be fatal but
thiamin, if started early enough, produces
dramatic improvement.

Central pontine myelinolysis occurs in alcoholics.
There is widespread destruction of myelin in the
pons involving all the long tracts. The picture
usually develops suddenly with tetraparesis,
dysphagia and anarthria and is often terminal.

Cerebellar lesions. Ataxia of gait with little affection of the arms is due to degeneration of the anterior superior vermis of the cerebellum in alcoholics; if the patient continues to drink alcohol more widespread cerebellar dysfunction develops. The contributions of dietary deficiency and the toxic effect of alcohol are not clearly defined but withdrawal of alcohol and giving vitamins result in marked improvement.

Spinal cord lesions. VITAMIN B_{12} DEFICIENCY. *Subacute combined degeneration of the spinal cord* is characterised by demyelination affecting particularly the posterior columns and corticospinal tracts of the spinal cord. There is usually involvement of the peripheral nerves. The condition is associated with Addisonian pernicious anaemia and rarely follows gastrectomy. It usually develops gradually in the middle-aged. The most common presenting symptoms are paraesthesiae of the toes and, later, of the fingers. Motor symptoms, notably weakness and ataxia, become progressively more severe as the spinal cord is more extensively involved.

The physical signs depend on the degrees of involvement of the peripheral nerves and of the posterior and lateral columns of the spinal cord. Glove and stocking impairment of superficial sensation is almost invariable. Calf tenderness is often increased. Position and vibration sense are usually markedly impaired in the legs. The tendon reflexes may be brisk but commonly the ankle jerks are lost. The plantar responses are usually extensor. Occasionally there may be an associated toxic confusional state. It responds to treatment, but without it, dementia follows. Diagnosis should be confirmed by the estimation of vitamin B_{12} in the serum.

The treatment of vitamin B_{12} deficiency comprises large doses of hydroxocobalamin, $1000\,\mu g$ daily for a week, weekly for 3 months and monthly thereafter. The response to treatment depends on the stage at which it is initiated. The signs due to a peripheral neuropathy often recover completely; ataxia may markedly improve; severe spasticity and dementia often persist.

It is likely that severe folic acid deficiency will cause a clinical picture similar to subacute combined degeneration of the spinal cord, but this is less common and less well documented.

TROPICAL SPINAL ATAXIA occurs mainly in West Africa and is caused by cyanide in unprocessed cassava in times of food shortage due to drought. Normally cyanogenic glucosides are removed by soaking or other processes.

LATHYRISM. The consumption of peas, a common constituent of Indian diets, may produce an acute or slowly progressive spastic paraplegia if the pulses include *Lathyrus sativus* which contains a neurotoxin.

Peripheral nerve lesions. Deficiency of one or more of the vitamins of the B complex leads to neuropathy. Thiamin, nicotinic acid and pyridoxine deficiencies may cause a symmetrical, mixed sensory-motor neuropathy. In many instances, particularly in alcoholics and in the burning feet syndrome in the elderly, there are combined deficiencies of these vitamins. If treated early, nutritional polyneuropathy re-sponds well to a mixed diet and generous doses of the vitamin B complex. Vitamin E deficiency, usually due to a malabsorption syndrome, can be associated with both peripheral neuropathy and loss of myelin within the central nervous system.

DISEASES OF THE SPINAL CORD AND PERIPHERAL NERVES

COMPRESSION OF THE SPINAL CORD OR NERVE ROOTS

Aetiology and pathology. The more important causes of spinal cord compression are:

1. *In the vertebral column:* crush fracture of a vertebral body; posterior protrusion of an intervertebral disc; secondary carcinoma (from breast, prostate, bronchus or other sites); myelomatosis and tuberculous disease of the spine.

2. *In relation to the spinal meninges:* epidural abscess; tumours (meningioma, neurofibroma; infiltration with lymphomatous and leukaemic deposits); syphilitic meningitis.

3. *In the spinal cord:* tumours (gliomas, ependymoma and metastatic deposits).

Tumours, disc protrusions and trauma account for the majority of cases of spinal cord compression. It is convenient in practice to divide the tumours into those arising outside the spinal cord (extramedullary), which constitute about 80%, and those arising within (intramedullary).

A space-occupying lesion within the spinal canal may involve nerve tissue directly by pressure, or indirectly by interfering with the blood supply. Oedema from venous obstruction impairs the function of the neurones. Ischaemia from arterial obstruction leads to necrosis of the spinal cord. The earlier stages are reversible but severely damaged neurones do not recover so it is most important to diagnose and treat spinal compression without delay.

Clinical features. The onset of symptoms of spinal cord compression is usually slow but it may be acute with trauma or metastases, especially if there is arterial occlusion. Pain localised over the spine or in a root distribution is the most common initial symptom. It may be aggravated by spinal movement or by coughing, sneezing or straining at the toilet which cause temporary elevation of spinal fluid pressure. Paraesthesiae and numbness or cold sensations may also develop early, especially in the lower limbs. Motor symptoms, which usually appear later, consist of heaviness, stiffness or weakness of a limb. Urgency or hesitancy of micturition, leading eventually to urinary retention is usually a late manifestation.

The signs found on examination vary according to the structures involved. There may be a local kyphosis if there is vertebral disease, and local tenderness may be present with this or with extradural abscess. A bruit may be heard with a stethoscope over the site of an angioma.

Involvement of the posterior root gives rise to hyperaesthesia and later to sensory loss over the appropriate dermatome. When the anterior roots are affected there are signs of a lower motor neurone lesion at the corresponding level.

Interruption of ascending fibres in the spinal cord causes sensory loss below the level of the lesion which may be of superficial sensation or of proprioceptive sense, according to which tracts are mainly involved (Fig. 15.3). Light touch, however, is often affected early. Interruption of descending fibres gives rise to upper motor neurone signs below the level of the lesion and control of the sphincters may be lost.

The *Brown-Séquard syndrome* results if damage is confined to one side of the cord. On the side of the lesion there is a band of hyperaesthesia with below it loss of proprioceptive sense and upper motor neurone signs. On the other side there is loss of spinothalamic sensation (pain, warmth and cold) as fibres of that tract decussate soon after entering the cord.

The distribution of these signs varies with the level of the lesion. Lesions above the fifth cervical segment give signs of an upper motor neurone lesion and sensory loss in upper and lower limbs (tetraplegia). A lesion between the fifth cervical and first thoracic segments gives signs of a lower motor neurone lesion and segmental sensory loss in the upper limbs and signs of an upper motor neurone lesion in the lower limbs. A lesion in the thoracic cord causes a spastic paraplegia with sensory loss having a horizontal upper level on the trunk. A lesion in the lumbosacral cord gives signs of a lower motor neurone lesion in the appropriate segments of the lower limbs and sensory loss. Spinal lesions lower than the first lumbar vertebra cannot damage the spinal cord but may damage the roots of the cauda equina.

Investigation. Patients with a short history of advancing spinal cord compression should be investigated urgently. Plain radiographs of the spine may reveal bony or soft tissue abnormalities, but myelography is necessary for localisation and characterisation of the lesion in most cases. CSF may be taken for analysis at the time of myelography, and in cases of spinal block shows a normal cell count, very elevated protein and xanthochromia (*Froin's syndrome*). Withdrawal of fluid may alter the pressure balance above and below the lesion and cause rapid neurological deterioration. It is preferable to alert neurosurgical help before such procedures are undertaken.

Treatment and prognosis. Surgical relief of the compression is a matter of great urgency since recovery from severe paralysis is unlikely. A delay of even a few hours may be critical in extradural abscess. Exploration is also often required to ascertain the pathological nature of the lesion. If a benign extramedullary tumour is found, it may be removed. In malignant tumours, leukaemic infiltration, and in most intramedullary lesions decompression helps little if at all. Radiotherapy may halt the course of the disease and may be of help in the relief of pain.

Prognosis depends on the severity and duration of the compression before it is relieved. In addition, the nature of the cause must be taken into account. Thus decompression for a malignant lesion may be undertaken though it will be of only temporary benefit.

Paraplegia

This may result from many causes, e.g. tumours, trauma and other forms of spinal compression, multiple sclerosis, subacute combined degeneration of the cord and, in India, lathyrism.

Treatment must be directed to the cause but management of the paraplegia itself is most important if complications, which may in themselves lead to death, are to be avoided. Pressure sores, urinary infections, renal calculi, faecal impaction and contractures can all be prevented.

SKIN. The skin is liable to be damaged with the formation of pressure sores because of the loss of sensation, diminished blood supply and the immobility. The patient must be nursed on a specially made rubber mattress and every 2 to 4 hours should be turned to a position which will avoid pressure on bony prominences such as the sacrum and heels. This is most easily done by nursing the patient in a Stryker frame.

The skin must be kept dry and clean. If a pressure sore forms, the patient must not lie on the affected side and scrupulous asepsis must be observed until healing takes place. Skin grafting may be required. Nutrition must be maintained by a well-balanced diet containing adequate amounts of protein, vitamin C and iron.

BLADDER. If retention occurs, aseptic intermittent catheterisation must be carried out. An indwelling catheter may then be inserted and attached to a water-seal drainage bottle. It should be clipped and allowed to drain at regular intervals to establish reflex emptying of the bladder. As the rhythm becomes established the catheter is withdrawn and the patient trained to micturate reflexly at fixed times. Emptying of the bladder should be assisted by manual compression of the lower abdomen by patient or nurse.

A permanent indwelling urinary catheter is not desirable since it predisposes to infection, reduces bladder capacity and promotes calculus formation. Some paraplegic patients who do not establish an automatic bladder can be taught intermittent self-catheterisation, or, if this is not feasible, a urinary

diversion procedure with an abdominal stoma and collecting bag can be considered.

It is not advisable to give antibiotics prophylactically but if infection develops, it must be treated promptly. An adequate consumption of fluid should be ensured. Frequent turning and early ambulation where possible are the best measures for reducing the dangers of urinary stagnation and calculus formation.

BOWEL. Constipation must be prevented by suitable diet and laxatives. If it occurs it must be relieved by enemas; otherwise the faeces will become hard and impacted and may require to be removed manually.

PARALYSED PARTS. Spasticity readily leads to the development of flexor spasm and contractures in the limbs. This danger can be reduced by regular passive movement of the limbs and by nursing the patient in such positions as will discourage flexion of the joints. The weight of the bedclothes should be taken from the lower limbs by a cradle to reduce reflex stimulation and prevent drop-foot deformity. If there is no hope of recovery, flexor spasms may be abolished by intrathecal injection of phenol in glycerine or by section of anterior nerve roots.

REHABILITATION. When the cause of paraplegia is not progressive, a great deal can be done by rehabilitation. Patients may learn to walk with calipers or to use a wheel-chair. They may thus be able to care for themselves and may even follow suitable occupations and take part in a variety of recreational activities.

There is hope that computer-programmed muscle electrical stimulation will enable paraplegic patients to obtain limited muscle function sufficient to permit standing or even walking. These techniques are not yet fully developed, but it is likely that they will become more effective.

Cervical disc herniation and cervical spondylosis

Degenerative changes occur in the cervical intervertebral discs in the same manner as in the lumbar region (p. 660) and may lead to herniation. This may affect one disc only, most commonly that between the sixth and seventh cervical vertebrae, or there may be involvement of several discs with secondary osteoarthrosis. The latter changes (cervical spondylosis) are liable to interfere with the blood supply to the spinal cord, and thus lead to further damage.

Clinical features. The syndromes of acute cervical disc protrusion and chronic cervical spondylosis may occur at different times in the same patient. Acute herniation is usually laterally situated and causes compression of a nerve root but does not typically involve the spinal cord. The chronic degeneration of discs may be associated with midline herniation and so spinal cord compression may result.

ACUTE PROTRUSION OF A CERVICAL INTERVERTEBRAL DISC may occur at any age, usually without apparent trauma to the neck. The patient complains of attacks of pain in the neck which may be referred to the skin segmental area of one of the lower cervical nerve roots and to the muscles, bones and joints which it supplies. Hyperaesthesia and hyperalgesia may be found in the affected segment but sensory loss sometimes occurs. Depression of tendon reflexes utilising the affected root is common and lower motor neurone paresis of root distribution is also an occasional finding. The neck is held stiffly, and pain is produced by its movement.

CERVICAL SPONDYLOSIS. The highest incidence is in the decade 60 to 70. The symptoms are of two types depending on whether the protrusion is lateral or dorsomedial.

1. Lateral herniation of discs, with secondary calcification and osteophytes encroaching on the intervertebral foramina, causes radicular symptoms like those of the acute disc syndrome, but the onset may be subacute or insidious and involvement of more than one root on one or both sides is common.

2. Dorsomedial herniation of discs which become calcified results in transverse bars which cause pressure on the spinal cord and on the anterior spinal artery which supplies the anterior two-thirds of the cord. The onset is insidious. Upper motor neurone weakness involves one or more limbs and the legs may be spastic before the upper limbs are involved. Sensory loss is most common in the upper limbs where it has a dermatome pattern. Involvement of the spinothalamic ᵗⁱ͏cts may cause disturbance of pain and tempera-

ture sensation in the lower limbs, and in some cases muscle-joint sense is also defective. Pain and limitation of movement of the neck are not marked features unless a particular posture causes nipping of a nerve root.

Investigation. Radiological examination shows narrowing of the disc spaces and osteophyte formation with loss of the normal cervical lordosis. Oblique views show encroachment by osteophytes on the intervertebral foramina. The CSF is normal unless its circulation is obstructed, when the protein may be raised. It may be necessary to confirm the diagnosis by myelography but this is indicated only if surgical treatment is being considered (e.g. to relieve cord compression) or if the diagnosis is in some doubt.

Treatment. The acute syndrome is treated by rest in bed or by intermittent neck traction followed by immobilisation of the neck in a light metal or plastic collar.

Chronic cervical spondylosis can usually be managed conservatively, since symptoms of radiculopathy often settle spontaneously. If they do not, or if the features of cord compression are present, surgical decompression and intervertebral fusion can be considered.

The lumbago-sciatica syndrome

Lumbago is pain in the lower part of the back; sciatica is pain in the distribution of the sciatic nerve. They are not, therefore, disease entities but symptoms and they are often associated.

Aetiology and pathology. The most common cause is herniation of an intervertebral disc. Other causes are much rarer but important to recognise. They include spinal tumour (neurofibroma and meningioma), ankylosing spondylitis, malignant disease in the pelvis, and tuberculosis of the vertebral bodies. Degenerative changes in the intervertebral discs may appear as early as 20 years of age, but herniation is often precipitated by trauma such as twisting the spine, lifting heavy weights while the spine is flexed or during childbirth. The nucleus pulposus may bulge or rupture the annulus fibrosus, giving rise to lumbago by pressure on nerve endings in the spinal ligaments and by producing changes in the vertebral joints, and to sciatica by causing congestion of, or pressure on, the nerve roots.

Clinical features. The onset may be sudden or gradual, and may follow closely upon trauma to the back. Attacks of lumbago may precede sciatica by months or years.

Lumbago is characterised by sudden severe low back pain when the patient is bending, preventing straightening. The sciatic pain is felt in the buttock and radiates down the posterior aspect of the thigh and calf to the outer border of the foot. It is exacerbated by coughing or sneezing which raises the pressure in the veins and the spinal subarachnoid space. Paraesthesiae and later numbness may be felt over the distribution of the involved nerve root, most often the first sacral. In severe cases, weakness of the calf muscles or foot-drop may occur, according to which roots are involved. The signs associated with prolapse of an intervertebral disc may be divided into two groups.

Signs due to altered mechanics of the lumbar spine. Muscle spasm causes flattening of the lumbar curve and scoliosis at the level of the prolapsed disc. Tenderness may be found when pressure is applied to the side of the vertebral spines in the region of the affected disc.

Signs due to pressure on the nerve root. Involvement of the *first sacral* root causes loss of the ankle jerk, weakness of eversion and plantar flexion of the foot, and sensory loss over the outer border and sole of the foot. The glutei may be wasted on the affected side. Involvement of the *fifth lumbar* root causes weakness of dorsiflexion of the toes, eversion of the foot, and sometimes foot-drop. Sensory loss occurs on the dorsum of the foot and the lateral aspect of the leg over the fifth lumbar dermatome. The ankle jerk is not affected but the hamstring jerk is depressed. Involvement of the *fourth lumbar* root causes weakness of inversion of the foot and of the quadriceps muscle and loss of the knee jerk. Sensory loss is over the medial aspect of the leg.

A valuable sign of root pressure is limitation of flexion of the thigh on the affected side if the straight leg is raised (Lasègue's sign). If the third or fourth lumbar roots are involved, straight leg raising may be normal, but pain in the back may be induced by hyperextension of the hip with the knee flexed (femoral nerve stretch test).

Investigation. Causes of sciatic pain other than disc herniation can usually be excluded by pelvic examination and radiological examination of the lumbosacral spine. There may be no apparent radiological change in acute disc herniation, or there may be narrowing of the disc space with osteophyte formation at the margins of the vertebral bodies. Myelography is required only if the diagnosis is in doubt or for purposes of localisation before operation.

Treatment. The initial treatment in all cases is rest in bed on a firm mattress supported by fracture boards. Rest must be absolute with prohibition of the sitting position. Compromise in this respect and permission to leave bed for toilet purposes are the usual reasons for failure of this treatment. The roots most commonly involved are the first sacral and the fifth lumbar, in which case the patient should be kept supine and no rotation of the spine permitted; but in disc protrusion involving the fourth lumbar root the lateral position with flexion of the hips is best suited to relax tension on the affected root and hence to relieve pain. Bed-rest is continued for 2 to 4 weeks, after which gradual mobilisation with back-strengthening exercises is carried out over a further period of 10 to 14 days. For middle-aged or elderly patients with chronic residual backache and a tendency to acute attacks of lumbago, a spinal support may be of value. Cases which do not respond to rest, or in which there are progressive or severe neurological deficits, require surgery. Central disc prolapse with bilateral symptoms and signs, and disturbance of sphincter function demands urgent surgical decompression.

PERIPHERAL NEUROPATHY

The cells of origin of peripheral nerves lie in the anterior horns of the spinal cord and the dorsal root ganglia. Axons represent elongated processes of these cells. They are enveloped by a series of Schwann cells which form the fatty myelin sheath. Pathological processes which primarily affect cell bodies may first manifest themselves at the distal ends of axonal processes.

Many diseases affect peripheral nerves whose pathological reactions may be (1) parenchymal where the lesion affects (a) nerve cells and their axons, or (b) the myelin sheath; (2) interstitial where the pathological process primarily affects the connective tissue or blood vessels of nerves. Although these rather stereotyped reactions do not lead to distinctive clinical features, a knowledge of the pathological nature of a neuropathy is helpful in assessing its prognosis. The clinical classification of peripheral nerve lesions comprises involvement of one or more individual peripheral nerves or a generalised polyneuropathy.

Mononeuropathy

Affection of a single nerve is commonly due to trauma or to diabetes mellitus (p. 483). Sustained pressure or stretching of nerve occurs in a variety of situations. The radial nerve is implicated as, for instance, in the 'Saturday night' palsy which results from bizarre sleeping postures caused by drunkenness. The ulnar nerve at the elbow and common peroneal nerve at the head of the fibula may be compressed. The signs are those of lower motor neurone paresis and sensory loss in the distribution of the respective nerves. Complete recovery of function in 4 to 6 weeks is almost invariable.

ENTRAPMENT NEUROPATHY. Nerves may be compressed whenever they pass through or near rigid anatomical structures, particularly fibro-osseous tunnels; this is one of the most frequent affections of peripheral nerves.

Compression of the median nerve in the carpal tunnel is the commonest example and occurs mainly in middle-aged women unaccompanied by other disease. It may also be a complication of pregnancy, myxoedema, acromegaly or rheumatoid arthritis. The patient complains of pain, numbness, tingling or an 'electric shock' feeling in thumb and fingers supplied by the median nerve, especially after using the hand or in bed at night when it may waken the patient from sleep. There is sometimes objective sensory loss of the radial three and a half digits and there may be weakness and wasting of abductor pollicis brevis and opponens pollicis muscles. The condition is often bilateral. The diagnosis can usually be confirmed by nerve conduction studies, which show motor and sensory impairment across the carpal tunnel.

Rest and splinting at night should be tried.

Local injection of a corticosteroid (p. 560) is sometimes effective if there is no muscular wasting. Thyroxine relieves the carpal tunnel syndrome in myxoedema. The syndrome occurring in pregnancy usually disappears in the puerperium but until then may be controlled by diuretics. If these measures are unsuccessful the condition can be relieved by surgical decompression of the nerve in the carpal tunnel.

The *lower trunk of the brachial plexus* may be compressed at the thoracic outlet, especially if there is a cervical rib or more often a fibrous band passing between the C7 transverse process and the first rib. Nocturnal pain in the arm and sensory-motor disturbance in the C8-T1 distribution are accompanied by wasting of the thenar and other intrinsic hand muscles. There may be tenderness and a bruit at the supraclavicular fossa. Minor symptoms often settle with rest and physiotherapy, but operative intervention is indicated if muscle wasting and weakness is established.

The *lateral cutaneous nerve of the thigh* may be entrapped at the inguinal ligament giving rise to paraesthesiae and pain over the anterolateral aspect of the thigh (meralgia paraesthetica).

Mononeuritis multiplex

In this condition several spinal nerves are involved concurrently or serially. Clinically signs are limited to discrete neural territories. Leprosy is a common cause in some geographical areas (p. 756). Polyarteritis nodosa, rheumatoid arthritis (p. 558) and other connective tissue disorders, diabetes mellitus (p. 483) and sarcoidosis may also give rise to mononeuritis multiplex.

Localised radiculopathy

Neuralgic amyotrophy. Demyelination of a localised group of nerve roots sometimes follows vaccination or inoculation; an immunological mechanism may be responsible. It may also occur after infection, injuries or operations.

The patient complains of severe pain over one shoulder, sometimes spreading up the neck or down the arm. Simultaneously, or 2 or 3 days later, paralysis develops in the painful muscles.

These are usually supplied by the fifth and sixth and less commonly the seventh cervical roots so that the deltoid, spinati, and serratus anterior muscles are usually involved, and frequently also the muscles of the upper arm. Wasting is rapid. Sensory loss is slight or absent and is often confined to the upper outer arm in the territory of the axillary nerve. Pain usually subsides in 1 to 2 weeks. Recovery from paralysis usually takes several months. Corticosteroids may be tried in the early stages.

Polyneuropathy

When the causal lesion lies in the nerve cell body the first manifestations are at the distal end of the longest nerves. This gives rise to the typical picture of a generalised polyneuropathy with distal paraesthesiae first affecting the feet and later the hands, and progressing proximally up the limbs. These sensory symptoms are associated with diminution of superficial sensation over 'stocking' and 'glove' areas. There is also distal weakness with diminished or absent tendon reflexes. There are variations of this stereotyped picture, e.g. the Guillain-Barré syndrome.

Aetiology. There are a large number of causes; some of the most important are listed:

GENETICALLY DETERMINED NEUROPATHIES: the peripheral types of peroneal muscular atrophy; progressive hypertrophic polyneuritis; hereditary sensory neuropathy.

DEFICIENCY NEUROPATHIES: deficiencies of vitamins B_1, B_2, B_6, B_{12} and E; folate deficiency.

TOXIC NEUROPATHY: lead, arsenic, mercury, triorthocresylphosphate; a variety of organic chemicals such as carbon tetrachloride, acrylamide and aniline dyes; a large number of drugs including chloroquine, phenytoin and vinca alkaloids; solvent abuse.

NEUROPATHIES ASSOCIATED WITH INFECTIONS: leprosy is true infective neuropathy; polyneuropathy may complicate a number of infections including influenza, measles, HIV and typhoid fever; some neuropathies are due to exotoxins notably diphtheritic polyneuropathy; the Guillain-Barré syndrome.

CONNECTIVE TISSUE DISORDERS: polyarteritis nodosa; rheumatoid arthritis, systemic lupus erythematosus and occasionally giant cell arteritis.

METABOLIC NEUROPATHIES: diabetes mellitus; renal and hepatic failure; acute intermittent porphyria, paraproteinaemia and amyloidosis.

MALIGNANT DISEASE: carcinoma of the bronchus and other malignant tumours including lymphomas and myelomatosis.

Descriptions of the many neuropathies listed above would be repetitive. Diabetic neuropathies (p. 483) illustrate the various clinical patterns. The Guillain-Barré syndrome is a relatively common and life threatening disease which is discussed in more detail here.

Acute inflammatory polyneuropathy (the Guillain-Barré syndrome)

About two-thirds of patients with this acute demyelinating peripheral neuropathy have had an infection 1–4 weeks before its onset. This and other features indicate an immunological pathogenesis involving the myelin sheaths of spinal roots and peripheral nerves. A wide variety of viral and bacterial illnesses may trigger the disorder, and attacks may follow immunisation procedures.

The presenting clinical features vary. Pain in the back is common. There may be tingling affecting the distal part of the limbs and ascending proximally. In about 50% of patients motor symptoms predominate, with weakness which may be profound and rapidly progressive and which often affects proximal more than distal limb musculature. Facial muscles are commonly involved. The most striking findings on examination are diffuse weakness and widespread loss of reflexes. The rate of spread is variable. Occasional patients will develop quadriparesis with respiratory failure within a few hours of the initial symptoms. In other cases there will be a progression for 1 to 2 weeks.

The protein content of the cerebrospinal fluid is markedly raised in most patients at some time during the illness though it may be normal during the first ten days. There is usually no rise in cells.

During the initial stages of the illness careful monitoring of respiratory function is essential. A deterioration in respiratory function tests or subjective feelings of dyspnoea should lead to early tracheostomy and the institution of intermittent positive pressure respiration. Steroid or immuno-suppressive therapy is not indicated in typical acute cases, but may benefit patients who show a chronic or relapsing course. Trials of plasma exchange in the acute disorder have produced equivocal results, but there may be a place for this treatment in early cases showing rapid deterioration.

The prognosis is good providing respiration is maintained. Approximately 90% of patients will recover completely within 3 to 8 weeks; 5% will die and 5% will be left with residual paralysis.

ACUTE INTERMITTENT PORPHYRIA may cause a neuropathy similar to that of the Guillain-Barré syndrome. Acute intermittent porphyria is characterised by attacks of unexplained colicky abdominal pain, constipation and psychiatric disturbances, notably confusion and emotional lability. Tachycardia and hypertension are frequent. The condition is due to a dominantly inherited deficiency of an enzyme in the pathway of haem biosynthesis (p. 495). An attack may be precipitated by phenobarbitone, oral contraceptives, sulphonamides, pentazocine, methyldopa, chlorpropamide, alcohol and other drugs. The diagnosis is confirmed by the finding of porphobilinogen in the urine (p. 376).

Diagnosis, prevention and treatment of polyneuropathy

Diagnosis. The clinical picture will usually localise the lesions to the peripheral nerves. Nerve conduction studies will, in most cases, confirm the presence of impaired conduction. This will be gross in most cases of peripheral segmental demyelination and relatively minor in lesions affecting nerve axons. Occasionally, particularly in those with interstitial neuropathies, a sural nerve biopsy will establish the cause. Sometimes the pattern of the clinical picture, as in the Guillain-Barré syndrome, will indicate the likely diagnosis.

Although the presence of a polyneuropathy is easily established clinically, the definition of a cause may be difficult or impossible. The presence of associated diseases, drug ingestion or exposure to toxic chemicals should be sought in each case.

The possibility of diabetes mellitus should always be excluded.

Prevention and treatment. Any new drug which is liable to cause neuropathy must be used with care and industrial hazards should be avoided by protective clothing, exhaust ventilation and other techniques advised by the industrial medical officer.

When polyneuropathy is due to a toxic substance the first step is to remove the patient from further exposure to it. When the cause is nutritional every effort should be made to restore the original body weight; plenty of protein is desirable supplemented by generous doses of the vitamin B complex. If the cause is metabolic the appropriate treatment must be initiated without delay, e.g. for diabetes.

In severe cases bed-rest is essential since the nervous control of the heart may be defective and cardiomyopathy is sometimes associated. The limbs should be supported in the optimum position, and passive movements carried out several times a day. A cage should protect the feet from the weight of the bed-clothes. Respiratory insufficiency may require tracheostomy or institution of intermittent positive pressure respiration. When recovery begins, active movements should be carried out under the supervision of a physiotherapist.

DISEASES OF MUSCLE

Diseases of muscle are not diseases of the nervous system, but as some of their manifestations may be readily confused with neurological conditions myasthenia gravis and myopathy are described here.

MYASTHENIA GRAVIS

This condition is characterised by progressive failure to sustain a maintained or repeated contraction of striated muscles.

Aetiology and pathology. Nicotinic receptors of acetylcholine in the post-junctional membrane of neuromuscular junctions are blocked or lysed by a complement-mediated autoimmune reaction between receptor protein and antiacetylcholine receptor antibody. The antibody is produced by B lymphocytes defectively controlled by T lymphocytes because of a disorder of the thymus gland. About 15% of cases, mainly of late onset, have an encapsulated or locally invasive thymoma. The majority, including all young cases, have one of a number of thymic abnormalities, the most characteristic being germinal centres in the medulla of the gland. The latter group has a marked personal and familial relationship with other autoimmune diseases (p. 27), and many have inherited an immunoreactive gene which is linked to some of the HLA haplotypes; in a North European population these are HLA-B8 and DRw3. Inheritance of this gene is not obligatory for myasthenia and nothing is known about possible triggering factors for the spontaneous disease. Penicillamine may be one such breaker of immunological tolerance.

Clinical features. The disease usually appears between the ages of 15 and 50 and females are more often affected than males. It tends to run a remitting course especially during the early years. Relapses may be precipitated by emotional disturbances, infections, pregnancy and severe muscular effort.

The cardinal symptom is abnormal fatiguability of muscles; movement, though initially strong, rapidly weakens. Intensification of symptoms towards the end of the day or following vigorous exercise is characteristic.

The first symptoms are usually intermittent ptosis or diplopia but weakness of chewing, swallowing, speaking or of moving the limbs also occurs. Any muscle of a limb may be affected, most commonly those of the shoulder girdle, so that the patient is unable to undertake work above the level of the shoulder, such as combing the hair, without frequent rests. Respiratory muscles may be involved and respiratory failure is a not uncommon cause of death. Asphyxia occurs readily as the cough may be too weak to clear foreign bodies from the airways. Muscle atrophy may occur in long-standing cases. There are no signs of involvement of the central nervous system.

Investigation. An invaluable diagnostic aid is the increase in muscle strength produced by an intravenous injection of a short-acting anticholinesterase, edrophonium hydrochloride. An initial dose of 2 mg is injected and a further 8 mg given half a minute later if there are no undesirable reactions such as fasciculation, sweating and colic. Improvement in muscle power occurs within 30 seconds of the injection and usually persists for 2 or 3 minutes. Ptosis or defects in eye movements are the most convenient parameters of improvement but diminution of dysarthria or increase of power in the limbs can also demonstrate a response to edrophonium.

Tests of electromyographic function during repetitive nerve stimulation may show characteristic decremental responses. Serum antibody to skeletal muscle acetylcholine receptors is present in more than 80% of cases.

Treatment. The principles of treatment are: (1) to maximise the activity of acetylcholine released at the remaining receptors in the neuromuscular junctions by nerve impulses and (2) to limit or abolish the immunological attack on motor endplates.

The duration of action of liberated acetylcholine is greatly prolonged by inhibiting its hydrolysing enzyme, acetylcholinesterase. The most commonly used anticholinesterase drugs, pyridostigmine and neostigmine, are chosen for rapid action lasting 2–8 hours (wide individual variation). Longer acting drugs are cumulative and even moderate overdosage so prolongs acetylcholine half-life as to cause depolarisation block of motor endplates and also of muscarinic endings, leading to muscular fasciculation and paralysis, pallor, sweating, excessive salivation and persistently small pupils; the last is the most valuable sign of this *cholinergic crisis*. Smaller doses cause diarrhoea, colic and other autonomic effects. These can be controlled by propantheline (15 mg as required) or, on occasion, by atropine (0.6 mg parenterally). These anticholinergic drugs are best avoided as they dilate the pupils and so remove the best marker for impending cholinergic crisis. Pyridostigmine is the anticholinesterase of choice, 60–120 mg given orally at intervals determined by supervised trial (2–8 hours). For exceptional muscular effort, neostigmine (15–30 mg) acts more promptly but for a shorter time. It may be given intravenously in an emergency but parenteral administration requires experience and is rarely necessary.

Sudden exacerbations of myasthenic or cholinergic weakness may require intermittent positive pressure respiration to save life. Early intubation before a crisis has developed will normally remove the need for a tracheostomy.

The immunological disorder is treated by various procedures. Thymectomy should be performed as soon as feasible in any patient with myasthenia not confined to the extraocular muscles, unless the disease has been established for more than 7 years; the indication for surgery is the stage of myasthenia gravis, not the presence of a thymoma.

Plasma exchange (plasmapheresis), by removing antibody from the blood, may give marked improvement but, as this is usually brief, such therapy is normally reserved for myasthenic crisis or for pre-operative preparation. Corticosteroid treatment may cause rapid improvement but this is commonly preceded by marked exacerbation of myasthenic symptoms and should be initiated only in a hospital with ventilation equipment. Various high and low dose, daily or alternate day dosage schedules are in use with apparently similar results. As it is usually necessary to continue treatment for months or years, with the possibility of adverse effects, corticosteroids are not recommended for first line management. In an attempt to reduce these risks, trials of azathioprine and other immunosuppressant drugs or of radiation of lymphoid tissues are being made. No anti-immunological therapy has yet proved superior to thymectomy, an operation with practically no mortality when performed early.

Prognosis is variable. Remissions sometimes occur spontaneously. When myasthenic affection is confined to the eye muscles prognosis for life is normal and disability slight. Rapid progression of the disease more than 5 years after its onset is uncommon. Thymectomy, perhaps followed by high dosage steroid treatment, often leads to marked improvement so that disability is minimal and life expectancy normal. When the disease is associated with a thymoma, even though this is removed, the outlook is markedly worsened.

MYOPATHY

Myopathy is a generic term comprising all primary diseases of muscle. It may be subdivided into genetically determined, congenital, metabolic and drug-induced myopathy. Inflammatory myopathy (polymyositis) is described on page 577. There are obvious exceptions, but it is a useful generalisation that myopathy affects mainly the proximal muscles of the limbs whereas neuropathic disease (polyneuropathy or motor neurone disease) affects mainly the distal muscles.

Genetically determined myopathy

Progressive muscular dystrophy is a group of hereditary disorders characterised by progressive degeneration of groups of muscles without involvement of the nervous system. The wasting and weakness are symmetrical, there is no fasciculation, tendon reflexes are preserved until a late stage and there is no sensory loss. Several clinical types have been described; from a prognostic viewpoint there are three major groups.

The *Duchenne type* is transmitted by an X-linked recessive gene and occurs almost exclusively in males (p. 12). The disease usually appears within the first 3 years of life, beginning in the pelvic girdle and lower limbs and later spreading to the shoulder girdle. About 80% of cases show an initial pseudohypertrophy. The affected muscles are larger and firmer than normal, but are nevertheless weak. The weakness gives rise to a characteristic waddling gait, and when rising from the supine position, the child rolls on to his face and then uses his arms to push himself up. Death occurs from inanition or respiratory infection by the middle of the second decade. Antenatal diagnosis is discussed on page 15.

Limb girdle type (juvenile scapulohumeral type of Erb). The gene carrying this disorder is inherited as an autosomal recessive, affecting both sexes. It usually appears in the second or third decade. It starts in either the shoulder or pelvic girdle and later spreads to involve both. The rate of progression is variable; it may be slow, with long periods of arrest, but severe disablement usually occurs within 20 years and the patient does not survive to middle age.

The facio-scapulo-humeral type is inherited by an autosomal dominant gene so that several siblings of both sexes may be affected. It appears at any age, first in the facial muscles and then in the shoulder girdle. After many years the pelvic girdle may also be involved. The disease progresses very slowly with periods of arrest and is compatible with a long life.

The *diagnosis of muscular dystrophy* is readily confirmed by electromyography (EMG) or muscle biopsy. Aldolase, or creatine kinase and other enzymes which are usually intracellular, are increased in the serum, especially in the rapidly advancing Duchenne type. Serum enzyme changes may be found before other clinical signs, enabling early detection of the disease in siblings. Less severe changes of the same type are found in women who carry the abnormal gene of the Duchenne type.

Treatment. No effective treatment is known. Deterioration may occur with excessive confinement to bed. Physiotherapeutic and orthopaedic measures may be required to counteract deformities and contractures.

Myotonia. This consists of slow relaxation of muscles due to hyperexcitability of the muscle cell membrane.

Myotonia congenita (Thomsen's disease) is inherited as an autosomal dominant and appears in early childhood. The only symptom is the slow relaxation of a muscle if it is contracted voluntarily or by mechanical stimulation. The patient may be unable to relax the grasp or to open the eyes if they have been closed tightly. The muscles may be unusually powerful in early life.

Dystrophia myotonica is also autosomal dominant and appears between the ages of 20 and 30 years. There is wasting of the facial and temporal muscles, sternomastoids, shoulder girdle, forearms, quadriceps and leg muscles, and all these and the tongue show myotonia after voluntary contraction or after percussion of the muscle. Ptosis is prominent. Unlike most muscular diseases, distal muscles are more severely affected than proximal. There is also cataract, frontal baldness and gonadal atrophy leading to impotence and sterility in men and amenorrhoea in women.

The disorder progresses at a variable rate, but many patients die in middle life usually from respiratory failure. Disorders of cardiac conduction are also common and may result in syncopal attacks; many such patients require a cardiac pacemaker.

Treatment. There is no treatment for the muscular dystrophy, but if myotonia is troublesome it can be relieved by procainamide, 0.5–1.0 g q.i.d., quinine sulphate 300–600 mg t.i.d. or phenytoin 100 mg t.i.d.

Congenital, metabolic and drug-induced myopathy

Congenital myopathies are rare and present in infancy with muscular weakness and limpness. Serum enzymes tend to be normal or slightly raised. The EMP is usually myopathic. The mode of inheritance is variable. They are named according to the type of structural abnormality found in the skeletal muscle fibres. Most cases are non-progressive or only slowly progressive.

Metabolic myopathy. *Thyrotoxic myopathy.* Mild weakness of the proximal muscles of the limbs is a common feature of thyrotoxicosis. In a few patients muscular wasting and weakness predominate, and the other manifestations of hyperthyroidism may not be obvious. Treatment of the hyperthyroidism results in recovery from the myopathy. Hypothyroidism may also cause myopathy.

Corticosteroid myopathy. Weakness of the pelvic girdle may occur in Cushing's syndrome and as a result of treatment with corticosteroids.

Familial periodic paralysis is characterised by attacks of profound weakness, lasting for several hours and often occurring after exertion or after a heavy carbohydrate meal. In the common variety the attacks of weakness are accompanied by a fall in the serum potassium level.

Drug-induced myopathy. A wide variety of drugs may cause disorders of muscle. Often muscle cramps and mild weakness are the first symptoms. Lithium or beta-blockers may cause mild symptoms which disappear when the drug is withdrawn. Alcohol may cause a spectrum of muscle diseases varying from a mild, proximal weakness to severe muscle necrosis.

Neurological and myopathic complications of carcinoma

Metastases. Cerebral invasion or spinal compression may be the presenting feature of a metastasis from an unsuspected primary neoplasm or may augment the disability already caused by tumours arising elsewhere in the body, particularly in bronchus and breast. More than half of all cerebral tumours are secondary deposits and this high incidence emphasises the need for a careful search for a primary neoplasm in those patients who present with an intracranial space-occupying lesion.

Paraneoplastic syndromes (p. 104) may arise at a distance from a primary carcinoma in the absence of metastases. Neural disturbances may occur at any stage during the development of the primary lesion and may antedate the symptoms directly attributable to the carcinoma by weeks or months. They may affect singly, or in combination, muscles and peripheral nerves as well as central neural structures and the brain. The syndromes presented are most conveniently categorised anatomically.

Myopathy, myositis and myasthenia. A proximal weakness of late onset, usually first affecting the legs may be due to a non-specific myopathy or polymyositis. Sometimes the weakness is markedly exacerbated by exertion producing a myasthenic-like syndrome and may be improved by an intravenous injection of edrophonium hydrochloride.

Peripheral neuropathy is probably the commonest of the distant neurological complications of carcinoma. Clinically the neuropathy is usually of mixed sensory-motor type. The cerebrospinal fluid protein content is often raised.

Spinal cord affection. Carcinomata may produce a picture which resembles motor neurone disease with loss of anterior horn cells, accompanied sometimes by upper motor neurone signs. Necrosis affecting the cells and the tracts of the spinal cord, maximal in the thoracic segments, is a rare complication of carcinoma.

Subacute degeneration of the cortical layers of the cerebellum is an uncommon manifestation of distant carcinoma characterised by ataxia and nystagmus. The course is often rapidly progressive.

Encephalopathy has occasionally been found in patients suffering from carcinoma. The most common presentation is an insidious and progressive dementia with memory disorder. This may be accompanied by features of brain stem involvement and upper motor neurone signs.

Treatment of the paraneoplastic syndrome is that of the primary lesion. Improvement, and occasionally complete remission, of a myasthenic-myopathic syndrome may occur with removal of the primary tumour but this is by no means invariable. In most instances the response of the neurological complications is unpredictable.

PROSPECTS IN NEUROLOGY

In previous editions, this section has stressed the potential value of neuroimaging, such as CT and magnetic resonance imaging, and these are now part of neurological practice in advanced centres. Their value to the neurosurgeon and others requiring localisation of gross lesions of the nervous system is unquestionable; they are rapidly replacing older radiological techniques, but they are of more limited value in medical neurology where disorders of neural function rather than macroscopic structure are frequent. Electrodiagnostic techniques are again advancing with stimulators for specific sensory modalities, signal averaging, and magneto-encephalography promising to improve the recording of cerebral electrophysiology.

Neurotransmitter research has moved from catecholamines to peptides and 'second messengers' and the enzymology of some genetic disorders is now known. These findings must soon influence neuropharmacology. Antiviral agents are now in regular use for herpes group infections but their clinical advantage is not yet well defined. Advances in immunopathology continue to improve understanding of muscle and nervous system disease, but the therapeutic follow-up is disappointing. The viral and immunological aspects of neurological disease have new urgency with the rapid spread of AIDS and the concentration of research on this plague will certainly advance treatment of other viral and immunology-associated disease of the nervous system.

Identification of the gene locus of Duchenne muscular dystrophy, myotonic dystrophy and Huntington's chorea has been imminent for 2 years and cannot be long delayed, but the nature of the gene products, necessary for potential therapy, is still for the future. Nevertheless, the time is long past when chronic 'degenerative' diseases of the nervous system were regarded as untreatable and hopeless. Even Alzheimer's disease may be capable of solution along the same lines, and with the same limitations, as Parkinson's disease.

J.A. SIMPSON
R.E. CULL

FURTHER READING:

Cull R E 1986 In: Macleod J, Munro J (eds) Clinical examination, 7th edn. Churchill Livingstone, Edinburgh. Contains an account of the examination of the nervous system designed to be read in conjunction with this chapter

Ross Russell R W, Wiles C M 1985 Integrated clinical science: neurology. Heinemann, London. An up-to-date account of common neurological disorders, with an approach based on the pathophysiology. Written for undergraduates, but of a level suitable for postgraduate study. Well illustrated

Matthews W B 1982 Diseases of the nervous system, 4th edn. Blackwell Scientific Publications, Oxford. A concise, readable account of neurological disorders intended for undergraduates

Bannister Sir Roger 1984 Brain's Clinical neurology, 6th edn. Eminently suitable for undergraduates, this book is popularly known as 'little Brain'

Brain Lord, Walton Sir John 1985 Diseases of the nervous system, 9th edn. Oxford University Press, London. A comprehensive text primarily for postgraduate students

Jennett W B 1977 An introduction to neurosurgery, 3rd edn. Heinemann, London. A succinct and clearly written introduction to surgical neurology

Weller R D, Swash M, McLellan D L, Scholtz C L 1983 Clinical neuropathology. Springer Verlag, Berlin. A valuable short account of pathological processes related to clinical neurology. It includes clear accounts of biochemical disorders of the nervous system

16

Psychiatry

Psychiatry is the study and treatment of disorders of the mind and of behaviour. The mind, or psyche, is usually defined as the part of the person consisting of the thoughts, the feelings and the function of willing. Psychiatric disorder, therefore, can be viewed to occur whenever there is an impairment of thinking (cognition), feeling (affect) or willing (volition). In a paranoid reaction, for instance, the patient wrongly thinks he or she is being persecuted by an ill-intentioned acquaintance; in depressive psychosis the patient is incapacitated by a persistent feeling of intense gloom; and in schizophrenia some patients are inactive, ineffectual and lacking in volition.

Psychiatry is the proper concern of all doctors, not only of psychiatrists. Only a small proportion of the psychiatric illness in the community is seen and can be treated by psychiatrists. In a country with as many doctors as Britain only 1 in 20 cases of psychiatric disorder is treated by psychiatrists. The epidemiological evidence makes it clear that the great proportion of psychiatric morbidity falls in the clinical domain of non-psychiatrists — general practitioners mainly but also physicians, surgeons, obstetricians and gynaecologists. Neurologists should also be singled out, for they treat many psychiatric patients.

Patients with emotional disorders tend to consult their doctors more often than patients with physical diseases and complain of a wider variety of symptoms. As a result, they are often referred to a succession of clinics for specialist investigation and commonly undergo minor or major surgery without avail. This involves a waste of both doctors' and patients' time, which could be avoided if the psychological disorder had been recognised at an earlier stage. Another reason for requiring all doctors to be psychiatrically informed and skilled is that psychiatric disorder and physical illness frequently occur in the same patient.

It follows that the priority is to ensure that psychiatric knowledge and skills, and professional attitudes appropriate to adequate provision of psychiatric care, are part of the clinical equipment of all doctors. They must know the symptoms, signs and syndromes in psychiatry, and they should all be aware of the psychological, pharmacological and physical treatments that are effective in psychiatric illness.

The basic skills are the ability to take a psychiatric history and to examine the mental state; such technical competence enables the doctor to elicit the clinical features of psychiatric disorder presented by the patient. This constitutes the psychiatric examination which is described on page 675.

MENTAL HEALTH

As a basis for understanding the abnormal, all doctors must know what constitutes mental as well as physical health. Before defining this it is necessary to consider the development of personality and the mechanisms of psychological defence.

Personality development. Personality is socially acquired, given its genetic basis, over the course of time. The individual arrives at an adult psychological state after passing successively through a series of maturational stages. A baby is born into a family, which provides immediate social support and responses. From the start the baby's 'personality' consists of the totality of its actions, but also of the reactions made particularly to the caring parent.

1. During the stage of *primary attachment* the baby is helpless and receptive, dependent utterly on succour; such total care occurs as a result of nurturing impulses in the mother, fostered from the first days by the relationship and the interactions which develop in the nursing couple. The baby's cries, its smiles after some weeks, its need of nourishment and the relative satisfaction or distress deriving from its alimentary experiences, its fear of strangers from 8 months, all combine to bring out the protectiveness of the parental family. During this first stage, the baby is perforce relatively passive; its needs are for care and nourishment.

2. During the *stage of initial socialisation*, from 9 months to 2 years of age, the infant comes to gain sphincter control and to become more socialised as a member of the family in other ways also, starting to learn the language and its usage, and coming to grasp the rules of the parental household.

3. The *stage of family role identification* extends from 2 to 6 years of age. One of its characteristics is that the child now has sufficient awareness of family interactions and social norms to want to become informed about such matters as the difference between the sexes, where babies come from and how they are made. Boys begin to imitate and assimilate aspects of their father's behaviour and character, while girls also become less concentrated in their attachment to the mother; they can show the most intense affection for their fathers, a passion that apparently needs recognition and an affectionate response for proper personality growth between 2 and 6 years.

During the *oedipal phase* (as this third stage is called in the psychoanalytic literature), the child is often intensely frustrated by diminutive size, puny strength and subservience to the powerful parents at a time when perception, knowledge and mastery of the environment evolve rapidly as physical and mental abilities develop.

4. *At 6 years, the child enters the social world outside the home*. The child is socially obliging, very actively adapting to school life and is becoming increasingly an independent personality, able to be away from the parents for substantial portions of the day. If the parents are not seriously deficient as culture carriers, through neurotic illness or crippling social handicaps, the child now comes closely to grips with the norms, the roles, the stereotypes and the obvious and prevailing cultural values. The child is extremely impressionable, as advertisers on television well know, eager to add to personality and experience by observing and borrowing from the behaviour and ideas of others.

5. At *puberty* the child's personality can enter a period of relative flexibility, when it may be given 'a second chance' and can set aside some trait patterns and in their place substitute new attitudes and beliefs. With the bodily and sexual changes of this period come demands for new orientations and relationships; a special requirement is for a friend. Children, just before entering their teens, either do succeed in achieving a close friendship or else they may suffer from a sense of unpopularity or loneliness.

The early teenage years are when *identity formation* either occurs or else fails to happen, when identity diffusion will result. Then the youngsters continue in a state of not knowing what they want to be or what aims their capacities and potential may permit. The boy may be timid and lacking in confidence, or compensatorily brusque and hostile; the girl may inwardly bewail her female state, be perturbed at having menstrual periods and feel uncertain and wretched in social relationships especially as these relate to the future prospect of being courted. When identity formation does occur successfully, the adolescent decides on life goals and works towards them more or less hopefully, while feeling common cause with enough agemates to be a member of a group.

6. At about 18 years, the late adolescent becomes capable of *intimacy*, able to regard the welfare of another loved person as no less important than one's own. Then adulthood follows, with the capacity for *generativity*, with the intention and the potential to provide responsibly and reliably for others.

When the question of psychological normality of a patient is at issue, this chronological and subjective progression through biographical epochs has to be borne in mind. Psychological theory holds that each of these different stages is not obliterated by the one succeeding it but, like layers of an onion, one developmental phase superimposes the challenges (and the person's solutions to them) over and around the earlier solutions achieved. The residues of past developmental periods persist to give individuality to the person. When particularly upsetting setbacks (psychologically traumatic experiences) are encountered, a *fixation* may result, the person not negotiating developmental challenges but instead remaining unduly preoccupied with the issues of that earlier life epoch. Often the facts about the psychic trauma are not remembered, as when a small boy is parted from his parents for a surgical operation he does not comprehend.

Jean Piaget was a pioneer in discovering that intellectual development also proceeds in stages, and that in the early years of life unrealistic thinking prevails. Only in middle childhood, from 7 to 8 years onwards, does the child acquire logical thinking, and even then abstract thinking and reasoning is not possible until about 13 years of age. Thus the first four stages of emotional development described above take place in parallel with magical, prelogical modes of thought.

This information makes it clearer why there are infantile psychic remnants in the thinking of many disturbed adults. Although knowledgeable about sex, a woman can fear she is pregnant despite intercourse not having occurred; a man can be distressed that he 'caused' the death of his mother by behaving harshly to her when she was terminally ill. Thinking that departs from reality or distorts it is often related to early demands which the child found unmanageable, or to distress which was intolerable emotionally at that time of life, such as the loss of a parent through death, or the family breaking up.

Adults, when handicapped by a persistence of immaturity, need not constantly manifest distortion of thinking or feeling in their behaviour. Only when a fresh setback occurs in adult life may they decompensate in behaviour and *regress* to act in extreme variance from their everyday demeanour,

for example with dependency and passivity (as when confronted by major surgery), or with obstinacy or hostility.

Mechanisms of defence. As a consequence of excessive strains occurring early in life with which the personality was insufficiently mature to cope, the person can make use of psychological devices, 'mental tricks', to alter the inner environment or the surrounding reality and create an illusion of safety and predictability. A girl, unable to clarify sexual issues at the age of 5 years, perhaps lacking a reassuring relationship with a kindly father, may use *denial* excessively. There are women who remain unaware of their sexual impulses and behave like school-girls forever — 'pregenital' personalities, some writers name them. A person may *overcompensate* — a timid, insecure boy setting out to acquire the outward characteristics of a tough male when he reaches adulthood. A boy who copes with upsetting homosexual desires at puberty by means of *repression*, in later life can be in greater emotional difficulty should he use the mechanism of *projection*; if psychotic, such a man may have an auditory delusion that other people are alleging he is a homosexual. A sexually deprived single woman, using the same mechanisms, may be profoundly distressed, in the course of a paranoid reaction, by her erroneous beliefs that neighbours view her as sexually promiscuous; her own suppressed wishes are not admitted to her awareness but are exteriorised so that she believes others falsely suspect her of immorality.

There are other psychological mechanisms in the range of distortions and evasions to which troubled people can have recourse in extremity. By *reaction formation* we imply that individuals give forth the opposite of facts they cannot acknowledge about themselves: the son dominated by his father often becomes not a domineering man, but a timid, ingratiating, subservient adult — perhaps overwhelmed by an intimidating wife. However, such a man can change character drastically and turn on his oppressor; the bedroom is the commonest setting for matrimonial murder when the victim is the wife; the husband dies often in the kitchen.

Of course, psychological defence mechanisms rarely present so dramatically, and for clinical purposes more precise observation of smaller cues is required. We all use defence mechanisms at times of great stress: the surgeon's matter-of-fact manner is sometimes seen as necessary suppression of sympathetic emotions which could impair his competence, and his *selective inattention* to pathetic life circumstances may be altogether appropriate in an emergency. A civilian disaster is not the time for anguish over the human condition, if one is a surgeon with an operation to carry out.

The defences which a person assumes psychologically can be of much social value to others. A latently homosexual youth leader may be a boon to a neighbourhood—until his *sublimation* no longer serves, perhaps if he drinks excessively and loses his customary mental controls. School teachers and clergymen who interfere sexually with boys are in this category, and some doctors who become sexually involved with patients.

In the course of clinical work, we judge a patient to assess whether he or she is spontaneous and unconstrained, or whether in contrast the patient when troubled denies mental conflict and imaginatively but unknowingly distorts surrounding reality in order to gain psychological relief.

Psychological normality

In common with medical practice generally, individuals are often considered psychiatrically normal if no evidence of disorder is clinically present. An epidemiologist doing a population survey may use an *empirical definition of normality* and regard as normal everybody who has not seen a psychiatrist nor consulted a general practitioner for any nervous ailment during the preceding year.

Another concept of normality at times invoked is an *ideal norm*, conveying an aspiration towards a desired state of well-being (such as is expressed in the preamble to the World Health Organization constitution), devoutly to be wished but not to be found in this world: 'Health is a state of complete physical, mental and social well-being and not merely the absence of disease or infirmity'.

Psychiatrists occasionally write about normality, or aspects of it, in such inspirational terms that only too evidently they are not describing people as they are but as they would be, if a theoretical schema or 'mental health' blueprint were to become actual.

The third concept is a *statistical norm*, implying the state of most people contained in the community of which the patient is a member. In this sense, without straining after the ideal, we can indicate features characteristic of psychiatric normality in mature adults. Each of these can be readily identified, especially when the doctor has additional background information from prior acquaintance with the patient or members of the family.

Individuals who have successfully negotiated the sequence of stages in personality development are *appropriately autonomous*; they can manage their own affairs and tasks without undue reliance on others and can be depended on to meet obligations and to discharge responsibilities appropriate to their occupation, social circumstances and interests. The statement that a mature person can work, love and play perhaps reflects this capacity for autonomy.

A second feature of normality is *accurate self-perception*, the person not overestimating nor belittling his or her abilities. A third characteristic is correct *reality-testing*, the environment being perceived in an undistorted way. A fourth feature is *adjustment*, the person taking things as they are and making the best of them. The final two qualities of maturity are *integration* (relative coherence of the parts of the personality in contrast to gross self-contradictions), and *achievement*, the person using skills and interests in such a way that efforts are productive.

DIAGNOSTIC DECISION-MAKING

The doctor's first consideration when examining a patient for psychiatric disorder, is to question whether the patient may be suffering from a psychosis, one of the serious disorders to which the term 'insanity' used to be applied. The psychoses are the serious illnesses which interfere with a patient's perceptions, thinking and feelings so profoundly that, at times, what is said to others no longer makes sense to them and that person is regarded as insane. The doctor scans the understanding obtained by means of history-taking and examination of the mental state, perhaps augmented — when the patient is uncooperative — by information from a relative or other informant. The doctor judges whether the syndrome presenting indicates an illness of psychotic quality and severity. Syndrome identification is of course possible only if the doctor has knowledge about the signs and symptoms of the two main classes of psychoses: the organic psychoses due to cerebral impairment, and the functional psychoses presumed to be related to an as yet undiscovered disturbance of cerebral biochemistry.

The major disorders (the psychoses)

Organic mental disorders. In these organic brain syndromes the functioning of the brain is impaired either by a physical lesion (trauma, tumour or infection) or by a toxic or degenerative process. Organic brain syndromes when acute are known as *delirium*. Examples are the toxic confusional states occurring with brain trauma, cerebral anoxia, infection, or intoxication with barbiturates, amphetamines or alcohol.

The chronic organic psychoses, where there is an irreversible brain lesion, are the *dementias*. The commonest are those associated with ageing: atherosclerotic and senile dementia. Mild degrees of dementia make the patient forgetful, easily confused, irritable and emotional; more severe dementia results in disorientation, gross loss of memory and deterioration in personal habits.

Functional psychoses are the major psychiatric illnesses occurring without brain disease or impairment. It is postulated that a neurophysiological or neurochemical aetiology will be found, resulting from the operation of complex causes. The two most common forms are *major depressive illness*, in which the principal symptom is a profound disturbance of the patient's mood, and the *schizophrenias* in which patients' thoughts become bizarre and disorganised, so that they lose contact with their fellows and surroundings.

The major disorders are discussed further on pages 679 to 684.

The minor disorders

The second step in the decision-making process towards a psychiatric diagnosis, having excluded the presence of psychosis, is for the doctor to determine whether the patient suffers from a 'minor' psychiatric disorder. The following forms of minor disorder are differentiated:

1. **The psychoneuroses.** Clinical recognition of one of the forms of psychoneurosis depends on the doctor knowing the signs and symptoms of each syndrome and of being able to elicit the relevant clinical data from the patient. The psychoneuroses are the most common forms of psychiatric illness encountered in general medical practice. They are subdivided into *anxiety, hysterical, obsessive, depressive* and *phobic psychoneurosis* and are discussed on pages 684 to 691.

2. **Personality disorder.** This term is used to describe patients whose personalities differ markedly from the normal population.

The third diagnostic rule, after the presence of possible psychosis or of psychoneurosis has been considered, is to make an appraisal of the personality of the patient. An individual's personality is regarded as normal if his or her actions and reactions are not grossly different from customary behaviour in society. When a personality is diagnosed as disordered, the implication is that the person deviates observably in behaviour, presenting a type of abnormal personality which is well recognised clinically. The abnormal personality manifests in recurrent disturbance in relationships with other people. In addition to their social difficulties, such people can be recognised to have traits (e.g. hostility, passivity) not found to the same degree in the personalities of normal people. Patients with moderate degrees of personality disorder are distressed by their inability to get on constructively with others and often seek treatment; otherwise they do so when they are further disabled by psychoneurosis or psychosomatic illness. Those with gross degrees of disorder (sociopathy) interfere disruptively in the lives of their relatives and associates and may come into conflict with the law; they may not regard themselves as abnormal and reject any efforts to treat them.

It is by no means unusual, indeed it is usual, for psychiatric illness and personality disorder to coexist. When the associated illness is of psychotic dimensions, the symptoms may so distort behaviour that a reliable estimate of the pre-illness personality will be possible only after recovery from the insanity. When the illness is a neurotic reaction, however, the functioning personality remains sufficiently intact for a personality diagnosis to be made at the same time as the illness is appraised. A personality disorder may also be associated with sexual deviation, alcoholism, drug dependency or psychosomatic illness.

3. **Alcoholism and drug dependency.** An alcoholic is an excessive drinker who is unable to stop although to do so has become necessary because of health impairment, marital strife or difficulties at work. An addict is physically or psychologically dependent on a drug which is used repetitively, and suffers distressing side-effects when deprived of it.

4. **Psychosexual disorders.** People not conforming sexually to the prevailing norm most often consult (or are brought to) their doctor only when their abnormality has become seriously disturbing to their relatives or has put them into conflict with the law. Some, however, are themselves distressed by their deviation and may on occasion need psychiatric treatment for complicating psychiatric disorder, such as a depressive illness or paranoid reaction. Now that sexual relations between consenting adults is no longer a crime in many countries, homosexuals are less vulnerable socially.

5. **Psychosomatic disorders.** The term is applied to the extremely common physical illnesses, such as some cases of asthma, peptic ulcer, dermatitis or ulcerative colitis, which emotional factors help to precipitate or to prolong.

Personality disorders, drug dependency, and psychosexual and psychosomatic disorders are discussed further on pages 691 to 695.

Mental handicap

The fourth and final diagnostic decision is to be clear about a patient's intellectual status. Mental subnormality is an impairment of the intellect present from birth or an early age, unlike psychiatric illnesses which supervene after a more or less normal psychological development. Two categories are distinguished:

1. *Mild mental retardation* (IQ 50 to 70). Although the intelligence level is below normal (I.Q. 85 to 115), the child may benefit from special teaching and social training.

2. *Severe mental retardation* (IQ 49 and below) refers to those so handicapped that they require very considerable attention and support and are incapable of leading an independent existence. The most common single cause of severe subnormality is Down's syndrome. A definite cause of subnormality is found only in a minority of cases, and then various clinical conditions can be responsible, e.g. phenylketonuria or hypothyroidism. Patients who are mentally subnormal may also suffer from other mental illnesses. They may, for example, become depressed or schizophrenic, but when this happens the symptoms of their mental illness will be modified by their basic handicap of mental retardation.

THE PSYCHIATRIC EXAMINATION

It must be emphasised that attention should be paid to the patient's emotional state not only when a frank psychiatric illness is suspected, but in the course of any thorough clinical examination. Psychiatric disorders can be elicited while taking the history and while examining the patient's mental state. The procedures for conducting these two aspects of the psychiatric examination are described in *Clinical examination* (p. 700) and will be indicated only briefly here.

The psychiatric history. Taking a history is one of the chief clinical skills in psychiatry. The technique differs from history-taking in internal medicine, being rather less directive, the doctor to a greater extent, perhaps, allowing the patient to raise apparently unconnected subjects and expand in directions initiated by the patient rather than the clinician. In internal medicine there may be a course of enquiry which the doctor wants to pursue; this is also so with psychiatric history-taking, but inevitably the patient will have personal information to give which may be unexpected. Hence the clinician is well advised to be especially receptive and to encourage disclosures which the patient initiates. Psychiatric disorder is most commonly missed because the doctor fails to attend to and understand what the patient communicates.

The following areas need to be explored in the course of taking the history:

1. The reason why the patient is seeking help.

2. The presenting complaints and the patient's detailed account of the present illness.

3. The patient's parental family: an account of father, mother, each brother and sister (with patient's birth order in the sibship), and the home atmosphere.

4. The personal history, including early childhood; schooling and other education; sexual development and experience; work record; friendships; marriage.

5. Previous illnesses, physical and psychiatric.

6. The personality before illness, with an account of the patient's interests, social activities, traits and such other information about subjective experiences and life events as the patient can provide.

Taking the history is also the first therapeutic step. Psychological treatment begins the moment that the patient and doctor meet. The doctor's attitude to the patient and to the illness should be powerful therapeutic factors which operate immediately. If history-taking is done patiently, thoroughly and objectively the individual feels a personal interest is being taken and that his or her problem is being understood. A spontaneous account of the illness by the patient should be encouraged.

Examining the mental state. As the interview proceeds, the doctor already is observing the patient's current mental functioning. The examination of the mental state is carried out in a systematic manner, paying attention in turn to the separate aspects of observable behaviour which disclose the state of mind.

Appearance and behaviour. The appearance of the patient may be immediately informative, a dejected posture suggesting depressive illness; if the gestures the patient makes are tense and restless, clues may be provided which guide the doctor to enquire after further evidence of anxiety.

Mood. Whether the patient feels cheerful or depressed, confident or fearful, suspicious or bewildered, will become evident when the doctor asks the appropriate questions. 'How do you feel in yourself?' may be enough, but many patients need some help before they can unburden themselves of fears, anxieties or feelings of intense unhappiness. Some patients are ashamed to mention emotional disturbances, such as a phobia, i.e. unreasonable intense anxiety experienced in certain settings, e.g. in open or confined spaces. The patient may show a lack of emotional response; a very gross failure in rapport should alert the doctor to the possibility that the patient may have schizophrenia.

Thought processes. The way a patient thinks is evident in the patient's talk, which may be abnormal through incoherence, changes of topic, or bewildering shifts from one topic to another; all these can be features of schizophrenia. The patient may speak very rapidly, with puns and rhymes, as occurs in mania. Talk may be laboured, slow and flat and indicate a depressive state. Repetitive thoughts characterise obsessional psychoneurosis, an important feature of which is an *obsession*, a persistent idea which the patient cannot get rid of; the repetitiveness may be extremely distressing even when the patient recognises the idea as absurd.

Perceptions of environment. The doctor next ascertains if the patient's perceptions are accurate. A girl may be unduly sensitive to glances or chance remarks. The patient may suffer from *illusions*, misinterpretations of sensations arising from real stimuli: a patient with delirium tremens may misinterpret furniture as menacing persons. *Hallucinations* are sense perceptions, such as visions, which occur in the absence of any kind of external stimulus. *Delusions* are false beliefs, such as that one is being slowly put to death, to which the patient adheres even when demonstrably wrong; a schizophrenic man may be firmly of the belief that he has changed sex.

Intellectual functions. While listening to the account, the clinician can at the same time pick up clues about the patient's intellectual level from the choice of words and from the ease or difficulty of expression. The best clues to the basic intellectual level are given by the patient's scholastic record and by the type of job performed in adult life.

If there is reason to suspect that there may be intellectual impairment, one can test general information by posing simple questions, such as asking the patient to name the head of state, the capitals of large countries, or to perform simple sums of mental arithmetic. The clinician notes whether a man knows the date and time of day, and recognises where he is and to whom he is talking: this tests orientation for time, place and person.

Impairment of mental function is commonly shown by inability to concentrate and hence to remember recent events. This may become apparent during the interview or it may be elicited by asking the patient to remember a name and address or a telephone number and then asking for it to be repeated after an interval of 1 or 2 minutes. The final step in the examination of the mental state is an assessment of the patient's degree of insight; for example, does a man recognise that he is ill or is he wrongly convinced that it is his environment and his fellows that are at fault?

When the history has been taken and an examination of the mental state completed, a thorough *physical examination* should be carried out and, following this, appropriate investigations when required. Such intervention needs to be handled well. Investigations which are necessary must be carefully planned, and quickly executed, and then a halt must be called. The pernicious habit of 'just having one more test' must be avoided as it undermines the confidence of the patient in the certainty of the diagnosis; the practitioner must be able to decide how much evidence is required to elucidate the nature and the cause of the disorder and, having obtained it, must act upon it.

Diagnosis and formulation. The doctor is now in a position to make a formal *diagnosis*, deciding from which psychiatric syndrome the patient suffers, i.e. whether the patient's illness falls in the general class of organic mental illness, functional psychosis, psychoneurosis or personality disorder.

The next step is the *formulation*, a brief statement in which is summarised the doctor's understanding of the disorder and the person suffering from it, including the main setbacks or conflicts with other people, in the sequence in which they occurred.

PSYCHIATRIC INTERVIEWING

When the clinician undertakes to see the patient for a series of interviews, particularly when psy-

choneurosis or a personality disorder is present, a more detailed investigation of the psychological state is embarked upon. To do so, the clinician must acquire the necessary skills by receiving training in psychiatric interviewing, and must gain theoretical understanding of the common developments which occur as the therapeutic relationship is established and progressively extended. The clinician has available four well-documented theoretical approaches to interviewing on which to base his or her own style and approach; at times a combination of approaches is best suited to a particular patient.

1. The *descriptive approach* is most akin to medical history-taking and examination and leads to syndrome identification. As in other branches of medicine, it is appropriate in psychiatry to think in terms of disease entities, that is, to assume that the patient is suffering from a particular illness with its specific aetiology, pathology, signs and symptoms, which can be elicited by history-taking and examination.

2. The *analytical approach* enables the doctor to elicit any relevant complexes or pathogenic ideas of which the patient may be partially or totally unaware. The name 'dissociation' is given to the process by which distressing thoughts, memories or ideas disappear from awareness, and then reappear in disguised form, e.g. as a dream or a physical symptom.

In addition to their symptoms, patients can also be found to have disturbances in their relations with people close to them. These self-defeating patterns of behaviour in personal relationships have been learned by life experience; the early life of the neurotic or psychosomatic patient has included some painful, frustrating or damaging experiences which disturbed peace of mind and continue to interfere with performance. Moreover, the minor psychiatric disorders differ from diseases by being biographically meaningful. We can often understand why that man became ill in that way at that particular time as we come to understand the course of his life and to comprehend his dilemma in relation to the people of importance to him. A psychoneurosis, in this sense, symbolises a personal predicament of the patient.

3. A third interview procedure is the *inter-*

personal approach, the doctor now exploring a patient's significant interpersonal relationships; much psychiatric illness, as we shall see, accompanies difficulties patients currently have in their associations with the people most important to them.

4. Finally, the *phenomenological approach* is the method whereby doctors, by an effort of imagination, use their own life experience to enable them intuitively to grasp what the patient is suffering; such empathic perception of the patient's present predicament in living calls on the clinician to attempt a feat of fellow-feeling by which understanding of the patient derived from the other three approaches can be extended.

Professional attitudes of the doctor

Three habits of mind are relevant to psychiatric work, in addition to those clinical attitudes which are necessary for the practice of medicine in general.

1. First, the clinician needs, for purposes of comprehensive interviewing, to surrender temporarily the relative detachment and authority appropriate to the practice of internal medicine, and instead to adopt a more receptive, less directive, clinical style. Much of the patient's experiences relevant to the psychiatric illness are locked up in the patient and get disclosed only if security, trust and some hope of being helped can be aroused in the patient. A paranoid patient who believes that there is a plot against him may conclude the doctor is part of the plot, unless by warmth and encouragement the doctor reassures the patient and brings him out of himself; a phobic patient may consider a fear of open spaces too ridiculous to disclose to the doctor, especially if already that doctor seems abrupt and critical.

Michael Balint wrote, in *The Doctor, His Patient, and the Illness* (1968), that medical training handicaps many clinicians for psychological work. He had in mind that when a person becomes a doctor that person sets aside to some extent the innate perceptiveness, readiness to be informed by the patient and to be led by him into unexpected avenues. The question-and-answer interviewing technique in medicine, and the professional status as the expert who knows what course the clinical

discussion should take, often constrains the patient. The 'small but necessary personality change' the doctor has to make, for purposes of psychiatric interviewing, is to be more passive, less decided in advance about matters to be explored, and more ready to receive private disclosures from the patient. Indeed, at first patients often impart a 'cover story', a version of the illness and personal troubles which they hope will not offend the doctor; only when they confirm for themselves that the doctor is not censorious and remains open to receive further revelations will patients give utterance to more distressing facts.

2. The second professional attitude of importance in psychiatric work is related to a skill which has already been indicated. The doctor must practise minimal intervention and allow the patient to be the more active.

3. Third, the doctor doing psychiatric work requires an orientation of self-scrutiny, reflecting constantly on the impact exerted on the patient and asking oneself whether the patient is being influenced as intended. A readiness continuously to study one's own personality in clinical action and the responses made to patients enables the doctor progressively to increase knowledge about the life experiences of others, skills for alleviating personal distress, and capacity for gaining self-knowledge. The doctor's personality is the chief clinical tool. It is always to this personal attribute that the psychiatrically ill patient will respond, over and above the clinical expertise the doctor exercises when engaged on the exploration, diagnosis and management of any disorder of the patient's mind or personality.

PSYCHIATRIC DISORDERS

Classification of psychiatric disorders

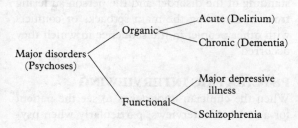

'Minor' disorders   Psychoneuroses (Anxiety, hysterical, obsessional, depressive and phobic neurosis)
Personality disorders (Obsessional, schizoid, hysterical and sociopathic)
Alcoholism and drug dependency
Psychosexual disorders
Psychosomatic disorders

Mental handicap (mental retardation)

THE ORGANIC MENTAL DISORDERS

Psychiatric symptoms may arise in the course of physical illnesses which either primarily or secondarily affect the brain. The mental symptoms of general paresis or the occurrence of delirium during the course of febrile illnesses are two well-known examples. It is important to recognise the particular mental symptoms which occur in organic mental syndromes, since their presence should lead to the search for physical factors which may not otherwise have declared themselves.

The organic mental disorders can be divided into two groups: *delirium*, which is an acute syndrome, and *dementia* which is a chronic disease. Generally speaking the acute form is potentially recoverable, being the result of temporary effects on the brain from toxic processes or disorders of metabolism, while the chronic form is the expression of more severe and progressive tissue changes in the brain and is thus not reversible. The mental symptoms of each of these organic syndromes are not specific to the causative disease and will be the same whatever may be the underlying physical disorder producing the delirium or dementia.

The terminology now used in the United States is similar, since the introduction in 1980 of the American Psychiatric Association's third edition of the *Diagnostic and Statistical Manual of Mental Disorders* (DSM-III).

Delirium

This acute syndrome may be produced by such varied conditions as (1) drug intoxication (alcohol, LSD), (2) physical disease such as infections (encephalitis, typhoid fever), (3) diseases of the brain, (4) electrolyte imbalance (uraemia), (5) metabolic disorders (hepatic failure, acute porphyria), (6) vitamin deficiency (Wernicke's encephalopathy), and (7) cerebral hypoxia (severe respiratory or heart failure).

In addition to the physical symptoms appropriate to the primary disorder there are often found slurred speech, tremor, nystagmus, diplopia and sluggish pupillary reactions. The characteristic mental symptoms are: insomnia and restlessness; disorientation; impairment of the sensorium (clouding of consciousness) so that alertness and attention are diminished; confusion; hallucinations, particularly in the visual sphere; ideas of persecution (paranoid ideas); and a feeling of fear or terror. All the symptoms and particularly the level of consciousness are variable. The patient may be in a state of restlessness varying from simple tossing and turning to such activities as aimlessly searching in the bed-clothes or agitation. The patient may appear orientated for time and place and be able to recognise visitors at one moment, only to be quite confused soon after. The easiest answer is often given to a question without regard to the truth and faulty memory and perception may be compensated for by invention (confabulation), as when a large meal is described in detail, when in fact nothing has been eaten.

Visual hallucinations are characteristic of delirium, and are usually vivid and may be terrifying. Many are based on illusional misinterpretations of objects seen in the room; thus patterns on the wallpaper may become an advancing army of hideous and menacing reptiles. Hallucinations of other senses may occur.

Doubt and suspicion are readily induced by the impaired mentality leading to misinterpretations and may blossom for a short time into transient and rather ill-defined delusions of persecution.

An acute organic syndrome is commonly precipitated by withdrawal of alcohol, or of barbiturates, from patients who have become habituated to taking them in substantial amounts. When the syndrome is due to alcoholism it is known as delirium tremens (p. 695), but its features do not greatly differ from those of delirium from other causes.

The course and prognosis of delirium depend, of course, on the underlying physical disease, and treatment of this in most cases clears up the mental symptoms completely. Sometimes, however, delirium may be an episode in a progressive dementia.

Treatment. The use of chlorpromazine (25–50 mg t.i.d. by mouth or 100 mg i.m.) has transformed the management of acute delirium, enabling the majority of patients to be cared for in a side-room of the medical or surgical ward where their primary disease is being treated. Thioridazine in similar doses has less hypotensive effect.

In all these conditions the patient can be helped by explanations and friendly support; patients who are frightened and bewildered tend to regress to a state of childlike dependency and welcome a firm reassurance from someone whom they are willing to trust. They cannot, however, be kept calm if staff changes expose them to many strange faces or if they are bewildered by too many novel events.

Some patients have catastrophic reactions following operations on the eyes, when they must submit to being blindfolded, and others have reacted adversely to the accompaniments of cardiac resuscitation or renal dialysis. These acute psychoses contain an element of panic. Nitrazepam (5–10 mg) or dichloralphenazone (1–4, 650 mg tablets) are suitable hypnotics.

Dementia

This chronic organic syndrome is very prevalent, affecting one person in 20 by the age of 70 and one person in five over the age of 80. Dementia may be caused by a wide variety of diseases of the brain. The most common of these are Alzheimer's disease (presenile and senile dementia) and cerebrovascular disease, the latter referred to also as 'multi-infarct dementia'. Other important causes include cerebral trauma, inflammations (neurosyphilis, encephalitis), multiple sclerosis, intoxications and deficiency disorders (alcoholism, pellagra, vitamin B_{12} deficiency), myxoedema, prolonged hypoglycaemia, carbon monoxide poisoning, cerebral neoplasm, and degenerative disorders such as Huntington's chorea.

It will be noted that some conditions (encephalitis, alcoholism, vitamin deficiencies) may also cause delirium. The cerebral changes brought about at first by these factors result in delirium and can be reversed by treatment, but if they are allowed to continue unchecked too long, permanent cerebral damage occurs, giving rise to dementia.

The clinical picture of dementia varies to some extent with the cause, the previous personality of the patient, the age of onset, and the rate of progression, but in all cases the mental symptoms are seen to involve the intellect, memory, emotions and behaviour, although the actual degree of impairment depends on the factors mentioned above. Insomnia is often an early symptom and may lead to nocturnal restlessness and confusion as the disease advances. Judgement and reasoning are involved early, and the disability caused by this will depend on the extent to which these faculties are utilised in the patient's daily life and work; it will be more noticeable in a teacher than in an unskilled labourer.

Impairment of memory is the most prominent finding, particularly in relation to recent events, and in the later stages this may combine with defective perception to produce disorientation in place and time. Impairment of higher control leads to emotional instability and outbursts of violence or sexual aberrations at variance with the patient's previous character. There may be wide fluctuations of mood with euphoria or depression but finally, as mood flattens, the patient sinks into apathy. Delusions are common, and may be either centred on the patient, when they are grandiose or self-condemnatory and hypochondriacal according to the mood, or centred on others, when they tend to be paranoid.

As the structure of the personality disintegrates, patients neglect their appearance and become lax in personal cleanliness; careless incontinence occurs. Focal neurological signs may be found, e.g. dysphagia, apraxia, agnosia, hemiplegia, and epileptic attacks, either focal or generalised.

Computed tomography reveals the increase in the size of the ventricles and in the width of the sulci present in brain atrophy. Dementia in the elderly is usually due either to cerebral atherosclerosis or is of senile type. Table 16.1 shows the differences between the two syndromes.

Table 16.1 Dementia in the elderly.

	Cerebrovascular	Senile
Age of onset	From 45 onwards	After 65
Impairment of intellect	Late in illness	Early
Deterioration of personality	Late	Early
Course	Steplike	Progressive
Brain damage	Focal	Global
Physical symptoms	Present	Absent
Physical signs	Present	Rare and late
CT scan	May show multiple infarcts	Cortical shrinkage and dilatation of ventricles

FUNCTIONAL PSYCHOSES

Major depressive illness

Depression is a mood which all of us experience from time to time, usually as a result of some distressing circumstance. In contrast, patients suffering from major depressive illness complain of a prolonged dejected state. They seem to have become ill for no reason they can identify, their low spirits and subjective misery causing them to feel altogether different as people. Such patients are suffering from depressive psychosis. Also known as endogenous depressive illness, in the American classification (DSM-III) the condition is called major affective disorder.

The patient may have been subject previously to mood swings or have had an over-scrupulous rigid personality following too strict upbringing. Major depressive illness may be induced by physical illness such as influenza or by drugs, notably corticosteroids and oral contraceptives. There is a genetic predisposition, particularly in bipolar illness when both depressive and manic episodes occur. Like the less severe psychoneurotic depressive reaction (p. 690), major depressive illness may be precipitated by external events particularly those which impart a sense of loss, separation or disappointment. Much more often it arises without detectable external influences. It is commoner in patients of middle age or older, but certainly does occur in the young and also in children.

Clinical features. In addition to a mood varying from mild depression to black despair the manifestations are: insomnia of a type character-

ised by early waking after 2 to 3 hours sleep; diurnal variation of mood, in which the depression often lifts considerably towards evening; slowness of thought and inability to make decisions; ideas of guilt, unworthiness and self-blame which are often delusional in intensity, i.e. they are impervious to reasoned argument or demonstration of their falsity; and various somatic manifestations such as anorexia, loss of weight, amenorrhoea, pressure headache, backache, constipation, retardation of physical activity (more rarely aimless overactivity or agitation), and hypochondriacal delusions. Such a patient may sit bowed and immobile on the edge of a chair obviously in the depths of misery, weeping silently, and answering questions in slow monosyllables. In the earlier stages the physical appearance is much less striking and the diagnosis depends on the doctor's ability to elicit the symptoms described above.

Severe depressive psychosis, especially when associated with restlessness and agitation (p. 699), with delusions of unworthiness and preoccupation with thoughts of death, is an extremely distressing condition and fraught with risks of suicide. This is the main hazard and the risk is often greatest at the onset of major depressive illness or when treatment begins to relieve the depression and reduce the accompanying psychomotor retardation. Severe cases should be admitted to psychiatric care in hospital.

In *manic-depressive psychosis*, the bipolar form, patients can suffer from morbid elation and hyperactivity in addition to attacks of depression. They look excessively cheerful, speak rapidly, shifting from one idea to another, often joking, teasing, making puns and paying poor attention to the environment. They are overconfident, over-optimistic and overimportant. They may suffer from grandiose delusions and behave in an extravagantly spendthrift way. They usually do not realise they are ill, and may react with violence if crossed or restrained. Failure to diagnose mania can have very serious consequences for patients, who can run up vast debts or jeopardise their social position drastically by ill-judged, embarrassing or boisterously inappropriate and undesirable behaviour.

Treatment. The first task after diagnosing major depressive illness is to proceed without delay to treat the patient with one of the potent antidepressant drugs. One has to bear in mind, however, that these do not take effect until after some 6 to 14 days. There are two principal groups of antidepressant drugs:

1. Tricyclic drugs (e.g. imipramine, amitriptyline and trimipramine), the monoamine reuptake inhibiting drugs.

2. The monoamine oxidase inhibitor (MAOI) drugs (e.g. phenelzine, mebanazine and tranylcypromine).

1. *Tricyclic drugs* constitute the treatment of choice for most cases of major depressive illness. In order to be effective, they have to be given in sufficient dosage. It is usual to prescribe 25 mg t.i.d. for 1 week, and 50 mg or more t.i.d. subsequently. Trimipramine may be given as a single dose (50–100 mg) at night. Amitriptyline is also available in 50 or 100 mg sustained-release tablets for use at night. A course of tricyclic drugs should be taken for 3 to 6 months; if they are stopped too soon the symptoms of depression may recur. A patient who fails to respond to one drug may benefit from another.

Tricyclic drugs give rise to some disagreeable anticholinergic effects, for example on the eyes, causing difficulty in focusing. They may cause tachycardia and should be given with caution to patients with heart disease such as myocardial infarction. Imipramine may make the patient feel even more on edge and restless during the first few days and it may also cause some difficulty in micturition. Amitriptyline tends to make some patients feel uncomfortably drowsy and causes dryness of the mouth. These side-effects usually recede with continued use and become quite easily tolerated once the patient begins to experience a lifting of the mood and a return of former energy.

2. *The monoamine oxidase inhibitors* are especially helpful in the treatment of 'atypical' depression (or prolonged phobic symptoms), occurring in patients with good previous personalities. Patients on MAOI drugs should be warned not to partake of substances rich in tyramine (such as cheese, chianti and some types of beer) because these may interact with the drug to provoke a hypertensive crisis, with splitting headaches and a risk of subarachnoid haemorrhage. The MAOI drugs also potentiate other drugs, including pethidine, opiates, barbiturates, phenothiazines,

amphetamine and alcohol, all of which should be avoided while a patient is taking this form of antidepressant. Caution is needed when changing from a MAOI drug to a tricyclic or vice versa: a drug-free interval of a week is advisable.

Electroconvulsive therapy (ECT) administered under intravenous anaesthesia and modified by muscle-relaxant drugs may be indicated if the patient has not improved after antidepressant medication has been given for about 4 weeks. It is a rapidly effective treatment free from adverse effects apart from transient amnesia in some patients.

Lithium carbonate is effective in controlling manic-depressive states. The patient needs to be in hospital at the start of treatment. It may also prevent the recurrence of manic attacks when used as maintenance therapy, in daily doses of 800–1600 mg, out-patients returning for weekly estimation of plasma lithium (p. 000) and a check on adverse effects which include nausea, vomiting, tremor, myopathy, polyuria and cardio-respiratory symptoms.

Manic attacks, except when mild, require treatment in hospital, sometimes compulsorily. Haloperidol (10–15 mg/d) or trifluoperazine (15–30 mg/d) will usually calm the patient. Benzhexol (p. 650) should be given if extrapyramidal side-effects of the antipsychotic drugs occur.

Rehabilitation. As a general rule, it is wise to postpone any practical decisions about business, change of work or domestic matters until the patient has regained a normal mood. Once the patient has responded to drugs or ECT it is essential to review personal circumstances and to help make plans to cope with the difficulties which may have precipitated the illness. Moreover, the patient may need to know that the illness sometimes takes a recurring form and that advice must be sought if symptoms return. However, major depressive illness, once of gloomy prognosis, is now eminently treatable, and with appropriate care few such patients become chronic hospital inmates.

Schizophrenia

Schizophrenia is the illness with symptoms corresponding most closely to the popular conception of madness. The personality becomes disintegrated, and detached from the social environment. The mental life becomes split up. The cardinal features are: disorder of thinking, which becomes incoherent, disjointed and rambling; incongruity of emotion; impulsive actions and utterances; and hallucinations (most commonly, in the form of threatening or unfriendly voices). Patients express bizarre delusions with little or no appreciation of why it is that their ideas are unacceptable to those around them.

Delusions and hallucinations may also occur in other forms of mental illness, such as severe depressive illness, mania, or delirium, but certain other features are especially suggestive of schizophrenia. These include (1) *passivity feelings*, in which the patient is convinced that his (or her) actions are controlled by some alien power, (2) *thought insertion* and *thought broadcasting*, in which he feels that other people put thoughts into his mind, and are able to read his thoughts, and (3) *paranoid delusions* in which he believes that he is surrounded by hostile forces which watch him and secretly intervene to do him harm.

Patients with depressive illness may also develop paranoid ideas, but these are coloured by their all-pervading feelings of guilt. For example, a depressed patient may believe that he is being watched by secret police because they have found out that he has committed a terrible crime. The paranoid schizophrenic, on the other hand, is quite sure that it is his unseen enemies who are the hostile villains, and he their innocent victim.

Schizophrenic patients tend to have little insight into the fact that they are ill and in need of treatment. When their behaviour is becoming alarming, it may be necessary, in their own interests, to admit them compulsorily to hospital. In Britain application is made by the patient's nearest relative supported by recommendations by the patient's family doctor and a psychiatrist. The patient's case must be reviewed after 28 days. In many cases he will continue in hospital voluntarily. A mentally ill patient who is a danger to himself or others may also be admitted compulsorily as an emergency for 3 days in England and Wales and 7 days in Scotland. This certificate is signed by only one doctor and can be used when the patient is already in hospital.

The features indicated above are the more florid manifestations of schizophrenia. The patient's functioning declines, in regard to the capacity for work, social relations and self-care. Milder signs, less easy to recognise, include instances of unexpected rudeness or tactlessness, and abrupt and inexplicable behaviour with a marked withdrawal from ordinary social contacts. Such persons may be considered awkward or unsociable and it is only when they reveal quite bizarre ideas, shout back at their hallucinatory voices, or otherwise behave in a conspicuously strange manner, that one realises that they are not merely eccentric, but mentally ill.

Treatment. Phenothiazine drugs such as chlorpromazine, and the butyrophenones (e.g. haloperidol) have changed the prognosis of schizophrenia but it should be remembered that even before there was any specific drug treatment for this illness, many cases made a spontaneous recovery from the stage of the psychosis in the course of 3 to 9 months. These drugs offer symptomatic relief of the patient's delusions, hallucinations and alienation from reality, rather than a radical cure of this little-understood disease. There is abundant evidence that the way in which the patient is treated, in hospital and in the community, will influence both the degree of recovery and the probability of a subsequent relapse.

Schizophrenic patients do badly if they are allowed to withdraw too completely from social contacts and practical activities; but they also do badly if they are involved in emotionally demanding relationships, to which they are unable to respond.

Many, if not most, schizophrenics must be regarded as having particularly vulnerable personalities and many emerge from the acute stage of their illness with some residual defects ('end states'). Those left with moderate or severe deficits, perhaps as many as a third, then lead impaired lives, and require skilled rehabilitation. These patients are not necessarily intellectually impaired — they may be highly intelligent — but they are seldom able to cope with positions of responsibility, particularly when they are required to supervise, or interact with other people. Many such partially recovered patients do best in tasks in which they can work on their own, with only rather formal contacts with their fellows.

Nowadays the great majority of schizophrenic patients, after discharge from hospital, can be treated at home, taking their prescribed drugs for at least the first year or two. The doctor should be ready to enlist the help of a community nurse or of a social worker if patients appear to be having difficulties either at work or in their domestic relationships.

During the acute stage of the illness, chlorpromazine or thioridazine is effective medication, 150–1000 mg being given each day in divided doses. About 60% of patients with acute schizophrenic symptoms can be expected to improve significantly within a matter of weeks. A suitable maintenance dose for a schizophrenic patient in remission is 50 mg twice daily. Chlorpromazine is also given by intramuscular injections (50–100 mg) in order to control stages of agitation or overexcitement. Postural hypotension is an important side-effect which is more marked with elderly patients, who should be given smaller doses. Haloperidol (up to 30 mg/d orally or i.m.) may be substituted for chlorpromazine.

A long-acting phenothiazine, fluphenazine decanoate (12.25–25 mg each 2–4 weeks) can be given intramuscularly on a maintenance basis for chronic schizophrenics treated as out-patients who are unreliable with oral medication.

All the phenothiazines can have adverse extrapyramidal effects, and antiparkinsonian drugs (p. 650) may also have to be taken. Restlessness and dystonia of the jaw and neck can occur. Another drug effect is tardive dyskinesia, continuous movements of the head and tongue, which may persist for years.

When the schizophrenic psychosis is of acute onset, and the previous personality relatively sociable and well-adapted, the outcome is better. It is important for doctors to know about the condition and recognise it when it occurs, because competent and early psychiatric treatment can spare the patient and the relatives extreme harm, through social catastrophe or accident.

THE PSYCHONEUROSES

There are two conditions to be met before the doctor can regard an illness as psychoneurotic.

First, one of the typical syndromes (to be described below) must be in evidence. Second, the person must have experienced a recent setback, usually a disturbance in his relationship with a person or persons important to him. Often, when the first condition applies, the doctor may need to act on the basis of a clinical diagnosis without having elicited the biographical corroboration, but it must be remembered that the omission exists and needs to be remedied, otherwise serious mistakes can be made. Symptoms resembling those of neuroses, e.g. hysterical states, can occur with cerebral trauma or disease or in a functional psychosis.

The interpersonal or social setback preceding the onset of psychoneurotic illness need not be gross. However, it will be highly charged emotionally, in the context of the patient's biography, sometimes fitting as a key does into a lock with an earlier similar setback. It then seems understandable that the recent miscarriage of a relationship (the dynamic cause) has disorganised the adaptation of a person previously sensitised by an earlier emotional trauma (the predisposing cause). A woman who becomes ill with psychoneurosis when afraid that she may be deserted on discovering that her husband has become attracted to another woman, may be found by further questioning to have lost her loved father through his death before her teens. The threat of the present loss is more understandably distressing in relation to the earlier deprivation.

Psychoneurosis, one of the 'minor' disorders, is an illness taking the form of one of the well-described syndromes in this category of disability: anxiety, hysterical, obsessional, depressive or phobic neurosis.

With all these characteristic syndromes the patient will be only partially disabled, many aspects of personality and social competence being unaffected. The man or woman can often cope with work and household responsibilities, and hence usually be treated as an out-patient. Reality testing is not impaired in any gross way, i.e. the misperceptions of the human and material environment characterising psychotic illness do not occur.

There is a great amount of psychoneurotic illness in every community, for psychoneurosis is much the most common psychiatric disorder. Many individuals will be mildly disturbed and may not need medical treatment. A man with a fear of heights is not disabled if he works on the ground in a community made up of low houses; the same man who moves for postgraduate work to New York, for example, where he may have to attend seminars in skyscrapers, can become seriously impaired. On the other hand, flying phobia developing in any member of aircraft personnel is instantly incapacitating.

Not all patients will accept with equanimity a diagnosis of psychoneurosis when their preferred concept of their illness is a physical one. This will often be evident from the initial reluctance with which some patients accept advice for psychiatric referral. A sickness of one's body is not regarded as a matter for which one is culpable. In contrast, a disturbance of one's mind could be regarded as an affliction of one's very self, and therefore a weakness in one as a person.

It has been demonstrated that the higher the social class of the patient, the more acceptable is a psychiatric diagnosis. The same correlation between socio-economic disadvantage and somatisation is evident in transcultural psychiatric studies: in the East and in Africa, patients in much greater numbers than in developed countries present psychogenic illness in the form of physical complaints. Indeed, as university health service experience with medical and other students has shown, even sophisticated patients often tend to complain first about somatic symptoms such as headache or stomach discomfort (and many doctors are more receptive about physical illnesses), and only afterwards proceed to relate a personal problem or to describe emotional distress.

The most important clinical rule is the need not only to elicit any psychoneurotic syndrome which may be present, but also to uncover the intrapersonal emotional conflict preceding the onset of the illness.

Anxiety neurosis

Anxiety is a state of fear, manifesting with a feeling of inner tension and somatic symptoms such as sweating, tremor and tachycardia. Anxiety neurosis is the most common form of psychoneurosis. Although anxiety is a symptom of many psychological disorders, in this syndrome it dominates the clinical picture and other symptoms such as depression are but minor features of the total illness.

Aetiology. Hereditary factors play a part, although a relatively small one, in the genesis of anxiety neurosis, manifestations of anxiety being found in 15% of parents and siblings of patients, which is more than in the population as a whole (5%). Twice as many women as men are affected.

In addition to the genetic trait, even more important aetiologically are emotionally disturbing experiences during the formative years. Often it is found that the patient's early years were attended by prolonged insecurity. For example, a parent may have been so burdened by problems that the child felt unloved, if not unwanted; a brother or sister may have seemed to get preferential treatment; or a mother's own profound anxieties may have imparted an excessive timidity to her child, gravely undermining the child's self-confidence.

This emotional trauma may not be apparent for several years, particularly if the experiences of school life and early adolescence prove free from alarming or painful incidents, but a setback in early adult life may precipitate adult emotional illness. Painful events, such as a bereavement, a reverse in a love affair, disappointment in one's career, being obliged to contend with disagreeable or frankly hostile people at work, or being involved in prolonged domestic strife, may cause a vulnerable individual to succumb to feelings of anxiety which interfere materially with the ability to cope with the daily routine. The adult setback will often be found to have been similar in quality to the earlier childhood emotional trauma.

Clinical features. The illness may take many forms. It may occur as an acute anxiety attack, often severe in intensity, referred to in the United States classification (DSM-III) as panic disorder. Another form is a chronic anxiety state, known as generalized anxiety disorder in DSM-III. It is present since adolescence in mild degree, but subject to periodic exacerbations occurring at the time of social setbacks, disappointments in close relationships, or work stresses.

The outstanding feature of all forms is anxiety, with its accompanying feeling of inner tension and unpleasant anticipation. Sometimes the anxiety is fear of a potential danger but often it is a diffuse dread. The fear and foreboding fluctuate in intensity, being sometimes mild tension or nervousness, and at other times a state of panic, in which the patient may be overwhelmed by a feeling of terror, which is no less disturbing because the reason for it is not apparent to the patient.

A *phobia* implies that anxiety is associated with a specific form of activity such as travelling in a bus or train, and so much may this be dreaded that the patient is eventually house-bound through being unable to travel at all. The state of anxiety gives rise to other symptoms. The ability to concentrate is impaired and decisions are difficult to make. There may be a continuous state of restlessness or extreme irritability. The patient may fear becoming insane or committing suicide though, in fact, both are extremely rare in anxiety neurosis. Preoccupation with bodily functions (*hypochondriasis*) and fear of serious illness (e.g. *cancerophobia*) are frequently manifested. Continued stress exhausts the patient who, lacking energy and perseverence, may be unable to continue at work.

Somatic symptoms are also prominent. There is a general tenseness of muscles, with hyperactivity, especially of the hands. A fine tremor of the fingers is often present and profuse perspiration, particularly of the palms and forehead, is common. The pulse rate is raised, the blood pressure labile and overactivity of smooth muscle commonly manifests by frequency of micturition or of defecation. Breathing is often rapid and feelings of nausea and flatulence occur; headaches of tension type (p. 626), dizziness and unsteadiness are frequent. The patient sleeps badly, finding it difficult to get off to sleep and being easily disturbed. Appetite is poor, and loss of weight may be a pronounced feature. Disturbances of menstruation are common.

Not infrequently the patient omits mention of the distressing emotional state and complains to the doctor only of the somatic accompaniments of anxiety; unnecessary special investigations can be initiated or diagnostic errors made if the doctor omits to ask about the state of the patient's mood.

Treatment. PSYCHOTHERAPY. When the formulation of the case indicates that emotional factors are prominent, some form of psychotherapy is required; the patient needs an opportunity for exploration and clarification, and for gaining greater insight into the nature of his (or her) difficulties. Simply informing the patient that there is nothing wrong with him, or that he must pull himself together, is useless. Even telling the patient that his difficulties are psychological and identifying the emotional problems in his life is unlikely to be of benefit, because although he may acquiesce verbally, his emotional tension will not be thereby lessened.

A series of interviews, for which periods of at least half an hour or longer should be set aside, are needed when the patient is encouraged to talk about his difficulties. Initially, the discussions should be allowed to proceed in any direction the patient desires; subsequently, aspects of his problems which come to seem relevant may be suggested by the doctor as themes for more detailed discussion. The error that is commonly made with this form of psychotherapy is for the doctor to talk too much and give advice. In order that the patient may achieve a better knowledge of himself, it is essential that he should do most of the talking, the doctor saying little, but maintaining an attitude of interest and expectation. If the patient's flow of talk is arrested, encouragement can often be given, without diverting him from his present theme. Thus, if he says 'I wasn't able to cope at work', and then becomes silent, after giving him ample time to resume spontaneously, the doctor may say, 'You found the job too much for you?', which starts the patient off again.

The effect of this approach is first that the patient feels better for having talked to someone about his troubles. A second effect is that frequently the patient comes to grasp more accurately the nature of his problems, and will, at that stage, often accept suggestions and interpretations which, if given earlier, would have been rejected. What emerges is that the patient is having difficulties with a person of importance: a spouse, a parent, or an employer, for example, and that there is a need for an improvement in the patient's own participation in the relationship. Thus a man may be too dependent on his wife, too docile to his parent, or too subservient to his employer — in which case his interviews should encourage greater assertiveness.

When the psychoneurotic illness takes the form of somatic symptoms and fear of bodily disease is prominent, it is not sufficient to tell the patient that there is no evidence of organic pathology. It is necessary to let him know that his distress and his symptoms are recognised as genuine and need exploration. It is often possible to use events in the patient's own experience to illustrate the influence of emotion on bodily functions. Many people can recognise what it feels like to be sick with excitement, to be aware of a pounding of the heart in moments of fear or to experience frequency of micturition when keyed up before an examination.

Patients are helped greatly when they can go one stage farther, to confront the painful situation and to master it, e.g. the patient can say to his employer that he considers he is being exploited and his abilities insufficiently recognised. When this is done, there is commonly an immediate, even if temporary, relief from the distressing symptom, together with a sense of accomplishment which encourages the patient to persevere with further efforts of self-discovery.

In the treatment of all forms of neurotic illness it is important to decide what can best be done, within the limitations of resources for treatment and in the circumstances of each individual patient.

Brief psychotherapy focuses upon recent events in the patient's personal experience and explores their emotional significance. By this method, many patients can be helped to reconstitute the way of life which, for the particular person, represents normal mental health.

Explorative psychotherapy, which calls on patients to take stock of their relationships with people close to them and to modify some of their habitual patterns of behaviour, is more time-consuming and aims to produce personality change as well as relief from the symptoms of the illness.

Relaxation training can be of considerable benefit in milder cases, but not when anxiety is severe.

DRUG THERAPY. Drugs can be particularly helpful in tiding a neurotic patient with anxiety over an especially difficult period of subjective distress. They do not, however, do anything to resolve the causes of the patient's symptoms, and unless this is altered either through psychotherapy or through a significant change in personal circumstances, the symptoms will tend to recur and the patient may become dependent on the palliative drug.

The use of drugs to obtain reduction of distressing mood disturbance is often a necessary preliminary to effective psychotherapy. A very anxious patient will not be able to concentrate sufficiently to benefit more than partially from clarification of conflicts discussed during an interview. Diazepam (5 mg b.d. for mild cases and 10 mg t.i.d.in more severe cases) and chlordiazepoxide (10–60 mg/d) are effective anxiety-reducing drugs. The phenothiazines, though widely used (up to 150 mg/d), are more likely to give rise to lethargy or drowsiness but thioridazine, in the same dosage, can be of value when the patient is both fearful and restless.

Adrenergic blocking agents, such as propranolol, are effective when palpitations are troublesome. Like all medication in treatment of psychoneurotic illness, it is no more than a part of a therapeutic approach in which the doctor's ongoing participation is crucial.

Hysterical psychoneurosis

Hysterical psychoneurosis is a protean group of disorders, commonly encountered in all branches of medicine. Essentially a hysterical neurosis consists of the production of the symptoms or signs of a 'physical' illness by a patient for some personal purpose, without being fully aware of the motive in doing so. Familiar examples are sudden 'blackouts' or 'loss of memory' by which a patient deals with a particularly painful or humiliating occurrence.

Aetiology. Heredity is even less important in the development of hysterical neurosis than it is in anxiety neurosis. Environment, by contrast, provides those situational factors which precipitate the development of hysterical symptoms. Lack of emotional security in the early years can encourage and prolong a state of child-like dependency. The lack of development of confidence to tackle practical difficulties makes a person rely on others to solve problems and such a person may later react with hysterical illness. Gross hysterical symptoms occur frequently in association with educational and intellectual disadvantage, and are a particularly common occurrence in developing countries.

Conversion hysterical neurosis. This type of psychoneurosis includes the illnesses in which the patient presents with a physical symptom, such as sudden blindness, or paralysis of one or more limbs, or total loss of sensation in a part of the body. Neurological examination will often reveal that the disability does not correspond to the anatomical areas served by motor or sensory nerves; instead, the lesion illustrates the patient's own idea of what it is like to lose the power of the right hand, or to be unable to walk. In many cases, the patient has acquired a concept of a particular affliction as a result of seeing someone who was similarly handicapped. The form the symptom takes may be determined by identification with another person, as when the daughter, after her mother's death, develops the symptoms of her mother's last illness.

The grosser forms of conversion symptoms are not so common today as they were a generation ago, but still occur particularly frequently as a complication of injuries where a compensation award enters the picture. A striking feature of conversion hysterical neurosis is that although apparently quite severely incapacitated by the symptoms, the patient is remarkably unconcerned about them. This is because the disability due to the illness has in fact intervened to remove a cause of anxiety, so that the patient feels strangely relieved, although not aware of the reason for being so calm.

The list of conversion hysterical symptoms and signs is extensive, for there are few clinical features which may not be encountered in the many forms of this diverse disorder. Some features, however, occur more commonly than others and may be arbitrarily divided into two groups, sensory and motor. *Sensory symptoms* may be of the special senses, such as blindness and deafness, or in the somatic sphere, when cutaneous and deep sensibility in their various forms are lost. The sensory loss does not obey anatomical or physiological laws but follows the patient's concept of disability. Cutaneous sensory loss may have a sharp horizontal upper margin on the limb. In monocular blindness, the patient may on occasion see with the 'blind' eye and the light reflex is preserved. There may also be subjective sensory symptoms such as headache, pain or tinnitus.

Motor symptoms consist of aphonia, mutism and paralysis and rigidity of movements. Positive clinical features in the motor sphere consist of tremors, tics and explosive utterances, spasm of ocular muscles, and fits. These fits may vary from simply falling to the ground to bizarre attacks with wild movements of arms and legs. Carpopedal spasm and other manifestations of tetany may result from hysterical hyperventilation.

In the 1980 United States classification (DSM-III) this illness is named conversion disorder and considered a subtype of the 'somatiform disorders', which have as essential features symptoms suggesting organic illness for which there are no demonstrable physical findings to explain the symptoms.

Dissociative hysterical neurosis. The second type of hysterical psychoneurosis includes the numerous altered states of awareness, such as faints, fits, amnesias, trances, twilight states and forms of multiple personality. A fugue state is one in which the patient wanders away from home in a condition of altered awareness. Hysterical stupor, when the patient lies motionless showing no reaction to the environment, is sometimes seen; in pseudodementia (seen on occasion in a prison setting) the patient behaves as if insane. The term 'dissociative disorder' is used in DSM-III.

Anorexia nervosa. In this condition, classified with the hysterical psychoneuroses, patients aim to become very slim and to stay so. The determination to diet is a disorder of motivation. Exertion of the will, so that over-riding priority is given to a stubborn and obsessive pursuit of thinness, is the chief feature of the illness.

Young girls are mainly affected, and boys much more rarely. If questioned suitably, the patients often reveal preoccupations (sometimes so distorted as to reach delusional proportions) relating to sex, sometimes following misinformation by parents; however, these patients also give evidence of great fear at growing up and accepting mature responsibilities. They are often in a hostile relationship with their mothers. Frequently there have been upsetting life experiences, such as separation from or death of a parent. In addition to dread of sexual development, girls with anorexia nervosa often show athletic preoccupations and are overactive physically. Teasing about being plump may be a precipitating factor. The usual mood state is cheerful high spirits, but depression can occur. Patients usually show unconcern about their physical deterioration even though they are emaciated.

Those anorexics who in addition induce vomiting and use purgation have a worse prognosis. Increasingly often, patients present with *bulimia* characterized by orgies of overeating followed at once by self-induced vomiting.

Amenorrhoea is a prominent feature as a result of a reversible disorder of the hypothalamic-pituitary-gonadal axis. Hypogonadism, hypercortisolism and other endocrine abnormalities can be demonstrated.

Treatment is often rejected and must be very firmly advised. Psychotherapy to achieve emotional maturation is usually necessary in hospital in addition to correction of the eating disorder.

Diagnosis of hysterical psychoneurosis. This can be the most difficult in medicine. Three steps are required: the first is to identify the psychoneurotic syndrome on the basis of its characteristic symptomatology, as described above. The second step to be taken, should any doubt still exist, is to demonstrate that there is no organic disease which can account for the symptoms and signs. Error in diagnosing hysterical psychoneurosis would be infrequent, however, if the diagnosis were not made until the third step was also taken: this consists of discovering what disappointment or setback preceded the development of symptoms. The precipitating cause of an hysterical illness is usually an emotionally charged experience, with unpleasant consequences socially or personally to the patient who excludes it from consciousness and replaces it with symptoms.

If evidence of previous hysterical breakdowns can be uncovered, the diagnosis is more firm. It should be kept in mind, however, that the stress of organic disease may provoke a superadded hysterical reaction in a person so disposed. An axiom worth remembering is that suspected hysterical neurosis appearing for the first time in a stable person in middle life has almost always an organic basis.

Treatment may be a difficult problem. Removal of a symptom can often be achieved by a prolonged interview in which intense persuasion is used; but if the precipitating situation is unaltered, relapse is usual. The method may be justified, however, in certain circumstances as when aphonia prevents discussion, or when loss of memory in hysterical amnesia prevents identification or revelation of the events which precipitated the illness.

The principles described for psychotherapy in the treatment of anxiety neurosis are also relevant in hysterical psychoneurosis. When hysterical personality disorder is also present, special aspects of management become necessary, as described on page 694.

Obsessional psychoneurosis

An *obsession* is a constantly recurring thought which the patient recognises as his own, but of which he tries to rid his mind because it is foolish or repugnant. In spite of his efforts to dismiss the thought, it persists in returning so that in the end he becomes tormented by it. A *compulsion* is a similarly insistent urge to perform, or to repeat, some act which the patient consciously repudiates as meaningless or troublesome; he struggles against the urge, but finds himself experiencing very acute anxiety, which is allayed only by giving in and performing the compulsive act.

Obsessive-compulsive symptoms may occur as episodes of illness in otherwise normal individuals. They may become aggravated during an episode of psychiatric illness. Sometimes obsessions and/or compulsions are the outstanding, if not the only, symptoms of which a patient complains. In this condition the patient, although perfectly lucid and in contact with the environment, may be severely handicapped by the unrelenting pressure of unwelcome thoughts and impulses. The illness is also remarkable in that a person almost incapacitated by obsessional symptoms can appear normal to the external observer, until the appallingly repetitive thoughts are disclosed.

Aetiology. Obsessive-compulsive neurosis has an hereditary factor: one-third of the parents of obsessional patients and one-fifth of their siblings have obsessional traits. Many observers believe that the meticulous, rigid routine imposed by such parents is more conducive to obsessional neurosis in the child than the hereditary endowment itself. Environmental factors, other than the influence of obsessive parents during the formative years, appear to contribute less to the causation of obsessional neurosis than is the case with the other syndromes of neurosis.

Clinical features. Obsessions may be arbitrarily divided into ideas (or images), impulses and ruminations. The *ideas* consist of thoughts, images (often obscene) and strings of words and phrases, which constantly recur to the patient despite resistance to them, and recognition that they are absurd and meaningless.

Impulses are urges to some act such as killing offspring, or jumping under a train, or to less fearsome activities like laughing at sorrow or arranging objects in a certain set manner. Fears of some act may accompany impulses. A fear of knives develops from an impulse to use them for murderous ends. Likewise, a patient may not be troubled by obscene thoughts but rather by the fear that he may have such thoughts; he fills his mind with neutral thoughts lest obscenity should intrude.

Ruminations comprise the practice of constantly turning over problems in the mind, seeking an answer to a question. Religious scruples are of this order, when the patient has repeatedly to examine and re-examine his conscience, uncertain as to whether he has offended or not.

These symptoms are often intermingled one with another, and may be of all degrees of intensity. Sometimes they are merely a nuisance, not interfering seriously with life, but preventing enjoyment and causing tension. In other cases they become so severe as to arrest all activity and make the ordinary daily round an impossible task. Thus a patient who was a house painter stood for three hours, unable to paint a crack on the wall until he had the 'right' thoughts in his mind. A housewife may spend all her time washing her hands for fear they should be contaminated, and so be unable to do her housework.

When the obsessions are severe they cause great anxiety and tension, the patients becoming increasingly agitated as they fight against the compulsion. In addition, they frequently become depressed, since life becomes so difficult and escape from the obsessions seems to be impossible. Suicide is, however, relatively uncommon except when depressive symptoms complicate the illness.

Treatment. The patient with obsessional illness does not respond well to treatment, but often the condition is self-limiting, at least in its acute phases. The patient should be encouraged by being given the assurance that the doctor knows that irrational, obscene or murderous thoughts are not indicative of that person's true nature, and that they are harmless. Behaviour therapy based on learning theory is sometimes helpful. The patient should be encouraged to avoid situations which foster the development of the obsessions and should diversify interests as much as possible. The best antidote for obsessive ruminations is for the patient to keep at work, occupied with practical tasks which demand attention.

Severe obsessional symptoms may be helped by a tricyclic antidepressant drug. Clomipramine has been used, 75–450 mg daily in divided doses, particularly when depressive symptoms are also present.

Depressive psychoneurosis

This type of illness is at times also named *reactive depression*. Characteristically the morbidly depressed state comes on after a personal setback which often takes the form of a loss of a person important to the patient, for example through death or separation as occurs with a divorce or a broken engagement. Careful exploration will show that the recent disappointment reflects one that occurred earlier in the patient's life. A typical example is the onset of depressive neurosis after a woman is left by her husband, and further interviewing discloses that she had lost a beloved father as a child. When the illness corresponds to an abnormal grief response after the death of a significant person, the term 'bereavement reaction' is sometimes used.

Mixtures of depressive symptoms with anxiety reaction occur frequently; some neurotically depressed patients are also hypochondriacal.

Treatment. Only occasionally is admission to a psychiatric hospital required, the patient often responding well to out-patient psychotherapeutic interviews.

It may be confusing but it is nevertheless of the greatest importance to emphasise that mixtures of depressive psychoneurosis and major depressive illness are extremely common. The clinical task is to scrutinise any case of depressive illness to determine the presence and amount of any component of 'endogenicity', i.e. so-called biological features including loss of energy, sleep disturbance, loss of appetite, constipation, impairment of libido, and—in severe cases—gross self-blame. In such mixed states antidepressant drugs are indicated, and good practice calls for a combined psychotherapeutic and pharmacological approach.

The 1980 United States classification omits the term depressive psychoneurosis, contending that these patients can be assigned to one or another illness entity, depending on the main clinical features.

Phobic psychoneurosis

These widely prevalent illnesses consist of unjustified fear which is firmly related to a precise stimulus, either a place or an object. The patient may be terrified at being in a supermarket, a bus, an open space (*agoraphobia*), or a closed place (*claustrophobia*). Fear of flying can be a nuisance to a housewife and may deter the family from taking overseas holidays, a major handicap to a business executive, and an occupational disaster to a pilot or other member of an air crew.

The phobic place or object can be so innocuous as to seem ridiculous, and dreading ridicule the patient may not be able to summon the courage to disclose the affliction to the doctor. Direct questioning may be needed to explore clues which are offered, such as a patient never coming unaccompanied to consult the doctor.

Phobias can at times be referred to parts of the body, hence the use at times of such terms as 'cardiac neurosis' and 'cancerophobia'. Patients can be terrified that they may have an urge to urinate when a toilet may not be accessible; when afflicted with this syndrome, patients know exactly the locus of every public lavatory in their neighbourhood.

The subjective benefit to the patient of suffering from a phobic state (rather than, say, an anxiety reaction or an obsessional illness) is that life can be perfectly manageable as long as the phobic stimulus is avoided. A person with a dog phobia need only find a dogless route to work, if one exists.

Treatment. Antianxiety medication, such as chlordiazepoxide or diazepam, can assist such patients greatly, in association with psychotherapeutic interviewing which encourages the patient to 'go against the phobia'. Monoamine oxidase inhibitors reduce agoraphobic symptoms, but there is often relapse when the antidepressant drug is stopped. A requisite of treatment is that the doctor should comprehend the terror experienced by the patient (often related to childhood traumatic experience) and avoid a belittling response even when the patient's fear is grotesquely unjustified.

Behaviour therapy has a high rate of success. It is based on devising for the patient a hierarchy of experiences relating to the phobic object or situation, in which increasing exposure is gradually built up, always avoiding excessive anxiety. Someone with a dog phobia may look with the doctor or clinical psychologist at canine pictures, starting with a benign species and coming at length to an Alsatian; then real dogs can be introduced to the interview, first a docile, aged pet and perhaps later quite daunting beasts encountered on a walk can be approached with due circumspection.

PERSONALITY DISORDERS

In every large community there are a number of people who do not conform to the prevailing norm. Statistically speaking, a person can be outside the range of normal either by being exceptionally gifted or by being so grossly under-endowed as to be an eccentric or a social misfit. It is the latter who are more likely to come to medical attention.

The personality disorders began to gain notice only late during the development of psychiatry as a medical discipline; they have been recognised increasingly as the out-patient responsibilities of psychiatrists have extended, and as psychiatric units have developed in general hospitals. The diagnostic differentiation between psychiatric illness and personality disorder is the more necessary because very often the two coexist. Indeed, clinical convention has it that hysterical psychoneurosis commonly supervenes in individuals with hysterical personality, obsessional neurosis in those with obsessional personality disorders, etc. In addition to their presentation with psychotic illnesses and psychoneuroses, people with abnormal personalities often appear clinically with psychosomatic disorders and may be chronic hospital attenders.

Abnormal personalities may not enter the medical ambit at all, but be encountered in penal settings. Still others may continue unrecognised in the community and escape anonymity only when widespread screening of the population occurs, as in a wartime when obligatory intake to the armed forces exposes all adults to clinical scrutiny.

The central feature of abnormal personality is some degree of persistent abnormality of behaviour which is frequently, but not necessarily, antisocial in its manifestations. The abnormality varies considerably in degree, ranging in severity from schizoid and hysterical people who are often valuable if somewhat unstable members of the community, to psychopaths who are socially destructive.

In the 1980 United States classification the personality disorders are classified on a separate axis from the psychiatric illnesses, encouraging multiple diagnoses wherever possible.

Obsessional personality disorder

Obsessional persons give scant regard to the emotional aspects of a situation or an interaction. They are rigid rather than flexible, overattentive to details rather than to the wider scope of an event or encounter, and prefer to have everything predictable and orderly. They often appear officious, sometimes so pedantically that they can be comical, and not only control themselves excessively but also attempt to dominate others. They appear to behave in an unduly egotistical manner, and respond in an overriding way when involved in a venture calling for co-operation. They are over-careful, methodical, punctual and overorganised, to the extent of becoming uncomfortable and even upset if their routines are disturbed by an unexpected development. They have a set of fixed standards and points of view, from which they can deviate only with great difficulty. They are uninfluenced, therefore, by the wishes, needs, opinions or views of other people.

The meticulousness and preservation of sameness extends to the person's mode of dress, which can be scrupulously neat. They can be overconscientious, and often work compulsively. Such persons, in consequence, can be of particular usefulness in bureaucratic posts calling for scrupulous concern with minutiae. They may be highly obstinate when faced by any requirement that they should deviate from the straight and narrow path.

At times such persons appear to leave some loophole, so that the conformity, inhibition and rigidity is waived in some context or other. The precise, neat youngster, who must have everything in place, may for example permit himself to have his clothes cupboard in disorder, or may periodically forget thrift to overspend in a foolish self-indulgence which rationally is at odds with his habitual miserliness.

The gross form of the disorder is easy to recognise. The milder forms may be less obtrusive, and may be particularly evident only at times of pressure, as when an examination is looming for a youngster or when a house-proud woman has relatives coming to stay in her home.

Schizoid personality disorder

Schizoid persons are essentially solitary. They are aloof in their loneliness, detached and distant from other people. The term 'introverted' is applied to this disorder in the 1980 United States classification. Such individuals have few close relationships, and may be much more preoccupied with some impersonal activity in the realms of electronics, physics, mathematics or engineering. Often the engrossing venture is a personal fad or invention, which may be of negligible application in ordinary life, but may be pursued with a single-minded devotion inappropriate to a mere hobby or interest.

Cold, quiet and shy, the person's abnormality may already have been apparent early in childhood, from an inability or disinclination to mix, and a preference for solitary pursuits. The lack of friendships may have been upsetting to the parents; as schizoid individuals grow up, they can themselves be distressed by their incapacity for any intimacy in their association with others.

The person may appear odd or eccentric and in awkward isolation may be seen as a figure of fun or seem excessively secretive. Schizoid people are often solitary workers, who cannot function satisfactorily in a team. Bookish, reserved, out of touch with others, relatively blind to social cues, their personal lives may appear barren. However, this remote exterior may belie the strong emotions which some schizoid people cannot express. Others find a vehicle for their private feelings, and may keep a diary, or indulge in day-dreaming, or succeed in establishing some relationship in which the expression of emotion is allowed.

Schizoid persons are rigid and brittle. They have little empathy with other people, of whose intentions, feelings and wishes they remain unaware. When attempting to appraise others intuitively, they are often wildly wrong, thereby complicating their already attenuated relationships. They can be made profoundly uncomfortable when well-meaning but misguided mentors or doctors attempt to have them mix more, or urge them to become intimate with other persons, perhaps other isolates as lacking in interpersonal skills as themselves.

Schizoid persons are at times mistrustful, seeing slights where none is intended. Suspicion can become the prevailing response to others, in the belief that they are being exploited, misused or disparaged. Some clinicians would differentiate this development separately, diagnosing such a personality as *paranoid*.

Hysterical personality disorder

People of this type can be identified on the basis of a constellation of behaviours: they seek to please and influence others; they crave attention; they are insincere; and they are given to excessive displays of emotion. They were often victims of inadequate maternal care in childhood.

Hysterical individuals appear to be exploitative, with an eye always on others. They talk for effect, not to convey any honestly felt opinion. One feels their need for appreciation, and their readiness to express themselves with that aim in view. They over-react in order to evoke a response from others.

Psychiatrists probably over-diagnose this type in abnormal women, attaching the label very much less often to men. The person is showy, histrionic in manner and dress, with a quality of spuriousness and exaggeration, even theatricality, in what she does. The condition is named 'histrionic personality disorder' in DSM-III. The exhibitionism appears intended to impress others, even to shock them. Speech is superficial, with plentiful hyperbole ('heavenly', 'ghastly'), which only heightens the effect of shallowness. Women of this type suffer from sexual timidity and frigidity, the more distressing to them because their frequently seductive manner and provocative dress invites advances with which they cannot cope; hysterical men also have difficulty in establishing a close relation with one woman, and may seek intimacy in a series of attachments of short duration.

The management of an hysterical personality disorder is discussed on page 694.

Sociopathy

Sociopaths suffer from the most severe form of abnormal personality. Because of serious defects in the capacity for feeling, they are often described as 'affectionless'. Lacking in conscience they have great difficulty in realising that other people are harmed when they behave antisocially. The name for the condition in DSM-III is 'antisocial disorder'. Loveless, indifferent and destructive, they cannot form satisfactory relationships, and major failures repeatedly occur in marriage, work and social life. They come into conflict with the norms, customs and laws of the community.

Impulsiveness is usually evident, sociopaths dismaying those associated with them by uncontrolled, often destructive outbursts in the absence of sufficient provocation. Such precipitate and deplorable action has been spoken of as 'short circuit reactions', to indicate that often the person is aware of the build-up to the outburst and will often admit after the aggressive or destructive episode to feeling calmer and relieved of tension.

Sociopaths do not show ability to modify destructive behaviour reactions, or to learn from even drastic setbacks; they may be punished repeatedly for the same unacceptable behaviour, and yet continue it; the individual's antisocial patterns are often monotonously repetitive. Kleptomania, gambling or physical assaults may each be associated with excitement which the sociopath seeks and indulges repeatedly; the antisocial behaviour can be seriously destructive to others, as in cases of sadistic attacks on children or of fire-raising.

The lack of regard for the possible consequences of their actions is also impressive, sociopaths appearing not to care about the outcome, and being inconsiderate even of persons on whom their welfare depends. They disregard their obligations to others. The lack of concern amounts often to callousness. The Mental Health Acts in Britain allow for the compulsory hospitalisation of the 'seriously irresponsible' sociopath, and so does the legislation of many other countries.

Social relationships are shallow and transient. Sociopaths are not loyal to individuals or to groups. They have poor judgement of situations, and often lie their way out of complications. They are indifferent to the welfare of others. Swindling and deception are frequent features.

Two types of sociopathy are distinguished:

Aggressive sociopath. The hostility displayed in attacks on other people, damage to property, thefts and fraud may bring the sociopath to legal attention.

Passive sociopath. Persons of this type are seriously inadequate and cannot adapt to social requirements; they are chronically inept, passive and dependent. Many are placid and responsive; others are cold, withdrawn and apathetic. They may exist as aimless drifters, to be found in places where hoboes congregate. Even if supported in a family or protective environment such as a halfway house or hostel, such people may be further incapacitated by the complications of drug addiction or alcoholism.

Management implications of personality disorders

The chief medical relevance of personality disorder, in terms of the doctor-patient relationship, is that patients respond to the clinician in accordance with their particular personality deviation. For this reason, diagnosis of the personality type permits the management to be planned realistically, so that the doctor does not expect a degree of co-operativeness which the patient is not equipped to provide. In addition, the doctor will be better able to predict the patient's pattern of behaviour in the future.

For example, the long-term management of a woman with an hysterical personality disorder has much in common with that of a frightened or petulant child. It consists in convincing her that you are on her side, even while refusing to comply with some of her requests. Treating a patient with such personality disorder is often a test of nerve; in the face of dramatic protestations and apparently alarming social crises, one must quietly but firmly insist upon facing the painful realities from which the patient has taken flight. If one has succeeded in gaining her confidence, helplessness and distress will sometimes disappear with dramatic suddenness, but all too often they are replaced by subsequent turmoil. The hysterical patient finds it difficult to abandon the defences against alarming feelings which she has been using since her early adolescence. In addition these patients are especially prone to develop an emotional dependence upon their doctors, which must be recognised and brought to their attention kindly but firmly. The family doctor can give helpful advice to other people in the patient's immediate environment, warning them that hysterical acting-out behaviour only becomes aggravated if too much attention is paid, and encouraging them to avoid entering into the patient's pattern of self-deception. It is usually much easier for the onlookers than for the patient herself to see the real motivation of her symptoms, but of course, it is no use simply telling her — she has to discover for herself why she behaves in the way she does.

The achievement of a long-term cure of an hysterical personality disorder is a formidable task since it requires the patient to mature emotionally. Not surprisingly, both patients and their doctors often tacitly agree not to attempt it. Instead, the doctor may concentrate upon dealing with the most pressing difficulties of the patient's immediate predicament and may settle for her remaining a somewhat demanding and dependent patient. In that case, the goal for each consultation can be to ensure that the patient departs calmer and with more self-esteem than when she arrived. The doctor helps the patient discover some modifiable aspect in a problem which she had considered insoluble.

ALCOHOLISM AND DRUG DEPENDENCE

Addiction to alcohol or drugs represents a form of psychological dependence and indicates that the patient has been unable to attain adequate satisfaction or self-esteem in his or her personal life. Addictions to drugs and to alcohol are associated with a high risk of suicide. The underlying lack of self-confidence is often so deep-seated that prolonged treatment and rehabilitation is necessary once the drug or alcohol has been given up. In the 1980 United States classification these conditions are named 'substance use disorders'.

Alcohol. Alcoholics are often brought reluctantly to their doctors by close relatives who can see more clearly than the patients how seriously their lives are being interfered with by the addiction. These unwilling patients are particularly difficult to treat; but the prospect is very different when the patient is distressed by the dependence and is anxious for change.

Alcoholism is one of the most serious public health problems in all developed countries. Mental disorders due to alcoholism are responsible for a large proportion of admissions to Scottish mental hospitals. It is an insidious condition, because the enjoyment of alcohol is socially accepted and even encouraged. There is a relationship between alcohol consumption in a country and rates of alcoholism; alcohol consumption has been increasing steadily in countries such as Britain, the United States (32% higher in 15 years), West Germany (61%) the Netherlands (83%) and Finland (50%). The Irish have a high alcoholism rate, while Chinese and Jews are rarely alcoholic.

The process by which an occasional drinker becomes an excessive drinker, and finally dependent on drink, can be gradual; acquaintances, and even friends are reluctant to draw attention to a man's excessive drinking because the alcoholic is liable to fear being shunned and is prone to take offence. Here, however, doctors have a clear responsibility because often an intercurrent illness, alimentary symptoms or haematemesis, or even a street accident will bring the patient to medical care, and a carefully taken history (especially if supplemented by information from others in the patient's family) will reveal the increasing dependence upon alcohol. Other conditions which may prove to be due primarily to an alcohol problem (p. 700) include cirrhosis of the liver (p. 353), pancreatitis (p. 298), cardiomyopathy (p. 181), neuropathy (p. 662) and myelinolysis, encephalopathy and dementia (p. 656).

Sometimes an unexpected hospital admission, interrupting a sustained high intake of spirits, results in the onset of *delirium tremens* which compels attention to the seriousness of the drinking problem. This acute psychosis is characterised by gross peripheral tremors, great restlessness, confusion, misidentification of people and places and delusional ideas. These delusions may be agreeable but much more often they are threatening or even terrifying, especially when accompanied by hallucinatory visions. Because of these complications, hospital admission may be necessary when starting to treat an alcoholic.

The fully established syndrome of alcoholism is characterised by: (1) a need for alcohol as for a drug, customary activities being difficult to perform without it; (2) taking of alcohol apart from social occasions; (3) tolerance, the person being able to drink increasing amounts without becoming incapacitated; (4) the abstinence response, i.e. unpleasant symptoms occurring as the blood alcohol level falls, e.g. tremor, sweating, wakefulness and tension; (5) loss of tolerance; becoming incapacitated before imbibing the amount of alcohol needed; (6) restitution, i.e. the rapid development of the entire syndrome after drinking is resumed following a period of abstinence.

Treatment of alcohol addiction. This consists initially of 'drying out', which often calls for hospital admission. Withdrawal symptoms can be controlled by phenothiazines, diazepam, haloperidol or chlormethiazole. The last is an hypnotic related to thiamin. It is probably the drug of choice in severe alcohol withdrawal syndromes including delirium tremens. In these circumstances it should not be used for longer than 1 week because of the danger of dependency. Vitamins B and C intravenously may also be of value.

The next phase of treatment, once the patient is abstinent, is to explore, by means of a series of interviews, the personal and other problems which require attention. Psychiatric assistance is needed if obvious psychological disorder is apparent once the drinking has stopped. Those abstinent alcoholics who consider themselves in danger of relapse can ensure their sobriety by taking disulfiram (0.5 g/d) or citrated calcium carbimide; when on these drugs, the patient will have an unpleasant reaction after taking only a small amount of alcohol.

The main requirement of treatment is that the alcoholic should become totally abstinent. Many alcoholics are active and valuable members of society and can maintain this necessary abstinence if given appropriate medical supervision.

Alcoholic women who are pregnant require urgent and skilled care to avoid damage to the fetus. The *fetal alcohol syndrome* is characterised by impairment of growth, mental retardation and dysmorphic features. Women who drink alcohol only socially would be well advised not to do so during pregnancy.

Morphine. Dependence is seen in doctors, nurses, pharmacists and dentists, and at times in patients who become addicted through therapeutic use. The desired euphoric effect can be achieved by subcutaneous injection, but as tolerance grows intravenous injections are used. Hypodermic tattooing of the skin, thrombosed veins and pinpoint pupils are indications of the condition.

Treatment, such as substitution with methadone, is best done at a centre with the necessary facilities.

Heroin. Dependence is increasing rapidly in incidence, and many addicts are young people. The drug has a marked euphoriant effect; it acts quickly and its desired action also dissipates quickly. The abstinence syndrome is particularly unpleasant. Many addicts cannot be cured, and their management then is by supplies of the smallest dose of the drug preventing the withdrawal symptoms, or by substitution of methadone in place of heroin.

Cocaine. Those addicted to cocaine take the drug in the form of snuff, smoke or intravenously. It is a stimulant, like amphetamine. The most well-known toxic symptom is formication, the sensation of insects crawling under the skin. Use occurs mainly in those addicted also to heroin, the effect of cocaine alone being unsatisfactorily brief. Physical effects are anorexia, emaciation, nausea, insomnia arrhythmias and convulsions.

By the Drug Addiction Act of 1968, issue of heroin and cocaine is limited in Britain to named doctors, usually psychiatrists in designated treatment centres. Social complications are damaging, disorganised behaviour leading to loss of friends and inability to work, and to trouble with the law because of possession, purchase or sale of the drug.

Lysergic acid diethylamide (LSD) is used mainly by young people. Taken by mouth, it has dramatic effects lasting about 6 hours. Illusions occur, colour is intensified, mood changes include euphoria, awe or anxiety, a curious blurring between the individual and the environment is experienced, and phantasy thoughts, flight of ideas and delusions serve to heighten the mystical nature of the 'trip'.

Physical dependence does not occur, but some users become psychologically dependent. Proponents of the drug as a 'mind expander' sometimes overlook the serious hazards. These include psychotic reactions with paranoid delusions which can last many weeks, and non-psychotic reactions chiefly terror; both can result in self-injury or suicide. A bad LSD experience can be cut short by chlorpromazine, used intramuscularly in severe cases.

Cannabis (hashish, marihuana, 'pot') is also used very commonly by the young, sometimes only a few times; there is no evidence that occasional use is harmful. At first the user feels 'high', and then drifts into a peaceful, drowsy state heightened by unusual mental images. Skin flushing, rapid pulse and dilated pupils may convey that a person has taken cannabis, usually by smoking a 'joint'. Many addicts use more than one drug. That physical dependence can occur is doubted, but marked psychological dependence is common.

Barbiturate. Many middle-aged or elderly women come to rely upon a nightly dose of sleeping tablets and some of them find that if they take two or three during the day, this helps to relieve tension and anxiety. Gradually, they begin to show the signs of chronic barbiturate over-dosage, namely, slight ataxia, absent-mindedness amounting at times to confusion as to time and place, defective judgement, loss of emotional control, slurred speech and tremor of the fingers. A sudden cessation of barbiturates can be followed by a major epileptic fit. The withdrawal syndrome can be alarming, with headaches, insomnia and vomiting, and a delirious state with delusions. Small doses of barbiturates may need to be administered. A patient cured of one addiction, e.g. alcoholism, may start using another drug, e.g. barbiturate, which is erroneously regarded as innocuous.

Another pattern of usage is in young people who obtain the drug illicitly and take it often with their associates and with other drugs.

Amphetamine formerly used in the treatment of obesity and still used for narcolepsy, soon came to be abused, particularly by teenagers, either alone or combined with barbiturate to provide a rapid lifting of the spirits and feeling of well-being. The use of amphetamine readily gives rise to a psychological dependency, when the daily dose taken can increase vastly, tolerance developing with continued use. The amphetamine addict has an impression of increased mental and physical drive and competence. There are also restlessness, irritability and excitability. Amphetamine can give rise also to an acute psychotic reaction with auditory and visual hallucinations and delusions of persecution. These features can be clinically indistinguishable from those of paranoid schizophrenia, but they clear up in about 3 weeks time after withdrawal of the drug. Since the Misuse of Drugs Act (1971), amphetamines are listed as controlled drugs in Britain, special regulations applying to prescribing them. The drug is justified medically only in occasional cases of narcolepsy.

Volatile substances (glue sniffing; solvent abuse) have received publicity because of their abuse by children and adolescents particularly in deprived communities. The most widely used is toluene, but benzene, lacquers, cigarette lighter fluids, paint thinners and xylene have been employed. The glue is sniffed from smears on rags, from plastic bags, or directly from tubes. This practice promotes stimulation ('jags'), but tolerance develops, and amounts are sniffed which lead to damage to the brain and other organs. Volatile solvents are among the most dangerous of the psychoactive substances to which users can become addicted.

Multiple drug abuse is frequent. Those who misuse alcohol also regularly make non-medical use of other drugs, e.g. benzodiazepines. This occurs especially in those with access to medicines, such as doctors, nurses or pharmacists but members of the general public, from adolescents to those in middle age, also frequently have poly-dependency, tobacco and pharmaceutical agents complicating, say, a drinking problem.

PSYCHOSEXUAL DISORDERS

These include sexual deviation (paraphilia) and conditions such as premature ejaculation and vaginismus.

Sexual deviation

Sexual deviants are people who are unable to obtain physical and emotional satisfaction in normal sexual intercourse, but can do so only in ways which to a greater or lesser degree are socially condemned. Practices which alarm, threaten or injure other persons, such as *exhibitionism* (exposing the genitals to a stranger), *paedophilia* (having sex with immature partners of either sex) or *sadism* (deriving sexual pleasure from inflicting pain) are still regarded as antisocial and are punishable by law. On the other hand, public opinion has become somewhat more tolerant of deviant practices which do not interfere with other people. The change of opinion found expression in the Sexual Offences Act 1967, which, for the first time in English history, excluded homosexual acts, carried out in private by consenting adults, from any legal sanction.

Homosexuality. People who are responsive erotically to partners of the same sex are frequent in the population. 4% of adult men are exclusively homosexual, and another 13% are so for years of their lives. For women the rates are half as much. During the 1970s increasing numbers of homosexuals have 'come out' and publicly declared their sexual orientation. After debate and public pressure the American Psychiatric Association in 1974 ruled that homosexuality as such would no longer be listed as a mental disorder, creating instead a new category of 'sexual orientation disturbance'.

Forms of deviant sexual behaviour also include *transvestism* (deriving gratification from wearing the clothing of the opposite sex) and *fetishism* (when the person becomes sexually stimulated by parts of the body not usually experienced as erotogenic — e.g. the feet — or by articles of clothing or other objects). These conditions seem to be the result of distorted experiences at the stage of development when boys and girls learn their sexual roles. The significance of hormones in determining such gender identity still remains debatable; there is no firm evidence for any hormonal difference in homosexuality.

Deviant forms of sexual gratification often prove very resistant to change. If the patient suffers because of them — and many sexual deviants appear to be content with their lot — treatment often has to be limited to damping down the intensity of the sexual drive, e.g. by the administration of oestrogens to males or to helping the patient (and perhaps also the spouse) to accept the condition.

PSYCHOSOMATIC DISORDERS

These are the physical illnesses which are caused in part by psychological factors or, when present, are maintained by psychological factors. Examples of such conditions are many cases of peptic ulcer, bronchial asthma, colitis and various forms of dermatitis. The implication of the term 'psychosomatic' is that tension arising from a long-standing emotional conflict can induce changes in bodily function (e.g. excessive secretion of gastric acid; bronchospasm) which, when repeated over a period of time, can in turn lead to actual tissue damage.

For many years, attempts have been made to delineate particular personality types associated with different forms of psychosomatic illness. A review of this literature, however, fails to reveal a specific type of personality in relation to each of these disorders. Instead, psychosomatic subjects tend to be characterised by relatively constant emotional elements, the chief of which are dependency, anger or fear, which appear to be the most harmful when they are denied conscious expression. Repressed dependency needs have been particularly associated with peptic ulcer and ulcerative colitis, repressed anger with asthma and hypertension.

Individual cases, however, when studied in depth, are not easily fitted into any common mould. Modern psychosomatic theory has, therefore, retreated to the more general observation that all patients with physical illness accompanied by a conspicuous psychological component have long-standing problems in the control of their own internal emotional experiences, and in the conduct of their relationships with people who matter in their private lives. It is probable that genetic factors, which have endowed some of us with a particularly vulnerable organ, will dictate both the occurrence of a psychosomatic illness and the choice of the organ which is affected.

Treatment of the emotional disturbance and disregard of the local physical factors, or vice versa, will seldom lead to benefit for the patient, and an assessment must be made in each case of the relative importance of both factors, so that whichever appears to have the greater aetiological significance can be the main target for therapy, while the lesser factor is in no way neglected. The family doctor is often in the best position to know the unrealised ambitions, the frustrations at work or at home, or the marital unhappiness which may form the background to the patient's physical illness. A knowledge of the family history may also reveal that hereditary predisposition plays a part in determining the form of the illness, as for example in migraine.

PSYCHIATRIC DISORDERS IN RELATION TO AGE

The individual is confronted with new problems in adaptation at all the main stages of change, namely puberty, adolescence, pregnancy or following childbirth, at the menopause and on retirement. Mental disorders occur particularly at these times.

Childhood. Psychiatric disorder in children is now a major subspecialty of psychiatry. In childhood very significant phases in the development of personality are taking place; the child is at the mercy of the environment, utterly dependent on the adequacy of the parents and the provisions they make. In addition to behaviour disorders including untoward fear, aggressiveness, jealousy, stealing, school phobia and truancy, children require treatment for such distressing syndromes as enuresis, soiling (involuntary defecation), psychoneurotic illnesses, psychotic disorders including early infantile autism, and the handicaps such as stammering, dyslexia, extreme hyperactivity and organic brain damage.

The doctor responsible for the health of the child needs to collaborate closely with the child psychiatrist, with institutions which may be involved including the school, and with professional colleagues who contribute in any treatment, especially the clinical psychologist and the social worker. The parents must always be implicated clinically. The outcome of a programme of management often depends crucially on the comprehensiveness and adequacy of the co-operation between those involved.

Adolescence. Psychoses are rare until adolescence, when they increase in frequency; psychotic illnesses thereafter are increasingly common with advance of age. At adolescence, the period between puberty and young adulthood, the young person has to cope with more complex social involvement, sexual commitment and occupational challenge, while also separating from parents and detaching from their domestic arrangements. The personality changes of normal adolescence may be upsetting to some parents, teachers or other adults; a period of turmoil when the adolescent is aggressive, defiant or rebellious may precede the achievement of a stable adult personality. A previously polite child may become rude and sarcastic in the course of developing assertiveness and independence.

Often the youngster surmounts troublesome behaviour if the family, school and community are understanding, encouraging and tolerant but certain disturbances of adolescence require clinical attention. These include delinquent behaviour, deviant sexual practices with consequences which are harmful socially or damaging to the young person, inadequate school attainment, mood disturbance such as depression sometimes with attempts at suicide, withdrawal, social isolation and apathy, and, of course, bizarre behaviour with psychotic features such as delusions or hallucinations which may signal the onset of schizophrenic illness.

Adolescents can develop any of a range of psychiatric disorders, such as the adjustment reaction of adolescence, psychoneuroses, the functional psychoses, personality disorders, acute organic psychoses, drug and alcohol misuse and psychosomatic disorders.

Adulthood. Mental disorder may be associated with pregnancy or the puerperium. Puerperal psychoses may be schizophrenic in type or, more rarely, manic-depressive. Psychoneurotic illnesses also occur in the postpartum period.

The majority of patients receiving psychiatric treatment are middle-aged. However, when the numbers of first hospital admissions are calculated in relation to the proportion of the general population in each group, the psychiatric admission rate to hospital rises steadily with increasing age, particularly after the sixth decade. In middle age, depressive psychosis is sometimes accompanied by intense anxiety, resulting in the syndrome of *agitated depressive psychosis*. The patient is characteristically restless, overwrought, hopeless, with extreme self-blame and low self-regard, and expressing nihilistic, guilty or hypochondriacal delusions. The previous personality in such patients is often characterised by over-conscientiousness or obsessionality.

Retirement from work can be a source of anxiety, especially for people who derived particular satisfaction, status, or esteem from working with others. Depressive illnesses with a sense of worthlessness or apathy can be a real burden for some at this stage of life. Women are often at risk in earlier middle life when their children leave home and make their separate existences, especially when mothering formed a predominant role in the woman's pattern of adjustment, unaccompanied by additional interests and commitments.

The elderly. The care of the elderly plays an increasingly large part in contemporary society. Dementia has been discussed on page 000 but of great clinical importance is the fact that many elderly people with dementia can also become depressed. It is a most serious omission to fail to recognise this common illness in the elderly, who may be incapacitated by such superadded psychiatric disability, but become able to cope again when relieved of the morbid gloom and apathy by antidepressant therapy.

What is also not widely appreciated is the fact that episodes of neurotic illness, with anxiety states, phobias, hysterical symptoms or compulsions are also encountered in this age group, and are no less amenable to simple psychotherapy than at other ages. In the after-care of these older patients it is important to remember that social isolation is an important threat to their mental well-being. This becomes even more important when physical disability or deafness further restricts their opportunities of making contact with other people. Here voluntary agencies as well as local authority welfare and preventive services can do useful prophylactic work, but the family doctor is often in the best position to recognise when an ageing (and perhaps recently bereaved) patient is in special need of help.

Elderly patients easily develop delirium, and then adapt poorly to sudden changes of scene and bewildering happenings. It is helpful for them if they can be visited by only a few nurses and doctors who take pains to identify themselves; their sick-room should be well lit and they should be encouraged to keep a few familiar possessions on their bed-side table. Since patients with even very slight clouding of consciousness are prone to misunderstand what is happening round about them, any changes of routine or new procedures should be explained to them in advance, in simple terms and if necessary more than once.

Conclusion

Psychiatric disorder can present diverse problems throughout an individual's life and also clinical challenges not only to psychiatrists but to all who practise medicine.

HENRY WALTON

FURTHER READING:

Walton H J 1986 In: Macleod J, Munro J (eds) Clinical examination, 7th edn. Churchill Livingstone, Edinburgh. For a detailed description of the pyschiatric examination

Trethowan W H 1979 Psychiatry, 4th edn. Baillière Tindall, London. A useful text for undergraduates

Kendell R E, Zealley A K (eds) 1983 Companion to psychiatric studies, 3rd edn. Churchill Livingstone, Edinburgh. A postgraduate textbook written mainly by Edinburgh teachers

Shepherd M (ed) 1983-85 Handbook of psychiatry. Cambridge University Press, Cambridge. An authoritative and comprehensive text in 5 volumes

Crammer J, Barraclough B, Heine B 1982 Use of drugs in psychiatry, 2nd edn. Gaskell, London

Royal College of Physicians 1987 The medical consequences of alcohol abuse: a great and growing evil. This report reviews the physical damage resulting from the social problem of alcohol misuse.

Edwards G, Grant M 1980 Alcoholism treatment in transition. Croom Helm, London

Bancroft J 1983 Human sexuality and its problems. Churchill Livingstone, Edinburgh. Sets out the range of sexual difficulties and their clinical management

Periodicals:

The British Journal of Psychiatry and the American Journal of Psychiatry should be consulted for recent advances

17

Acute poisoning

Self-poisoning is a very common and urgent medical problem. The number of patients admitted to hospital because of it has increased steadily in Britain over the last 30 years, so much so that this type of behaviour has become endemic in our society. In England and Wales, there were 33 600 hospital admissions due to acute poisoning in 1962, whereas in recent years the figure has been well in excess of 100 000, representing 10 to 30% of all admissions to acute medical units in Britain with a general average of 15%. These hospital statistics are formidable, but the true incidence is probably much higher. Many symptomless children and up to 40% of adults who reach accident and emergency departments may be sent home because the physical effects are mild. Many patients, estimated to be about 30%, are not even referred to hospital but are treated at home by their general practitioners. In Britain, therefore, it is more likely that the true incidence of poisonings is over 300 000 per annum.

The mortality due to acute poisoning in Britain has fallen in recent years but according to official statistics approximately 4000 deaths occur due to poisoning each year. It has been estimated, however, that about 80% of all deaths from acute poisoning occur outside hospital and so it is important that hospital statistics should not be considered alone as an index of the physical consequences of poisoning in the community. The fall in mortality has occurred, despite the increase in incidence, for two main reasons. Carbon monoxide poisoning has become rare since the relatively non-toxic natural gas replaced coal gas in domestic supplies, and prescriptions for barbiturates have been much reduced with the substitution of safer hypnotics such as benzodiazepines. Improved methods of treatment have also played their part, and in any good district hospital the mortality resulting from acute poisoning should be less than 1%.

The major causes of death by poisoning are now dextropropoxyphene, barbiturates, tricyclic antidepressants, salicylate and paracetamol. Perhaps as a result, there are two peaks in mortality; the first occurs in the 15 to 25 age group mainly from analgesics, and the second in patients over 65 due to barbiturates with, in addition, coexisting physical disease. At all ages the number of females who die tends to be greater than males, but this is probably a reflection of the fact that acute poisoning is commoner in women than in men. Among the 25 to 30-year-olds, suicides constitute one in 10 of all deaths, and in doctors, death from acute poisoning is as common as death from carcinoma of the lung.

The problem of acute poisoning is not restricted to Britain but is experienced in all the developed and many developing countries of the world. In the United States of America five million poisonings occur every year and the number is increasing. Acute poisoning is the fourth most common cause of accidental death in that country and the reported mortality is over 5000 per annum. Poisoning is the most common medical emergency in paediatric hospitals. At all ages it accounts for 10% of all emergency home visits and 5 to 10% of adult medical admissions. In most European

701

countries a similar problem exists, but direct comparison, especially in terms of mortality statistics, is difficult due to the wide variations in which deaths from poisoning are recorded and coded. Morbidity statistics are subject to even greater discrepancy and much more standardised information is required before the true international situation can be assessed.

This chapter deals with the clinical features, diagnosis, treatment and prevention of acute poisoning. Food poisoning is discussed on page 751. Brief reference is made to industrial and agricultural poisons. The effects of exposure to ionising radiation are discussed on page 531.

Classification and causes of acute poisoning

Acute poisoning can be accidental or intentional.

Accidental poisoning. Death from accidental poisoning has increased almost three-fold in the past 30 years, women being more likely than men to die in this way. In Britain the mortality from this cause is approximately 15 per million population; in other European countries there is considerable variation. In Scandinavia, for example, the rate is about 20 per million. Except in children, it is doubtful if the official statistics reflect the true incidence of accidental poisoning. For example, it is difficult to believe the official figures that more adults die each year from accidental barbiturate poisoning than from suicidal poisoning by these drugs. Certification is often purposely made inaccurate to save family feelings. Confused elderly patients may develop acute accidental poisoning because they are often given many medicines and they are prone to make mistakes in the dosage and frequency of the administration of drugs. This is particularly the case when inappropriate psychotropic therapy is prescribed.

SUBSTANCES INVOLVED IN ACCIDENTAL POISONING. Children are most frequently involved due to the careless storage of medicines and household products. Common causes include ingestion of medicine (e.g. aspirin, tricyclics, antihistamines or iron), a wide range of household substances (e.g. paraffin, detergents or bleach) weed killers (e.g. paraquat) and, rarely, poisonous berries. Inhalation of organic solvents (e.g. glues and cleaning fluids) and carbon monoxide from incomplete combustion due to faulty gas appliances or motor car exhaust pipes, also occurs.

Accidental poisoning may also be caused by arthropods (e.g. common insects, scorpions, spiders, and ticks), marine animals (e.g. poisonous and stinging fish and cone shells), snakes, fungi (mushrooms) and vegetables (pp. 706–711).

Intentional poisoning. This is due to a wide variety of causes ranging from a minority of patients who are determined on self-destruction, i.e. *suicidal poisoning*, to a large group who indulge in *self-poisoning* which some prefer to call *parasuicide*. The term *attempted suicide* is best discarded as it implies a motive to an act of self-administered poisoning, which is frequently incorrect. The majority of people who deliberately take poison do not wish to die; in fact, they often take positive precautions to ensure that help will be available. Self-poisoning is usually a conscious, often impulsive act undertaken to manipulate a situation or a person and secure redress of circumstances which have become intolerable. Frequently relatives and society rally to help and the situation which has caused so much distress is rectified. Mistakes, however, do occur through misjudgement of dosage or a lack of available help, and an act which was committed primarily to draw attention to a particular situation may end in death. Self-poisoning often occurs in a setting of poverty or alcoholism and with a background of a broken home in childhood. The alarming increase in the incidence of acute poisoning is largely due to self-poisoning which accounts for approximately 90% of all adult poisoned patients admitted to hospital. Such behaviour now constitutes a major social problem. This is the case particularly in areas of dense conurbation and is less marked in small towns and rural communities.

Homicidal poisoning, which is another form of intentional poisoning, is rarely encountered now in hospital practice.

SUBSTANCES AND METHODS USED IN INTENTIONAL POISONING. *Self-poisoning.* Perhaps the most important cause for the increase in self-poisoning is the ready availability of drugs in the community. There is no doubt that the dramatic increase in the frequency and size of individual prescriptions over the last 35 years in Britain, in the National Health Service, has tended to encourage the mistaken belief in the community that the taking of pills is the answer for all life's ailments.

Almost any substance may be used for self-poisoning, but evidence of the importance of availability is the changing pattern of drugs taken in overdosage over the years. Ten years ago 60% of admissions were due to barbiturates and other hypnotics, notably methaqualone. As a result of campaigns and voluntary restrictions by doctors in prescribing, the incidence of these drugs in acute overdosage is now very low. In contrast, psychotropic drugs, especially sedatives and anti-depressants, which are now commonly prescribed, are frequent causes of poisoning. Benzodiazepines account for 40% of poisonings and tricyclic anti-depressants 13%. Salicylates and paracetamol amount to 10%. The incidence of acute salicylate poisoning, particularly in children, has been reduced in recent years. This is due to an increased awareness of the toxicity of salicylates in overdos-age, resulting in more careful prescribing habits together with the provision of child-proof con-tainers and individually wrapped tablets. For similar reasons acute poisoning with the analgesic combination of paracetamol and dextropropoxy-phene, has become less common.

Combinations of drugs are taken in about 60% of overdoses and alcohol is involved in 70% of poisonings in men and about 50% in women. These combinations may cause problems in assessment of the severity of poisoning and in treatment; chemical analysis also may be difficult.

Suicide. The methods adopted for deliberate self-destruction vary from country to country and between sexes. In Britain women most often use drugs, with drowning second choice. Self-injury, such as hanging, is most common in men with drug overdosage second. In America, shooting is the first choice in males, but takes second place to drugs in women. For reasons stated, coal gas poisoning, which was previously common, now seldom occurs.

Diagnosis of acute poisoning

Information service. The impact made by poisoning on medical services has led to increasing demands for information regarding the toxicity of substances and drugs. In the last 25 years, therefore, there has been a proliferation of poisons information and poison control centres in many countries. Information can be obtained immedi-ately on a 24-hour basis regarding the ingredients of a substance and the approximately fatal dose of a poison. In many of these centres the best method of treatment can be discussed with a physician trained in clinical toxicology. In order to provide as comprehensive, accurate and up-to-date information as possible with ready accessi-bility, much of the data has been computerised, especially in the United States where, in addition to regional centres, extremely comprehensive information may be obtained at national level.

Clinical features. For the majority of poisons the clinical features are non-specific. Fortunately, the diagnosis is usually apparent from the history obtained from the patient, relatives or friends or on circumstantial grounds such as finding tablets beside the patient. Difficulty arises when there is no such information and the physician is faced with the diagnosis of the unconscious patient. It is helpful to remember that in the age group 15–40 years acute poisoning is the commonest cause of unconsciousness in the absence of head injury.

Pinpoint pupils, vomiting and depressed respi-ration suggest overdosage of morphine and related alkaloids or of cholinesterase inhibitors. In young people in particular, a history of marked and sometimes rapid changes in level of consciousness with associated respiratory and perhaps cardiac arrest is often associated with dextropropoxy-phene poisoning, especially if taken with alcohol. Widely dilated pupils, bladder distension, absent bowel sounds, cardiac arrhythmias and upper motor neurone involvement characterise tricyclic antidepressant toxicity. Sweating, tinnitus, deaf-ness and hyperventilation strongly suggest acute salicylate poisoning.

In general, however, it is impossible to provide clear clinical diagnostic guidelines because the range of substances available for poisoning is so great and their potential toxic effects are so vari-able in an individual patient. Too much import-ance is often placed on the state of the pupils, changes in limb reflexes and other neurological features. For example, inequality of pupil size, abnormalities of eye movements and nystagmus, which may have great significance in patients with primary neurological diseases, may all be due to drug effects. In patients with acute poisoning, therefore, assessment of the level of consciousness, which for many poisonings is the most practical means of determining the severity of toxicity, is best kept as simple as possible as in the Edinburgh method: grade 0 — fully conscious; grade 1 — drowsy but responsive to vocal command; grade 2 — unconscious but responsive to minimal painful stimuli; grade 3 — unconscious but just responsive to strong painful stimuli and grade 4 — unconscious with no response to stimuli.

Other useful clinical features are evidence of self-injury especially on the flexor aspects of the arms and wrists and on the face and hands. Also all patients suspected of self-poisoning should be examined carefully for venepuncture marks, abscesses or skin ulceration on the arms, hands and feet, which suggest recent 'mainlining' by a drug addict. Many household products, such as volatile hydrocarbons and solvents, have characteristic smells which aid diagnosis when they are ingested or inhaled. There may be buccal damage after the ingestion of strong acids or alkalis, phenols and cresols, although with some serious poisonings, such as paraquat, this may not become apparent for up to 36 hours after ingestion.

Identification of poisons. More secure identification has now become possible by the marking of an increasing number of tablets and capsules with a code letter and number. Others can be recognised by their characteristic appearance or with the help of a coloured diagram.

Laboratory analysis. The only conclusive identification of acute poisoning is laboratory analysis using specimens of blood, gastric aspirate or urine as appropriate. Simple, rapid screening methods using thin layer chromatography are available for approximately 90% of common poisonings and can be of considerable help to the clinician. Confirmatory and more precise quantitative measurement is usually done by gas chromatography which is sometimes combined with mass spectrometry. Although these analyses can be carried out, the results seldom influence treatment but may be of value for medico-legal purposes. Simple clinical methods of analysis are available for salicylates and paracetamol.

General therapeutic measures

Treatment should not be delayed by spending excessive time in attempting to identify precisely the poison involved, since the essential immediate management of poisoning is dependent on the application of well-established basic therapeutic principles.

The major considerations are the establishment and maintenance of adequate respiration and circulation. Removal and inactivation of the poison should also be achieved where possible. The first-aid treatment is often the responsibility of the general practitioner outside hospital and if carried out effectively, contributes substantially to reducing both mortality and serious morbidity. Particular care should be taken during the transport of an unconscious patient to hospital.

Maintenance of respiration. A clear airway is essential. Dentures, vomitus, foreign bodies and excess secretions should be carefully removed from the mouth and fauces. An oropharyngeal or cuffed endotracheal tube should be inserted if the patient is unconscious. All such patients who do not have the protection of an endotracheal tube should be transported or nursed in the semiprone position. Artificial respiration is required if respiration is depressed. Mouth to mouth respiration should be given, but, where facilities are available, more effective ventilation is achieved by administering oxygen using an Ambu bag and Water's cannister through a face mask or endotracheal tube. When significant respiratory depression persists more elaborate methods of mechanical ventilation become necessary (p. 213). Antibiotics should be given only if there is good evidence of aspiration or respiratory infection.

Maintenance of circulation. Serious cardiac arrhythmias should be treated by the administration of antiarrhythmic drugs (p. 135), particular attention being paid to the pharmacological actions of the poisoning to guard against adverse interactions with the therapy. The details of the treatment of acute circulatory failure are described on page 143. The foot of the bed should be raised, heat loss prevented and high flow oxygen given. A catheter should be inserted into the bladder of all 'shocked' patients in order to monitor urinary output with a urimeter. Otherwise catheterisation should be avoided unless bladder distension cannot be controlled by intermittent suprapubic manual compression. Cardiac resuscitation may be required (p. 135).

Removal or inactivation of the poison. Patients with gassing must be removed to fresh air as quickly as possible. When a liquid or solid poison capable of cutaneous absorption is in contact with the patient's clothes these must be removed and any poison on the skin washed off. Care should be taken during these procedures to avoid personal contamination. When the poison has been swallowed within the previous hour, conscious patients should be given orally 50–100 g of activated charcoal.

EMESIS; GASTRIC ASPIRATION AND LAVAGE. A decision as to whether emesis or gastric aspiration and lavage should also be undertaken will depend on three factors: (1) the substance ingested, (2) the state of consciousness of the patient, and (3) the length of time since the poison was ingested.

1. *Nature of substance ingested.* The only contra-indication to inducing vomiting or passing a stomach tube is the knowledge that paraffin oil (kerosene) or other petroleum distillates have been swallowed, as the entry of even a small quantity of these substances into the lungs results in a severe pneumonia. Great care must be exercised in passing a stomach tube in corrosive poisoning, in alcoholics, in patients who have had gastric surgery and in the very young and elderly.

2. *Level of consciousness.* Fully conscious patients should be made to vomit by giving syrup of ipecacuanha (30 ml followed by 200 ml of water). The limitation of this emetic is a delay in its onset of action. The dose may be repeated on one further occasion if vomiting does not result after 20 minutes. Emesis is the treatment of choice in young children as, apart from the trauma involved, a sufficiently large tube cannot be passed to achieve effective removal of gastric contents.

In a semiconscious patient, emetics are to be avoided in view of the danger of aspiration pneumonia, but gastric aspiration and lavage can be employed provided the cough reflex is still present. In the deeply unconscious patient, gastric lavage is particularly important, but, as the cough reflex may be absent, it is a highly dangerous procedure unless the lungs can be first protected by the insertion of a cuffed endotracheal tube.

3. *Time since ingestion.* If 4 hours have passed since ingestion very little or no recovery of the poison will be achieved by inducing vomiting or by gastric lavage. In salicylate poisoning these procedures are of value up to 24 hours after the poison has been taken. In the case of tricyclic drugs a worthwhile recovery may be achieved up to 12 hours after ingestion.

Technique of gastric aspiration and lavage. With the foot of the trolley raised about 0.5 m and the patient lying on the left side a wide-bore Jacques stomach tube, English gauge 30, should be passed. Rubber tubes are most suitable for routine use, but if there is any suspicion that the patient may have hepatitis, not uncommon in drug addicts, disposable plastic tubes should be used and appropriate precautions taken by staff. A gag may be necessary to prevent biting on the tube. After insertion the position of the tube in the stomach is verified by aspiration of stomach contents or by blowing a little air through it and auscultating over the abdomen when a bubbling sound will be heard.

Aspiration is best achieved by lowering the funnel to which the stomach tube is attached, to a level well below the patient's head. Aspiration is advisable prior to lavage as initial lavage will drive some of the stomach contents into the duodenum and promote absorption. When no further material can be aspirated, repeated careful lavage with tepid water should be undertaken, using the same apparatus and no more than 300 ml for each single washout. Lavage should be continued until the returning fluid is clear. Except in the specific instances given on pages 706–711 little is achieved by employing lavage fluid other than water.

On occasions, after lavage, some further impairment of consciousness may occur. In general, therefore, the stomach should be left as empty as possible in view of the dangers of subsequent aspiration pneumonia, especially if an endotracheal tube has not been inserted.

OTHER METHODS OF ELIMINATION OF POISONS. If considerable absorption has occurred the patient may be gravely ill; hence measures to enhance elimination of the poison may be required. These can be carried out only in hospital because of the technical skill and special apparatus required; they include forced diuresis (p. 709), peritoneal dialysis, haemodialysis and haemoperfusion.

Haemoperfusion. Attempts have been made to develop safer ways of increasing removal of toxic substances from the body. The most effective of these is haemoperfusion whereby heparinised blood from the patient is passed through a column containing charcoal coated with synthetic acrylic hydrogel or alternatively ion-exchange resins. These methods may be life-saving for some severe poisonings, such as those due to medium and short-acting barbiturates, glutethimide, methaqualone and meprobamate for which previous techniques of elimination were inadequate. Haemoperfusion, however, is still not free from risk and therefore is indicated only in seriously ill patients in whom intensive supportive therapy fails.

ANTIDOTES. It is widely but erroneously believed that for each toxic substance there is a specific antidote. There are, in fact, no antidotes for the majority of substances producing poisoning. Certain pharmacological antagonists are, however, of value, and can be life-saving. Examples are naloxone (opiate poisoning), cobalt edetate (cyanide poisoning), desferrioxamine (iron poisoning) and n-acetylcysteine (paracetamol poisoning). Details of the use of these are given on pages 706–711.

Other therapy. *Hypothermia.* A rectal thermometer which records low temperatures is required for the accurate assessment of hypothermia. Since it reduces the oxygen demands of the tissues, a moderate degree of hypothermia is not a deleterious feature provided the patient is nursed in a space blanket and in a warm moist environment. If, however, the rectal temperature is below 35°C, it may cause hypotension, sludging of the blood, confusion, coma and cardiac arrest.

The patient with hypothermia below 35°C should be rewarmed rapidly by external methods (e.g. immersion of one forearm in water at 43°C) and oxygen given. If there is hypotension or increased peripheral vasoconstriction, warm fluids are administered intravenously. Metabolic acidosis is controlled by sodium bicarbonate (p. 95).

Epileptiform convulsions should be treated with diazepam (p. 620).

· *Fluid and electrolytes* require careful monitoring and appropriate replacement therapy as necessary.

Psychiatric assessment. As most instances of poisoning in adults are deliberate acts of self-poisoning it is very important that all patients, whether suffering from apparent accidental or intentional poisoning, should have a psychiatric assessment. Self-poisoning is often an important feature of various psychiatric disorders and of depression in particular. It is greatly to the benefit of the patient if the initial psychiatric interview takes place as soon as possible after the act before the patient and the relatives have time to discuss the event and thereafter present the same rationalised and often false picture. The incidence of repeated acts of self-poisoning has been shown clearly to be reduced by early psychiatric consultation.

Notes on clinical features and treatment of poisoning and envenomation by specific agents *(including common insect stings and poisoning by marine animals, mushrooms, scorpions, snakes, spiders, ticks and vegetables)*

The following descriptions are directed primarily towards adults. For children, appropriate adjustments in doses of drugs suggested in treatment regimens would require to be made.

Amphetamine group. *Clinical features.* Alertness, excitement, tremor and insomnia are common. Confusion, aggressiveness, hallucinations and even homicidal tendencies may occur. Initial excitement may give way to lethargy and depression. Brisk reflexes, tachycardia and hypertension occur and nausea, vomiting, diarrhoea and abdominal colic may be severe. In very heavy overdosage convulsions and deep unconsciousness are characteristic.

Treatment (1) General measures. (2) Droperidol (5–15 mg) or haloperidol (5–10 mg) by slow intravenous injection are the recommended treatments. Alternatively, chlorpromazine 100 mg intramuscularly. (3) In severe poisoning, forced diuresis using intravenous ammonium chloride to make the urine acid.

Barbiturates. *Clinical features.* Absorption is unpredictable but drowsiness and coma develop rapidly. The duration of cerebral depression varies greatly with the type of barbiturate taken, the dose and the tolerance of the patient. In general a large dose of short- or medium-acting barbiturate causes more severe poisoning than long-acting phenobarbitone. Changes in the pupils and limb reflexes are very variable and are unreliable guides to the severity of the poisoning. Withdrawal features such as restlessness, insomnia, delirium and convulsions may occur. Ventilatory depression and hypotension may be severe. Hypothermia is common and if severe may be associated with renal failure. Bullous lesions occur in 6% of patients with acute barbiturate overdosage especially with short- or medium-acting drugs.

Treatment. (1) General measures with particular emphasis on respiratory and cardiovascular support. (2) When these measures fail, haemodialysis for phenobarbitone and barbitone, and charcoal haemoperfusion for short- and medium-acting barbiturates.

Benzodiazepines. *Clinical features.* Drowsiness, ataxia, dizziness, hypotension and ventilatory depression may all occur, but the toxic effects are usually surprisingly mild.

Treatment. General supportive treatment is adequate in almost all cases.

Beta-adrenoceptor antagonists. *Clinical features.* Bradycardia and hypotension with low output cardiac failure. Bronchospasm. Cardio-respiratory arrest may occur. Drowsiness, delirium, fits and hallucinations. Hypoglycaemia.

Treatment. (1) Gastric aspiration and lavage if appropriate and intensive supportive measures. (2) When bradycardia is severe, atropine 0.6 to 3 mg intravenously (50 µg/kg in children), followed if necessary by isoprenaline 2 mg diluted in 500 ml normal saline or 5% dextrose at a rate of 20 to 40 drops per minute depending on the response. A cardiac pacemaker should be inserted. (3) If significant hypotension occurs, the inotropic action of glucagon is beneficial—50 to 150 µg/kg intravenously over 1 minute, followed by an infusion of 1 to 5 mg/h. In severe cases dobutamine infusion 2.5 to 20 µg/kg/min may be effective. (4) For bronchospasm, salbutamol by nebuliser. Intravenous salbutamol or aminophylline may be required. (5) Intravenous glucose for hypoglycaemia.

Corrosives. *Clinical features.* Stains and burns of the mouth, lips and fauces. Abdominal pain, shock and hepatic or renal damage.

Treatment. (1) General measures. (2) Gastric lavage is contraindicated in severe poisoning. (3) Neutralise acid or alkali. Milk by mouth is often the most effective available treatment. (4) Analgesics, blood transfusion and correction of acid-base balance all may be required.

Cyanides and hydrocyanic acid. *Clinical features.* Odour of bitter almonds with shallow breathing; pink colour of skin and mucosae; widely dilated pupils and shock.

Treatment. This is very urgent. (1) General measures. (2) Cobalt edetate 600 mg in 20 ml intravenously over 1 minute. (3) If no recovery in the next minute, repeat 300 mg cobalt edetate. (4) If ingested, gastric lavage with 50% sodium thiosulphate. (5) Correct acidosis with i.v. sodium bicarbonate.

Dextropropoxyphene. See opium alkaloids.

Digoxin. (p. 138).

Dinitro-ortho-cresol weedkillers. *Clinical features.* These may develop very rapidly. Yellow skin and burns of the lips and mouth. Anxiety, restlessness, fatigue, convulsions and coma. Tachypnoea, pulmonary oedema, hyperpyrexia and intense sweating are common. Acute renal and liver failure may result.

Treatment. (1) Wash exposed skin. (2) Sedation with chlorpromazine 100 mg intramuscularly. (3) General measures. (4) Tepid sponging to reduce temperature.

Domestic bleach. *Clinical features.* Local irritation if in contact with skin. If inhaled, cough and possible pulmonary oedema. If ingested, burning sensation of mouth and fauces, nausea and vomiting.

Treatment. (1) Gastric lavage with 2.5% sodium thiosulphate or alternatively with milk. If severely ill sodium thiosulphate (1%) 250 ml intravenously.

Ethanol. See page 696; blood levels page 814.

Fish and other marine animals. Poisonous fish are numerous and widely distributed around the world. In some areas they are a common source of poisoning.

CIGUATERA POISONING. This is common, particularly in the Indo-Pacific and the Caribbean. It occurs sporadically after eating reef-dwelling fishes, which are popular items of diet. It is impossible to identify fish which are poisonous from others which are not and the toxins responsible are unaffected by all forms of preparation and cooking. Ciguatoxin is the cause of poisoning and the primary source is thought to be an alga (*Gambierdiscus toxicus*) eaten by herbivorous fish such as parrot fish and surgeon fish. Ultimately carnivorous fish such as barracuda also become poisonous.

Clinical features. The onset of symptoms is usually 1–6 hours after eating toxic fish, but may vary from a few minutes to 30 hours. Numbness and paraesthesiae of the lips, tongue and throat are common, followed by abdominal pain, diarrhoea, headache, arthralgia and myalgia. In 20% of patients, dyspnoea, hypotension and paresis occur.

Treatment. Principally symptomatic with bed-rest and analgesics. Most patients recover after about 3 days, but sometimes arthralgia and myalgia may be prolonged.

SCROMBOID FISH POISONING. The flesh of scromboid fish, such as mackerel, tuna, bonito and skipjack, has a high free histidine content. Many bacteria decarboxylate histidine to histamine and, if fish become contaminated by these organisms, large amounts of histamine accumulate in the flesh.

Clinical features. Flushing, headache, dizziness, abdominal cramps and symptoms of gastroenteritis occur. These usually develop 30 minutes after ingestion and the upset lasts for about 4 hours.

Treatment. Symptomatic.

SHELLFISH POISONING. Paralytic shellfish poisoning results from eating filter-feeding shellfish such as mussels, clams, oysters and scallops contaminated by the toxic protozoa, *Gonyaulax catanella* and *G. tamarensis*. The neurotoxin involved is called saxitoxin. These protozoa tend to colour the sea when present in numbers and fishing communities are well aware that it is dangerous to eat molluscs when the tide is red, blue or green. Food poisoning due to infected shellfish is described on page 751.

Clinical features. Circumoral paraesthesiae, a 'floating' feeling, headache, nausea, vomiting and diarrhoea are common with, in severe cases, weakness, dysarthria and respiratory depression.

Treatment. (1) Gastric aspiration and lavage. (2) Symptomatic and supportive therapy. A less severe, but similar, poisoning results from eating shellfish contaminated by another dinoflagellate, *Gymnodinium breve*. The resultant illness is self-limiting, requiring only symptomatic treatment.

TETRODOTOXIC POISONING. This is generally known as 'puffer fish poisoning'. These fish are found in all warm and tropical seas. In Japan the detoxicated puffer fish ('fugu') is a popular delicacy. The mortality is as high as 50% because tetrodotoxin is one of the most powerful neurotoxins known.

Clinical features. Early symptoms are circumoral paraesthesiae, malaise, hypotension, dizziness and a feeling of 'floating in air'. In severe poisoning, ataxia, dysphagia and profound descending neuromuscular paralysis develop.

Treatment is symptomatic as there is no known antidote.

VENOMOUS MARINE ANIMALS. Serious illness from venomous marine creatures is rare in temperate waters. Poisoning by sea snakes is described under snake bites.

VENOMOUS FISH. Although many species occur, only two major groups are of real significance, the sting-rays and scorpion fishes. All sting-rays inhabit warm or tropical coastal waters with the exception of one fresh water variety in South America. These fish will sting only if stood upon by mistake. Scorpion fish include the zebra fishes, the true scorpion fishes and the stone fishes. The spines of these fish are their offensive weapons and they are all capable of aggressive stinging. The stone fishes are particularly poisonous and zebra fishes are becoming popular for domestic aquaria.

Clinical features. Immediate intense pain and swelling at the site of the sting. Severe tissue necrosis may occur and systemic features include nausea, vomiting and diarrhoea. Cardiac arrhythmias may occur.

Treatment. (1) Analgesics and local anaesthesia if pain severe. (2) Careful cleansing of the wound and surgical removal of the sting sheath if it has been retained. (3) The venoms are heat- labile and if possible the wound should be immersed in water as hot as can be borne for 1 hour. (4) In the case of stone fish antivenoms are available.

VENOMOUS MOLLUSCS. Only two members of this very large species are venomous to man. These are the cone shells and the octopuses. The cone shells are not uncommon causes of poisoning as the colourful shells are eagerly collected. These predatory gastropods catch their prey by shooting out a dart-like tooth attached to a muscular venom gland. The only octopuses of importance are the small blue ringed octopuses of Australia which have toxic saliva and this may flow into wounds made by the beak of the octopus.

Clinical features. There is a local inflammatory response with generalised paraesthesiae. This is rapidly followed by muscular paresis which in severe poisoning may result in respiratory failure. Fatalities have occurred.

Treatment. Symptomatic and supportive therapy.

VENOMOUS COELENTERATA. These include the hydroids, jelly-fish, sea anemones and corals. Although many of these animals may cause painful and at times disfiguring stings, few fatalities have resulted. The most important are the Portuguese man-of-war (*Physalia physalis*), sea wasps (*Cubomedusae*) and the true jellyfishes *Chironex fleckeri* and *Chiropsalmus quadrigatus*. Some authors suggest that only *Chironex* should be considered truly lethal. The precise toxins are not yet fully identified but haemolytic, dermatonecrotic and cardiotoxic substances have all been isolated.

Clinical features. All species cause intense pain at the site of envenomation and large wheals appear which may become necrotic, leading to extensive scar formation. Severe abdominal and generalised pains may result. In severe poisoning the patient rapidly loses consciousness with cyanosis and hypotension. Death may occur quickly or be delayed for some hours.

Treatment. (1) Analgesics and local anaesthesia if pain severe. (2) Any tentacles must be carefully removed with adhesive tape. The bare hand should not be used as the tentacles may still be capable of causing stings for many hours after removal from the water. Vinegar can be used to inactivate adhering tentacles, but alcohol solutions should not be used as this may stimulate further stinging. (3) Antivenom for sea-wasp stings is available.

At certain seasons 'Irukandji stings' affect bathers in the sea off N.E. Australia. They are caused by minute *Carybdeid* (simple sea-wasps). Acute poisoning develops in a few minutes characterised by violent abdominal and generalised pains, vomiting and prostration. After a few days of acute illness, full recovery always occurs.

Insect stings. Stings from ants, wasps, hornets and bees usually result only in local pain and swelling, unless the sting is on the mouth or tongue when local oedema may cause respiratory distress. Occasionally deaths may result from very extensive stings or more commonly due to severe anaphylaxis in individuals previously sensitised particularly to bee stings.

Clinical features. (1) Local pain and oedema. (2) Severe cases may become shocked; local tissue necrosis, acute haemolysis and acute nephritis may occur.

Treatment. Bee stings are acid and wasp, hornet and ant stings are alkaline. Local application is soothing, e.g. bicarbonate for bee, vinegar for wasp; systemic antihistamines may be helpful. The barbed bee stings should be removed as soon as possible as the gland attached continues to release venom. In severe sensitivity reactions, subcutaneous adrenaline (0.5 ml) and hydrocortisone (100 mg) intravenously may be life-saving. Allergic patients should carry adrenaline for immediate self-injection. In some, desensitisation has proved helpful.

See also scorpion, spider and tick.

Iron salts. *Clinical features.* These are more severe in children but this poisoning is potentially dangerous at all ages. It occurs in three stages. The predominant initial features are epigastric pain, nausea and vomiting. Haematemesis is frequent and may cause shock. Respiration and pulse are rapid. These symptoms may settle after a few hours and there may then be a quiescent period lasting for up to several days, suggesting that all is well, but then frequent black and offensive stools may be passed, followed by acute encephalopathy and circulatory failure. Most deaths occur in this second stage, but even if the patient survives, acute liver and renal failure may develop later and both carry a high mortality.

Treatment. Speed is essential. (1) An intramuscular injection of 2 g desferrioxamine is given immediately (1g in a child). (2) Gastric lavage is performed following which 100 ml 5% sodium bicarbonate is left in the stomach. (3) This is followed by an intravenous infusion of desferrioxamine in saine, dextrose or blood. The amount should not exceed 15 mg/kg body weight/hour up to a maximum of 80 mg/kg in 24 hours. (4) Full supportive treatment for convulsions, shock, acidosis, blood loss and electrolyte disturbance.

Mushrooms. Serious poisoning is uncommon in Britain. Considering the many types of fungi, a relatively small number are poisonous. The difficulty is that identification of these harmful species is not easy and often dangerous mushrooms grow in the same places as edible varieties. The commonest types of mushroom poisoning result from eating species containing heat-labile toxins, many of which have not been identified. These cause acute and sometimes severe abdominal colic with diarrhoea, nausea and vomiting developing about two hours after ingestion. Occasionally the features are those of muscarine toxicity with parasympathetic stimulation which can be counteracted with atropine 0.6–2.0 mg in the adult. If the patient is excited or disorientated, atropine should not be given and chlorpromazine prescribed instead. The Common Ink Cap (*Coprinus atramentarius*) contains coprine which has a disulfiram-like action and, if taken with alcohol, provokes acute vomiting.

A trend amongst adolescents has been to ingest 'Magic' mushrooms (*Psilocybe semilanceate*) and *Panaeolus foenisecii* containing psilocybin and psilocin, which are hallucinogens. The amount required to obtain a 'trip' varies greatly from individual to individual and so some develop acute toxic effects. Acute gastroenteritis may result with visual hallucinations lasting up to 6 hours. Occasionally the symptoms last for several days and acute psychiatric upset has been reported continuing for weeks.

DEATH CAP (AMANITA PHALLOIDES). This mushroom accounts for 90% of all deaths due to mushroom poisoning in Britain. It contains two types of toxin; phallotoxins, which cause severe gastroenteritis within 6–12 hours of ingestion, and amatoxins, which also may cause gastric upset, but the major effect is delayed and results in liver and renal tubular damage. These toxins are heat-stable and may survive cooking.

Clinical features. After an initial delay of 6–12 hours and occasionally as long as 24 hours, acute and usually severe gastroenteritis with abdominal colic. The patient may then seem to improve before the onset of liver and renal damage.

Treatment. (1) If possible the mushrooms eaten should be identified, ideally by an expert in mushrooms. It is useful to remember that the later the onset of abdominal symptoms, the more likely it is to be a serious poisoning. (2) Gastric aspiration and lavage. (3) Careful medical care for liver and renal failure if these develop. Haemodialysis and haemoperfusion are ineffective in removing the toxins but the former may be required for renal failure and the latter for liver failure.

Other species of mushroom which produce similar toxic effects to *A. phalloides* are the North American *Deadly Agaric (A. verna), A. virosa* and some types of *Galerina*.

Opium alkaloids (dextropropoxyphene). *Clinical features.* Pinpoint pupils, pallor, nausea and vomiting, depressed respiration and coma are characteristic. These effects are potentiated by alcohol and the combination may cause sudden respiratory and cardiac arrest which may occur even in previously healthy young people.

Treatment. (1) General measures. (2) If ingested gastric lavage with very dilute potassium permanganate — 1 in 10 000. (3) Naloxone 0.4 mg intravenously and 0.8 mg repeated intravenously three minutes later, if required. In heavy overdosage larger quantities may be necessary. The patient should be kept under close observation and naloxone repeated if required.

Nsaids. *See* anthranilic acid derivatives.

Organophosphorus compounds. *Clinical features.* These insecticides are very toxic. Being cholinesterase inhibitors, the symptoms and rationale of treatment are explained by excess cholinergic activity. Clinical features include constricted pupils; cold perspiration; salivation, nausea, vomiting and diarrhoea; twitching, which may go on to convulsions; bradycardia; bronchospasm, intense bronchorrhoea and pulmonary oedema.

Treatment. (1) Remove contaminated clothing and wash skin, but take care to wear protective gloves. (2) General measures including meticulous care of the airway. (3) Atropine 2 mg intravenously, but if cyanosis is present this must first be corrected by oxygen therapy. The atropine is repeated at 5 to 10 minute intervals to achieve full atropinisation and this is maintained for at least 2–3 days. (4) Pralidoxime should be given in addition to atropine in a dose of 30 mg/kg intravenously at a rate not exceeding 500 mg per minute and repeated every 30 minutes as necessary. More recently obidoxime 3 mg/kg body weight by intramuscular injection has been reported to be more effective than pralidoxime as it has a faster action and crosses the blood-brain barrier. When these cholinesterase reactivators take effect the dosage of atropine should be reduced to avoid atropine toxicity.

Paracetamol (acetaminophen). *Clinical features.* Nausea and vomiting initially, but at first symptoms are often non-specific. After 36 hours in severe poisoning (plasma paracetamol levels above 200 μg/ml at 4 hours after ingestion) more serious toxic effects may develop including hypotension, hypothermia, metabolic acidosis, hypoglycaemia, bleeding tendency and delirium. The main danger, however, is acute liver failure which tends to occur several days after ingestion and carries a high mortality.

Treatment. (1) General measures. (2) In moderate or severe poisoning (likely over 20 × 500 mg tablets) the liver damage may be prevented provided the following treatment is given within 12 hours of the poisoning. An initial dose of n-acetylcysteine 150 mg/kg in 200 ml 5% glucose is given intravenously over 15 minutes, followed by an infusion of 50 mg/kg in 500 ml 5% glucose in 4, 8 and 8 hours (total 300 mg/kg in 20 hours). (3) Intravenous glucose may be required to correct hypoglycaemia. (4) The best investigation to assess impending acute liver failure is the prothrombin time ratio. If this rises above 3.0 full medical prophylaxis to combat hepatic encephalopathy must be started. (5) Charcoal haemoperfusion for fulminant liver failure. (6) Haemodialysis for acute renal failure.

Paraffin and petroleum distillates. *Clinical features.* Pallor; vomiting and diarrhoea; cough and dyspnoea.

Treatment. (1) Do not wash out stomach (p. 705). (2) Antibiotics if aspiration has occurred. (3) General measures.

Salicylates. *Clinical features.* Young children are much more susceptible to the toxic effects of salicylates than adults, particularly to the complex and altering metabolic disturbances which occur. Coma is common in children, in contrast to adults in whom coma is seen only in very severe poisoning. In adults, plasma salicylate levels above 3.6 mmol/l (50 mg/100 ml) indicate moderate or severe poisoning. In this situation, characteristic features are tinnitus, deafness and blurring of vision. Restlessness, sweating and increased metabolic rate also occur. Hyperventilation results in respiratory alkalosis. There may be vomiting and this, together with hyperventilation and profuse sweating, often results in severe dehydration. Hypokalaemia is common. The initial respiratory alkalosis is frequently followed by a metabolic acidosis, which may be severe, especially in children. Despite these formidable fluid, electrolyte and acid-base disturbances the patients may seem less ill than they really are. Marked acidosis should be regarded as a very serious feature as it may herald sudden respiratory or cardiac arrest.

Treatment. (1) General measures, but gastric aspiration and lavage should be done in all patients when practicable. (2) In moderate or severe poisoning *forced alkaline diuresis* should be given. The following should be mixed together and given intravenously at a rate of 2 litres hourly for 3 hours:

Saline (0.9%)	0.5 litre
Glucose (5%)	1 litre
Sodium bicarbonate (1.26%)	0.5 litre
Potassium chloride	3 g

If this regimen of diuresis cannot be given because of renal or cardiac impairment, peritoneal dialysis or haemodialysis are effective. Careful monitoring of fluid replacement, electrolyte and acid-base status must be carried out during this treatment.

Scorpion stings. Many genera of scorpions are found in the tropics and subtropics. Stings can cause dangerous poisoning. In Mexico, for example, 1000 deaths occur per year. Paired poison glands are situated in the terminal segment of the jointed tail.

Clinical features. (1) Intense local pain occurs immediately around the single puncture site, followed by erythema, swelling and sometimes ecchymosis. (2) Severe systemic features may follow, especially in children, such as sweating, salivation, nausea, vomiting and respiratory depression. Disseminated intravascular coagulation may occur, and in Trinidad, acute but usually reversible pancreatitis is a feature of stings from the scorpion, *Tityus trinitatis*.

Treatment. (1) A firm pressure bandage should be applied to limit the spread of the neurotoxic venom. (2) Analgesics and general supportive therapy. (3) In children, antivenom (5 ml i.m.) should be given if available. (4) Specific treatment of disseminated intravascular coagulation, if present.

Snake bite. In Britain there is only one indigenous poisonous snake, the adder (*Vipera berus*) which seldom causes significant poisoning. Serious snake bites may still occur as dangerous snakes are kept in zoos and by amateurs, often in less than ideal circumstances. There are three families of medically important venomous snakes. All have fangs at the front of their mouths whereby they inject venom from the parotid glands. The *Elapidae* (cobras, mambas, kraits, tiger snakes, and coral snakes) are found in all parts of the world except Europe. They have short fangs and are land snakes, the venom of which produce neurotoxic features. Local tissue necrosis may occur, a feature characteristic of venom of Asian cobras and the African spitting cobra. The *Hydrophidae* (sea snakes), which abound in the Asian-Pacific coastal waters, also have short fangs and characteristic flattened tails. The venom of these snakes is myotoxic. The *Viperidae*, which have long erectile fangs, are divided into *Viperinae* (true vipers) such as the European adder, Russell's viper and Carpet viper. These occur in all parts of the world except America and the Asian-Pacific area. The second sub-group is the *Crotalidae* (pit vipers) such as rattlesnakes, Fer-de-lance and Malayan pit viper which have a small heat-sensitive pit between eye and nostrils. The venom of the *Viperidae* is vasculo-toxic.

At least 50% of people bitten by snakes suffer few or no toxic effects as little or no venom has been injected. By contrast, if the dose of venom is high mortality without effective treatment is 10% in *Elapidae* poisoning within 5 to 20 hours of the bites, 10% for sea snakes within 15 hours and 1 to 15% in *Viperidae* within 2 days. In the early stages snake bite is very unpredictable and all patients must be carefully monitored for at least 12 hours.

First aid measures. Firm pressure bandaging of the bite area and immobilisation of the part substantially delays spread of the venom. Patients are often very apprehensive and should be reassured and sedated if necessary.

Clinical features. Local pain and fang marks are very variable and of no help in diagnosis.

Viperidae. Local swelling starts almost immediately. This is also a feature of poisoning in bites by Asian cobras and the African spitting cobra, but may not develop for up to 2 hours. Early signs of systemic poisoning, which may develop within 15 minutes of the bite include vomiting, hypotension and signs of abnormal bleeding from or into any site. Later signs include increase in local swelling which may become massive over 48 to 72 hours with associated bruising. Blister formation around the site of the bite is common and spreading blisters suggest a large dose of venom and may precede necrosis. Local tissue necrosis with an offensive putrid smell is typical of cobra bites. Shock may occur and haemorrhage into a vital organ which is often fatal may occur up to a week after the bite if antivenom has not been given.

Elapidae. There is seldom any local swelling. Vomiting, hypotension and a polymorph leucocytosis suggest systemic envenomation. More specific signs of muscle weakness such as ptosis, glossopharyngeal palsy and cough indicate severe poison-ing and may be delayed for 10 hours after the bite. There is a danger of respiratory paralysis and ECG changes and rises in cardiac enzymes occur.

Hydrophidae. The early features are similar to *Elapidae*.

More specific signs are generalised myalgia, with the appearance of myoglobinuria 3 to 5 hours later. Paresis of the limbs may follow with respiratory paralysis within a few hours of the bite, although it may be delayed for up to 60 hours. Hyperkalaemia may result in cardiac arrest and acute renal failure may occur.

Treatment. (1) The site of the bite should be cleansed and then left strictly alone; otherwise the risk of infection is increased. If skin necrosis occurs, sloughs should be excised with skin grafts applied as appropriate. (2) General measures, including intravenous fluids, should be given to support vital functions. (3) Sedatives are required if the patient is apprehensive. (4) Appropriate antitetanus prophylaxis should be given taking account of the patient's immune state. (5) Antivenoms should be given only if there is clear evidence of systemic poisoning. Some local effects, however, especially necrosis, may be avoided or minimised if antivenom is given within 4 hours of the bite. This is the case in bites by Asian cobras, African spitting cobras, puff adders and rattlesnakes. In *V. berus* bites, the only poisonous snake in Britain, adult patients may have prolonged and painful local swelling which can be effectively treated by Zagreb antivenom if given within the first few hours. All antivenoms may cause severe allergic reactions which may be fatal. Appropriate precautions, therefore, are mandatory. The potency of the antivenom should be checked by first making sure that it is clear and has no opacities. Depending on the severity of poisoning, 20–100 ml antivenom is diluted in 2 to 3 volumes of isotonic saline. This is then given by slow intravenous infusion (15 drops per minute). Adrenaline (1:1000 solution) must be immediately available. If a reaction occurs the drip is stopped temporarily and 0.5 ml adrenaline injected intramuscularly. Provided the adrenaline is given at the first sign of anaphylaxis, it is rapidly effective and the drip can be restarted with care. Several injections of adrenaline may be indicated. There is marked variation in the requirements of different patients for antivenom. Therefore it is important to give sufficient antivenom to counteract the toxic effects of the poisoning and children require the same doses of antivenom as adults. This is especially important in neurotoxic poisoning.

Spider bite. Only a few genera of spiders are harmful to man. *Lactrodectus* species are found only in warm climates. The Black Widow Spider (*L. mactans*) is the most dangerous and occurs only in the tropics. The Funnel Web Spider (*Atrax Robustus*) also quite often causes venomous bites. These spiders are shy, inhabiting dark corners of sheds, basements and foundations of houses and outside privies. Death may occur in up to 6% of cases, especially in young children.

Clinical features. (1) Burning of the bite site. (2) After about 1 hour, generalised muscular pain, which may simulate an acute abdomen, nausea and vomiting. (3) Pyrexia, sweating and shock.

Treatment. (1) 10–20 ml calcium gluconate (10%) by slow intravenous injection. (2) Analgesics. (3) If severe systemic toxicity give specific antivenom if available.

In the South States of America, Central and South America, the Brown Recluse Spider (*Loxosceles reclusa*) and related species may be found in houses and outbuildings. The spider often crawls into clothing and bed-clothes. Poisoning is relatively uncommon but important as it results in necrosis at the site of the bite, which is slow to heal. Fever, vomiting and rashes may occur and occasionally haemolysis and thrombocytopenia. Analgesics should be given as required and antihistamines and corticosteroids are considered helpful.

Theophylline. *Clinical features.* Nausea, vomiting, abdominal discomfort, diarrhoea, thirst, polyuria and agitation are common. The development of cardiac arrhythmias, hypotension and convulsions indicate severe poisoning with a poor prognosis, especially in elderly patients.

Treatment. (1) General supportive measures. (2) Gastric aspiration and lavage. (3) Intravenous diazepam (5–10 mg) to control convulsions. (4) Charcoal haemoperfusion if severe poisoning (plasma level > 60 m g/1).

Tick bite. Tick paralysis is due to venom in the saliva of certain hard ticks. If such a tick remains attached to the skin for some days there is increasing and spreading paralysis with a danger of respiratory failure and mechanical ventilation may be required. If the tick is removed in time the patient recovers.

Tricyclic antidepressants. *Clinical features.* These features appear 1 to 2 hours after ingestion, but seldom last longer than 18–24 hours. Dry mouth, dilated pupils, urinary retention and absent bowel sounds are common. Varying degrees of loss of consciousness result but deep coma is not common. Hallucinations and loquacity occur. Cardiac arrhythmias may be severe, especially in children, and hypotension may result. Torticollis and ataxia may be pronounced in children, but at all ages brisk reflexes are common and tonic-clonic movements occur. Ventilatory depression, on occasions, is severe.

Treatment. (1) General measures. (2) Gastric lavage is effective up to 12 hours after ingestion. (3) Supportive therapy is all that is required in the great majority of patients but, if inadequate, physostigmine salicylate (1–3 mg) by slow intravenous injection will abolish the central nervous system effects and some of the cardiac complications. If necessary, the injection may be repeated after 10 minutes. (4) Cardiac arrhythmias may respond to 40 mEq sodium bicarbonate by rapid intravenous infusion over 20 minutes. If this is ineffective, appropriate antiarrhythmics should be given.

Vegetable toxins. The harmful effects of the ingestion of aflatoxin (p. 720), cassava (p. 657) and bush teas (p. 361) are mentioned elsewhere.

EPIDEMIC DROPSY (ARGEMONE POISONING). This is seen mainly in India and in Indian communities elsewhere when curried dishes are prepared with mustard oil contaminated by extracts from the seeds of the poppy weed, *Argemone mexicana*, which contain the toxin, sanguinarine. This substance interferes with the oxidation of pyruvic acid, which accumulates and causes dilatation of capillaries and small arterioles. Haemangiomas may develop.

Clinical features. Nausea, vomiting, diarrhoea and fever occur followed by the development of peripheral oedema and cardiac failure. There is erythematous mottling of the skin and raised haemangiomas may appear. Severe glaucoma may result.

Treatment. All contaminated mustard oil must be identified and further exposure avoided. Supportive therapy for cardiac failure is effective, but the response may be slow.

VOMITING SICKNESS OF JAMAICA (ACKEE POISONING). The unripe fruit of the common West Indian and South American tree, *Blighia sapida*, contains a water-soluble toxin, capable of blocking gluconeogenesis in the liver. If eaten, especially by undernourished children, severe and prolonged hypoglycaemia may result. Vomiting, loss of consciousness and convulsions are common. Continuous intravenous infusion of glucose should be started as soon as possible. Without treatment the mortality is high.

Industrial and agricultural poisoning

Lead, cyanide (p. 707), mercury, beryllium (p. 258) and cadmium are potential causes of industrial poisoning. In agriculture many highly toxic weedkillers, including paraquat and the dinitro-ortho-cresol group, and organophosphorus insecticides have been developed in recent years. They have been responsible for only a small number of cases of acute poisoning in Britain owing to effective legislation for controlling their use. In some countries, however, they have caused many deaths.

PREVENTION OF ACUTE POISONING

An indication of the size and complexity of the problem has been given in the introduction to this chapter. Thus, in Britain, acute poisoning now accounts for approximately 15% of all acute medical admissions to hospital. The scope for preventive action is clear.

About 60% of patients consult their doctors in the month prior to taking the overdosage and many do so within a week of their action. Also a considerable number poison themselves again after discharge from hospital or during active treatment for psychiatric conditions such as depression. There can be no doubt, therefore, that doctors can make a very important contribution to the prevention of poisoning by learning to recognise the danger signs of imminent overdosage and take appropriate preventive action. General practitioners are particularly well placed for this purpose as not only can they assess the personality concerned, but also the social and family circumstances which are often the main cause of the problem. For example, it has become apparent that some poisoning incidents in young children occur as an expression of abuse by their parents. Improvements are required in the social services in order that their response to such difficulties should be more immediate and effective; but even now doctors should make more use of agencies such as the Marriage Guidance Council, Alcoholics Anonymous and the Samaritans.

At all ages a major predisposing factor is the ready availability of medicaments and toxic household products. In the prevention of poisoning in children, the best method is to keep all medicines in a locked cupboard. Poisoning by household preparations is also common in children under the age of 5 years and is likely to continue as long as these articles are stored in places accessible to inquisitive toddlers. A potentially very dangerous practice is the storage of toxic chemicals such as weedkillers in old lemonade or beer bottles.

Another important factor in acute poisoning is that many tablets and capsules are supplied in a variety of attractive colours and shapes, often similar to popular sweets and therefore very appealing to children. This danger is increased by parents who, often with the best intentions, encourage their children to take medicines by suggesting that the tablets are in fact sweets. Also, many potent and dangerous drugs are dispensed as pleasant elixirs and syrups with an increased danger of overdosage in the unwitting youngster. An effective preventive measure has been the development of drug containers which children find difficult to open. An increasing number of drugs are also being supplied in individual wrapping, a useful deterrent for patients inclined to impulsive self-poisoning. These measures may add substantially to the price of production of drugs, but when one considers the cost of hospital and social care, the additional expense is justified on that basis alone.

The major cause of acute poisoning incidents is intentional self-poisoning which, as has been stated, is usually of an impulsive and conscious type. The availability of drugs is particularly relevant in this group. Patients should therefore be constantly encouraged to dispose of unused drugs from previous prescriptions and it follows that doctors should make every effort to prescribe numbers of tablets carefully calculated for the immediate needs of the patients. Also, sedative and psychotropic drugs should be prescribed only when there is a clear and genuine medical indication. In the recent past the numbers of prescriptions in Britain for these types of drugs rose in a most dramatic way and there is no reason to suspect that serious psychiatric illness had undergone any major increase in the same time. This suggests that much prescribing of sedative and antidepressant drugs was inappropriate and

was given often for psycho-social problems rather than significant psychiatric disorder. On the other hand, patients who are significantly depressed must be kept under careful observation when therapy is commenced because the antidepressant may cause partial improvement, but also make these patients capable of taking active measures towards self-destruction.

There have been various attempts in the field of health education with the aid of schools, national press and television to make the general public aware of the need for preventive measures, but these campaigns are often of limited duration and quickly lose their impact. The medical profession as a whole has not played a very direct role in these educational exercises and much more could be done in this regard. In Britain, poison information services answer questions only from members of the medical profession, but experience in other countries suggests that the scope of these services could be widened with benefit to the community. In the United States, for example, poison control centres have provided information and advice direct to the general public and fulfilled a valuable educational role whereby, for example, parents have become more aware of the importance of keeping drugs and household products out of the reach of toddlers. As a result in many parts of the United States, the incidence of childhood poisoning has fallen substantially.

Considering the large number of people involved and the vast range of possible toxic substances used in industry, accidental industrial poisoning is uncommon in Britain. This is largely due to the vigilance and initiative of industrial medical officers and to the effectiveness of legislation which regulates the safe storage, transport and use of potentially toxic substances. Also, many essential processes in industry involving the use of dangerous poisons have been made safer by the introduction of automatic mechanical techniques which avoid exposure of workers to the risk.

Inevitably, the management of patients with acute poisoning rests with the medical profession and the social services, and it is easy to criticise their apparent inability to improve the situation. The basic problem, however, lies within the community. Until a more responsible attitude emerges with a willingness to be more supportive towards the emotional problems of individuals, there seems little doubt that acute self-poisoning will continue to be an expression of a plea for help to correct a situation which for the individual has become intolerable.

A.H. LAWSON

FURTHER READING:

Practical manuals for rapid consultation in an emergency:
Vale J A, Meredith T J (eds) 1981 Poisoning: diagnosis and treatment. MTP Press, Lancaster
Proudfoot A T 1982 Diagnosis and management of acute poisoning. Blackwell Scientific Publications, Oxford
Polson C J, Green M A, Lee M R 1983 Clinical toxicology, 3rd edn. Pitman, London
Haddad L M, Winchester J F 1983 Clinical management of poisoning and drug overdose. Saunders, Philadelphia

Dreisbach R H 1983 Handbook of poisoning, 11th edn. Lange Medical, Los Altos

Specialist sources written primarily for the postgraduate, but suitable for reference by the undergraduate:
Gilman G A, Goodman L S, Gilman A (eds) 1980 The pharmacological basis of therapeutics, 6th edn. Macmillan, New York
Clayton G D, Clayton F E (eds) 1981–82 Patty's Industrial hygiene and toxicology, 3rd edn, vols 2A, 2B & 2C. Toxicology. Wiley, New York
Habermehl G G 1981 Venomous animals and their toxins. Springer Verlag, Berlin
Hayes W J 1982 Pesticides studied in man. Williams and Wilkins, Baltimore
Department of Health and Social Security 1983 Pesticide poisoning. HMSO, London
Cooper M R, Johnson A W 1984 Poisonous plants in Britain and their effects on animals and man. HMSO, London
Frohne D, Pfander H J 1984 A colour atlas of poisonous plants. Wolfe Scientific, London
Sax N L 1984 Dangerous properties of industrial materials, 6th edn. Van Nostrand Reinhold, New York

18

Tropical diseases and climatic disorders

Many factors affect the patterns of disease around the world. Important among them are climate, which helps determine the range of pathogenic microbes in the environment, and wealth which provides the means to avoid and control the microbes through education, development, sanitation and health services. The majority of tropical countries are hot, humid and poor. They cannot feed themselves and have rudimentary health services that cannot educate or protect their exploding populations. Infectious diseases and malnutrition are rife, especially among children. Cosmopolitan diseases, such as measles or diarrhoea may take on special significance, while others like malaria (p. 770) or sleeping sickness (p. 779) are confined to certain areas for climatic reasons. Disease due to infection is the main determinant of childhood mortality, the strength of the working man, the health of the mother and the pattern of systemic disease including neoplasia.

This chapter considers the patterns of disease seen in tropical countries and describes some of them. Diseases due to infection, with particular reference to those encountered in the tropics, are described in Chapter 19. The rapid economic growth of the developed nations and the ubiquity of air travel mean that no country of the world can be considered remote any more, nor its diseases exotic. Rich and poor countries are becoming increasingly interdependent and doctors should be aware of the health problems of countries other than their own. Worldwide travel has also led to a rapid increase in the importation of tropical diseases into temperate countries, by refugees, immigrants, tourists and businessmen. British students should be familiar with these diseases.

PATTERNS OF DISEASE IN TROPICAL AND DEVELOPING COUNTRIES

Patients in the tropics suffer from disorders of all the major systems and psyche, as they do in temperate and developed countries. In tropical countries, however, the aetiological factors may be different, especially in the case of infectious disease which still represents the greatest problem. The genetic constitution of patients in many parts of the world makes them resistant to certain conditions and predisposes them to others. The battle against acute disease is often a single episode in a long campaign against chronic infection and malnutrition. Clinical patterns of illness in the tropics, therefore, differ in many ways from those in temperate zones. Although the principles of diagnosis and treatment will be the same, multiple pathologies and diagnoses are the rule rather than the exception and treatment may need to be modified in the light of the background factors. The preponderance of children in the tropics and the high incidence of diarrhoeal and parasitic disease and malnutrition create special problems.

THE BACKGROUND TO DISEASES IN THE TROPICS

Climate. A large number and variety of microbial agents and parasites flourish in the moist heat of the tropics and subtropics. Insects and other arthropods abound and many of them serve as vectors of infections. Numerous species of animals, especially rodents, live close to man and are reservoirs of disease. Close contact with animals exposes man to a wide range of zoonotic diseases. Venomous animals are relatively common, as are toxic plants and fungi that may contaminate foodstuffs. Desert and mountain people suffer fewer infectious diseases. Heat (p. 722) and altitude (p. 725) impose special physiological demands on the body.

Genes and race. The best example of genetically determined disease is sickle-cell anaemia in which homozygous producers of haemoglobin S become anaemic and often die in infancy. The heterozygous carrier of haemoglobin S, on the other hand, is healthy and enjoys a measure of protection against the severe complications of malaria. Other examples of racially determined responses to disease are seen in leprosy, which is worse in Caucasians and Mongolians than in blacks, and in tuberculosis, Indians having more glandular and intestinal lesions than Europeans.

Nutrition and agriculture. The presence or absence of malnutrition depends on the availability of food, its cost and the correctness of its use and also on infection, especially gastrointestinal. Traditional practices and taboos may limit the use of available food, e.g. the banning of eggs and milk in pregnancy. Malnutrition impairs both the cellular and humoral components of the immune response and predisposes children to infection which further drains the body's nutritional reserves and retards growth. Moderate degrees of undernutrition are much commoner than the gross malnutrition syndromes and may be overlooked.

Dietary toxins are found in some areas and produce conditions such as tropical spinal ataxia from cassava in Africa (p. 657), veno-occlusive liver disease from seneccio alkaloids in Jamaica and elsewhere (p. 361) and hepatoma from aflatoxin in badly stored nuts and cereals (p. 720).

Infections. Acute infectious diseases, especially respiratory infections, measles and gastro-enteritis, still account for the high infant mortality in some parts of the tropics where up to 40% of children die before the age of 5 years. Acute infections may precipitate the syndromes of malnutrition, which may then be complicated by further infection, for example measles leading to kwashiorkor and cancrum oris.

Many of the decimating diseases of the past are now controlled by vaccination (yellow fever), vector control (malaria and sleeping sickness) and general improvement of living standards (plague and relapsing fever), but control is imperfect and the diseases reappear as, for example, malaria in the Indian subcontinent and relapsing fever among refugees. Other epidemic diseases such as cholera in Asia and meningococcal meningitis in Africa remain largely uncontrolled and still kill hundreds of thousands of people annually. Efficient vaccines exist for many diseases, such as yellow fever, poliomyelitis, measles and tetanus, but they have made little impact because of the cost and practical difficulty of administering them.

Chronic infections do serious damage to important organs, such as the liver or kidneys in schistosomiasis, the heart in trypanosomiasis cruzi (Chagas' disease), the lungs, bones and lymph nodes in tuberculosis, the bone marrow reserves of iron in ancylostomiasis and of folate in malaria, the small bowel in strongyloidiasis and the nerves in leprosy. These organs may then fail prematurely if increased demand is imposed on them by work, pregnancy or additional disease. Such infections produce chronic ill-health in millions of children and even more so in adults. Amyloidosis is common. Very often the degree of suffering is not sufficient to take people to hospital, even if one is available, but the ceaseless pruritus and gradually failing vision of onchocerciasis, the persistent diarrhoea of schistosomiasis mansoni and the immobilising cellulitis of the guinea worm are examples of conditions sufficiently debilitating to reduce performance, deepen poverty and lead to malnutrition. These chronic infectious diseases are enormous economic burdens on the nation as well as on the patient and the family.

Epidemiological factors. The distribution, prevalence, incidence and endemicity of a disease, especially if it is infectious, determine its pattern in the community. In many places, especially the urban slums, the lack of a supply of clean water and absence of any hygienic system for disposal of sewage and refuse, ensure the prevalence of infections transmitted orally from faeces. Endemic malaria, poliomyelitis and viral hepatitis affect the indigenous children, who either die or become immune so that adults suffer less from these diseases. Non-immune adults, such as tourists, invading soldiers or refugees are, however, fully susceptible unless specifically protected. Particular requirements of organisms, vectors, hosts or intermediate stages of parasites determine the distribution of disease. Thus rabies is sporadic, meningococcal meningitis is particularly common in the Sudan savanna, cholera is riverine, scrub typhus is rural, Chagas' a poverty disease and hookworm affects the bare-footed where sanitation is non-existent. Cooking and eating habits determine the prevalence of paragonimiasis, clonorchiasis and tapeworm infection.

Immunity and autoimmunity. The natural insusceptibility of animals to some human infection such as smallpox, which has only man for its host, has enabled this disease to be abolished, whereas the eradication of yellow fever is prevented by the susceptibility of monkeys to it. Natural immunity of individuals may possibly explain why some people do not suffer certain infections, but immunity acquired in childhood is a more usual explanation. Leprosy, for example, commonly causes subclinical but immunising infections in children living in an endemic area, so that clinical disease is seen mainly in teenagers and young adults in whom naturally acquired immunity has failed.

Most human infections are terminated or controlled by an efficient immune response. When the response is inefficient the organism multiplies unchecked, causing either death, or chronic disease as in lepromatous leprosy or onchocerciasis. Immunity is usually accompanied by hypersensitivity, which often causes more damage than the organism itself, as in tuberculoid leprosy or hepatosplenic schistosomiasis. Sometimes the immune response seems to be inappropriate, as in the tropical splenomegaly syndrome of chronic malaria, or to be grossly exaggerated, as with the hyperglobulinaemia of trypanosomiasis. In sharp contrast with their prevalence in temperate countries, autoimmune diseases are relatively uncommon in the tropics.

Poverty, politics and progress. The poverty of so many tropical countries is often tragically deepened by the strife that accompanies attempts to progress. Development itself may introduce new health problems. The construction of dams and irrigation canals may create breeding sites for the vectors of malaria, yellow fever, schistosomiasis or onchocerciasis. Penetration into forests uncovered Lassa and Marburg viruses (p. 732) in Africa, and has caused much mutilation from espundia (p. 779) in Brazil. New settlements in the Middle East are plagued by cutaneous leishmaniasis (p. 778).

Variations within the tropics. As well as the gross but general differences between patterns of disease in tropical underdeveloped and temperate developed countries, there are many variations within the tropics. A certain condition may be present in only one climatic belt, continent or even community, but be very important there; examples are loiasis in the West African rain forest and Chagas' disease in South America.

GEOGRAPHICAL INFLUENCES ON DISEASES OF THE MAIN SYSTEMS

Diseases due to infection are considered in Chapter 19; their distribution throughout the world is shown in Figure 18.1.

CARDIOVASCULAR DISEASE

Acclimatisation to a hot, humid environment demands a 20% increase in cardiac output and later an increase in plasma volume. A diseased heart is less able to acclimatise.

Rheumatic heart disease is worldwide, especially where there is overcrowding due to urbanisation and industrialisation. In Mexico, one tenth of all deaths is due to rheumatic heart disease. A restrictive cardiomyopathy (p. 182) due to endomyocardial fibrosis is just as important in children and young adults in parts of East and West Africa, Sri Lanka and Southern India, Brazil and Colombia. In West Africa restrictive cardiomyopathy may be a sequel to the hypereosinophilia of a filarial infection. Cardiomyopathy is due to alcohol in parts of Africa and to thiamine deficiency in parts of S.E. Asia and Southern Africa. In some countries cardiomyopathy is a common cause of heart failure as is anaemia due to hookworms, sickle-cell disease or kwashiorkor.

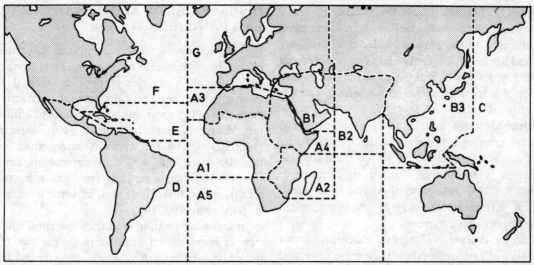

Fig. 18.1 Geographical distribution of disease due to infection. (Based on information supplied by the Ross Institute of Tropical Hygiene, London.)

	Area											
	Africa					Asia and Pacific				America		Europe
Disease	A1	A2	A3	A4	A5	B1	B2	B3	C	D	E	F	G
Malaria	††	††	*	†	*	†	††	††	†	†	*		
Schistosomiasis	†	†	*	††	*	*	1	†		†	*		
Trypanosomiasis 2	†	†		*	*					†			
Leishmaniasis	*	3, †	3, *	†	*	†	†	*		†	†		*
Cholera 4	*	*	*	*		*	††	†			*		
Amoebiasis	†	†	†	†	†	†	††	††	†	††	†	*	*
Typhoid fever	†	†	†	†	*	††	††	††	*	†	†	*	*
Leprosy	††	††	†	††	*	*	††	††	†	†	*	5	5
Onchocerciasis	††	†		†		6, *				6, *			
Lymphatic filariasis	††	††		†			†	††	††	†	*		
Paragonimiasis	*						7, *	††	7, *				
Clonorchiasis								††					

*Endemic.
†Highly endemic.
††Very highly endemic.

1. Small foci in B2, near Bombay and Madras.
2. Sleeping sickness in A, Chagas' disease in D.
3. Visceral in A2, both in other areas.
4. Situation varies with gradual spread of seventh pandemic.
5. Only a few small residual foci in F and G.
6. Yemen only in B1, north of equator in D.
7. Nepal and Sri Lanka in B2, Korea in C.

Infective endocarditis is often secondary to skin sepsis but is no more common than in temperate climates whereas pericarditis is much more frequent and is usually either pyogenic or tuberculosis. Chagas' disease, which accounts for 10% of all necropsies in Brazil, is an outstanding cause of myocarditis; other causes in the tropics are African trypanosomiasis, typhoid

fever, diphtheria, rickettsial infections and acute schistosomiasis.

In some rural tropical communities blood pressure does not increase with age. The 'normal' blood pressure is usually lower than in temperate communities, essential hypertension is rare and pregnancy hypertension less frequent, but in other communities, essential hypertension is becoming common. Atherosclerotic and especially coronary heart disease is virtually unknown in many rural populations, whose plasma cholesterol levels are low and fibrinolytic activity high, but is increasing in affluent groups in cities. Cor pulmonale is also rare in the tropics except where schistosomiasis is highly endemic.

Other forms of arterial disease are rare, but primary arteritis of the aorta, which can affect any of its major branches and of which the Takayasu syndrome is an example, is relatively common in Japan, S.E. Asia and parts of Africa. In East and Central Africa an arteritis of unknown origin causes peripheral gangrene.

With the exception of tropical phlebitis, venous diseases such as haemorrhoids, varicose veins and deep vein thrombosis with its complication of pulmonary embolism are rare in the tropics.

TROPICAL PHLEBITIS of uncertain origin occurs in tropical Africa. Vascular granulation tissue is laid down, especially in the wall of the vein which becomes thrombosed and painful. Splenic vein thrombosis may cause necrotic infarction and liquefaction in the spleen. The patient is usually febrile. The venous lesion gradually resolves and the circulation is re-established. Treatment is symptomatic.

RESPIRATORY DISEASE

Acute respiratory infection is the commonest cause of childhood death all over the world, especially where measles is still prevalent. Most adult respiratory diseases in the tropics are also due to infection. Pneumococcal pneumonia and tuberculosis are commonest, followed by histoplasmosis in parts of South America, paragonimiasis in S.E. Asia, filariasis (pulmonary eosinophilia) in India and the pulmonary complications of hepatic amoebiasis and schistosomiasis. Chronic bronchitis is rare in most rural areas, although common in North and Central India and parts of New Guinea where it is attributed to woodsmoke in huts. In countries that are starting to become industrialised, diseases such as silicosis and byssinosis are appearing.

DISEASE OF THE ALIMENTARY TRACT AND PANCREAS

Diarrhoea is the second commonest cause of death in childhood the world over and the most frequent in infancy in countries of poor hygiene if the mother is not breast feeding. In adults, infectious diseases are the most important causes of alimentary disorders, especially acute gastro-enteritis, giardiasis (p. 776), typhoid and other salmonelloses (p. 750), ileocaecal tuberculosis, amoebic and bacillary dysentery (p. 753), schistosomiasis mansoni (p. 784) and, in some countries, tropical sprue (p. 719).

In many developing countries the rural diet is rich in hand-milled grain fibre (bran) which is not only nutritious in vitamins, protein and iron and helps protect against deficiency diseases such as beriberi, but also makes a bulky soft stool which is passed two or three times daily. This bowel habit is associated with a virtual absence of appendicitis and diverticular disease. Other diseases which are rare in the tropics include Crohn's disease and ulcerative colitis. Cholecystitis is infrequent except as a complication from biliary flukes (p. 786). The prevalence of peptic ulcers varies greatly between different regions; when it is high, gastric outlet obstruction is common. In certain parts of the tropics calcifying pancreatitis is common in children and young adults and may be related to protein deficiency associated with a highly alkaline vegetarian diet. In others it may be associated with alcohol.

Acute gastroenteritis

Ten million people die each year from acute gastroenteritis, especially infants and children in the tropics. Many infectious agents may be responsible, including rotavirus, coronavirus, other enteroviruses, enterotoxogenic *Escherichia coli*, *Salmonella* and *Giardia lamblia*. Attacks are often associated with bottle, as opposed to breast, feeding, and with weaning. Most attacks are self limiting within a few days, but if diarrhoea and vomiting are severe and treatment is not available, death may follow dehydration as in cholera (p. 754). Infantile diarrhoea is also the single most important cause of malnutrition in the tropics.

Treatment is by rehydration. Mothers can be taught to make up glucose electrolyte solutions (p. 755) from prepared packs and give it to their children to drink, thus reducing the need for intravenous rehydration in hospital.

Tropical sprue

Tropical sprue is due to malabsorption occurring in a patient in or from the tropics, in the absence of other intestinal disease or parasites. Its manifestations resemble those of coeliac disease (nontropical sprue, p. 304).

Aetiology. This is unknown but the prevalence of sprue in certain well-defined tropical countries and localities, and its epidemiological pattern, suggest that an infective agent may be involved initially. In established sprue the jejunal contents are grossly overpopulated with aerobic enterobacteria which seem to play a role in maintaining the disease. Sprue is not due to gluten or any other demonstrable sensitivity and there is usually no evidence of preceding malnutrition, but folate deficiency, as in pregnancy, may precipitate the disease. Not all cases necessarily have the same aetiology, which may account for occasional reports of sprue from Africa and elsewhere where the disease is not usually encountered.

Sprue occurs mainly in Asia, including Sri Lanka, Southern India, Malaysia, Indonesia, Hong Kong and China, some Caribbean Islands, Puerto Rico and parts of South America. It is a problem of European residents in Asia and in the indigenous populations. It is common among travellers returning to Europe overland from India and Nepal.

Pathology. The changes closely resemble those of coeliac disease, although they tend to be less advanced. The jejunal villi are blunted or, rarely, absent and there is a subepithelial infiltration with plasma cells and lymphocytes. In severe cases the ileum is also affected. These changes are associated with malabsorption of fat, protein, carbohydrate and vitamins and the presence of diarrhoea which may lead to depletion of water, electrolytes, iron and calcium. A macrocytic anaemia is common with megaloblastic change in the bone marrow due to folate deficiency. Vitamin B_{12} deficiency takes longer to develop.

Mild changes in the jejunal mucosa are common in asymptomatic indigenous peoples, without gross malabsorption, throughout the tropics (*tropical enteropathy*).

Clinical features. Although the onset of sprue may be acute with explosive diarrhoea and occur within a few weeks of arrival in the tropics, it is more often insidious with increasing lassitude, apathy, anorexia and flatulence. Remissions and relapses are a characteristic feature. In severe cases 10 stools or more may be passed daily, especially in the morning or during the night. The stool is bulky, frothy, pale and fatty, loose, foul-smelling and floats in the lavatory pan and is difficult to flush away. Vomiting may occur with nausea, abdominal distension and borborygmi. The tongue becomes sore, red, fissured and painful, and there may be difficulty in swallowing. The patient loses weight and may become emaciated.

Continued malabsorption leads to specific deficiencies; follicular keratosis, angular stomatitis (vit. B), osteomalacia and tetany (vit. D), bleeding (vit. K) and hypoproteinaemic oedema, but peripheral neuropathy is rare. Loss of fluid and electrolytes causes dehydration, muscular weakness and cramps.

Diagnosis. The clinical features and the history of residence in an area noted for tropical sprue will suggest the correct diagnosis. Evidence of malabsorption should be sought. Macrocytosis occurs early. Erythrocyte folate levels are low. Anaemia may also be hypochromic from defective absorption of iron. Jejunal biopsy shows partial villous atrophy which is not specific for tropical sprue. Jejunal mucus and fluid is examined to exclude parasites. Barium meal and follow through examinations are necessary only to exclude other disease.

Differential diagnosis is from other forms of steatorrhoea. Additional causes in the tropics are infections of the intestine with *Giardia intestinalis*, *Strongyloides stercoralis* or *Capillaria philippinensis*. Early symptoms of sprue may erroneously be attributed to amoebiasis or neurosis.

Treatment. Dehydration and potassium deficiency must be corrected. Tetracycline, 1 g daily in divided doses for 28 days, will usually eliminate the jejunal bacterial overpopulation, reduce diarrhoea and improve absorption. In addition folic acid, 5 mg daily (10 mg intramuscularly in severe cases), is given as this seems to improve absorption as well as to relieve symptoms due to folate deficiency. The jejunal mucosa soon returns to normal. It has not yet been established whether to give a small prophylactic dose of folic acid daily to prevent a relapse in patients remaining in the tropics or to administer folic acid only if a relapse occurs.

Deficiencies of B_{12} and other vitamins and iron should be corrected. It is often helpful to give a multivitamin preparation containing 10 mg thiamin, 5 mg riboflavin and 50 mg nicotinamide twice daily for a few weeks.

Complicated diets are no longer advised but the diet initially should be bland and appetising, limited in fat and carbohydrate and high in protein. After recovery, the diet should contain meat, liver and green vegetables which are rich in folate. Folic acid supplements should be given to women who have had sprue should they become pregnant. Often, after apparently successful treatment, mild diarrhoea and flatulence may persist. These are usually due to secondary hypolactasia and respond to a lactose-free diet.

DISEASE OF OTHER SYSTEMS

Liver disease. This is a serious cause of disability and death throughout the tropics and subtropics. The microscopic structure of liver from a normal person in tropical Africa differs from that in a European. The hepatocytes are irregular in size and staining and frequently contain more than one nucleus. Portal tracts are infiltrated with mononuclear cells and a variable degree of fibrous tissue. Black pigment may be present in Kuppfer cells or portal tracts. These changes probably reflect the insults to which the liver is exposed in the tropics, including protein and vitamin malnutrition, alimentary infections and toxins, and systemic infections, notably malaria and schistosomiasis. The effects of protozoal and helminthic infections on the liver are discussed on page 361.

In most areas where hygiene is poor, type A viral hepatitis is endemic and especially affects children. Cirrhosis of the liver and hepatoma are common in adults and a relationship has been shown with hepatitis B virus which is extremely common in some parts of Africa where the prevalence exceeds 10% of the population. Aflatoxins, produced by fungi from badly stored groundnuts and grains can cause hepatoma.

Genito-urinary disease. Schistosomiasis haematobium (p. 784), which is the commonest cause of haematuria in endemic areas, may grossly damage the bladder and ureters. Skin infection with streptococci is a frequent precursor of acute glomerulonephritis. Pyelonephritis is common and in males often follows a gonococcal stricture of the urethra. *Plasmodium malariae* (p. 772) is an important cause of the nephrotic syndrome in children. Lepromatous leprosy (p. 756) may also result in glomerulonephritis. Bancroftian filariasis (p. 794) is a frequent cause of orchitis, epididymitis and hydrocele in endemic areas and schistosomiasis of damage to the female genital tract (p. 784).

Endocrine and metabolic disease. The prevalence of chronic fluoride poisoning is high in some areas (p. 60). Diabetes mellitus seems to be common throughout the tropics, but with few cardiovascular complications. The prevalence of other endocrine disorders is less certain though goitre is endemic in some localities (p. 60).

Blood disease. In many tropical countries anaemia is common and often severe. This is largely explained by the high frequency of protozoal, helminthic and bacterial infections and the prevalence of malnutrition. The aetiology of anaemia in the tropics varies from one country to another, and from one area to another, and effective management can only follow the clear appreciation of local patterns of disease, nutrition and social custom.

Ancylostomiasis (p. 792) is a major cause of iron deficiency anaemia. Although Addisonian pernicious anaemia occurs in all races, it is relatively uncommon in tropical countries where megaloblastic anaemia is much more frequently due to nutritional deficiency.

The various types of haemolytic anaemia which occur in temperate climates are also encountered in tropical countries. Haemolytic anaemia in the tropics is frequently due to malaria. In addition two types of genetic abnormality resulting in haemolytic anaemia are also particularly common, namely deficiency of the enzyme glucose-6-phosphate dehydrogenase, and the haemoglobinopathies. Haemolysis also occurs in acute bartonellosis (p. 755) and may be caused by the venom of certain snakes (p. 710) and spiders.

Onyalai is a thrombocytopenic purpura of unknown origin which occurs sporadically in Africa. Large haemorrhagic bullae on the tongue and buccal mucosa are conspicuous features.

Connective tissue disease. Autoimmune disease is rare in most tropical countries. The incidence of dermatomyositis, scleroderma, lupus erythematosus and rheumatoid arthritis is low, but differs between races. In Malaysia lupus erythematosus is commoner in Chinese than in Malays. Acute tropical polyarthritis, of obscure aetiology, is a common self-limiting disorder. Reiter's disease is frequent in Africa and Papua New Guinea and causes much disability.

Disease of muscle. Painful tender muscles, but without suppuration, are a feature of several systemic infections, notably dengue fever (p. 735), trypanosomiasis (p. 781) and relapsing fever (p. 764), and are characteristic of trichinosis (p. 799) and cysticercosis (p. 788).

TROPICAL MYOSITIS. The cause of suppurative myositis in the tropics is uncertain. Abscesses explored early are sterile but, later, culture of the pus usually yields *Staph. aureus*. Pyomyositis starts with fever and painful induration of one or more of the large muscles, mostly in the lower limbs. The indurated area subsequently suppurates and a large abscess may form and be associated with a swinging temperature and leucocytosis. The affected area is swollen, hot and tender. When the pus is superficial, fluctuation can be detected.

Diagnosis of tropical myositis is usually not difficult although meningitis or peritonitis may be simulated. The differential diagnosis includes Calabar swellings (p. 794), sparganosis (p. 789), scurvy and an underlying osteomyelitis. When an abscess has formed, it should be incised, the pus evacuated and an appropriate antibiotic given.

Disease of the nervous system. Infections still cause much of the neurological disease throughout the tropics, e.g. pyogenic and tuberculous meningitis, rabies and arthropod-borne viral encephalitis, malaria, tetanus, poliomyelitis, cysticercosis and hydatid disease. In some African countries as many as 1% of children suffer an attack of paralytic poliomyelitis. Locally important neurological diseases include trypanosomiasis in Africa, bartonellosis and Chagas' disease in South America, and eosinophilic meningitis in the Far East. Leprosy is the commonest cause of peripheral neuritis in the world and Chagas' disease of systemic autonomic neuropathy. Tuberculoma is a frequent and amoebic abscess a rare cause of an intracranial space-occupying lesion. In some tropical communities cerebrovascular accidents and trauma are becoming the chief causes of neurological disease. Certain diseases, such as tabes dorsalis, multiple sclerosis, parkinsonism and vitamin B_{12} neuropathy are rare. In countries where undercooked pork is eaten cysticercosis is a common cause of epilepsy.

There are several syndromes, due to dietary deficiencies or toxins, which are locally important. These include beriberi in the poorer areas of S.E. Asia, Wernicke's encephalopathy among the Bantu in Southern Africa and pellagra among maize eaters.

Tropical spinal ataxia may be caused by cyanide in unprocessed cassava (p. 657). Causes of spastic paraplegia in the tropics include lathyrism in India and the horn of Africa, Burkitt's lymphoma in African adolescents, schistosomiasis in Africa, hydatid disease in the Middle East, and, commonest of all, spinal tuberculosis.

Ophthalmic disease. Eye disease is a major cause of suffering and poverty in the tropics; it often proceeds to blindness as in vitamin A deficiency (p. 62). The other most frequent causes are keratitis, glaucoma and cataract which commonly occur as complications of neonatal ophthalmia, trachoma, onchocerciasis, malnutrition and leprosy. In Zambia, for example, 3 per 1000 of the population are blind.

Psychiatric disease. The prevalence of psychiatric diseases in the tropics is similar to that in temperate countries, but some of the precipitating factors and symptom-complexes are different. Included among the causes of organic confusional states are alcoholism, meningitis, syphilis, malaria, trypanosomiasis and typhoid fever.

Functional psychoses present in the same ways as in temperate countries, but acute emotional disturbances, especially in Africans, often present with schizophrenic features such as hallucinations and paranoia; the prognosis is, however, good. Fear, implanted by witchcraft, may have profound effects and, in addition, the subject may have been made to swallow potent poisonous charms. Neuroses are especially common in people from underdeveloped countries who are suddenly moved to a strange environment. Symptoms are often florid and usually hysterical, the patient having little understanding of their cause.

Malignant disease. Patterns of malignant disease vary greatly between different communities. Some tumours are rare — for example, carcinoma of the colon or lung in Africa and Asia — and some extremely common locally. Hepatoma is frequent in parts of Africa and in the Singapore Chinese. Carcinoma of the mouth is the commonest cancer in India and Sri Lanka and carcinoma of the nasopharynx associated with the Epstein Barr virus is frequent in Kenya and among Chinese in S.E. Asia. Four of the commonest tropical neoplasms, hepatoma, nasopharyngeal carcinoma, Burkitt's lymphoma and Kaposi's sarcoma are due to viruses, probably in association with another carcinogen.

KAPOSI'S SARCOMA, or idiopathic multiple haemorrhagic sarcoma of the skin, is a multifocal malignancy composed of new blood vessels and large spindle cells. It presents as firm, bluish-brown nodules in the skin, usually on the limbs. It is common in parts of tropical Africa and occurs in Western societies in homosexual males with the syndrome of acquired immunodeficiency (p. 726).

FURTHER READING:

Manson-Bahr P E C, Apted F I C 1982 Manson's tropical diseases, 18th edn. Baillière Tindall, London
Parry E H O 1984 Principles of medicine in Africa, 2nd edn. Oxford University Press, Oxford
Cook G C 1980 Tropical gastroenterology. Oxford University Press, Oxford
Greenwood B M, Whittle H C 1981 Current topics in immunology series. 14. Immunology of medicine in the tropics. Arnold, London

DISORDERS DUE TO CLIMATE

Acclimatisation to heat and heat injury; exposure to strong sunlight; solar keratosis; prickly heat; tropical anhidrotic asthenia; heat exhaustion; heat hyperpyrexia; cold injury; high altitude acclimatisation and deterioration; mountain sickness

Acclimatisation to heat and heat injury

In cool climates heat production in the body is balanced by loss from the surface chiefly by radiation and convection. When the atmospheric temperature is above that of the body, evaporation of sweat is all-important in the maintenance of a stable body temperature, assisted to a minor degree by insensible loss through the skin.

Acclimatisation to heat is an essential preparation for workers exposed to excessive heat in certain industries in cool climates as well as for people who go to the tropics. This can be achieved by undertaking exercise daily under artificially produced or natural hot weather conditions for 10 to 14 days. The total volume of circulating fluid increases and is accommodated in the expanded vascular bed; this is accompanied by a diminished pulse rate and an increased cardiac output. Salt excretion by the kidneys and in sweat is reduced, mainly as a result of increased production of aldosterone. The sweat glands also become more active, responding more rapidly and efficiently to increases in body temperature; consequently the rise in body temperature in response to exercise diminishes. With these adjustments the individual is better able to work and remain well under conditions of high atmospheric temperature provided an adequate intake of water and salt is maintained.

Heat syncope occurs in people dressed in unsuitable clothes in a warm atmosphere with poor air circulation, during exercise or on suddenly standing up.

Sunburn. This is caused by exposure to ultraviolet light. The skin of those with fair complexions, green eyes and red hair is especially sensitive to strong sunlight. Natural tolerance to the sun may be won by gradual exposure which enables the skin to acquire protective pigmentation.

Short periods of unaccustomed strong sunlight produce erythema and itch. Prolonged exposure causes pain, oedema and bullae, accompanied by malaise, headache and nausea. Severe cases may suffer from prostration and even acute circulatory failure. When a large area of skin has been damaged, this may interfere seriously with sweating and predispose to heat hyperpyrexia (p. 723).

No treatment is needed for mild sunburn, but for severe cases rest in bed in a cool room is required with sedatives to relieve the pain. Shock and dehydration must be corrected. Large blisters should be pricked. Calamine lotion should be applied to intact skin. Antihistamine drugs given by mouth help to relieve pruritus. Some protection is afforded by creams or lotions containing 5% para-aminobenzoic acid which absorbs ultraviolet light.

Solar keratosis. After prolonged residence in the tropics atrophic patches are liable to develop on exposed parts of the body. The backs of the hands, the neck and the forehead are most commonly affected. These areas may later develop small patches of hyperkeratosis which occasionally progress to carcinoma. This process is most severe in albinos.

The skin should be protected as far as possible from the sunlight by clothing and creams. Hyperkeratotic areas can be removed by the application for one week of 5% fluorouracil ointment.

Prickly heat. (*Miliaria rubra*). Many Europeans living in the tropics, especially when humidity is high, suffer from prickly heat. This arises from blockage of sweat ducts within the prickle cell layer of the epidermis so that sweat escapes into the epidermis and causes severe irritation. The lesions consist of numerous minute papules, surrounded by erythema, which become vesicular or pustular. The pus is sterile, although scratching may lead to secondary pyogenic infection. The lesions are most numerous on covered parts of the body.

The principles of treatment are to reduce sweating to a minimum and to overcome the blockage of the sweat ducts. If the patient can be transferred to a cool environment such as an air-conditioned room, the blocked ducts may become patent within a week or two. In severe cases it may be necessary to move to a cooler climate. Calamine lotion relieves the irritation.

In prevention, excessive washing and irritation from clothing should be avoided and a bland soap containing hexochlorophane used. Clothing must be loose fitting, changed frequently and thoroughly rinsed after washing. Obese patients must lose weight. Curries, condiments and alcohol, which cause sweating, should be avoided.

Tropical anhidrotic asthenia. The majority of patients with this disorder have suffered from prickly heat which has left extensive areas of skin, especially on the trunk and limbs, incapable of sweating properly. The condition develops insidiously towards the end of the hot weather, with headache, giddiness, lack of energy, diminished sweating and often marked polyuria, the dilute urine containing chloride. Fever is common and hyperpyrexia may develop. The patient must live in a cool climate for several months until the skin has recovered and sweating has returned to normal.

Heat exhaustion. This is brought on by a period of great heat or by extra effort in hot weather, when the patient has not taken enough fluid and salt to balance the increased loss by sweating. The amount of fluid lost as sweat during a working spell in a hot environment may be as much as 6 to 8 litres and even in persons fully acclimatised to heat, this may entail a loss of approximately 2 g sodium chloride per litre of sweat. Ill-health, especially gastrointestinal disturbances with vomiting and diarrhoea, will increase the risk of heat exhaustion.

Warning signs include headache, giddiness, loss of appetite, nausea, cramps and irritability. Lack of thirst may disguise the severity of dehydration until tachycardia, hypotension and a cold clammy skin develop (the 'cold moist man', c.f. the hot dry man, p. 724). A cool environment and cold drinks with added sodium chloride (10 g/l) are adequate for mild cases; others require intravenous rehydration. When heat exhaustion is not recognised and treated, the patient may pass into heat hyperpyrexia.

Heat hyperpyrexia (heat stroke)
This occurs in those exposed for considerable periods to unusually high environmental temperatures, independent of exposure to direct sunlight.

Unacclimatised people are more liable to suffer, but a prolonged period of very high temperature may affect even those who are fully acclimatised, including local inhabitants. The disorder is always associated with cessation of sweating, and the rectal temperature may reach 42°C to 43°C or even higher. Predisposing factors are those which interfere with the production and evaporation of sweat—unsuitable clothing, poor ventilation and heavy work in conditions of high temperature and humidity. Old people and those with congenital absence of sweat glands, with cystic fibrosis or skin diseases are particularly vulnerable. Hyperpyrexia may follow heat exhaustion when dehydration leads to cessation of sweating.

Pathological and clinical features. The most important changes are in the central nervous system. There is general congestion of the brain with increased pressure of the cerebrospinal fluid. Microscopic examination may show degeneration of nerve cells, particularly in the hypothalamic region and base of the brain.

The onset is usually dramatic with no warning in a person who appears to be neither dehydrated nor deficient in salt, but who may have noticed that perspiration has diminished. Loss of consciousness is rapid and may be preceded by prodromal signs of cerebral irritation. On examination a dry burning skin is found (the 'hot dry man'). When the temperature reaches between 41° and 42°C unconsciousness supervenes and without treatment the patient dies. Hyperpyrexia may be complicated by acute circulatory failure, hypokalaemia, acute renal or hepatic failure and haemorrhage.

Treatment. The aim is to reduce the temperature as quickly as possible in order to prevent permanent damage to vital structures. In the field, the patient is moved into the shade, the clothing removed and the skin kept wet and fanned vigorously. In hospital this is done by spraying the naked patient with water or loosely wrapping the individual in a cool wet sheet and promoting evaporation by fanning. Ideally the water should be at 15°C and the airstream at 30–35°C. The use of iced water, or immersion in cold water causes vasoconstriction and hinders heat loss. Cooling should be stopped when the rectal temperature has fallen to 39°C. The airway must be maintained and oxygen given.

Potassium deficiency should be corrected and severe haemorrhage controlled by blood transfusion. Acute circulatory failure (p. 143), acute renal failure (p. 401) or hepatic failure (p. 349) may require treatment. Parenteral antimalarial therapy (p. 773) should be given concurrently if malaria is a possibility. With energetic treatment 90% of patients recover.

Prevention of ill-effects of heat. Careful selection should be made of those required to work under hot atmospheric conditions. General physical fitness, youth, mental stability and acclimatisation are important. Fever, gastrointestinal disease, obesity, alcoholic excess and lack of sleep all predispose to the ill-effects of heat. It is highly important that the skin should be healthy and that sweating should be normal.

When the atmospheric temperature is very high, leading to excessive sweating, even the fully acclimatised require to take extra fluid and salt. A daily intake of up to 15 litres of cool drinking water and 30 g of sodium chloride (3 flat teaspoonfuls of salt) per person may be needed to prevent water and salt depletion. The extra salt is taken with food and in the drinking water or in enteric coated tablets.

In addition, everything possible should be done to improve working conditions by arranging for a free circulation of air and for a reduction of high temperature and excessive atmospheric humidity by air-conditioning. Clothing should be light and loose fitting. Hard or prolonged manual work should not be undertaken when atmospheric conditions are exceptionally unfavourable. Off-duty living conditions should be made as cool and comfortable as possible.

Cold injury

Frostbite. Dry cold, below 0°C, freezes poorly insulated tissues such as fingers, especially in people exercising at altitudes where oxygen demand is high and availability low. The warning sign is intense pain in fingers or feet. Superficial frostbite causes blistering of skin, and deep frostbite necrosis of tissues leading to gangrene. Frostbite is treated by rapidly rewarming the whole patient with good insulation and hot drinks, and by warming the affected part in water at 40°C.

Accidental hypothermia. This can be due to sudden immersion in a cold pond or sea, or to gradual but steady heat loss from exposure or from evaporation off the wet clothes of a poorly clad hill walker on a rainy day. The old and the sick become hypothermic if they are not well insulated at night. Clinical features and treatment are described on page 706.

High altitude acclimatisation and deterioration

The partial pressure of atmospheric oxygen decreases with altitude (p. 495). Physiological acclimatisation starts at about 7000 ft (2100 m) and most people feel the need to acclimatise by about 12 000 ft (3650 m). Pulmonary ventilation and perfusion increase, plasma volume decreases and renal excretion of bicarbonate increases. These and other changes serve to maintain arterial oxygen tension until erythrocyte production raises the haemoglobin and haematocrit. Above 14 000 ft (4270 m) heart rate and cardiac output increase and pulmonary artery pressure rises. Physically fit young people acclimatise best and do better with each ascent. Lowlanders, however, never attain the performance of highlanders. Lack of acclimatisation is shown by increased respiration, Cheyne-Stokes respiration, mild headache and irritability, easy fatiguability and sleeplessness.

Acclimatisation continues successfully up to 17 500 ft (5330 m) above which arterial oxygen saturation falls and physical performance starts to decline. Short bursts of work can be undertaken, but at the risk of the production of an exaggerated lactic acidosis. Prolonged residence above this height causes anorexia, weight loss, decreasing mental and physical capacity and increasing susceptibility to infection. There are no permanent human habitations above 15 000 ft (4575 m).

Acute mountain sickness is experienced by people who go up too high too quickly; some suffer at 8000 ft (2440 m), others reach 19 000 ft (5795 m) without trouble. The earliest symptoms are headache, nausea and vomiting, followed by lassitude, muscle weakness, breathlessness, dizziness, rapid pulse and insomnia. Retinal haemorrhages may occur.

The symptoms are probably due to intracellular oedema and may herald the onset of two severe, possibly fatal, complications: pulmonary oedema and, less commonly, cerebral oedema. Paradoxically the robust young man is prone to pulmonary oedema, probably due to overconfidence. Cerebral oedema causes drowsiness, irritability, confusion, fits and coma. Its presence may be confirmed by the detection of papilloedema.

These complications are prevented by ascending gradually and by acetazolamide which probably acts by causing a metabolic acidosis and an increased drive to ventilation. They are treated by descending rapidly and by giving oxygen. Frusemide (40–120 mg), or morphine (15 mg) is the treatment for pulmonary oedema, and dexamethasone (p. 623) for cerebral oedema.

Venous thromboses, which may lead to pulmonary embolism, may afflict the partially acclimatised; they are due to increased viscosity of blood and are prevented by adequate hydration and exercise.

Chronic mountain sickness is due to alveolar hypoventilation and chronic hypoxia and may affect highlanders as well as acclimatised lowlanders. It causes cyanosis, cardiac failure, pulmonary hypertension and neuropsychiatric symptoms. It is treated by taking the patient down to sea level.

A.D.M. Bryceson

FURTHER READING:

Dickinson J G 1982 Terminology and classification of acute mountain sickness. British Medical Journal 285: 720

Heath D, Williams D R 1981 Man at high altitudes, 2nd edn. Churchill Livingstone, Edinburgh

Bardwell A R et al 1986 Effect of acetazolamide on exercise performance and muscle mass at high altitude. Lancet 1: 1001–1005

Ellis F P 1976 Heat illness. Transactions of the Royal Society of Tropical Medicine and Hygiene 70: 402–411

19

Diseases due to infection

with particular reference to those encountered in the tropics

In Chapter 3, 'Infection and disease', general topics relating to infection and its treatment were discussed. In Chapter 18, the importance of infection in tropical and developing countries has been stressed. In this chapter, an account is given of diseases due to infection other than those that are more appropriately described in the system mainly involved. These include infective endocarditis, pneumonia and other respiratory infections, viral hepatitis, infections of the kidney and genitourinary tract, infectious mononucleosis and infections of the nervous system.

The sequence in this chapter is determined by the infecting agent and consists of diseases due to:

1. Viruses (below)
2. Chlamydiae (737)
3. Rickettsiae (p.737)
4. Bacteria (p.741)
5. Spirochaetes (p.761)
6. Fungi (p.766)
7. Protozoa (p.770)
8. Helminths (p.782)
9. Arthropods (p.800)

The chapter concludes with a section on advice to travellers about the prevention of disease.

DISEASES DUE TO VIRUSES

No single classification of viral diseases is entirely satisfactory for the clinician, whether by viral structure and nomenclature, by method of transmission or by type of disease. Viruses are divided into two groups according to whether they contain DNA or RNA in their genome, and are subdivided further into families according to their structure (Table 19.1).

The diseases due to viruses described in this section are: *human T immunodeficiency infection and AIDS ,measles, rubella, mumps, herpes simplex and cytomegalovirus infections, chickenpox, smallpox, rabies, Lassa fever, Marburg and Ebola viral diseases, other haemorrhagic fevers, arboviral infections (yellow fever, dengue, Rift Valley fever and Japanese B encephalitis).*

HUMAN IMMUNODEFICIENCY VIRAL INFECTION (INCLUDING AIDS)

Aetiology. The occurrence in 1981 of severe and often fatal pneumonia caused by the opportunist pathogen *Pneumocystis carinii* in apparently healthy male homosexuals in the United States led to the recognition of the acquired immune deficiency syndrome (AIDS). Two years later the infectious agent causing this apparently new disease was identified as a previously unknown retrovirus which was first called the human T cell lymphotrophic virus (HTLV III). It was also known as the lymphadenopathy associated virus (LAV). The agreed name is now human immunodeficiency virus (HIV). This virus has a tropism particularly for helper T lymphocytes which play a crucial role in regulating the immune system (p. 23). Damage to, or destruction of, helper lymphocytes leads to the development of a cellular

Table 19.1 Classification of viruses causing disease in man.

Nucleic acid	Virus family	Examples of disease
RNA Single stranded	**(Ortho) myxoviruses** (Gr. *orthos* = correct, *myxa* = mucus, i.e. true virus with affinity for mucus)	Influenza
	Paramyxoviruses (Gr. *para* = alongside, i.e.resembling myxoviruses)	Parainfluenza, measles, mumps, respiratory syncytial disease of infants
	Rhabdoviruses (Gr. *rhabdo* = rod)	Rabies
	Retroviruses	AIDS and related disorders. Rare form of leukaemia
	Arenaviruses (L. *arena* = sand, as seen by electronmicroscopy)	Lymphocytic meningitis, Lassa fever, Bolivian and Argentinian haemorrhagic fevers
	Coronaviruses (like rings in EM)	Coryza
	Picornaviruses (L. *picollo* = small + RNA)	1. **Enteroviruses** include poliomyelitis, Coxsackie (pleurisy, myocarditis and pericarditis) and ECHO viruses (meningitis) 2. **Hepatitis A** virus 3. **Rhinoviruses** cause the common cold
	Togaviruses (L. *toga* = cloak)	Rubella and most arbovirus infections (p. 733)
	Bunyaviruses	Some arboviral infections (p. 734)
RNA Double stranded	**Reoviruses** (Respiratory Enteric Orphan virus)	1. **Rotaviruses** cause infantile diarrhoea 2. **Orbiviruses** cause Colarado tick fever
DNA Single stranded	**Parvoviruses** (L. *Parvus* = small)	Rubella-like illness; transient arthralgia in adults, aplastic crises in sickle-cell disease
DNA Double stranded	**Poxviruses**	Smallpox and vaccinia
	Papovaviruses (papilloma inducers)	Warts
	Adenoviruses (Gr. *aden* = gland)	Respiratory infections (p. 215)
	Herpesviruses	Herpes simplex, varicella-zoster, infectious mono- nucleosis and cytomegaloviral infections

Agents causing hepatitis B, Marburg and Ebola viral diseases and the slow viral encephalitides are not yet classified.

immunodeficiency disease rendering the patient susceptible to a wide variety of infections but particularly to those caused by viruses, protozoa, fungi and intracellular bacteria. Patients suffering from AIDS also develop various malignancies, most notably Kaposi's sarcoma and also lymphomas. The HIV virus also attacks cells of the nervous system including the brain.

HIV infection is most commonly a sexually transmitted disease amongst homosexual males but it can also be transmitted heterosexually and by blood and blood products such as factor VIII. The routes of transmission are therefore similar to those of virus B hepatitis and infected persons include drug addicts and haemophiliacs. Infection can also be transmitted transplacentally and at delivery.

Clinical features. The initial infection with HIV is usually subclinical although a very small number of patients can develop an infectious mononucleosis-like illness with fever, lymphadenopathy and rash within 2 to 3 weeks of infection. The large majority, however, remain symptom-free. After an incubation period of between 2 months and 5 years about 70% of these will develop one of the following syndromes:

1. AIDS. This syndrome is associated with profound cellular immunodeficiency, serious opportunistic infections, especially *Pn. carinii* pneumonia (p. 220) and, commonly, Kaposi's sarcoma (p. 722). It has been estimated that about 40% of HIV infected persons will develop the full AIDS syndrome.

2. Persistent generalised lymphadenopathy (PGL) or AIDS-related complex (ARC) will develop in about a further 30% of those infected. PGL has a relatively good prognosis especially if the patient is symptom-free, although a small number will eventually develop AIDS. Patients with ARC are always symptomatic and may have weight loss, diarrhoea, candidosis and fever along with leucopenia and depletion of helper T cells. They have a high possibility of developing AIDS and ARC is known also as prodromal AIDS.

3. Brain involvement. Dementia, psychosis or chronic encephalitis may be due either to the

human immunodeficiency virus or to opportunistic infection.

4. Thrombocytopenic purpura (p. 498).

The diagnosis of HIV infection is confirmed by the demonstration of serum antibodies to the virus. Current knowledge suggests that the virus persists in the body for life and a patient who is HIV antibody positive must therefore be considered to be infectious.

Treatment. There is no specific therapy for HIV infection although certain antiviral drugs, such as zidovudine (p. 46), will suppress the virus. The management of AIDS therefore depends on supportive measures and the treatment of secondary infection. No vaccine is yet available.

Prevention of transmission of infection depends on (1) modification of sexual practices particularly with regard to promiscuity and anal intercourse, (2) screening of donated blood and also blood products for HIV antibody, and (3) the counselling of persons found to be antibody positive. Transmission of the virus has very rarely followed needlestick injury involving medical or nursing staff, although none have developed AIDS. HIV is readily inactivated by heat and by disinfectants such as glutaraldehyde.

At the end of 1986 over 26 000 cases of AIDS had been diagnosed in the United States, approximately 4000 in Western Europe and over 600 in Britain. In East and Central Africa AIDS is now epidemic where it is spreading heterosexually. 80% of patients with AIDS have died within 2 years of diagnosis.

MEASLES

Measles is caused by a paramyxovirus which spreads by droplet infection. One attack confers a high degree of immunity. Most people suffer from measles in childhood, and a mother who has had the disease confers passive immunity on her infant for the first 6 months of life. Measles is very severe with a high mortality in many tropical countries. The incubation period is about 10 days to the commencement of the catarrhal stage.

Clinical features. *Catarrhal stage.* Measles commences in much the same way as a common cold. There is a febrile onset, with nasal catarrh, sneezing, redness of the conjunctivae and watering of the eyes. In addition cough, hoarseness of the voice due to laryngitis, and photophobia usually appear by the second day.

At this stage, a diagnosis of measles may be made from the presence of Koplik's spots on the mucous membrane of the mouth. These are small white spots surrounded by a narrow zone of inflammation. Though often numerous on the inside of the cheeks, they may be sparse and confined to the region around the opening of the parotid duct. The disease is highly infectious during the catarrhal stage and the child is miserable and irritable.

Exanthematous stage. After 3 or 4 days the diagnostic Koplik's spots disappear while the dark red macular or maculopapular rash develops first at the back of the ears and at the junction of the forehead and the hair. Within a few hours there is invasion of the whole skin and as the spots rapidly become more numerous they fuse to form the characteristic blotchy appearance of measles. The face is ordinarily the most densely covered area. When the rash is fully erupted, usually in 2 or 3 days, it tends to deepen in colour and then fade into a faint brown staining followed by a fine desquamation. The malaise and the fever subside as the rash fades.

Complications. Fits occur in young children and are commonest as the rash is appearing. Secondary infection may cause otitis media or pneumonia. Persistent conjunctivitis may be followed by corneal ulceration which, if neglected, may result in impairment of vision. Stomatitis, gastroenteritis, appendicitis and encephalitis may also occur. In the undernourished child, measles may precipitate kwashiorkor.

Treatment. The patient should be isolated if possible and excluded from school for 10 days from the appearance of the rash. Most cases, in spite of the high temperature, remain uncomplicated, and antibiotics should be prescribed only for unequivocal bacterial complications.

Prevention. ACTIVE IMMUNISATION. One injection of live attenuated measles virus should be given subcutaneously in children over 1 year old who have not had the disease. In the United States an aggressive immunisation programme has led to the virtual eradication of measles.

PASSIVE IMMUNISATION. Human normal

immunoglobulin, given intramuscularly, is recommended for the prevention or attenuation of measles, for contacts under 18 months of age and for debilitated children, especially those with malignant disease. The dose is 250 mg for children under 1 year old and 500 mg for those over this age.

RUBELLA (GERMAN MEASLES)

Rubella is caused by a togavirus which spreads by droplet infection. One attack confers a high degree of immunity. It tends to affect older children, adolescents and young adults and spreads less readily than measles. The disease in children is trivial. In adults the illness may be more severe, but of short duration and of little importance except when it develops in a woman during the first 4 months of pregnancy. In such cases the child may be born with a congenital malformation such as a cardiac or mental defect, cataract or deafness. The risk of damage to the fetus by the rubella virus varies from over 70% during the first 4 weeks of pregnancy to virtually zero after the end of the fourth month. The incubation period is usually about 18 days.

Clinical features. In children the constitutional symptoms are so slight that the illness is rarely suspected until the rash is seen. The spots are pink macules which appear first behind the ears and on the forehead. The rash spreads rapidly, first to the trunk and then to the limbs. Tender enlargement of the suboccipital lymph nodes is usual. Sometimes many groups of lymph nodes are affected and the tip of the spleen may be palpable. In adolescents and adults the onset may be acute with fever and generalised aches, but even then the illness lasts for only 2 or 3 days. Polyarthritis is the commonest complication. Encephalomyelitis and thrombocytopenic purpura are very rare. Complete recovery from all of them is the rule. Serological studies are usually necessary for definitive diagnosis.

Treatment and prevention. No treatment is available. If infection is known to have occurred during the first 16 weeks of pregnancy there is such a high chance of fetal abnormality that termination should be recommended. It is therefore advisable to immunise all girls between their 11th and 13th birthdays who have not had the disease as shown by the absence of serum antibodies to the virus. Women of child-bearing age who are found to be serologically negative should also be offered vaccine provided that they are not pregnant and are willing to avoid pregnancy for 12 weeks after vaccination.

MUMPS

Mumps is caused by a paramyxovirus which spreads by droplet infection and affects mainly children of school age and young adults. The infectivity rate is not high and there is serological evidence that 30–40% of infections are clinically inapparent. The incubation period is about 18 days.

Clinical features. Malaise, fever, trismus and pain near the angle of the jaw is soon followed by tender swelling of one or both parotid glands. Parotid swelling alone is often the first feature. The submandibular salivary glands may also be involved. The swollen glands subside in a few days, and may be succeeded by swelling of a previously unaffected gland. Orchitis occurs in about one in four males who develop mumps after puberty; it is usually on one side only, but if it is bilateral, sterility may be a sequel. Obscure abdominal pain may be due to pancreatitis or oöphoritis. Acute lymphocytic meningitis is another mode of presentation. Encephalomyelitis is rare.

Most cases of mumps can be diagnosed on clinical grounds alone, but the diagnosis can be confirmed in doubtful cases by the demonstration of specific antibodies, or the virus may be cultured from the saliva, or from the cerebrospinal fluid in meningitis.

Treatment. Oral hygiene is important when the mouth is very dry due to lack of saliva. Apart from the relief of symptoms as they appear, no other treatment is necessary. Orchitis can be relieved by prednisolone (40 mg daily for 4 days). Cases of mumps should be isolated until the gland last affected has subsided.

HERPES SIMPLEX INFECTIONS

Herpes simplex (Herpesvirus hominis) is a common DNA virus which frequently causes non-specific illness; hence many people have serum antibodies to the organism. It has assumed greater importance as a cause of serious, and sometimes fatal, infections in immunocompromised patients. There are two strains of *Herpesvirus hominis*, type 1 and type 2, the latter being principally responsible for sexually transmitted anogenital infections (p. 420). Infections caused by these viruses can be categorised as primary or recurrent.

Primary infections include ulcerative stomatitis (commonest in infants), keratitis (dendritic ulcer), finger infections (often in nurses), vulvo-vaginitis and encephalitis. In neonates and the immunosuppressed the infection may be disseminated, involving many organs and tissues, and can be fatal. The newborn may contract the infection from the mother's genital tract during birth and active genital *H. simplex* infection is therefore an indication for Caesarean section.

Recurrent *H. simplex* infections are commonest on the lips and adjoining skin (herpes labialis or 'cold sore'). The lesions start as macules, become vesicular and then pustular. Attacks of herpes labialis may be precipitated by various stimuli including sunlight, menstruation and viral and bacterial infections. Genital lesions also commonly recur.

The virus can readily be cultured from lesions and infection is confirmed by rising serum antibody titres.

The *H. simplex* virus is susceptible to idoxuridine and acyclovir although most infections resolve spontaneously. Drops containing idoxuridine or acyclovir are effective in eye infections and intravenous acyclovir is indicated for disseminated infections in immunocompromised patients. Acyclovir is also indicated for *H. simplex* encephalitis, which has a mortality of up to 80%. An oral preparation of acyclovir has been made available for the treatment of infections of the skin and mucous membranes. Acyclovir will not eradicate the *H. simplex* virus from posterior root ganglia and recurrent attacks cannot therefore be prevented.

CYTOMEGALOVIRAL INFECTION

Cytomegaloviral (CMV) infection is very common all over the world. The name refers to a characteristic enlargement of involved cells. Although most CMV infections are symptomless, this herpesvirus can also cause severe congenital abnormalities, a disease resembling infectious mononucleosis (p. 522) and disseminated infection in immunocompromised patients. The virus may be isolated from the urine and a specific antibody response occurs.

CHICKENPOX

Chickenpox (varicella) is caused by a herpesvirus (varicella-zoster virus) which spreads by droplets from the upper respiratory tract or by contamination from the discharge from ruptured lesions of the skin or through contact with herpes zoster (p. 645). Herpes zoster is due to reactivation of infection with the varicella-zoster virus and may be accompanied by a varicelliform rash.

Chickenpox is highly infectious and chiefly affects children under 10 years of age. Most children tolerate this disease well but, as often happens with viral infections, adults may develop a more severe illness. In patients with leukaemia or immunocompromised, the disease may be severe or even fatal. The incubation period is 14–21 days.

Clinical features. Constitutional symptoms are usually brief and mild, and the first sign of the disease is often the rash. Lesions are sometimes present on the palate before the characteristic rash appears on the trunk on the second day of the illness. Then the face and finally the limbs are involved. The spots reach their maximum density upon the trunk, and are more sparse on the periphery of the limbs. Macules appear first and within a few hours the lesions become papular and then vesicular and, within 24 hours, pustular. The vesicles and pustules are fragile and may be ruptured by the chafing of garments. Damage from scratching is also frequent, since itching may be troublesome. Whether or not the pustules rupture, they dry up in a few days to form scabs. The spots appear in crops, so that lesions at all stages of development are seen in any area at the same time.

The course of the disease is usually uneventful but secondary infection may occur. Serious complications, which are rare, include chickenpox pneumonia (p. 219), myocarditis, proliferative glomerulonephritis (p. 384), and acute demyelinating encephalomyelitis (p. 648).

Treatment. No treatment is required in the majority of cases but acyclover (p. 46) can be used in the immunocompromised patient. If there is secondary infection a local antiseptic should be applied to the skin, e.g. chlorhexidine. If bacterial infection progresses, an antibiotic should be prescribed. Immunocompromised children who have been in contact with chickenpox or shingles should have an injection of human anti-varicella gamma-globulin (zoster immune globulin).

SMALLPOX

As a result of the WHO programme of case detection and vaccination, it is confidently believed that smallpox has been eradicated. Apart from two laboratory-acquired infections in 1978, the last known case occurred in Somalia in 1977. Major smallpox produces a severe constitutional disturbance associated with a peripherally distributed rash with lesions which, in any one area, progress in unison from macules through papules to pustules. The mortality rate may be as high as 40%.

A similar virus causes *monkeypox* in primates in jungle areas of Central Africa, with lesions resembling those of smallpox. Some human cases have occurred in those in contact with infected primates but inter-human spread is exceptional.

The virus of smallpox is being maintained in two designated laboratories, in order to be able to differentiate such diseases as monkey-pox from smallpox. Only staff employed in these designated laboratories, of which there are none in Britain, now require to be vaccinated against smallpox. Limited stocks of smallpox vaccine are available for this purpose and in case, contrary to all expectation, the disease should reappear.

RABIES

Rabies is caused by a rhabdovirus which infects central nervous tissue and salivary glands. It affects a wide range of animals and is conveyed by bites and licks on abrasions or on intact mucous membranes. Transmission by droplets in confined spaces has also been demonstrated. In Europe the maintenance host is the fox and in recent years the disease has spread from Poland westwards through Germany and has progressively penetrated through France. Man is most frequently infected from dogs but cats and other animals may be responsible. In the USA skunks are an important host and may infect man, while in Central and South America vampire bats also cause death of domestic animals and occasionally man. There have been several cases of rabies transmitted by corneal grafts taken from people who had died of undiagnosed rabies.

Clinical features. The incubation period, during which the virus is spreading centripetally along axons to the brain, varies in man from a minimum of 9 days to many months but is usually between 4 and 8 weeks. Severe bites, especially if on the head or neck are associated with short incubation periods.

Although only a proportion of people bitten by a rabid animal develop the disease, once it is manifest it is almost invariably fatal. At the onset there may be insidious fever and a return of pain or paraesthesia at the site of the bite. After a prodromal period of from 1 to 10 days, during which anxiety may be increasingly evident, the characteristic fear of water, responsible for the alternative name of 'hydrophobia', becomes evident in many cases. Although the patient is thirsty, attempts at drinking provoke violent contractions of the diaphragm and other inspiratory muscles and thereafter the sight or even the sound of water may precipitate these distressing spasms and attacks of panic. Delusions and hallucinations may develop accompanied by spitting, biting and maniacal behaviour, with lucid intervals in which the patient is acutely anxious. Cranial nerve lesions develop and terminal hyperpyrexia is common. Death ensues, usually within a week from the onset of symptoms.

In a small proportion of cases there is an ascending paralysis without mental excitement and these patients survive, on average, 12 days. This type is particularly associated with bites from vampire bats.

During life the diagnosis is usually made on clinical grounds but rapid immunofluorescent techniques to detect antigen in corneal impression smears or skin biopsies have been successfully employed.

Treatment. A few patients with rabies have survived. All received some post-exposure prophylaxis. Intensive care is needed with facilities to control cardiac and respiratory failure. Usually only palliative treatment is possible once symptoms have appeared. The patient should be heavily sedated with diazepam 10 mg 4–6 hourly, supplemented by chlorpromazine 50–100 mg, if necessary. Nutrition and fluids should be given intravenously or through a gastrostomy.

Prevention. *Pre-exposure prophylaxis* is required by those who handle professionally potentially infected animals, those who work with rabies virus in laboratories and those who live at special risk in rabies endemic areas. Protection is afforded by two intradermal injections of 0.1 ml human diploid cell strain vaccine given 4 weeks apart, followed by yearly boosters.

Post-exposure prophylaxis. The wound should be thoroughly cleaned, preferably with a quaternary ammonium detergent or soap; damaged tissues should be excised and the wound left unsutured. Rabies can usually be prevented if treatment is started within a day or two of biting. Delayed treatment may still be of value. For maximum protection hyperimmune serum and vaccine are required.

The safest antirabies antiserum is human rabies immune globulin. The dose is 20 i.u./kg body weight, once. Half is infiltrated around the bite and half is given intramuscularly at a different site from the vaccine. The dose of hyperimmune animal serum is 40 i.u./kg. Hypersensitivity reactions, including systemic anaphylaxis are common.

The safest vaccine, free of complications, is human diploid cell strain vaccine; 1.0 ml is given intramuscularly on days 0, 3, 7, 14, 30 and 90. In developing countries, where human rabies globulin may not be obtainable, 0.1 ml of vaccine should be given intradermally into eight sites on day 1, with single boosters on days 7 and 28. Where human products are not available and when risk of rabies is slight (licks on the skin, scratches or abrasions, or minor bites of covered arms or legs) it may be justifiable to delay starting treatment up to 5 days while observing the confined animal or awaiting examination of its brain rather than use the older vaccine.

The biting animal should be confined, if possible. If it is healthy after 5 days, it does not have rabies and treatment is stopped. If it dies, or is killed, the brain is examined by immunofluorescence for Negri bodies. If positive, or if the animal escapes, treatment is continued.

Control of spread. Human rabies is an infrequent disease even in endemic areas. Its fearful manifestations, however, justify stringent attempts being made to prevent its spread. In endemic areas household dogs should have a yearly dose of a Flury canine (live) vaccine, and stray dogs killed. Importation of all animals into uninfected countries should be strictly controlled, with isolation in quarantine for a minimum of 6 months. Vigilance and appropriate measures of control over infected maintenance hosts, such as the fox, are urgently required where areas of endemicity are extending.

LASSA FEVER

This disease, first observed in 1969, is due to an arenavirus, a group which also includes the viruses responsible for Argentine and Bolivian haemorrhagic fevers. Outbreaks have so far been limited to subsaharan West Africa where serological studies have shown that the infection is widespread. The natural reservoir is the multi-mammate rat and spread is probably through urine. The mode of human infection is unknown but case to case transmission in hospital occurs through direct inoculation and possibly inhalation.

Clinical features. The disease has the general features of a viral infection, high fever, intercostal myalgia, bradycardia, a low blood pressure and leucopenia. Adherent yellow exudates on the pharynx are particularly characteristic. The fever lasts between 7 and 17 days. In severe cases liver and renal failure, electrolyte imbalance, haemorrhage and acute circulatory failure develop. Mortality rates of overt infections have been as high as 50% but mild and subclinical infections also occur.

The virus may be isolated, or antigen detected, in maximum security laboratories from serum, pharynx, pleural exudate and urine but diagnosis will usually be established from 'paired sera', the later specimens being taken 6–8 weeks after the onset of infection. The diagnosis should be considered in Britain in patients presenting with fever within 21 days of leaving West Africa.

Treatment and prevention. Strict isolation and general supportive measures, preferably in a special unit, are required. Ribavirin is given intravenously (100 mg/kg, then 25 mg/kg/d for 3 days and 12.5 mg/kg/d for 4 days). The administration of convalescent immune plasma has been followed by recovery and is therefore recommended for prophylaxis after accidental exposure to infection.

MARBURG AND EBOLA VIRAL DISEASE

In Marburg, West Germany, in 1967 a severe infectious illness broke out among laboratory workers who had handled tissues from a batch of vervet monkeys imported from Uganda. In 1976 outbreaks of the disease occurred in Sudan and Zaîre from a focus on the Ebola River. The viruses causing these two outbreaks have a unique identical structure but are antigenically distinct. Sporadic cases have occurred elsewhere in Africa. The natural animal reservoir of these viruses is not known nor is the usual mode of spread, but man-to-man transmission can take place. In these outbreaks the mortality has varied from 25% of treated patients to over 90% in the untreated, but successive human passage seems to reduce virulence.

After an incubation period of 5 to 9 days, the illness presents suddenly with fever, severe myalgia and diarrhoea. By the fourth or fifth day the fauces become inflamed and a bright red, follicular rash appears on the extensor surfaces of the limbs; it spreads to the trunk and face, becomes maculopapular and finally confluent and livid. There may be lymphadenopathy. About the sixth day, in severe cases, bleeding associated with thrombocytopenia starts usually in the gastro-intestinal tract. The virus also attacks the brain, kidneys and lungs. Fatal complications, often between the sixth and tenth days of the illness, include haemorrhage, secondary infection, encephalitis, renal failure and pneumonia.

Treatment consists of supportive measures, replacement of blood and the management of complications. Immune plasma may be beneficial if given at an early stage. No vaccine is available.

OTHER HAEMORRHAGIC FEVERS

The term haemorrhagic fevers is increasing in popularity but covers too wide a field of medicine to be of much value. Infections due to many different organisms may cause bleeding, and through several different mechanisms. Common among them are certain arboviral infections (yellow fever, dengue, Kyasanur forest disease, Omsk haemorrhagic fever, chikungunya, Crimean haemorrhagic fever), Marburg-Ebola viral disease, Rocky Mountain spotted fever, relapsing fever, meningococcal septicaemia, plague and other Gram-negative septicaemias, and trypanosomiasis, all of which are described elsewhere in this book. There still remain a number of other viral infections that are commonly associated with severe haemorrhage.

Bolivian and *Argentinian haemorrhagic fever* are caused by Machupo virus and Junin virus, respectively. Both are arenaviruses, like that of Lassa fever. Both have a reservoir in *Calomys* rodents which excrete the virus in urine. Both cause epidemics in rural workers, characterised by fever, with severe haemorrhage developing about the fifth day. Treatment with convalescent plasma greatly reduces the mortality.

Haemorrhagic fever with renal syndrome has occurred in outbreaks in Korea, Manchuria and Eastern Europe. The virus (Hantaan virus) normally infects certain small rodents that pass it in their faeces. The infection causes severe capillary congestion, leakage and haemorrhage, especially in the renal medulla, so that oedema and acute renal failure develop, with oliguria and the passage of cells and protein in the urine. Untreated the mortality is about 30%, but with proper treatment for acute renal failure (p. 401) and blood transfusion if necessary, all patients should recover. A less severe form of the disease, nephropathia epidemica, is found in Scandinavia.

ARBOVIRAL INFECTIONS

Classification. So called because they are *ar*thropod-*b*orne, the hundred or so arboviruses are divided into groups according to their antigenic characters.

Group A are togaviruses all of which are transmitted by mosquitoes. The group includes three important causes of encephalitis in the New World, Eastern, Western and Venezuelan equine encephalitis, and several important fevers of Africa (Chikungunya, O'nyong-nyong, Sindbis and Semiliki Forest fevers), South America and Australia (Ross River fever).

Group B are also togaviruses, many of which cause encephalitis or haemorrhagic fevers. Yellow fever, dengue, Japanese B encephalitis, and West Nile, St Louis and Murray Valley fevers are transmitted by mosquitoes. Russian and European spring-summer encephalitis, Omsk haemorrhagic fever, Kyasanur forest disease of India and louping ill of Britain are transmitted by ticks.

Bunyamwera group of bunyaviruses, all of which are mosquito borne, are responsible for a large number of fevers, especially in the New World, including California encephalitis.

The remaining arboviruses, many of which are bunyaviruses, are placed in small groups or are ungrouped. Included here are the sandfly fevers, Rift Valley fever, and the haemorrhagic fevers of Crimea, Congo and Korea.

Clinical features. Arboviruses often cause epidemics. Clinically many infections are mild; even with the potentially serious ones, subclinical cases outnumber severe cases one hundred or one thousand times. The immunity that follows is often life-long and is an important determinant of the pattern of disease in the exposed community. Normally immunity protects and prevents further epidemics, but in the case of dengue, it may also sensitise and predispose to more severe disease if the person is infected with a different, but cross-reacting type.

The incubation period is usually less than a week. The presentation is with fever which may disappear after a few days, either permanently or to return accompanied by the clinical features and complications characteristic of the particular infection. In many arbovirus infections there is a maculopapular rash, conjunctival suffusion, photophobia and orbital pain. Arthralgia and myalgia are common; pain may be severe and immobilising. Lymphadenopathy is found in a few infections.

The most serious complications of arboviral infections are encephalitis and haemorrhage. When inoculated into mice most arboviruses cause encephalitis, but relatively few do so in man. The important ones are listed above, but their distribution is wider than their names suggest. The clinical features of encephalitis are described on page 643.

The causes of haemorrhage in arboviral infections are not fully understood. In some, such as dengue, disseminated intravascular coagulation is important; in others, notably yellow fever, haemorrhage follows severe hepatitis when deficiency of prothrombin and other coagulation factors develops. Thrombocytopenia occurs in many arboviral infections, and may contribute. Acute circulatory failure may follow haemorrhage, or occur on its own, possibly due to increased capillary permeability, as in dengue.

Diagnosis may be possible on clinical grounds during the course of an epidemic. For virological confirmation blood is transported on ice for inoculation into mice or tissue culture. It may be possible to isolate virus from cerebrospinal fluid if there are signs of encephalitis. Serological diagnosis depends on demonstrating rising titres of antibodies, usually by complement fixation or haemagglutination-inhibition. Such antibodies are, however, usually only group specific. Neutralising antibodies may be genus specific, but are more time consuming and expensive to assay.

Prevention rests mainly on vector or reservoir control, but vaccines are available for some, including yellow fever, Kyasanur forest disease, European Spring-Summer encephalitis and Japanese B encephalitis.

Yellow fever

Yellow fever is caused by a togavirus. It is normally a zoonosis of monkeys that inhabit tropical rain forests in West and Central Africa and South and Central America, among whom it may cause devastating epidemics. It is transmitted by mosquitoes living in tree tops. *Aedes africanus* is the vector in Africa and *Haemagogus* species in America. The infection is brought down to man either by infected mosquitoes when trees are felled, or by monkeys raiding human plantations. In the latter case *Aedes simpsoni*, which breeds in the axils of banana plants, may transmit the disease to man. In towns yellow fever may be transmitted between humans by *Aedes aegypti* which breeds efficiently in small collections of water. The distribution of this mosquito is far wider than that of yellow fever and poses a continual risk of spread.

Man is infectious during the viraemic phase which starts 3 to 6 days after the bite of the infected mosquito and lasts for 4 to 5 days. Mosquitoes become infectious 8 to 12 days after biting a patient and remain so for the rest of their 6 to 8 week life span. They may pass on the virus transovarially.

Pathology. In the liver, acute mid-zonal coagulation necrosis leads to deposits of hyalin called Councilman bodies (p. 342), and intranuclear eosinophilic inclusions called Torres bodies; another characteristic feature is the absence of inflammatory infiltrate. The kidneys show tubular degeneration, which may partly be due to reduced blood flow. Widespread petechial haemorrhages are most marked in the stomach and duodenum. Haemorrhage is due to liver damage and disseminated intravascular coagulation.

Clinical features. Yellow fever is often a mild febrile illness lasting less than a week. The classical disease starts suddenly with rigors and high fever, after an incubation period of 3–6 days. Backache, headache and bone pains are severe. Nausea and vomiting start. The face is flushed and the conjunctivae injected. Bradycardia and leucopenia are also characteristic of this phase of the illness, which lasts 3 days and is followed by a remission lasting a few hours or days. The third stage is characterised by a return of fever, and the onset of jaundice, petechial haemorrhages in the mucosae, ecchymoses, haematemesis and oliguria. Death, often preceded by a brief coma, occurs in many patients, usually in the third stage.

Diagnosis and treatment. An outbreak of fatal jaundice in an endemic area should suggest the diagnosis. The differential diagnosis includes other viral causes of hepatitis (p. 342), other causes of haemorrhagic fever, malaria, typhoid and leptospirosis. Diagnosis is confirmed by isolation of virus from the blood (p. 334) during the first 4

days of the illness, or by serological examination of acute and convalescent sera. Histology of liver taken by needle biopsy post mortem may also provide the diagnosis.

Patients should be nursed under a mosquito net until the viraemic stage has passed. Treatment is supportive, with meticulous attention to fluid and electrolyte balance, urine output and blood pressure. Blood transfusions, plasma expanders and peritoneal dialysis may become necessary.

Prevention. A single vaccination with the 17 D non-pathogenic strain of virus, available at internationally recognised centres, gives full profor at least 10 years (p. 802). The vaccine does not produce appreciable side-effects in adults, unless they are allergic to egg protein. Vaccination is not recommended in children under 9 months of age because of a slight risk of encephalitis. No ill-effects have as yet been observed from vaccination during pregnancy.

Only travellers possessing valid certificates of vaccination against yellow fever are allowed to proceed from an endemic area to 'receptive areas', by which is meant countries free from the disease but in which the potential vectors exist. In this way the disease has not yet entered Asia. Mosquito control of airports should be maintained. The urban disease can be eradicated by the abolition of the breeding places of *Aedes aegypti*, by the use of residual insecticides in houses and by mass vaccination in endemic areas. Vaccination is the only means to prevent human disease being transmitted from forest reservoirs.

Dengue

Four types of dengue virus have been described. Man is the reservoir and the virus is transmitted by mosquitoes, chiefly *Aedes aegypti*. Infectivity is as in yellow fever.

The disease is a risk in many tropical and subtropical countries, especially in coastal areas. It is most prevalent during the hot season when the mosquitoes are numerous and many large epidemics have occurred. One attack usually gives immunity for about 9 months and after several attacks a considerable degree of permanent immunity is attained. Some cross-immunity exists between dengue and other members of the B group of arboviruses, including the virus of yellow fever.

Clinical features. The incubation period is usually 5 to 6 days. The disease varies considerably in its severity. It may be mild or an illness with marked constitutional symptoms and signs lasting for 7 to 10 days. Subclinical infections are common. A prodrome of malaise and headache for 2 days may precede the acute onset, characterised by fever, generalised pains and intense backache. Painful movement of the eyes, photophobia, conjunctival injection and lachrymation, anorexia, nausea, vomiting, prostration, insomnia and depression are typical. In severe cases the temperature may remain elevated for 7 to 8 days. An afebrile interval lasting 24 to 48 hours may intervene at the end of the third day when symptoms subside temporarily, to be followed with a recurrence of symptoms and a further febrile period of a day or two ('saddleback fever'). There is bradycardia, cervical lymphadenopathy and leucopenia.

A scarlet, morbilliform rash may appear, especially during the second febrile period. It usually begins on the dorsum of the hands and feet and spreads up the arms and thighs to the trunk. After the temperature has fallen, depression and prostration often persist.

Dengue haemorrhagic fever occurs in S.E. Asia, rarely elsewhere. After 3 to 4 days of fever bleeding starts with petechiae, ecchymoses, epistaxis and melaena, and proceeds to acute circulatory failure. Even with treatment of these complications, 10% of patients die. Disseminated intravascular coagulation and complement activation which leads to vascular damage are thought to be triggered by hypersensitivity to the virus.

Diagnosis is usually easy in an endemic area when a patient has the characteristic symptoms and signs. However, mild cases may resemble other viral diseases and a severe attack may be mistaken for anicteric yellow fever, but the absence of urinary changes will help to differentiate it. The virus can be recovered from the blood and antibody titres rise.

Treatment and prevention. There is no specific treatment. The severe pains can be relieved by paracetamol, but occasionally opiates are required. Fluid replacement, blood trans-

fusions and corticosteroids are indicated in the haemorrhagic varieties.

The patient is nursed under a mosquito net. Breeding places of *Aedes* mosquitoes should be abolished and the adults destroyed by insecticides. Vaccines against each serotype are being tested.

Rift Valley fever

This disease is caused by an arbovirus which normally infects sheep and goats in East and South Africa. It is usually conveyed by a culicine mosquito, especially *Culex pipiens*. Cattle and other domestic animals may act as amplifying hosts. Sporadic infections have followed direct contact with infected meat and from inhalation. In 1975 an outbreak occurred in South Africa with 12 cases of encephalitis, 4 fatal. Since 1977 there have been large outbreaks in Egypt with four clinical types characterised by: (1) uncomplicated fever resembling dengue, (2) retinal changes, (3) haemorrhages and jaundice and (4) meningo-encephalitis. Deaths occurred in the last two groups. There is no specific treatment.

Japanese B encephalitis

This arbovirus is transmitted to man by the bites of infected culicine mosquitoes which have fed on infected animals or birds, notably nestling herons. Pigs and other domestic animals are important sources of infection acting chiefly as amplifiers of the virus brought to them by mosquitoes. The virus is widespread in the Pacific Islands from Japan to Guam, in the Philippines, Taiwan, Borneo, Malaysia and Singapore and is spreading slowly west across the Indian subcontinent. Devastating epidemics, with a high mortality rate, have occurred. In endemic areas, serological surveys indicate a high incidence of subclinical infection and only sporadic cases may be encountered. Inflammatory and degenerative changes are found in the brain.

Clinical features. Many infections are subclinical but overt disease may occur at any age, although children are particularly susceptible. With the development of encephalitis the patient experiences a very severe headache, fever, often with rigors, and vomiting. The physical signs in severe cases are neck rigidity, dilated retinal veins, imperfectly reacting pupils, muscular twitching and tremors; and, in severe cases, cranial nerve palsies and coma. The cerebrospinal fluid is under raised pressure and an increase of cells and protein appears within several days. The acute illness may last from a few days to 2 weeks or longer and convalescence is prolonged. Persistent neurological damage is common. The mortality rate in overt disease varies from 15 to 40%.

The virus has only rarely been recovered from the blood or cerebrospinal fluid but in fatal cases may sometimes be obtained from the brain. A rise in antibody titre is the usual basis for diagnosis.

Treatment and prevention. There is no specific treatment. Skilled nursing for the patient in coma may be life-saving. The elimination of breeding places of the vector mosquitoes, the control of piggeries, and the use of insecticides, where practicable, should be instituted. A vaccine, made in Japan and available in Britain, is safe and effective.

DISEASES DUE TO CHLAMYDIAE

Chlamydiae cause psittacosis and ornithosis (p. 219), urethritis (p. 418), lymphogranuloma venereum (p. 419) and trachoma.

TRACHOMA

Trachoma is a specific communicable kerato-conjunctivitis caused by *C. trachomatis*. Transmission is usually by contact or from fomites in unhygienic surroundings. Some infections occur during birth from infected genital passages.

Vast numbers of people suffer from trachoma in the hot dry dusty areas of the subtropics and tropics but it is also present in Southern Europe, and among immigrants in Britain. The disease varies markedly in incidence and in severity in different geographical areas. In endemic areas the disease is commonest in children.

Pathology. The infection lasts for years, may be latent over long periods and may recrudesce. The conjunctiva of the upper lid is first affected with combined vascularisation and cellular infiltration; pannus, spreading to the cornea causes opacity and impairment of vision.

Clinical features. The onset is usually insidious and infection may not be apparent to the patient. Early symptoms include conjunctival irritation, and blepharospasm, but the problem may not be detected until vision begins to fail. Trachoma may also present as an acute ophthalmia neonatorum.

The early follicles of trachoma are characteristic, but clinical differentiation from conjunctivitis due to other viruses may be difficult at this stage. Scarring of the lids causes entropion. Intracellular inclusions may be demonstrated in conjunctival scrapings by staining with iodine or immunofluorescence. Chlamydia may be isolated in chick embryo or cell culture.

Treatment and prevention. Local ophthalmic ointment or oily drops of 1–3% tetracycline may be used twice daily for 3 months. In mass therapy in endemic areas such topical application twice daily for 3 to 6 consecutive days each month for 6 months has given good results. An oral sulphonamide daily for 3 weeks is a useful addition. Deformity and scarring of the lids, corneal opacities, ulceration and scarring require surgical treatment, after control of local infection.

Personal and family cleanliness should be improved. Proper care of the eyes of newborn and young children is essential. The finding of a case, particularly in a child, should lead to examination of the whole family. Population surveys should lead to discovery and treatment of asymptomatic infections. Trachoma clinics are required in areas of high endemicity.

DISEASES DUE TO RICKETTSIAE

Typhus fevers; rickettsialpox, trench fever; Q fever.
Rickettsiae are natural inhabitants of the cells of the intestinal canal of arthropods. Some species may parasitise higher mammals including man. Infection is usually conveyed to man through the skin from excreta of arthropods but the saliva of some biting vectors is infected. Transovarian infection in arthropods to the next generation occurs in ticks and mites, which serve as reservoirs as well as vectors of infection.

Pathological and clinical features. In man

rickettsiae multiply in vascular endothelial cells especially of capillaries, producing lesions in the skin, central nervous system, heart, lungs, kidneys and skeletal muscles. Endothelial proliferation, associated with a perivascular reaction (nodules of Fraenkel) may cause thromboses and small haemorrhages. In epidemic typhus the brain and in scrub typhus the cardiovascular system and lungs are particularly attacked.

The common clinical findings are fever, severe prostration, mental disturbance and often a rash. The rash in epidemic, endemic and scrub typhus is at first central, but in tick typhus it starts peripherally. In Q fever a sparse rash is occasionally seen.

An eschar is often found in tick and scrub typhus and in rickettsialpox, but not in epidemic and endemic typhus or in Q fever. An eschar is a necrotic sore, often scabbed, at the site of the bite and is due to vasculitis following immunological recognition of the inoculated organism. Regional lymph nodes often enlarge.

Diagnosis. The Weil-Felix reaction, which is the non-specific agglutination by the patient's serum of the strains of organisms Proteus OX 19 or OXK, helps in the differentiation of human infections (Table 19.2). A fourfold rise in titre is diagnostic.

Table 19.2 Weil-Felix reaction

Disease	Vector	Weil-Felix reaction	
		OX 19	OXK
Epidemic typhus	Louse	+ + +	negative
Endemic typhus	Flea from rat	+ + +	negative
Rocky Mountain spotted fever	Tick	+	negative
Other forms of tick typhus	Tick	+	variable
Scrub typhus	Larval mite	negative	+ + +
Q fever	None or tick	negative	negative
Rickettsialpox	Mite from mouse	negative	negative
Trench fever	Louse	negative	negative

Species-specific antibodies may be detected by complement fixation, microagglutination and fluorescence in specialised laboratories. Rickettsiae may be isolated from the blood in the first week of illness by intraperitoneal inoculation into male guinea-pigs, mice or voles.

TYPHUS FEVERS

There are epidemic (louse-borne), endemic (flea-borne), tick-borne and scrub (mite-borne) typhus fevers.

Epidemic typhus fever

Louse-borne or epidemic typhus is caused by *R. prowazeki* and is transmitted by infected faeces from the human body louse, *Pediculus humanus* usually through scratching the skin, or sometimes by inhalation. Patients suffering from epidemic typhus infect the lice which leave when the patient is febrile. In conditions of overcrowding the disease spreads rapidly. During interepidemic periods the disease may be maintained by inapparent or latent cases or perhaps by infected fleas and rats. The disease is prevalent in parts of Africa especially Ethiopia and Rwanda, the South American Andes and Afghanistan. Large epidemics have occurred in Europe, usually as a result of war.

Clinical features. The incubation period is usually 12 to 14 days. There may be a few days of malaise but the onset is more often sudden with rigors, fever, frontal headaches, pains in the back and limbs, constipation and bronchitis. The face is flushed and cyanotic, eyes congested, and the patient soon becomes dull and confused.

The rash appears on the fourth to the sixth day and often resembles measles. In its early stages it disappears on pressure but soon becomes petechial with subcutaneous mottling. It appears first on the anterior folds of the axillae, sides of the abdomen or back of hands, then on the trunk and forearms. The neck and face are seldom affected.

During the second week symptoms increase in severity. Sores collect on the lips, and the tongue, dry and brown, becomes shrunken and tremulous. The spleen is palpable, the pulse feeble and the patient stuporous and delirious. If the patient recovers, the temperature falls rapidly at the end of the second week and convalescence ensues. In fatal cases the patient usually dies in the second week from general toxaemia, cardiac or renal failure or pneumonia.

Common complications are bronchopneumonia, parotitis, venous thrombosis and gangrene of fingers, toes, nose or genitalia. In endemic areas indigenous people may suffer relatively mildly. A mild relapse (Brill's disease) may occur after many years.

Diagnosis and treatment. The clinical features are diagnostic when there is an epidemic of the disease but in mild cases may be less distinctive. Laboratory aids to diagnosis are discussed on page 738 and treatment on page 740.

Endemic typhus fever

Flea-borne or 'endemic' typhus caused by *R. mooseri* is endemic world-wide. Man is infected when, by scratching, he introduces the faeces or contents of a crushed flea which has fed on an infected rat. The incubation period is 8 to 14 days. The symptoms resemble those of a mild louse-borne typhus. The rash may be scanty and transient. Laboratory aids to diagnosis are discussed on page 738 and treatment on page 740.

Tick-borne typhus fevers

1. Rocky Mountain spotted fever

The causal organism, *R. rickettsi* is transmitted by the bite of hard (*Ixodid*) ticks which carry the infection to rodents and dogs and on occasion to man. It is widely distributed and increasing in western and south-eastern states of the USA and also in South America. The pathological changes are similar to those in epidemic typhus. Haemorrhages and gangrene of the genitalia, ears and digits are more common.

Clinical features. The incubation period is about 7 days. There may be an eschar at the site of the bite, with enlargement of the regional lymph nodes. Symptoms closely resemble those of louse-borne typhus. The rash appears about the third or fourth day, at first like measles, but in a few hours the typical maculopapular eruption develops. Each day it becomes more distinct and papular and finally petechial. The rash first appears on the wrists, forearms and ankles, spreads in 24 to 48 hours to the back, limbs and chest and lastly to the abdomen where it is least pronounced. The fully developed rash often affects also the palms, soles and face. Petechiae may appear in crops. Cutaneous and subcutaneous haemorrhages of considerable size may appear in severe cases. The liver and spleen become palpable. Complications are as in louse-borne typhus. Untreated, the course of the disease may be mild or rapidly fatal.

Diagnosis and treatment. There may be a history of a bite by a tick. The character of the rash, appearing first at the periphery, is helpful. Laboratory aids to diagnosis are discussed on page 738 and treatment on page 740. Detection of organisms by immunofluorescence in frozen sections of skin biopsies is quick and efficient.

2. Other forms of tick-borne typhus fever

The causal agents of African tick-borne typhus are *R. conori* and a substrain *R. conori pijperi*. They cause typhus in South and East Africa, the reservoir hosts being dogs and rodents. 'Fièvre boutonneuse' of the Mediterranean is similar, as is also the infection in Queensland where *R. australis* is the causal organism. Infected hard ticks may be picked up by walking on grasslands, or dogs may bring the ticks into the house. An eschar and lymphadenitis are usual. A maculopapular rash may cover the trunk and limbs and affect the palms and soles but may be scanty. There are no haemorrhages into the skin. There may be delirium and meningeal signs in severe infections but recovery is the rule except in the debilitated.

Scrub typhus fever

Mite-borne or 'scrub' typhus is caused by *R. tsutsugamushi* transmitted by the bite of infective larval trombiculid mites. It occurs in the Far East, Assam, Burma, Pakistan, Bangladesh, India, Indonesia, S. Pacific Islands and Queensland.

Pathological and clinical features. The pathology is similar to that of louse-borne typhus, but lesions in the lungs are more prominent. In most cases one or more eschars develop, surrounded by an area of cellulitis and enlargement of regional lymph nodes.

The incubation period is about 9 days. The onset of symptoms is usually sudden with headache, often retro-orbital, fever, malaise, weakness and cough. In severe cases the general symptoms increase, with apathy and prostration. An erythematous maculopapular rash often appears on about the fifth to the seventh day and spreads to the trunk, face and limbs including the palms and soles with generalised painless lymphadenopathy. The rash fades by the fourteenth day. The temperature rises rapidly and continues as a remittent fever with sweating until it falls by lysis about the twelfth to the eighteenth day. In severe cases the patient is prostrate with cough, pneumonia, confusion and deafness. Cardiac failure, renal failure and haemorrhage may develop. Convalescence is often slow and tachycardia may persist for some weeks. Mild subclinical cases are common.

Diagnosis and treatment. In endemic areas diagnosis is often possible on the clinical findings. Laboratory aids to diagnosis are discussed on page 738 and treatment below.

OTHER RICKETTSIAL DISEASES

Rickettsialpox is due to *R. akari*, transmitted from the domestic mouse by a mite. It appears to be restricted to New York and Philadelphia where mice are now adapted to live in communal rubbish chutes of apartment houses.

The illness starts with a papule, which develops into an eschar, and is followed a week later by the sudden onset of fever, sweating, backache and a rash, maculopapular at first but which soon vesiculates and crusts, healing without scarring.

Trench fever is caused by *R. quintana* and is spread to man by louse faeces. It was prevalent in the First World War among troops in the trenches and again in the Second World War in the USSR. The disease is otherwise rare.

The incubation period is 10 to 20 days. The onset is sudden with headache, severe pains in trunk and limbs. The temperature rises sharply and remains raised for 5 to 7 days. The initial illness is like a mild case of typhus fever but febrile relapses are common, usually at intervals of 5 to 6 days and may be debilitating.

Treatment of the rickettsial diseases. The various fevers due to rickettsiae vary greatly in severity but respond to tetracycline or chloramphenicol. Tetracycline is given in a dose of 500 mg 4 times daily. The fever usually settles within 2 or 3 days. As there is a tendency to relapse tetracycline should be continued for 2–3

days after the patient is afebrile. In endemic areas good results have been obtained in louse-borne typhus and scrub typhus by a single dose of 100 mg doxycycline.

Patients suffering from louse- or flea-borne typhus are a danger to others unless they have been disinfested. Nursing care is important, especially in epidemic typhus. Sedation may be required for delirium and blood transfusion for haemorrhage. Relapsing fever and typhoid are common intercurrent infections in epidemic typhus, and pneumonia in scrub typhus. They must be sought and treated. Convalescence is usually protracted especially in older people.

Prevention. For louse- and flea-borne typhus and in trench fever steps should be taken to get rid of all lice and fleas and their faeces. An insecticide powder can be insufflated into the undergarments of those at risk without their undressing; 5% carboryl or 0.5% malathion are replacing 2% gamma-benzene hexachloride and DDT to which lice are becoming resistant. Residual insecticide powder on floors and bedding kills hatching fleas. To prevent flea-borne typhus, food stores and granaries should be protected from rats. Rats and their fleas must be destroyed.

Attendants on patients with louse-borne typhus should wear protective clothing smeared with an insect repellent such as dimethylphthalate (DMP). The patient should be washed, and an insecticide applied all over, especially to the hairy parts. Clothing should be disinfested with insecticide in plastic bags, or sterilised in a domestic tumble drier or autoclaved.

To guard against tick-borne typhus, dogs should be regularly disinfested of ticks with forceps and should not be allowed to sleep in bedrooms. Protection of the legs when walking through grasslands may reduce the risk of picking up infected ticks. The early removal of ticks and cleansing the site of the bite are also important. Floors of log cabins in the USA should be creosoted annually.

Mite-borne typhus is acquired when man enters scrub country in endemic areas. Protection against the larval mite can be secured by wearing suitable clothing, the inside of which has been smeared once a week with a mite-repellent such as DMP. Mites can be destroyed by aerial spraying of infected areas with Aldrin or Dieldrin, repeated every 3 months.

Active immunisation. Those likely to be at risk can be protected by vaccines prepared from killed *R. prowazeki*, *R. mooseri* or *R. rickettsi* cultured in eggs. Three doses each of 1 ml should be given subcutaneously at intervals of 7 to 10 days and booster doses of 1 ml at 6-monthly intervals or yearly. No protective vaccine is available against mite-borne typhus.

Chemoprophylaxis. It is likely that doxycycline (100 mg/weekly) would protect those at risk.

Q FEVER

Q (Query) fever is caused by *Coxiella burnetii*, a rickettsia-like organism, which is widespread in nature and is highly resistant to drying. It is carried by many insects, ticks and animals, including cattle and sheep. The exact method of transmission of the organism to humans is unknown although air-borne spread is considered to be one important route and unpasteurised milk is another.

Clinical features. The incubation period of Q fever is from 7 to 14 days. The clinical features of the illness are protean ranging from subclinical infection to fatal encephalitis or endocarditis (p. 160). Acute Q fever usually starts like influenza with pyrexia followed by myalgia, headache and sweating. Many cases resolve without specific therapy. Some patients have a cough and radiological examination may reveal an atypical pneumonia. Less common features of Q fever include myocarditis, epidydimo-orchitis, hepatitis, iritis and osteomyelitis.

The diagnosis of Q fever should be especially considered in patients living in rural areas and those whose hobbies take them into the countryside. *C. burnetii* does not grow in the media used for routine blood cultures and it is therefore important to consider Q fever as a possible cause in patients with clinical evidence of endocarditis who have sterile blood cultures. The diagnosis of Q fever is confirmed by the detection of serum antibodies to the two polysaccharide antigens of *C. burnetii*; acute infection is confirmed by a fourfold rise in phase II antibody titres in paired specimens of blood taken at intervals of between 10 and 14 days. Phase I antibody titres rise more slowly than phase II and the persistence of both suggest chronic infection.

Treatment. *C. burnetii* is sensitive to the tetracyclines, clindamycin and chloramphenicol. Acute infections usually respond to one of the tetracyclines in a dose of 500 mg 4 times daily for 2–3 weeks. The treatment of chronic infections, especially if there is endocarditis, requires prolonged therapy with tetracycline plus clindamycin.

DISEASES DUE TO BACTERIA

Streptococcal infections; staphylococcal infections; diphtheria; tetanus; anthrax; meningococcal infections; gonococcal infection (p. 417); whooping cough; brucellosis; plague; tularaemia; melioidosis; salmonella infections (typhoid and paratyphoid fevers, food poisoning); campylobacter infection; bacillary dysentery; cholera; bartonellosis; leprosy; mycobacterial ulcer

STREPTOCOCCAL INFECTIONS

A numer of different streptococci cause disease in man. These include *Streptococcus pyogenes* (scarlet fever, impetigo and erysipelas), *Strep. faecalis* (pyelonephritis and endocarditis), *Strep. sanguis* (endocarditis), anaerobic streptococci (liver abscess and pulmonary infections) and Group B streptococci (neonatal infections). All can cause septicaemia which may be rapidly fatal. The present section describes infections caused by Group A haemolytic streptococci (*Strep. pyogenes*).

Haemolytic streptococcal infection results in features which vary with the invasiveness of the organism, its capacity to produce toxins, the site involved and the reaction of the host. If the resistance is low and the invasive properties of the haemolytic streptococcus are high, a rapidly spreading erysipelas, cellulitis, lymphangitis or bacteraemia, may result. The haemolytic streptococcus may produce a specific exotoxin causing a widespread punctate erythema. When the infection is associated with such a rash the syndrome is known as scarlet fever. The same type of streptococcus may produce in one person acute tonsillitis, in another scarlet fever and in a third erysipelas.

Scarlet fever

Although scarlet fever is at present a mild disease, it may not necessarily remain so, as fluctuations in its severity have been recorded for the past 300 years. The primary site of infection in scarlet fever is usually the pharnyx or the tonsils but the disease may follow haemolytic streptococcal infection in other sites, e.g. in the genital tract after childbirth or in wounds. It is transmitted by air-borne infection, or more rarely by milk or ice-cream contaminated by streptococci. The incubation period is about 2 to 4 days.

Clinical features. Scarlet fever occurs most commonly in children. It has a sudden onset and the more severe cases present with a sore throat, shivering, pyrexia, headache and vomiting. There is inflammation of the fauces; the tonsils are enlarged and may be covered with a follicular exudate. The exudate may be distinguished from the membrane seen in diphtheria by its yellow appearance and the ease with which it is wiped off. There is tender enlargement of the tonsillar lymph nodes. The rash, which usually appears first behind the ears on the second day, rapidly becomes a generalised punctate erythema. It is most intense in the flexures of the arms and legs. The face is not affected by the rash, though it is usually flushed due to fever, and the region round the mouth is pale. The tongue is initially furred but shows prominent red papillae. The rash fades in about 1 week and is succeeded by desquamation. A profuse growth of haemolytic streptococci can usually be obtained from a throat swab.

The complications are less common than formerly as a result of the mild form of the disease and the introduction of effective chemotherapy. Acute otitis media, cervical adenitis and sinusitis may occur. Rheumatic fever and glomerulonephritis are rare sequelae which develop 2 or 3 weeks after the onset of any haemolytic streptococcal infection.

Treatment and prevention. The treatment of scarlet fever is the same as for streptococcal sore throat. Most cases respond rapidly to phenoxymethylpenicillin (250 mg for children and 500 mg for adults t.i.d. for 7 days). An institutional epidemic calls for chemoprophylaxis with penicillin or erythromycin.

Erysipelas

Erysipelas is an acute haemolytic streptococcal infection of the skin, commoner in the elderly. The onset is abrupt with heat and pain in the infected skin together with a systemic upset. There is a rapidly spreading red patch of inflamed skin with underlying oedema of the subcutaneous tissues. The edge of the patch is palpably raised and clearly defined and the lymph nodes draining the area become enlarged and tender. As the oedema subsides vesicles and bullae appear in the central part of the affected area. The face is involved in at least 80% of all cases of erysipelas as a result of the spread of streptococci from the nose. Erysipelas is usually brought under control within 48 hours with penicillin; hence the prognosis is excellent for a disease which used to be very serious.

STAPHYLOCOCCAL INFECTIONS

Staphylococcus aureus is responsible for a wide variety of suppurative conditions such as infected lacerations, styes, boils, carbuncles, abscesses, osteomyelitis, pneumonia, endocarditis, umbilical cord sepsis, enterocolitis and bacteraemia with pyaemic abscesses. Many infections, particularly boils, carbuncles and abscesses, are due to autogenous infection as the organisms can be grown from the nasopharynx and skin of up to 30% of healthy persons. The staphylococcus is readily spread from these sites and from clothing to contaminate the dust in which it survives in the dry state for weeks or months. In hospital this organism is an important cause of wound infection, pneumonia and neonatal sepsis. Under suitable conditions it multiplies freely in food and milk to produce a heat-stable toxin which is an important cause of food poisoning (p. 751).

Staphylococcal endocarditis occurs in drug addicts and as a complication of septic thrombophlebitis associated with intravenous cannulae and lines. *Staphylococcus epidermidis* is a skin commensal organism which can cause serious infections in the immunosuppressed and in those with prosthetic heart valves and joint implants. Endocarditis due to this organism is particularly difficult to cure.

The *toxic shock syndrome* is a condition caused by the toxins of certain *Staph. aureus* strains and principally occurs in women using some types of tampon, the infection originating in the vagina and presenting with fever, rash and shock. The syndrome has also been described in men and women as a complication of staphylococcal infections of the skin, lungs and breasts.

Treatment. 90% of *Staph. aureus* strains are now resistant to penicillin which should be used only if the organism is known to be sensitive. If the illness is severe, treatment should be commenced with flucloxacillin (p. 40), unless the patient is known to be allergic to the penicillins when erythromycin (p. 44), fusidic acid (p. 44) or clindamycin (p. 44) should be given.

Staph. aureus strains resistant to all antibiotics except vancomycin (and sometimes also rifampicin) are causing outbreaks of hospital infection in many countries. Known as methicillin (or multiply) resistant *Staph. aureus* (MRSA), these organisms can cause serious and often fatal infections. Patients colonised by MRSA must be placed in isolation.

DIPHTHERIA

In many parts of the world diphtheria is still an important cause of illness. It is, however, very rare in Britain.

Infection with *Corynebacterium diphtheriae* occurs most commonly in the upper respiratory tract and sore throat is frequently the presenting feature. The disease is usually spread by droplet infection from cases or carriers. The organisms remain localised at the site of infection and the serious consequences result from the absorption of a soluble exotoxin which damages the heart muscle and the nervous system. The infection may occur rarely on the conjunctiva or the genital tract, or it may complicate wounds, abrasions or diseases of the skin.

The average incubation period is 2 to 4 days. Cases are isolated until cultures from six daily nose and throat swabs are negative.

Clinical features. The disease begins insidiously. The temperature is seldom much raised although tachycardia is usually marked. The diagnostic feature is the 'wash-leather' elevated membrane of variable extent on the tonsils with a well-defined edge and surrounded by a zone of inflammation. The membrane is firm and adherent. There may be swelling of the neck and tender enlargement of the lymph nodes. In the mildest infections, especially in the presence of a high degree of immunity, a membrane may never appear and the throat is merely slightly injected.

With anterior nasal infection there is also nasal discharge often tinged with blood. In laryngeal diphtheria there is a husky voice, a high-pitched cough, and a danger of respiratory obstruction which can be fatal if tracheostomy is not carried out. When the infection spreads towards the uvula, to the fauces and then to the nasopharynx, the patient is often gravely ill. The pulse is rapid and of poor volume and the blood pressure low. Death from acute circulatory failure may occur within the first 10 days. Those who survive the earlier toxaemia may later develop arrhythmias or cardiac failure. Electrocardiographic changes are common and are due to myocarditis. These are reversible and there is no permanent damage to the heart in those who survive.

Involvement of the nervous system sometimes occurs, and after tonsillar or pharyngeal diphtheria it usually commences with palatal palsy on about the tenth day of the illness. Paralysis of accommodation often follows and may be inferred from the patient's complaint of difficulty in reading small print. A week or two later, though somewhat rarely, weakness and paraesthaesia in the limbs due to polyneuritis may develop. Recovery from such neuritis is always ultimately complete.

Treatment. Upon making a clinical diagnosis of diphtheria, the case should be notified to the community medical authorities and sent urgently to a hospital for infectious diseases. Antitoxin should be injected intramuscularly without awaiting the report on a throat swab if the clinician considers that diphtheria is likely to be the cause of the illness. Delay increases the danger to the patient, because toxin, once fixed to the tissues, can no longer be neutralised by antitoxin. However, horse serum, in which antitoxin is contained, being a foreign protein, is liable to cause undesirable reactions. There may be an immediate anaphylactic reaction with dyspnoea, pallor and collapse or even death. Serum sickness, with fever, urticaria and joint pains may occur 7 to 12 days later. If there is a previous history of inoculation of horse serum, the symptoms commonly appear in 3 or 4 days. As anaphylaxis is potentially lethal, all patients must be asked whether they have ever had antiserum before and whether they suffer from any allergic disorder. In all cases a small test injection of serum should be given half an hour before the full dose.

When a reaction does occur after the test dose in an allergic subject, rapid desensitisation must be undertaken with extreme caution. An ampoule of 1/1000 adrenaline solution must be close at hand to deal with any immediate type of reaction (0.5–1.0 ml i.m.). An antihistamine is also given.

In a very severe case the risk of anaphylactic shock is outweighed by the mortal danger of diphtheritic toxaemia and up to 100 000 units of antitoxin should be injected intravenously if the test dose has not given rise to symptoms. For cases of moderate severity 16 000–32 000 units i.m. will suffice, and for mild cases 4000–8000 units.

Penicillin should be administered for 1 week to eliminate C. diphtheriae. Patients allergic to penicillin can be given erythromycin.

Prevention. Active immunisation should be given in accordance with the instructions on page 38.

If diphtheria occurs in a closed community, all close contacts should be given erythromycin which is more effective than penicillin in eradicating the organism in carriers. All contacts should also be advised to have active immunisation or a booster dose of toxoid.

TETANUS

This disease results from infection with *Clostridium tetani*, which exists as a commensal in the gut of man and domestic animals and is found in the soil. Infection enters the body through wounds, often trivial, such as those caused by a splinter, a nail in the boot or a garden fork or following septic infection such as a dirty abrasion. Tetanus is rare in Britain and occurs mostly in gardeners and farmers. By contrast the disease is common in many developing countries where dust contains spores derived from animal and human excreta. If childbirth takes place in an unhygienic environment *tetanus neonatorum* may result from infection of the umbilical stump or the mother may develop the disease.

In circumstances unfavourable to the growth of the organism, spores are formed and these may remain dormant for years in the soil. Spores germinate and bacilli multiply only in the anaerobic conditions which occur in areas of tissue necrosis or if the oxygen tension is low as a result of the presence of other organisms, particularly aerobic ones. The bacilli remain localised but produce an exotoxin with an affinity for motor nerve endings and motor nerve cells. Involvement of the former by direct spread causes local tetanus. The anterior horn cells are affected after the exotoxin has passed into the bloodstream and their involvement results in rigidity and convulsions. Symptoms first appear from 2 days to several weeks after injury — the shorter the incubation period, the more severe the attacks and the outcome may well be fatal with an incubation period of only a few days.

Clinical features. Much the most important early symptom is trismus — spasm of the masseter muscles which causes difficulty in opening the mouth and in masticating, hence the name, 'lockjaw'. This tonic rigidity spreads to involve the muscles of the face, neck and trunk. Contraction of the frontalis and the muscles at the angles of the mouth gives rise to the 'risus sardonicus'. There is rigidity of the muscles of the neck and trunk of varying degree. The back is usually slightly arched and there is a board-like abdominal wall.

In the more severe cases violent spasms lasting for a few seconds to 3 or 4 minutes occur spontaneously or may be induced by stimuli such as moving the patient, or making a noise. These convulsions are painful, exhausting and of very serious significance, especially if they appear soon after the onset of symptoms. They gradually increase in frequency and severity for about 1 week and the patient may die from exhaustion, asphyxia or aspiration pneumonia. In less severe cases convulsions may not commence for about a week after the first sign of rigidity and in very mild infections they may never appear. Autonomic involvement may cause cardiovascular complications such as hypertension.

Rarely the only manifestation of the disease may be *local tetanus* — stiffness or spasm of the muscles near the infected wound — and the prognosis is good if treatment is commenced at this stage.

The diagnosis is made on clinical grounds. It is rarely possible to isolate the infecting organism from the original locus of entry. Spasm of the masseters due to dental abscess, septic throat or other causes is painful, in contradistinction to tetanus. Conditions which can mimic tetanus include hysteria and phenothiazine overdosage.

Tetanus is still one of the major killers of adults, children and neonates in the tropics where the mortality rate can be nearly 100% in the newborn and around 40% in others.

Treatment. This should be begun as soon as possible. The essentials are as follows:

1. *Prevention of further absorption of toxin from the wound.* A single intravenous injection of immune serum containing 1000–3000 i.u. of antitoxin should be given immediately the diagnosis is suspected. Whenever possible human antitetanus globulin should be used. The wound requires to be thoroughly cleaned and drained if there is evidence of necrotic tissue, foreign body or sepsis. Surgery should not be undertaken until 1 hour after the injection of antitoxin. Metronidazole or benzylpenicillin should be administered.

2. *Control of spasms.* The patient should lie in a quiet room with subdued lighting and with the bedclothes supported by a cradle. All necessary manipulation of the patient should be done gently and with due warning, for unexpected stimuli are particularly liable to provoke spasms. Expert nursing, preferably in an intensive care unit, is of supreme importance.

In most cases spasms may be controlled by diazepam. In more serious cases curare should be given, but only when facilities for assisted respiration are available. The aim is to control spasms which are terrifying, exhausting and occasionally fatal.

3. *General measures.* Nutrition and fluids are of vital importance to enable the patient to survive an ordeal which may be prolonged. If oral treatment is impossible, intravenous feeding should be commenced without delay. Aspiration of bronchial secretions and antibiotic treatment of pneumonia may be necessary. It is vital that the patient should be repeatedly reassured that a complete recovery from this terrifying illness will be made.

Prevention. Active immunisation should be given (p. 38). Contaminated injuries must be treated by débridement. The immediate danger of tetanus can be greatly reduced by the injection of a dose of a long-acting preparation of penicillin followed by a 7-day course of oral penicillin. When the risk of tetanus is judged to be present, further protection may be given by a subcutaneous injection of 250 units of human tetanus antitoxin, and an intramuscular injection of toxoid which should be repeated 1 month and 6 months later. For those already protected only a booster dose of toxoid is required.

ANTHRAX

Anthrax is a disease of domestic animals which become infected by inhaling or ingesting spores of *Bacillus anthracis* passed in faeces. Grazing lands remain infective for years. In man anthrax is an occupational disease of farmers, butchers and dealers in hides, hair, wool and bone meal from endemic areas. Anthrax is endemic in communities where skins are used as sleeping mats, for clothing or for carrying water, and where diseased cattle are eaten. Inoculation of spores subcutaneously is more common than their spread by inhalation or ingestion.

Pathology. The primary lesion in man may be in the skin, nares, pharynx, larynx, lung or intestinal tract, from any of which sites the infection may spread to lymph nodes and lead to a bacteraemia and infection of spleen, lungs, meninges and brain. The microscopical changes are those of haemorrhagic inflammation with areas of necrosis and interstitial oedema. There is a neutrophil leucocytosis of the blood and infiltration in the tissues without abscess formation.

Clinical features. The incubation period is usually 1 to 3 days. A cutaneous lesion begins as an itching papule which enlarges and forms a vesicle filled with serosanguineous fluid surrounded by gross oedema—the 'malignant pustule'. The lesion is relatively painless and accompanied by slight enlargement of regional lymph nodes. The vesicle dries to form a thick black 'eschar' surrounded by blebs. Occasionally there are multiple lesions. In endemic areas patients may exhibit only slight constitutional symptoms and little oedema but in non-immune persons high fever, toxaemia and fatal septicaemia may develop.

When infected meat is eaten, an ulcer with much surrounding oedema may be seen in the pharynx or more commonly the infection causes a severe, fatal gastroenteritis. Older people may escape unscathed, presumably because of previously acquired immunity.

Those who acquire the infection by inhalation, 'wool-sorters' disease', may develop an acute laryngitis or a virulent haemorrhagic bronchopneumonia. Anthrax may also present as meningitis.

Diagnosis. The appearance of a cutaneous lesion and the environmental and occupational history should suggest the diagnosis. A stained smear of fluid taken from the edge of a malignant pustule demonstrates the organism, which may be confirmed in an atypical case by culture and pathogenicity tests in mice, rabbits or guinea-pigs. *B. anthracis* is also recoverable from laryngeal and pulmonary anthrax and from the CSF in meningitis. If a group of people who have feasted on an animal which has sickened and died are taken abruptly ill with fulminating gastroenteritis, anthrax should be suspected. *B. anthracis* may be cultured from the faeces. Post-mortem examination is dangerous and may spread the infection.

Treatment and prevention. Treatment is with penicillin. For mild cases 600 mg of procaine penicillin is given intramuscularly every 12 hours, but for severe cases up to 12 g of benzylpenicillin, intravenously may be necessary daily. The organism is also sensitive to sulphonamides, erythromycin, tetracycline, chloramphenicol and streptomycin.

The disease is controlled in cattle by slaughter and deep burial of the diseased animal and by vaccination of healthy animals at risk. Imports from endemic areas should be subject to strict control and sterilisation. Persons at risk through their occupation should be vaccinated.

MENINGOCOCCAL INFECTIONS

Infections caused by the Gram-negative diplococcus, *Neisseria meningitidis*, are serious and not infrequently fatal. In the Sudan savanna belt of Africa special climatic conditions predispose to annual outbreaks of 10 000 to 100 000 cases. Spread is by the air-borne route and epidemics occur, particularly in cramped living conditions or when the climate is hot and dry. The organism invades through the nasopharynx producing bacteraemia and usually also pyogenic meningitis. The meningococcus is the commonest cause of bacterial meningitis in Britain where an increasing proportion of meningococci have become sulphonamide-resistant; fortunately, all strains remain sensitive to penicillin.

Clinical features. The disease may present in a fulminating form with abrupt onset and prostration associated with shock and a widespread purpuric rash. The progression of the infection may be relentless even with specific therapy and the patient can die within hours of the first symptom. Disseminated intravascular coagulation (p. 551) can also occur in the course of meningococcal infections.

Meningitis (p. 638) is a much commoner presentation. Upper respiratory symptoms for 1 to 2 days are followed by fever, vomiting, headache and usually a petechial rash. This frequently starts with a few lesions on the buttocks spreading to involve limbs and trunk. The spots can remain petechial but occasionally large purpuric areas may form. The patient, often a child, is febrile and toxic, and signs of meningeal irritation are common. Convulsions may occur, especially in babies.

Chronic meningococcaemia is a rare condition in which the patient can be unwell for weeks or even months with recurrent fever, sweating, joint pains (p. 571) and transient rash.

Investigation. There is a polymorph leucocytosis. The CSF is turbid due to the presence of many neutrophils, the protein content is raised and the glucose reduced. Diagnosis is confirmed by culture of *N. meningitidis* from blood or CSF or by antigen detection (p. 639). Microscopic examination of CSF usually shows Gram-negative kidney-shaped diplococci in the polymorphs. However, in some cases, particularly if the patient has been treated with an antibiotic prior to admission to hospital, Gram stain and culture of CSF may be unhelpful and an early clinical diagnosis is therefore of the utmost importance in a disease which can be so rapidly fatal.

Treatment and prevention. Benzylpenicillin, given by intravenous injection, is the antibiotic of choice for meningococcal infection. The dosage used in meningitis is given on page 639. Treatment may also be required for shock (p. 48) or for disseminated intravascular coagulation (p. 551).

Close contacts of patients with meningococcal infections, especially children, should be given a 5 day course of tetracycline, or 2 days of rifampicin. Vaccines are available for the prevention of disease caused by meningococci of Groups A and C but not Group B which is the commonest serogroup isolated in many countries including Britain.

WHOOPING COUGH

Whooping cough (pertussis) is a highly infectious disease caused by *Bordetella pertussis*. It is spread by droplet infection. Clinical diagnosis in the early and most infectious stage is virtually impossible so that epidemics occur. The incubation period is 7 to 14 days. Whooping cough occurs at all ages but approximately 90% of cases are children under 5 years of age.

Clinical features. The first stage of whooping cough consists of a highly infectious upper respiratory catarrh lasting about 1 week during which conjunctivitis, rhinitis and an unproductive cough are present. The distinctive paroxysmal stage follows and is characterised by severe bouts of coughing. The number of such paroxysms in 24 hours varies from an occasional attack to 40 or 50 and they are more severe at night. Each paroxysm consists of a succession of short sharp coughs, gathering in speed and duration and ending in a deep inspiration during which the characteristic whoop may be heard. It may be absent in older children and in adults because the air passages are so much wider. The last paroxysm of a series frequently ends with vomiting. The paroxysmal stage lasts from 1 to several weeks and is followed by the stage of convalescence during which the cough becomes less frequent and the sputum less tenacious.

The most important complications of whooping cough are pneumonia and segmental or lobar collapse which may be followed by bronchiectasis. Fits may be induced by cerebral anoxia. Subconjunctival or periorbital haemorrhage, ulceration of the frenum of the tongue, and prolapse of the rectum are relatively unimportant results of the stress of coughing. Neonates are highly susceptible and the mortality is greatest in the first year of life.

The diagnosis of whooping cough is very difficult in the catarrhal stage when the disease is most infectious. It can be confirmed in the laboratory by the isolation of *Bordetella pertussis* taken from the posterior wall of the nasopharynx on small swabs passed along the floor of the nose. Examination of the blood shows a lymphocytosis which, however, may not develop until the disease is well established. The diagnosis is easy in the paroxysmal stage when the whoop has developed, but by this time the danger of transmission of infection has largely disappeared.

Treatment. Erythromycin may reduce the severity of the infection if given during the catarrhal stage. Antibiotics are of no value if the spasmodic stage has been reached and they should not be used unless secondary infection occurs. The milder case need not be kept in bed, and is better out of doors. A cough suppressant such as methadone may be helpful in controlling the severity of paroxysms. When the illness is of long duration and vomiting is frequent, skilled nursing will be required to maintain nutrition, especially in infants and young children. Feeds are usually accepted and retained if they are given immediately after the vomiting which frequently follows a paroxysm of coughing.

Prevention. Active immunisation (p. 38) can very rarely cause fits or neurological damage and adverse publicity regarding this had led to a marked decrease in the number of children who are immunised against the disease. However, the adverse effects of the vaccine have to be balanced against the risk of contracting a potentially serious disease, especially in young children. Many of the deaths from whooping cough occur in the first 3 months of life and hence very special care must be taken to avoid exposure of infants to the risk of contracting the disease.

BRUCELLOSIS

(Undulant fever; Malta fever; abortus fever)

Brucellosis is caused in Northern Europe by infection with *Brucella abortus* which is usually spread to man by the ingestion of raw milk from infected cattle. It is also an occupational hazard of veterinary surgeons, laboratory personnel and slaughterhouse workers. The infection has now been virtually eradicated from cattle in Britain. In Malta and many Middle East countries the disease is frequently due to *Br. melitensis* and is transmitted by infected goats or sheep. In the USA and the Far East *Br. suis* acquired from pigs may be the causative organism. The incubation period is about 3 weeks.

Clinical features. The disease commences as a bloodstream infection and the clinical manifestations are gradual in onset and variable. The symptoms in order of frequency are sweating, weakness, headache, anorexia, pain in limbs and back, rigors, and joint pains. The spleen may be palpable. The temperature characteristically shows undulations, during which febrile and afebrile periods alternate over periods of a week or so. In other cases the pyrexia may be continuous and sweating profuse. Arthritis, spondylitis, bursitis and osteomyelitis may occur (p. 572). Untreated, the disease may last for a few days or continue for many months, and in the latter case the patient often becomes extremely depressed. Neutropenia and lymphocytosis usually occur in the more severe cases.

Blood, cultivated under special conditions, usually yields the organism in acute cases. Brucella serology is unreliable: a fourfold rise in titre of agglutinating antibody may be diagnostic but cross reactions are common. Complement fixation

and radioimmunoassay are more useful, but seldom obtainable.

Treatment and prevention. Tetracycline 500 mg 6 hourly or co-trimoxazole 2 tablets twice a day for 4 weeks is usually effective. The addition of streptomycin, 1 g daily for the first 2 weeks, reduces the relapse site. The spread of brucellosis by milk is prevented by pasteurisation or boiling. Veterinary surgeons and others handling infected animals need to exercise scrupulous hygiene.

PLAGUE

Epidemics of plague, such as the Black Death, have attacked man since ancient times. Now, the disease is limited to rodents in the wild with occasional sporadic human cases or local outbreaks. The causative organism, *Yersinia pestis*, is a small Gram-negative bacillus. It is spread between rodents by their fleas and if domestic rats become infected then infected fleas may bite man. In the late stages of human plague *Y. pestis* may be expectorated and inter-human spread by droplets, 'pneumonic plague', may result. This can also be caused by the accidental inhalation of a laboratory culture or by hunters inhaling dust containing viable organisms from infected wild rodents or fleas. Recent outbreaks have predominantly been in Vietnam and East Africa with sporadic cases in USA and elsewhere.

Pathology. Organisms inoculated through the skin are phagocytosed and taken rapidly to the draining lymph nodes where they elicit a severe inflammatory response that may be haemorrhagic. If the infection is not contained, septicaemia ensues and necrotic, purulent or haemorrhagic lesions develop in many organs. Vascular damage and fluid loss may lead to oliguria and shock, and disseminated intravascular coagulation may result in widespread haemorrhage. Inhalation of *Y. pestis* causes alveolar damage and copious exudation.

Clinical features. The incubation period is short, 3 to 6 days, but less in pneumonic plague.

Bubonic plague. In this, the commonest form of the disease, the onset is usually sudden with a rigor, high fever, dry skin and severe headache. Soon aching and swelling at the site of the affected lymph nodes begin. The most common site of the bubo, made up of the swollen lymph nodes and surrounding tissue, is one groin. Some cases are relatively mild but in the majority toxaemia rapidly increases, with a rapid pulse, dilated heart and mental confusion. The spleen is usually palpable.

Septicaemic plague. Those not exhibiting a bubo usually deteriorate rapidly. Meningitis and pneumonia with expectoration of blood-stained sputum containing *Y. pestis* may complicate bubonic or septicaemic plague.

Pneumonic plague. The onset is very sudden with cough and dyspnoea. The patient soon expectorates copious blood-stained frothy, highly infective sputum, becomes cyanosed and dies. Radiographs of the lung show a lobar opacity.

Diagnosis. A report of deaths among rats should alert suspicion of an outbreak. Early diagnosis is urgent. An aspirate from a bubo, sputum, or the buffy coat is used to show the characteristic organism by staining with methylene blue, or by immunofluorescence. Blood, sputum and aspirate should be cultured. Plague is notifiable under the International Health Regulations.

Treatment. If the diagnosis is suspected on clinical and epidemiological grounds, treatment should be started as soon as, or even before, samples have been collected for laboratory diagnosis. Streptomycin should be given by intramuscular or intravenous injection every 6 or 12 hours, at a daily dose of 30 mg/kg for 10 days or tetracycline, 10 mg/kg every 6 hours orally or intravenously, is given for 10 days. Treatment may also be needed for acute circulatory failure, disseminated intravascular coagulation or hypoxia.

Prevention. This largely depends on preventing biting by fleas carrying plague. Rats should be controlled. Powders containing 1.5% Dieldrin or 2% Aldrin applied to floors and blown into rat holes kill all the fleas and remain active for 9 to 12 weeks. In endemic areas people should avoid handling and skinning wild animals.

A formalin-killed vaccine is available for those at occupational risk. Patients are isolated and attendants must wear gowns, masks and gloves. Contacts should be protected by tetracycline 2 g daily, or a sulphonamide 3 to 6 g daily for a week. Post-mortem examination is dangerous.

TULARAEMIA

Tularaemia is an infection due to *Francisella tularensis* transmitted to mammals and birds by the bites of infected blood-sucking flies and ticks. It is often seasonal. Man may be infected by ticks or accidentally in a laboratory or while skinning infected wild rabbits or hares. In Norway lemmings are another source. The micro-organisms enter through dermal abrasions, the conjunctiva or mouth. Contaminated water and infected meat are less common sources of human infection. The disease is found in the Americas, Japan, the USSR, and most European countries excluding Britain.

Pathological and clinical features. Focal areas of necrosis occur especially in lymph nodes, spleen, liver, kidneys and lungs. There may be cutaneous, oral or ophthalmic lesions when infection is by these routes. The commonest presentation is of a papule at the site of inoculation, which becomes swollen and painful and suppurates, causing an ulcer up to 2 cm in diameter. Regional lymph nodes become tender, enlarged and may suppurate. There may be a systemic illness with fever, often prolonged. Sometimes the conjunctiva is the site of entry, and is inflamed. Sometimes the presentation is only glandular.

Septicaemia is the rarest, but most severe form of the disease. There is a sudden onset of high fever, prostration, aching limbs, vomiting, diarrhoea and mental confusion. Pneumonia, pleurisy and pericarditis are serious complications.

The organism may be isolated with difficulty and danger by culture on special media or guinea-pig inoculation. An intradermal test using killed *F. tularensis* may be positive as early as the third day and positive agglutination and complement-fixation tests after 10 to 12 days.

Treatment and prevention. Streptomycin or gentamicin is the treatment of choice, though tetracycline (500 mg 6 hourly for 2 weeks) is also likely to be effective. Masks should be worn in the laboratory and gloves should be used when skinning rabbits and hares in endemic areas. Adequate cooking renders infected meat safe for eating.

MELIOIDOSIS

Melioidosis is caused by *Pseudomonas pseudomallei*, a micro-organism closely related to *Ps. mallei*, the cause of glanders, which is a rare disease of horses and grooms. *Ps. pseudomallei* is a saphrophyte found in puddles following recent rain. Infection is through abrasions of the skin. Diabetics and patients with severe burns are particularly susceptible. The disease is commonest in the Far East and S.E. Asia and occurs rarely in India, Africa, Australia and America.

Pathological and clinical features. A bacteraemia is followed by the formation of abscesses in the lungs, liver and spleen. There is high fever, prostration and sometimes diarrhoea with signs of pneumonia and enlargement of the liver and spleen. A chest radiograph resembles that of acute caseous tuberculosis. In more chronic forms multiple abscesses also recur in subcutaneous tissue and bone. Culture of blood, sputum or pus may yield *Ps. pseudomallei*. Except in fulminating infections, antibodies may be detected by indirect haemagglutination, direct agglutination, and complement-fixation tests.

Treatment. In acute cases prompt treatment, without waiting for cultural confirmation, with tetracycline 3 g daily and chloramphenicol 3 g daily, in divided doses, may be life-saving. Treatment is maintained for weeks or months until cavities have healed.

SALMONELLA INFECTIONS

There are approaching 2000 Salmonella serotypes. Most of these originate in animals, especially poultry, and are transmitted to man either directly or in food. The exception is *Salmonella typhi* which invariably has a human source. Salmonellae can cause:

1. Typhoid and paratyphoid fevers.
2. Food poisoning producing gastroenteritis, sometimes associated with septicaemia which may lead to metastatic abscesses or endocarditis.
3. An asymptomatic carrier state.

Typhoid and paratyphoid (enteric) fevers

In many countries where sanitation is primitive, typhoid and paratyphoid fevers, which are transmitted by the faecal-oral route, are an important cause of illness. Elsewhere they are relatively rare. Nevertheless, outbreaks occur from time to time and the infection may be contracted by persons travelling abroad.

Aetiology. The enteric fevers are caused by infection with *S. typhi* and *S. paratyphi A* and *B*. In Britain spread is usually by carriers, often food handlers, through the contamination of food, milk or water; infected shell fish are occasionally responsible for an outbreak. In carriers the bacilli may live in the gall bladder for months or years after clinical recovery and pass intermittently in the stools and less commonly in the urine. The incubation period of typhoid fever is about 10 to 14 days; that of paratyphoid is somewhat shorter.

Pathological and clinical features. After a few days of bacteraemia, the bacilli localise mainly in the lymphoid tissue of the small intestine. The typical lesion is in the Peyer's patches and follicles. These swell at first, then ulcerate and ultimately heal, but during this sequence they may perforate or bleed.

Typhoid fever. The onset may be insidious. The temperature rises in a stepladder fashion for 4 or 5 days. There is malaise, with increasing headache, drowsiness and aching in the limbs. Cough and epistaxis occur. Constipation may be present although in children diarrhoea and vomiting may be prominent early in the illness. The pulse is often slower than would be expected from the height of the temperature.

At the end of the first week the typical rash may appear on the upper abdomen and on the back as sparse slightly raised, rose-red spots which fade on pressure. It is usually visible only on white skin. About the seventh to tenth day the spleen becomes palpable. Often about this time constipation is succeeded by diarrhoea and abdominal distension with tenderness in the right iliac fossa. Bronchitis and delirium may develop. By the end of the second week the patient may be profoundly ill unless the disease is modified by antibiotic treatment. In the third week toxaemia increases and the patient may pass into coma and die.

Paratyphoid fever. The most common variety in Britain is due to *S. paratyphi B*. The course tends to be shorter and milder than that of typhoid fever but the onset is often more abrupt with acute enteritis. The rash may be more abundant and the intestinal complications less frequent.

Complications. Haemorrhage from or perforation of the ulcerated Peyer's patches may occur at the end of the second week or during the third week of the illness. Additional complications may involve almost any viscus or system as a result of the septicaemia present during the first week; these include cholecystitis, pneumonia, myocarditis, arthritis, osteomyelitis and meningitis.

Investigation. In the first week the diagnosis may be difficult as in this invasive stage with bacteraemia the symptoms are those of a generalised infection without localising features. A white blood count may be helpful as there is typically a leucopenia. In a suspected case, blood culture is the most important diagnostic method. The faeces will contain the organism more frequently during the second and third weeks. The Widal reaction detects antibodies to the causative organisms and can be useful in supporting a clinical diagnosis particularly when cultures are negative.

Treatment. The patient should be treated in bed and preferably in isolation. Special attention should be paid to the maintenance of nutrition and fluid intake, care of the mouth and the prevention of pressure sores. Scrupulous precautions must be taken against the spread of infection by the provision of special gowns and adequate washing facilities by the bedside.

Chloramphenicol should be given for 14 days initially in a dose of 1 g t.i.d. reducing to 500 mg 6 hourly. Co-trimoxazole (or amoxycillin) is an alternative to chloramphenicol in typhoid fever and is the drug of choice for paratyphoid fever. Pyrexia may persist for up to 5 days after the start of specific therapy. Even with effective chemotherapy there is still a danger of complications, of recrudescence of the disease and of the development of a carrier state. A second course of chemotherapy must be given in the event of a relapse and this usually produces good results. The chronic carrier should be treated for several weeks with co-trimoxazole, as chloramphenicol has proved ineffective; in some cases cholecystectomy may be necessary.

The treatment of haemorrhage is described on page 289. Prior to the introduction of chloramphenicol the treatment of perforation was by surgery, which carried a high mortality in the seriously ill. Such patients can be treated conservatively while chloramphenicol is continued, but advice from a surgeon should be sought as laparotomy may be indicated.

The patient should be considered as infective until six consecutive stools and urines are found to be negative on culture.

Prevention. Those who propose to travel to or live in countries where enteric infections are endemic should be inoculated with the monovalent typhoid vaccine (p. 802).

Food poisoning

Food poisoning includes a number of disorders, presenting with diarrhoea and vomiting, due to acute gastroenteritis developing up to 48 hours after the consumption of food or drink. It is customary not to include under this term the enteric fevers, dysenteries (p. 753) and cholera (p. 754) which are also spread by infected food and drink. In contrast to enteric fever which is relatively uncommon and cholera which has been almost unknown in Britain for the past 100 years, there is an increase in the reported incidence of bacterial food poisoning. Outbreaks affecting large numbers of persons occur in canteens, restaurants, hospitals and other institutions.

Food poisoning may also be due to intestinal allergy, e.g. to shell fish, or to children eating unripe fruit or other unsuitable foods. Rarely a poisonous substance may be eaten, e.g. *Amanita phalloides*, in mistake for a mushroom, or a chemical poison in food may be unwittingly consumed. Food which has been placed in a container previously used for holding a chemical poison may be contaminated. Placing acid fruit juices in cheap enamel or zinc vessels may result in the liberation of antimony or zinc.

Aetiology. Bacterial food poisoning is usually divided into the infective and toxic types.

INFECTIVE TYPE. The organisms mainly responsible are the Salmonella group and *Campylobacter jejuni*. Certain birds, rodents, cattle and less frequently reptiles, such as pet tortoises, are sources of Salmonellae. The domestic fowl is the commonest source and modern methods of poultry husbandry involving battery-rearing and deep-freezing of carcasses encourage the spread and transmission of infection.

Salmonella typhimurium is an important cause of food poisoning of the 'infective' type. Food may be contaminated with infected excreta of mice or rats, or the bacteria may be transferred by flies or by human carriers employed in the handling of food. The size of the infecting dose of bacteria bears a close relationship to the speed of onset of symptoms and to the severity of the illness. This indicates the dangers of bacterial multiplication which may take place when food is contaminated and thereafter remains warm for many hours or days. The types of food which are particularly likely to be affected are twice-cooked meat dishes, stews, soups, milk and synthetic cream. The danger of food poisoning is greatly reduced if such foods are kept in a refrigerator. Ducks tend to be carriers of salmonella organisms in the oviduct and alimentary tract, and ducks' eggs are not suitable for the preparation of lightly cooked foods.

Campylobacter jejuni is now the commonest bacterial cause of food poisoning in Britain. Sources of infection include poultry, dogs, water, and unpasteurised milk.

Bacillus cereus infection is a hazard of eating rice which has been cooked and then consumed at a later date. Infective gastroenteritis in adults may also be caused by viruses such as the *rotavirus* which is more commonly responsible for infantile gastroenteritis (p. 321).

TOXIN TYPE. Such poisoning is most commonly caused by the enterotoxin of *Staph. aureus*. This frequently originates from a food handler suffering from a septic lesion. Incubation at a suitable temperature leads to growth of the organism and production of toxin which is relatively heat resistant and may not be destroyed by cooking. Strains of *Clostridium welchii*, many of them relatively resistant to heat, may contaminate certain foods, particularly meat. Pre-cooking of stews and pies may not destroy all the spores and the keeping of such food will lead to the formation of heat-stable toxins which can give rise to gastro-enteritis, sometimes severe.

Clinical features. The simultaneous occurrence of symptoms in more than one member of a household or institution often simplifies diagnosis. The incubation period is a useful pointer to the aetiology. If vomiting starts within 30 minutes of the ingestion of suspected food, it is likely to be due to a chemical poison; if it arises 12 to 48 hours later, it is probably due to a salmonella or campylobacter infection. The incubation periods of staphylococcal and clostridial food poisoning are intermediate between these.

The principal symptoms are nausea, vomiting, diarrhoea and abdominal colic. Staphylococcal food poisoning may be associated only with vomiting while diarrhoea and abdominal pain are more prominent with *Cl. welchii* toxins. In severe cases there may be prostration, collapse and dehydration. In the chemical and toxin types of food poisoning the onset tends to be sudden and severe and the patient may rapidly become shocked. Recovery, however, usually occurs within 24 hours. In the infective type, symptoms develop more slowly and there is usually pyrexia and toxicity. The patient may be ill for several days. The stools are watery and offensive, and may contain blood and some mucus, in contrast to bacillary dysentery where there is also pus. Salmonella septicaemia may be associated with osteomyelitis, septic arthritis, endocarditis or meningitis.

Severe abdominal pain and blood in the stool are common in campylobacter infections. Rarely, septicaemia may complicate campylobacter gastroenteritis, and endocarditis has been reported. Campylobacter enteritis may be confused with ulcerative colitis and rectal biopsies can appear similar in both diseases.

Botulism is a rare form of bacterial food poisoning due to the ingestion of the toxin produced by *Cl. botulinum* in imperfectly treated tinned food or preserved fish contaminated with the organism. The clinical features differ from all other types of bacterial food poisoning and consist chiefly of vomiting and pareses of skeletal, ocular, pharyngeal and respiratory muscles. The mortality rate can be high.

Investigation. A specimen of the patient's stool or vomit together with the suspected food, if available, should be sent for culture. Campylobacter and organisms of the salmonella group can usually be readily isolated. In more severe cases blood should be sent for culture. Notification of salmonella infection and other types of food poisoning is compulsory in Britain.

Treatment. Most cases are mild and symptoms subside in a few days. Solid food should be withheld and the patient instructed to take fluids only. Fluid and electrolytes can usually be replaced orally, but special care is needed with young children. The solutions used in cholera are satisfactory (Table 19.3). Patients who are severely ill or dehydrated require intravenous fluid therapy. When acute symptoms cease, a semi-fluid low-roughage diet may be taken. Codeine phosphate or loperamide is useful in controlling diarrhoea.

Antibiotics should not be given routinely for acute diarrhoea and vomiting as they are ineffective and frequently exacerbate symptoms. If salmonella bacteraemia is suspected or confirmed, ampicillin, 1 g every 6 hours should be given by intramuscular or intravenous injection. Co-trimoxazole is a satisfactory alternative. Campylobacter enteritis is treated with erythromycin.

If the poisoning is thought to be due to a chemical or a poisonous food, the patient's stomach should be washed out with tepid water, using the technique described on page 705 and the stomach contents kept for analysis.

Prevention. In Salmonella food poisoning the carrier state persists on the average for about 14 days after infection but may be much longer. A reduction in the high incidence of food poisoning can best be achieved by improving the standards of personal hygiene, especially in those handling food, and by stressing the importance of hand-washing after using the lavatory. Low temperature storage is required for food which has to be kept for some hours or days before being consumed. It is essential to keep frozen poultry at room temperature for at least 12 hours before cooking or pathogens at the centre may survive unharmed.

DYSENTERY

Dysentery is an acute inflammation of the large intestine characterised by diarrhoea with blood and mucus in the stools. Its causes are bacillary or amoebic infection. The latter is described on page 775.

Bacillary dysentery

The bacilli belong to the genus *Shigella* of which there are three main pathogenic groups, *dysenteriae*, *flexneri* and *sonnei* the first two having numerous serotypes. In Britain the majority of cases of bacillary dysentery are caused by *Shigella sonnei* although in recent years there has been a significant increase in imported infections caused by *Sh. flexneri* whereas sonnei dysentery has decreased.

Epidemiology. Bacillary dysentery is endemic all over the world. It occurs in epidemic form wherever there is a crowded population with poor sanitation, and thus has been a constant accompaniment of wars and natural catastrophes. Spread may occur by contaminated food or flies but contact through unwashed hands after defecation is by far the most important factor. Hence the modern provision of handbasins, disposable towels and hot air driers goes a long way towards the prevention of the faecal-oral spread of disease. Outbreaks occur in mental hospitals, residential schools and other closed institutions. The disease is notifiable in Britain.

Pathology. There is inflammation of the large bowel which may involve the lower part of the small intestine. Sigmoidoscopy shows that the mucosa is red and swollen, the submucous veins are obscured and mucopus is seen on the surface. Bleeding points appear readily at the touch of the endoscope. Ulcers may form.

Clinical features. There is great variation in severity. Sonne infections may be so mild as to escape detection and the patient remains ambulant with a few loose stools and perhaps a little colic. Flexner infections are usually more severe while those due to dysenteriae may be fulminating and cause death within 48 hours.

In a moderately severe illness, the patient complains of diarrhoea, colicky abdominal pain and tenesmus. The stools are usually small, and after the first few evacuations, contain blood and purulent exudate with little faecal material. There is frequently fever, with dehydration and weakness if the diarrhoea persists. On examination there will be tenderness over the colon more easily elicited in the left iliac fossa. In sonne infection the patient may develop a febrile illness and diarrhoea may be mild or even absent; there is usually some headache and muscular aching. Arthritis or iritis may occasionally complicate bacillary dysentery as in Reiter's disease. Diagnosis depends on culture of faeces.

Treatment and prevention. Diarrhoea may be controlled by codeine or loperamide. A fluid or semifluid low-roughage diet should be given depending on the severity of the diarrhoea but if this is severe, formal replacement of water and electrolyte loss will be necessary (Table 19.3).

Bacillary dysentery is usually a self-limiting disease and antibiotics or sulphonamides are not indicated in most cases. In severe infections, especially those caused by dysenteriae or flexner strains, ampicillin 500 mg 6 hourly or trimethoprim two tablets twice daily should be given. In many countries including Britain the majority of shigellae are now sulphonamide-resistant.

The prevention of faecal contamination of food and milk, the isolation of patients, and the identification of carriers, are methods which are theoretically important but may be difficult to apply except in limited outbreaks. Hand washing is very important.

CHOLERA

Cholera is a severe acute gastrointestinal infection, caused by *Vibrio cholerae*. Its home is in the valleys of the Ganges and other great rivers of the Far East, where high humidity and population density have maintained the disease. In these valleys devastating epidemics have commenced, often following large religious festivals, and pandemics have spread throughout Asia and Europe even to North America. The present, seventh, pandemic began in 1961. Good hygiene has prevented its spread in Europe, but cholera is present in the Near East and Africa, where it has for the first time become endemic. The biotype of *V. cholerae*, El Tor, that is responsible for the pandemic, is more resistant than the classical vibrio, and amenable to more prolonged carriage following infection. In 1982 the classical vibrio began to re-establish itself in Bangladesh.

The organism is passed in stools, or vomit, of patients with cholera and the very much larger number of subclinical cases, who excrete it for a few days. Chronic carriage is rare. The organism survives up to 2 weeks in fresh water and 8 weeks in salt water. Transmission is normally through infected drinking water, though shell fish and contamination of food by flies and hands also occurs.

Pathology. Cholera vibrios multiply in the lumen of the small bowel and are noninvasive. They secrete a powerful exotoxin (enterotoxin) which stimulates the adenyl cyclase-adenosine monophosphate pathway of the mucosa, resulting in an outpouring of normal alkaline, small bowel fluid. Severe dehydration follows rapidly even though absorption of fluid by the bowel is hardly impaired. There may be acidosis and depletion of sodium and potassium with attendant complications, of which renal failure is the most important.

Clinical features. After an incubation period of a few hours to 5 days severe diarrhoea without pain or colic, followed by vomiting, begins suddenly. Fluid gushes effortlessly from the bowel and stomach. After the faecal contents of the gut have been evacuated the typical 'rice-water' material is passed. This consists of clear fluid with flecks of mucus. In severe cases an enormous quantity of fluid and electrolytes is rapidly lost. This soon leads to intense dehydration with agonising muscular cramps. The skin becomes cold, clammy and wrinkled and the eyes sunken. The blood pressure falls, the pulse becomes imperceptible, and the urine output falls. The patient, however, usually remains mentally clear. Unless fluid and electrolytes are replaced the patient may die from acute circulatory failure within a few hours. With proper treatment, however, improvement is rapid. Rarely anuria persists and may lead to death.

Although this is the classical picture of cholera, the majority of infections cause only a mild illness with slight diarrhoea. Occasionally a very intense illness, 'cholera sicca', occurs in which the patient is overwhelmed by the infection and the rapid loss of fluid into the dilated bowel kills the patient before typical gastrointestinal symptoms appear.

In children under 12 years the mortality rate is higher (15 to 17%) than in adults (4 to 6%). In paediatric practice adverse factors are water retention and pulmonary oedema from overtreatment, febrile reactions to therapy, pyrexial convulsions and encephalopathy, tetany, meteorism, hypoglycaemia, hypernatraemia and acidosis.

Diagnosis. During a cholera epidemic clinical diagnosis is usually easy. In other situations, it is important to confirm the diagnosis bacteriologically so that an outbreak may be brought rapidly under control. *V. cholerae* has a characteristic movement that can be seen under the microscope. Culture of the stool or a rectal swab is used to isolate and identify the organism. Other diseases such as acute bacillary dysentery, viral enteritis, *P. falciparum* malaria, food poisoning, including *Vibrio parahaemolyticus* infections from eating infected shell fish and certain chemical poisons may produce symptoms like those of cholera. Cholera is notifiable under the International Health Regulations.

Treatment. The chief aim is to maintain the circulation by replacement of water and electrolytes; the earlier this is started, the better the prognosis. A quick clinical assessment of the state of dehydration is made from the appearance of the patient, the pulse, blood pressure and skin turgor. In severe cases or when there is vomiting, fluids are given intravenously. A large needle is plunged into a large vein (the femoral can always be quickly found) and the fluid is run in as fast as possible until pulse and blood pressure return. The rest of the estimated deficit is replaced more slowly. If intravenous fluids or apparatus are unavailable, a nasogastric tube is passed and fluid is poured in remorselessly.

Vomiting usually stops once the patient is rehydrated and fluid should then be given orally every hour. Patients can be made to drink up to 500 ml hourly. The quantity of fluid required is calculated every 8 hours from the output of urine, stool, vomit and estimated insensible loss which may be as much as 5 litres in 24 hours in a hot humid climate. Total fluid requirements can be in excess of 50 litres over a period of 2 to 5 days. Accurate records are essential and are greatly facilitated by the use of a 'cholera cot' which has a reinforced hole under the patient's buttocks beneath which a graded bucket is placed. The ideal solutions are shown in Table 19.3.

Other satisfactory fluids include Ringer lactate (BP) or Hartman's solution and Darrow's solution, in which case supplements of potassium are given as 10 mmol/l of intravenous fluid or 2–4 g potassium chloride or citrate three times daily by mouth. Isotonic saline is better than nothing but every 2 litres should be alternated with 1 litre of isotonic sodium lactate (18.7 g/l) or bicarbonate (14 g/l) and added potassium. Acetate is a satisfactory substitute for bicarbonate, and more stable. The presence of glucose in the oral fluid has been shown to promote electrolyte absorption. Chlorpromazine, 50 mg 6 hourly, reduces intestinal secretion and fluid loss.

The use of correct fluids for replacement has done away with the need for estimation of plasma electrolytes or specific gravity. In children, the elderly, the anaemic and those with underlying heart disease overvigorous intravenous rehydration readily causes pulmonary oedema. Children require most careful attention to fluid balance. Ringer lactate is the fluid of choice. They are prone to hypoglycaemia. Any deterioration despite adequate rehydration is an indication for a bolus infusion of 25% glucose, 4 ml/kg and maintenance with 10 mg/kg/h. Renal failure is managed in the usual way (p. 401).

Three days' treatment with tetracycline 250 mg 6 hourly or co-trimoxazole one tablet daily reduces the duration of excretion of vibrios and the total volume of fluid needed for replacement.

Table 19.3 Ideal solutions for treatment of cholera.

Intravenous	g/l	mmol/l	Oral	g/l
Sodium chloride	5	Na 133	Commercial salt	3.5
		Cl 98	(NaCl)	
Potassium chloride	1	K 13	Potassium chloride	1.5
			or citrate	2.7
Sodium bicarbonate	4	HCO₃ 48	Sodium bicarbonate	2.5
			Glucose	20

Prevention and control. Personal prophylaxis means strict personal hygiene. Water for drinking should come from a clean piped supply or be boiled. Flies must not be allowed access to food. Vaccination with a killed suspension of *V. cholerae*. may provide some protection (p. 802).

In an epidemic, control of water sources and of population movement and public education are most important. Mass vaccination with a single dose of vaccine and mass treatment with tetracycline are valuable. Disinfection of infective discharges and soiled clothing and scrupulous hand washing by medical attendants reduces the danger of spread from treatment centres.

BARTONELLOSIS
(Carrión's disease; Oroya fever; Verruga peruana)

This disease is caused by *Bartonella bacilliformis*, transmitted by sandflies. It is prevalent in narrow hot valleys on the western slopes of the Andes at heights between 2000 and 10 000 ft (600–3000 m), in Peru, Ecuador, Bolivia, Colombia and Chile.

Clinical features. After an incubation period of 14 to 21 days fever and haemolysis develop suddenly, accompanied by pains in muscles and joints, nausea, vomiting and diarrhoea, delirium or coma. The spleen and liver are enlarged and tender. Bartonellae are present in large numbers in the erythrocytes and also in the endothelial cells lining small blood vessels. Untreated the mortality is over 90%. Secondary infection by salmonellae is a frequent cause of death.

Verruga peruana, the cutaneous form, usually follows 30 to 40 days later with crops of cherry-red haemangioma-like cutaneous nodules 2 to 10 mm in diameter. They are distributed peripherally on the head and limbs and occasionally on the mucosa of the mouth and pharynx and heal in 2 to 3 months.

Diagnosis is confirmed by the demonstration of bartonellae in the erythrocytes, blood cultures or skin lesions.

Treatment and prevention. In the early febrile stage, penicillin, streptomycin or tetracycline for 5 days gives good results. Blood transfusions, fluids and electrolytes may be required. The use of insecticides, insect repellents and sleeping under fine mesh nets are advisable for personal protection.

LEPROSY

Leprosy is the commonest cause of peripheral neuritis in the world. It is a chronic granulomatous disease caused by *Mycobacterium leprae*, an acid- and alcohol-fast bacillus that has a very slow multiplication time of 12–14 days. It is one of the most seriously disabling and economically important diseases of the world and it is estimated that 20 million people are affected. *Myco. leprae* will grow in mice and the armadillo, but not in artificial media. Local multiplication of the organism in the foot-pads of mice is a most useful technique for demonstrating the identity and viability of *Myco. leprae* and the existence of drug-resistant strains, for the screening of drugs and for studying vaccines. The most important mode of spread of *Myco. leprae* is by droplets from the sneezes of lepromatous patients whose nasal mucosa is heavily infected. The organism may enter the body through the nasal mucosa or by inoculation through the skin. The incubation period is usually between 2 and 5 years.

The disease is common in tropical Asia, the Far East, tropical Africa, Central and South America, and in some Pacific Islands. It is still endemic in Southern Europe, North Africa and the Middle East.

Pathology. The organisms show a predilection for peripheral nerves, skin and mucosa of the upper respiratory tract. The response of the host to their presence varies widely. The early infection, usually transient and self-healing, is called 'indeterminate'. The histological appearances are non-specific. If the infection does not heal it develops into one of the determinate types, tuberculoid, lepromatous and borderline or dimorphous leprosy, whose features reflect the balance between the host cell-mediated immune response and bacillary multiplication (Fig. 19.1).

In *tuberculoid leprosy* there is a marked response, indicative of vigorous cell-mediated immunity, around nerves, sweat glands and hair follicles. Caseation does not occur except occasionally in a nerve. Organisms are scanty, and found mainly in the vicinity of terminal nerve endings in the dermis. They are seen only after prolonged search or by the use of concentration techniques. Tuberculoid leprosy is probably non-infective.

In *lepromatous leprosy*, the infective form of

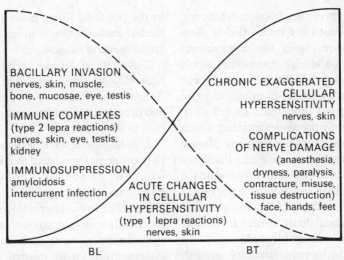

BACILLARY INVASION
nerves, skin, muscle,
bone, mucosae, eye, testis

IMMUNE COMPLEXES
(type 2 lepra reactions)
nerves, skin, eye, testis,
kidney

IMMUNOSUPPRESSION
amyloidosis
intercurrent infection

ACUTE CHANGES
IN CELLULAR
HYPERSENSITIVITY
(type 1 lepra reactions)
nerves, skin

CHRONIC EXAGGERATED
CELLULAR
HYPERSENSITIVITY
nerves, skin

COMPLICATIONS
OF NERVE DAMAGE
(anaesthesia,
dryness, paralysis,
contracture, misuse,
tissue destruction)
face, hands, feet

BL   BT

Fig. 19.1 Leprosy: mechanisms of damage and tissues affected. Mechanisms under the broken line are characteristic of disease near the lepromatous end of the spectrum and those under the solid line of the tuberculoid end. They overlap in the centre where, in addition, instability predisposes to type 1 lepra reactions. At the peak in the centre neither bacillary growth nor cell-mediated immunity has the upper hand. BL = borderline lepromatous; BT = borderline tuberculoid.
(From Bryceson A, Pfaltzgraff R E 1979 Leprosy, 2nd edn. Churchill Livingstone, Edinburgh.)

the disease, there is no cell-mediated immune response to *Myco. leprae*. Organisms are present in great abundance in the dermis, eventually replacing the normal architecture. They are mainly grouped in 'globi', which are large macrophages, often showing foamy degeneration, containing 50 or more organisms, and found in nerve tissue, the erectores pilorum muscles and the endothelial cells of blood vessels but rarely in the cells of the epidermis itself. They are carried in the bloodstream to the peripheral nerves, eye, and mucosa of the nose and upper respiratory tract, the testes and small muscles and bones of the hands, feet and face, in which they multiply. Nephritis and amyloidosis are common late complications.

Borderline or dimorphous leprosy. Between these two 'polar' types of leprosy, there is a spectrum of manifestations grouped under the terms 'borderline' or 'dimorphous'. The host reaction varies from the near-lepromatous to the near-tuberculoid. *Myco. leprae* are demonstrable in varying numbers. In the centre of the spectrum the disease is unstable. Immunity may diminish (downgrading) in untreated patients, especially in pregnancy or other times of stress and the disease becomes more lepromatous. Alternatively immunity may increase (upgrading or reversal),

especially in response to successful chemotherapy, and the disease becomes more tuberculoid.

Lepromin test. Lepromin is a suspension of dead *Myco. leprae*. The test is performed like the tuberculin test, but is read after 4 weeks. The result indicates the degree of cellular hypersensitivity in a patient. Positive reactions are obtained in tuberculoid leprosy, negative responses in lepromatous leprosy and negative or weak positive responses in borderline leprosy. This test is of no value in establishing the diagnosis of leprosy since positive results are also found in many normal people, but it is useful in helping to classify the disease, and so determine treatment and prognosis.

Lepra reactions. Any determinate form of leprosy may undergo an acute exacerbation or *reaction* which is caused by an episode of acute allergic inflammation. In lepromatous disease the reaction, *lepra reaction type 2*, is due to immune complex mediated vasculitis. In borderline and tuberculoid disease the reaction, *lepra reaction type 1*, is due to a sudden increase in cellular hypersensitivity. Borderline reactions are often associated with upgrading or downgrading.

Leprosy damages the body in three main ways:

1. Peripheral neuritis leads to loss of sensory, motor and autonomic functions. Sensory loss

permits trauma from pressure, friction, burns and cuts, the effects of which are intensified if there are abnormal pressures from the contractures following muscular paralysis. Autonomic nerve damage causes dry skin which cracks easily and heals slowly. Secondary bacterial infection in an anaesthetic, unprotected limb leads to cellulitis, osteomyelitis and gross tissue destruction which produces the deformities with which the disease is still, so unnecessarily, associated. Paralyses result in claw hand and dropped foot from damage respectively to the ulnar and peroneal nerves. A combination of fifth and seventh cranial nerve damage exposes an anaesthetic cornea to trauma and sepsis, so the eye is easily blinded.

2. In lepromatous leprosy bacillary growth insidiously damages the infiltrated organs and renders them liable to type 2 lepra reactions. Bones of hands and feet are easily fractured.

3. Acute lepra reactions may destroy nerves overnight, or cause severe eye damage.

Clinical features. The onset is usually gradual. The most common first symptom is a small but persistent area of impaired sensation or numbness. In other cases the first noticeable feature may be macules, which are usually hypopigmented and erythematous. The disease may also present acutely, in a lepra reaction, with neuritis, iritis or erythema nodosum leprosum.

The macule of *indeterminate leprosy* is an inconspicuous lesion 2 to 3 cm in diameter, situated anywhere on the body, exhibiting slight pigmentary and sensory changes. This lesion usually heals spontaneously.

Tuberculoid leprosy is characterised by one or a few solitary lesions in skin and peripheral nerves. Skin lesions are macular or raised as plaques or as rings whose flat centres indicate central healing. The lesion is hypopigmented in dark skins, coppery in pale skins, with a well-defined margin. Its surface is dry, often scaly, and usually anaesthetic unless the lesion is on the face. Lesions are of almost any size and occur anywhere on the body, especially on outer surfaces of arms, legs or buttocks. The nerve twig supplying the skin lesion or a large peripheral nerve at one of the sites of predilection may be enlarged, i.e. the ulnar nerve above the elbow, the median above the elbow or at the wrist, radial at the wrist, common peroneal in the popliteal fossa, posterior tibial around the medial malleolus, and great auricular across the sternomastoid muscle.

Tuberculoid leprosy tends spontaneously to heal slowly, often without residual disability. Sometimes its course is punctuated by a reaction and occasionally it downgrades into the borderline part of the spectrum.

Lepromatous lesions of the skin are described as they progress from early to late, as being macular, infiltrative or nodular. Lepromatous macules are numerous, hypopigmented and erythematous. They differ from tuberculoid macules in that they are small, widely scattered on the body, usually symmetrically, and with margins that merge imperceptibly with normal skin. Sensation in them is not impaired. They are often inconspicuous except to the trained eye. As the disease advances, the macular lesions become infiltrated and succulent; in advanced lepromatous leprosy nodular lesions appear, especially on the ears and face, and eyebrows are lost. A less common manifestation of lepromatous leprosy is diffuse symmetrical thickening of the skin, often with thickened brow and lobes of the ear, producing the 'leonine facies'.

Clinical evidence of nerve damage appears relatively late in lepromatous leprosy. Anaesthesia and anhidrosis are first detected in the dorsal aspects of the forearms and lower legs, later in a 'glove and stocking' distribution and eventually over the trunk and face, although the palms, soles, axillae and groins may be spared. Muscular weakness results from bacillary infiltration as well as from nerve damage.

The testes may be destroyed and gynaecomastia ensue. The mucous membranes of the nose, mouth and trachea may ulcerate; necrosis of the cartilage and bones may result in late deformities of the phalanges and of nose and oral cavity and loss of the upper incisor teeth. Adjacent lesions may spread into the eye but, more commonly, this is infected through the bloodstream. The most frequent lesions in the eye are miliary lepromata on the iris and superficial punctuate keratitis. Untreated lepromatous leprosy gradually gets worse.

Borderline or dimorphous leprosy may present with lesions intermediate in character between lepromatous and tuberculoid, or as a mixture of them. Skin lesions are often bizarre. The eyes and nose are spared. Nerve lesions are more numerous than in tuberculoid disease. In Asia, the majority of patients have borderline lepromatous leprosy. In Africa the majority have borderline tuberculoid leprosy. If the disease upgrades, nerve damage may increase with severe residual disability.If it downgrades the complications of extensive bacillary multiplication are added to those of widespread nerve damage. In either event the patient is liable to undergo reactions.

LEPRA REACTIONS. These may be defined as episodes of acute inflammation in pre-existing lesions of leprosy. Sometimes a reaction is the first clinical manifestation of the disease. One half of patients with lepromatous leprosy and one quarter with borderline lepromatous disease will be likely to suffer *type 2 lepra reactions* at some time during the course of their disease, most commonly in their second year of treatment. These reactions are characterised by fever and the appearance of crops of painful roseolar papules or nodules, called *erythema nodosum leprosum*, which may necrose and discharge sterile pus, before subsiding. In addition deeper subcutaneous nodules, iritis, orchitis, lymphadenitis, nerve pain and tenderness, and oedema of hands and feet may develop. Such reactions may threaten eyes and nerves and a succession of them may be extremely debilitating.

Type 1 lepra reactions are especially common in borderline tuberculoid patients. They occur spontaneously or may be precipitated by treatment. Skin and nerve lesions become acutely inflamed, painful and tender. Nerve function is rapidly lost, irretrievably so unless the reaction is promptly treated. Rarely lesions in the skin ulcerate and in nerves caseate.

Diagnosis. Lepromatous and borderline lepromatous disease ('multibacillary leprosy') is diagnosed by demonstration of *Myco. leprae* in material obtained by a slit skin smear. The skin is pinched between finger and thumb to expel blood, incised with the point of a scalpel and the exposed dermis scraped with the flat of the blade. The tissue juice obtained is smeared on a microscope slide and stained by a modified Ziehl-Neelsen's method. Smears are made from skin lesions, earlobes and dorsum of the ring or middle finger — sites in which bacilli multiply readily and persist. Nasal mucus may also contain the organisms in lepromatous leprosy and this is a good indication of infectivity. *Myco. leprae* are less readily demonstrable in skin smears in borderline tuberculoid disease and are undetectable in tuberculoid disease.

In borderline, and especially tuberculoid disease ('paucibacillary leprosy'), the cardinal signs of leprosy are enlarged nerves and anaesthesia. Nerves are usually enlarged at sites of predilection asymmetrically and irregularly; they may be tender. Loss or diminution of sensation, or misreference (the inability to locate accurately the site stimulated) may be detected in a skin lesion or in the distribution of a large peripheral nerve. Biopsy of skin or nerve is seldom necessary.

Treatment of leprosy is long and often complicated. The physician must gain the patient's confidence. The patient must understand the disease and its complications, comply and persevere in the treatment and learn to look after anaesthetic limbs, control fear and cope with any stigma that exists in the community. Admission to hospital for a few days is useful to establish rapport and start education.

SPECIFIC CHEMOTHERAPY. The essential features of the available drugs are given in Table 19.4.

Patients with multi-bacillary disease (lepromatous and borderline lepromatous) are preferably isolated until they are rendered non-infectious, which takes only a few days with rifampicin. Ideally treatment should be with three drugs, rifampicin, clofazimine and dapsone, to prevent the emergence of dapsone resistance. Rifampicin, the most expensive but most efficient bactericidal drug, need only be given monthly, because of the long generation time of *Myco. leprae*. It is most effective if given for two consecutive days in a daily dose of 600 mg, or 450 mg for patients under 35 kg in weight. Clofazimine is given in a dose of 50 mg daily, or 100 mg three times in the week (totalling 6 mg/kg/week for children). Dapsone is given in a dose of 2 mg/kg daily, not exceeding 100 mg. For mass treatment campaigns, when compliance is often poor, WHO recommends that rifampicin be given in a single supervised monthly

Table 19.4 Main features of drugs available to treat leprosy.

Drug	Dose (mg)	Peak serum level/MIC*	Duration of MIC: days	Bactericidal activity
Dapsone	100	100–500	4–12	+
Acedapsone	225	16	200	−
Rifampicin	600	30	1	+ + +
Clofazimine	100	(Stored in R.E. cells, possible depot)		?
Ethionamide	500	60	1	+ +
Thiacetazone	150	8	1	−

*MIC = minimum inhibitory concentration.

dose of 600 mg, and that a supervised monthly dose of clofazimine 300 mg be given in addition to the self-administered daily dose of clofazimine and dapsone. Treatment is continued for at least 2 years, preferably until bacilli can no longer be demonstrated in slit skin smears.

Patients with paucibacillary disease (indeterminate, tuberculoid and borderline tuberculoid) are treated with rifampicin once monthly and dapsone daily for 6 months.

The duration of treatment now recommended with triple therapy is much shorter than with the previous regimes using dapsone alone. Relapse rates are imperfectly known in many parts of the world. Patients should be followed up for 5 years.

Side-effects of dapsone are rare. They include psychosis, dermatitis and haemolytic anaemia. Should they occur the drug is temporarily withheld, and resumed at half the dose. Thiacetazone is a cheap reserve drug; it is weak, and cross-resistance may develop with the more useful ethionamide. Acedapsone is an injectable repository of dapsone that has sometimes been used in control schemes.

Secondary dapsone resistance occurs in up to 15% of lepromatous patients treated, often intermittently or in low dosage, for 10–20 years with dapsone alone. It presents as the re-emergence of solitary nodules or as a more generalised relapse. In the last 5 years primary dapsone resistance has been emerging as a new and increasing problem in several countries. Resistance is confirmed by mouse footpad inoculation, or by supervised full dose dapsone treatment. It is treated either by clofazimine alone, to which no resistance has yet appeared, or by combined treatment with daily ethionamide and rifampicin given on the first two days of each month. Clofazimine is a red-brown dye that gradually colours the skin and all bodily secretions and is therefore not always acceptable to a pale-skinned patient. It does, however, reduce the incidence of lepra reaction type 2. Doses in excess of those recommended may cause severe abdominal pain.

TREATMENT OF REACTIONS. *Type 1 lepra reactions*, in borderline or tuberculoid disease, causing pain or tenderness in nerves are treated with corticosteroids, such as prednisolone in a dose of 40–80 mg initially, followed by 20 mg daily for a few weeks until the inflammation is settling, then tailing off the drug over several months. Mild reactions, limited to skin lesions, are treated with aspirin 600 mg and chloroquine 150 mg base three times daily. Chemotherapy for leprosy is continued.

Type 2 lepra reactions in lepromatous patients respond rapidly to thalidomide in a dose of 100 mg four times daily. The dose is reduced slowly over weeks or months. This drug must never be given to premenopausal women because of its disastrous teratogenic effects. If thalidomide is contra-indicated or unavailable, other anti-inflammatory drugs are used; reactions threatening nerve damage or extensive skin ulceration or orchitis require prednisolone in an initial dose of 20–40 mg/d. Increasing the dose of clofazimine to 200 mg or 300 mg daily for a few weeks will help control the reaction and permit prednisolone to be reduced or withdrawn. Iritis is a dangerous complication and can usually be managed by local measures, namely the instillation of 1% hydrocortisone drops or ointment (or the subconjunctival injection of a depot preparation of methyl predniso-lone), and the twice daily instillation of 1%

atropine drops.

MANAGEMENT OF NERVE DAMAGE. In the event of acute paralysis complicating reactional neuritis, the affected limb is splinted and exercised passively each day until function begins to return when active exercises can be added. A patient with an anaesthetic limb must be taught to accept the limitations it imposes, to adjust life accordingly, to inspect that limb daily for trauma or infection and to learn how not to damage it.

Tarsorrhaphy helps protect an exposed anaesthetic cornea. Secondary sepsis is treated with appropriate antibiotics and osteomyelitis and its sequelae are managed in the most conservative manner possible. Patients with plantar ulcers are confined to bed, or given crutches or a walking plaster until healing is complete. Shoes must fit and protect anaesthetic feet against trauma and must be made specially if there is added deformity.

Prevention and control. In endemic areas the disease is commonest among intimate contacts of patients, and children and young adults are especially susceptible. *Myco. leprae* is easily spread and two-thirds of contacts undergo subclinical immunising infections within 2 years of regular exposure. Of the small proportion of contacts (about 1%) that develop clinical disease only about 2% will be lepromatous. It is at present impossible to identify this small group at risk and logical prophylaxis is impossible. No specific vaccine is available. BCG is of some value, especially in Africa, and should be given to all child contacts of lepromatous patients. Dapsone may be given for 2 years to infant contacts of lepromatous patients. Neither measure is a substitute for 6-monthly examination of contacts.

Mass prophylaxis is impossible, but mass treatment and follow-up of all cases identified during a population survey reduces deformity and lowers the incidence of leprosy. With improvement of socio-economic conditions the disease tends to disappear. The rapid spread of dapsone resistance poses a great problem to existing control schemes.

MYCOBACTERIAL ULCER

This condition, first accurately described in Australia and New Guinea, later named Buruli ulcer from its frequency in the Nile valley of Uganda, is caused by *Mycobacterium ulcerans*. The epidemiology is unknown. It begins as a single small subcutaneous nodule situated commonly on the leg or forearm. The skin over the centre of the nodule ulcerates and, untreated, the ulcer extends to involve a progressively larger area. Histologically there is much necrosis of subcutaneous fat and *Myco. ulcerans* are abundant in the necrotic tissue in the base of the ulcer.

If suspected before ulceration, the nodule should be excised and healing readily follows. Ulcers require to be excised and skin grafted. Antimycobacterial chemotherapy is disappointing.

DISEASES DUE TO SPIROCHAETES

Leptospirosis; syphilis (p. 415); yaws; endemic (non-venereal) syphilis; pinta; relapsing fevers; rat-bite fevers; tropical ulcer; cancrum oris; Lyme disease (p. 572).

LEPTOSPIROSIS

Although over 100 serotypes of leptospires have been identified only *Leptospira icterohaemorrhagiae* and *L. canicola* have been shown to cause human disease in Britain.

The natural host of *Weil's disease*, caused by *L. icterohaemorrhagiae*, is the rat and other rodents. Infected urine contains spirochaetes which can penetrate the skin or mucosa of man. Abbatoir and farm workers, veterinarians, and vagrants are most at risk. It has become uncommon in sewer workers, fish cleaners and miners because of better working conditions. Immersion in canals or stagnant water may result in sporadic infection. In patients dying from Weil's disease, there is a combination of hepatic, renal and cardiac failure.

Infection by *L. canicola*, which is contracted from dogs and pigs, usually presents as aseptic meningitis or pyrexia of unknown origin. It is not often associated with jaundice and is less severe than Weil's disease.

Clinical features. The average incubation period is 10 days, the range being 4 to 21 days. A high proportion of infections are subclinical or cause a mild undiagnosed fever. In the more severe infections the illness begins abruptly with headache, severe myalgia, pyrexia, conjunctival suffusion, anorexia and vomiting. Infrequently, there are rashes or petechiae and enlargement of the liver and spleen.

After about a week leptospiral antibodies appear in the blood. The temperature falls by lysis and is usually normal for 2 or 3 days. In the majority of patients, there is further pyrexia for a few days and transient meningism followed by prompt recovery. In other cases, especially those caused by *L. icterohaemorrhagiae*, during this phase, hepatitis, renal tubular necrosis, myocarditis and meningitis may occur. The condition may progress to acute liver necrosis. Renal tubular necrosis may lead to acute renal failure. Myocarditis is suggested by tachycardia, fall in blood pressure and cardiac enlargement. The development of profound hypotension, arrhythmias and cardiac failure are ominous signs. Meningitis causes severe headache, neck stiffness and a positive Kernig's sign and is the usual clinical picture in *L. canicola* infections.

By the third and fourth week of the illness, the majority of patients enter the convalescent phase. When there has been serious involvement of the liver, kidneys and heart, mortality in Weil's disease is in the region of 15 to 20%. Those who recover do so completely.

Investigation. Most patients with leptospirosis show a polymorphonuclear leucocytosis. When there is liver involvement, liver function tests indicate a mild hepatocellular jaundice with an intrahepatic obstructive element; bilirubin and urobilinogen are present in the urine. In patients with renal failure the urine contains protein, red blood cells and cellular and granular casts; in severe cases the rise in blood urea is progressive. Meningitis is characterised by an increase of lymphocytes in the cerebrospinal fluid with little or no rise in protein; xanthochromia may be observed in the jaundiced patient.

The diagnosis is made by culturing the organism from the blood in the first week or from the urine in the second and third weeks. Alternatively, blood or urine specimens may be inoculated into a guinea-pig. From the second week onwards, a rising titre of specific leptospiral antibodies is found. The titre may not reach diagnostic levels in those cases treated promptly.

Treatment. Leptospires are sensitive to penicillin in vitro. Benzylpenicillin, 600 mg 6 hourly for 7 days is effective provided it is given early enough and in adequate doses; it shortens the average illness and reduces the incidence of complications. Penicillin is of doubtful value if treatment is initiated late in the infection. Appropriate fluid replacement is important during the period of acute illness. In severely affected patients supportive treatment for acute liver necrosis, acute renal failure, arrhythmias and cardiac failure may be required.

YAWS

Yaws is a granulomatous disease mainly involving the skin and bones and caused by *Treponema pertenue*, morphologically indistinguishable from the causative organisms of syphilis and pinta. The three infections induce similar serological changes and possibly some degree of cross immunity. Organisms are transmitted by bodily contact from a patient with infectious yaws through minor abrasions of the skin of another person, usually a child. Infection is most likely to take place in huts at night when the temperature and humidity are high and families use communal sleeping mats. The mass campaigns by WHO in the 1950–1960 treated over 60 million people and eradicated yaws from many areas, but the disease has persisted patchily throughout the tropics and there has been a resurgence in the 1980s in West and Central Africa.

Pathology. At the site of the inoculation a proliferative granuloma develops containing numerous treponemes. This primary lesion is followed by eruptions, the most characteristic being multiple papillomatous lesions of the skin with a histology similar to the primary lesion. In addition there may be hypertrophic periosteal lesions of many bones with underlying cortical rarefaction. All these lesions of 'early yaws' heal without appreciable scarring or deformity unless there has been secondary infection. After a variable interval 'late yaws' may develop, characterised by destructive lesions which closely resemble the osteitis and gummas of tertiary syphilis and which heal with much scarring and deformity.

Clinical features. *Early yaws.* The incubation

period is 3 to 4 weeks. The primary lesion or 'mother yaw' is usually on the leg or buttocks. The secondary eruption usually follows a few weeks or months later, sometimes before the primary lesion has healed. The most typical are the 'papillomas', often very numerous, consisting of exuberant tissue covered with a whitish-yellow exudate, and more prolific in the moist flexures and around the mouth. There may be successive crops of lesions which are highly contagious. Sometimes a lesion erupts through the palm or sole, when walking becomes painful, 'wet crab yaws'. The bones of all the fingers distal to the carpus, except the terminal phalanges, particularly in children, may rarify and be surrounded by periosteal deposits. There may be a swelling of a long bone and also of the nasal bones (goundou). The distorted tibia may remain as the 'sabre tibia' but most of the lesions of early yaws will eventually subside, even if untreated.

Latent yaws. Following the spontaneous resolution of 'early yaws' serological changes may persist, to be followed by further manifestations of 'early yaws', or, after an interval of as much as 5 to 10 years, by the tertiary lesions of 'late yaws'.

Late yaws. Solitary or multiple nodular lesions develop. They ulcerate and spread superficially and also, in places, penetrate deeply into the underlying tissue. In this way gross disfigurement may be caused with distressing ulceration and deformity. The lesions tend to heal with scarring in one part while the ulcer is extending in another. Osteitis and periostitis present as localised swelling of bones over which tissue may ulcerate. Lesions in the hand, skull, nose and palate are common. Gross mutilation making the nose and mouth one open cavity ('gangosa') is one of the most tragic results still compatible with life. Other late lesions include hyperkeratosis with fissuring of the palms and soles 'dry crab yaws', hydrarthrosis, bursitis and juxta-articular nodules consisting of painless, firm, subcutaneous fibrous deposits about the elbows, hips and knees. Unlike tertiary syphilis, yaws does not affect the internal viscera or the cardiovascular and nervous systems.

Serological tests (VDRL, TPHA and FTA-ABS, p. 416) are positive.

Treatment and prevention. Lesions of early and late yaws respond rapidly to the intramuscular administration of 750 mg of procaine penicillin on two occasions at an interval of 1 week, or to tetracycline 1 to 2 g daily for 5 days. Early yaws heals completely but late yaws may leave deformity.

With improved housing and cleanliness the disease disappears. In few fields of medicine have chemotherapy and improved hygiene achieved such dramatic success as in the control of yaws.

ENDEMIC (NON-VENEREAL) SYPHILIS

In certain tropical countries, where lack of hygiene prevails, this treponematosis occurs as a family disease. The causative organisms are regarded as modified strains of *Treponema pallidum*, with which they are morphologically identical but biologically distinct.

Congenital infections are rare and sexual transmission unusual. The common mode of infection is through an abrasion, the disease being transmitted from one child to another and occasionally from a child to a parent. Sometimes it spreads in a closed community by the use of common drinking vessels and possibly mechanically by flies. The poor social conditions in which the disease prevails are similar to those where yaws is found but the clinical lesions resemble those of juvenile syphilis.

In contrast to venereal syphilis the primary lesion is rarely seen, except when a child has inoculated the nipple of the mother during suckling, in which case the lesion presents as an ulcerative papule without regional adenitis. The secondary and tertiary lesions include all the common types of skin, mucosal and bone manifestations of syphilis. Serological tests cross-react with venereal syphilis.

The disease responds to treatment by penicillin in the same way as venereal syphilis (p. 417). Prevention depends on the development of improved social and economic conditions and the mass treatment of affected communities.

Pinta

Pinta is a clinical and geographic variant of endemic syphilis caused by the related organism *Treponema carateum*. It is endemic in localised areas in Central and South America and in some West Indian and South Pacific Islands.

The incubation period is 14 to 20 days. There is a primary scaly papular lesion on an exposed part, usually the leg. The lesion enlarges slowly, up to 10 cm in diameter and is surrounded by smaller papules. Regional lymph nodes enlarge and like the primary lesion contain treponemes. The second stage is manifest 5 to 12 months later and consists of a generalised eruption of macules and miliary papules, 'pintids', pinkish and slightly scaly. Most of these heal but others coalesce and form hyperpigmented patches, commonly on the face and exposed parts. The secondary lesions may persist for years and may be accompanied by hyperkeratosis of palms and soles. In the tertiary stage the affected patches become atrophic and depigmented. In the secondary and tertiary stages there are serological changes closely resembling those of syphilis. Treatment is by a long-acting penicillin (p. 417).

THE RELAPSING FEVERS

The relapsing fevers are a group of diseases due to infections by spirochaetes of the genus *Borrelia* transmitted by body lice or soft (*Argasid*) ticks. The louse-borne *Borrelia recurrentis* infects only man and is not transmitted from a louse to its progeny. This disease appears in epidemics particularly during wars or famine when refugees are crowded together in conditions under which infestation with the human body-louse is frequent. It may accompany louse-borne typhus. The disease is endemic in Ethiopia from where recently recorded epidemics have probably arisen.

Species of *Borrelia* that cause tick-borne relapsing fever, are transmitted by various species of the genus *Ornithodoros*. Ticks live for years and once infected remain so for life and may convey the infection to the offspring. Tick-borne relapsing fever is thus an endemic disease.

Louse-borne relapsing fever

Lice cause itching. Borreliae are liberated from the infected louse when it is crushed during scratching which also inoculates the borreliae into the skin.

Pathology. The borreliae multiply in the blood, where they are abundant in the febrile phases, and invade most tissues, especially the liver, spleen and meninges. Hepatitis causing jaundice is frequent in severe infections and there may be petechial haemorrhages in the skin, mucous membranes and serous surfaces of internal organs. Thrombocytopenia is marked. The urine frequently contains protein and sometimes there is frank haematuria.

Clinical features. After an incubation period varying from 2 to 12 days there is a sudden onset of fever. The temperature rises to 39.5° to 40.5°C and is accompanied by a rapid pulse, headache, generalised aching, injected conjunctivae and frequently a petechial rash, epistaxis and herpes labialis. As the disease progresses, the liver and spleen frequently become tender and palpable and jaundice is common. There may be severe serosal and intestinal haemorrhage. Mental confusion and meningism may occur. The fever ends by crisis between the fourth and tenth day, often associated with profuse sweating, hypotension, circulatory and cardiac failure. There may be no further fever but, in a proportion of cases, after an afebrile period of about 7 days there may be one or more relapses which are usually milder and less prolonged. In the absence of specific treatment the mortality rate may be as high as 40%, especially among the elderly and malnourished.

The organisms are demonstrated in the blood during fever either by dark ground illumination of a wet film or by staining thick and thin films.

Treatment and prevention. The problems of treatment are to eradicate the infection and to minimise the severe Jarisch-Herxheimer reaction (p. 780) which inevitably follows successful chemotherapy and to prevent relapses. The safest treatment is with procaine penicillin 300 mg intramuscularly followed the next day by 0.5 g tetracycline. Tetracycline alone is effective and prevents relapse, but gives rise to a worse reaction. Doxycycline, 200 mg once by mouth, as an alternative to tetracycline has the advantage of being curative also for typhus, which often accompanies epidemics of relapsing fever.

Treatment is followed within a half to 3 hours by a chill or rigor, a brisk rise of temperature to 40–42°C, tachypnoea, tachycardia and often cough, confusion, distress, delirium and, occasionally, convulsions and coma. This phase is rapidly followed by profound hypotension and vasodilatation which may last from 8–12 hours and may be complicated by cardiac failure. The patient must be confined strictly to bed for 48 hours after treatment, carefully observed and managed as complications demand. Tepid sponging for fever over 41°C, careful attention to hydration, preferably by oral fluids, and prompt treatment of cardiac failure are required.

The patient, clothing and all contacts must be freed from lice as in epidemic typhus (p. 740).

Tick-borne relapsing fever

This disease is conveyed by a variety of soft ticks and its endemicity is governed by the presence of the vector. In the Mediterranean area *Ornithodoros tholozani* is responsible; in the Middle East, Iran, Afghanistan and India and in the New World there are other vectors. These ticks can become infected from rodents or bats as well as by congenital transmission and man is only an incidental host. In Central and East Africa, however, where *O. moubata* is the vector of *Borrelia duttoni*, man is probably the only important mammalian host. The disease in these areas is thus confined to old camp sites, old houses and their surroundings where *O. moubata* lives in dried mud floors and walls.

The pathological changes resemble those of louse-borne relapsing fever but with late neurological lesions.

Clinical features are similar to those of louse-borne relapsing fever. The febrile bouts, although severe, last usually only for 3 to 5 days, and the apyrexial periods may also be shorter. Relapses are, however, more frequent and may be as numerous as 10. Iritis and neurological complications, including cranial nerve palsies, optic atrophy, localised palsies and spastic paraplegia, may develop during these later relapses.

The methods used in diagnosis are similar to those for louse-borne relapsing fever. *Bor. duttoni* are, however, scantier in the peripheral blood but young mice are readily infected.

Treatment and prevention. As many strains are resistant to penicillin, tetracycline 1 g daily for 7 days is given and the course repeated after an interval of a week. Except for the Jarisch-Herxheimer reaction (p. 780), good results follow a single dose of 200 mg doxycycline. Ticks can be killed by lindane applied to the inside of the walls, floors and across the entrance to houses.

OTHER SPIROCHAETAL INFECTIONS

Rat-bite fevers

There are two rat-bite fevers, one caused by *Spirillum minus*, the other by *Streptobacillus moniliformis*. The latter, in addition to being transmitted by a rat-bite, has also occurred as an epidemic due to infected milk (Haverhill fever) and in other cases also there has been no known contact with rats or mice. Both infections are world-wide.

Pathological and clinical features. The manifestations of both fevers are very similar. In *Sp. minus* infection (Sodoku) the bite wound usually heals. After 5 to 21 days it suddenly becomes inflamed, indurated, purplish and painful; it may ulcerate and is accompanied by lymphangitis, regional lymphadenitis, leucocytosis, splenomegaly and fever. After a week the local and general reactions subside but recur after a further few days. Without treatment, periods of fever lasting 24 to 48 hours may recur for weeks and the patient becomes anaemic. A macular or maculopapular dusky red rash, sparse over the trunk and extremities, appears during the febrile phases.

In streptobacillus fever the incubation period is 1 to 5 days. The rat-bite usually heals well but occasionally an abscess forms. Regional lymphadenopathy is not marked. The general symptoms resemble those of *Sp. minus* infections but there is frequently painful arthritis and it is unusual to have recurrences of fever after the initial bout which lasts only 48 to 72 hours.

Diagnosis and treatment. *Sp. minus* can be demonstrated in the exudate from the inflamed bite or in fluid aspirated from a lymph node, either by examination under darkground illumination or by inoculation intraperitoneally into an uninfected mouse. Blood inoculated into mice or guinea-pigs will yield *Sp. minus* in the peritoneal fluid 5 to 14 days later. There are serological cross reactions with syphilis. In *Strep. moniliformis* infections agglutinating antibodies are demonstrable after

10 days. A titre of 1 in 80 or a rising titre is considered diagnostic but the serological tests for syphilis are negative. The organism can be recovered from the blood or, more easily, from an effusion into an inflamed joint. Both infections are readily cured by penicillin, streptomycin or tetracycline.

Tropical ulcer

Tropical ulcer is a specific infection with *Borrelia vincenti* and an anaerobic bacterium occurring especially in adolescent males. Minor injury in the presence of undernourishment, poor hygiene and debilitating disease are predisposing factors.

Clinical features. The initial lesion of a tropical ulcer is a bleb filled with sanguineous fluid. It may be painful and itchy with some constitutional upset. Soon the bleb ruptures, and a green-grey moist slough is exposed which rapidly spreads in the skin and subcutaneous tissue up to a diameter of 5 cm or more. In a few days these tissues slough and liquefy releasing an offensive discharge. After about a week there is usually no further spread and the necrotic tissue separates, exposing an ulcer.

In a chronic ulcer the edges are raised and slope sharply. The damage may be limited to the skin and superficial fascia, but in severe cases deep structures, e.g. tendons, nerves, blood vessels and periosteum, may be invaded. Bone is rarely involved. Tropical ulcers generally affect the parts of the body exposed to trauma, especially the lower third of the leg and the foot. The ulcer is usually solitary and heals slowly with a tissue-paper-like scar which breaks down easily. Big ulcers lead to scarring and deformity or fail to heal and may develop malignant changes after many years. General constitutional effects of a tropical ulcer are slight, and lymphadenitis is not found except as a result of secondary infection.

Treatment and prevention. Local treatment consists in thorough cleaning of the ulcer with hypertonic magnesium sulphate. Procaine penicillin 300 mg i.m., metronidazole 400 mg t.i.d., or tetracycline 2 g daily for 7 days gives good results. Chronic ulcers are excised and grafted. Ulcers over 5 cm diameter also need grafting.

Where tropical ulcers are a risk, abrasions should be cleansed and covered. The provision of a good diet, washing facilities and a first-aid service have abolished tropical ulcers from labour forces on well-run estates.

Cancrum oris

Cancrum oris is now rare except in poorly nourished children in the tropics. It is characteristically preceded by an infective illness, especially measles. The pathology is that of a rapidly developing gangrene, beginning inside the mouth and penetrating through the lips and cheek resulting in severe disfigurement. Untreated it frequently causes death. However, with or without treatment, gangrene becomes demarcated and ulceration follows. *Bor. vincenti* and an anaerobic bacterium are frequently found in the ulcer.

Penicillin or sulphonamides arrest the infection but do not prevent gangrene of already diseased tissue. Coexistent malnutrition, anaemia or dehydration should be corrected. Subsequently skilled plastic surgery may do much to overcome the hideous defects. Prevention depends on improved nutrition and hygiene in the community and on control of acute infectious diseases.

DISEASES DUE TO FUNGI (MYCOSES)

Dermatophytes; candidosis; pityriasis versicolor; mycetoma; zygomycosis; chromomycosis; rhinosporidiosis; sporotrichosis; histoplasmosis; coccidioidomycosis; paracoccidioidomycosis; blastomycosis; cryptococcosis.

Pathogenic fungi are ubiquitous; their importance varies between different parts of the world. Some fungi are opportunistic and will not normally invade unless the defence mechanisms are impaired, as in the immunocompromised host. Fungal infections are transmitted by spores or hyphae, and normally enter the body through the lungs or skin, where they may cause disease, or from where they may disseminate to other parts of the body. Fungal infections tend to be chronic, and often require prolonged chemotherapy. For some infections there is still no effective treatment. Fungi also cause disease through allergy (p. 241) and toxins such as ergot, muscarine and aflatoxin

(p. 720).

Fungal infections commonly present as skin disease, as subcutaneous swellings or as systemic infections.

CUTANEOUS FUNGAL INFECTIONS

An intact healthy skin is especially important in the tropics, where fungal infections are common. Extensive infections may impair sweating and heat loss, and cause misery through irritation. Scratching leads to secondary pyogenic infection.

Dermatophytes. This large group of fungi infect keratinised tissues and are responsible for ringworm of the body and scalp, 'dhobi's itch' in the inguinal folds, and infection of the hair and nails. *Trichophyton rubrum* is the commonest cause and most difficult to treat. Tinea imbricata *(T. concentricum)*, characterised by multiple concentric rings, causes widespread disabling infections in some Pacific Islands and in S.E. Asia. *T. schoenleinii* produces a mass of creamy white material, with an offensive odour, on the scalp, known as favus. Many dermatophytes are primarily parasites of domestic and farm animals. Dermatophytes are treated with topical antifungal ointments if mild, or if severe with griseofulvin 500 mg twice daily or ketoconazole 200–400 mg daily, by mouth.

Candidosis (moniliasis). A yeast, *Candida albicans* is the commonest fungus of medical importance. Infections of skin or nails may resemble those caused by dermatophytes. Infections of skin folds and on the buttocks of babies are common. Mucosal infection (thrush) is also frequent, especially in the mouth (p. 277), in diabetic women, on the vulvae (p. 483) and in hypocalcaemia, of the nails (p. 447). Chronic mucocutaneous or disseminated candidosis occurs in immunocompromised individuals. Superficial infections may respond to topical treatment with gentian violet or nystatin, but otherwise ketoconazole (p. 46) is given orally in a dose of 200–600 mg daily according to severity. Amphotericin (p. 769) is required for systemic infections.

Pityriasis versicolor is due to a yeast that causes a widespread very superficial infection, especially of the chest, back and upper arms.

SUBCUTANEOUS FUNGAL INFECTIONS

Mycetoma (madura foot)

Mycetoma, in this restricted sense, is a chronic fungal infection of the deep soft tissues and bones, most commonly of the limbs, but also of the abdominal or chest wall or head. It is produced by members of two groups of organisms classified as *Eumycetes* and aerobic *Actinomycetes*. A feature common to both groups is the formation of grains which are colonies of matted organisms with characteristic colours, ranging from 60 microns to 3 mm in diameter. The incidence appears to be related to climate, being especially high when an arid hot season ends in rains. The more common species of fungi causing mycetoma, as defined above, are shown in Table 19.5. The fungus can be identified by the microscopic appearances of the tissue and grains and confirmed by culture. Antibodies can usually be demonstrated by precipitation.

Table 19.5 Fungi causing mycetoma.

Species	Type of grains
Eumycetoma	
Madurella mycetomatis	Brown or black (big)
Madurella grisea	Black or brown (big)
Exophiala jeanselmei	Black
Petriellidium boydii	White or yellow (big)
Acremonium spp.	White or yellow
Actinomycetoma	
Actinomadura madurae	White, yellow, red (big)
Actinomadura pelletieri	Red (small)
Streptomyces somaliensis	White or yellow (big)
Nocardia brasiliensis	White, yellow (microscopic)

Pathological and clinical features. The lesions may occur in any part of the body but as the fungus is usually introduced by a thorn they are more common in the foot and leg in those who walk bare-footed. At the site of implantation the mycetoma begins as a painless swelling which grows and spreads inexorably within the soft tissues causing swelling and eventually penetrates bones.

The histology is that of a chronic granuloma with a fibrous stroma and cyst-like spaces in which lie the characteristic grains. Nodules develop under the epidermis and these rupture revealing sinuses through which mucopus containing the coloured grains is discharged. Some sinuses may heal with scarring while fresh sinuses appear elsewhere.

There is little pain and usually no fever, but progressive disability. Secondary pyogenic infection does not usually penetrate far down the sinuses, possibly because of antibiotic activity of the fungi. It is unusual for the fungus to reach the lymph nodes unless there has been surgical interference. When the lesion is in the scalp, the skull may be affected but the dura mater appears to be an effective barrier. Apart from involvement of bones by a spreading mycetoma, intraosseous lesions may be found in the metaphysis of a long bone, especially at the upper end of the tibia and sometimes there may be an encapsulated periosteal mass. *Nocardia brasiliensis* often affects the skin of the back. It is seldom localised and may spread widely.

Diagnosis is confirmed by demonstration of fungal grains in pus or tissue biopsy. Culture is usually necessary for species identification, although serology may be helpful.

Treatment. The difference between *Eumycetes* and *Actinomycetes* is crucial in that there is no drug of proven efficacy for the former. Sporadic successes with griseofulvin against *Eumycetes* have been reported, but the results have been mostly disappointing and eumycetoma requires to be excised. It has a strong tendency to recur.

The treatment of actinomycetoma is more hopeful. It consists of rifampicin (4 mg/kg/d by mouth) or streptomycin (14 mg/kg/d i.m.) for 3 months plus oral dapsone (1.5 mg/kg b.d.) or oral co-trimoxazole for 4–24 months. *Nocardia* infection may respond to dapsone alone. Precipitating antibodies disappear if treatment is successful.

Other subcutaneous mycoses

Zygomycosis (phycomycosis) is caused by one of several species of fungi. Subcutaneous swellings of the face or proximal limbs are the commonest presentations. Systemic infections are occasionally seen in immunocompromised or diabetic patients. Treatment is with potassium iodide 1.5–3.5 g daily or amphotericin (p. 769) according to the species of fungus.

Chromoblastomycosis is one of the causes of mossy foot. These pigmented fungi are acquired on splinters from decaying timber and give rise to a warty condition of the foot and also rarely affect the face, and upper limbs. The diagnosis is confirmed by the recognition of dark-brown spheroid bodies 4 to 8 microns in diameter in biopsy specimens or by culture. Treatment is oral flucytosine 30–50 mg/kg body weight 6 hourly for several months. Blood levels are monitored, especially when renal function is poor.

Rhinosporidiosis is caused by *Rhinosporidium seeberi* and occurs in South America, India, Sri Lanka, and East Africa. This organism forms a cyst which on rupture discharges spores which spread by lymphatics to connective tissue. It produces polypi in the nose and localised swellings on the cheek and elsewhere. The characteristic sporangia and spores are recognised histologically. The organism has not yet been cultured. Treatment is surgical.

Sporotrichosis is caused by *Sporothrix schenckii*. The infection occurs throughout the world and is prevalent in Central and Southern Africa. It causes swellings resembling a gumma or a chancroid type of ulcer. Affected lymphatic vessels may be thickened and palpable as a chain of nodules. Uncommonly dissemination takes place into lungs, bones, the central nervous system and elsewhere. The fungus can be cultured from discharges or biopsy material. Potassium iodide up to 10 g daily should be given orally until after apparent clinical cure. Widely disseminated infections respond to amphotericin.

SYSTEMIC FUNGAL INFECTIONS

Histoplasmosis

Histoplasmosis is caused by *Histoplasma capsulatum (Darling)* which is a yeast in its parasitic phase but is a filamentous fungus of soil at other times. A variant, *Histoplasma duboisii*, is found in parts of tropical Africa. The spores of *Histoplasma* remain viable for years in the soil and infection is by inhalation of infected dust. Occasionally infection passes through the buccal or intestinal mucosa or through the skin. The disease attacks dogs, rats and mice, and the fungus multiplies in soil enriched by the droppings of chickens, pigeons and bats. The infection is a hazard for explorers of caves.

Histoplasma capsulatum

This is found in all parts of the United States of America, especially in the East Central States, and less commonly in Latin America from Mexico to Argentina, in Europe, North, South and East Africa, Nigeria, Malaysia, Indonesia and Australia.

Pathological and clinical features. The parasite in its yeast phase multiplies mainly in monocytes and macrophages and produces areas of necrosis in which the parasites may abound. From these foci the bloodstream may be invaded leading to metastatic lesions in the liver, spleen and lymph nodes. Pulmonary histoplasmosis may produce pathological changes similar to those of tuberculosis.

Probably 90% of pulmonary infections are benign producing no symptoms, but more severe infections may closely simulate pulmonary tuberculosis, including the production of a primary complex with enlarged regional lymph nodes, multiple small discrete lesions and occasionally cavitation. Healed lesions may calcify. Lesions of the skin or mucosa may be found on the rare occasions when infection has entered that way.

Disseminated histoplasmosis is characterised by enlargement of the liver, spleen and lymph nodes, irregular pyrexia, anaemia and leucopenia. Addison's disease may be produced by caseation in the adrenals. When the mucosa of the mouth and gastrointestinal tract become infected, the predominant symptoms may be vomiting and diarrhoea. Occasionally the central nervous system is invaded. The severity of the symptoms of histoplasmosis varies from, in the majority of cases, a slight fever of short duration, like influenza, to a severe and prolonged pyrexial illness which ultimately proves fatal.

Diagnosis. In an area where the disease occurs, histoplasmosis should be suspected in every obscure infection in which there are pulmonary signs or where there are enlarged lymph nodes with or without hepatosplenomegaly. Tissue is obtained by biopsy for impression-smear, histology, culture and animal inoculation. Radiological examination in long-standing cases may show calcified lesions in the lungs, spleen or other organs. In the more acute phases of the disease single or multiple soft pulmonary shadows with enlarged tracheo-bronchial nodes may be seen.

Delayed hypersensitivity to the intradermal injection of histoplasmin develops in patients with either active or healed infections but is usually negative in the rapidly progressive form of the disease. Complement-fixing antibodies are detected within 3 weeks of the onset of an acute primary infection and increase in titre as the disease progresses. Precipitating antibodies may also be detected.

Treatment. Specific treatment with amphotericin is indicated only in severe infections. The dosage is 0.5 mg/kg, in 500 ml of 5% glucose given intravenously over a 6-hour period, gradually increasing to a maximum of 1.0 mg/kg. Treatment is given on alternate days. If badly tolerated, the dosage may have to be reduced. Side-effects are anorexia, nausea, fever, headache and venous thrombosis. These may be controlled by the addition of 10 mg prednisolone to the intravenous solution. Plasma urea rises and haemoglobin falls during treatment, but later return to normal. Amphotericin may have to be continued for up to 3 months or longer, depending on the clinical response. Recovery from generalised histoplasmosis is rare.

Histoplasma duboisii

Histoplasma duboisii, the fungus of African histoplasmosis, is considerably larger than the classical *H. capsulatum*. It is found throughout East, Central and West Africa.

This disease differs in several ways from *H. capsulatum* infection. The bones, skin, lymph nodes and liver develop granulomatous lesions or cold abscesses resembling tuberculosis, but the lungs are seldom involved. The visceral form with liver and splenic invasion is often fatal, while ulcerative skin lesions and bone abscesses follow a more benign course.

Radiological examination may show rounded foci of bone destruction sometimes associated with abscess formation. Multiple lesions of the ribs are common and the bones of the limbs may also be involved. Diagnosis is by isolation of the fungus. Immunodiagnostic tests are helpful.

The disease is treated in the same way as *H. capsulatum* infections. A solitary lesion in bone may require only local surgical treatment.

Other systemic mycoses

Aspergillosis is the most common respiratory mycosis in Britain and is discussed on page 233.

Coccidioidomycosis is caused by *Coccidioides immitis* and found in Southern United States, and in Central and South America. The disease is acquired by inhalation. In 40% of cases it affects the lungs, lymph nodes and skin. Rarely it may be carried by the bloodstream to the bones, adrenals, meninges and other organs. In 60% of cases the infection is asymptomatic. Infections, including subclinical attacks, are followed by immunity. The fungi grow readily on culture media but as they are highly infective, diagnostic investigations are usually limited to intradermal, complement-fixation and precipitin tests. Some localised pulmonary lesions can be treated by surgery. Amphotericin or ketoconazole may be beneficial.

Paracoccidiodomycosis is caused by *Paracoccicidiodes brasiliensis* and occurs in South America. Mucocutaneous lesions occur early. Involvement of lymphatic nodes and the lungs is prominent and the gastrointestinal tract may also be attacked. Most cases respond to ketoconazole (200 mg/d for at least 6 months, monitoring liver function). Otherwise sulphonamides or amphotericin may be used.

Blastomycosis. *North American blastomycosis* is caused by *Blastomyces dermatitidis*. It also occurs in Africa. Systemic infection begins in the lungs and mediastinal lymph nodes and resembles pulmonary tuberculosis. Bones, skin and the genito-urinary tract may also be affected. Treatment is with amphotericin (p. 769).

Cryptococcosis is caused by *Cryptococcus neoformans*. Its distribution is world-wide. It causes local gummatous-like tumours and granulomatous lesions of the lung, bones, brain and meninges. The cerebrospinal fluid often contains the fungus when the nervous system is affected. The diagnosis is made by culture or recognition of spores in the cerebrospinal fluid, biopsy and serological detection of antigen. Amphotericin should be given intravenously and flucytosine orally (p. 768). Surgical removal of local pulmonary lesions may be necessary. Recovery may be monitored by fall in antigen titre.

DISEASES DUE TO PROTOZOA

Malaria; amoebiasis; giardiasis; balantidiasis; leishmaniasis; trypanosomiasis; toxoplasmosis

MALARIA

Human malaria is caused by *Plasmodium falciparum, P. vivax, P. ovale* and *P. malariae*. It is transmitted by the bite of anopheline mosquitoes, in which the parasite undergoes a cycle of development which is temperature-dependent. Malaria is therefore predominantly a disease of hot wet climates, but it used to occur in Europe as far north as England and Denmark. Malaria may also be transmitted by blood transfusion or inoculation. Transplacental infection may occur in the child of a non-immune mother.

Malaria is endemic or sporadic throughout most of the tropics and subtropics below an altitude of 1500 m, excluding the Mediterranean littoral, the USA and Australia. One hundred million people are attacked annually of whom 1% die, mainly children. As the result of WHO sponsored campaigns of prevention and more effective treatment, the incidence of malaria was greatly reduced in 1950–60 but since 1970 there has been a resurgence. In the 1980s *P. falciparum* has become resistant to chloroquine over a steadily increasing area (Table 19.6). Most serious is the emergence of resistance in East Africa, now spreading through Central Africa towards West Africa. Malaria due to this parasite is more severe than that due to the sensitive parasite. Because of increased travel and neglect of chemoprophylaxis about 2000 cases are imported annually into Britain. Most are due to *P. vivax* from Asia. One in five, usually from Africa, is due to *P. falciparum* and of these 1% die because of late diagnosis. A few people living near airports in Europe have acquired malaria

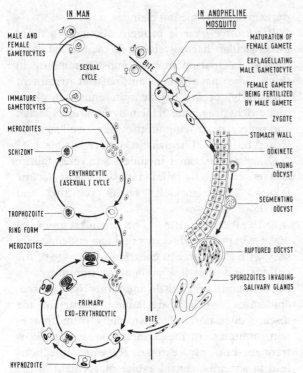

Fig. 19.2 Life cycle of malarial parasites.

from accidentally imported mosquitoes.

Pathogenesis. LIFE CYCLE OF PARASITE (Fig. 19.2). The female anopheline mosquito becomes infected when it feeds on human blood containing gametocytes, the sexual forms of the malarial parasite. The development in the mosquito takes from 7–20 days. Sporozoites inoculated by an infected mosquito disappear from human blood within half an hour. After 5^1 days in *P. falciparum* malaria, 8–15 days or occasionally longer for the other species, 'merozoites', leave the liver and invade red cells where further cycles of multiplication take place producing schizonts. Rupture of the schizont releases more merozoites into the blood and causes fever. Each cycle in the red cells takes 48 hours in the case of *P. vivax* and *P. ovale* and results in a 'tertian' fever, the temperature rising on alternative days; *P. malariae* takes 72 hours resulting in a 'quartan' fever, while the cycle in *P. falciparum* takes rather less than 48 hours, is less well-synchronised and the fever is continuous rather than periodic.

P. vivax and *P. ovale* may persist in liver cells as dormant forms, hypnozoites, that are capable of developing into merozoites months or years later. Thus the first attack of clinical malaria may occur long after the patient has left the endemic area, and the disease may relapse after treatment with drugs that kill only the erythrocytic stage of the parasite.

P. falciparum and *P. malariae* have no persistent exo-erythrocytic phase but recrudescences of fever may result from multiplication in the red cells of parasites which have not been eliminated by treatment and immune processes.

EFFECTS ON RED CELLS AND CAPILLARIES. Malaria is always accompanied by haemolysis and in a severe or prolonged attack anaemia may be profound. Haemolysis is most severe with *P. falciparum* which invades red cells of all ages, but especially young cells. *P. vivax* and *P. ovale* invade reticulocytes, and *P. malariae*, normoblasts, so that infections remain lighter. Uninfected red cells are also destroyed by components of complement, activated in the circulation, adhering to them. Splenomegaly causes red cell sequestration with premature destruction and also haemodilution. Chronic malaria depletes folates stores especially during pregnancy.

In *P. falciparum* malaria, red cells containing schizonts adhere to the lining of capillaries in brain, kidney, liver, lungs and gut. The vessels become congested and the organs anoxic. Rupture of schizonts liberates toxic and antigenic substances which may cause further damage. Thus the main effects of malaria are haemolytic anaemia and, with *P. falciparum*, widespread organ damage.

P. falciparum does not grow well in red cells that contain haemoglobin F, C or especially S. Haemoglobin S heterozygotes (AS) are protected against the lethal complications of malaria. *P. vivax* cannot enter red cells that lack the Duffy blood group. West African negroes and black Americans are protected.

Clinical features. MALARIA IN THE NON-IMMUNE. This is the pattern in children in an endemic area once they have lost the protection conferred by maternal antibodies, or in visitors of any age from a non-endemic area. The incubation period is often longer than the pre-erythrocytic cycle and may be up to several weeks for *P. falciparum* or months for *P. vivax*.

P. vivax and P. ovale malaria. In many cases the illness starts with a period of several days of continued fever before the development of classical bouts of fever on alternate days. Fever starts with a rigor. The patient feels cold and the temperature rises to about 40°C. After half to 1 hour the hot or flush phase begins. It lasts several hours and gives way to profuse perspiration and gradual fall in temperature. The patient feels comfortable, but the cycle is repeated 48 hours later. Gradually the spleen and liver enlarge and may become tender. Anaemia develops slowly. Herpes simplex is common.

P. malariae infection is usually associated with mild symptoms and bouts of fever every third day. Parasitaemia may persist for many years without producing any symptoms. *P. malariae* causes glomerulonephritis and the nephrotic syndrome in children.

Relapses are characteristic of vivax, ovale and malariae infections. They seldom occur more than 2 years after the patient has left the malarious area although much longer intervals are recorded with *P. malariae*.

P. falciparum infections are more dangerous than other forms of malaria. The onset, especially of primary attacks, is often insidious with malaise, headache and vomiting. Cough and mild diarrhoea are common suggesting influenza. The fever has no particular pattern and does not usually rise quite so high as in the other forms. The cold, hot and sweating stages are seldom found. Jaundice is common, due to hepatitis and haemolysis. The liver and spleen enlarge and become tender. Anaemia develops rapidly.

A patient with falciparum malaria, apparently not seriously ill, may suddenly develop serious complications. Children may die rapidly without any special symptoms other than fever. In pregnancy immunity is impaired, and abortion from parasitisation of the maternal side of the placenta is frequent. Splenectomy increases the risk of severe malaria.

Mixed infections with more than one species of malaria parasite may occur.

COMPLICATIONS OF FALCIPARUM MALARIA. *Cerebral malaria* is the most urgent complication and is manifested either by the onset of coma, usually without localising signs, or by hyper-pyrexia or acute mental changes.

Blackwater fever is brought about by a rapid intravascular haemolysis. It is associated with chronic falciparum malaria, most commonly in those who have taken antimalarial treatment irregularly, or are deficient in glucose-6-phosphate dehydrogenase. Haemolysis is unexpected and severe, destroying uninfected as well as parasitised red cells. The urine is dark red or black.

Other complications include acute renal failure and less commonly pulmonary oedema or hepatic failure. There may be severe vomiting and diarrhoea.

ENDEMIC MALARIA. The manifestations of malaria in people who grow up in an endemic area vary with the degree of endemicity, the age of the patient and the development of immunity. In hypoendemic areas little immunity is acquired, epidemics of malaria are liable to occur and the disease does not differ materially from that in non-immunes. In mesoendemic areas malaria is frequent but only seasonal. Repeated infections lead to anaemia, considerable enlargement of the spleen with danger of its rupture, and chronic ill-health with bouts of fever. The growth and development of children may be retarded.

In hyperendemic areas malaria transmission takes place throughout the year, but with seasonal increases, and adults develop considerable immunity. Although they may have palpable spleens and parasitaemia, malaria causes only occasional short bouts of fever. In holoendemic areas malarial transmission is intense throughout the year and adults do not suffer from the infection, although they support a low parasitaemia, and the spleen becomes impalpable.

In hyperendemic and in holoendemic areas malaria may kill up to 15–20% of children below the age of 5 years. The regular taking of antimalarial drugs prevents the manifestations of chronic malaria but may impair the development of immunity.

TROPICAL SPLENOMEGALY SYNDROME. In some hyperendemic areas gross splenomegaly is associated with an exaggerated immune response to malaria and is seen, unexpectedly, in adults who have high antibody titres to malaria and low parasitaemias. The condition, which is commoner in females and in certain racial and family groups is characterised by enormous overproduction of IgM, levels reaching 3 to 20 times the local mean value. Much of the IgM is aggregated with other immunoglobulin or complement and precipitates in the cold, *in vitro*. IgM aggregates are phagocytosed by reticuloendothelial cells in the spleen and liver, and the demonstration of this by immunofluorescence in a liver biopsy section is diagnostic. Light microscopy of the liver usually shows sinusoidal lymphocytosis. Anaemia and lymphocytosis can be confused with leukaemia. Portal hypertension may develop.

Diagnosis. If a febrile patient is in a malarious locality or has recently left such an area, malaria should be considered. Besides malaria there are many causes for acute febrile splenomegaly in the tropics. Gross enlargement of the spleen may also result from tuberculosis, visceral leishmaniasis, schistosomiasis mansoni and japonicum and chronic brucellosis as well as leukaemia and lymphoma. Well-stained blood films, thick and thin, should be examined and repeated if necessary. *P. falciparum* parasites may be very scanty, especially in those who have been partially treated. With *P. falciparum* only ring forms are normally seen in the early stages. With the other species all stages of the erythrocytic cycle may be found. Gametocytes appear after about 2 weeks. In semi-immunes in endemic areas malaria may coexist with other diseases and not be the cause of the illness.

Treatment. CHEMOTHERAPY OF THE ACUTE ATTACK. The drug of choice is chloroquine. The usual course of treatment is 600 mg of the effective base (4 tablets) followed by 300 mg base in 6 hours then 150 mg base twice daily for 3 to 7 more days. The initial dose for children is 5–10 mg/kg. For semi-immunes a single dose is usually adequate. Infections with *P. falciparum* from a chloroquine-resistant area (Table 19.6) should be treated with quinine dihydrochloride 650 mg (10 mg/kg) three times daily for 5 days by mouth, followed by a single dose of sulfadoxine 1.5 g combined with pyrimethamine 75 mg, i.e. 3 tablets of Fansidar. If quinine toxicity develops, dosage is reduced to twice daily. If quinine is not tolerated, amodiaquine may be used in the same dosage as chloroquine, or quinidine in the same dosage as quinine.

TREATMENT OF COMPLICATED P. FALCIPARUM MALARIA. Patients with 'cerebral malaria'

or other severe manifestations, or non-immunes with more than 1% of red cells infected, are medical emergencies. The immediate administration of chloroquine or quinine is indicated, the drug being given as an intravenous infusion over 2–4 hours to avoid acute circulatory failure or acute encephalopathy. Quinine is indicated if a chloroquine-resistant infection is at all likely. The dose of chloroquine is 5 mg/kg and of quinine 10 mg/kg. The dose should be repeated at intervals of 12 hours until the patient can take drugs orally. The drugs may instead be given intramuscularly but chloroquine may cause convulsions (especially in undernourished children) and quinine may cause necrosis of muscle; the hydrochloride is less irritant than the dihydrochloride. In a comatose patient lumbar puncture may be indicated to exclude coexisting bacterial meningitis.

Severe anaemia requires transfusion with packed red cells. In blackwater fever prednisolone (20 mg) may prevent further haemolysis. If oliguria develops, frusemide or an infusion of mannitol may forestall renal failure. Intravenous fluid, if necessary, should be monitored by the central venous pressure, because pulmonary oedema develops easily and total fluid should be restricted to less than 2 litres daily. Exchange blood transfusion has proved life-saving in very heavy infections (over 10% of red cells infected).

The prognosis is good if correct treatment is given early, but poor if diagnosis is late, parasitaemia is high or organs are failing.

TREATMENT OF TROPICAL SPLENOMEGALY SYNDROME. Splenomegaly and anaemia usually resolve over a period of months of continuous treatment with proguanil 100 mg daily, which should be continued for life to prevent relapse. Complicating folate deficiency is treated with folic acid 5 mg daily.

RADICAL CURE OF MALARIA DUE TO *P. vivax* and *P. ovale*. Relapses can be prevented by taking one of the antimalarial drugs in suppressive doses. Radical cure can be ensured by a course of primaquine (15 mg/d for 14 days) which destroys the hyponozoite phase in the liver. Haemolysis may develop in those who are G6PD deficient. Cyanosis due to the formation of methaemoglobin in the red cells is more common but not dangerous.

Causal prophylaxis and suppression. Clin-

Table 19.6 Chemoprophylaxis of malaria.

Area	Antimalarial tablet	Adult prophylactic dose
Chloroquine resistance present***	Pyrimethamine 12.5 mg plus dapsone 100 mg (Maloprim)*	One tablet weekly
	OR	
	Progunail 100 mg plus chloroquine 100 mg, 150 mg or 300 of base	200 mg daily 300 mg weekly
Chloroquine resistance absent	Chloroquine 100 mg, 150 mg or 300 mg of base	300 mg weekly
	OR	
	Proguanil 100 mg	100–200 mg daily**

*Chloroquine should be taken in addition where high *P. vivax* transmission is present (East and Central Africa, Brazil, Papua New Guinea, S.E. Asia, Indian subcontinent).
**200 mg in sub-Saharan Africa or other areas of intense transmission.
***South America. S.E. Asia including Southern China, Indonesia, Malaysia, Phillipines, Papua New Guinea. Bangladesh, N.E. India, Nepal. East and Central Africa, Cameroun.

ical attacks of malaria can be prevented by drugs such as proguanil and pyrimethamine which attack the pre-erythrocytic form ('causal prophylaxis'), or by drugs such as chloroquine which act on the parasite after it has entered the erythrocyte ('suppression'). Maloprim (pyrimethamine 12.5 mg and dapsone 100 mg) and Fansidar (pyrimethamine 25 mg and sulfadoxine 500 mg) contain two compounds which block two successive enzymes in the parasite's folate pathway.

Tables 19.6 and 19.7 give the recommended doses for protection of the non-immune. Chemoprophylaxis is begun 1 week before entering the malarious area, and is continued until 4 weeks after leaving it. Resistance to the cheap and well-tolerated drugs proguanil and pyrimethamine is increasing and frequently coincides with the much more serious spread of chloroquine resistance. Resistance to Maloprim and Fansidar is also reported. Chloroquine should not be taken continuously as a prophylactic for over 5 years, as it may cause irreversible retinopathy. Infants under 8 weeks of age should not be given Maloprim or Fansidar. Pregnant and lactating women may take proguanil or chloroquine safely. Fansidar should be avoided by those sensitive to sulphonamides; allergic rashes are common and deaths have occurred, e.g. from agranulocytosis or Stevens-Johnson syndrome (p. 45). Amodiaquine should

not be used for prophylaxis.

Table 19.7 Doses of antimalarials for children—weight is preferable to age.

Dose in relation to adult dose	Weight range	Age range
One-quarter	under 5 kg	under 1 year
One-half	5–20 kg	1–5 years
Three-quarters	20–40 kg	6–12 years
Adult dose	over 40 kg	over 12 years

Prevention. Control of anopheline mosquitoes, especially by the spraying of houses with residual insecticides, has greatly reduced or abolished the risk of malaria in many areas. However, unless eradication is complete, all visitors should take regular prophylactic drugs. Chemoprophylaxis alone may not be sufficient to prevent malaria. It is also important to avoid anopheline mosquitoes, which bite at night. Outside the house, long sleeves and trousers should be worn. Repellent creams and sprays can be used. Screened windows and the use of a mosquito net also reduce the risk.

AMOEBIASIS

Amoebiasis is usually caused by *Entamoeba histolytica*, a potentially pathogenic intestinal amoeba that is propagated between humans by its cysts, 10 microns or more in diameter. *Ent. histolytica* must be distinguished from other species which are non-pathogenic, notably *Ent. hartmanii* and *Ent. coli*. In addition two amoebae of genera *Naegleria* and *Acanthamoeba* which inhabit polluted surface water and swimming pools all over the world are causes respectively of fulminating meningitis and granulomatous encephalitis.

Pathogenesis. Cysts of *Ent. histolytica* survive well outside the body and are ingested in water or uncooked food which has been contaminated by human faeces. Lettuce is a common vehicle of infection. The disease is occasionally acquired in Britain.

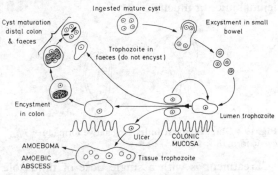

Fig. 19.3 Amoebiasis. Life cycle of *Entamoeba histolytica*. (Adapted from Knight R 1982 Parasitic disease in man. Churchill Livingstone, Edinburgh.)

In the colon the vegetative trophozoite forms emerge from the cysts (Fig. 19.3). While they remain free in the colon the condition is symptomless but some genetic strains, that can be distinguished enzymatically, may invade the mucous membrane of the large bowel. The lesions, which are usually maximal in the caecum but may be found as far down as the anal canal, are flask-shaped ulcers varying greatly in size and surrounded by healthy mucosa. A localised granuloma (*amoeboma*), presenting as a palpable mass in the rectum or causing a filling defect in the colon on radiography, is a rare complication. Since it responds well to antiamoebic treatment it is important that it should not be mistaken for a carcinoma.

Amoebae may find their way into a vein and be carried to the liver where they multiply rapidly and destroy the parenchyma causing an amoebic abscess. The liquid contents at first have a characteristic pinkish colour which later may change to chocolate brown. Amoebic ulcers only rarely penetrate through the muscular coat of the colon but may cause severe haemorrhage. Cutaneous amoebiasis presents as progressive genital or perianal ulceration, usually in homosexuals, or around abdominal surgical wounds. The incubation period varies from 2 weeks to many years.

Clinical features. *Intestinal amoebiasis*, or *amoebic dysentery* usually runs a chronic course with grumbling pains in the abdomen and two or more rather loose stools a day. Periods of diarrhoea alternating with constipation are a frequent feature. Mucus is usually passed, sometimes with streaks of blood, and the motions often have an offensive odour. There may be tenderness along the line of the colon, usually more marked over the caecum and pelvic colon. The right iliac pain may simulate acute appendicitis. Particularly in the aged, in the puerperium and with superadded pyogenic infection of the ulcers there may be more acute bowel symptoms, with very frequent motions and the passage of much blood and mucus, simulating bacillary dysentery or ulcerative colitis.

Hepatic amoebiasis often occurs without a history of recent diarrhoea. It is common in the tropics and an important cause of imported fever in Britain. Early symptoms may be local discomfort only and malaise; later a swinging temperature, sweating and an enlarged tender liver, cough and pain in the right shoulder are characteristic, but symptoms may remain vague and signs minimal. In particular, the less common abscess in the left lobe may not be diagnosed. There is usually a neutrophil leucocytosis and a raised diaphragm with diminished movement on the right side. A large abscess may penetrate the diaphragm and rupture into the lung from where its contents may be coughed up. Rupture into the pleural cavity, the peritoneal cavity or pericardial sac is less common but more serious.

Diagnosis. A careful naked-eye inspection of a freshly passed motion should be made. Any exudate is examined at once under the microscope for motile trophozoites which are about 30 microns in diameter, with a clear ectoplasm and a granular endoplasm, and usually contain red blood cells. Movements cease very soon as the preparation cools. Sigmoidoscopy may reveal typical ulcers and a scraping should be examined for *Ent.*

histolytica. In chronic amoebiasis several stools may need to be examined before cysts are found. The presence of cysts in the faeces does not equate with invasive amoebiasis: in endemic areas one-third of the population are symptomless passers of amoebic cysts.

An amoebic abscess of the liver is suspected from the clinical and radiographic appearances and confirmed by radionuclide or ultrasonic scanning. Aspirated pus from an amoebic abcess has the characteristic appearance described above but only rarely contains free amoebae.

Antibodies are detectable by immunofluorescence in over 95% of cases of hepatic amoebiasis and intestinal amoeboma but in only about 60% of dysenteric amoebiasis. Precipitin tests are less sensitive but become negative in a few months after cure.

Treatment and prevention. Invasive intestinal amoebiasis responds quickly to oral metronidazole (800 mg t.i.d.for 5 days), or tinidazole (single doses of 2 g daily for 3 days). Furamide 500 mg should be given orally t.i.d. for 10 days after treatment to eliminate luminal cysts. Stools are re-examined 4 weeks later.

Early hepatic amoebiasis responds quickly to treatment by metronidazole or tinidazole as above, or to chloroquine 300 mg base b.d. for 2 days, followed by 150 mg b.d. for 14 days. Furamide is given to eliminate the intestinal infection. If the abscess is large or threatens to burst, or if the response to chemotherapy is not prompt, aspiration is also required and repeated if necessary. If culture of the 'pus' indicates that there is secondary bacterial infection, treatment will be required with an appropriate antibiotic. Rupture of an abscess into the pleural cavity, pericardial sac or peritoneal cavity necessitates immediate aspiration or surgical drainage. Small serous effusions resolve without drainage.

Personal precautions against contracting amoebiasis in the tropics and subtropics consist of not eating fresh uncooked vegetables or drinking unboiled water.

GIARDIASIS

Infection with the flagellate *Giardia intestinalis* (Fig.19.4), known also as *G. lamblia*, is world-wide but commoner in the tropics. It particularly affects children in endemic areas, tourists and patients in mental hospitals and is the parasite most commonly imported into Britain. The flagellates attach to the mucosa of the duodenum and jejunum and cause inflammation and partial villous atrophy. Recurrent attacks of urgent diarrhoea with abdominal discomfort and explosive loose pale stools are characteristic. There may be severe malabsorption. Lethargy, flatulence, abdominal distension, epigastric pain and nausea are frequent. Giardiasis is diagnosed by recognising the cysts in stools or the flagellate form in jejunal juice or mucus.

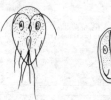

Fig. 19.4 Giardia intestinalis. Vegetative form ($14 \times 7\,\mu$); cystic form ($8 \times 12\,\mu$).

Treatment is with a single dose of tinidazole 40 mg/kg in the range 0.5 g to 2 g, repeated after 1 week. Metronidazole 200–400 mg t.i.d. for 14 days is less efficient.

BALANTIDIASIS

Balantidium coli is a ciliate that causes dysentery in pigs and occasionally infects man in whom the disease resembles amoebic dysentery. Treatment is with tetracycline 10 mg/kg four times daily for 10 days or metronidazole 200–400 mg according to age three times daily for 7 days.

LEISHMANIASIS

This group of diseases is caused by protozoa of the genus *Leishmania*, conveyed to man by female phlebotomine sandflies in which the flagellate (promastigote) forms of leishmania develop. In man the leishmaniae are found in cells of the monocyte-macrophage system as oval forms known as amastigotes or Leishman-Donovan bodies (Fig. 19.5). Leishmaniasis may take the form of a generalised visceral infection, kala-azar, or of a purely cutaneous infection, known in the Old World as oriental sore. In South America

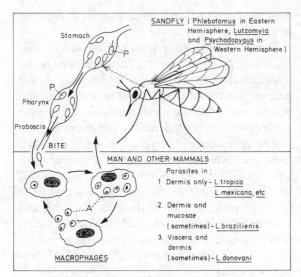

Fig. 19.5 Leishmaniasis. Life cycle of *Leishmania*.
A = amastigote (Leishman-Donovan body);
P = promastigote. (Adapted from Knight R 1982 Parasitic disease in man. Churchill Livingstone, Edinburgh.)

cutaneous leishmaniasis may remain confined to the skin or metastasise to the nose and mouth.

Visceral leishmaniasis (kala-azar)

Visceral leishmaniasis is caused by *Leishmania donovani* and is prevalent in the Mediterranean and Red Sea littorals, Sudan, parts of East Africa, Asia Minor, mountainous regions of Southern Arabia, eastern parts of India, China and South America. In India, where the disease is epidemic, man appears to be the chief host. In most other areas, including the Mediterranean, dogs and foxes are the main reservoirs of infection. Here the disease is endemic and occurs chiefly in young children or tourists. In Africa various wild rodents provide the reservoir, and the disease is rural occurring in older children and visiting hunters and soldiers. Transmission has also been reported to follow blood transfusion in Northern Europe. The disease has presented unexpectedly in immunosuppressed patients, for example after renal transplantation.

Pathology. Multiplication, by simple fission, of leishmaniae takes place in monocytes and macrophages in various organs, especially the liver and spleen, which becomes greatly enlarged, the bone marrow, lymphoid tissue and the small intestinal submucosa. The disease is accompanied by malnutrition and immunosuppression which is both specific to leishmania and non-specific. Acute intercurrent infection or tuberculosis are common complications. Granulocytopenia and thrombocytopenia occur. Anaemia is due to haemolysis, hypersplenism and marrow depression. Serum albumin is low and globulin, mainly IgG, high, but hepatocellular damage and bleeding are late complications.

Clinical features. The incubation period is usually about 1 or 2 months but up to 10 years has been recorded. The onset is usually insidious with a low-grade fever, the patient remaining ambulant, or it may be abrupt with sweating and high intermittent fever, sometimes showing a double rise of temperature in the 24 hours. The spleen soon becomes enlarged, often massively. Hepatomegaly is less marked. If not treated, the patient will become anaemic and wasted, frequently with increased pigmentation especially on the face. Lymphadenopathy is common and rarely is the only clinical finding.

After recovery post kala-azar dermal leishmaniasis sometimes develops. It may present first as hypopigmented or erythematous macules on any part of the body or as a nodular eruption, especially on the face. Amastigotes are scanty.

Diagnosis is established by demonstrating the parasite in stained smears of aspirates of bone marrow, lymph node, spleen or liver, or by culture of these aspirates. Antibody is detected by immunofluorescence or enzyme-linked immuno-absorbent assay early in the disease. The leishmanin skin test is negative; it is performed and read in the same way as the tuberculin test, using a suspension of killed promastigotes as antigen.

Treatment and prevention. The response to treatment varies with the geographical area in which the disease has been acquired. In Europe and Asia the disease is readily cured, but in the Sudan and East Africa it is more resistant. Pentavalent antimonials are the drugs of choice. Sodium stibogluconate contains 100 mg Sb/ml, meglumine antimoniate contains 85 mg Sb/ml. Children are given 20 mg Sb/kg i.v. or i.m. daily for 20 to 30 days. The adult dose is 10–20 mg Sb/kg to a maximum of 850 mg.

Intercurrent infection is sought and treated.

Rarely blood transfusion is needed for anaemia or bleeding. Measurement of spleen size, haemoglobin and serum albumin are useful in assessing progress. A small proportion of patients relapse, and should be re-treated for 2 months. Second line drugs for patients who fail to respond to antimonials include pentamidine (p. 780) and amphotericin (p. 46).

· In an endemic area where they are the reservoir, infected or stray dogs should be destroyed. Sandflies should be combated. They are extremely sensitive to insecticides. The ordinary mosquito net sprayed with an insecticide will keep out the tiny sandfly. Insect-repellent creams may be helpful.

Early diagnosis and treatment of human infections reduces the reservoir and controls epidemic kala-azar in India. Serology is useful for case detection in the field. There is no vaccine.

Cutaneous leishmaniasis of the Old World (oriental sore)

In the Old World, cutaneous leishmaniasis is found around the Mediterranean littoral, throughout the Middle East and Central Asia, as far as Pakistan, and in sub-Saharan West Africa and Sudan. It is caused either by zoonotic *L. major*, a parasite of gerbils and other desert rodents, or by the arthroponotic *L. tropica*, in towns. In the highlands of Ethiopia and Kenya a third parasite, of hyraxes, *L. aethiopica* is the cause. The disease is commonly imported into Britain. On inoculation the parasites are taken up by dermal histiocytes in which they multiply and around which lymphocytes and plasma cells accumulate. With time, the histology becomes more tuberculoid and the overlying epidermis crusts and may ulcerate centrally. Healing is accompanied by subepidermal fibrosis.

Clinical features. The incubation period is from 2 weeks to 5 or more years but usually is from 2 to 3 months. Lesions, single or multiple on exposed parts of the body, start as small red papules which increase gradually in size, reaching 2–10 cm in diameter. A crust forms, overlying an ulcer with a granular base. Tiny satellite papules are characteristic. Untreated, the lesion heals in 3 months to 3 years, or longer. Healing produces a depressed mottled scar which may be disfiguring or disabling.

Forms of cutaneous leishmaniasis occur that do not heal spontaneously. In diffuse cutaneous leishmaniasis (*L. aethiopica*) an immune defect permits the disease to spread all over the skin, and in recidivans (lupoid) leishmaniasis (*L. tropica*) apparently healed sores relapse persistently.

The appearance of a typical lesion in a patient from an endemic area suggests the diagnosis. Leishman-Donovan bodies can be demonstrated by inserting a dry needle into the margin of the ulcer, or making a slit skin smear (p. 759) and staining the material obtained with Giemsa's stain or culturing it. The leishmanin skin test is positive except in diffuse cutaneous leishmaniasis. Serology is unhelpful.

Treatment and prevention. The local application of heat by infra-red, hot water or a thermostatically controlled pad at 40°C may accelerate healing. When the lesions are multiple or in a disfiguring site it is better to treat the patient by parenteral injections of pentavalent antimonials (p. 777), but *L. aethiopica* is not sensitive to antimonials. Diffuse cutaneous leishmaniasis is treated with pentamidine (p. 780).

In addition to those prophylactic measures described under visceral leishmaniasis against animals and sandflies, a lasting immunity can be achieved by deliberate inoculation of a living culture of *L. major* on the upper arm, which produces a typical sore but protects against a subsequent, possibly disfiguring, lesion.

Cutaneous and mucocutaneous leishmaniasis of the New World

In South and Central America, cutaneous leishmaniasis is endemic and mostly caused by parasites of the *L. mexicana* and *L. brasiliensis* groups, which occur in hot, moist, forest regions and are conveyed to man from a variety of rodents by several species of sandflies (Fig. 19.5). *L. mexicana* is responsible for chiclero's ulcer, the self-healing sores of Mexico, Guatemala and Honduras, and for some of the sores in the north of South America, including diffuse cutaneous leishmaniasis (*L. m. amazonensis*). *L. brasiliensis* extends widely from the Amazon basin as far as Paraguay and Costa Rica and is responsible for self-healing sores and for mucocutaneous leishmaniasis. A third variety of the disease occurring in the Peruvian Andes is known as 'uta' and is caused by *L. peruviana*, dogs providing the reservoir.

Pathological and clinical features. The microscopic appearances of the skin lesions may be similar to oriental sore. Mucocutaneous lesions begin as a perivascular infiltration; later endarteritis may lead to destruction of the surrounding tissues (see below). Clinically, lesions of *L. mexicana* and *L. peruviana* closely resemble those seen in the Old World, but lesions on the pinna of the ear are common and are chronic and destructive.

The primary lesions of *L. braziliensis* are similar but in some areas up to 80% develop 'espundia', i.e. metastatic lesions in the mucosa of the nose or mouth. Mucosal lesions either accompany the skin lesions or appear some years later. The nasal mucosa becomes congested and later all tissues of the nose ulcerate except for the bone. The lips, soft palate and fauces may be invaded and destroyed leading to terrible suffering and deformity. Secondary bacterial infection is common. Two subspecies, *L. b. guyanensis* and *L. b. panamensis* are thought not to cause espundia.

Diagnosis depends on the history and clinical appearance, confirmed by demonstration of the parasites in smears, culture or histological section. As parasites are not easily found the leishmanin test is of value and serology may be useful.

Treatment. Purely cutaneous disease may be successfully treated by sodium stibogluconate given as recommended for visceral leishmaniasis (p. 777) but in established espundia amphotericin (p. 46) is sometimes necessary.

AFRICAN TRYPANOSOMIASIS (SLEEPING SICKNESS)

African sleeping sickness is caused by trypanosomes conveyed to man by the bites of infected tsetse flies of either sex. The disease is naturally acquired only in Africa between 12°N and 25°S. Two trypanosomes affect man, *Trypanosoma brucei gambiense* conveyed by *Glossina palpalis* and *G. tachinoides* and *T. b. rhodesiense* transmitted by *G. morsitans*, *G. pallidipes*, *G. swynnertoni* and *G. palpalis*.

Gambiense trypanosomiasis has a wide distribution in West and Central Africa reaching to Uganda and Kenya; rhodesiense trypanosomiasis is found in parts of East and Central Africa where it is currently on the increase. In West Africa trypanosomiasis transmission is mainly at the riverside, where the fly rests in the shade of trees. Animal reservoirs of *T. b. gambiense* have not been identified although pigs may harbour it. *T. b. rhodesiense* has a large reservoir in numerous wild animals and transmission takes place in the shade of woods bordering grasslands. Devastating epidemics of both types have occurred. Trypanosomiasis of cattle, caused mainly by *T. b. brucei*, is also widespread and seriously reduces grazing land and the production of meat and milk.

Pathological and clinical features. Only a low percentage of tsetse flies are infected. A bite by a tsetse fly is painful and commonly becomes inflamed but, if trypanosomes are introduced, the site of the bite may again become painful and swollen about 10 days later ('trypanosomal chancre'), and the regional lymph nodes enlarge. Within 2 to 3 weeks of infection the trypanosomes invade the bloodstream.

In *gambiense infections* the disease usually runs a slow course over months or years with irregular bouts of fever and enlargement of lymph nodes. These are characteristically firm, discrete, rubbery and painless and are particularly prominent in the posterior triangle of the neck. Sometimes during these early weeks transient circinate erythematous eruptions can be seen and there is tachycardia. The spleen and liver may become palpable. After some months, in the absence of treatment, the central nervous system is invaded. This is shown clinically by headaches and changed behaviour, insomnia by night and sleepiness by day, mental confusion and eventually tremors, pareses, wasting, coma and death. The histological changes in the brain are similar to those found in viral encephalitis but trypanosomes are scattered in the substance of the brain and large mononuclear (morula) cells are found whose cytoplasm contains globules of IgM.

In *rhodesiense infections* fever is higher and more constant than in gambiense infections, so that within days or a few weeks the patient is usually severely ill and may have developed pleural effusions and signs of myocarditis or hepatitis. There may be a petechial rash. Enlargement of lymph nodes is usually less than in gambiense infections. The clinical manifestations of involvement of the nervous system may not be obvious but within a few weeks of infection the cerebrospinal fluid will be abnormal and in the untreated case death ensues from toxaemia or heart failure. If the illness is less acute, drowsiness, tremors, and coma may be prominent.

Diagnosis. In any febrile patient from an endemic area trypanosomiasis should be considered. In rhodesiense infections the trypanosomes can often be detected by microscopic examination of a wet blood film in which agitation of red cells by the trypanosomes is seen. Thick and thin blood films stained as for the detection of malaria, will reveal trypanosomes (Fig. 19.6).

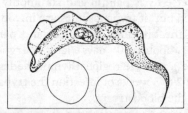

Fig. 19.6 Trypanosome in blood film.

In the earliest stages of gambiense infections the trypanosomes may be seen in the blood or from puncture of the primary lesion but it is usually easier to demonstrate them by puncture of a lymph node.

Concentration methods include buffy coat microscopy and miniature anion exchange chromatography. Animal inoculation is sometimes used for the detection of rhodesiense infections. Serological tests are employed in field work. If the central nervous system is affected the cell count and protein content of the cerebrospinal fluid are increased and the glucose diminished and sometimes trypanosomes may be found by centrifugation. Very high levels of serum IgM or the presence of IgM in the cerebrospinal fluid are suggestive of trypanosomiasis.

Treatment. If treatment is begun early, before the brain has been invaded, the prognosis is good. For this purpose either suramin or pentamidine isethionate may be used, the latter being employed only for gambiense infections. After the nervous system is affected an arsenical will be required.

Suramin is given intravenously. An initial trial dose of 200 mg tests for sensitivity. This is followed on the next day by 1g dissolved in 10 ml of distilled water repeated at intervals of 3 to 5 days to a total dosage of 5 to 10 g. Children are dosed according to weight. Toxic effects include dermatitis, nausea, vomiting, diarrhoea, peripheral neuritis and nephritis. The urine should be examined before each injection and the drug temporarily discontinued if red cells and casts appear.

Pentamidine isethionate is less toxic than suramin, but may cause diabetes. It is painful when given intramuscularly but intravenous administration causes profound hypotension. The dose is 3 to 5 mg/kg to a maximum of 250 mg dissolved in 5 ml distilled water, on alternate days for 10 injections. When used to treat leishmaniasis (p. 778), less frequent injections for a longer period are preferred.

Melarsoprol is a combination of the trivalent melarsan oxide and dimercaprol administered intravenously. It has proved highly efficacious in advanced rhodesiense infections, which were formerly fatal, and for other resistant and relapsing cases. The main danger is encephalopathy due to a Jarisch-Herxheimer reaction following the death of many trypanosomes and encephalopathy due to arsenic which kills 10% of cases. Before commencing treatment the patient's condition may be improved by a few preliminary injections of suramin. The initial dose of melarsoprol is assessed on the patient's general condition rather than on the weight. Patients who are severely ill may only tolerate 0.5 ml and the initial dose must never exceed 2 ml. Further injections are given on the second and third days. The maximum dose is 3.6 mg/kg, i.e. 5 ml for a man of 50 kg. There then follows a rest period of 1 to 2 weeks followed by a second series of three injections. If the initial dose was very small, additional courses may be required during the next 4 or 5 weeks. The total dosage aimed at is 30 ml.

Nitrofurazone is liable to produce haemolytic anaemia in those whose red cells are deficient in G6PD and peripheral neuritis, but it has been used successfully in cerebral trypanosomiasis in a dose of 10 mg/kg t.i.d. for 10 days.

Prevention. Against *T. b. gambiense* a single intramuscular injection of 250 mg pentamidine gives protection for 6 months because of the slow excretion of the drug. As the protection against *T. b. rhodesiense* is less sure and shorter in duration, chemoprophylaxis is not advised in rhodesiense areas. In endemic gambiense areas various measures may be taken against tsetse flies and field teams detect and treat early human infection. In rhodesiense areas control is difficult.

AMERICAN TRYPANOSOMIASIS (CHAGAS' DISEASE)

The cause of Chagas' disease is *Trypanosoma cruzi* transmitted to man from the faeces of a reduviid bug in which the trypanosomes have a cycle of development before becoming infective to man. The bugs are liable to fly down from the ceilings of primitive houses on to the faces of those sleeping below. Infected faeces from the bug are rubbed in through the conjunctiva, mucosa of mouth or nose or through an abrasion of the skin. Dogs and cats are the sources of infection for bugs in houses although in nature opossums and armadillos and other animals are commonly infected. Acute illness has also followed blood transfusion.

The trypanosomes travel by the bloodstream and develop into amastigote forms in the tissues. These multiply in many sites, especially in the myocardium causing pseudocysts, in muscle fibres, and also in the ganglion cells of the autonomic nervous system, giving rise to the changes described below. Chagas' disease occurs widely in South and Central America.

Clinical features. The entrance of *T. cruzi* through an abrasion produces a dusky-red firm swelling with enlargement of regional lymph nodes. A conjunctival lesion, though less common, is more characteristic; the unilateral firm reddish swelling of the lids may close the eye and constitutes 'Romana's sign'. Young children are most commonly affected. In a few cases evidence of a generalised infection soon appears, with fever, lymphadenopathy and enlargement of the spleen and liver. Neurological features include personality changes and signs of meningoencephalitis. Only infants die readily in the acute infection

from encephalitis or myocarditis. Indeed in most cases the early infection is silent.

After a latent period of many years features of the chronic infection appear, notably damage to Auerbach's plexus with resulting dilatation of various parts of the alimentary canal, especially the colon and oesophagus. Dilatation of the bile ducts and bronchi are also recognised sequelae. Invasion of the myocardium causes a cardiomyopathy characterised by cardiac dilatation, arrhythmias, partial or complete heart block and sudden death. Autoimmune processes may be responsible for much of the damage.

Diagnosis. In the acute illness *T. cruzi* may be seen in a blood film. In chronic disease it may be recovered by xenodiagnosis in which infection-free, laboratory-bred, reduviid bugs are fed on the patient; subsequently the hind gut or faeces of the bug is examined for parasites. Complement-fixation, direct agglutination and fluorescent antibody tests are positive in 95% of cases.

Treatment and prevention. Nifurtimox is given orally. The dosage, which has to be carefully supervised to minimise toxicity while preserving parasiticidal activity, is: under 10 years, 15–20 mg/kg and 10–17 years, 12.5–15 mg/kg for 90 days; over 17 years, 8–10 mg/kg for 120 days. Cure rates of 80% in acute disease and 90% in chronic disease are obtained. Temporary side-effects include anorexia, nausea, vomiting and epigastric pain; insomnia, headache, vertigo and excitability; myalgia and arthralgia.

Preventive measures include improved housing and destruction of reduviid bugs by spraying of houses with lindane or other insecticides. Blood taken for transfusion in endemic areas is treated with gentian violet.

TOXOPLASMOSIS

Toxoplasmosis is a world-wide infection caused by *Toxoplasma gondii*. Transmission from a mother infected during pregnancy to the fetus causes congenital toxoplasmosis. Infection after birth results from the ingestion of cysts excreted in the faeces of infected cats or from eating undercooked beef or lamb. Immunocompromised patients are particularly at risk.

Pathology. In the congenital form the organism is widespread in the central nervous system, eyes, heart, lungs and adrenals. If the infant survives, the parasite soon disappears from most organs except the central nervous system and retina. The brain shows large areas of necrosis with cyst formation and patchy calcification; the spinal cord may be similarly affected. In the acquired disease the organism commonly invades lymph nodes and spleen and less commonly liver and myocardium.

Clinical features. The manifestations in congenital infections are mainly cerebral. There may be hydrocephalus or microcephaly associated with convulsions, tremors or paralysis. Radiological examination may show patches of calcification in the brain. Microphthalmos, nystagmus and chorioretinitis are common. The cerebrospinal fluid is often xanthochromic with increased protein and mononuclear cells. An enlarged liver, jaundice, diminished thrombocytes and purpura may also be found. Congenital infections are usually fatal, and if the child survives it is usually disabled and blind.

Many acquired infections are symptomless. In the acute form there may be pneumonia with fever, cough, generalised aches and pains, profound malaise, a maculopapular rash and rarely jaundice and myocarditis. In the more chronic infections, often afebrile, there may be only enlargement of the lymph nodes with a lymphocytosis showing atypical mononuclear cells similar to those present in infectious mononucleosis. Toxoplasmosis is a cause of chorioretinitis and ivitis in adults.

Diagnosis. Serological tests are of value. Antibodies detectable by fluorescence or the dye test appear early in the disease and persist for years. Complement-fixing antibodies are late to appear and decline more quickly. A rise in titre or IgM antibodies indicates acute infection. Antibodies may not be detectable in adult ocular toxoplasmosis. Biopsy material from a lymph node may be inoculated into a laboratory animal, or show characteristic histological changes.

Treatment. Most patients with acquired toxoplasmosis do not require specific therapy as the infection usually resolves spontaneously. Patients for whom treatment is essential include infants, the immunosuppressed and those with eye involvement. A combination of a sulphonamide 1 g 6-hourly and pyrimethamine 25 mg on alternate days for 2–6 weeks should be administered. If this fails or causes adverse effects tetracycline (250 mg 6-hourly) is given for 4 weeks. For iritis and choroidoretinitis corticosteroids are given in addition.

DISEASES DUE TO HELMINTHS

Infections caused by the commoner helminths, or worms, are described in this section, grouped according to the three zoological classes which parasitise man: (1) trematodes or flukes, (2) cestodes or tapeworms and (3) nematodes or roundworms. Much morbidity is caused in the tropics by helminths, and they are an important cause of imported disease in temperate countries.

The only prevalent parasitic helminth of humans in Britain is the nematode *Enterobius (Oxyuris) vermicularis* or threadworm. Other worms which may be acquired in Britain include the roundworms, *Ascaris lumbricoides*, *Toxocara canis*, *Trichuris trichiura* (whipworm) and *Trichinella spiralis*. *Taenia saginata* (beef tapeworm), *Echinococcus granulosus* causing hydatid disease and *Fasciola hepatica*, an endemic fluke infecting sheep, are occasionally acquired in Britain.

Many helminths have a complicated life cycle, often involving one or more intermediate host. Only *Strongyloides stercoralis* can complete its life cycle within man. Disease may be caused by invasive larval stages (e.g. tropical pulmonary eosinophilia), adult worms (e.g. hookworms) or their progeny, either eggs (e.g. schistosomiasis) or microfilariae (e.g. onchocerciasis). Adult worms may be present in the body before, or without, producing disease. Sometimes larval stages that normally develop in intermediate hosts cause disease in man (e.g. cysticercosis). Man may also suffer from invasion by larval stages of worms that normally only infect other animals (e.g. hydatid disease).

1. DISEASES DUE TO TREMATODES (FLUKES)

Schistosomiasis; paragonimiasis; liver flukes; fasciolopsiasis

Schistosomiasis (bilharziasis)

Schistosomiasis is one of the most important causes of morbidity in the tropics and is being spread by irrigation schemes. Schistosome eggs have been found in Egyptian mummies dated 1250 BC.

There are three species of the genus *Schistosoma* which commonly cause disease in man, *S. haematobium*, *S. mansoni* and *S. japonicum*. *S. haematobium* was discovered by Theodor Bilharz in Cairo in 1861 and the genus is sometimes called *Bilharzia* and the disease bilharziasis. The ovum is passed in the urine or faeces and gains access to fresh water where the ciliated miracidium inside it is liberated and enters its intermediate host, a species of fresh water snail, in which it multiplies. Large numbers of fork-tailed cercariae are then liberated into the water where they may survive for 2 to 3 days. Cercariae can penetrate the skin or the mucous membrane of the mouth of their definitive host, man. They transform into schistosomulae and moult as they pass through the lungs and are carried by the bloodstream to the liver and so to the portal vein where they mature (Fig. 19.7). The male worm is up to 20 mm in length and the more slender cylindrical female, usually enfolded longitudinally by the male, is rather longer. Within 4 to 6 weeks of infection they migrate to the venules draining the pelvic viscera where the females deposit their ova. The eggs of *S. haematobium* pass mainly through the walls of the bladder and rectum. The eggs of *S. mansoni* and *S. japonicum* pass mainly through the lower bowel wall.

Pathology. Penetration of the skin by the cercariae may produce a papular eruption which may later become vesicular. A similar cutaneous eruption may follow invasion of the skin by cercariae of non-human schistosomes. During the migration of the immature schistosomes, transitory lesions may be produced, including areas of pneumonia. At this stage there is usually an eosinophilia (p. 498) but the count falls progressively after the disease is established. Adult worms do not normally cause disease, unless they lodge in unusual sites. Schistosome eggs are responsible for most of the lesions. In a heavy infection ova may be found widely distributed in many tissues, but each species has a special territory for

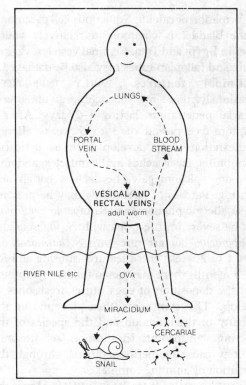

Fig. 19.7 Schistosoma life cycle.

maximum egg deposition.

Eggs pass through the wall of the bowel or bladder early in the infection causing inflammation and bleeding. Some eggs travel with the bloodstream to the liver or other organs. Later in the infection passage of eggs is held up by the immune response, and a granuloma forms, composed of epithelioid cells, lymphocytes and eosinophils. The eggs die and may become calcified especially in the bladder wall or give rise to fibrosis, particularly in the liver.

In schistosomiasis mansoni and japonicum periportal fibrosis leads to portal hypertension; egg deposition in the lungs may cause pulmonary hypertension. In the colon, early inflammation is followed by the appearance of papillomas, and thickening of the bowel wall, sometimes with stenosis.

In schistosomiasis haematobium egg deposition causes bleeding and the appearance of 'sandy patches' seen at cystoscopy. Later papillomas may develop. Fibrosis causes a small bladder and obstructive uropathy with hydronephrosis which predispose to secondary bacterial infection and the formation of calculi. Squamous cell carcinoma of the bladder is common in relatively young males in Egypt and Iraq. Seminal vesicles, vagina, cervix and fallopian tubes may also be damaged.

Clinical features. EARLY INFECTION. Occasionally there may be itching at the site of cercarial penetration, lasting 1–2 days. After a symptom-free period of 3 to 5 weeks allergic manifestations may develop such as urticaria, eosinophilia, fever, aches in the muscles, abdominal pain, splenomegaly, headaches, cough and sweating. Patches of pneumonia may be present. These allergic phenomena (*Katayama syndrome*) may be severe in infections with *S. mansoni* and *S. japonicum* but are rare with *S. haematobium*. After 1 to 2 weeks these features subside and for 2 or 3 months there may be no further symptoms until the deposition of eggs causes fresh ones to develop. The symptoms then depend on the intensity of the infection and the species of the infecting schistosome. In addition, schistosomiasis may cause glomerulonephritis, through the deposition of immune complexes.

SCHISTOSOMIASIS HAEMATOBIUM. Man is the only natural host. *S. haematobium* is highly endemic in Egypt, the east coast of Africa and the adjacent islands and occurs throughout most of Africa, in Iran, Iraq, Syria, Yemen, South Arabia, Lebanon and Israel. It also occurs in Turkey, Cyprus and in solitary foci in Portugal and the Maharashtra State of India.

Painless terminal haematuria is usually the first and commonest symptom. Frequency of micturition follows, due to the contracted fibrosed or calcified bladder. Pain is often felt in the iliac fossa or in the loin, passing down to the groin. In advanced cases, pyelonephritis, hydronephrosis or pyonephrosis may be accompanied by hypertension or uraemia. Disease of the seminal vesicles may lead to haemospermia. Females may be sterile and schistosomal lesions of the cervix may be mistaken for carcinoma. Intestinal symptoms may result from lesions in the bowel wall.

The severity of *S. haematobium* infection varies greatly, and many with light infections suffer little. However, as adult worms can live for 20 years or more and lesions may progress, treatment should always be given (p. 785).

SCHISTOSOMIASIS MANSONI. Man is the only natural host of importance although the infection is also found in baboons. *S. mansoni* is endemic in the Nile Delta and Libya, Southern Sudan, East Africa continuing as far south as the Transvaal and in West Africa from Sénégal and Gambia to Cameroun, throughout Zaïre and also Arabia. It is also found in South America in Venezuela, Brazil and in the West Indian Islands of the lesser Antilles, Puerto Rico and Dominica.

The characteristic symptoms of local disease begin 2 months or longer after infection. They may be slight or consist of abdominal pain and frequent stools which contain blood-stained mucus. With severe advanced disease increased discomfort from rectal polypi may be experienced. The early hepatomegaly is reversible but portal hypertension may cause massive splenomegaly, fatal haematemesis from oesophageal varices or progressive ascites. Jaundice and hepatic failure are uncommon. *S. mansoni* infections predispose to the carrier state of *S. typhi*. Eggs may be deposited in the spinal cord and cause paraplegia.

SCHISTOSOMIASIS JAPONICUM. The adult worm parasitises, in addition to man, the dog, rat, field mouse, water buffalo, ox, cat, pig, horse and sheep. *S. japonicum* is prevalent in the Yellow River and Yangste-Kiang basins in China where the infection is a major public health problem. It also has a focal distribution in Japan, the Philippines, Celebes, Laos, Thailand, Vietnam and the Shan States of Burma.

The histopathology of *S. japonicum* is similar to that of *S. mansoni* but as this worm produces more eggs the lesions tend to be more extensive and widespread. The small bowel as well as the large may be affected, and hepatic fibrosis with splenic enlargement is usual. Deposition of eggs or worms in the central nervous system, especially in the brain, causes symptoms of cerebral irritation or compression in about 5% of infections. Evidence of cerebral involvement includes Jacksonian epilepsy, hemiplegia, blindness and paraplegia. The clinical features of schistosomiasis due to *S. japonicum* otherwise resemble those of very severe infection with *S. mansoni*. The morbidity and mortality rate in *S. japonicum* infections is greater than from either of the other species.

Diagnosis. A history of residence in an endemic area with characteristic symptoms will indicate the need for investigation. In *S. haematobium* infection dip-stick urine testing shows blood and albumin. The terminal spined egg can usually be found by microscopical examination of the centrifuged deposit of terminal stream urine, especially late in the morning or after exercise. The eggs may also be found by microscopic examination of the stools or of an unfixed rectal snip: a fragment of unstained rectal mucosa removed through a proctoscope. A radiograph may show calcification in the wall of the bladder while intravenous urography or ultrasound scanning may show stenosis or dilatation of the ureters, reduction in capacity of the bladder, or hydronephrosis.

In a heavy infection with *S. mansoni* or *S. japonicum* the characteristic egg with its lateral spine can usually be found in the stool. When, however, the infection is light or old a rectal snip should be examined. Cystoscopy or sigmoidoscopy may show characteristic changes. Biopsies should be examined for ova. Serological tests (enzyme-linked immunosorbent assay or immunofluorescence) are useful as screening tests, but diagnosis rests on demonstration of ova. The bowel symptoms and barium enema appearances of *S. mansoni* and *S. japonicum* infection may resemble those associated with amoebiasis or a neoplasm of the large bowel.

Treatment. The object of specific treatment is to kill the adult schistosomes and so stop egg laying. In mass treatment campaigns in communities where reinfection is likely, it may not be possible or desirable to kill all adult worms, but a reduction in egg output of around 90% is often achieved and this significantly reduces morbidity, and possibly transmission, without impairing what little acquired immunity there may be.

Niridazole, 25 mg/kg daily, orally in 3 divided doses, for 7 days is highly effective in haematobium schistosomiasis but rather less so in mansoni schistosomiasis. The drug colours the urine brown and may cause anorexia, vomiting, headache and psychosis, especially in the presence of portal hypertension. It has largely been replaced by the following three newer but more expensive drugs.

Praziquantel is normally the drug of choice for all forms of schistosomiasis. For *S. haematobium*

and *S. mansoni* a single dose (40 mg/kg) is given by mouth. Cure rates are of the order 90–100% in the former and 60–90% in the latter, depending to some extent on the intensity of infection. Egg production is reduced by over 99%. Ideally, treatment is repeated a month later. For *S. japonicum* infections 2 doses each of 30 mg/kg are given in 1 day, or better 10 mg/kg thrice daily for 2 days. Side-effects are uncommon and mild, and include nausea, headache, giddiness and drowsiness.

Oxamniquine orally in a dose of 15 mg/kg twice daily for 2 days cures over 95% of cases of *S. mansoni*. It is safe in the chronic hepatic forms of the disease, though it may cause fever for a few days.

Metrifonate is an organophosphorus inhibitor of cholinesterase, and paralyses the worm. It is effective against *S. haematobium* only, and is given in a dose of 7.5 mg/kg once every 2 weeks for three doses. Higher or more frequent doses cause abdominal pain, nausea or vomiting. A simple, cheap and efficient treatment for *S. haematobium* is a single dose of metrifonate 10 mg/kg, combined with a single dose of niridazole 25 mg/kg; this reduces the egg output by over 90%.

Surgery may be required to deal with residual lesions but large vesical granulomas usually respond well to chemotherapy. In cases of chronic *S. haematobium* infection, ureteric stricture and the small fibrotic urinary bladder may require plastic procedures. For rectal papillomas removal by diathermy or by other means may give the patient relief. Granulomatous masses in the brain or spinal cord may call for neurosurgery if the manifestations do not yield to chemotherapy and corticosteroids.

Prevention. This presents great difficulties, and so far no really satisfactory means of controlling schistosomiasis has been established. If the ova of the schistosome in the urine or faeces are not allowed to contaminate fresh water containing the snail host, then the life cycle is terminated. The provision of latrines and of a safe water supply remains a major problem in rural areas throughout the tropics. In the case of *S. japonicum*, moreover, there are so many hosts besides man that the proper use of latrines would be of little avail. Mass treatment of the population helps against *S. haematobium* and *S. mansoni* but this method has so far had little success against *S. japonicum*. Attack on the intermediate host, the snail, presents many difficulties and has not on its own proved successful on any scale.

Personal protection. Contact with infected water must be avoided. Accidental immersion or contact should be followed by a shower and vigorous towelling. Storage of water, free of snails, for three days will usually kill cercariae.

Paragonimiasis (endemic haemoptysis)

There are several species of the flukes of the genus *Paragonimus* which may affect man, the commonest being *P. westermani*. The adult flukes measuring 10×6 mm live in small 'nests' in the lung and elsewhere. The sputum contains ova, some of which may be expectorated and the others swallowed and passed in the faeces. From these eggs myracidia emerge in water and seek the first intermediate host, a freshwater snail. Larvae emerging from the snail encyst as metacercariae in freshwater crabs or crayfish. If man or certain other mammals eat these crustacea raw or inadequately cooked, they become infected. Human infections are most frequent in the Far East but there are also endemic foci in South America, West Africa, Somalia and India.

Pathological and clinical features. The adults lie in cysts up to 1 cm in diameter, containing reddish-brown fluid, situated chiefly in the lung. There are seldom more than 20 such cysts present. In heavy infections, cysts may also be present in the pleural or peritoneal cavities, in the brain, muscles, skin or elsewhere.

The first symptoms are slight fever, cough and the expectoration of brown or black sputum. Occasionally there are bouts of frank haemoptysis with severe pain in the chest. Increasing signs in the chest may simulate pneumonia or pulmonary tuberculosis which may coexist. When the parasites lodge in the abdomen there may be symptoms of enteritis or hepatitis. If they settle in the abdominal wall they may produce sinuses which discharge through the skin. Cysts in the central nervous system may cause signs of cerebral irritation, encephalitis or myelitis. The disease may be very chronic as the adult worms may survive for 20 years.

Ova may be found on microscopic examination of the faeces, sputum, or a discharge. The radiological appearances of affected lungs are variable but the lesions are usually situated close to the pleural surfaces. Extrapulmonary lesions are diagnosed by biopsy.

Treatment and prevention. Praziquantel is given in a dose of 25 mg/kg twice daily for 2 days. Less effective is bithionol given in a dose of 30 mg/kg daily in three divided doses on alternate days for 15 days. Lesions localised to or maximal in one lobe of a lung may be treated surgically.

In an endemic area crab or crayfish should not be eaten unless adequately cooked. Immersion of crustaceans in wine, vinegar or brine does not kill the parasites.

Liver flukes

Table 19.8 sets out the main features of the diseases caused by flukes which infect the bile ducts of man. In the Far East and S.E. Asia, liver flukes are an important cause of ill-health. Severe acute infections cause anorexia, abdominal pain, diarrhoea, eosinophilia and increased serum levels of liver enzymes. Chronic infections cause recurrent febrile jaundice from cholangitis, and rarely cirrhosis and biliary carcinoma. Many people with light infections remain symptom free.

Fasciolopsiasis

Fasciolopsis buski is the largest fluke to infect man. The adults, 2–7.5 cm long, inhabit the small intestine of man, pigs and dogs. The infection is common in Central and S. China and among Chinese in S.E. Asia. It is spread from ova passed in the faeces into water. The intermediate hosts are snails. Man becomes infected by ingesting metacercariae encysted on water plants, particularly when he uses his teeth to peel them.

Light infections are symptomless. Heavy infections give rise to epigastric pain and loose motions. Very heavy infections may be fatal. The diagnosis is made by detecting ova or adult worms in the faeces.

Praziquantel is given in a single dose of 15–25 mg. Prevention is by the proper disposal of

Table 19.8 Diseases caused by flukes in the bile ducts.

Disease	Clonorchiasis	Opisthorciasis	Fascioliasis
Parasite	*Clonorchis sinensis*	*Opisthorcis felineus*	*Fasciola hepatica*
Other mammalian hosts	Dogs, cats, pigs	Dogs, cats, foxes, pigs	Sheep, cattle
Mode of spread	Ova in faeces into water	As for *C. sinensis*	Ova in faeces on to wet pasture
1st intermediate host	Snails	Snails	Snails
2nd intermediate host	Freshwater fish	Freshwater fish	Encysts on vegetation
Geographical distribution	Far East, esp. S. China	Far East, esp. N.E. Thailand	Cosmopolitan incl. Britain
Pathology	*Esch. coli* cholangitis, liver abscesses, biliary carcinoma	As for *C. sinensis*	Toxaemia, cholangitis, eosinophilia
Symptoms	Often symptom-free, recurrent jaundice	As for *C. sinensis*	Obscure fever, tender liver, may be ectopic subcut. fluke
Diagnosis	Ova in stool or duodenal aspirate	As for *C. sinensis*	*As for C. sinensis* also immunofluorescence
Prevention	Cook fish	Cook fish	Avoid contaminated watercress
Treatment	Praziquantel 25 mg/kg 8-hourly for 2 days	As for *C. sinensis* but 1 day only	Bithionol 30 mg/kg daily for 10–15 days

faeces. Edible water plants can be made safe by immersing them in boling water.

2. DISEASES DUE TO CESTODES (TAPEWORMS)

Taenia saginata; Taenia solium and cysticercosis; Echinococcus granulosus and hydatid disease; Multiceps multiceps; Diphyllobothrium latum; Diphyllobothrium mansoni; Dipylidium caninum; Hymenolepis nana

Cestodes are ribbon-shaped worms which inhabit the intestinal tract. They have no alimentary system and absorb nutrients through the surface. The anterior end, or scolex, is provided with suckers for attachment to the host. From the scolex arises a series of progressively developing segments, the proglottides, which when shed may continue to show active movements for some time. Cross-fertilisation takes place between segments. Ova, present in large numbers in mature proglottides, remain viable for weeks and during this period they may be consumed by the intermediate host. Larvae liberated from the ova pass into the tissues of the intermediate host. Man gets tapeworms by eating undercooked beef infected with *Cysticercus bovis*, the larval stage of *Taenia saginata* (beef tapeworm), undercooked pork containing *Cysticercus cellulosae*, the larval stage of *T. solium* (pork tapeworm), or undercooked freshwater fish containing larvae of *Diphyllobothrium latum* (fish tapeworm). Usually only one adult

tapeworm is present but up to 10 have been reported. The lifecyles of *Diphyllobothrium mansoni, Dipylidium caninum* and *Hymenolepsis nana* are different (p. 790). *Echinococcus granulosus* is a tapeworm of dogs.

Taenia saginata

This worm may be several metres long. The scolex, the size of a pin head, has four suckers; mature segments 1.3 cm × 1 cm, contain a central-stemmed uterus with 15 to 20 lateral branches which are easily seen if the segments are left in water for 24 hours (Fig. 19.8). The ova of both

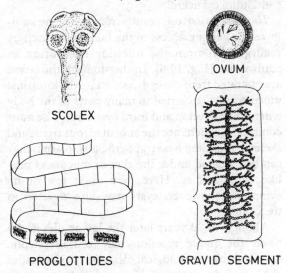

SCOLEX

OVUM

PROGLOTTIDES

GRAVID SEGMENT

Fig. 19.8 Taenia saginata (ova 30–40 μ)

T. saginata and *T. solium* are spherical and indistinguishable microscopically. The thick outer shell has radial striations and the ovum contains six hooklets.

Infection with *T. saginata* occurs in all parts of the world, including Britain. The adult worm produces little or no intestinal upset in human beings, but knowledge of its presence, by noting segments from it in the faeces or on underclothing, may distress the patient. The segments should be identified. Ova may also be found in the stool.

Treatment and prevention. Praziquantel is the drug of choice, in a single dose of 10 mg/kg. Less effective is niclosamide; 2 tablets of the drug, each containing 0.5 g, are chewed and swallowed with a little water. One hour later a further 2 tablets are similarly taken. There are no side-effects. Prevention depends on efficient meat inspection or the thorough cooking of beef.

Taenia solium and cysticercosis

T. solium, the pork tapeworm, was formerly cosmopolitan in distribution but is now rare except in Central Europe, South Africa, South America and in parts of Asia. It is not so large as *T. saginata*, and the uterus usually has less than 14 lateral branches. The scolex has, in addition to suckers, two circular rows of hooklets anterior to the suckers. The adult worm is found only in man following the eating of undercooked pork containing cysticerci.

Human cysticercosis results from ova being swallowed or gaining access to the human stomach by regurgitation from the intestine harbouring an adult worm (Fig. 19.9). In the stomach the larvae are liberated from the eggs, penetrate the intestinal mucosa and are carried to many parts of the body where they develop and form cysticerci. The most common locations are the subcutaneous tissue and skeletal muscles; when superficially placed they can be palpated under the skin or mucosa as pea-like ovoid bodies. Here they cause few or no symptoms; however, cysts may also develop in the brain.

About 5 to 20 years later the larvae die; in the brain the tissue reaction may cause epileptic fits, obscure neurological disorders, personality changes and occasionally internal hydrocephalus.

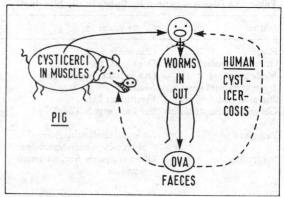

Fig. 19.9 Cysticercosis. Life cycle of *Taenia solium*.

After death of the larvae in muscles the cysts calcify and this enables them to be recognised radiologically. In the brain, however, much less calcification takes place and larvae are only occasionally demonstrated radiologically. CT scanning usually shows them. Epileptic fits starting in adult life should suggest the possibility of cysticercosis if the patient has lived in an endemic area. The subcutaneous tissue should be palpated and any nodule excised for histology. Radiological examination of the skeletal muscles for calcified cysts must be made and repeated after intervals of 6 months if at first negative.

Treatment and prevention. *T. solium* can be destroyed by praziquantel or niclosamide (p. 787). Praziquantel improves the prognosis of cerebral cysticercosis — 50 mg/kg in 3 divided doses daily for 10 days. Prednisone, 10 mg every 8 hours is also given for 14 days, starting one day before the praziquantel. In addition antiepileptic drugs should be given to tide the patient over the period until the reaction in the brain has subsided. Operative intervention is indicated if hydrocephalus develops.

Prevention of *T. solium* infection consists in cooking pork well before eating it. Cysticercosis is avoided if food is not contaminated by ova or segments. Patients with pork tapeworm probably get cysticercosis from ingesting ova from contaminated fingers, rather than from regurgitation of segments. Great care must be taken by nurses and others while attending a patient harbouring an adult worm.

Echinococcus granulosus (Taenia echinococcus) and hydatid disease

The dog, and certain wild canines, are the definitive host of the tiny tapeworm *E. granulosus*. The larval stage, a hydatid cyst, normally occurs in sheep, cattle and other animals, including camels, that are infected from contaminated pastures or water. Man, by handling a dog or drinking contaminated water, may ingest eggs (Fig. 19.10). The embryo is liberated from the ovum in the small intestine and gains access to the bloodstream and thus to the liver. The resultant cyst grows very slowly. It may calcify or may rupture giving rise to multiple cysts. The disease is common in the Middle East and North and East Africa, Australia and Argentina. Foci of infection persist in rural Wales and Scotland. A variant, *E. multilocularis* which has a cycle between foxes and voles, causes a similar but more severe infection, 'alveococcosis' which invades the liver like cancer.

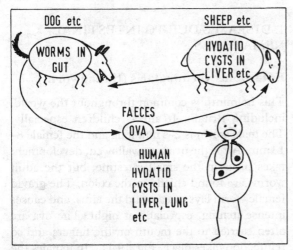

Fig. 19.10 Hydatid disease. Life cycle of *Echinococcus granulosus*.

In man a hydatid cyst is typically acquired in childhood and it may, after growing for some years, cause pressure symptons. These will vary, depending on the organ or tissue involved. In nearly 75% of patients with hydatid disease the right lobe of the liver is invaded and contains a single cyst. In others a cyst may be found in lung, brain, or elsewhere. The diagnosis depends on the clinical, radiological, and ultrasound findings in a patient who has lived in close contact with dogs. Complement-fixation and immuno-fluorescent tests usually give support to the diagnosis.

Treatment and prevention. Hydatid cysts should be excised. Great care is taken to avoid spillage and cavities are sterilised with 2% formalin, 0.5% silver nitrate or 2.7% sodium chloride. Albendazole (400 mg b.d.) has been used for inoperable disease. The most effective dosage and duration of treatment have not yet been established.

Prevention is difficult when man lives in close association with dogs and sheep. Better personal hygiene, meat inspection and deworming of dogs can greatly reduce the prevalence of disease.

Other tapeworms

Multiceps multiceps. This tapeworm of dogs occurring in sheep-grazing areas of East and Southern Africa has a similar life cycle to *Echinococcus granulosus*. Only its larval stage, *Coenurus serialis*, is known in man. It is liable to cause a space-occupying cyst in the brain, especially in the posterior fossa.

Diphyllobothrium latum is relatively common in Finland and the Scandinavian countries but is also acquired from rivers and lakes of many other countries, including some in Africa and Asia. The ova are excreted in the faeces of an infected man or other fish-eating animal. The larval stages take place first in a small freshwater crustacean, *Cyclops* or *Diaptomus*, which in turn is swallowed by a fish. The infections are usually symptomless. Occasionally there are signs of allergy and in a small percentage of cases a megaloblastic anaemia develops, the worm competing with the host for vitamin B_{12}. The diagnosis is made by finding ova in the stool and treatment is by praziquantel or niclosamide (p. 787).

Diphyllobothrium mansoni (Spirometra erinacei). The adult worms are harboured by cats and dogs. The second larval stage, a sparganum, is occasionally found in the subcutaneous tissues of man. The Masai in East Africa probably become infected by ingestion of the first intermediate host, a *Cyclops*, from well water and the patient presents with a painful swelling usually in the lower limbs. In the Far East ocular *sparganosis* arises from the migration of a sparganum from a split frog applied as a traditional poultice. Sparganosis also occurs in the USA. Surgical removal is required.

Dipylidium caninum is a short tapeworm of dogs and cats. The ova are passed in the faeces and the larva has to undergo development in a flea or louse before being swallowed by the definitive host. Children are occasionally infected by picking up and ingesting an infected flea from a dog. The diagnosis is made by finding segments or ova in the stools. Treatment, in appropriate doses for a child, is by niclosamide in a single dose of 1–2 g depending on age.

Hymenolepis nana. This dwarf tapeworm is unusual in not requiring an intermediate host. It is a common infection in children living in insanitary conditions in the tropics and subtropics. In a heavy infection enteritis and allergic phenomena may develop. The diagnosis is made by recognising the ova in the faeces. Treatment is with praziquantel in a dose of 20 mg/kg once or niclosamide 0.5–2 g, depending on age, daily for a week.

3. DISEASES DUE TO NEMATODES (ROUNDWORMS)

Nematode infections of man may be divided into three groups:

1. INTESTINAL NEMATODES. The commonest that cause disease are *Enterobius vermicularis*, *Ascaris lumbricoides*, *Trichuris trichiura*, *Necator americanus*, *Ancylostoma duodenale*, *Strongyloides stercoralis* and *Capillaria philippinensis*. Others, notably *Trichostrongylus*, are not pathogenic.

Adult male and female worms live in the lumen of the gut and do not normally invade tissues. They often have complex life cycles and may cause a syndrome of fever, cough and eosinophilia during the stage of larval invasion. Eggs or larvae are passed in the faeces and the worm does not normally complete its life cycle in man. *Strongyloides*, however, breaks both these rules and is potentially the most dangerous.

2. TISSUE-DWELLING HUMAN NEMATODES. These are the filarial worms (*Wuchereria bancrofti*, *Brugia malayi*, *Loa loa*, *Onchocerca volvulus*, and some others with a more restricted distribution), and the guinea worm *Dracunculus medinensis*.

These worms have complex life cycles, with an intermediate host that is also a vector. Disease may be due to the presence of the adult worms or to their progeny, the microfilariae, which migrate in the blood or tissues, provoking a massive eosinophilia; but often the infection is long lived and well tolerated.

3. NEMATODES OF OTHER ANIMALS that cause ectopic infections in man. The most important are *Toxocara canis*, *Ancylostoma brasiliensis*, *Oesophagostomum* species, *Angiostrongylus cantonensis*, *Trichinella spiralis*, *Gnasthostoma spinigerum* and *Anisakis marina*.

The infective larvae of these worms are unable to 'home' to their normal site for development into adults, in their abnormal host. They may wander or may become trapped in a particular organ. They tend to provoke severe inflammatory reactions characterised by eosinophilic granulomas.

1. DISEASES DUE TO INTESTINAL NEMATODES

Enterobius vermicularis (threadworm)

This helminth is common throughout the world, including Britain. It affects children especially. The male worm is 2–5 mm long and the female 8–13 mm. After the ova are swallowed, development takes place in the small intestine, but the adult worms are found chiefly in the colon. The gravid female worm lays ova around the anus, and causes intense itching, especially at night. The ova are often carried to the mouth on the fingers and so reinfection takes place (Fig. 19.11). In females the genitalia may be invaded. The adult worms may be seen moving on the buttocks or in the stool. Ova are detected by applying the adhesive surface of cellophane tape to the perianal skin in the morning. This is then examined on a glass slide under the microscope.

Treatment. A single dose of one of the drugs in Table 19.9 is given and repeated after 2 weeks to control auto-reinfection. Where infection constantly recurs in a family, all members should be treated with mebendazole 100 mg twice daily for 3 days repeated after 10 days. During this period

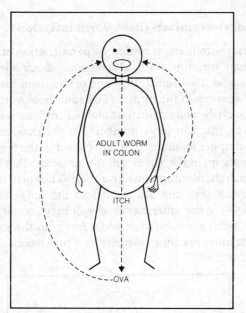

Fig. 19.11 Threadworm. *Enterobius vermicularis* life cycle.

all night clothes and bed linen are laundered and finger nails are scrubbed before meals.

Ascaris lumbricoides ('roundworm')

This pale-yellow worm is 20–35 cm long. Man is infected by eating food contaminated with mature ova. These hatch in the duodenum and the larvae migrate through the lungs, where they moult, ascend the bronchial tree and trachea and are swallowed. They mature in the small intestine. In heavy infections, larvae in the lung may cause pulmonary eosinophilia (p.240).

Adult worms commonly cause abdominal discomfort or colic. Sometimes a worm is vomited or passed *per rectum*. In children with severe infections a tangled mass of worms may cause intestinal obstruction. Many worms competing with a child for nourishment may contribute to malnutrition. Other complications include block-

Table 19.9 Relative activity of drugs used for the common gut nematodes.

	Ascaris	Hookworm	Enterobius	Trichuris	Strongyloides
Piperazine salts 100 mg/kg	+++	+	+++	--	--
Pyrantel pamoate 10 mg/kg	+++	++	+++	--	--
Oxantel pamoate 10 mg/kg	--	--	--	+++	--
Mebendazole 100 mg (any age)	++	++	+++	++	+
Albendazole 400 mg	++	++	+	+	+
Thiabendazole 25 mg/kg	(++)	(++)	(++)	(+)	+++
Levamisole 5 mg/kg	+++	+	+	--	--
Pyrvinium 5 mg/kg	+	--	+++	--	--

Size of single dose is given. Activities given in parenthesis indicate that the drug is not used for that species. Piperazine is cheap and safe, but with a limited range. Mebendazole given twice daily for 3 days is completely safe and eradicates most infections. Thiabendazole has a wide spectrum; it is absorbed and effective against many tissue-dwelling nematodes, but toxic, causing dizziness, headache, anorexia, vomiting and drowsiness. A single dose antihelmintic is ideal for mass treatment and control schemes. Levamisole is the first choice for roundworms, and has a useful action against hookworms. A single dose of pyrantel pamoate and oxantel pamoate or of albendazole is used for multiple infections. (Adapted from Knight R 1982 Parasitic disease in man. Churchill Livingstone, Edinburgh.)

age of the bile or pancreatic duct and obstruction of the appendix by adult worms.

The diagnosis is made by finding ova in the faeces or by observing an adult worm (Fig. 19.12). A solely male infection is usually revealed only after the giving of an antihelmintic to a patient with an unexplained eosinophilia. Occasionally the worms are demonstrated radiographically by barium.

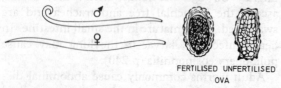

FERTILISED UNFERTILISED
OVA

Fig. 19.12 Roundworm. *Ascaris lumbricoides* (ova $16 \times 45 \mu$ fertilised; $90 \times 40 \mu$ unfertilised).

Treatment. See Table 19.9. If obstruction occurs and fails to respond to nasogastric suction and sedation, surgery is required, when the worms are 'milked' past the obstruction, or removed by enterostomy.

Trichuris trichiura (whipworm)

Under unhygienic conditions, infections with whipworm are common all over the world. Infection takes place by the ingestion of earth or food contaminated with ova which have become infective after lying for 3 weeks or more in moist soil. The adult worm is 3–5 cm long and has a coiled anterior end resembling a whip (Fig. 19.13).

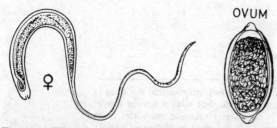

OVUM

Fig. 19.13 Whipworm. *Trichuris trichiura* (ova $50 \times 22 \mu$).

Whipworms inhabit the caecum, lower ileum, appendix, colon and anal canal. There are usually no symptoms, but intense infections in children may cause persistent diarrhoea or rectal prolapse. The diagnosis is readily made by identifying ova in faeces. Treatment is with mebendazole in doses of 100 mg twice daily for 3–5 days or a single dose of oxantel (Table 19.9).

Ancylostomiasis (hookworm infection)

Ancylostomiasis is caused by parasitisation of the small intestine with *Ancylostoma duodenale* or *Necator americanus*. It is one of the main causes of anaemia in the tropics. The adult hookworm is a greyish-white nematode about 1 cm long which lives, often in large numbers, in the duodenum and upper jejunum. Eggs are passed in the faeces. In warm, moist, shady soil the larvae develop and reach the filariform infective stage. They penetrate human skin and are carried to the lungs (Fig. 19.14). After entering the alveoli they ascend the bronchi, are swallowed and develop in the small intestine, reaching maturity in 4 to 7 weeks after infection.

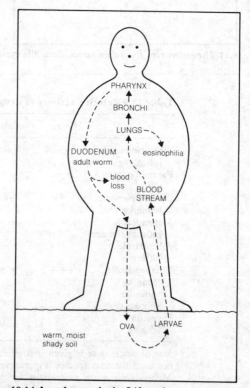

Fig. 19.14 Ancylostomiasis. Life cycle.

Hookworm infection is widespread under insanitary conditions in the tropics and subtropics and used to be common in mines in Europe. *A. duodenale* is endemic in the Far East and Mediterranean coastal regions and is also present in Africa. *N. americanus* is endemic in West, East and Central Africa and Central and South America as well as in the Far East.

Pathology. At the site of entry through the skin the larvae may cause allergic inflammation. When infection is heavy, the passage through the lungs may cause pulmonary eosinophilia (p. 240). In the small·intestine the worms attach themselves to the mucosa by their buccal capsule and withdraw blood. The mean daily loss of blood from one *A. duodenale* is 0.15 ml and for *N. americanus* 0.03 ml. The degree of iron and protein deficiency which develops depends not only on the load of worms but also on the nutrition of the patient and especially on the stores of iron, so that in a light infection there may be no anaemia. In the early stage of infection eosinophilia is common.

Clinical features. In a well-nourished person with a light established infection there may be no symptoms. At the time of infection hookworm dermatitis (ground itch) may be experienced, usually on the feet. An itchy erythema appears first and soon develops through papules and vesicles to pustules. In a heavy infection the passage of the larvae through the lungs causes a paroxysmal cough with blood-stained sputum, associated with patchy pulmonary consolidation. When the worms have reached the small intestine, vomiting and epigastric pain, like that of a duodenal ulcer, may ensue. Sometimes frequent loose stools are passed, the condition then resembling early sprue or giardiasis. In the undernourished, anaemia and hypoproteinaemia may develop. In children mental and physical development may be retarded.

The characteristic egg can be recognised in the stool. If hookworms are present in numbers sufficient to cause anaemia, tests of the stool for occult blood will be positive and ova will be present in large numbers.

Treatment. See Table 19.9. Mebendazole twice daily for 3 days is preferred, but for single-dose treatment pyrantel is the best choice. Anaemia associated with hookworm infection responds well to oral iron. When it is severe enough to cause heart failure blood should be transfused slowly, with frusemide 20 mg in each unit.

Strongyloidiasis

Strongyloides stercoralis is a very small nematode (2 mm × 0.4 mm) which parasitises the mucosa of the upper part of the small intestine in large numbers. The eggs hatch in the bowel and only larvae are passed in the faeces. In moist soil they moult and become the infective filariform larvae. After penetrating human skin they undergo a development cycle similar to that of hookworms but the female worms burrow into the mucosa and submucosa. In the intestine some larvae may develop into filariform larvae which may then penetrate the mucosa or the perianal skin and lead to auto-infection and a very persistent infection. Man is the natural host, but dogs may also be infected. Strongyloidiasis is world-wide in the tropics and subtropics and is especially prevalent in the Far East.

Pathology. There may be a dermatitis at the time of entry of the larval worms. In the intestine the female worm burrows into the mucosa and sets up an inflammatory reaction; with very heavy infections the mucosa may be severely damaged leading to malabsorption. Granulomatous changes, necrosis, and even perforation and peritonitis may also occur. Eosinophilia commonly persists. Actively motile larvae are passed in the faeces. Immunosuppression may lead to fatal systemic strongyloidiasis.

Clinical features. An itch may be produced during invasion of the skin. With slight infections there will be no intestinal symptoms, but in more severe cases abdominal pain and diarrhoea may be produced, which is on occasion severe. Urticaria, arthralgia, wheeze, anaemia, weakness and emaciation may also be present as well as signs of malabsorption.

Penetration of the skin about the anus or the intestinal wall by filariform larvae may lead to extremely itchy, linear, urticarial weals that may travel 3 or 4 cm in an hour, and are known as 'larva currens' to distinguish them from the creeping eruption 'larva migrans' (p. 799). The weals subside in a few hours and recur in a new site. Skin lesions may be the only sign of the infection.

Systemic strongyloidiasis causes diarrhoea, pneumonia and sometimes meningoencephalitis; it is rapidly fatal unless diagnosed and promptly treated.

Diagnosis and treatment. Motile rod-shaped larvae can be seen on microscopic examination of the faeces and occasionally in the sputum. Excretion is intermittent so repeated examinations or jejunal aspiration may be necessary. Filarial serology is positive in 15% of patients (p.795).

Thiabendazole is given orally in a dose of 25 mg/kg body weight twice daily for 2 to 4 days, according to tolerance. A second course may be required. For systemic strongyloidiasis the drug is given by nasogastric tube for a longer period.

Capillariasis

Infection with *C. philippinensis* suddenly appeared as an epidemic in the Philippines in the 1960s and in Thailand. Adult worms 2–4 mm long invade the jejunal mucosa, causing abdominal pain with severe diarrhoea and malabsorption. Eggs resembling those of *Trichuris* are passed in the faeces. Freshwater fish are intermediate hosts. Untreated, mortality is high, but mebendazole (200 mg b.d. for 2 weeks) is effective.

Control of intestinal nematode infections

Most of these worms are transmitted through contaminated soil or unwashed hands. Safe disposal of faeces, the provision of clean drinking water and strict personal hygiene form the basis of control. Mass treatment at yearly intervals is also useful (Table 19.9). Capillariasis is controlled by cooking fish.

2. DISEASES DUE TO TISSUE-DWELLING HUMAN NEMATODES

Filariases

A number of different nematodes of the family *Filariidae* affect man. The adults are thin worms varying from 2 to 50 cm in length and the larvae, or microfilariae, are easily visible under the low power of the microscope (Fig. 19.15). The adults of the species *Wuchereria bancrofti* and *Brugia malayi* inhabit and tend to block lymphatic vessels. Adult filariae of the species *Loa loa* wander in the subcutaneous tissue and cause 'Calabar' swellings. The adults of *Onchocerca volvulus* may be surrounded by fibrous tissue in subcutaneous nodules but it is their larvae which cause a dermatosis and

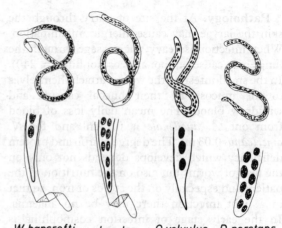

W. bancrofti   Loa loa   O. volvulus   D. perstans

Fig. 19.15 Microfilariae (170–320 × 3–10 μ) Second row shows tails (greatly enlarged).

eye lesions. The larvae of *Dipetalonema streptocerca* may produce a similar but milder dermatosis but *Dipetalonema perstans* and *Mansonella ozzardi*, the larvae of which circulate in the blood, are non-pathogenic. The microfilariae have distinguishing morphological appearances (Fig. 19.15). Filarial infections are commonly associated with a marked eosinophilia.

Bancroftian filariasis

Wuchereria bancrofti is conveyed to man by the bites of infected mosquitoes of a number of different species, the most common being *Culex fatigans*. The adult worms, 4 to 10 cm in length, live in the lymphatics, and the females produce microfilariae which at night circulate in large numbers in the peripheral blood. In the mosquito ingested microfilariae develop into infective larvae. As *Culex fatigans* bites at night the nocturnal periodicity of the microfilariae facilitates the spread of the infection. In some of the Pacific islands there is a non-periodic strain of *W. bancrofti* maintained by mosquitoes which bite in the daytime. When not circulating in the peripheral blood, the microfilariae are chiefly in the capillaries in the lungs and can cause pulmonary eosinophilia (p. 240). The infection is widespread in tropical Africa, the North African coast, coastal areas of Asia, Indonesia and Northern Australia, South Pacific Islands, West Indies and also in North and South America.

Pathology. Light infections are likely to be associated with an eosinophilia. In more intense and repeated infections the presence of mature worms in the lymphatic vessels and nodes leads to allergic inflammation around the lymphatics and to temporary lymphatic obstruction. Eventually, after repeated attacks, in some of which secondary bacterial infections may play a part, permanent obstruction of a main lymphatic trunk may be produced. Progressive enlargement of the limb or region below the obstruction then follows with thickening and fibrosis of the tissues.

Clinical features. After an incubation period of not less than 3 months there are bouts of fever accompanied by pain, tenderness and erythema along the course of inflamed lymphatic vessels. Inflammation of the spermatic cord, epididymitis and orchitis are common. After a few days the fever abates and the symptoms and signs subside.

Further attacks follow and temporary oedema from obstructed lymphatics tends to become more persistent, and some enlargement of regional lymph nodes may remain. The lymphatics draining the lower limbs, the scrotum and the upper limbs are most frequently affected, mainly or only on one side, and often accompanied by the formation of superficial lymph varices and the production of hydroceles. Progressive enlargement, coarsening, corrugation and fissuring of the skin and subcutaneous tissue, with warty superficial excrescences, develops gradually causing irreversible 'elephantiasis', which may also occur in an upper limb, the scrotum, vulva or breast. The scrotum may reach an enormous size. Obstruction of the abdominal or thoracic lymphatics may lead to chyluria, chylous ascites or a chylous pleural effusion (p. 263). Eventually the adult worms may die but the lymphatics remain obstructed. The interval between infection and the onset of elephantiasis is usually not less than 10 years and elephantiasis develops only in association with repeated infections in highly endemic areas.

Diagnosis. In the earliest stages of lymphangitis the diagnosis is made on clinical grounds, supported by eosinophilia and sometimes by positive serology. After about a year from the time of infection microfilariae appear in the blood at night and can be seen moving in a wet blood film (Fig. 19.15) or by microfiltration of a sample of lysed blood. They are usually present in hydrocele fluid which may on occasion yield an adult filaria. By the time elephantiasis develops microfilariae become difficult to find. Calcified filariae may sometimes be demonstrable by radiography. An initial exaggeration of symptoms following the administration of diethylcarbamazine suggests a filarial infection.

Immunodiagnosis. Indirect fluorescence detects antibody in over 95% of active cases and 70% of established elephantiasis. Cross-reactions occur in 15% of cases of strongyloidiasis and 5% of other intestinal nematodes. The test becomes negative 1–2 years after cure. Complement fixation is rather less specific and sensitive. Intradermal tests of immediate hypersensitivity are positive and persist for life. None of these tests distinguishes between the different filarial infections.

Non-filarial elephantiasis, usually affecting one or both legs, occurs in certain geographical areas which are free from filariasis. It is attributable to damage to lymphatics by silicates absorbed from soil derived from volcanic rocks.

Treatment. Diethylcarbamazine kills microfilariae and adult worms. The dosage is 9 to 12 mg/kg daily in three divided doses for 21 days orally. The full dosage should only be reached slowly, starting with 50 mg (one tablet) and doubling daily if no untoward allergic responses ensue. This course may be repeated twice at intervals of 4 to 6 weeks. To control allergic phenomena antihistamines or corticosteroids may be required. In established elephantiasis plastic surgery is indicated. Great relief may be obtained by removal of excess tissue but recurrences are probable unless new lymphatic drainage is established. Tight bandaging, or bed-rest with suspension or raising of the affected part or the nightly use of pneumatic stockings, may control the swelling to some extent.

Prevention. In endemic areas treatment of the whole population with diethylcarbamazine, 100 mg for adults (50 mg for children) three times daily for 7 days, has reduced but not eliminated the infection. Children are given such a course on starting and just before leaving school. This mass treatment should be combined with control of the vector by insecticides. Early chemotherapy prevents later elephantiasis. Individuals should avoid being bitten by mosquitoes (p. 774).

Brugia filariasis

Brugia malayi resembles *W. bancrofti* closely. The microfilariae usually exhibit nocturnal periodicity but a semiperiodic form, which may affect man, commonly infects animals. A similar filaria, *Brugia pahangi*, is found chiefly in animals but has been transmitted to man. It may be responsible for some cases of tropical pulmonary eosinophilia (p. 241). The vectors of *B. malayi* are mosquitoes mostly belonging to the genus *Mansonioides*. *B. malayi* is found in Indonesia, Borneo, Malaysia, Vietnam, South China, South India and Sri Lanka. A distinct, closely related, species, *B. timori* occurs in Timor.

The pathology, clinical manifestations, treatment and personal prophylaxis are the same as for *W. bancrofti* except that elephantiasis is usually limited to the legs. A selective weed-killer, phenoxylene, has been used with success to rid ponds of the water hyacinth upon which the larvae of *Mansonioides* are dependent.

Loiasis

Loiasis is caused by infection with the filaria *Loa loa* (Fig. 19.15). The adults, 3 to 7 cm × 0.4 mm, parasitise chiefly the subcutaneous tissue of man. The larval microfilariae circulate harmlessly in the peripheral blood in the daytime. The vector is *Chrysops*, a day biting, forest dwelling, fly.

Pathology. The adult worms move about in the subcutaneous tissues and other interstitial planes. Usually there is little evidence, apart from an eosinophilia, of a reaction of the host's tissues but from time to time a short-lived, inflammatory, oedematous swelling (a *Calabar swelling*) is produced, presumably around an adult worm. Heavy infections may rarely cause encephalitis, especially when treated.

Clinical features. The incubation period is commonly over a year but is often as short as 3 months. The infection is often symptomless. The first sign is usually a Calabar swelling. This is an irritating tense localised swelling which is painful if it is near a joint. The swelling is generally on a limb; it measures a few centimetres in diameter but sometimes is more diffuse and extensive. It usually disappears after a few days but may persist for 2 or 3 weeks. A succession of such swellings may appear at irregular intervals, often in nearby sites. Sometimes there is some urticaria and pruritus elsewhere. Occasionally a worm may be seen wriggling under the skin, especially of an eyelid and may cross the eye under the conjunctiva, taking many minutes to do so. When an adult worm is moving in retro-orbital tissues, severe unilateral headache resembling migraine is experienced.

Diagnosis is made be demonstrating microfilariae in the blood, but they may not always be found in patients with Calabar swellings. The filarial indirect fluorescent antibody test is positive in 95% of cases and there is an eosinophilia. Occasionally a calcified worm may be seen on a radiograph.

Treatment and prevention. Diethylcarbamazine (p. 795) is curative, gradually increased to a dose of 9 to 12 mg/kg daily and continued at that dosage for 21 days. In patients with a heavy microfilaraemia treatment may precipitate a severe reaction characterised by fever, joint and muscle pain and encephalitis and should be given under steroid cover.

Protection is afforded by siting houses away from trees and by having dwellings wire-screened against the fly. Protective clothing and repellents are also useful. Mud flats where *Chrysops* is breeding should be treated with Dieldrin or other chemicals to destroy the larvae and pupae. Treatment of the population with diethylcarbamazine will diminish the infective rate of the vector.

Onchocerciasis (river blindness)

Onchocerciasis is the result of infection by the filaria *Onchocerca volvulus* (Fig. 19.15). Although only about 0.3 mm in diameter, the adult female may be as long as 50 cm, the male being much shorter. The infection is conveyed by flies of the genus *Simulium* which inflict a painful bite. In West Africa the vector is *S. damnosum*, in Northern Nigeria also *S. bovis* and in East Africa and Zaïre *S. neavei*. The flies breed in rapidly flowing well-aerated water, the larvae being attached to submerged vegetation and rocks. The larvae of *S. neavei* may be attached to crabs and mayfly nymphs. Adult flies bite during the daytime both inside and outside houses. Man is the only known definitive host.

Onchocerciasis is endemic in well-defined areas throughout tropical Africa, in Southern Arabia and also in South Mexico, Guatemala, Colombia, Venezuela and Brazil. It is estimated that over 20 million people are infected. In parts of West and Central Africa it affects the whole adult population and blindness rates of 10% are common, reaching 35% in some parts of Ghana. Because of onchocerciasis huge tracts of fertile land lie virtually untilled.

Pathology. Infective larvae of *O. volvulus* are introduced into the skin by the bite of an infected *Simulium*. The worms mature in 2 to 4 months and live for up to 17 years in small colonies in subcutaneous and connective tissue. At sites of trauma, over bony prominences and around joints, fibrosis may form nodules around adult worms which otherwise cause no direct damage. In these nodules, in the adjacent tissues and widely distributed in the skin, innumerable microfilariae, discharged by the female *O. volvulus*, move actively and may invade the eye.

Live microfilariae elicit little tissue reaction, but dead microfilariae may cause severe allergic inflammation leading to hyaline necrosis and loss of collagen and elastin. In the eye, death of microfilariae causes conjunctivitis, sclerosing keratitis with pannus formation, iritis which may lead to glaucoma and cataract and, less commonly, choroidoretinitis and optic neuritis.

Clinical features. The infection may remain symptomless for months or years. The first symptom is usually itching at first localised to one quadrant of the body and later becoming generalised and involving the eyes. In Europeans evanescent oedema of part or all of a limb is an early sign, followed by papular urticaria spreading gradually from the site of infection. This is difficult to see on dark skins in which the commonest signs are papules excoriated by scratching, spotty hyperpigmentation from resolving inflammation and more chronic changes of a rough, thickened skin or inelastic wrinkled skin. Superficial lymph nodes enlarge and may hang down in folds of loose

skin at the groins. Hydrocele, femoral hernias and scrotal elephantiasis occur. In chronic infections, firm subcutaneous nodules (onchocercomas) are palpable, 1 or more cm in diameter.

Eye disease is commonest in some highly endemic areas and is associated with chronic heavy infections and nodules on the head. Early manifestations include itching, lachrymation, conjunctival injection and evidence of the features listed under pathology. Classically, 'snow flake' deposits are seen in the edges of the cornea.

Diagnosis. The finding of nodules or characteristic lesions of the skin or eyes, in a patient from an endemic area, associated with eosinophilia is suggestive. Aggravation of the dermatosis after a test dose of 50 mg of diethylcarbamazine supports the diagnosis. A skin snip or shaving, repeated if necessary from calf, buttock and shoulder is placed in saline under a cover slip on a microscope slide and examined after 1 hour. In all but the lightest infections microfilariae are seen wriggling free. Microfilariae can also sometimes be seen moving in the anterior chamber of the eye examined with a slit-lamp or identified in a conjunctival snip. A nodule may be removed and incised, showing the coiled threadlike adult worm. Filarial antibodies may be detected by immunofluorescence in 95% of cases.

Treatment and prevention. Any nodules detected should be removed. Diethylcarbamazine (p. 795) rapidly kills the microfilariae and this causes an allergic reaction for the first few days of treatment. The itch increases, eye lesions are aggravated and there may be accompanying fever with pain in the joints, hypotension and respiratory distress. Only a small dose should be given initially, 25 mg on the first day, this being gradually increased as the drug is tolerated until, if possible, a dose of 12 mg/kg is reached. This dose should be continued for 21 days. An antihistamine, such as chlorpheniramine maleate, may alleviate mild reactions but corticosteroids, locally as drops to the eyes and systemically, are needed to control severe reactions. Ideally the patient should be in bed for the first 24 hours of treatment.

Ivermectin, in a single dose of 100 to 200 μg/kg, kills microfilariae and prevents their return for up to 9 months. It is non-toxic and does not trigger severe reactions. It is likely to be marketed in

1987. Adult worms are killed by suramin (1 g i.v. weekly for 5–6 doses). In endemic areas where reinfection is inevitable, and in patients with little or no eye involvement, repeated courses of diethylcarbamazine or long-term suppression with 50 mg daily may be preferred to the potential toxicity of suramin.

Mass treatment is impossible at present. The *Simulium* can be destroyed in its larval stage by the application of insecticide to streams or the adult flies can be attacked by spraying vegetation near streams. Dimethylphthalate applied to skin or clothing will repel the fly for several hours. Long trousers or skirts and sleeves discourage the fly from biting.

Other filariases

Dipetalonema streptocerca. Microfilariae and adult worms of this parasite have been identified in the skin in Ghana, Cameroun and Zaïre. The microfilariae may produce a mild dermatosis of the trunk, usually less irritating than in onchocerciasis. This filariasis also responds to a course of diethylcarbamazine.

Dipetalonema perstans is a filarial parasite of man which is usually non-pathogenic. In endemic areas microfilariae of *D. perstans* are commonly found in the peripheral blood (Fig. 19.15). The adults inhabit chiefly the retroperitoneal and perirenal tissues and have been found in the pericardial sac. The intermediate hosts and vectors are the midges *Culicoides austeni* and *C. grahami*. This filaria is found throughout equatorial Africa as far south as Zambia, and also in Trinidad and parts of northern and eastern South America.

D. perstans has never been shown to cause disease but it may be responsible for a persistent eosinophilia and occasional allergic manifestations. *D. perstans* is resistant to diethylcarbamazine and the infection may persist for many years.

Mansonella ozzardi is non-pathogenic and is found in the West Indies and South America. The adults inhabit the mesentery and subperitoneal tissues. The microfilariae circulate in the blood. Diethylcarbamazine is ineffective.

Dracontiasis (Guinea worm infection)

The female *Dracunculus medinensis*, which measures over a metre in length, 0.9 to 1.7 mm in diameter, lives in the interstitial and subcutaneous tissues of man. The male worm, which is rarely seen, is only 2.5 cm long and dies earlier. Man is infected by ingesting a small crustacean, *Cyclops*, which inhabits the bottom of wells and ponds and which contains the infective larval stage of the worm.

When the cyclops is ingested by man the mature larvae penetrate the intestinal wall and migrate through the connective tissue of the host. After 9 to 18 months the fully mature female seeks the surface of the skin where a vesicle is raised, soon ruptures and exposes the anterior end of the worm. The distended uterus then ruptures and discharges its larvae externally. The worm is attracted to the surface by cooling, hence the larvae are likely to be expelled into water and complete the life cycle. Man is the most important host but *D. medinensis* has been found in dogs and cats.

The disease can be extremely disabling and is especially liable to affect women and children who collect water at water-holes or farmers at the beginning of the rains and thus seriously interfere with planting. It is found in West, Central and East Africa, the Sudan, Arabia, Iran, Turkey, Pakistan, Central India, Burma, the Caribbean Islands and the northern parts of South America.

Clinical features. The adult may sometimes be felt beneath the skin. Some hours before the head of the worm emerges from the skin there is usually some local inflammation. There may also be erythema, giant urticaria, nausea, vomiting and diarrhoea. These symptoms usually subside as soon as the vesicle has ruptured and the larvae begin to be discharged. This is usually complete in 3 to 4 weeks, after which the worm is often spontaneously extruded and healing takes place.

The vesicle commonly appears in the lower part of the leg or in any area which has been kept moist and relatively cool. If the worm dies or is broken during extraction there will be a marked allergic inflammation. The patient is immobilised by pain and swelling. Secondary infection is common and causes severe cellulitis, arthritis or septicaemia. Tetanus is a well-recognised complication. Multiple infections may occur and reactions around aberrant worms may cause serious lesions, exceptionally spinal cord compression.

Diagnosis is usually easy from the appearance of a vesicle, the protrusion of a worm and the recognition of the discharged larvae. A radiograph occasionally shows calcified worms.

Treatment and prevention. Traditionally the protruding worm has been extracted by winding it out gently over several days on a sterile match stick. Niridazole in doses of 25 mg/kg daily in 2 divided doses for 10 days, or mebendazole 100 mg b.d. for 7 days, may reduce inflammation and aid the extraction of the worm. Antibiotics for secondary infection and prophylaxis of tetanus are also required.

The provision of a satisfactory water supply would eradicate the infection. Where this is impracticable, wells and ponds may be protected or treated chemically.

3. DISEASES DUE TO ANIMAL NEMATODES

Toxocara canis. This is a common intestinal worm of dogs. The eggs are passed in the animal's faeces. Children who are in close contact with infected puppies are particularly liable to ingest ova of *Toxocara canis*. Larvae, liberated in the stomach, then migrate through the body and may cause allergic phenomena such as asthma, eosinophilia and also splenomegaly ('visceral larva migrans'). The worms do not usually mature in the human host. Occasionally a granuloma develops around a dead larva in the eye, resembling a neoplasm and causes blindness. Serology may aid diagnosis. Larval worms can be killed by diethylcarbamazine (9–12 mg/kg daily for 3 weeks). Granulomas may require surgical treatment.

Hookworms causing larva migrans. *Ancylostoma braziliense and A. caninum* are intestinal parasites of dogs with a similar life cycle to *A. duodenale*, but in man they cause a creeping eruption or cutaneous larva migrans. The larva burrows between the corium and stratum granulosum and progresses irregularly at about 1cm in 24 hours. The skin at the advancing end is erythematous and the older part of the burrow

discoloured and scaly. Itching may be intense. The larva may remain active for months. Treatment is topical. One 0.5 g tablet of thiabendazole is ground into 5 g petroleum jelly and rubbed in twice daily. Symptoms are relieved and the larva dies in a day or two.

Oesophagostomiasis. Species of the genus *Oesophagostomum*, a nematode related to hookworms, may cause a granuloma of the wall of the small intestine resembling a neoplasm. It has been reported chiefly from Uganda and is diagnosed at laparotomy.

Angiostrongylus. *A. cantonensis*, a nematode affecting the lungs of rodents, has a larval stage in molluscs and freshwater shrimps. In the Far East and the Pacific, where infected crustacea are eaten or infected slugs on vegetables are inadvertently swallowed, the larvae may cause a serious eosinophilic meningitis and immature worms may be found in the cerebrospinal fluid. Thiabendazole is effective but patients often recover spontaneously.

Trichinella spiralis. This parasite of rats and pigs is transmitted to man by eating partially cooked infected pork, usually as sausage or ham. Symptoms result from invasion of the body by larvae produced by the adult female worm in the small intestine and from their encystment in striated muscles. Outbreaks have occurred in Britain as well as in other countries where pork is eaten. Polar bear meat is another source.

The clinical course of trichinosis depends largely on the number of larvae. If there are only a few worms present there may be no symptoms but many worms may cause nausea and diarrhoea 24 to 48 hours after the infected meal. Soon, however, these symptoms are overshadowed by those associated with larval invasion, namely fever and oedema of the face, eyelids and conjunctivae. Invasion of the diaphragm may lead to pain, cough and dyspnoea; involvement of the muscles of the limbs, chest and mouth causes stiffness, pain and tenderness in the affected muscle groups. Pyrexia may reach 40°C with daily remissions. Larval migration may cause acute myocarditis and encephalitis. An eosinophilia is usually found after the second week. An intense infection may prove fatal, but those who survive recover completely.

It is not uncommon for a group of persons who

have eaten infected pork from a common source to develop symptoms about the same time. When suspected, biopsy from the deltoid or gastrocnemius after the third week of symptoms may reveal encysted larvae. Precipitin and intradermal tests are also helpful.

Thiabendazole, 25 mg/kg b.d. for 2 days, may relieve muscle pain. Given early in the infection it may kill adult worms in the gut. Corticosteroids are given to control the serious effects of acute inflammation.

Gnathostomiasis. *G. spinigerum* is a nematode of dogs and cats. In the Far East the third stage larva is acquired by man eating inadequately cooked infected fish or by swallowing water containing infected *Cyclops*. The immature worm usually migrates to the subcutaneous tissue where it causes recurrent swellings. The full grown adult worm, which may be as long as 3 cm, may be visible through the skin when it can be excised. In deeper tissues the worm may cause injury to the brain, kidney, lung, eye or other organs. Eosinophilia is usually pronounced. Diagnosis is easy when the adult worm is visible. Otherwise serological tests are performed. Treatment is not satisfactory but some success has been obtained with bithionol used as for paragonimiasis (p. 786).

Anisakiasis (herring worm disease). *A. marina* parasitises herrings and other marine animals. Human infections occur in Holland and Japan from the consumption of raw herrings. An eosinophilic granuloma forms in the intestine and may give rise to colic, fever and intestinal obstruction. An indirect haemagglutination test has been used for diagnosis. Surgery may be required.

DISEASES DUE TO ARTHROPODS

Infections conveyed by arthropods; lice infestation; scabies; tungiasis; myiasis; porocephalosis

Arthropods may be responsible for disease in three ways. They may act as vectors of infectious agents (Table 19.10). They may envenomate through stings or bites (p. 706), or they may infest or even infect the human body directly.

Lice. As well as transmitting serious diseases, the body louse *Pediculus humanus corporis* causes dermatitis and sleeplessness through itching, especially in poor crowded communities in cold countries (for control see p. 740). The head louse, *Pediculus humanus capitis*, is cosmopolitan and increasing in prevalence in British schools. It makes the child itch and alarms parents and teachers. Tiny white oval eggs, 'nits', are seen attached to the base of hairs on the scalp. The crab louse (p. 421) is transmitted while sharing beds. A single treatment with gammabenzene hexachloride (BHC) shampoo or lotion is usually

Table 19.10 Infections conveyed by arthropods.

Name	Genus	Disease
House fly	Musca	Dysenteries, enteric fevers, salmonelloses, ?cholera, ?trachoma, ?tropical ulcer
Horse fly	Tabanidae	?anthrax, tularaemia
Oscinid fly	Hippelates	?yaws, streptococcal dermatitis and nephritis
Tsetse fly	Glossina	African trypanosomiasis
Mosquito	Anopheles	Malaria, some arboviruses, Bancroftian and Brugia filariasis in some areas
	Aedes	Yellow fever, dengue, and other arboviruses
	Culex	Bancroftian and Brugia filariasis, Japanese B encephalitis and other arboviruses
Black fly	Simulium	Onchocerciasis
Midges	Culicoides	Dipetolema perstans, D. streptocerca, Mansonella ozzardi
Soft ticks	Ornithodoros	Tick-borne relapsing fever, Lyme disease
Hard ticks	(Ixodidae), Rhipicephalus, etc.	Some typhus fevers, ?Q fever, Kyasanur Forest disease, tularaemia
Sandflies	Phlebotomus	Leishmaniases, sandfly fever, bartonellosis
Lice	Pediculus	Epidemic typhus fever, louse-borne relapsing fever, trench fever, Dipylidium caninum
Mites	Leptotrombidium	Scrub typhus fever
	Allodermanyssus	Rickettsialpox
Winged Bug	Triatoma	Chagas' disease
Fleas	Xenopsylla	Plague, endemic typhus fever
	Ctenocephalides	Dipylidium caninum

curative. In countries, such as Britain, where resistance is developing to BHC, malathion or carbaryl is preferred.

Scabies is due to the mite *Sarcoptes scabei*; it is common all over the world. It causes itching, initially between the fingers or on the buttocks or genitals where the mite burrows, and later all over the body. In the tropics secondary streptococcal infection is an important cause of rheumatic fever and glomerulonephritis. The diagnosis of scabies is confirmed by finding the causative mite in a burrow. Scabies is treated by a single application of gammabenzene hexachloride 1% to the whole body below the neck or by three daily applications of benzyl benzoate 15%.

Tungiasis (Jiggers) is due to infestation with *Tunga penetrans* (the chigoe or jigger flea). It is widespread in tropical America and Africa. Man and pigs are important hosts. The pregnant female flea burrows into the skin about the toes and soles and grows as large as a pea, packed with eggs which are subsequently discharged on to the surface. The burrows irritate and become inflamed but the chief danger is from secondary pyogenic infection or tetanus. The chigoe and egg sac should be removed with a sterile needle and a mild antiseptic ointment applied. Massive infestations, such as may be seen in neglected children and in senile persons, may be treated by immersing the feet in an aqueous solution containing benzene hexachloride 5% and cetrimide 0.8%.

Myiasis is an infestation of various tissues of man by the larvae of flies.

CUTANEOUS MYIASIS. A common cause of cutaneous myiasis is *Cordylobia anthropophaga* (Tumbu fly) which lays its eggs on laundry spread on grass. The larvae penetrate the skin and produce lesions like boils with central orifices through which they breathe. On reaching maturity they emerge. A drop of thick oil or petroleum jelly usually brings a larva out in search of air and facilitates its removal. Occasionally the common warble fly (*Hypoderma bovis*) may infest man.

MYIASIS OF WOUNDS, SORES AND CAVITIES. The larvae of many flies may infest necrotic tissue in open wounds or ulcers and occasionally invade living tissue. *Chrysomya bezziana* is found in Africa, India and South Vietnam. It may penetrate the nasal sinuses and cause great destruction. The application of 10% chloroform in a light vegetable oil is the treatment of choice for infested wounds.

INTESTINAL MYIASIS. In the tropics especially, vague digestive disturbances or abdominal cramps with diarrhoea and vomiting may be caused by fly larvae in the intestinal canal, the eggs having been ingested with food.

Porocephalosis is invasion of the body by 'tongue worms', degenerate arthropods of which *Armillifer armillatus*, *A. moniliformis* and *Linguatula serrata* occur in man. Adult *Armillifer* parasitise the trachea and bronchi of snakes. Man is infected by ingesting ova on uncooked vegetables or by eating undercooked snakes. The condition is usually symptomless in man but calcified nymphs may be seen in the radiographs of the chest and abdomen.

Halzoun is the name given in the Middle East to a form of acute dysphagia and laryngeal obstruction from pharyngitis and oedema of the larynx. It is due to the ingestion of nymphs of *Linguatula serrata* in undercooked liver and lymph nodes of sheep and goats. Foxes and dogs are the definitive hosts. Antihistamines and a local anaesthetic spray may be helpful.

ADVICE TO TRAVELLERS

A map illustrating the distribution of the most serious tropical diseases is shown in Figure 18.1.

Yellow fever is the only infection for which immunisation is currently required by International Health Regulations. Information about this and about other medically recommended immunisations is given in Table 19.11.

In addition, it is important that all visitors to the tropics and subtropics should take all appropriate measures to avoid malaria and also take prophylactic antimalarial drugs regularly from the week before travel and continue until 4 weeks after returning to a non-malarious area. Details are given on page 774. Neglect of this advice has been responsible for fatalities. Other common problems that the traveller should take steps to avoid include diarrhoea, hepatitis, insect bites, venereal disease, AIDS, disorders due to climate and jet lag.

Table 19.11 Medically recommended immunisations for travellers.

Inoculation	Where advised	Course programme	Validity	Minimum age advised	Other comments
Yellow fever	Central Africa 15°N to 10°S Panama State to 15°S	1 subcutaneous injection	After 10 days for 10 years	1 year	The only immunisation currently *required* by International Health Regulations
Cholera	Entering or transiting a cholera zone	2 subcutaneous injections, 4–6 weeks apart	After 6 days for 6 months	1 year	Poor protection. Very few countries *require* it
Typhoid	Everywhere	2 subcutaneous injections, 4–6 weeks apart	Booster injection every 3 years	2 years	0.1 ml intradermal adequate for booster, less toxic
Tetanus	Everywhere	3 subcutaneous injections 4–6 weeks and 6 months apart	Booster injection every 10 years	None	See also page 38
Poliomyelitis	Everywhere	3 oral doses of attenuated virus at monthly intervals	Booster every 5 years, 3 doses better than 1	None	See also page 38
Rabies	Endemic countries	3 subcutaneous or intradermal injections 4 weeks 4–6 months apart	Over 5 years	1 year	Groups at risk, using human diploid cell vaccine
Plague	Parts of S.E. Asia, E. Africa, USA	2 injections at 10–20 day intervals, 3rd 6 months later	6 months	1 year	Only special groups at risk
Typhus	Parts of S.E. Asia, Ethiopia, etc.	2 injections at 7–10 day intervals, 3rd 6 months later	1 year		Only special groups at risk
Hepatitis B	Endemic countries	3 intramuscular injections 4 weeks and 6 months apart	Over 5 years	1 year	Special groups at risk, resident expatriates
Gamma Globulin for type A hepatitis	Countries where sanitation is poor	Intramuscular injection 250 mg or 500 mg. Age under 10 years, halfdose	4–6 months	10 years	Also protects against measles, rubella

Malaria prophylaxis, see page 774.
Diphtheria and pertussis, see page 38.

Global aspects of the prevention of disease and the promotion of health are discussed in the next chapter.

A.D.M. BRYCESON
A.M. GEDDES

FURTHER READING:

General:

Christie A B 1980 Infectious diseases: epidemiology and clinical practice, 3rd edn. Churchill Livingstone, Edinburgh
Mandell G L et al (eds) 1985 Principles and practice of infectious diseases, 2nd edn. Wiley, New York
Mims C A 1982 The pathogenesis of infectious disease, 2nd edn. Academic Press, London

Walker E, Williams G 1985 ABC of healthy travel, 2nd edn. British Medical Association, London
Clinics in tropical medicine and communicable diseases 1987 Baillière Tindall, Eastbourne. A series of reviews of advances in these fields on an international basis

Parasitology:

Knight R 1982 Parasitic disease in man. Churchill Livingstone, Edinburgh
Muller R 1975 Worms and disease. Heinemann, London
Beaver P C et al (eds) 1985 Clinical parasitology, 9th edn. Lea and Febiger, Philadelphia

Leprosy:

Hastings E C (ed) 1986 Leprosy. Churchill Livinstone, Edinburgh

Malaria:
Bruce-Chwatt L J 1985 Essential malariology, 2nd edn. Heinemann, London

Amoebiasis:
Stamm W P 1976 Amoebiasis: a neglected diagnosis. Journal of the Royal College of Physicians of London 10: 294–298

20

The promotion of health and prevention of disease

Physicians of the utmost fame,
Were called at once; but when they came,
They answered as they took their fees,
'There is no cure for this disease.'

Hilaire Belloc

Unfortunately most doctors see their role as curing rather than preventing disease. However, despite the major advances that have occurred in medicine, there are still many diseases for which there is no cure and where immediate hope for the future lies in prevention. An example of this is the antenatal diagnosis of diseases such as Down's syndrome or neural tube defects. More recently new genetic techniques combined with chorion biopsy have raised the real possibility that conditions like muscular dystrophy, retinitis pigmentosa and polycystic kidney disease could be detected at an early stage in pregnancy. It is also possible to diagnose cystic fibrosis, the commonest lethal inherited disease, in utero. It is thus likely that major advances in the field of prevention will markedly affect the pattern of diseases that doctors will face in the next decade. Throughout this book special attention has been paid to prevention when individual diseases have been discussed. However, the importance of the topic is such that it is appropriate to conclude by giving a broader consideration to the allied questions of the promotion of health and prevention of disease. In this context we must obviously consider not just the problems of an affluent society but also put diseases into a global perspective. Physicians would do well to remember Sir Thomas Browne's full quotation: 'Charity begins at home, is the voice of the world'.

Needs of tropical and developing countries

A survey of patterns of disease in the tropics and developing countries has been made in Chapter 18 and methods of prevention of individual diseases have been discussed. The promotion of health and the prevention of disease are, however, related to fundamental principles sometimes far removed from medical therapeutics and prophylaxis.

Whereas obesity is a major problem in affluent communities, undernutrition and malnutrition are dominant in underdeveloped countries. Adequate nutrition depends primarily on preserving the fertility of the soil and making good use of its vegetable products and, if customs permit, of the animals which are themselves dependent on the vegetation. Preservation or construction of water supplies is also a fundamental need and afforestation and contour terracing may help to prevent the land becoming denuded by floods. Only if a poor country can become richer, can sustained improvement in health be expected. More efficient agriculture and animal husbandry will tend to lead to improved health and economy; further progress may follow the utilisation of mineral resources and the development of productive industries and tourism.

Much help has been given in starting these processes by outside agencies but in order that lasting benefit should accrue it must be accompanied by better education. It is of paramount importance that the people concerned must themselves be fully convinced of the value and practicability of the projects and desire their benefits. Progress may be slow when improvements in health necessitate changes in food habits and other traditional practices, and will be maintained only when projects become an integral part of the development programme of the country and are operated largely by local personnel. Training of local nationals is, therefore, essential.

Increases in food supplies may be outstripped by increases in population. Family planning is, thus, a priority in many developing countries and emphasis should be laid both on the successful rearing of healthy children and on the reduction of the population growth. Any progress can be vitiated by war or other political disturbance, hence the preservation of peace and law and order are crucial.

It will be clear that the medical practitioner's role in these measures will be chiefly that of an informed adviser. The relative values to community health of money spent, for example, on improved schooling as compared with eradication of malaria may be very difficult to assess, yet governments with limited resources have frequently to decide between such priorities. It has been shown in some areas that the provision of a protected water supply is the most economical way of improving health. Irrigation schemes may be essential to increase the areas of fertile land but expert advice may be required to prevent the spread thereby of malaria, schistosomiasis and onchocerciasis. The eradication of onchocerciasis and animal trypanosomiasis would lead, but at great expense, to the conversion of vast tracts of unused fertile land to pastoral and agricultural use.

In developing countries the provision of curative measures, which may also be important factors in prevention, involves the same principles as in affluent societies but their application is modified by the limitations of available finance and personnel. Priority should be given to measures which will improve the health and prospects of children and wage earners.

In order to reach the scattered rural population a chain of health centres, under-5-year-old clinics and peripheral aid posts have proved of great value. At the health centres, maternity and child welfare have priority and at all levels health education is actively pursued. Breast feeding of all children for at least the first 6 months should be the rule and importation of expensive foreign baby foods should be kept to a minimum. Breast feeding is probably the most important contraceptive in the world. Frequent suckling maintains high levels of prolactin and hence continuing secondary amenorrhoea and infertility. Thus the introduction of free milk powder with cessation of breast feeding has produced a population explosion in some countries.

Immunisation of children and, in the case of tetanus, of expectant mothers also, may do much to reduce mortality rates. Domiciliary visits from the centres increase the contact with outlying homesteads. The vulnerability of small children to gastroenteritis underlines the importance of education in cleanliness and the provision of pure water supplies, but may also necessitate the organisation of local facilities for rapid rehydration.

Making the best use of medical auxiliaries is essential if the health services are to become widely available. Peripheral clinics have to be related to district and central hospitals from which some degree of supervision can be exercised and to which patients can be referred if transport is available. Only minimal curative medicine is carried out at the peripheral clinics, but preventive measures must be seen to be related to curative medicine, otherwise little support for them will be forthcoming. The provision of specialised care, even in the central hospitals, should not be out of proportion to the general standard of medical care and medical education should include experience in both categories. Political pressure to divert effort and money into prestige units should be resisted.

The misuse of drugs in the developed countries is more than matched by that in the developing world. Thus scarce resources are often wasted because people are prescribed drugs which are not required and many expensive combinations are used. Because of this antibiotic resistance is common and drug side-effects present a major problem. What is tragic is that this abuse of drugs by one section of the population is associated with the lack of essential drugs for the majority. These problems can be solved only by educating doctors so that prescribing is improved, and by informing patients so that their demands for polypharmacy are reduced. Only then will all pharmaceutical companies realise that the Third World can no longer be used as a dumping ground for drugs with toxicity that has severely limited their use in more developed countries, or as an area to be exploited to maintain profit margins.

Organisation in disaster situations

If earthquakes, floods, drought or other disasters strike an area, help from outside is urgently needed to maintain food supplies and to prevent the spread of disease from sudden impairment of hygiene. When the disaster is war, a nuclear accident (p. 531), earthquakes or volcanic eruptions it may be difficult and dangerous to get supplies to the stricken areas. Failure of food and medicines to reach the people is often more the result of disorganisation than unavailability of supplies that can be flown in from international donors. Relief agencies from different countries often try to operate without adequate communication with local community leaders or with one another. Governments in countries where famine is recurrent should have civil servants permanently employed in keeping plans for famine relief up to date.

Needs of developed countries

The term 'developed' is used to denote wealthy communities, mainly industrial. It is not intended to imply that the acquisition of more material possessions is necessarily a desirable goal or that the way of life in developed societies does not contain defects, some of which are deleterious to health.

The role of the family doctor. National and local government bodies assume the responsibility for ensuring the availability of adequate food supplies, education, housing, health services and the prevention of environmental pollution but the family doctor plays an important role in encouraging people to make full use of preventive services and in advising them about healthy living.

All doctors must give much thought to finding means of enhancing the acceptance of health advice by individual patients.

Genetic counselling (p. 15), immunisation programmes and the early recognition and treatment of disease, the provision of iron and folic acid for expectant mothers and vitamins C and D for young children do much to ensure a good beginning in the building of a healthy nation. Where local mineral deficiencies exist, fluoridation of water to prevent dental caries and iodised salt to prevent goitre have proved their value.

The medical profession must continue to seek improvement in the working conditions in mines and factories and to draw attention to the special needs of persons in stressful occupations or doing repetitive work on mass production assembly lines. Industrial hazards and environmental risk factors such as lead must be identified and eliminated.

Screening for disease, such as tuberculosis, hypertension and diabetes mellitus, can be carried out readily by the family doctor and can be supplemented by the use of mass miniature chest radiography. Malignant disease of the breast and cervix can be detected at a very early stage, if apparently healthy young women are examined regularly. Self-examination of the breasts can be taught. For those in the middle years of life, medical reviews, at intervals of no longer than 2 years, facilitate the early recognition of disease such as hypertension, diabetes and malignancy.

The needs of the elderly may include prophylactic measures such as the use of vitamins C and D. There is also a requirement to assess and treat the multiple disabilities frequently overlooked in this age group, to provide social support and community services for the isolated and to find suitable accommodation for those whose need is for continuing care.

For patients of all ages it is the doctor's duty to encourage healthy living habits in matters such as exercise and diet with emphasis on an energy value appropriate to the needs of the individual, an ample content of dietary fibre, and, more contentiously, moderation in the intake of saturated fat.

The dietary guidelines in Scandinavia for the general public were introduced in 1968 and have since been followed, with local modifications, in several major industrial countries: 'The supply of calories (energy) in the diet should in many cases be reduced to prevent overweight. The total consumption of fat should be reduced from 40% (the present figure) to between 25 and 35% of energy. The use of saturated fat should be reduced and consumption of polyunsaturated fats increased (p. 811). Consumption of sugar and sugar-rich products should be reduced. The consumption of vegetables, fruit, potatoes, skimmed milk, fish, lean meat and cereal products should be increased'. Food additives are rightly kept under regular and careful review by responsible governments.

From the medical and nutritional standpoint the importance of taking regular exercise from an early age, particularly for those who have mainly sedentary occupations, should also be emphasised. What has been lightheartedly called the runner's 'high' or the daily exercise 'fix' may well be due to a surge of opioid peptides. Regular exercise is also beneficial for the elderly.

In 1604, King James, son of Mary Queen of Scots, described tobacco smoking as a custom loathsome to the eye, harmful to the brain and dangerous to the lungs. Since then many other adverse features have been described but nevertheless much more positive action is required by individuals and the community. A constant awareness is also necessary about the dangers of the consumption of alcohol and other addictive drugs.

The role of promiscuity amongst male homosexuals in spreading the virus responsible for the acquired immunodeficiency syndrome (AIDS) is now clear. It is important that doctors should keep up to date on this distressing condition as it raises major moral and ethical issues in addition to the medical problems. Drug addicts who share syringes are frequently infected with the AIDS virus as well as hepatitis B. It is more sensible to provide free syringes than to allow spread in this way.

Hepatitis B virus infection is widespread in both developed and developing countries. It has been suggested that 170 million people in the world are persistently infected with this virus with about 800 000 chronic carriers in the United States. Infection is linked to the development of chronic liver disease and liver cancer. An effective vaccine is now available but the cost of widescale immunisation is prohibitive. Doctors thus need to identify those people with a high risk of exposure to the virus.

Much can be done to promote mental health by doctors listening attentively to patients and thus helping individuals to contend with their psychological problems while also detecting those with psychiatric disturbances. In this area the prevention of intentional self-poisoning in modern society presents a major challenge (p. 711). There is increasing evidence that good mental health retards physical deterioration in mid-life. Many people think that for full health some form of 'belief' may be necessary to satisfy man's need to feel he belongs to the cosmos and is part of something outside himself. In the words of John Donne, 'No man is an island, entire of itself'.

Conclusion

In all communities, there should be continuing demands for improvement in housing standards and in food hygiene particularly for those in the lower socio-economic group whose vulnerability is often increased by unemployment and by inadequate access to health resources. In many societies the morbidity and mortality from road traffic accidents is rapidly increasing and is related to the abuse of alcohol and drugs. In urban areas there are growing problems in regard to corruption, crime, violence, baby and wife battering, rape, sexual promiscuity and heroin addiction. But there are even greater potential hazards. Man has now the capacity to destroy himself not only with nuclear weapons but by using up the natural resources of the planet so fast and by polluting the environment so thoroughly that he is in danger of precipitating his own doom. Everyone, especially doctors, economists, agriculturists and statesmen, is involved in this challenge and the response to it is vital.

C. R. W. EDWARDS
I. A. D. BOUCHIER

FURTHER READING:

Black D, Morris J N, Smith C, Townsend P 1982 In: Townsend P, Davidson N (eds) Inequalities in health: the Black report. Penguin, Harmondsworth. A critical analysis of health in Britain in comparison with other industrialised countries, containing many recommendations for improvement

Howe G M, Lorraine J A (eds) 1980 Environmental medicine, 2nd edn. Heinemann, London. Wide-ranging reviews by experts on environmental and social threats to health

Morley D 1973 Paediatric priorities in the developing world. Obtainable at low cost from the Institute of Child Health, 30 Guildford Street, London WC1

Robinson D A (ed) 1984 Epidemiology and community control of disease in warm climate countries, 2nd edn. Churchill Livingstone, Edinburgh

21

Appendices

CONTENTS

Diets

Desirable weights

Biochemical values

Haematological values

Drug nomenclature and prescription

DIETS

The diet sheets that follow have been constructed to illustrate the quantitative and qualitative aspects of diets required for the treatment of obesity and diabetes mellitus. The quantities given in a standard diet sheet will obviously require some modification in relation to the size, age, sex, and occupation of the patient. In the dietetic treatment of most diseases it is unnecessary to weigh accurately the amounts of the different foods eaten. Under these circumstances sufficient accuracy will be secured by the use of household measures as illustrated in Diet 1 and by the terms 'small', 'medium' or 'large' helping for meat, fish or chicken. A small helping weighs approximately 30–60 g (1 to 2 oz), a medium helping 60–90 g (2 to 3 oz) and a large helping 120 g (4 oz) or more.

The qualitative content of the diet, i.e. the actual food consumed, will vary widely. The examples detailed here are suitable for persons whose food habits are those of the Western world. If they are to be effective therapeutically, diet prescriptions must be carefully adapted to take account of national, cultural and local eating habits.

The subcommittee on Metrication of the British National Committee for Nutritional Sciences of the Royal Society recommended in 1972 that kilojoules should be used in place of the kilocalories. 1 kcal = 4.184 kJ, so that the calorie conversion factors (heat of combustion; available energy) for carbohydrate, fat, protein and alcohol are 16, 37, 17 and 29 kJ/g. Useful practical approximations are: 950 kcal = 4000 kJ; 1450 kcal = 6000 kJ; 2850 kcal = 12 000 kJ

1. LOW ENERGY (CALORIE) DIET

Suitable for adults with obesity with or without diabetes.

Approximately: Protein 60 g. Carbohydrate 100 g. Fat 40 g. Energy 1000 kcal (4184 kJ)

Early morning	Cup of tea, milk from allowance, if desired.
Breakfast	1 egg or 30 g (1 oz) grilled lean bacon (2 rashers) *or* cold ham *or* breakfast fish. 20 g (⅔ oz) white or brown bread, *or* exchange, with butter from allowance. Tea or coffee, with milk from allowance.
Mid-morning	Tea or coffee, with milk from allowance, or 'free' drink from Group A3. 1 cream cracker or water biscuit
Mid-day meal	Clear soup, tomato juice or grapefruit, if desired Small helping, 60 g (2 oz) lean meat, ham, poultry, game or offal *or* 90 g (3 oz) white fish (steamed, baked or grilled) *or* 2 eggs *or* 45 g (1½ oz) cheese. Salad or vegetables from Group A1 as desired. 40 g (1⅓ oz) bread (white or brown) *or* exchange, with butter from allowance if desired. 1 portion of fruit from bread exchange list below. Tea or coffee with milk from allowance.

Mid-afternoon   20 g ($\frac{2}{3}$ oz) white or brown bread, *or exchange*, with butter from allowance.

Evening meal   Clear soup, meat or yeast extracts, tomato juice or grapefruit, if desired.

Small helping, 60 g (2 oz) lean meat, ham, poultry, game or offal *or* 90 g (3 oz) white fish (steamed, baked or grilled) *or* 1 egg *or* 45 g (1$\frac{1}{2}$ oz) cheese.

Salad or vegetables from Group A1 as desired.

40 g (1$\frac{1}{3}$ oz) bread (white or brown) *or* exchange, with butter from allowance if desired.

1 portion of fruit from list below.

Tea or coffee with milk from allowance.

Before bed   Tea or coffee with milk from allowance.

1 cream cracker or water biscuit.

Allowance for day: 200 ml ($\frac{1}{3}$ pint) milk with the cream poured off the top.

15 g ($\frac{1}{2}$ oz) butter or margarine.

Exchanges for 20 g ($\frac{2}{3}$ oz) bread ($\frac{1}{2}$ slice from a large cut loaf):

2 cream crackers	1 potato (the size of a hen's egg)
1$\frac{1}{2}$ of any crispbread	1 portion of fruit (from list below)
2 water biscuits	
1 oatcake	

Exchanges for 40 g (1$\frac{1}{3}$ oz) bread (1 slice from a large cut loaf):

4 cream crackers	2 potatoes
3 Ryvita	4 water biscuits
2 oatcakes	

Fruit list: 1 medium apple, 1 orange, 1 pear, 1 small banana, 10 grapes.

Group A: foods which may be taken as desired

1. *Vegetables*

Artichoke, asparagus, aubergine, French beans, runner beans, broccoli, Brussels sprouts, cabbage, carrots, cauliflower, celeriac, celery, chicory, courgette, cucumber, endive, leeks, lettuce, mushrooms, mustard and cress, onions, parsley, pumpkin, radishes, salsify, seakale, spinach, swede, tomatoes, turnip tops, vegetable marrow, watercress.

2. *Fruits* (stewed without sugar, or raw)

Gooseberries, grapefruit, lemon, melons (cantaloupe, water or honeydew), rhubarb, blackcurrants, red currants, blackberries, strawberries and raspberries.

3. *Drinks*

Water, soda water, tea or coffee (without milk or sugar) lemon juice, tomato juice, diabetic fruit squash, clear soup (chicken or beef cubes may be used).

4. *Miscellaneous*

Saxine, saccharine or any proprietary sweetening agents (except Sucron and sorbitol) salt, pepper, mustard, vinegar, herbs, spices, gelatine. Flavourings and colourings may be used.

Group B: foods to be avoided

All fried foods.

Sugar (brown or white), glucose, sorbitol.

Sweets, toffees, chocolates, cornflour, custard powder.

Jam, marmalade, lemon curd, syrup, honey, treacle.

Tinned, frozen or bottled fruits.

Dried fruits, e.g. dates, figs, prunes, apricots, sultanas, currants, raisins, bananas, grapes.

Cakes, buns, pastries, pies, steamed or milk puddings.

Sweet or chocolate biscuits, scones.

Cereals, e.g. rice, sago, macaroni, barley, spaghetti.

Breakfast cereal, porridge.

Ice cream, fresh or synthetic cream. Table jelly.

Evaporated or condensed milk.

Peas, parsnips, beetroot, sweetcorn, haricot beans, butterbeans, broad beans, lentils.

Nuts.

Salad cream, salad dressing, mayonnaise.

Tomato and brown sauce or any thickened sauce.

Sweet pickles and chutney.

Thickened soups, gravies.

Alcoholic drinks, e.g. beer, wine, sherry, spirits.

Sweetened fruit juices, fruit squash, Coca Cola and other sweet, fizzy, 'soft drinks'.

Starch-reduced products, 'diabetic' foodstuffs.

Sausages.

All foods must be served without thickened gravies and sauces. All foods may be baked, grilled, boiled or steamed — *but not fried.*

2. MEASURED DIABETIC DIET

Method of constructing a diet restricted in carbohydrate containing approximately 1800 kcal (7560 kJ) with 230 g carbohydrate, 72 g protein and 66 g fat suitable for adults with diabetes mellitus.

Use is made of the Atwater calorie conversion factors of 4, 4 and 9 kcal/g for carbohydrate, protein and fat respectively. Each *carbohydrate exchange* contains approximately 10 g carbohydrate, 1.5 g protein and 0.3 fat. Calorie value is about 50 (equivalent to 20 g bread).

Each *protein exchange* contains approximately 7 g protein and 5 g fat. Calorie value is about 70 (equivalent to 30 g meat).

Each *fat exchange* contains approximately 12 g fat and almost no carbohydrate or protein. Calorie value is about 110 (equivalent to $\frac{1}{2}$ oz butter). One pint of milk contains approximately 30 g carbohydrate, 18 g protein and 24 g fat. Calorie value is about 410.

In practice, for quick construction of a diabetic diet it is usually only necessary to work in terms of grams of carbohydrate and total calories. Thus, a diet prescription for 230 g carbohydrate, 1800 kcal would be calculated as follows:

1. The daily intake of carbohydrate (230 g) represents 23 carbohydrate exchanges.

2. The daily allowance of milk is decided, either on the basis of the patient's food habits or special requirements. In this example it is 400 ml ($\frac{2}{3}$ pint), which contains 2 carbohydrate exchanges, leaving 21 for distribution throughout the day.

3. The daily allowance of protein is then decided. Four protein exchanges will provide 280 kcal.

4. The calories allocated so far amount to 1590; a further 220 kcal are needed to bring the total up to approximately 1800 kcal. This must be provided by fat. As one fat exchange provides 110 kcal, two are needed.

Exchanges	Grams of carbohydrate	kcal
400 ml ($\frac{2}{3}$ pint) milk = 2 carbo- hydrate exchange	20	260
21 carbohydrate exchanges	210	1050
4 protein exchanges	—	280
Total	280	1610
2 fat exchanges	—	220
GRAND TOTAL	230	1810

5. Finally, the exchanges (23 carbohydrate, 4 protein and 2 fat) are distributed throughout the day according to the eating habits and daily routine of the patient.

Useful CHO exchanges

Each item on this list = 1 CHO exchange (10 g CHO): $\frac{1}{2}$ slice bread from a large loaf, 1 large digestive biscuit, 2 cream crackers, 8 tablespoons natural unsweetened orange juice or grapefruit juice, 1 medium-sized eating apple or orange, 10 grapes, 1 small banana, $\frac{1}{3}$ pint milk, 1 teacup cooked porridge, 1 teacup of cream or tinned soup, $\frac{2}{3}$ teacup cornflakes, 1 small packet of crisps, one small potato.

3. UNMEASURED DIABETIC DIET

Patients who are unable to measure their diet or for whom this is unnecessary, are given a list of foods which are grouped into three categories.

I. *Foods to be avoided altogether:*

1. Suger, glucose, jam, marmalade, honey, syrup, treacle, tinned fruits, sweets, chocolate, lemonade, glucose drinks, proprietary milk preparations and similar foods which are sweetened with sugar.

2. Cakes, sweet biscuits, chocolate biscuits, pies, puddings, thick sauces.

3. Alcoholic drinks unless permission has been given by the doctor.

II. *Foods to be eaten in moderation only:*

1. Breads of all kinds (including so-called 'slimming' and 'starch-reduced' breads, brown or white, plain or toasted).

2. Rolls, scones, biscuits and crispbreads.

3. Potatoes, peas and baked beans.

4. Breakfast cereals and porridge.

5. All fresh or dried fruit.

6. Macaroni, spaghetti, custard and foods with much flour.

7. Thick soups.

8. Diabetic foods.

9. Milk.

III. *Foods to be eaten as desired:*

1. All meats, fish, eggs.

2. Cheese.

3. Clear soups or meat extracts, tomato or lemon juice.

4. Tea or coffee.

5. Cabbage, Brussels sprouts, broccoli, cauliflower, spinach, turnip, runner or French beans, onions, leeks or mushrooms, lettuce, cucumber, tomatoes, spring onions, radishes, mustard and cress, asparagus, parsley, rhubarb.

6. Herbs, spices, salt, pepper and mustard.

7. Saccharine preparations for sweetening.

For overweight diabetics butter, margarine, fatty and dried foods must be restricted.

4. FAT-MODIFIED DIET

Low in saturated fats and cholesterol with increased amounts of polyunsaturated fat.

Foods to be avoided:

Butter and hydrogenated margarines. Use polyunsaturated margarine, e.g. 'Flora'.

Lard, suet, shortenings and cakes, biscuits and pastries made with these.

Fatty meat and visible fat on meat. Meat pieces, sausages and luncheon meats.

Whole milk and cream.

Chocolate, ice cream (except water ices). Cheese, except low fat cottage cheese.

Coconut and coconut oil.

Eggs — no more than 1 to 2 egg yolks per week, including that used in cooking.

Organ meats — liver, kidneys and brain.

Shellfish and fish roes.

Fried foods unless fried in polyunsaturated oil (like sun-flower or corn oil).

Potato crisps and most nuts.

Gravy unless made with polyunsaturated oil, and tinned soups.

Salad dressing unless made with polyunsaturated oil.

Use:

Polyunsaturated margarine, e.g. Flora instead of butter.

Polyunsaturated oil, e.g. Sunflower or corn oil in place of lard.

Further reading about dietetics and additional diets:

Passmore R., Eastwood M.A. (1986) Davidson's Human nutrition and dietetics, 8th edn. Churchill Livingstone, Edinburgh. A well-established standard textbook.

DESIRABLE WEIGHTS

Table 21.1 Weight for age: birth to 5 Years.[1] Sexes combined.[2]

Age (months)	Weight (kg) Standard	80% Std	60% Std	Age (months)	Weight (kg) Standard	80% Std	60% Std
0	3.25	2.6	1.95	31	13.45	10.8	8.1
1	4.15	3.3	2.5	32	13.65	10.9	8.2
2	4.95	4.0	3.0	33	13.85	11.1	8.3
3	5.7	4.6	3.4	34	14.05	11.2	8.4
4	6.35	5.1	3.8	35	14.15	11.3	8.5
5	7.0	5.6	4.2	36	14.35	11.5	8.6
6	7.5	6.0	4.5	37	14.55	11.6	8.7
7	8.0	6.4	4.8	38	14.7	11.8	8.8
8	8.5	6.8	5.1	39	14.9	11.9	8.9
9	8.9	7.1	5.3	40	15.05	12.0	9.0
10	9.2	7.4	5.5	41	15.2	12.2	9.1
11	9.55	7.6	5.7	42	15.4	12.3	9.2
12	9.85	7.9	5.9	43	15.5	12.4	9.3
13	10.1	8.1	6.1	44	15.7	12.6	9.4
14	10.35	8.3	6.2	45	15.85	12.7	9.5
15	10.55	8.4	6.3	46	16.05	12.8	9.6
16	10.75	8.6	6.45	47	16.15	12.9	9.7
17	10.95	8.8	6.6	48	16.35	31.1	9.8
18	11.15	8.9	6.7	49	16.5	13.2	9.9
19	11.35	9.1	6.8	50	16.6	13.3	10.0
20	11.5	9.2	6.9	51	16.8	13.4	10.1
21	11.7	9.4	7.0	52	16.95	13.6	10.2
22	11.85	9.5	7.1	53	17.1	13.7	10.3
23	12.05	9.6	7.2	54	17.25	13.8	10.4
24	12.25	9.8	7.35	55	17.45	14.0	10.5
25	12.25	9.8	7.35	56	17.55	14.1	10.5
26	12.45	10.0	7.47	57	17.7	14.2	10.6
27	12.65	10.1	7.6	58	17.85	14.3	10.7
28	12.85	10.3	7.7	59	18.0	14.4	10.8
29	13.05	10.4	7.8	60	18.2	14.6	10.9
30	13.25	10.6	7.95				

[1]Based on: A growth chart for international use in maternal and child health care 1978. WHO, Geneva.

[2]On average boys are 0.3 kg heavier and girls 0.3 kg lighter than the mean standard but the differences are smaller than this in the first 2 months and from 50–60 months.

Table 21.2 Guidelines for body weight in adults (men and women)

Height without shoes m	Approx. ft	Approx. in	Significantly underweight (80% of lower end of Acceptable)	Acceptable	Obese	Grossly obese
			Weight (kg) without clothes			
1.45	4	9	34	42–53	63	84
1.48	4	10	35	44–55	66	88
1.50	4	11	36	45–56	68	90
1.52	5	0	37	46–58	69	92
1.54	5	1	38	47–59	71	95
1.56	5	1	39	49–61	73	97
1.58	5	2	40	50–62	75	100
1.60	5	3	41	51–64	77	102
1.62	5	4	42	52–66	79	105
1.64	5	5	43	54–67	81	108
1.66	5	5	44	55–69	83	110
1.68	5	6	45	56–71	85	113
1.70	5	7	46	58–72	87	116
1.72	5	8	47	59–74	89	118
1.74	5	9	48	61–76	91	121
1.76	5	9	50	62–77.5	93	124
1.78	5	10	51	63–79	95	127
1.80	5	11	52	65–81	97	130
1.82	6	0	53	66–83	99	132
1.84	6	0	54	68–85	102	136
1.86	6	1	55	69–86	104	138
1.88	6	2	57	71–88	106	141
1.90	6	3	58	72–90	108	144
1.92	6	4	59	74–92	111	147
BMI			< 16	20–25	> 30	> 40

The body mass index (BMI) is used to define nutritional status. It is derived from the formula, weight(kg)/height(m)^2. The acceptable (normal) range is 20–25. Obesity is taken to start at a BMI of 30 and gross obesity at 40. The grading of starvation is given on page 54. The standards are the same for men and women.

BIOCHEMICAL VALUES

Table 21.3 Venous blood: approximate adult reference values.

Analysis	Reference values	
	S.I. units	*Other units*
Acid phosphatase (unstable enzyme)	*	0.1–0.4 i.u./l†
Alanine aminotransferase (ALT) (glutamic-pyruvic transaminase (GPT)	*	10–40 i.u./l
Alkaline phosphatase	*	40–100 i.u./l
Amylase	*	50–300 i.u./l
α_1-Antitrypsin	2–4 g/l	
Ascorbic acid—serum	23–57 μmol/l	0.4–1.0 mg/dl
—leucocytes	1420–2270 μmol/l	25–40 mg/dl
Aspartate aminotransferase (AST) (glutamic-oxaloacetic transaminase (GOT)	*	10–35 i.u./l
Bile acids		
Cholate—fasting	<3 μmol/l	
—2 h post prandial	<9 μmol/l	
Chenodeoxycholate—fasting	<3 μmol/l	
—2 h post prandial	<13 μmol/l	
Bilirubin (total)	2–17 μmol/l	0.3–1.0 mg/dl
Caeruloplasmin	1–2.7 μmol/l	15–40 mg/dl
Calcium (total)	2.12–2.62 mmol/l	8.5–10.5 mg/dl
Carbon dioxide (total)	24–30 mmol/l	24–30 meq/l
β-Carotene	0.9–5.6 μmol/l	50–300 μg/dl
Chloride	95–105 mmol/l	96–105 meq/l
Cholesterol (fasting)	3.6–6.7 mmol/l	145–270 mg/dl
Copper	11–24 μmol/l	100–128 μg/dl
Creatinine	55–150 μmol/l	0.6–1.7 mg/dl
Creatinine clearance		90–130 ml/min
Creatine kinase (CK)—males	*	30–200 i.u./l
—females ‡	*	30–150 i.u./l
Ethanol—marked intoxication	65–87 mmol/l	0.3–0.4 g/dl
—stupor	87–109 mmol/l	0.4–0.5 g/dl
—coma	>109 mmol/l	>0.5 g/dl
Ferritin—males	§	6–186 μg/ml
—females	§	3–162 μg/ml
α-Fetoprotein	2–6 units/ml	<30 ng/ml
γ-Glutamyl transferase (γ-GT)—males	*	10–55 i.u./l
—females	*	5–35 i.u.l
Glucose (fasting)	3.9–5.8 mmol/l	70–110 mg/100 ml
Immunoglobulins (Ig): IgA	0.5–4.0 g/l (40–300 i.u./l)	
IgG	5.0–13.0 g/l (60–160 i.u./l)	
IgM—males	0.3–2.2 g/l (40–270 i.u./l)	
—females	0.4–2.5 g/l (50–300 i.u./l)	
Iron—males	14–32 μmol/l	77–178 μg/dl
—females	10–28 μmol/l	56–156 μg/dl
Iron binding capacity (total)	45–72 μmol/l	250–400 μg/dl
Iron binding capacity (saturation)		14–47%
Lactate	0.4–1.4 mmol/l	3.6–13.0 mg/dl
Lactate dehydrogenase (LD)	*	100–300 i.u./l
Lead	0.5–1.9 μmol/l	10–40 μg/dl
Lipids—*see* Cholesterol and Triglycerides		
Magnesium	0.75–1.0 mmol/l	1.8–2.4 mg/dl
5′ Nucleotidase	*	1–11 i.u./l
Osmolality	285–295 mOsm/kg	285–295 mOsm/kg water

Tables 21.3 (*continued*)

Analysis	Reference values	
	S.I. units	Other units
Phosphatase *see* acid and alkaline		
Phosphate	0.8–1.4 mmol/l	2.5–4.5 mg/dl
Potassium	3.3–4.7 mmol/l	
Proteins—total	62–82 g/l	6.2–8.2 g/dl
—albumin	36–47 g/l	3.6–4.7 g/dl
—globulins	24–37 g/l	2:4–3:7 g/dl
—electrophoresis (% of total)		
albumin 52–68		
globulin α_1 4.2–7.2		
α_2 6.8–12		
β 9.3–15		
γ 13–23		
Pyruvate—fasting	35–80 μmol/l	
—after 50 g glucose—60 m	<110 μmol/l	
—90 m	<120 μmol/l	
Sodium	132–144 mmol/l	
Triglyceride (fasting)	0.6–1.7 mmol/l	40–145 mg/dl
Urate—males	0.12–0.42 mmol/l	2–7 mg/dl
—females	0.12–0.36 mmol/l	2–6 mg/dl
Urea‖	2.5–6.6 mmol/l	15–40 mg/dl
Vitamin A	0.7–1.7 μmol/l	20–50 μg/dl

*Enzyme activity in the SI system is measured in nmol sec^{-1}/l^{-1} and this unit is known as the katal. Only conventional units are given here as the katal is not used widely in clinical practice. There is, however, a constant relation between the international unit (i.u.) and the katal (1 i.u. = 16.6 nkatal).

†Representing the prostatic isoenzyme.

‡CK–MB (myocardial isoenzyme) is normally <10 i.u./l unless CK activity is very high (>500 i.u./l) when CK–MB should be <5% of total activity to make myocardial damage unlikely

§Measured against a British standard preparation.

‖Urea × 0.4665 = Urea nitrogen   Urea nitrogen × 2.14 = Urea

Note. The normal adult reference values given above are largely those of the Department of Clinical Chemistry, Royal Infirmary, Edinburgh. Methodology varies between laboratories, and clinicians should be guided by the normal reference ranges for the laboratories they use; this applies especially to the results of enzyme assays and the reference ranges of some enzymes vary greatly, particularly acid phosphatase, alkaline phosphatase, amylase and lactate dehydrogenase. The above estimations can be made in plasma or serum; serum is required for plasma protein electrophoresis and is preferable for radio-immunoassays.

The normal reference values of laboratory procedures used in the Massachusetts General Hospital are published in the New England Journal of Medicine 1986 314 (1): 39 and 315 (25): 1606.

Table 21.4 Miscellaneous approximate adult reference values.

Arterial blood analyses

Analysis	Reference values	
	S.I. units	Other units
Ammonia	11–35 μmol/l	20–63 μg/dl
Hydrogen ion	36–44 nmol/l	pH 7.37–7.45
Carbon dioxide (PaCO$_2$)	4.8–6.0 kPa	36–45 mmHg
Plasma bicarbonate	22–26 mmol/l	22–26 mEq/l
Oxygen (PaO$_2$)	11–13 kPa	83–98 mmHg

Cerebrospinal fluid (Lumbar puncture)
Cells: 5/mm^3 (all mononuclear cells)
Chloride 120–170 mmol/l
Glucose: 2.5–4.0 mmol/l (45–72 mg/dl) — 50 to 70% of
    plasma concentration
Immunoglobulin G: 20–50 mg/l
Protein (total): 100–400 mg/l
Pressure: 5–15 cmCSF

Gastrointestinal, pancreas and liver
Faecal fat: <18 mmol/24 h (<5 g/24 h)
Stool weight (wet): <200 g/24 h
D-Xyloseexcretion (25 g dose): 33–53 mmol/5 h
    (5–8 g/5 h) Serum Xylose: 1.7– 2.7 mmol/l at
    1 h (25–40 mg/dl)
Pancreatic exocrine function (secretin stimulation)
    Juice volume: >2 mg/kg/h
    Bicarbonate—output: >10 mmol/h
        —concentration: >80 mmol/l
Liver: Copper <50 μg/g dry weight
    (Wilson's disease >250 μg/g dry weight)
Iron 40–60 μg/100 mg dry weight
    Haermochromatosis >1000 μg/100 mg dry weight)

Sweat (pilcarpine iontophoresis)
Sodium <85 mmol/l
Potassium <25 mmol/l
N.B. Minimum sweat sample 50 mg

NOTES ON INTERNATIONAL SYSTEM OF UNITS (SI UNITS)

Examples of basic SI units

Length	metre (m)
Mass	kilogram (kg)
Amount of substance	mole (mol)
Energy	joule (J)
Pressure	pascal (pa)

Examples of decimal multiples and submultiples of SI units

Factor	Name	Symbol
10^6	mega-	M
10^3	kilo-	k
10^{-1}	deci-	d
10^{-2}	centi-	c
10^{-3}	milli-	m
10^{-6}	micro-	μ
10^{-9}	nano-	n
10^{-12}	pico-	p
10^{-15}	femto-	f

Volume. The basic SI unit of volume is the cubic metre (1000 litre). Because of its convenience the litre is used as the unit of volume in laboratory work.

Amount of substance ('molar') concentration (e.g. mol/l, μmol/l) is used for substances of defined chemical composition. It replaces equivalent concentration (mEq/l), which is not part of the SI system. For univalent ions such as sodium, potassium, chloride and bicarbonate the numerical value is unchanged. For divalent ions such as calcium and magnesium the numerical value is halved.

Mass concentration (e.g. g/l, μg/l) is used for all protein measurements, for substances which do not have a sufficiently well defined composition and for serum vitamin B$_{12}$ and folate measurements. The numerical value in SI units will change by a factor of 10 in those instances previously expressed in terms of 100 ml.

Haemoglobin is an exception. It is generally expressed in terms of g/dl although the International Committee for standardisation in Haematology recommended in 1982 that the unit for haemoglobin should be g/l.

SI units are not employed for enzymes nor usually for immunoglobulins.

Table 21.5 Hormone concentrations in plasma; approximate adult reference values. Peptide hormone concentrations vary between different assays according to the standards used. The following values are based on the current WHO international reference preparations.

Analysis	Conditions	Reference Values S.I. units	Other units
Adrenocorticotrophin (ACTH) 09:00	Avoid stressful venepuncture	10–80 ng/l	
22:00	Separate and store at −20°C immediately	<10	
Cortisol (RIA) 09:00	Avoid stressful venepuncture	190–550 nmol/l	7.0–20 µg/100 ml
22:00		<190	<190
Follicle-stimulating hormone (FSH)			
Male			1.5–9.0 U/l
Female, early follicular			3.0–15.0 U/l
Female, post-menopausal			30–115 U/l
Gastrin	Collect after overnight fast. Separate and store immediately at −20°C	60–200 pg/ml	
Growth hormone (GH)	Avoid stressful venepuncture		often <1.0 mU/l but variable
Insulin	Collect after overnight fast Separate and store immediately at −20°C		5–25 mU/l, but variable
Luteinising hormone (LH)			
Male			1.5–9.0 U/l
Female, early follicular			2.5–9.0 U/l
Female, post-menopausal			30–115 U/l
Oestradiol			
Male		<150 pmol/l	<4 ng/100 ml
Female, early follicular		80–250	2–7
luteal		400–900	11–24
post-menopausal		<85	<2
Parathyroid hormone (PTH)	Separate and store at −20°C immediately	Values depend upon antiserum specificity	
Prolactin (PRL)	Avoid stressful venepuncture		60–390 mU/l
Progesterone			
follicular		<2 nmol/l	<62 ng/100 nl
mid-luteal		22–88	690–276
post-menopausal		<0.5	<16
Testosterone			
Male		10–30 nmol/l	290–860 ng/100 ml
Female		0.8–2.8 nmol/l	23–81 ng/100 ml
Thyroid-stimulating hormone (TSH)			<5.7 mU/l
Thyroxine		70–150 nmol/l	5.5–12 µg/100 ml
Triiodothyronine		1.1–2.8 nmol/l	70–180 ng/100 ml

Table 21.6 Urine: approximate adult reference values.

Analysis	Reference Values	
	S.I. units	Other units
Amylase		35–260 Somogyi units/l
Calcium (low calcium diet)	1.2–3.7 mmol/24 h	50–150 mg/24 h
Copper	<1 μmol/24 h	<100 μg/24 h
Cortisol (early morning specimen)	9–50 μmol/mol creatinine	
5-Hydroxyindole-3-acetic acid	10–45 μmol/24 h	2–9 mg/24 h
4-Hydroxy, 3-methoxy mandelic acid	<30 μmol/24 h	8 mg/24 h
Metadrenalines	<7 μmol/24 h	
Osmolality	70–1200 mOsm/kg	
Phosphate (normal diet)	15–50 mmol/24 h	
Porphyrins—coproporphyrins	150–230 nmol/24 h	
—uroporphyrins	<40 nmol/24 h	
Potassium	25–100 mmol/24 h	
Protein	<100 mg/24 h	
Sodium	100–200 mmol/24 h	

Table 21.7 Therapeutic concentrations of drugs in blood.

Drug	Blood concentration		Conditions
	S.I. units	Other units	
Antiepileptic drugs			
Carbamazepine	34–51 μmol/l	4–10 μg/ml	4–6 h after last dose
Ethosuximide		50–85 μg/ml	
Phenobarbitone	65–170 μmol/l	15–40 μg/ml	
Phenytoin	40–80 μmol/l	10–20 μg/ml	>10 d after start of therapy
Primidone	18–55 μmol/l	4–12 μg/l	
Digoxin		1–2.6 ng/ml	6–18 h after last dose
Gentamicin		Peak: <10 μg/ml	1 h after intravenous injection
		Trough: <2 μg/ml	Pre-dose
Lithium	0.8–1.2 mmol/l		12–18 h after last dose
Procainamide	17–42 μmol/l	4–10 μg/ml	just before next dose
Salicylate	up to 1.8 mmol/l	up to 250 mg/l	just before next dose

Note: Monitoring the concentration of a drug in the blood is not a substitute for a careful clinical assessment but is helpful (1) if toxic effects occur when dosage is only slightly greater than that required for a therapeutic effect as in the case of phenytoin or digoxin, (2) when renal function is impaired, and (3) if there is uncertainty about the patient taking the drug. Peak and trough measurements are helpful if there is a risk of accumulation of a drug as in the case of gentamicin. Lithium can be measured as easily as other electrolytes and its level should be monitored regularly when it is used in the treatment of manic-depressive states.

Table 21.8 Haematological values.

	S.I. units	Other units
Bleeding time (Ivy)	Up to 11 min	
Body fluid (total)		50% (obese)–70% (lean) of body weight
Intracellular		30–40% of body weight
Extracellular		20–30% of body weight
Blood volume		
Red cell mass, men	30 ± 5 ml/kg	
women	25 ± 5 ml/kg	
Plasma volume (both sexes)	45 ± 5 ml/kg	
Total blood volume, men	75 ± 10 ml/kg	
women	70 ± 10 ml/kg	
Erythrocyte sedimentation rate (Westergren)		0–6 mm in 1 h normal
(Figures given are for patients under		7–20 mm in 1 h doubtful
60 years of age. Higher values in older		>20 mm in 1 h abnormal
persons are not necessarily abnormal)		
Fibrinogen	1.5–4.0 g/l	150–400 mg/dl
*Folate—serum	2–20 µg/l	2–20 ng/ml
—red cell	>100 µg/l	>100 ng/ml
Haemoglobin—men	130–180 g/l	13–18 g/dl
—women	115–165 g/l	11.5–16.5 g/dl
Haptoglobin	0.3–2.0 g/l	30–200 mg/dl
Leucocytes—adults	4.0–11.0 × 10⁹/l	4000–11000/µl
		4.0–11.0 × 10³/mm³
Differential white cell count		
Neutrophil granulocytes	2.5–7.5 × 10⁹/l	40–75%
Lymphocytes	1.0–3.5 × 10⁹/l	20–45%
Monocytes	0.2–0.8 × 10⁹/l	2–10%
Eosinophil granulocytes	0.04–0.4 × 10⁹/l	1–6%
Basophil granulocytes	0.01–0.1 × 10⁹/l	0–1%
Mean corpuscular haemoglobin (MCH)	27–32 pg	27–32 µµg
Mean corpuscular haemoglobin		
concentration (MCHC)	30–35 g/dl	30–35%
Mean corpuscular volume (MCV)	78–98 fl	78–98 μ^3 or μm^3
Packed cell volume (PCV) or		
haematocrit—men	0.40–0.54	40–54%
—women	0.35–0.47	35–47%
Platelets	150–400 × 10⁹/l	150 000–400 000/µl or/mm³
Prothrombin time	11–15 s	
Red cell count—men	4.5–6.5 × 10¹²/l	4.5–6.5 × 10⁶/µl or mm³
—women	3.8–5.8 × 10¹²/l	3.8–5.8 × 10⁶/µl or mm³
Red cell life span (mean)	120 days	
Red cell life span T$_\frac{1}{2}$ (⁵¹Cr)	25–35 days	
Reticulocytes (adults)	10–100 × 10⁹/l	0.2–2%
*Vitamin B₁₂ (in serum as cyanocobalamin)	160–925 ng/l	160–925 pg/ml or µµg/ml

*Also measured by radioassay; normal range of reference values should be obtained from the laboratory carrying out the estimation.

DRUG NOMENCLATURE AND PRESCRIPTION

In this book the names that have been given for drugs have almost invariably been those approved for use in Britain. These are devised or selected by the British Pharmacopoeia Commission and published by the Health Ministers at regular intervals. It must be realised, however, that many countries have their national non-proprietary names, and that the World Health Organization also has its own list. Usually these various names are similar, but there are significant differences; for example, paracetamol (BP) is listed as acetaminophen in the United States Pharmacopoeia. Proprietary names are given in this book only in exceptional circumstances, but can usually be found in the British National Formulary, the Data Sheet Compendium and as an addendum to some textbooks. There may be many totally different names for the same substance and this can cause confusion. Doctors must also be prepared to interpret the jargon used by addicts about drugs of dependence and their effects.

Abbreviations used in relationship to the administration of drugs are i.m. (intramuscular injection), i.v. (intravenous injection), s.c. (subcutaneous injection), b.d. (twice daily) and t.i.d. (thrice daily). The dosage given is a guide for use in adults of average build and should be checked against that in a national formulary or in the manufacturer's instructions. It is particularly important to confirm that a dosage given in mg/kg body weight is, indeed, correct, and great care must be taken to ensure that no error occurs in the quantity of a drug prescribed for an infant or child.

Some drugs, e.g. in the chemotherapy of malignant disease, are prescribed in weight of drug per square metre of body surface. With the use of a nomogram, the body surface area can be calculated from the height in centimetres and the weight in kilograms.

Patient compliance (i.e. the taking of medicines as prescribed) is improved if instructions are simple and specific, especially for the elderly. Polypharmacy should be avoided if possible, one reason being the danger of interaction between drugs. Some (e.g. rifampicin) induce liver enzymes (p. 000) which may increase the metabolism of concurrently administered preparations (e.g. corticosteroids, oral contraceptives, oral anticoagulants, oral hypoglycaemic drugs, dapsone and phenytoin). Conversely elimination of compounds metabolised in the liver by oxidation (e.g. oral anticoagulants, phenytoin and diazepam) can be prolonged by the action of other drugs (e.g. cimetidine). All drugs, whenever possible, should be avoided during the early months of pregnancy.

STANDARD REFERENCE BOOKS:

British National Formulary 1987 The British Medical Association and The Pharmaceutical Society of Great Britain.
Martindale — the extra pharmacopoeia 1983 28th edn. Pharmaceutical Press, London.

FURTHER READING ABOUT DRUGS:

Avery G S (ed.) 1987 Drug treatment, 3rd edn. Churchill Livingstone, Edinburgh.
Girdwood R H (ed.) 1984 Clinical pharmacology, 25th edn. Baillière Tindall, London.

Index